PROBLEMS IN *Pediatric* DRUG THERAPY

FOURTH EDITION

NOTICES

The inclusion in this book of any drug in respect to which patent or trademark rights may exist shall not be deemed, and is not intended as, a grant of or authority to exercise any right or privilege protected by such patent or trademark. All such rights or trademarks are vested in the patent or trademark owner, and no other person may exercise the same without express permission, authority, or license secured from such patent or trademark owner.

The inclusion of a brand name does not mean the editors, the authors, or the publisher have any particular knowledge that the brand listed has properties different from the other brands of the same drug, nor should its inclusion be interpreted as an endorsement by the editors, authors, or publisher. Similarly, the fact that a particular brand has not been included does not indicate the product has been judged to be in any way unsatisfactory or unacceptable. Further, no official support or endorsement of this book by any federal or state or provincial agency or pharmaceutical company is intended or inferred.

The nature of drug information is that it is constantly evolving because of ongoing research and clinical experience and is often subject to interpretation. Readers are advised that decisions regarding drug therapy must be based on the independent judgment of the clinician, changing information about a drug (e.g., as reflected in the literature and manufacturers' most current product information), and changing medical practices.

The editors, the authors, and the publisher have made every effort to ensure the accuracy and completeness of the information presented in this book. However, the editors, the authors, and the publisher cannot be held responsible for the continued currency of the information, any inadvertent errors or omissions, or the application of this information.

Therefore, the editors, the authors, and the publisher shall have no liability to any person or entity with regard to claims, loss, or damage caused, or alleged to be caused, directly or indirectly, by the use of information contained herein.

PROBLEMS IN *Pediatric* DRUG THERAPY

FOURTH EDITION

Edited by

Louis A. Pagliaro
MS, PharmD, PhD, FPPR
Former Professor of Pharmacy and Pharmaceutical Sciences
Professor of Pharmacopsychology

Ann Marie Pagliaro
BSN, MSN, PhD Candidate, FPPR
Professor of Nursing

University of Alberta • Edmonton, Alberta, Canada

American Pharmaceutical Association • Washington, D.C.

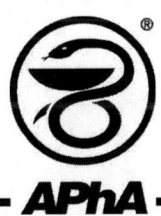

Editor: L. Luan Corrigan
Acquiring Editor: Julian I. Graubart
Layout and Graphics: Northeastern Graphic Services, Inc.
Cover Design: Jim McDonald
Proofreading: Publications Professionals LLC
Indexing: Lillian R. Rodberg

©2002 by the American Pharmaceutical Association
©1979, Drug Intelligence Publications
©1987, 1995, Drug Intelligence Publications, Inc.

Published by the American Pharmaceutical Association
2215 Constitution Avenue, N.W.
Washington, DC 20037-2985
www.aphanet.org

To comment on this book via e-mail, send your message to the publisher at aphabooks@aphanet.org.

All rights reserved.

No part of this book may be reproduced, stored in a retrieval system, or transmitted in any form or by any means, electronic, mechanical, photocopying, recording, or otherwise, without written permission from the publisher.

Library of Congress Cataloging-in-Publication Data

Problems in pediatric drug therapy / edited by Louis A. Pagliaro, Ann Marie Pagliaro.—4th ed.
    p. ; cm.
Includes bibliographical references and index.
ISBN 1-58212-001-3
   1. Pediatric pharmacology—Handbooks, manuals, etc. 2. Drugs—Handbooks, manuals, etc. I. Pagliaro, Louis A. II. Pagliaro, Ann M.
   [DNLM: 1. Drug Therapy—Child—Handbooks. 2. Drug Therapy—Infant—Handbooks.
WS 39 P962 2002]
RJ560 .P76 2002
615.5′8′083—dc21
                                                                2002025876

How to Order This Book
Online: www.pharmacist.com. By phone: 800 878-0729 (from the United States and Canada). Visa®, MasterCard®, and American Express® cards accepted.

Dedicated to the Promotion and Maintenance of
Health for
All Neonates, Infants, Children, and Adolescents,
and to the
Pediatric Clinicians
Who Work to Achieve This Goal
through the Provision of
Optimal Pediatric Drug Therapy

Special Dedication

The fourth edition of *Problems in Pediatric Drug Therapy* is specially dedicated to Dr. Gloria Niemeyer Francke. . . . In recognition of the long positive working relationship that we had over the past twenty-five years as she gave tirelessly of herself, as the owner and publisher of Drug Intelligence Publications, to the first three editions of *Problems in Pediatric Drug Therapy*. Gloria is a true pioneer and leader in the field of clinical pharmacy who has received many well-deserved accolades and awards, including U.S. pharmacy's highest award, the Remington Medal, for her significant contributions. It has been our honor and pleasure to have known and worked with her as both colleague and friend.

LAP/AMP

CONTENTS

Preface xi
Acknowledgments xiii
Contributing Authors xv
Pediatric Advisory Committee xvii

1. Administering Drugs to Infants, Children, and Adolescents
   Ann Marie Pagliaro 1
   Drug Administration 2
   General Developmental Considerations for Drug
      Administration (Table) 3
   Special Considerations 6
   Oral Dosage Forms 7
   Rectal Dosage Forms 19
   Vaginal Dosage Forms 22
   Ophthalmic Dosage Forms 23
   Otic Dosage Forms 27
   Intranasal Dosage Forms 28
   Inhalation Dosage Forms 31
   Topical Dosage Forms 36
   Injectable Dosage Forms 42

2. Drugs as Human Teratogens and Fetotoxins
   Louis A. Pagliaro and Ann Marie Pagliaro. 87
   Maternal Pharmacotherapy and Other Drug Use during
      Pregnancy 88
   Factors Affecting Teratogenesis 89
   Teratogenesis Drug Monographs 96

3. Drugs Excreted in Human Breast Milk
   Neeta Bahal O'Mara and Milap C. Nahata 201
   Absorption 202
   Metabolism and Excretion 202
   Drugs Excreted in Human Breast Milk (Table) 203

4. Pediatric Poisoning
    Wendy Klein-Schwartz and Gary M. Oderda . . . 245
        General Considerations 247
        Treatment of Common Pediatric Poisonings 253

5. Adverse Drug Reactions in Neonates, Infants, Children, and Adolescents
    Michael J. Rieder 283
        Classification of ADRs 283
        Risk Factors 284
        Establishing ADRs 285
        Drugs Commonly Required by Infants, Children, and
            Adolescents: Associated ADRs and
            Clinical Comments (Table) 291

6. Pediatric Drug Interactions
    Philip D. Hansten 315
        Sites of Drug Interactions 315
        Drug Interactions and QT Prolongation 316
        Drug Interactions Involving Hepatic Cytochrome P-450
            Isoenzymes (Table) 317
        Drug Interactions in Pediatric Patients 319

7. Abusable Psychotropic Use among Children and Adolescents
    Ann Marie Pagliaro 347
        Interactive Model of Abusable Psychotropic Use 349
        Abusable Psychotropic Variables 354
        Pattern-of-Use Variables 370
        Treatment 373

8. Intravenous Drugs for Neonates, Infants, Children, and Adolescents: Preparation, Storage, and Administration
    Dawn R. Butler, Carla Wallace,
    Tamara K. Hutson, and John J. Piecoro, Jr. 387
        General Considerations 387
        Intravenous Drug Administration Guidelines for Infants and
            Children (Table) 390

9. Pediatric Immunizations
David W. Scheifele 433
General Cautions 433
Active Immunization Schedules and Monographs for Vaccines and Toxoids 437

10. Pediatric Pharmacokinetics
Clarence T. Ueda and Eric B. Hoie 459
Pharmacokinetic Factors and Drug Effect 459
Pharmacokinetic Principles 463
Altered Pharmacokinetics in Disease States and with Concurrent Drug Therapy 468

11. Pediatric Pharmacogenetics
J. Steven Leeder 475
Pharmacogenetic Principles 475

12. Pediatric Antineoplastic Drug Therapy
Norman J. Lacayo, Tina Baggott, and Branimir I. Sikic 493
Pediatric Considerations 495
Guidelines for Use 501
Antineoplastic Drug Dosing for Children and Adolescents (Table) 507

13. Drug Dosing for Neonates
Robert P. Lemke 531
Recommended Drug Dosing for Neonates (Table) 532

14. Drug Dosing for Infants, Children, and Adolescents
Louis A. Pagliaro and Ann Marie Pagliaro 555
Drug Dosages for Infants, Children, and Adolescents 556
Recommended Drug Dosing for Infants, Children, and Adolescents (Table) 558

Appendices 779
Appendix A: Abbreviations and Symbols 781
Appendix B: Normal Pediatric Laboratory Values 785

Index 789

PREFACE

A number of health and social care professionals, including advanced practice nurses, child and adolescent clinical and health psychologists, clinical pharmacists, family practice physicians, general practitioners, pediatricians, pediatric nurse practitioners, and social workers are actively involved in the promotion and maintenance of the health of neonates, infants, children, and adolescents. This text is written for these pediatric clinicians and for students, interns, and residents who require knowledge of pediatric drug therapy. Its purpose is to present an authoritative, concise, referenced, and easily accessible compilation of human clinical and empirical evidence concerning the use and effects of drugs in the fetus, neonate, infant, child, and adolescent.

This fourth edition of *Problems in Pediatric Drug Therapy* attempts to build on the well-received style and method of presentation characteristic of the previous three editions. Specifically, the concise, thoroughly referenced format (more than 3000 cited references), which utilizes an integration of narrative, figures, and tables, has been retained. Each of the original chapters from the third edition has been extensively and comprehensively revised, reviewed, and edited to reflect current, optimal pediatric drug therapy research, knowledge, and practice. A major change has been the expansion of the handbook from twelve to fourteen chapters to include new chapters dealing with "Pediatric Pharmacogenetics" and "Pediatric Antineoplastic Drug Therapy." The inclusion of these additional chapters should prove to make the text even more comprehensive and useful to pediatric clinicians. The Pediatric Advisory Committee has been retained and its membership expanded to enhance and complement the coverage of the various chapters and to ensure the highest possible standard of quality in relation to the accuracy, timeliness, and comprehensiveness of the topics discussed.

Each chapter deals with a major, potentially problematic, area of pediatric drug therapy. Thus, each chapter provides the necessary information pediatric clinicians and students may require to effectively avoid or minimize the occurrence of these problems. The contributing authors of the various chapters have been carefully chosen for their demonstrated clinical experience, expertise, and interest in pediatric drug therapy. The varied backgrounds and expertise of these clinicians, educators, and researchers provide this handbook with an added depth and dimension that exemplify the optimization of drug therapy that can be achieved only by an interdisciplinary pluralistic and increasingly transdisciplinary approach. The references cited by the authors are primarily original human studies. However, general review articles and texts have been included to allow further study by interested readers. Evaluations and recommendations based on each author's personal experience and interpretation of the literature are included in the chapters. These comments reflect the opinions of the respective author(s) solely and may not reflect the opinion of the editors, the members of the Pediatric Advisory Committee, or the publisher.

The drugs discussed in this text and listed in the Index are referred to by their nonproprietary (generic) USAN names. Cross-references are provided for common proprietary or trade (brand) names that are used in Canada and the United States. All dosages included in this book are average dosages and are, therefore, approximate. In all cases, variability in drug response because of environmental, genetic, maturational, pathologic, or physiologic differences may necessitate alterations in dose or dosage regimen. Accepted guidelines for the use of each drug (e.g., drug information center guidelines; product package inserts) should be consulted whenever there is a further question about the use, dose, or dosage regimen of a particular drug.

We hope that, by using the information presented in this text, pediatric clinicians and students, who are involved in promoting and maintaining the health of neonates, infants, children, and adolescents, will be better able to provide the maximal benefits of drug therapy to their patients, with minimal adverse effects, as they work toward the goal of promoting and maintaining optimal pediatric health.

LAP/AMP
May 2002

ACKNOWLEDGMENTS

The editors gratefully acknowledge the assistance of a number of people whose hard and diligent work made this project possible. First, all of the contributing authors who took the time and effort necessary to prepare and revise each of the chapters and the members of the Pediatric Advisory Committee who extensively reviewed the chapters in order to ensure that the highest possible standards were met. Pediatric clinicians and their patients owe all of the contributing authors and advisory committee members a great debt, and the editors are most grateful.

Last, but certainly not least, we wish to thank Julian Graubart, director of books and electronic publishing, for his support of this project and patience and faith in our abilities to see it to completion; Luan Corrigan, our production editor, for her assistance and friendship; and the staff at the American Pharmaceutical Association for their diligence and hard work in the production of this text. The constructive feedback received from the editorial and production staff during the entire revision process and their patience, support, and encouragement have helped to make this edition of *Problems in Pediatric Drug Therapy* the very best possible.

Finally, the following quotation, which was paraphrased from Adlai Stevenson and used in the previous edition, continues to be the best sentiment that summarizes the feelings that have guided all who have worked on and contributed to this text:

We have not done as well as we should have liked to have done, but we have done our best, honestly and forthrightly. No one can do more and you [the reader] are entitled to no less.

CONTRIBUTING AUTHORS

Tina Baggott, RN-CS, MSN, PNP, is Nurse Practitioner, Lucile Salter Packard Children's Hospital at Stanford, UCSF-Stanford Health Care, Stanford, California.

Dawn Butler, PharmD, is Clinical Pharmacy Specialist, Neonatal Intensive Care, Cincinnati Children's Hospital Medical Center, Cincinnati, Ohio.

Philip D. Hansten, PharmD, is Professor and Acting Chairman, Department of Pharmacy, University of Washington, Seattle, Washington.

Eric B. Hoie, PharmD, is Associate Professor, College of Pharmacy, The University of Nebraska Medical Center, Omaha, Nebraska.

Tamara Hutson, PharmD, is Clinical Pharmacy Specialist, Pediatric Intensive Care, Cincinnati Children's Hospital Medical Center, Cincinnati, Ohio.

Wendy Klein-Schwartz, PharmD, MPH, is Coordinator of Research and Education, Maryland Poison Center, and Associate Professor, School of Pharmacy, University of Maryland, Baltimore, Maryland.

Norman J. Lacayo, BA, MD, is Staff Physician, Lucile Salter Packard Children's Hospital at Stanford, and Clinical Instructor, Department of Pediatrics, Division of Hematology-Oncology, Stanford University School of Medicine, Stanford, California.

J. Steven Leeder, PharmD, PhD, is Chief, Section of Developmental Pharmacology and Experimental Therapeutics, Division of Clinical Pharmacology and Toxicology, The Children's Mercy Hospital, and Associate Professor of Pediatrics and Pharmacology, The University of Missouri, Kansas City, Missouri.

Robert P. Lemke, MD, BMSc, FAAP, FRCPC, is Neonatologist, Section of Newborn Services, Royal Alexandra Hospital and Stollery Children's Health Centre, and Assistant Clinical Professor of Pediatrics, Faculty of Medicine, University of Alberta, Edmonton, Alberta.

Milap C. Nahata, PharmD, is Professor of Pharmacy and Pediatrics, College of Pharmacy, The Ohio State University, Columbus, Ohio.

Gary M. Oderda, PharmD, MPH, is Professor and Chairman, Department of Pharmacy Practice, College of Pharmacy, University of Utah, Salt Lake City, Utah.

Neeta Bahal O'Mara, PharmD, is Assistant Editor, *Pharmacist's Letter and Prescriber's Letter*, Skillman, New Jersey.

Ann Marie Pagliaro, RN, BSN, MSN, PhD Candidate, FPPR, is Professor of Nursing, Faculty of Nursing, and Director, Substance Abusology Research Unit, University of Alberta, Edmonton, Alberta.

Louis A. Pagliaro, MS, PharmD, PhD, CPsych, FABMP, FPPR, is former Professor of Pharmacy and Pharmaceutical Sciences and current Professor of Pharmacopsychology, Department of Educational Psychology, University of Alberta, Edmonton, Alberta.

John J. Piecoro, Jr., MS, PharmD, is Professor, Division of Pharmacy Practice and Science, College of Pharmacy, University of Kentucky, Lexington, Kentucky.

Michael J. Rieder, MD, PhD, FRCPC, is Professor of Paediatrics, Pharmacology and Toxicology and Medicine, University of Western Ontario, and Head of the Section of Paediatric Clinical Pharmacology, Children's Hospital of Western Ontario, London, Ontario.

David W. Scheifele, MD, is Director, Vaccine Evaluation Center, B.C. Children's Hospital, and Sauder Professor of Pediatric Infectious Diseases, Faculty of Medicine, University of British Columbia, Vancouver, British Columbia.

Branimir I. Sikic, BS, MD, is Professor, Faculty of Medicine, Stanford University, Stanford, California.

Clarence T. Ueda, PhD, is Professor and Dean, College of Pharmacy, The University of Nebraska Medical Center, Omaha, Nebraska.

Carla Wallace, PharmD, BCPS, is Clinical Pharmacy Specialist, Hematology/Oncology, Cincinnati Children's Hospital Medical Center, Cincinnati, Ohio.

PEDIATRIC ADVISORY COMMITTEE

Jacob V. Aranda, MD, PhD, FRCP(C), FAAP, is Chief of Pediatric Clinical Pharmacology, Children's Hospital of Michigan, Wayne State University, Detroit, Michigan.

Joseph A. Carcillo, MD, is Assistant Professor, Center for Clinical Pharmacology, Department of Anesthesiology, Critical Care Medicine, and Pediatrics, Children's Hospital of Pittsburgh, University of Pittsburgh, Pittsburgh, Pennsylvania.

Jeffrey M. Daly, MD, is Staff Physician, Department of Outpatient Psychiatry, Four Winds Hospital, Saratoga Springs, New York.

Samir M. Douidar, MD, PhD, is Clinical Associate Professor and Director of Pediatric Emergency Center, University Community Hospital, Tampa, Florida.

William E. Evans, PharmD, is Chairman and First Tennessee Professor, Pharmaceutical Department, St. Jude Children's Research Hospital, Memphis, Tennessee.

William D. Figg, PharmD, is Senior Investigator, National Cancer Institute, Bethesda, Maryland.

David A. Flockhart, MD, PhD, is Associate Professor of Medicine and Pharmacology, and Director, Pharmacogenetics Core Laboratory, Division of Clinical Pharmacology, Georgetown University Medical Center, Washington, D.C.

Reginald F. Frye, PharmD, PhD, is Assistant Professor, Department of Pharmaceutical Sciences, School of Pharmacy, University of Pittsburgh, Pittsburgh, Pennsylvania.

James M. Gallo, PharmD, PhD, is Director, Department of Pharmacology, Fox Chase Cancer Center, Philadelphia, Pennsylvania.

Lewis R. Goldfrank, MD, is Director, Emergency Services, Bellevue Hospital Center and New York University Medical Center, Associate Professor of Clinical Medicine, New York University School of Medicine, and Medical Director, New York City Poison Control Center, New York, New York.

Dennis M. Grasela, PharmD, is Associate Director, Department of Human Pharmacology, Bristol-Myers Squibb Pharmaceutical Research Institute, Princeton, New Jersey.

Joseph R. Hageman, MD, is Medical Director, Inpatient Pediatrics, and Division Chief, Pediatric Critical Care Program, Evanston Hospital, and Associate Professor of Pediatrics, Northwestern University Medical School, Chicago, Illinois.

Shinya Ito, MD, is Associate Director, Department of Pediatrics, The Hospital for Sick Children, Toronto, Ontario.

Ralph E. Kauffman, MD, is Marion Merrell Dow/Missouri Chair of Medical Research, and Professor of Pediatrics and Pharmacology, The Children's Mercy Hospital, Kansas City, Missouri.

Gregory L. Kearns, PharmD, FCP, is Marion Merrell Dow/Missouri Professor of Pediatric Clinical Pharmacology, Professor of Pediatrics and Pharmacology, University of Missouri, Kansas City, and Chief, Section of Pediatric Clinical Pharmacology and Experimental Therapeutics, Children's Mercy Hospital, Kansas City, Missouri.

Deborah Kupecz, MSN, NP, is Adult Nurse Practitioner, Department of Veterans Affairs, Outpatient Clinic at Fitzsimmons, Aurora, Colorado.

Timothy Madden, PharmD, is Director, Pharmaceutical Research, University of Texas, Department of Pediatrics, M.D. Anderson Cancer Center, Houston, Texas.

Armen P. Melikian, PharmD, is Associate Director, Department of Clinical Pharmacology, Berlex Laboratories, Montville, New Jersey.

Michael V. Miles, PharmD, is Professor of Pharmacy and Pediatrics, Children's Hospital Medical Center, Cincinnati, Ohio.

Ellen P. Morgan, RN, BSN, MPH, is Child Health Nurse, Berkeley County Health Department, Moncks Corner, South Carolina.

Gail M. Murphy, MD, is Director of Clinical Pharmacology, Merck Research Laboratories, Blue Bell, Pennsylvania.

Stephanie J. Phelps, PharmD, is Professor, College of Pharmacy, University of Tennessee, Memphis, Tennessee.

Michael D. Reed, PharmD, FCCP, FCP, is Professor of Pediatrics, School of Medicine, Case Western Reserve University, and Director, Pediatric Clinical Pharmacology and Toxicology, Rainbow Babies and Children's Hospital, Cleveland, Ohio.

Amelia Wall, PharmD, is Post Doctorate Fellow, Pharmaceutical Department, St. Jude Children's Research Hospital, Memphis, Tennessee.

Robert M. Ward, MD, FAAP, is Professor of Pediatrics and Neonatology, University of Utah School of Medicine, Salt Lake City, Utah.

Donald B. Wiest, PharmD, is Associate Professor, Department of Clinical Pharmacy, Medical University of South Carolina, Charleston, South Carolina.

1

Administering Drugs to Infants, Children, and Adolescents

Ann Marie Pagliaro

Drug therapy is commonly required during infancy, childhood, and adolescence to promote and maintain health and to prevent and treat disease. Immunization against communicable diseases and the management of common medical conditions, such as acute, self-limiting respiratory infections, often introduce infants, children, and adolescents to pediatric healthcare and drug therapy. Some pediatric patients may require drug therapy for the management of asthma, cystic fibrosis, insulin-dependent diabetes mellitus, or other chronic medical conditions. Others may require drug therapy for the treatment of accidental injuries, such as burns and bone fractures, and for life-threatening diseases, such as childhood cancers and acquired immune deficiency syndrome (AIDS).[1] This chapter presents an overview of drug formulations for pediatric use and their methods of administration (Table 1-1). Attention also is given to the factors (age, developmental level, general health status) that may affect the selection and use of a particular formulation for a pediatric patient.

Optimal pediatric drug therapy demands a multidisciplinary approach that respects each patient's self-medication abilities in relation to both short- and long-term drug therapy. It also requires attention to any fears or concerns that the patient may have about any aspect of drug therapy (Table 1-2). In addition, optimal pediatric drug therapy requires a respect for the abilities and contributions of parents[2] and others (day-care personnel, residential treatment staff, teachers) who may be responsible for, or involved with, drug therapy (e.g., administration, monitoring). In this regard, prescribers and other pediatric clinicians are responsible for adequately prepar-

---

1. The appropriate use of universal precautions (i.e., treating all pediatric patients as if they have been infected with the human immunodeficiency virus [HIV]) is recommended for drug administration procedures that expose pediatric clinicians or others involved with drug administration to blood and other body fluids. The use of protective gloves, gowns, and masks may be required for selected patients, depending on their prescribed drug therapy and clinical condition. Clinicians are reminded that basic hand washing is essential in preventing the transmission of disease and remains an important component of all drug administration procedures.

2. The term "parent" is used throughout this book to signify the infant's, child's, or adolescent's legal guardian or the person responsible for his or her general health and well-being.

TABLE 1-1
Major Routes of Pediatric Drug Administration and Associated Dosage Forms[a]

ROUTE OF ADMINISTRATION	DOSAGE FORMS
Inhalation	Solutions: for use with compressed-air nebulizer, for delivery by metered-dose inhaler
	Powders: for insufflation
Injectable	
Subcutaneous	Aqueous solutions, suspensions
Intramuscular	Aqueous solutions, emulsions, suspensions
Intravenous	Aqueous solutions, oil-in-water emulsions (e.g., *Diprivan®*)
Intraosseous	Aqueous solutions, suspensions
Intranasal	Creams
	Drops: solutions, suspensions
	Ointments
	Rhinyles: solutions
	Sprays
Ophthalmic	Drops: solutions, suspensions
	Inserts (not commonly used by pediatric patients)
	Ointments
Oral	Liquid oral dosage forms: elixirs, emulsions, oils, solutions, suspensions, syrups
	Solid oral dosage forms: capsules, granules, lozenges, microencapsulated beads, tablets
Otic	Drops: solutions, suspensions
Rectal	Enemas, large- and small-volume: oils, solutions, suspensions
	Gels, ointments
	Suppositories
Topical	
Local	Aerosol sprays, creams, gels, jellies, lotions, ointments, pastes, powders, shampoos, soaps, solutions, suspensions
Transdermal	Transdermal drug delivery systems (TDDSs) (not commonly used by pediatric patients)
Transmucosal	Buccal adhesive tablets (not commonly used by pediatric patients)
	Chewing gums
	Lozenges (e.g., *Fentanyl Oralet®*)
	Sublingual tablets (not commonly used by pediatric patients)
Vaginal	Creams, foams, gels, jellies, ointments, solutions, suppositories, tablets

[a] Selection of a dosage form should be based on individual needs, including age, general state of health, and developmental abilities. Attention to the pediatric patient's personal preference for taste, color, and texture, or that of caregivers in regard to ease of administration (e.g., oral suspension versus having to crush a solid oral dosage form for administration with an appropriate vehicle), should likewise be considered.

ing pediatric patients prior to administering required drug therapy and ensuring, as appropriate, that they, and their parents, understand the correct administration of a required drug and its safe handling, storage, and disposal. Attention to these aspects of pediatric drug therapy helps achieve optimal therapeutic benefit with a minimum of adverse drug effects, missed doses, incorrect administration, inadvertent overdosages, and accidental poisonings (*see also* Chapters 4 and 5).

Drug Administration

The ability of children and adolescents and their parents to influence drug therapy is an important aspect of pediatric healthcare. Even young children make choices regarding drug therapy and can assist with drug administration. The administration of drugs to pediatric patients can be difficult and challenging. For example, getting an infant to swallow an unpleasant-tasting drug; encouraging a toddler to remain still for the instillation of eye drops; obtaining a preschooler's cooperation with the insertion of a rectal suppository; securing a child's cooperation with the intradermal, subcutaneous, or intramuscular injection of drugs and vaccines; or obtaining an adolescent's cooperation with the insertion of a venous access device for the injection of an intravenous drug takes time, patience, and clinical know-how.

Pediatric clinicians should not forget that many pediatric patients react negatively to intrusive procedures because these procedures

(Continued on page 6)

TABLE 1-2
General Developmental Considerations for Drug Administration

INFANTS (1–12 MONTHS)

General Development: Infants are in Freud's (1964a, 1964b) oral stage of development, Erikson's (1950, 1963) stage of trust versus mistrust with a lasting outcome of drive and hope, and Piaget's (1950, 1963, 1969) stage of sensorimotor perception. Basic trust, according to Erikson (1950, 1963), who extended Freudian theory, is thought to develop during infancy. It is during this time that infants become attached to their mother or primary care provider. Feelings of familiarity are important to infants, and consistency, continuity, and sameness of experience encourage infants to trust themselves (i.e., cope with their own urges) and others. They are increasingly able to remember painful experiences (e.g., injections) and associate these experiences with other stimuli (e.g., white uniforms or laboratory coats).

Application: Infants as young as 4 months may fear strangers and separation from their parents or usual care providers. When hospitalization is required, needlessly separating infants from their parents or usual care providers should be avoided. Flexible visiting hours and rooming-in or care-by-parents programs should be encouraged. As appropriate, parents should be taught how to administer their infant's drugs and then encouraged to do so whenever possible. Provide appropriate guidance and supervision, ensuring that parents understand the purpose of drug therapy and drug administration procedures. The pediatric clinician should encourage them to ask questions and should answer their questions honestly and sensitively. If, for whatever reason, parents are unable to assist with drug administration, the infant should be given an opportunity to become familiar with the pediatric clinician. Transitional objects, such as a favorite blanket or stuffed toy, should be kept nearby. Infants should be spoken to softly and in high-pitched tones. They should be handled gently and should be held and cuddled before and after drug administration. These basic approaches to drug therapy are particularly important when procedures are painful or intrusive.

TODDLERS (1–3 YEARS)

General Development: Toddlers are in the anal stage of Freudian development and Erikson's (1950, 1963) stage of shame versus doubt with a lasting outcome of self-control and willpower. According to Piaget (1950, 1963, 1969), they are in the early stage of preoperational thought and continue to be egocentric and use magical thinking as they develop separation-individuation. They have little concept of body integrity and have no conception of mass. Their major fears generally include separation from their parents or primary care provider and loss of control or autonomy. Toddlers are gradually developing language skills and the ability to think in images and symbols. They can understand more than they can verbalize and they are highly literal. They can communicate their needs and wants. Toddlers are concerned only with the present and can focus on only one aspect of an event at a time. They do not have a well-developed concept of time, and they can perceive direct interaction as threatening.

Application: Toddlers should be prepared only a few minutes before drugs are administered to prevent prolonged anxiety, which may occur when preparation is given too far in advance. When toddlers are prepared for drug administration, they should be given simple explanations in a depersonalized manner, using dolls or stuffed toys for demonstration. Toddlers should be allowed to explore drug administration equipment (e.g., plastic drug cup, intravenous tubing), which should then be used during therapeutic play sessions following drug administration. Therapeutic play can help toddlers deal with their feeling that drug therapy and illness are forms of punishment. For example, toddlers can give "medicine" to their teddy bear or doll. This approach not only helps them visualize what to expect, but also can help them maintain control during threatening situations. Large or unusual equipment can increase anxiety and is best introduced during therapeutic play *after* rather than before intrusive procedures are performed. Undue physical restraint can cause increased fear and protesting, and should be avoided when drugs are administered to toddlers. Toddlers should be approached calmly and with confidence, and the drug should be administered promptly.

Pediatric clinicians should be truthful and help the toddler cope with frightening, intrusive, or painful procedures in a positive way, keeping in mind that toddlers can react negatively to such procedures and often remember them. Toddlers should be allowed to object to their drug therapy, and their anger should be accepted. Aggression should be redirected (e.g., by encouraging play with a wooden or plastic hammer and peg board), rather than punished. In in-patient settings and clinics, separation from parents should be minimized, and parents should be allowed and encouraged to administer drugs whenever possible. Active participation by the parents meets the toddler's developmental needs and presents an opportunity for the

TABLE 1-2 *continued*

clinician to teach drug administration techniques and develop the parents' abilities. When parents are not available to administer a toddler's drugs, transitional objects should be kept close by. Such objects also can be used for demonstrating administration procedures to prepare the toddler for therapy and during therapeutic play after drug administration.

PRESCHOOLERS (3–5 YEARS)

General Development: Preschoolers are in Freud's (1964a, 1964b) stage of genital development and Erikson's (1950, 1963) stage of initiative versus guilt—the stage of the castration complex—with a lasting outcome of direction and purpose. They are in Piaget's (1950, 1963, 1969) preoperational stage of cognitive development. Preschoolers fear abandonment, the unknown, the dark, and loss of control. They are egocentric and imaginative. Magical thinking and animism are characteristic of preschoolers who have well-developed communication and self-care abilities. However, they are not capable of abstract thinking and have a limited understanding of the inside of the body. Preschoolers have difficulty differentiating "good hurt" (e.g., injection) from "bad hurt" (e.g., injury). They also may interpret words literally, and they use words they have heard but do not understand, often creating their own explanations and definitions. The preschooler has a limited concept of time and may have primitive ideas about body integrity and disease causation. For example, preschoolers may fear that their insides will leak out if a bandage is not applied after they receive an injection. They also have castration and mutilation fantasies.

Application: Preschoolers can participate actively in many aspects of drug therapy. Explanations regarding drug therapy should be kept simple and concrete and wording should be carefully chosen. Because verbal explanations usually are inadequate, simple drawings of the body, body outlines, simple anatomical models, and drug administration equipment should be used in explaining drug therapy. Descriptions of familiar body parts and what the preschooler will see, hear, feel, smell, and taste should be provided.

Preschoolers usually will take an oral dosage form after a simple explanation and a little encouragement. A positive approach is important. Preschoolers should be approached as if they are expected to take the drug; they should never be threatened or bribed. To provide them with a sense of control over the situation, they should be given a choice whenever possible. For example, a preschooler might be given a choice of how to take a drug (e.g., as a liquid from a plastic drug cup or an oral syringe, as a liquid diluted in a favorite compatible beverage, or as a chewable tablet) and where to take it (e.g., sitting on a parent's lap or in a favorite chair). When changes in the drug therapy plan are required, the pediatric clinician should be honest in explaining why, thus maintaining the child's trust.

It also is important that preschoolers be allowed and encouraged to help with various aspects of drug administration. A preschooler could, for example, go with the pediatric clinician to get the drug and needed supplies, take a tablet (or other solid oral dosage form) out of a plastic drug cup, and dispose of the cup (or other equipment) safely with supervision. Preschoolers often enjoy being referred to as helpers and such activities increase their sense of control.

Some preschoolers need help with certain aspects of drug administration, particularly intrusive procedures that are frightening or painful. When preschoolers cannot cooperate with drug administration, they should be reassured that they will be helped during the procedure and that they have done nothing wrong and are not being punished.

Such sensitivity on the part of the pediatric clinician will help preschoolers deal with the feelings of guilt and blame associated with their primitive concept of illness causation. Positive reinforcement should be given for their assistance and cooperation with any aspect of drug administration. For example, the preschooler might be told something like "that was good—holding still—I know that was hard for you to do" even if gentle manual restraint of the extremity or cuddling by the parent or another clinician was necessary to keep the child in a required position. Preschoolers like colorful stickers and adhesive bandages, which can be used as rewards.

Pediatric clinicians need to choose their words carefully. Confusing "dye" with "die," for example, or hearing phrases such as "he has no veins" or "I need to draw blood," can cause undue distress among preschoolers. Terms such as "with your breakfast," "after lunch," and "before you go to sleep" should be used to explain dosage schedules. The need for drug therapy should be explained each time it is required; it cannot be assumed that a preschooler will remember information provided earlier.

Preschoolers may fear that their insides will leak out after they have received an injection; clinicians should always offer to apply a colorful bandage to injection sites. To ascertain their understanding and per-

TABLE 1-2 *continued*

ceptions regarding drug therapy, preschoolers should be asked to repeat the information they've been told to the clinician or parent, or to a doll. Therapeutic play is particularly helpful for preschoolers. The pediatric clinician should be attentive to what the child says when playing and should emphasize that the drug is to help her/him get better faster or be healthier. To promote feelings of pride and increased self-esteem, preschoolers should be praised when they demonstrate an understanding of the reasons for their drug therapy and for cooperating with drug administration procedures. For example, a preschooler might be told, "Yes, the medicine is to help your tummy not hurt so much" or "Thank you for drinking your medicine in one gulp." To prevent confusion, preschoolers should not be told that they are "good" for ingesting a drug; rather, they should be told that they are "good medicine takers."

SCHOOL-AGE CHILDREN (6–12 YEARS)

General Development: School-age children are in Freud's (1964a, 1964b) stage of latency and Erikson's (1950, 1963) stage of industry versus inferiority with a lasting outcome of method and competence. According to Piaget (1950, 1963, 1969), they are in the stage of concrete operations. The major fears of school-age children are loss of control; bodily injury and mutilation; not being able to live up to the expectations of adults, particularly parents, teachers, and pediatric clinicians; and death. Although school-age children begin to think logically and can reason, they continue to have a tendency to be literal and may have vague or false ideas about illness, body construction (i.e., anatomy), and function (i.e., physiology) or may have no ideas about them at all. School-age children have a good understanding of the concept of time and an increasing awareness of the significance of various illnesses, potential hazards of treatment, life-long consequences of injury, and death. Although they have an increasing ability to understand the relationship between illness and treatment, they continue to have misconceptions about disease causation, believing that illness can be caused by misdeeds or "bad" behavior. School-age children have a tendency to nod as if they understand what they have been told when, in fact, they do not. They may be reluctant to ask questions or admit that they do not know something they think they should know. They enjoy peer interaction.

Application: Body diagrams, age-appropriate anatomical models, teaching dolls, and drug administration equipment should be used to demonstrate and explain drug therapy. Pediatric clinicians can build on the school-age child's knowledge of the human body and provide basic physiologic descriptions. Metaphors (e.g., nerves are like telephone wires) can be used in explanations. However, to prevent undue anxiety, explanations should be limited based on the school-age child's age and maturity and on what he or she wants to know at a particular time (as indicated by questions and behavior). School-age children should be involved in making decisions about their care whenever possible and should participate in appropriate aspects of the drug administration process (e.g., selecting required equipment, tearing tape to secure their venous access device). This approach helps to prevent regression to a less mature state, a problem sometimes encountered when school-age children feel threatened. Providing school-age children with a choice often helps to increase their feelings of control and self-esteem and, thus, enhances their cooperation with their drug therapy.

Activities that school-age children can participate in despite their illness should be stressed to decrease their sense of feeling different from healthy children. School-age children should be reassured that they have done nothing wrong and that the need for drug therapy is not a punishment for misdeeds. When cooperation is difficult to obtain, as with painful or frightening procedures, pediatric clinicians should explain that they understand how difficult the situation is and they know the child is trying to do his or her best. It is important that school-age children be praised for helping with any aspect of the procedure. As with younger children, age-appropriate colorful stickers and adhesive bandages and small, safe toys can be used as rewards. To prevent misunderstandings, school-age children should be asked to repeat the information they are given. Peer-group teaching sessions also are effective.

ADOLESCENTS (13–17 YEARS)

General Development: Adolescents are in Erikson's (1950, 1963) stage of identity versus role confusion with a lasting outcome of devotion and fidelity, and Piaget's (1950, 1963, 1969) stage of formal operations. Adolescents fear altered body image, loss of control, and separation from their families and peers. Although they need to demonstrate independence from their parents, they alternate between needs for independence and dependence. They are concerned with sexual development and have a need for privacy.

Adolescents generally are concerned that others will think they are dumb if they do not understand something they are expected to know and then fear that their feelings of inadequacy, dependency, and

TABLE 1-2 continued

confusion will be discovered. Formal operational thought and the ability to reason and think abstractly continue to develop during adolescence.

Adolescents are interested in scientific explanations and understand analogies and proverbs. However, they generally have little understanding of the structure and function of their bodies. Some magical thinking (e.g., feeling guilty for their illness), egocentrism, and castration anxiety still exist in this age group. Although they are generally oriented to the present, adolescents can project to the future and see long-term consequences. They may be overly sensitive to pain; thus their reactions to intrusive procedures may not always seem appropriate. They also may have an exaggerated response to even simple procedures. Peer groups are important to adolescents.

Application: Adolescents need accurate information about their drug therapy. However, they can become anxious when information is threatening. Thus, clinicians need to be sensitive when giving information, as adolescents react not only to what they are told, but also to how information is communicated to them. Adolescents' knowledge about drugs and the need for drug therapy should be explored and assessed carefully.

Adolescents should be involved in making all decisions about their care. When discussing drug therapy, pediatric clinicians should stress ways in which adolescents can participate. Medical terminology and diagrams that illustrate anatomy and physiology can be used to explain drug therapy. Printed information and instructions should be made available to adolescents. The importance of compliance and the consequences of not following planned drug therapy should be discussed truthfully.

Whenever possible, adolescents should be prepared in advance of procedures. Being prepared in advance will enhance their ability to cope and cooperate with required drug therapy. Preparation for subcutaneous or intramuscular injections, intravenous infusions, and other invasive procedures should be planned individually in relation to the adolescent's coping style and the type of drug therapy required. As with preschool and school-age children, age-appropriate play, including creative writing and expressive art, can be used to help adolescents cope with and communicate their perceptions and concerns.

Adolescents can receive support from peers who have had similar experiences; teaching and discussion sessions regarding drug therapy should include peers whenever possible. Adolescent support groups also can be used as a forum for expressing feelings and voicing complaints and worries.

---

may be frightening or be perceived as painful invasions of their bodies. Thus, it is essential that, whenever possible, each pediatric patient be adequately prepared for drug therapy according to age, developmental abilities, and coping style. Previous experiences with drug therapy, both positive and negative, also must be considered. To assist clinicians with this task, guidelines using developmental theory and current recommendations for the administration of various dosage formulations are presented in Table 1-2. The use of these guidelines and recommendations can assist clinicians in assessing the needs and abilities of pediatric patients in regard to drug therapy and can assist in planning approaches to secure cooperation, prevent undue injury, and promote active participation. The approach used has the potential to affect the patient's knowledge about health and illness, reaction to diagnostic and treatment procedures, and willingness to participate in drug therapy.

The importance of individually assessing each infant, child, and adolescent prior to explaining drug therapy or administering drugs as well as the importance of establishing rapport and trust cannot be overemphasized. The use of evidence-based recommendations for drug administration can assist pediatric clinicians with the selection and administration of dosage forms.

Special Considerations

Pediatric patients who are confused, mentally retarded, or have other mental disorders (e.g., attention-deficit/hyperactivity disorder [A-D/HD], autism, childhood or adolescent schizophrenia) can present a special challenge to pediatric clinicians in relation to drug administration and often require time and patience. Clinicians may have to resort to creative and individualized approaches reflective of the specific needs or concerns of the patient, who may react negatively to such procedures as the instillation of eye, ear, and nose drops; the insertion of suppositories; or the administration of injections and venipuncture. These procedures can be painful and frightening for these patients who may misinterpret them as an attack. In addition, confused, mentally retarded, or psychotic patients may have a hyper-responsiveness to pain. Thus, their reactions to intrusive procedures involved in drug therapy may not always seem appropriate. They may have a magnified response to even simple procedures. Advance preparation and appropriate timing for procedures may enhance their ability to cope and cooperate. Preparation for injections, intravenous therapy, and other intrusive procedures should be planned in relation to the patient's cognitive and mental abilities, coping style, physical abilities, and previous drug therapy experiences. The maintenance of patient dignity, including personal rights and freedoms, and the prevention of injury are major concerns.

The confused, mentally retarded, or psychotic patient should be approached calmly and with confidence, and the drug should be administered promptly. Undue physical restraint should be avoided because it can increase combativeness, fear, and protest. Pediatric clinicians should acknowledge the patient's fear or confusion. Depending on mental age, a warm touch or hug after completion of the procedure, if appropriate, can be effective. A caring and understanding approach is essential. Patients should be allowed to object, and their anger should be accepted. However, they must be protected from harming themselves and others. Aggression should be redirected and not punished or "treated" with undue use of physical or chemical restraints.

With the confused, mentally retarded, or mentally disordered patient, explanations regarding drug therapy should be kept simple and concrete. Teaching sessions should be completed in areas where there are few distractions and noise is minimal. To enhance verbal explanations, body diagrams, simple models, and the actual equipment required for drug therapy should be used along with demonstrations. These patients may require continued reminders and re-explanations each time the drug is administered.

The confused, mentally retarded, or psychotic patient will usually take the required drug after a simple explanation and with a little encouragement. A positive approach is important. To maintain independence, patients should be allowed and encouraged to make decisions regarding aspects of their drug therapy as appropriate for their cognitive and mental abilities. For example, although a confused, mentally retarded, or psychotic person may not have a legal say regarding required drug therapy, he or she may be able to choose how the drug will be ingested (e.g., in a particular beverage or soft food, in tablet or liquid form) and where it will be ingested (e.g., at the dispensary, in the television room, sitting in a favorite chair in the residence).

To promote appropriate participation, confused, mentally retarded, and psychotic patients should be acknowledged for demonstrating an understanding of any aspect of their drug therapy and for cooperating in any way. For example, they could be told: "The medicine helps you not to shake and to walk better"; "Yes, the medicine helps your hands to feel better and your fingers to move easier"; or "Yes, your *Thorazine*® at this higher dosage helps you get along better with the other boys on your unit." Psychotic or confused patients should be treated not condescendingly, but in a warm, respectful, and understanding way. They should not be told that they are "good" for taking their drugs; rather, they should be acknowledged and thanked for making an effort to participate in their drug therapy.

Oral Dosage Forms

Many common pediatric drugs are available in liquid and solid oral dosage forms (Table 1-1). Although oral dosage forms have several advantages, including stability, portability, and convenience, they have several disadvantages. For example, liquid and solid oral dosage forms may be associated with irritating effects on the GI system, resulting in nausea, vomiting, or diarrhea. Also, the ingredients used in the formulation of a particular oral dosage form may cause allergic-type reactions among susceptible pediatric patients.[3] In addition, the willingness of pediatric patients to follow their prescribed drug therapy may be adversely affected by an unpleasant taste (e.g., chloral hydrate *[Noctec®]*), smell (e.g., phenytoin *[Dilantin®]*), or texture (various liquid antacids).[4]

The absorption of oral dosage forms varies because of the gastric emptying rate, the transit time through the GI tract, and the pH of gastric and intestinal fluids. These factors, in turn, may be influenced by food or liquids in the GI tract or by the actions of other drugs (e.g., drugs that have anticholinergic actions, such as antidepressants, may increase intestinal transit time by slowing bowel motility). In addition, the type of oral dosage form selected (e.g., capsule or tablet) and the differences between "identical dosage forms" manufactured by different drug companies may significantly affect absorption of the drug and its effects (*see* Chapter 10). However, despite these limitations, oral dosage forms continue to be the most commonly used dosage form for pediatric patients, and therefore it is important to understand factors involved with their use.

Generally, oral dosage forms should be prescribed so that the dosing schedule is as simple as possible (e.g., once-daily dosing) without compromising therapeutic efficacy. Prescribers also should be attentive to individual patient preferences for taste, odor, and texture and should accommodate these preferences whenever possible. For example, chlorpromazine *(Largactil®, Thorazine®)* is formulated as capsules, tablets, oral suspension, flavored or unflavored syrups, and concentrated oral solution that can be selected according to patient needs and preferences.

Although oral dosage forms are convenient and offer options for individualizing pediatric drug therapy, they are contraindicated for pediatric patients who are sedated, struggling, vomiting, undergoing gastric or intestinal suction, unconscious, or unable for any other reason to ingest foods or liquids by mouth (e.g., fasting for laboratory tests, religious observances, surgery).

All oral dosage forms require safe storage in the clinical setting, home, or residential facility so they cannot be inadvertently accessed by others. Expiration dates must be checked to ensure that oral formulations are not outdated. Any expired drugs require safe disposal (e.g., return to the dispensing pharmacy for disposal). The manufacturer's storage recommendations (e.g., protect from moisture and light, store under controlled room temperature)[5] should be followed to avoid or minimize drug deterioration, which can adversely affect therapy.

Liquid Oral Dosage Forms

Elixirs, oils, solutions, suspensions, and syrups are available for most pediatric drugs. Such liquid dosage forms are commonly prescribed for infants and children younger than 5 years and for older children and adolescents who have difficulty swallowing solid oral dosage forms such as capsules and tablets (*see* Solid Oral Dosage Forms). All liquid oral dosage forms are less portable and less convenient to ingest than solid oral dosage forms (e.g., they generally require the use of a measuring device such as a calibrated dropper, they may require refrigeration). In addition, solutions and elixirs can be particularly irritating to the gastric mucosa and may be associated with such

---

3. For example, sulfites may cause an allergic-type reaction (anaphylaxis, hives, itching, wheezing) among pediatric patients, particularly those who have a history of asthma.

4. Specific drug examples, including both generic and brand or trade names, have been included throughout the chapter to assist in making the related concepts more meaningful. Unless specifically noted, the concepts that apply to a specific generic drug apply to all brand or trade name formulations of that generic drug and not solely to the brand or trade names listed. The specific brand or trade names listed are provided simply as examples and not as an exhaustive list.

5. The bathroom is a common, but inappropriate, place to store drugs. Advise patients and their parents to avoid storing drugs in the bathroom because high temperature and humidity contribute to drug decomposition. Instruct them to safely store drugs according to manufacturer recommendations in a locked cabinet or drawer in a cool, dry room.

adverse drug reactions (ADRs) as nausea and vomiting. Concern also has been raised regarding the stability of liquid dosage forms for pediatric patients (Nahata, 1999).

Some liquid oral dosage forms have high sodium concentrations while others, such as syrups and some elixirs, are sweetened to make them more palatable. These oral formulations may present a potential problem for pediatric patients who require dietary regulation of salt (e.g., children who have cardiovascular disorders [congestive heart failure, hypertension], nephrotic syndrome) or sugar (e.g., children who have diabetes mellitus), particularly when chronic, long-term use is required. The alcohol content of elixirs and some syrups (e.g., butabarbital elixir, which contains 7% alcohol; morphine oral syrup *[M.O.S.®]*, which contains 5% alcohol; phenobarbital elixir, which contains 10% alcohol) also may preclude their use for pediatric patients who have histories of alcohol use, are receiving disulfiram *(Antabuse®)*, or cannot tolerate the additional CNS depression associated with these alcohol-containing formulations. Prescribers and other pediatric clinicians should be aware of the alcohol, sodium, and sugar content of liquid oral dosage forms as well as other nonmedicinal ingredients when selecting a product. For example, amprenavir *(Agenerase®)* oral solution contains a large amount of propylene glycol and is contraindicated for neonates, infants, and children younger than 4 years.

Oral suspensions (e.g., amitriptyline *[Elavil®])*, including those formulated as powders or granules for reconstitution with purified water prior to dispensing, are often available for drugs that are insoluble or, when in solution, are unstable or unpalatable. Other suspension products are formulated as ready-to-use liquids (e.g., *PediaProfen®* [ibuprofen]). Because they tend to precipitate, oral suspensions must be shaken well to ensure that the correct dose is measured and ingested. Syrups (other than cough syrups, which may be used for both their local and systemic effects) should be ingested with an appropriate amount of water or other compatible liquid chaser to ensure that the drug is evenly distributed in the suspension and that the correct dose has been swallowed. The oral syrup formulation of meperidine *(Demerol®)* also should be ingested with sufficient water (30–60 ml) to lessen its topical anesthetic effect, unless it is prescribed for this indication.

Oil formulations (e.g., castor oil, cod liver oil, mineral oil) generally are not recommended for pediatric use because they are unpleasant to ingest and their use has been associated with diminished nutrient and vitamin absorption, with anal leakage and pruritus, and with lipid pneumonia as a result of inadvertent aspiration.

Palatability. Unpleasant tasting liquids can be made more palatable by diluting them in a small amount of water or other compatible beverage (cold fruit juices, soft drinks) or soft food (cold applesauce, pudding). Many liquid oral dosage forms have been specially formulated to make them more acceptable to infants, children, and adolescents. For example, liquid oral dosage forms of ampicillin are available in vanilla-pineapple, fruit, and cherry flavors. Amoxicillin is available in strawberry, banana, and bubble gum flavors. Ibuprofen suspension is available in orange and berry-vanilla flavors. Some oil formulations also are flavored and can be administered over ice or in juice to further improve their palatability. Most pediatric patients will ingest unpleasant-tasting liquid oral dosage formulations if they are made more palatable by mixing them in small amounts of compatible liquids (e.g., fruit juices, cold drinks such as ginger ale) or cold soft foods (e.g., applesauce, pudding). However, attention to potential incompatibilities of liquids and soft foods is needed to avoid potential drug interactions that could adversely affect therapeutic benefit.[6]

For example, children and adolescents who require liquid oral dosage formulations because they cannot swallow solid oral dosage

---

6. Prescribers and other pediatric clinicians also must ensure that patients are aware of which beverages and soft foods should be avoided when diluting liquid oral dosage forms, because pH incompatibilities or the formation of precipitates may affect drug potency.

forms may be more compliant if the dose is diluted in a small amount of compatible beverage instead of water. For example, haloperidol *(Haldol®)* solution can be mixed in apple, orange, or tomato juice or in cola drinks before ingestion. It should not, however, be diluted with coffee or tea. Children and adolescents who require chlorpromazine *(Largactil, Thorazine)* may prefer ingesting each dose mixed in orange juice from frozen concentrate, lemon-lime soda, or apricot, grapefruit, prune, tomato, or a mixed vegetable juice. However, it should not be diluted with apple juice, coffee, cola, diet ginger ale, root beer, or tea. In addition, although fluphenazine oral concentrate *(Permitil® Oral Concentrate)* may be diluted with tomato or fruit juices, milk, and noncaffeinated soft drinks, it should not be diluted with beverages that contain caffeine (e.g., coffee, cola drinks), tannins (e.g., tea), or pectinates (e.g., apple juice) because of physical incompatibilities. Both product labeling and a pharmacist should always be consulted about beverage and food compatibilities when liquid oral dosage forms need to be made more palatable for pediatric patients.

In addition to making liquid oral dosage forms more palatable for pediatric patients, the selection of concentrated oral liquid formulations (i.e., concentrated oral liquid dosage forms that are dosed in small volumes) may be another alternative. Several drugs are (or will be) available as concentrated oral liquid formulations *(Intensol®* products for chlorpromazine, dexamethasone, diazepam, hydrochlorothiazide, morphine, prednisone, propranolol, thioridazine; Roxane Laboratories, Columbus, Ohio). They are relatively tasteless and are compatible when mixed with most beverages and soft foods. *Intensol* products can be ingested with small amounts of juices, soft drinks, applesauce, or pudding. These products and other concentrated oral liquid dosage forms are suitable for pediatric patients who require fluid restriction or nutritional formulas by gastric or nasogastric tubes, or who have difficulty swallowing (e.g., a child with cerebral palsy). They also may be helpful for pediatric patients who have difficulty ingesting solid oral dosage forms.

Measuring devices. Several devices facilitate both the measurement and administration of liquid oral dosage forms, including plastic calibrated drug cups, spillproof liquid drug spoons, and oral syringes and droppers. Plastic drug cups are usually calibrated in 5-ml increments, teaspoons, tablespoons, and ounces, and they accommodate up to 30 ml. Plastic oral syringes are calibrated in 1-ml increments, usually accommodate up to 10 ml, and have no needle. They are commonly used in pediatric in-patient settings and clinics. Oral drug syringes (e.g., Monoject Oral Drug Syringe®) are manufactured by several companies and are sold in many pharmacies for home use. They are available with both clear plastic and amber-colored barrels for non-light-sensitive and light-sensitive drugs, respectively.

The use of drug dispensing cups provided with pediatric liquid cough and cold products and pediatric analgesics (e.g., acetaminophen elixir) has been associated with measurement errors at home. These measurement errors resulted from the parent's difficulty differentiating between teaspoon and tablespoon abbreviations on the dispensing cup and from the incorrect assumption that the full dispensing cup was the dose to be ingested by the infant or child. Another concern for pediatric clinicians is the possibility that the 30-ml plastic drug cups commonly used in pediatric clinical settings to provide more accurate drug measurement could cause dose measurement errors in the home setting if used by children, adolescents, and their parents without adequate instruction.

Some concentrated liquid oral dosage formulations, including those for chlorpromazine *(Largactil),* diazepam *(Valium®),* morphine *(M.O.S.),* and thioridazine *(Mellaril®),* are supplied with calibrated droppers that always should be used to measure the required dose of the product. These devices should not be used interchangeably for measuring different liquid oral drug products because the viscosities may be different, thus affecting the accuracy of the dose significantly. Pediatric patients and their parents, as appropriate, should be taught to use measuring devices correctly. Such instruction is particularly important when patients/parents are measuring doses of the highly concentrated oral liquid dosage forms (e.g., *Intensol* products) or other drugs that have a narrow therapeutic index, such as anticonvulsants (e.g., phenytoin *[Dilantin]*), antidysrhythmics (e.g., digoxin *[Lanoxin]*), and bronchodilators (e.g., theophylline *[Aquaphyllin®]*). Although the *Intensols* and other concentrated drug products offer pediatric clinicians and their patients an important alternative to other oral liquid drug therapy (i.e., they can be administered in small amounts, they are generally odorless and tasteless, they are generally compatible with most foods and beverages), they are **concentrated** drug products that require particular attention to use and storage to prevent inadvertent overdosage and poisoning.

The standard teaspoon, thought to hold 5 ml, is not generally recommended for measuring oral liquid dosage forms because of variability associated with the style of the teaspoon, the viscosity of the liquid measured, and the person measuring. Generally, the oral drug syringe should be used for measuring liquid dosage forms when drugs have a narrow therapeutic index (e.g., digoxin *[Lanoxin]*, lithium *[Eskalith®, Lithane®]*) or when several different people are administering the drug (e.g., family members, residential care personnel, teachers). When used correctly, the oral drug syringe ensures a more accurate and consistent dose. Pediatric patients and their parents should be shown the correct use of the oral drug syringe. In addition, they should routinely check expiration dates on liquid formulations and safely store liquid oral formulations in a cool, dark place, preferably in a locked drawer or cabinet to prevent inadvertent ingestion by others.

Pediatric clinicians must be aware that all measuring devices for liquid oral dosage forms have the potential for error. To prevent errors, clinicians should be familiar with the drug products they prescribe and administer, particularly those dispensed with droppers or other special measuring devices, and they should have the actual drug formulation required or a sample drug container for demonstrating correct drug measurement and administration.

The accuracy of the dose of an oral liquid drug formulation delivered from a unit-dose container has been questioned because of the substantial volume of residual liquid left in the container after the dose has been ingested. However, because unit-dose products are customarily overfilled to achieve delivery of the proper dose, pediatric patients should ingest their dose directly from the liquid unit-dose container. They should be advised not to fill the container with water and ingest the residual drug, unless they are specifically directed to do so in the product labeling or by their pharmacist. They also should be told not to transfer the drug to another container or device (e.g., oral drug dosing syringe) for ingestion.

Solid Oral Dosage Forms

Tablet and capsule solid oral dosage forms generally offer greater drug stability and dosing accuracy than liquid oral dosage forms. However, these solid oral dosage forms have some disadvantages, including the potential for esophageal irritation or injury.[7] In addition, the bioavailability of a solid oral dosage form may be less than that obtained from an equivalent dose of a liquid oral dosage form (*see* Chapter 10). Solid oral dosage forms also may present problems for those children and adolescents who have difficulty swallowing them (e.g., children and adolescents with cerebral palsy). To obtain the desired maximal benefit, solid oral dosage forms must be ingested according to their specific design, intended use, and pharmacologic action.

Tablets. Tablets are the most widely used solid oral dosage form because of their convenience, compactness, dosing accuracy, ease of administration, economy, portability, and stability. Tablets are generally differentiated by color, flavor, shape (e.g., oval, rectangular, round, square, triangular), type of coating (e.g., enteric, film, thin sugar), and size

---

7. "Pill-sticking injury" may occur if a solid oral dosage form sticks to the mucosa of the esophagus after it is swallowed. The tablet or capsule may cause discomfort and local irritation as the tablet or capsule dissolves.

(large, small).⁸ Some tablets have been reformulated as caplets (e.g., aspirin [Anacin® Caplet], lactase [LactAid® Caplet]) to facilitate drug transit through the esophagus. Caplets can be swallowed whole or chewed before swallowing, depending on the manufacturer's instructions (e.g., Anacin Caplets are nonchewable, whereas LactAid Caplets can be chewed). There also are chewable tablets, including children's chewable vitamins (e.g., Bugs Bunny®, Flintstones®, Garfield®, Sesame Street®).

Chewable tablets (e.g., chewable acetaminophen [Children's Anacin-3®] and mebendazole [Vermox®]) are commonly used in pediatric drug therapy. These tablets require thorough chewing before swallowing to ensure complete disintegration of the tablet, drug release, and proper drug absorption. If chewable tablets are not chewed completely before swallowing, some chewable tablets (e.g., calcium carbonate antacids [e.g., Tums®]) may have limited effectiveness and may also cause serious ADRs (e.g., GI obstruction requiring surgical intervention). However, other tablets (e.g., phenazopyridine [Pyridium®]) should not be allowed to dissolve in the mouth, nor be chewed. These tablets should be swallowed whole because of adverse effects if chewed (e.g., staining of the teeth).

Controlled-release, extended-release, prolonged-release, and sustained-release tablets also are available for pediatric use (e.g., codeine [codeine Contin®], metformin [Glucophage XR®], methylphenidate [Ritalin-SR]). These oral tablets gradually release their active drug ingredient into the GI tract for up to 24 hours. These tablets, likewise, should not be chewed. To simplify drug dosing schedules for children and adolescents, several drugs (e.g., clorazepate [Tranxene-SD®], methamphetamine [Gradumet Sustained-Release Desoxyn®], methylphenidate [Ritalin-SR®], oxycodone [OxyContin®]) have been formulated as sustained- or extended-release tablets that reduce the need for frequent dosing. To ensure that these tablets dissolve at the correct rate and to prevent dangerous ADRs associated with "dumping" the full dose, the patient should not chew or crush controlled-, extended-, and sustained-release tablets.⁹

A 24-hour controlled-release osmotic tablet (e.g., nifedipine [Procardia XL® extended-release tablet]) has been developed. This tablet form maintains constant plasma concentrations over 24 hours, which greatly simplifies dosing regimens and, in doing so, greatly promotes compliance. This controlled-release tablet is formulated as a two-layer system (i.e., drug layer and osmotic driving agent layer). GI fluid is pulled into the osmotic layer of the 24-hour controlled-release tablet through its semipermeable membrane. The pressure increases in the osmotic layer, causing the drug layer to release drug through a precision laser-drilled orifice in the tablet.

The composition of the dosage form and the mechanism of drug release appear to be important in determining the effect of the absence or presence of food in the stomach on drug release and absorption. As with other controlled-, extended-, and sustained-release tablets, the 24-hour controlled release tablets should be swallowed whole, not cut, crushed, chewed, or dissolved in the mouth.

Another controlled-release product that uses osmotic release technology is the Concerta® (methylphenidate) extended-release tablet. The Concerta tablet is dosed once a day, in the morning, without regard to meals, and provides 12-hour sustained blood concentrations. It is a capsule-shaped tablet composed of three separate compartments. Once ingested, one end is "pushed" to activate the system. The drug is then released at a controlled rate through an "exit port" at the other end of the tablet. As with other osmotic tablets, Concerta tablets should be swallowed whole. Chewing, crushing, or breaking the tablet destroys the delivery mechanism. The tablet shell does not dissolve and may appear intact in the stool. Pediatric patients and their parents, as

---

8. Tablet size generally depends on the amount of drug binders, excipients, fillers, and other nonmedicinal ingredients used.

9. Sustained- or extended-release tablets that are scored may be cut or broken along the score mark, if necessary (e.g., to adjust the dosage, to facilitate ingestion), and will retain their sustained-release properties.

appropriate, should be advised that the appearance of this "ghost" in the stool is normal and not a cause for concern.

Effervescent tablets (e.g., *Alka-Seltzer®, K-Lyte®*) should be dissolved in water before ingestion according to the manufacturer's instructions that accompany the product. To minimize the possibility of ingesting bicarbonate, children and adolescents should be instructed not to drink the drug solution until the effervescence has subsided. They also should be cautioned against ingesting effervescent tablets before dissolving them.

Orally disintegrating, or "quick-dissolve," tablets (e.g., loperamide *[Imodium Quick-Dissolve®]*, mirtazapine *[Remeron SolTab®]*, olanzapine *[Zyprexa Zydis®]*) also are used for pediatric patients. The tablets can be swallowed whole, with or without water, chewed before swallowing, or allowed to dissolve on the tongue and then swallowed. These tablets usually dissolve in 30 seconds.

Rather than being orally ingested, buccal and sublingual tablets and some lozenges (e.g., *Fentanyl Oralet®*) are placed inside the cheek, under the tongue, or sucked (not chewed) for dissolution and transmucosal absorption. Other lozenges are used for their local oropharyngeal effects (e.g., benzocaine lozenges *[Vick's Children's Chloraseptic®]* for the relief of a sore throat).

Enteric-coated tablets also are used by pediatric patients. Tablets that have no coating (e.g., penicillin G), film coatings (e.g., amitriptyline *[Elavil]*), or thin sugar coatings (e.g., mesoridazine *[Serentil®]*) dissolve readily in the stomach when ingested. Enteric-coated tablets, however, are formulated to dissolve in the alkaline environment of the small intestine, where the drug is then released. As a direct result of their formulation, enteric-coated tablets can either protect the mouth, throat, esophagus, and stomach from the irritating effects of some drugs (e.g., aspirin *[Entrophen®, Novasen®]*, bisacodyl *[Dulcolax®]*, sulfasalazine *[Azulfidine EN-Tabs®]*, valproic acid *[Depakote®]*) or protect the drug (e.g., divalproate sodium *[Epival®]*) from degradation by the acidic secretions of the stomach.[10] To take advantage of enteric-coated tablets, children and adolescents should be advised to swallow enteric-coated tablets whole. These tablets should not be cut in half, chewed, crushed, or dissolved in the mouth. Also, they generally should not be ingested with antacids or milk, which can theoretically raise the pH of the stomach contents and, consequently, dissolve the enteric coating prematurely.

Other oral tablets not only should be swallowed whole, but also should be ingested with food or a meal to increase their bioavailability. For example, finofibrate oral tablets are absorbed slowly and variably when ingested on an empty stomach. When ingested with a meal, their bioavailability increases significantly. The micronized capsule formulation *(Lipidil Micro®)* offers even greater bioavailability when ingested with a meal; even further increased bioavailability can be achieved with the newer microcoated tablet formulation *(Lipidil Supra®)*.

If a child or adolescent cannot swallow whole a tablet that should not be broken, chewed, crushed, or dissolved in the mouth, an alternative oral dosage form (i.e., liquid oral dosage form) or method of administration (e.g., intramuscular or rectal) should be used. This recommendation also applies when unscored tablets must be cut in half or in quarters to obtain the correct dose, particularly when a drug has a narrow therapeutic index (e.g., lithium *[Eskalith, Lithane, Lithotabs®]*).[11]

---

10. The ingestion of enteric-coated tablets with food may delay their therapeutic action because of delayed gastric emptying and absorption. Thus, when rapid onset of action is required, enteric-coated microformulations (i.e., enteric-coated micropellets) of the particular drug should be used. These formulations release the micropellets in the stomach; because of their smaller size, gastric emptying is possible during the interdigestive and the digestive period. Attention to this predictable drug–food interaction is encouraged. In addition, it is also advised that if concomitant intake of food and enteric-coated tablets is unavoidable, and a rapid onset of drug absorption is necessary, micropellet formulations should be used. In addition, when the therapeutic effect is insufficient, drug dosage formulation and timing of drug administration should be assessed before a change in drug therapy is made.

11. In this case, lithium syrup could be substituted for lithium tablets.

Capsules. Many drugs are formulated for oral administration as hard or soft gelatin capsules, gelatin-filled capsules, soluble elastic capsules, and soft elastic capsules. Delayed-release capsules also are available.[12] Capsules can be prepared in various ways so that their drug contents can be ingested more easily. For example, hard gelatin capsules usually can be taken apart and their contents (e.g., powder or time-released beads) gently mixed in a small amount (5 ml [teaspoonful]) of compatible soft food such as cold applesauce or pudding. Powder contents must be adequately mixed to avoid inhaling the powder into the lungs, resulting in lung irritation (e.g., aspiration pneumonia, granuloma formation) or toxicity. Patients also should not chew timed-release beads (e.g., divalproex [*Depakote® Sprinkle*]) that have been sprinkled on or gently mixed into soft foods. These drug–food mixtures should be ingested immediately; they should not be prepared and stored for later use. Also, to ensure that the entire dose is swallowed completely, it should be followed with a glassful of cool water or other compatible beverage.

Soft gelatin capsules contain liquid forms of drug (e.g., chloral hydrate *[Noctec]*, docusate sodium *[Colace®]*, vitamin E). These capsules generally cannot be taken apart, nor should they be pierced or cut, which can result in drug loss. Most soft gelatin capsules can be dissolved in a small amount of water and ingested as a liquid. This procedure ensures that the entire dose is ingested. Some soft gelatin capsules (e.g., valproic acid [*Depakene®* 500 mg]) are enteric coated and should not be dissolved. If necessary, chloral hydrate *(Noctec)*, can be moistened with water and inserted rectally in the same way as a suppository. Generally, however, if a soft capsule cannot be swallowed whole or dissolved in a small amount of water, an alternative dosage form should be selected.

Powders and granules. A few drugs are available for pediatric use as powders and granules. For example, pancrelipase *(Viokase®)* is a powder that can be ingested with meals by pediatric patients who have cystic fibrosis. To avoid possible irritation to the respiratory tract, these patients should be cautioned against inadvertently inhaling the powder. They also should be cautioned against holding the powder in the mouth because the proteolytic activity of the pancrelipase enzyme may irritate the oral mucosa.

Administering solid oral dosage forms. Several factors affect the transit of solid oral dosage forms through the esophagus: size, shape, type of coating, and other physical properties; volume of the liquid "chaser"; body position while swallowing; and esophageal function (e.g., presence of a motility disorder, mechanical obstruction). Capsules or tablets that become lodged in the esophagus dissolve and release their contents in a concentrated form, causing localized inflammation, stricture, or perforation and hemorrhage. Therefore, children and adolescents should be advised to swallow all solid oral dosage forms, regardless of shape, size, or other factors, with a sufficient amount of liquid chaser (120–240 ml) while they are in a full-upright seated position or, preferably, standing. Patients should not ingest solid oral dosage forms while they are lying down or immediately before bedtime or naptime (i.e., immediately before reclining). In addition, to further reduce pill sticking, tablets and capsules can be ingested with food or meals, if not contraindicated, or chased with a few bites of a well-chewed banana or other soft food (e.g., bread).[13]

Before solid oral dosage forms are prescribed for or administered to a pediatric patient, the patient's ability to swallow them should be assessed. When these forms cannot be swallowed, various flavored syrups and

---

12. A newly approved product is the *Videx EC®* capsule (didanosine). This capsule contains enteric-coated beadlets which prevent the rapid degradation of the didanosine in the acidic pH of the stomach.

13. An often-missed sign or symptom of esophagitis related to tablet sticking is prolonged hiccups. If pediatric patients complain of feeling that a tablet is stuck or lodged in the throat, or if they present with prolonged hiccups, pill-induced esophageal injury should be suspected and patients should be further evaluated.

other vehicles, such as jam or pureed fruit, can be used to increase the palatability of crushed tablets, capsule contents, dissolved tablets, and other solid oral dosage forms prepared to promote ingestion. Commercial tablet crushers (e.g., Delux Medicrush #100, plastic crush cups #101 [Meltitech Medical]) are recommended to create fine powders that can be readily mixed with compatible foods and liquids and to avoid cross-contamination (e.g., leaving penicillin powder or another possible allergen behind).

When selecting appropriate vehicles for mixing a prepared drug for ingestion, attention must be given to individual preferences, dietary restrictions (e.g., sugar or salt restrictions), and drug incompatibilities. For example, penicillin G and erythromycin base deteriorate when mixed with acidic foods (e.g., applesauce) and certain acidic beverages (e.g., carbonated beverages, fruit juices). In addition, because of physical incompatibilities, tetracyclic antidepressants should not be ingested with carbonated beverages or grape juice. Coffee and tea should not be used as liquid chasers for haloperidol, lithium, or monoamine oxidase inhibitors (MAOIs), and cola drinks should be avoided with MAOIs. Applesauce or other pureed foods are commonly used as vehicles for mixing drugs for oral ingestion; they offer a consistency that allows ingestion without spills or drug loss. Pediatric patients, such as children and adolescents who have difficulty swallowing (e.g., have a brain tumor, have had a stroke), may find it easier to swallow drugs that are mixed with textured foods (e.g., custards, rice pudding, toast, yogurt) rather than applesauce.[14]

Although most oral tablets can be crushed and most oral capsules can be emptied without compromising drug efficacy if administered immediately in an appropriate vehicle, there are exceptions. Several brand-name suffixes are commonly used to identify these tablets, including CR (controlled release or continuous release), Dur (duration), EC (enteric coated), En-tab® or Entab® (enteric tablet), LA (long acting), SA (sustained action), SR (sustained release or slow release), TD (time delay), and XR (extended release). Children and adolescents, as well as their parents, should be taught the meanings of these common suffixes to help them better understand their drug therapy and its required method of administration. They also should be encouraged to seek clarification from their primary pediatric clinician or pharmacist when in doubt.

Powders and granules should be prepared according to their accompanying directions. Generally, to prevent aspiration or choking, powders should never be ingested without first moistening them with water or jam or mixing them in a small amount of compatible cold soft food. Psyllium fiber supplements (*Metamucil*® formulations) are available in several different oral formulations, including granules and powders, and are prepared by measuring a quantity of the product and slowly mixing it with a specified volume (e.g., 240 ml) of cool water, fruit juice, or other compatible beverage. These products should be ingested immediately after mixing and, after ingestion, should be followed by an additional glassful of water or other compatible beverage. Because of the risk for esophageal obstruction, they should never be ingested dry or without adequate liquid.

Children and adolescents sometimes refuse to ingest the required oral dosage form of a particular drug or refuse to follow their prescribed drug therapy. Pediatric clinicians should explore the child's or adolescent's reasons for refusing a particular drug or drug therapy and then address these reasons appropriately. Usually, all that is required is the selection of an alternative dosage form or method of administration. For example, a child or adolescent may refuse to ingest an unpleasant-tasting drug. Whenever possible, a flavored formulation of the drug that may be more acceptable to the child or adolescent should be selected. If a more palatable

---

14. Several commercially available products can be used to assist dysphagic patients in swallowing tablets and capsules that cannot be crushed (e.g., enteric-coated tablets). Tablets can be placed on the "built-in shelf" of the Drink-a-Pill® cup. The cup should be filled halfway with water or a compatible beverage. As the child or adolescent drinks, the liquid picks up the tablet or capsule and chases it down without triggering the gag reflex.

formulation is not available, unpleasant-tasting drugs should be mixed in the smallest amount of food or volume of liquid possible that will both mask the unpleasant taste and also ensure that the entire dose can be swallowed. Some children and adolescents may prefer to swallow an unpleasant-tasting drug straight and then chase it down with a favorite compatible beverage (ginger ale, orange juice). Individual patient preferences should be followed, and when children and adolescents are hospitalized, clinicians should identify and then follow drug administration procedures that have been used successfully at home, and should use familiar dosage forms (including brand names). Clinicians should discuss the required drug therapy with the child or adolescent and involve her or him appropriately with the various aspects of that therapy. Attention should always be given to the child's or adolescent's specific age and developmental level. (*See* the following discussion and Table 1-2.)

Integrating Developmental Theory

The developmental level of pediatric patients requiring oral dosage forms is more important than chronological age. Although gross developmental differences may be observed among infants, children, and adolescents, pediatric clinicians should note subtle differences within these age groups that may affect oral drug administration.

Infants. For administration of oral liquid dosage forms, young infants generally should be held in the same position as for breast- or bottle-feeding to prevent aspiration of the drug and to prevent it from running out of the corners of the infant's mouth. Because young infants have underdeveloped swallowing mechanisms unless they are sucking, oral liquids should be given through a plastic nipple to take advantage of their strong rooting and sucking reflexes. Administered through a plastic nipple, a liquid dosage form usually is readily ingested, particularly if the infant is hungry.

If the infant refuses the nipple, the drug can be given with the use of a plastic oral drug syringe. To prevent the infant from choking or drooling, small amounts of the drug (i.e., ≤0.5 ml at a time) should be placed inside the infant's cheek at the gums toward the back of the mouth. The infant should be allowed to swallow each portion of the drug and should not be laid down until the last portion has been completely swallowed. If necessary, the outside of the infant's throat can be gently stroked in a downward motion to facilitate swallowing. A gentle puff of air in the infant's face will elicit the Santmyer swallow reflex and also promote swallowing among healthy premature and full-term infants younger than 11 months.

Because it cannot be guaranteed that all of the bottle contents will be consumed, liquid drugs should never be added to an infant's bottle of juice, water, or formula. Mixing the liquid dosage form with an infant's formula or with essential foods may result in a taste aversion to the formula or food, so this technique of drug administration is not recommended. Honey or corn syrup should not be used as a vehicle for administering liquids to neonates; they may contain spores of *Clostridium botulinum* which causes botulism poisoning and may be fatal.

A plastic oral drug syringe or drug cup generally works better than a nipple for older infants (6–12 months), who can refuse or spit out liquids they dislike. Liquid oral dosage forms and crushed tablets or the contents of capsules also can be administered from a spoon after being mixed in a small amount of an appropriate vehicle. Applesauce is one of the first foods introduced to infants because allergies to it are rare. It offers a consistency that facilitates mixing of drugs and is easily ingested by infants with little spillage or drug loss. However, cultural variations must be considered because some infants, particularly infants who recently migrated to North America, may not be familiar with this pureed fruit. Safety precautions, including keeping drugs out of the reach of infants, are needed because fine motor development and mobility improve rapidly as infants grow older.

Toddlers. A calm but firm approach is recommended when administering oral dosage forms to toddlers, who may spit out unfamiliar or unpleasant-tasting liquids. Since toddlers tend to be ritualistic, pediatric clinicians should identify and follow successful home routines as much as possible. Many toddlers can drink from a plastic drug cup by themselves with supervision to prevent spilling or they will drink a liquid dosage form while someone holds the plastic drug cup for them. If preferred, a plastic oral syringe can be used for toddlers in the same general manner as for young infants. Although some toddlers are able to chew oral tablets thoroughly before swallowing, particularly when they have taken a particular drug over a long period, most toddlers require either a suspension or a crushed tablet mixed in an appropriate vehicle and given with a spoon.

After ingesting their "medicine," toddlers should be praised for their cooperation and be given the opportunity to express any fears and dislikes that they may have related to their drug therapy. When toddlers refuse their drugs, several strategies can be tried, including the selection of a therapeutically equivalent alternative dosage form. To reduce the risk of poisoning, toddlers (and other children) should never be told that a drug is candy (*see* Chapter 4) or be bribed to ingest a drug.

Preschoolers. Preschoolers usually can ingest liquid and solid oral dosage forms, but they may refuse oral dosage forms that "taste bad." Because of their developing concept of time, even young preschoolers can be told that the unpleasant taste will last only a minute. They might also be told that the medicine is necessary and that it can help them to get better even if it tastes bad and they do not like to take it. Encouraging the preschooler to wash the medicine down with a sip of water or a favorite compatible drink also is helpful.

School-age children and adolescents. School-age children and adolescents usually are able to swallow solid oral dosage forms if they are given proper instruction. Generally, children at these ages should be told to take a sip of water, place the tablet or capsule on the back of their tongue, and swallow it with another drink of water. To facilitate swallowing a solid oral dosage form, they should be instructed to keep their head and neck in a normal upright or slightly flexed position. School-age children and adolescents should be instructed to swallow solid oral dosage forms with a sufficient quantity of water or a compatible beverage (120–240 ml) in a standing position to prevent the pill from sticking in the esophagus. Before solid oral dosage forms are administered, school-age children and adolescents must be assessed for both their ability to swallow tablets and capsules and their understanding of any special directions that may be required (e.g., "chew it thoroughly," "swallow it whole"). For those who have difficulty swallowing, some solid oral dosage forms can be crushed and mixed with or dissolved in a soft, cold food. If available, liquid dosage forms or chewable tablets are preferable.

School-age children and adolescents who have common chronic childhood conditions (e.g., cystic fibrosis) take several drugs in solid oral dosage forms throughout the day. Many of these patients have developed the habit of taking their drugs in one gulp, a habit that should be discouraged. They should swallow solid oral dosage forms one at a time with an adequate volume of liquid as a chaser while standing to avoid aspiration and esophageal injury. Evening doses should be ingested at least 30 minutes before bedtime. In situations where school-age children and adolescents require fluid restriction (e.g., because of nocturnal enuresis), an alternative dosage form (e.g., oral liquid dosage form, oral quick-dissolve tablet) should be selected.

Other recommendations for the prevention of pill sticking include ingesting solid oral dosage forms with meals or immediately following the pill's ingestion with a few bites of thoroughly chewed banana or bread. As a precaution, the use of large tablets (e.g., co-trimoxazole *[Bactrim DS®, Septra DS®]*) or tablets or capsules containing potentially irritating drugs (e.g., doxycycline *[Vibra-Tabs®]*, tetracycline *[Sumycin®, Tetracyn®]*) generally should be avoided, particularly for children and adolescents who are bedridden or who have esophageal motility disorders or difficulty swallowing solid oral dosage forms. In these situations, an alternative dosage form (e.g., liquid oral dosage form) should be selected. In addition, any school-age child or adolescent who complains that a tablet or capsule is "stuck" or who presents with a history of prolonged hiccups should be evaluated for pill-induced esophageal injury.

Infants, children, and adolescents with special needs. Pediatric clinicians must adapt their approaches to oral drug administration to the special needs of patients, including those who are nonambulatory or bedridden, physically or mentally disabled, or require nasogastric or gastrostomy feeding.

Nonambulatory or bedridden patients. Children and adolescents who are nonambulatory or bedridden should be assisted with the administration of prepared solid and liquid oral dosage forms by being positioned as for feeding to prevent aspiration and loss of drug. To prevent aspiration and to enhance swallowing, the head should be tilted forward, with the chin toward the chest (slightly flexed), rather than tilted backward (hyperextended). An oral drug syringe, drug cup, or spillproof spoon can be used for liquid dosage forms. If an oral syringe is used, small amounts of the drug should be injected into the patient's cheek at the gums toward the back of the mouth. The patient should be allowed to swallow between each injection of the drug and should not be positioned in a lying (supine) or side-lying position until the drug has been completely swallowed. If necessary, the throat can be gently stroked in a downward motion to facilitate swallowing.

Patients with physical or mental disabilities. Infants, children, and adolescents who are physically or mentally disabled may require special approaches. Liquid oral dosage forms or solid oral dosage forms prepared by mixing with compatible beverages or soft, textured foods (e.g., custard, rice pudding, yogurt) generally are more readily swallowed than are solid oral dosage forms. To facilitate swallowing, these patients should be helped to assume their usual feeding position. The liquid oral dosage form should be administered from a plastic drug cup, spillproof spoon, or oral drug syringe, depending on the individual abilities and preferences of the infant, child, or adolescent. If a plastic oral drug syringe is used, small amounts of the liquid should be placed inside the cheek at the gums toward the back of the mouth. The infant, child, or adolescent should be allowed to swallow each portion and should not be placed in a supine position until the last portion has been swallowed.

Patients with nasogastric and gastrostomy feeding tubes. Drug therapy for infants, children, and adolescents who require enteral nutrition with nasogastric or gastrostomy feeding tubes requires special consideration. The type of feeding tube (e.g., large- or small-bore, polyethylene or other synthetic polymer, and nasogastric or gastrostomy), tube placement (e.g., in the stomach, duodenum, or jejunum), enteral nutrition (e.g., special diet for renal impairment), and feeding schedule (intermittent or continuous) have important implications for drug administration, drug absorption, and potential drug–nutrient interactions.

Generally, infants, children, and adolescents who have feeding tubes should ingest their drugs orally whenever possible. If oral administration is not possible, a liquid should be selected and administered through the nasogastric or gastrostomy tube. If liquid dosage forms are unavailable, a solid form can be prepared for administration (*see* Solid Oral Dosage Forms) through large-bore feeding tubes. Because of the risk for tube clogging, crushed tablets and capsule contents diluted in water should not be administered through small-bore feeding tubes. To prevent large-bore feeding tubes from clogging, tablets should be pulverized to fine powders using equipment such as the Pill Prep® tablet pulverizer or Deluxe Medi Crush®. Drug products that have been associated with tube occlusion (e.g., *Dyazide®* [triamterene and hydrochlorothiazide], ibuprofen *[Advil®, Motrin®]*, *Metamucil®* [psyllium], *Theo-Dur®* [theophylline]) should be avoided. Problems with tube clogging are minimized if the drug is prepared appropriately and the tube is flushed adequately both before and after drug administration.

Only liquid oral dosage forms should be administered through small-bore feeding tubes; flushing before and after drug administration is required to ensure drug delivery to the GI tract and to prevent tube clogging. Drugs that can cause gastric irritation at high concentrations should be diluted with warm water before administration. Highly viscous formulations (e.g., co-trimoxazole suspension [Bactrim, Septra]) also should be diluted before administration to prevent clogging of the tube. Liquid dosage forms should not be administered with formula, as they may increase the risk for formula clumping and tube clogging. When a liquid dosage form must be administered with a sterile enteral formula, sterile technique should be used to avoid contamination. The drug should be added slowly while the formula is stirred vigorously, and the mixture should be inspected for physical incompatibilities (e.g., creaming, flocculation, clumping) before administration.

Because tube occlusion is one of the most serious concerns associated with administering oral dosage forms through feeding tubes, several steps must be followed to help ensure tube patency. All feeding tubes should be flushed with warm water before and after the administration of drugs and enteral feedings. If more than one drug must be administered at the same time, the tube should be flushed with at least 5 ml of warm water between drugs. The possible drug–drug and drug–formula incompatibilities that could result in formula clumping and tube occlusion must be considered.

Drugs that should be taken on an empty stomach (e.g., astemizole [Hismanal®], didanosine [Videx]) should be given before feedings, a much simpler task for those infants, children, and adolescents who require intermittent feedings than for those who require continuous feedings. Continuous feedings should be discontinued 15 minutes before a drug is administered. Increasing the formula administration rate briefly can compensate for the interruption associated with drug administration and ensure that nutritional needs are met. Care must be taken to avoid drug interactions (e.g., tetracycline and di- or trivalent cations such as aluminum, calcium, or magnesium in antacids and mineral supplements). Caution should be used when administering drugs (e.g., digoxin, furosemide, phenytoin, theophylline) and formulas (e.g., Ensure®, Osmolite®) that increase the osmolality of GI contents, thus resulting in gastric irritation and osmotic diarrhea.

Correct placement of the nasogastric tube is verified by inserting 5 ml of air with a syringe, auscultating with a stethoscope placed over the gastric area for the characteristic sound, and gently aspirating or using gravity to withdraw gastric fluid. Then the drug is poured into the barrel of a syringe (5–50-ml syringe, depending on the size and condition of the pediatric patient and the volume of drug to be gavaged) from which the plunger has been removed and the tip has been inserted into the end of the tube. Drugs should not be forced into the tube using the syringe plunger; they should be administered by gravity. After the drug has been administered, 10–30 ml of warm tap water should be poured into the syringe barrel to flush it and the tube. The tube should then be clamped. The tube can be attached to a suction device (such devices typically are used between intermittent feedings) after 30 minutes, or continuous feeding can be resumed (unless it is contraindicated because of possible drug–formula interaction). To provide additional protection against tube clogging, the tube should be flushed again before the enteral feeding is resumed.

Feeding tubes made of polyurethane have a lower incidence of clogging than tubes made of other materials, so they should be used whenever possible. Although small-bore feeding tubes generally are more comfortable for children and adolescents than large-bore tubes are, they have a greater tendency to clog. Tube reinsertion is required when clogging occurs; it is generally uncomfortable and can cause tissue trauma. Thus, in addition to flushing, tubes should also be manipulated at least every 4–6 hours to keep formula from clumping. The instillation of enzyme solutions (e.g., pancrelipase adjusted to a pH of 7.9) within 24 hours after tube clogging has been recommended for dissolving tube obstructions.

Rectal Dosage Forms

The rectal route is used for drugs indicated for either local or systemic effects. Rectal creams, foams, ointments, and suppositories are available for pediatric use, as are various small-volume (micro or less than 20 ml) and large-volume (macro or 67.5 ml or more) enema solutions and suspensions. The rectal route of administration is generally not recommended for infants, children, or adolescents when systemic effects are required. However, some drugs (e.g., chlorpromazine *[Thorazine]*, hydromorphone *[Dilaudid®]*, pentobarbital *[Nova Rectal®]*) have been formulated as rectal suppositories or gels for use when the oral route is contraindicated (e.g., when pediatric patients are receiving continuous nasogastric suctioning, are unconscious, or are vomiting) or when immediate drug effects are required (e.g., diazepam *[Diastat®]*, to manage repetitive seizures [status epilepticus]; morphine *[MS Contin®]*, to provide immediate pain relief) and when other routes of administration are not available.

Although the rectal route is important for pediatric drug administration, the use of rectal suppositories, gels, enemas, and other rectal dosage forms is contraindicated when pediatric patients have inflammation or irritation of the anus or rectum, diarrhea, rectal bleeding, or other conditions (e.g., concurrent antineoplastic drug therapy) that would make them prone to rectal abscess or injury.

In the adolescent, the rectum comprises the distal 15–20 cm of the large intestine. It produces approximately 2–3 ml of mucous fluid secretions of pH 7–8. The 200–400-cm^2 surface area of the rectum has limited absorption capacity because it lacks villi and microvilli. Drug absorption can be affected by luminal pressure, degree of rectal motility, and the presence of feces. These factors, in turn, can be affected by age, trauma, disease, and other factors that can result in both erratic and unpredictable drug effects. Although the rectal route has several limitations, it also has some advantages. For example, it is independent of gastric emptying and intestinal transit time.

The blood supply to the upper and lower portions of the rectum differs; the upper portion of the rectum is supplied by portal circulation and the lower portion by systemic circulation.[15] Drugs absorbed from the upper part of the rectum are more likely to be affected by first-pass hepatic metabolism than are drugs absorbed from the lower part. Thus, when drugs are administered for their systemic effects, the extent of first-pass hepatic drug metabolism increases as the depth of drug insertion into the rectum increases.[16]

The rectal administration of drugs can be upsetting to young children because they may experience the procedure as an attack from behind. It also may be poorly accepted by older children and adolescents, who generally find insertion difficult, distasteful, or embarrassing. Thus, children and adolescents must be adequately prepared for rectal drug administration with sensitivity to their concerns and with age-appropriate explanations. They should be told about the correct procedure for rectal administration, and clinicians should not assume that the child or adolescent has any previous experience with rectal drug administration. Children and adolescents should be told the reason for the use of the enema, suppository, or other rectal dosage form and how it will be inserted. Of particular importance, they should know what they can do to help with insertion. Children and adolescents should notify a parent or their clinician if the dosage form (e.g., enema solution, suppository) is expelled prematurely, particularly if it was administered for its systemic effects.

Rectal Suppositories

Rectal suppositories (e.g., bisacodyl *[Dulcolax]*, glycerin) are formulated to melt or dissolve in rectal fluids. Suppositories usually should be refrigerated to prevent melting. To facilitate insertion, those formulated with synthetic oil bases should be warmed in the hands before the wrapper is removed. Polyethylene glycol base suppositories should be moistened with warm tap water prior to inser-

---

15. The major source of blood supply to the rectum is provided by the iliac vein and vena cava. The superior hemorrhoid vein drains directly into the portal vein, which then enters the liver.

16. The rectum is well supplied with lymphatic vessels and first-pass hepatic metabolism also is avoided when the drug is absorbed by these lymphatic vessels.

tion. If suppositories become too soft, they can be held under cold running tap water to harden them. Because the drug is not necessarily evenly distributed throughout a suppository base, when lower dosages are required, suppositories should not be cut. If the required dose is not available as a suppository, another rectal dosage form or route of administration should be selected. Suppositories should be retained in the rectum for at least 20–30 minutes to ensure melting or dissolution of the base and release and absorption of the drug. Synthetic oil-base suppositories may produce a slight laxative effect after use.

Administering Rectal Suppositories

Children and adolescents should evacuate their bowels prior to suppository insertion and should squat or bend forward to facilitate its insertion. They should be encouraged to hold onto a hand rail or stable piece of furniture to maintain their balance. Depending upon their age and mental and physical abilities, they should be told to reinsert a suppository that is inadvertently expelled.

Infants, toddlers, preschoolers, and children and adolescents who require assistance from a parent or pediatric clinician should be positioned on the left side with the upper leg flexed toward the chest and the lower leg extended. The parent or clinician should wear a glove or finger cot. The anal area should be assessed for any changes in skin integrity (e.g., bleeding, inflammation) and should be well-exposed to prevent injury during insertion. However, adequate draping is required to ensure privacy and minimize embarrassment. The clinician's sensitivity to these concerns is especially important for preschoolers (who are developing concerns regarding modesty) and for older children and adolescents. For children younger than 3 years, the external anal sphincter should be gently dilated with the fifth digit (the index finger should be used for school-age children and adolescents) before the suppository is inserted in order to assess the anal area and to ensure that the suppository will not be placed in feces. The suppository should be lubricated with tap water or a water-soluble jelly to facilitate insertion. To distract children and adolescents and help them to relax the external sphincter muscle, they should be told to take a deep breath or to bear down as the suppository is gently inserted (rounded end first). To ensure correct placement, the suppository should be inserted past the internal sphincter the length of the finger, at an angle toward the umbilicus. The buttocks should be gently held together until the child or adolescent no longer feels an urge to expel the suppository. This general technique must be adapted according to patient size and health state (e.g., the fifth digit is used for children and adolescents who are debilitated) and to the size and purpose of the suppository.

Older children and adolescents can learn to insert their own rectal suppositories. They should be provided with clearly printed instructions and illustrations and be supervised until they demonstrate the ability to correctly insert a suppository. Generally, children and adolescents should be taught to empty their bowels (unless the suppository is indicated for the relief of constipation), wash their hands with soap and water, remove the wrapper from the suppository, and gently and smoothly push the suppository into the rectum, with the rounded end first, while lying on one side with the bottom leg straight and the upper leg flexed toward the chest. A glove or finger cot can be used. The child or adolescent can squat or bend forward to facilitate insertion, if preferred.

Rectal Gels

Diazepam rectal gel *(Diastat)* is formulated as a nonsterile gel with benzyl alcohol, ethanol (alcohol, 10%), and propylene glycol. It is available in a prefilled unit-dose rectal delivery system that includes a plastic applicator with a flexible, molded tip, supplied in two lengths designated as pediatric (4.4 cm, 1.75 inches) and adult (6 cm, 2.36 inches).

Diazepam rectal gel is indicated for the symptomatic management of acute repetitive seizures among selected refractory pediatric patients, 2 years and older, who have seizure disorders and who are generally stabilized on other anticonvulsants. Such patients may require intermittent use of diazepam gel rectally to control acute episodes of repetitive seizures. Diazepam rectal gel can be administered at home by a parent during an acute repetitive seizure. It is generally recommended that diazepam rectal gel be used only once in any 5-day period for acute repetitive seizures and for no more than five such episodes per month.

Diazepam rectal gel should be administered only by parents who are, in the opinion of the clinician, able to meet the following criteria: (1) they are able to distinguish the distinct cluster of seizures (and/or the events presumed to herald their onset) from usual seizure activity, (2) they have received adequate instruction concerning the administration of diazepam rectal gel, (3) they have been evaluated as being competent to safely administer this gel, (4) they explicitly understand the indication for its administration (i.e., they can differentiate the types of seizure activity that should and should not be treated with diazepam rectal gel), (5) they can appropriately monitor the clinical response, and (6) they are competent to evaluate the response and determine when it is insufficient or inappropriate and immediate action is warranted (e.g., calling for emergency assistance).

Enemas

Small- and large-volume enemas are rectally administered solutions or suspensions usually used to stimulate bowel evacuation, although they can be used to deliver drugs locally or systemically for other actions. Small-volume enemas are used as a routine bowel preparation for certain medical and surgical procedures and for the relief of constipation. Small-volume enemas generally are contraindicated when pediatric patients have abdominal pain, have nausea, or are vomiting. They should not be used for pediatric patients who have cardiovascular disorders or severe dehydration because some solutions (e.g., *Fleet*® enema) are hypertonic electrolyte solutions that can adversely affect fluid and electrolyte balance.

Enemas generally can be stored at room temperature. Small- and large-volume enemas are administered similarly to rectal suppositories. The pediatric patient is positioned comfortably on the left side with both legs flexed or the lower leg straight and the upper leg flexed. The protective cap of the enema container should be removed and the prelubricated tip gently inserted a short distance into the rectum at an angle directed toward the umbilicus. If no discomfort or resistance is noted, the tip can be gently advanced as far as it will go comfortably. The plastic enema container is squeezed to deliver the desired amount of enema solution. The tip should then be slowly withdrawn and the buttocks gently held together until the urge to expel the enema passes. When enemas are used for their laxative effects, children and adolescents should be encouraged to retain the enema for 2–5 minutes or until they feel the urge to defecate. The enema should be retained for as long as possible when systemic effects are desired.

The administration of enemas can result in anorectal injury, especially when infants, children, or adolescents have preexisting perianal or rectal pathology. Serious injury, including perforation of the bowel and abdominal viscera, can result in infection and disruption of normal bowel and bladder function as well as pain and discomfort. Enema-induced injuries can be avoided. Regardless of indication, enemas should always be administered with care to infants, children, and adolescents. Pediatric clinicians should carefully observe an infant's response to the insertion of the enema container tip and the administration of the enema contents. When children and adolescents complain of pain or discomfort during insertion or at any time during a procedure, the procedure should be discontinued and the rectal area carefully inspected for injury before any attempt to repeat the procedure is made. When enemas are required at home, pediatric patients and their parents, as appropriate, should be advised to discontinue the administration of an enema if there is any pain or discomfort and to notify their clinician.

Vaginal Dosage Forms

Various drugs are formulated for vaginal use as creams, foams, jellies, ointments, suppositories, and tablets. Although vaginal drugs are used infrequently for infants and young children, school-age and adolescent girls may require them for vaginal infections and some adolescent girls may use them for contraception. Medicated douches and irrigation solutions also may be used. Vaginal formulations usually are dispensed with their own applicators.

Toddlers and preschoolers should be prepared carefully to minimize any psychological distress associated with the treatment of the vaginal area. Older children and adolescents likewise require an approach individualized to their developmental needs. An explanation of the purpose of the vaginal drug and how it will be administered is helpful. School-age and adolescent girls generally require information about the vagina and its functions. It is crucial that the clinician be sensitive to and understanding of any embarrassment or discomfort a patient experiences, particularly when vaginal drug therapy is required for an infection or injury associated with rape.

The following general information is provided for the **administration of vaginal dosage forms**. After the purpose for vaginal drug therapy and the required procedure have been explained, the girl should empty her bladder and position herself comfortably on her back with her knees flexed and her hips rotated laterally. Preschool, school-age, and adolescent girls can be told to press the small of the back down on the examination table or bed to help maintain this position. To allow inspection of the vaginal area and to prevent trauma to the area during vaginal drug administration, the labia should be gently spread so that the vaginal orifice can be clearly visualized. Held in the dominant hand, the applicator should be gently inserted approximately 3–4 inches (7.5–10 cm) along the posterior fornix or wall of the vagina (depending on the girl's age and size). Panty liners or perineal pads can be used to prevent the drug from soiling undergarments and clothing. Tampons should not be used, as they may absorb drugs that are administered vaginally, thus affecting the amount of drug available for therapeutic effect.

Older school-age and adolescent girls can insert their own vaginal drugs and care for the applicator, which should be washed in warm soapy water, rinsed well, and dried after each use. They also should be instructed to wash their hands before and after administering vaginal drugs.

Ophthalmic Dosage Forms

Infants, children, and adolescents often require ophthalmic drugs to prevent postoperative infections after various surgeries involving the eye or its related structures (e.g., strabismus correction) or for the medical treatment of common pediatric eye conditions (e.g., corneal abrasion, infection). Most ophthalmic drugs are available as drops (solutions or suspensions) in plastic bottles with dropper tips (i.e., ophthalmic squeeze bottles) or as ointments in tubes. These products should be individually dispensed for the treatment of each affected eye to prevent contamination and cross-infection.

Patient acceptability of liquid and ointment ophthalmic dosage forms has been limited by the relatively frequent dosing required and the way they must be administered. Infants and young children generally perceive the procedure as a frightening intrusion. Although several alternative ophthalmic dosage forms, such as ophthalmic inserts (e.g., hydroxypropyl cellulose ophthalmic insert *[Lacrisert®]*), have been developed, their use in the pediatric population has been limited. Other efforts have been aimed at developing more convenient and effective ophthalmic dosage forms that prolong drug contact. These forms include muco-adhesive products and drug-impregnated contact lenses.

Ophthalmic Solutions and Suspensions

Ophthalmic drops are formulated as sterile aqueous solutions or suspensions. Aqueous solutions undergo rapid dilution in tears and drainage from the eye after instillation, limiting contact time with the corneal surface. Ophthalmic suspensions are formulated to prolong drug action by increasing corneal contact time. However, they contain small drug particles that can be retained in the conjunctival sac and cause eye irritation and increased tear secretion. These effects result in drug dilution and loss through spillage over the eyelid margin or rapid drainage through the nasolacrimal apparatus. To enhance corneal contact and drug effects, factors associated with the protective physiologic functions of the eye and related structures (particularly tear volume, blinking, and nasolacrimal drainage) should be considered when ophthalmic drops are instilled.

Tear volume, blinking, and drug loss. The natural production of human tears affects the bioavailability of ophthalmic drops. Because the normal adult tear volume is approximately 7 µl and the precorneal surface of the human eye accommodates approximately 20 µl, any additional volume (such as ophthalmic drops instilled into the conjunctival sac) overflows from the eyelid margins or enters the nasolacrimal apparatus. Upon entering the nasolacrimal apparatus, the drug may drain into the nasal cavity and mouth, where it may be swallowed and then either degraded in the stomach or absorbed from the GI tract into the systemic circulation. Thus, children and adolescents may complain of a bad taste after the administration of an ophthalmic drug or the occurrence of unwanted systemic effects, as may occur with the administration of anticholinergic ophthalmic formulations (e.g., atropine *[Isopto®]*, cyclopentolate *[Cyclogyl®]*). In addition, whereas the nonblinking adult eye may accommodate an increased tear volume of up to 30 µl, excessive blinking can accelerate drug loss by increasing spillage from the eye and increasing drainage into the nasolacrimal apparatus.

The effect of an ophthalmic drug also can be influenced by the production rate of human tears, which are replaced continuously at approximately 15% per minute. Drug metabolism by the enzymes in tears, the cornea, and the aqueous humor also may affect corneal drug absorption and, thus, the action of an ophthalmic drug.

When ophthalmic drops are instilled, more than 90% of the drug is lost because of the limited capacity of the precorneal area in relation to the average drop volume (i.e., approximately 25–75 µl) delivered by a standard commercial eye dropper or ophthalmic squeeze bottle. This loss increases with blinking and also may be increased if the eye is rubbed. The ideal drug volume to instill is 5–10 µl. Unfortunately, studies have found that patients who used a dropper designed to deliver this smaller volume (5 µl) felt that insufficient drug had been administered and instilled extra drops in a misguided effort to ensure an adequate dose. Other strategies to address the issue of drop volume have included increasing the viscosity of ophthalmic drops with methylcellulose and increasing the drug concentration. These strategies generally have been unsuccessful because of difficulty with the formulation (i.e., poor flow characteristics of the methylcellulose formulation that made it inconvenient to use) and with eye irritation, respectively.

Other problems are encountered when multiple-drop therapy is required. For example, when drops are instilled in immediate succession, a large portion of the first drop is lost as a result of spillage from the eye and drainage through the nasolacrimal apparatus. As the number of drops instilled increases, the proportion of the administered dose absorbed decreases. Although the instillation of multiple drops at short intervals may avoid dilution of the drug in the precorneal tear film, at least a 5-minute interval between drop instillation is recommended to permit corneal absorption and to minimize drug loss through spillage and nasolacrimal drainage.

Nasolacrimal occlusion and eyelid closure. The nasolacrimal apparatus flushes tears and foreign material from the cul-de-sac of the eye to the vascular mucous membranes of the nasopharyngeal area. Systemic absorption across these membranes exceeds that following subcutaneous injection and, thus, may be clinically problematic when ophthalmic drugs, such as anticholinergics, are instilled into the conjunctival sac. Local adverse effects associated with nasolacrimal drainage after ophthalmic drug administration include dryness and irritation of the throat, postnasal drip, and nasal congestion. Systemic adverse effects also may be expected, depending on the drug instilled.

Nasolacrimal occlusion (NLO) is a technique in which gentle digital pressure is applied externally at the inner canthus to close the nasolacrimal drainage system. The use of both NLO and eyelid closure, which reduces the action of the nasolacrimal pump, for 5 minutes after ophthalmic drug instillation increases ocular bioavailability and reduces the incidence of local and systemic adverse effects. For example, NLO and eyelid closure reduce the incidence of common local and systemic adverse effects associated with anticholinergic ophthalmic drugs (e.g., atropine ophthalmic drops *[Isopto® Atropine]*), such as dryness of the mucous membranes, flushing, headache, tachycardia, and urinary retention.

Generally, NLO with eyelid closure immediately after instillation of the ophthalmic drops increases the amount of drug in the anterior chamber, decreases systemic absorption, and increases corneal contact time, which for some indications can significantly increase therapeutic ocular effects.

Ophthalmic Ointments

Ophthalmic ointments contain a drug dissolved or suspended in a petroleum-based vehicle formulated to melt at body temperature. Thus, ophthalmic ointments generally have greater bioavailability than their respective ophthalmic solution or suspension formulations. This greater bioavailability is associated with increased corneal contact time, prolonged drug release from the ointment vehicle, lower susceptibility to dilution by tears, and resistance to drainage into the nasolacrimal apparatus. However, upon application, the ophthalmic ointment formulation blurs vision and makes it difficult for children to open and close the affected eye(s). Thus, ophthalmic ointments should be administered before naps or at bedtime to prevent falls or other accidents associated with blurred vision as well as to maximize corneal contact time and increase therapeutic effect.

Ophthalmic Inserts

The ophthalmic insert offers older children and adolescents convenience and simplified dosing regimens for drugs required continuously (e.g., artificial tears). The small, wafer-like drug delivery system is inserted in the conjunctival sac, where it gradually releases the drug over 12–24 hours. Occasional loss of the insert from the eye and poor patient acceptability are factors that may limit its use. Older children and adolescents must be shown the correct procedures for insertion and removal of inserts and must check periodically throughout the day to verify that inserts are in the proper position.

Administering Ophthalmic Dosage Forms

Several precautions should be taken before ophthalmic drugs are administered. The concentration and expiration date of all products should be checked. In addition, ophthalmic solutions should be examined for cloudiness and discoloration, which may indicate contamination or deterioration. Ophthalmic suspensions should be thoroughly shaken to ensure that the drug is evenly distributed and that the correct concentration is delivered. It is particularly important to verify that the drug is intended for ophthalmic use, and not for otic, nasal, or any other use. Products intended for these other uses are commonly dispensed in containers similar in size and shape to those used for ophthalmic products.

Parents and school-age children and adolescents should be told not to share ophthalmic drugs with other people and to properly discard any unused product to minimize the transmission of infection. Ophthalmic drugs should be dispensed separately for the treatment of each patient and each eye, and any unused portion should be discarded after 1 week to minimize the transmission of infection. Steri-Dropper® bottles are available in 3-, 7-, and 15-ml sizes and have provided hospital pharmacists with a means to efficiently package and dispense small volumes of sterile ophthalmic drugs they prepare in-house.

Many infants and children (as well as some adolescents) find the administration of ophthalmic drugs uncomfortable and even frightening. Thus, age-appropriate information on the need for the drug and the correct procedures for administering it should be provided to decrease fear and promote the development of age-appropriate drug administration abilities. The young toddler or preschooler may require gentle manual restraint to prevent eye injury during ophthalmic drug administration. Proper preparation of children increases their ability to cooperate and prevents struggling (which can lead to eye injury) and crying (which can result in drug dilution or loss and diminution of therapeutic effect).

Ophthalmic solutions and suspensions. To ensure optimal therapeutic benefit, the administration of ophthalmic solutions and suspensions requires consideration of the appropriate formulation and its concentration, the number of drops to be instilled, the sequence of instillation when more than one ophthalmic drug must be instilled, and the frequency of instillation.

Ophthalmic solutions and suspensions may be stored under refrigeration to increase their shelf life and to prevent microbial growth. However, they should be warmed to room temperature before use to prevent excess blinking (which can encourage drug loss) and eye irritation. Infants and young children can be positioned on their backs with a small pillow placed under their shoulders to hyperextend their necks. This position helps to disperse the drug over the cornea. Older children and adolescents can tilt their heads back while remaining in a sitting position, if preferred. Generally, older children and adolescents can instill their own ophthalmic drops.

When instilling ophthalmic solutions and suspensions, sterile technique should be used to prevent the introduction of pathogens into the eye and the drug container. Hands should be washed before and after ophthalmic drugs are handled. The eyelid and eyelashes should be gently cleansed of any exudate. Care should be taken to prevent the dropper tip from coming into contact with the eye, eyelashes, or fingertips; microbial contamination can result if it does.

The lower lid should be gently retracted and the drop instilled into the conjunctival sac. Young infants can squeeze their eyes tightly closed and may need to have their eyelids gently separated using the fingertips of the index and second finger of the nondominant hand. After the drug has been instilled, the eyelid should be gently released to its original position. Children and adolescents should close their eyes gently rather than squeeze them shut and should avoid blinking and rubbing the eye. Nasolacrimal occlusion should be performed to prevent drainage of drug through the nasolacrimal apparatus. The recumbent position (or tilted head) should be maintained to maximize drug contact with the eye. Children and adolescents should be encouraged to move the eye from side to side under the closed eyelid to evenly distribute the drug. After 2 minutes, any excess drug solution or suspension can be gently wiped away with a clean tissue.

If preferred, an alternative procedure can be used. While sitting, children and adolescents should look up at the ceiling. The lower eyelid can then be grasped gently below the eyelashes with the thumb and index finger of the nondominant hand and pulled slightly forward to create a pocket for instillation. The eyelid should be maintained in this position for a few seconds until the instilled drop settles into the pocket. Children and adolescents should look down while the eyelid is released to its normal position, not squeeze the eye shut, and avoid blinking and rubbing the eye. The eye should remain closed with gentle NLO for at least 2 minutes.

Infants, children, and adolescents should be monitored carefully for systemic effects associated with ophthalmic drugs. These effects can be overlooked or misdiagnosed and treated inappropriately. For example, misdiagnosis and inappropriate treatment of psychosis associated with the instillation of anticholinergic ophthalmic drops in children and adolescents have been reported. Greater emphasis on NLO and eyelid closure is recommended for ophthalmic drugs associated with potentially serious systemic effects (e.g., timolol *[Timoptic®]*).

Ophthalmic ointments. Ophthalmic ointments are administered similarly to ophthalmic solutions and suspensions. The same body positions should be used. The lower eyelid should be gently retracted and a small amount of ointment (0.6–1.2 cm [¼–½ inch]) should be squeezed in a line along the conjunctival sac. The ointment tube can be rotated with a twisting motion to stop the ointment flow. The eyelid should be gently released and the child or adolescent should close the eye slowly and remain in the same position for a few minutes. To prevent both injury to the eye and microbial contamination of the ointment, the tip of the ointment tube should not come into contact with the eye, eyelashes, or fingertips. If ophthalmic ointment in addition to ophthalmic drops is required, the drops should be instilled first and the ointment applied 5–10 minutes later (*see previous section*).

Otic Dosage Forms

The basic ear structures include the external ear, middle ear, and inner ear. Systemic drug therapy is used to treat problems with middle and inner ear structures; topically applied otic drugs are usually used to treat conditions involving the external ear (and external tympanic membrane). Local infections, local inflammation, and accumulation of cerumen may require the instillation of otic drugs, which generally are formulated as solutions or suspensions in aqueous or oily vehicles (e.g., *Murine Ear Drops*®). Antibiotic formulations of ear drops (e.g., neomycin and polymyxin B) should be used with caution because of the potential for hypersensitivity. In addition, aminoglycoside formulations (e.g., gentamicin and neomycin) can cause hearing impairment or deafness if the tympanic membrane is ruptured and, thus, are contraindicated if the tympanic membrane is not intact.

For the **administration of otic dosage forms** sterile technique generally is not required because the ear canal is not sterile. If, however, the tympanic membrane is ruptured, or if there is drainage from the ear canal, sterile technique should be used. Liquid otic dosage forms stored under refrigeration should be warmed to room temperature before use to prevent common adverse effects associated with the administration of cold otic drug products (e.g., nausea, vertigo). Infants and young children should be gently placed on their sides with the affected ear up and exposed. Older children and adolescents usually can position themselves properly after the procedure has been explained to them. Infants and young children may require gentle manual restraint to keep them from moving their heads. Generally, young infants can be snugly wrapped in their blankets and positioned on their sides.

If there is cerumen in the ear canal, it should be gently removed before the drug is instilled. The outer aspect of the ear should be cleansed carefully of any crusting or drainage to prevent excoriation and to ensure adequate drug contact with treated surfaces. To prevent infection, the solution used to clean the outer ear structures (e.g., warm tap water or normal saline) should not be allowed to enter the ear canal.

The ear canal is cartilaginous and straight in infants and children younger than 3 years. To separate the walls of the canal for the instillation of liquid otic dosage forms, the pinna should be gently pulled downward and back (Figure 1-1A). For children older than 3 years, and for adolescents, the pinna should be pulled upward and back because the ear canal has more ossification and angles slightly (Figure 1-1B). The otic drug should be directed toward the side of the ear canal, not toward the tympanic membrane. Allowing otic drops to directly hit the tympanic membrane causes pain.

After an otic drug has been instilled, the tragus should be massaged gently to facilitate entry of the drug into the ear canal. Children and adolescents should remain on their sides for a few minutes so that the otic drug permeates to the tympanic membrane. Cotton pledgets can be placed loosely in the ear canal to prevent the drug from draining out. Children should be instructed not to put their fingers in their ears or remove the pledgets.

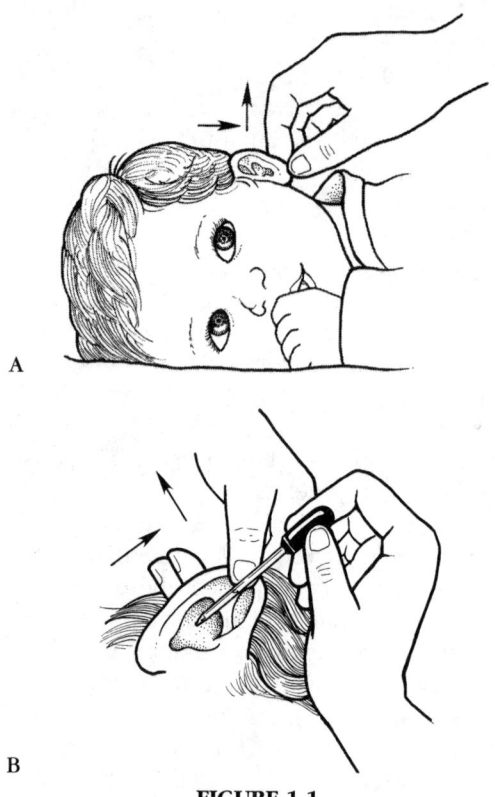

FIGURE 1-1
Administering Otic Dosage Forms
(A) The pinna is gently pulled downward and back for infants and children younger than 3 years.
(B) The pinna is gently pulled upward and back for children 3 years of age and older and adolescents.

Intranasal Dosage Forms

The nasal cavity is highly vascularized and consists of a central system, turbinates, and epithelial cilia and mucus, which assist in the removal of airborne particles and nasal debris. The intranasal route is an effective one for the delivery of drugs for both local (e.g., decongestant) and systemic (e.g., antidiuretic) effects. It is particularly useful for drugs that are unstable in the GI tract or that undergo rapid first-pass hepatic metabolism.

The nasal mucosa appears to be more permeable than other mucous membranes to peptides (e.g., desmopressin, oxytocin), which can be administered by injection or intranasally but cannot be readily administered by other routes. The nasal route offers a convenient alternative to the injectable route.

It is likely that more drugs, including growth hormone-releasing hormone, will be reformulated as intranasal dosage forms because of the usefulness of this route. Currently, the intranasal route is still used primarily for local conditions such as nasal congestion and rhinitis, although several intranasal corticosteroid products have been developed (e.g., budesonide *[Rhinocort®]*, flunisolide *[Nasalide®]*) for the management of seasonal or perennial allergic rhinitis.

Drug disposition in the nasal cavity is affected by dosage form and droplet size delivered (i.e., intranasal drops versus intranasal sprays). Intranasal drops readily spread across nasal surfaces throughout the nasal cavity. Intranasal sprays, which deliver droplets larger than 10 µl, tend to deposit a drug over a small area toward the front of the nose. Systems that deliver droplets smaller than 10 µl (e.g., metered-dose inhalers) enable the drug to penetrate further into the airways (see Inhalation Dosage Forms). Adequate retention has been reported for 60–80-µl intranasal spray droplets.

The initial clearance of intranasal drops and sprays is rapid. Approximately 30%–50% of the drug is lost within 10 minutes. Subsequent clearance appears to be much slower, particularly for sprays, probably because the drug is deposited in nonciliated regions (intranasal drops spread quickly across ciliated areas). Thus, intranasal spray formulations may be preferable to drops. Although the intranasal route offers promise for drug delivery, the rapid loss of drugs due to the mucociliary system limits its use and only a few drugs have been formulated as nasal sprays for systemic absorption. These drugs include butorphanol (*Stadol NS®*), an opiate analgesic, and nicotine (*Nicotrol NS®*), indicated for smoking cessation. Although intranasal butorphanol spray for cancer pain and intranasal nicotine spray for cigarette smoking cessation are becoming increasingly available for adults, reports of their use in the pediatric age group are limited.

Administering Intranasal Dosage Forms

Intranasal dosage forms include creams, ointments, solutions, sprays, and suspensions. Intranasal drops are probably the most commonly used nasal dosage form. The administration of intranasal dosage forms is a clean (but generally not a sterile) procedure. The outer nares should be cleansed to remove mucous crusts before intranasal dosage forms are administered. Hands should be washed before and after drug administration.

Intranasal Creams and Ointments

Intranasal creams and ointments are applied to the accessible surfaces of the nostrils to protect the skin from irritating nasal secretions, relieve chapping, or promote nasal breathing. Lanolin or lanolin-petrolatum formulations provide satisfactory relief from dryness and irritation when applied to the nostrils. Hypersensitivity to lanolin is possible, however, and should be ascertained before these products are used. Eczematous lesions may require the application of a corticosteroid formulated in a cream or ointment base. Intranasal creams and ointments should be applied to clean skin surfaces for maximal effect; previously applied cream and ointment should be gently removed before each application.

Intranasal Drops

Intranasal drops are used for the symptomatic treatment of the nasal cavity and to soothe swollen nasal mucous membranes. They also may be used to relieve nasal congestion among infants (infants are obligate nasal breathers) to facilitate breast- or bottle-feeding. Although intranasal drops are generally well tolerated, the use of oil-based formulations for infants and young children should be avoided because of the risk for inadvertent aspiration of the product and resultant lipid pneumonia.

Infants and young children often react negatively to the instillation of intranasal drops because they perceive the procedure as an invasion of their bodies. The instillation of intranasal drops also is associated with tickling sensations, difficulty breathing, and an unpleasant taste because the nares drain into the back of the mouth and throat. Thus, children should be carefully prepared for the instillation of intranasal drops. Gentle manual restraint may be required to stabilize the head and prevent injury.

Infants should be held with the closest arm positioned behind the parent's or pediatric clinician's back and the head tipped back over the parent's or clinician's nondominant arm. The nondominant hand can then be used to gently restrain the infant's other arm, and the intranasal drops can be administered with the dominant hand. If preferred, infants can be positioned on their backs with a small pillow placed under the shoulders to allow the head to tip back.

To facilitate the flow of drops into the nasal cavity, children and adolescents should be helped to assume a dorsal recumbent position after the procedure has been carefully demonstrated and explained. While in this position, a pillow is placed under the shoulders to allow the head to tip back. Alternatively, children and adolescents can hang their heads over the edge of a bed, if preferred; the head must be supported to avoid strain on the neck muscles. When the sinuses are being treated, the patient should be supine. The head should be maintained in a straight line (Proetz position) for treatment of the ethmoid and sphenoid sinuses and be turned to one side (Parkinson position) for treatment of the maxillary and frontal sinuses.

To prevent intranasal drops from running down the throat, the dropper or dropper bottle should be held just above the nostril and drops should be directed toward the midline of the superior concha of the ethmoid bone. To prevent nasal tissue injury and dropper contamination, touching the nasal mucous membranes with the dropper or dropper bottle tip should be avoided. Children and adolescents should maintain the required position for 5–10 minutes so the drug can be absorbed and maximal therapeutic benefit achieved. Residual liquid in the dropper should be discarded, and the dropper should be thoroughly cleaned in hot, sudsy water, rinsed under hot running tap water, and dried before being returned to the drug container. When possible, sterile disposable droppers (SYON Corp) should be used.

Intranasal Aerosols and Sprays

Intranasal aerosols and sprays usually are used for the treatment of nasal congestion (e.g., naphazoline *[Privine®]*, oxymetazoline *[Afrin®]*) and to provide symptomatic relief of seasonal or perennial rhinitis (e.g., azelastine *[Astelin®]*, beclomethasone *[Becanase®, Vancenase®]*, flunisolide *[Nasalide, Nasarel®]*, triamcinolone *[Nasacort®]*) among school-age children and adolescents. In addition, some children may require nasal hormone products for diabetes insipidus (e.g., desmopressin *[DDAVP® nasal spray]*). These products generally are available for administration by intranasal inhaler, intranasal pump, or intranasal spray devices.[17]

When intranasal aerosols or sprays are required, children and adolescents should sit or stand with the head straight or tilted slightly backward after the nasal passages have been cleared. If nasal passages are blocked, a topical nasal decongestant may be used 5–15 minutes prior to the corticosteroid to ensure adequate drug penetration. The outer portion of the nose should be cleaned with a damp tissue. Hands should be washed with soap and water and dried before the procedure.

The intranasal inhaler, pump, or spray container should be shaken. The cap should be removed and the bottle tip should be introduced into a nostril after the opposite nostril has been occluded by pressing with the index and second fingers of the nondominant hand. The aerosol or spray should be sniffed into the nostril as the inhaler, pump, or spray device is activated or squeezed. The child or adolescent should hold his or her breath for a few seconds and exhale through the mouth. If indicated, the procedure should be repeated for the other nostril using the recommended number of activations or sprays. Children must understand that overuse of intranasal decongestant aerosols and sprays can result in rebound congestion. Proper instruction and monitoring are essential because children and adolescents have been known to abuse such products. To avoid contamination after use, the inhaler, pump, or spray tip should be rinsed under warm running tap water and dried with a clean paper towel or tissue before it is recapped. The hands should be washed again.

Nicotrol NS® is a **nicotine nasal spray** that delivers a nicotine dose for the relief of the nicotine-withdrawal syndrome associated with tobacco smoking cessation. The product delivers a 0.5-mg nicotine dose per each 50-µl spray. Generally, a dose consists of two sprays, one in each nostril. Nicotine administered intranasally is rapidly absorbed. Peak levels are achieved within 10 minutes. This rapid nicotine absorption results in nicotine levels comparable to those produced by smoking a tobacco cigarette. The nasal spray is used whenever the patient has the urge to smoke (up to 40 doses per day). The most common ADRs associated with the nicotine nasal spray are cough, throat and nasal irritation, runny nose, sneezing, and watering eyes. Other ADRs include headache, increased heart rate, and lightheadedness. Unfortunately, addiction appears to be more common with *Nicotrol NS* than with other nicotine replacement products. Thus, adolescent patients require monitoring to ensure that they are not using excessive quantities or using the spray product longer than the recommended 6 months, when the incidence of addiction increases. The quantity of nicotine present in the nasal spray bottle can be toxic to a child or pet. Instruct adolescent patients to safely store the nasal spray out of the reach of younger siblings and pets.

Rhinyles (Rhinals). Desmopressin, a synthetic antidiuretic hormone used for central diabetes insipidus and primary nocturnal enuresis, may be administered intranasally either by intranasal spray or by the more unusual rhinyle (*DDAVP®* rhinal [rhinyle] tube). A rhinyle is a flexible plastic tube with volume gradation for measuring doses of intranasal drug solutions. After the rhinyle has been filled with the appropriate amount of drug solution, one end of the tube is inserted into a

---

17. Note that intranasal corticosteroid products are supplied as metered-dose products and often include a nasal adapter.

nostril and the other into the mouth. The dose is quickly blown into the nose through the tube. Although it is slightly more complicated to use than other intranasal dosage forms and drug delivery devices, the rhinyle allows more sensitive drug dosage adjustments for children and adolescents who can learn the more complex procedure.

Inhalation Dosage Forms

The therapeutic effect of drugs administered by inhalation, such as bronchodilators (e.g., albuterol [Ventolin®]), corticosteroids (e.g., beclomethasone [Beclovent®]), antivirals (e.g., ribavirin [Virazole®]), is optimized when adequate amounts of drug are deposited in the lower respiratory tract where they produce the desired pharmacologic effect on specific target cells (e.g., bronchodilation by relaxation of bronchial smooth muscle) or viruses (e.g., inhibition of respiratory syncytial virus). The site and extent of drug deposition are affected by many factors, including airway physiology, breathing pattern, and drug particle size. These factors must be considered when drugs are administered by inhalation to infants, children, and adolescents who have acute or chronic respiratory conditions (e.g., asthma, cystic fibrosis) managed with inhaled drugs.

Although inhalation provides a rapid effect and is well tolerated and convenient for certain respiratory conditions in the pediatric patient, it may be problematic in situations where infants, children, or adolescents are overly agitated, frightened, uncooperative, or in extreme distress. In such situations, an intramuscular, intravenous, or subcutaneous injection may be required. The following discussion provides current recommendations for the administration of inhaled drugs, with attention to common drug delivery systems used by inhalation, such as compressed-air and other nebulizers (e.g., hand bulb nebulizers, jet nebulizers, sidestream nebulizers, ultrasonic nebulizers), metered-dose inhalers (MDIs), and powder inhalers or insufflators.

Compressed-Air and Other Nebulizers

Compressed-air nebulizers (CANs) and other nebulizers are commonly used to provide aerosol treatments for infants, children, and adolescents who have various respiratory conditions (e.g., asthma, cystic fibrosis). CANs use compressed air or oxygen to deliver a drug solution as a fine aerosol mist. The use of CANs for the treatment of severe respiratory conditions is more common in hospital settings than in home settings, primarily because of the expense and limited portability. However, some children and adolescents do use CANs at home. Other nebulizers produce a fine spray or mist by rapidly passing air through a liquid or, as with ultrasonic nebulizers, by vibrating a liquid at a high frequency so that the particles produced are extremely small. These nebulizers can be used in hospital or home settings. While bronchodilators are often administered by CAN devices, antibiotics and other drugs can be administered by other nebulizers. Budesonide (Pulmicort Respules®) inhalation suspension has been approved for the treatment of asthma in infants as young as 12 months and for children. It is the first corticosteroid to be generally available as a nebulizer formulation in the United States.[18] The amount of drug delivered to the pediatric patient from a nebulizer is variable, depending on several factors, which include type of nebulizer (e.g., CAN, hand bulb, jet, ultrasonic), nebulization time (generally 10–20 minutes, with rest periods as needed), volume fill (generally 2–4 ml), inspiratory/expiratory ratio, tidal volume of the pediatric patient, use of face mask or mouthpiece, and condition of the equipment used.

There are several types of nebulizer devices. A commonly used nebulizer is the intermittent positive pressure breathing (IPPB) apparatus. Use of this device requires consideration of the sensitivity of the machine and the amount of pressure necessary to "trigger" it. Infants and young children can be frightened by the IPPB apparatus and the noise it makes when cycled. Older children and

---

18. Budesonide suspension (*Pulmicort Nebuamp®*), available in Canada, should not be used with an ultrasonic nebulizer because it is generally more difficult to nebulize than a solution.

adolescents may fear that they will be unable to breathe adequately during a treatment. In addition, many drugs delivered by the IPPB (e.g., acetylcysteine [*Mucomyst*®]) have an unpleasant taste or smell, which can affect reactions to and cooperation with therapy.

Children and adolescents, as well as their parents, require appropriate explanation of the need for and use of the IPPB and other nebulizer devices. An individualized approach ensures an understanding of the therapy and correct use of the device. When possible, the use of the device, using plain normal saline, should be demonstrated before the drug is administered.

The child or adolescent should be seated comfortably for the nebulizer treatment. Young children may be more cooperative if they are held by the parent during the treatment or if they are distracted with a game associated with the treatment (e.g., watching the gauge on the IPPB apparatus or making the gauge needle move with each cycle). Whenever possible, children and adolescents should hold the mouthpiece between their teeth and seal their lips tightly around the outer edges. If a mask is required, it can be attached directly to the top of the nebulizer assembly in place of the T-adapter and be comfortably placed over the nose and mouth. The mask should fit properly so that mist does not flow up into the eyes.

Children and adolescents should position themselves sitting upright in a straight-back chair for maximal airway ventilation and should inhale and exhale slowly through the mouthpiece using a normal rate and depth of respiration. Some children and adolescents may need a nose clip to prevent nasal breathing. Approximately every 10–15 breaths, the child or adolescent should be instructed to take a deep breath and hold it for 5–10 seconds; such a breathing pattern increases both drug deposition in the lower respiratory tract and the therapeutic effect. This process should be continued until all drug solution in the nebulizer cup or drug chamber has been aerosolized.

If children or adolescents become lightheaded or tired during therapy, they should pause and remove the mouthpiece for a few minutes. Although the nebulizer cup or drug chamber and assembly for most CAN and other devices compensate for inadvertent patient movement (which can result in drug spillage and loss), children and adolescents should be reminded to hold the mouthpiece horizontally to avoid spills.

When home use is indicated, parents should be provided with information regarding additional resources for obtaining required services and other equipment and supplies. In addition, because pediatric patients may require the inhalation of more than one drug by nebulization, and each treatment may require 15–20 minutes, every effort should be made to simplify regimens. The safe storage of drugs administered by nebulizers also should be emphasized.

Children and adolescents should be taught to disassemble the CAN or other nebulizer device and to assist with its daily care by rinsing each part (e.g., mask, mouthpiece) with warm water and allowing it to air dry on a clean paper towel. At the end of the day (or every 24 hours), the mask, mouthpiece, and tubing should be washed with a solution of warm water and liquid detergent and rinsed with warm water. The parts then should be immersed in disinfectant solution (e.g., white vinegar and distilled water), soaked for 30–60 minutes, rinsed in warm water, and allowed to air dry. To ensure proper functioning, the nebulizer assembly and tubing should be replaced at least once a month. Equipment should be replaced as needed.

Monitoring for excessive reliance on nebulizer therapy, which has been associated with asthma deaths, is recommended. Measurement of peak expiratory flow rate (PEFR), an indicator of the degree of resistance to airflow in the airways, is an inexpensive and nonintrusive means for monitoring response to therapy, both at home and in the hospital. Pediatric clinicians should ensure that children, adolescents, and parents use peak flow meters (e.g., Clement Clarke Meter®, Vitalograph®) correctly and consistently by providing written instructions for measuring PEFR at home and by asking them to demonstrate use of the meter. They also need to ensure that manufacturer's guidelines for use and care of the meter are being followed. In addition, a crisis plan should be provided for obtaining immediate assistance if the required PEFR response is not achieved or if the response provided by usual bronchodilator doses is not obtained.

Metered-Dose Inhalers

Metered-dose inhalers (MDIs) are metal canisters containing drug particles dissolved or suspended in a mixture of propellant (e.g., chlorofluorocarbons) and surfactant under high pressure. The canister has a metering chamber (usually with a 25–50-ml capacity) and is attached to a valve assembly. The MDI delivers up to 400 individual metered doses. MDIs are commonly used to administer bronchodilators (e.g., albuterol *[Ventolin]*), corticosteroids (e.g., beclomethasone *[Beclovent]*),[19] and anticholinergic drugs (e.g., ipratropium bromide *[Atrovent®]*) to pediatric patients who have asthma and other chronic obstructive pulmonary diseases.[20]

MDIs are generally well accepted and convenient for children and adolescents to use, but, despite instruction and practice, they often are used incorrectly. Questions regarding the accuracy of instructions provided by clinicians to patients also have been raised. Pediatric clinicians have been found to lack sufficient knowledge about the proper use of MDIs, which may result in their teaching incorrect technique to patients.

General recommendations for MDI use are to follow both the manufacturer's instructions and these basic steps. The canister should be properly connected to the valve assembly. The cap should be removed from the mouthpiece and the MDI shaken well to evenly distribute its contents. Children and adolescents should be taught to hold the MDI with the canister in a vertical position (i.e., the canister should be pointed up) and to fully exhale (i.e., breathe out). Tilting the head back and keeping the tongue and teeth from blocking the mouthpiece, they should place the mouthpiece between the teeth and activate the inhaler by pressing down the canister while inhaling slowly and deeply (i.e., breathing in).[21] After inhaling the aerosol, children and adolescents should hold their breath for at least 10 seconds, or for as long as is comfortable, and then exhale.

If more than one puff is required, the child or adolescent should wait 1 minute before

---

19. *Qvar®* is a newer beclomethasone inhaler that contains the propellant hydrofluoroalkane instead of the ozone-depleting chlorofluorocarbons. The new propellant helps produce smaller-sized beclomethasone particles, thus improving delivery of the drug to the smaller airways. This change in beclomethasone formulation may result in elimination of the need for a spacer for improved drug delivery. Pediatric patients whose *Beclovent* or *Vanceril®* MDI therapy is replaced with *Qvar* may require as little as half the dose of *Beclovent* or *Vanceril*. The *Qvar* dosage should be adjusted as necessary. As with other inhalation corticosteroids, pediatric patients will still require a reminder to rinse their mouths after use to prevent candidiasis (thrush).

20. A new soft mist inhaler, *Respimat®*, is available in Europe as an alternative to the more conventional pressurized MDIs. The Respimat slowly releases a metered dose of active substance as a soft mist with a high proportion of the dose in the fine particle fraction, leading to improved lung deposition after inhalation when compared with conventional MDIs. It reportedly doubles deposition of the administered drug in the lungs and significantly reduces oropharyngeal deposition compared to the use of a conventional MDI with a spacer device. The Respimat has been demonstrated to be effective for the delivery of fenoterol *(Berotec®)*, fenoterol in combination with ipratropium *(Duovent®)*, and flunisolide *(AeroBid®)*.

21. Previously recommended was an open mouth or two-finger technique in which the mouthpiece was placed 3–5 cm, or the width of two fingers, in front of the open mouth. The MDI was then activated and the aerosol inhaled slowly and deeply. This technique was recommended to decrease oropharyngeal deposition of aerosolized particles and to increase bronchodilation from bronchodilator MDI therapy. However, published research findings have been mixed regarding the effect of these methods on particle deposition and achievement of desired effect (bronchodilation). The closed mouth technique is currently recommended, particularly for drugs (e.g., ipratropium bromide *[Atrovent]*) that could cause local reactions to the eyes (e.g., blurred vision) and their related structures (e.g., aggravation of narrow-angle glaucoma) if inadvertent contact occurs as a result of improper aim.

repeating the procedure to allow the metering chamber to refill; this step ensures that the proper amount of drug is delivered with the next actuation. The waiting period also allows for maximal bronchodilation so that deeper lung penetration can be achieved with the second puff. The cap should be replaced on the MDI as soon as the treatment is finished, and the MDI should be stored safely in a clean, dry place.

Children and adolescents should be advised that the MDI functions best at room temperature and should not be stored in an extremely hot or cold place. If it is not used regularly, the MDI should be actuated once or twice prior to use to ensure that the metering chamber is full and that an accurate dose is delivered. If a bronchodilator and a corticosteroid are both required by MDI, the patient should use the bronchodilator first in order to dilate the bronchioles and increase the subsequent deposition of the corticosteroid in the small airways and alveoli. The mouth should be rinsed after corticosteroid use to reduce the occurrence of oral fungal infections.

In addition to instructions regarding the use of MDIs, patients need information on disposing of empty canisters. Canisters are pressurized and should not be punctured or incinerated. The pediatric clinician can estimate how long an MDI should last, when used as directed, by calculating the number of doses delivered by a particular unit and the number of times the MDI is used daily. Because receiving the correct amount of drug in each inhalation cannot be guaranteed when canisters are almost empty, refills should be obtained promptly. Children and adolescents should also be reminded not to exceed the prescribed dosage or discontinue the use of the MDI without first consulting with their clinician. The warning about abruptly discontinuing use is particularly important for corticosteroids.

The instructions provided by the manufacturer generally are not sufficient for teaching MDI use. Oral instruction and demonstration of MDI use by clinicians promotes correct use. Also, the patient's technique should be evaluated carefully and re-evaluated periodically. An audible signal (e.g., a horn) can be a helpful training or retraining aid. A device that records respirations can be used to demonstrate breathing patterns and promote better inhalation patterns and breath-holding technique. Improved patient understanding, correct administration technique, and optimal bronchodilation can be achieved when instruction and practice are provided and the patient is required to demonstrate the technique to his or her clinician.

To use the MDI, children and adolescents must be able to hold their breath and thereby achieve maximal therapeutic benefit from the aerosolized drug. A simple test of this ability is to ask the child or adolescent to hold his or her breath for 10 seconds. If he or she is unable to do this, a spacer or other device should be used with the MDI.

Spacers and Other Inhalation Devices

Spacer devices, aerosol-holding chambers, and reservoir systems (e.g., Inhal-Aid®, InspirEase®, Breathancer®, Aerochamber®, Aerochamber with Mask®), which are attached to the MDI, are used to improve drug delivery. The Aerochamber and InspirEase accommodate most MDIs, whereas the VentaHaler® and Nebuhaler® are intended for use with MDIs made by their manufacturer. Aerosolized particles from the MDI are held in a chamber long enough for the child or adolescent to take a slow deep breath or several normal breaths. Spacers and other inhalation devices improve drug delivery to the small airways, particularly for beta-adrenergic agonists (e.g., albuterol, terbutaline), which are used to relieve acute bronchospasm. Although inconclusive, the published research regarding the therapeutic efficacy of these devices generally indicates that the combined use of an MDI and an appropriate spacer device produces equivalent therapeutic benefit as the use of nebulizers. It should be noted, however, that significant variability has been observed in the amount of drug delivered by different spacer devices when used by pediatric patients.

Spacers and other devices have been effective in reducing the incidence of adverse local effects (e.g., candidiasis, hoarseness, unpleasant taste) and systemic effects (e.g., growth suppression from long-term daily use of corticosteroids). They also allow more time for evaporation of propellants and decrease aerosol velocity, thus minimizing drug deposition on the back of the throat and subsequent swallowing of the drug. In addition, spacers and other inhalation devices appear to facilitate the use of MDIs when children and adolescents have difficulty holding their breath for 10 seconds or have poor hand–lung coordination. Some pediatric clinicians prefer the use of spacer devices with MDIs to the use of MDIs alone. Although further research is required, spacer devices also provide a way for using MDIs for mechanically ventilated, intubated patients. Mask units (e.g., Aerochamber with Mask) have enabled infants and young children, for whom MDI use was previously impossible, to benefit from MDI drug therapy.

The Aerochamber has a one-way valve that allows the child or adolescent to breathe in and out through the device without losing the drug. The device should be washed in a mild soap and water solution once a week. The device usually should be replaced after 4–6 months, as the valve becomes brittle after that long. The Aerochamber has a whistle device that alerts the child or adolescent if the inspiratory flow rate is too rapid.

The InspirEase has a mouthpiece attached to a collapsible reservoir bag that collapses when the patient inhales and expands upon exhalation. Bags must be replaced every 2–3 weeks. The InspirEase also encourages proper breathing; slow inspiration causes the bag to deflate properly, whereas rapid inspiration triggers a warning sound that alerts the child or adolescent to breathe more slowly. Mouthpieces should be cleaned weekly with a mild soap and warm water solution.

Powder Inhalers

Powder inhalers, or insufflators (e.g., Diskhaler®, Rotahaler®, Spinhaler®, Turbuhaler®) deliver micronized (fine) drug particles to the lungs. These devices are breath activated and do not require hand–lung coordination. Except for the Turbuhaler, these devices require a high inspiratory flow rate to maximize particle deposition in the lower respiratory tract. Previously, limited availability of drugs as powders for inhalation and difficulty with the use of powder inhalers by children favored MDI use over powder inhaler use. However, because of continued reports of incorrect use of MDIs and the desire to avoid the hydrocarbon propellants in MDIs, interest in powder inhalers has been renewed. For example, the Ventolin Rotahaler was developed as an alternative albuterol inhalation device in response to these problems. Similarly, the Flovent Diskus® (fluticasone inhalation powder in a breath-activated delivery device) has been approved for children 4 years and older for the prophylactic management of asthma.

Diskhaler. Diskhalers were developed to overcome the humidity problems associated with the Rotahaler. Ventodisk® (albuterol) and Beclodisk® (beclomethasone) Diskhalers are multiple-dose devices that contain a cartridge disk with separate blisters for eight individual doses. Each disk is covered with foil and packaged under conditions that minimize environmental effects on the drug. When the device is actuated, a prong pierces the foil blister, releasing the drug for inhalation. Diskhalers have the advantage of having eight doses in an easy-to-load, easy-to-use device that has no additives or propellants.

Rotahaler. The Rotahaler breaks a gelatin capsule (Rotocap®), releasing the drug (e.g., albuterol, beclomethasone) for inhalation. The use of this device has been problematic because the capsules are affected by humidity, which causes the lactose filler and drug to clump. Clumping increases particle size, thereby decreasing the delivery and, thus, the effectiveness of the drug. Each capsule must be loaded individually, which can be a problem during an acute asthmatic attack. The device should be cleaned with a mild soap and water solution every 2 weeks. Because of their durability and simple design, Rotahaler devices rarely require replacement even with long-term regular use.

Spinhaler. The Spinhaler is designed for use with hard gelatin capsules containing a micronized (fine) drug powder (e.g., cromolyn sodium *[Intal®]*). This device pierces the capsule and releases the micronized drug particles, which are inhaled through the mouthpiece of the unit. Cromolyn sodium also is formulated for administration by MDI and CAN, but the Spinhaler is simpler to use. The major disadvantage of the powder inhaler is local irritation from drug deposition on the oropharyngeal mucosa. In addition, powdered cromolyn is formulated with lactose, which may cause GI disturbances among pediatric patients who have a lactose intolerance, if sufficient amounts of the lactose are swallowed.

Turbuhaler. Unlike the Spinhaler, the Turbuhaler and other powder inhalers (e.g., Rotahaler) were developed as multiple-dose units that do not require filling between doses. The Turbuhaler is a breath-activated device that contains 200 doses of micronized drug powder (e.g., terbutaline [Bricanyl Turbuhaler®]). After many children and adolescents found the powder irritating to the pharynx, the Turbuhaler was reformulated without fillers or excipients to reduce particle size, making it much less irritating. Children and adolescents need to be informed that they may not feel the powder in their throats even when the drug is being delivered. The Turbuhaler is convenient for children and adolescents to use. An indicator alerts the user when the device is empty.

Selecting CANs, MDIs, and Powder Inhalers

The wide range of dosage forms and devices available for drug administration by inhalation offers flexibility for individualizing drug therapy for pediatric patients. Availability, convenience, low cost, and high efficacy make the MDI the delivery system of choice for many children and adolescents. However, the CAN is the most effective device for emergency treatment of the severely dyspneic child or adolescent and for children and adolescents who are unable to use MDIs. The powder inhalers are breath actuated and do not require propellants or other additives. Pediatric clinicians should refer to the manufacturer's information for additional details about the use and care of these devices.

Topical Dosage Forms

Dermatologic topical dosage forms available for pediatric use include creams, foams, gels, lotions, ointments, pastes, powders, shampoos, soaps, solutions, and sprays. These formulations generally are used for their local effects on the skin or mucous membranes and are commonly indicated for the treatment of acne, burns, dermatitis, diaper rash, eczema, external parasitic infestations (e.g., pediculosis, scabies), psoriasis, and wounds among pediatric patients. Topical drugs also are used to decrease pruritus and to treat local skin infections. A more recently developed topical dosage formulation for the treatment of minor fungal infections involving the fingernails and toenails is *Penlac®* "nail polish," a ciclopirox-containing clear nail lacquer that is brushed onto affected nails. The topical product is less expensive than oral antifungals and apparently has no reported systemic adverse effects when used as directed.

Some drugs (e.g., nicotine, nitroglycerin, scopolamine) are specially formulated for transdermal or transmucosal absorption as lozenges, ointments, sprays, tablets, or transdermal drug delivery systems to produce systemic effects. Because of limited experience with patients in this age group, these topical dosage forms generally have not yet been approved for pediatric use by either the Food and Drug Administration (FDA) or Health Protection Branch (HPB). However, oral transmucosal fentanyl citrate in the form of a raspberry-colored and -flavored lozenge on a plastic handle that resembles a lollipop has been approved by the FDA. This product *(Fentanyl Oralet®, Actiq®)* is used as a premedication for children and adolescents who require anesthesia or monitored anesthesia care (i.e., it is used prior to painful procedures for children in healthcare settings where emergency resuscitation equipment and specially trained pediatric clinicians are available to monitor the patient).

Application of Topical Dermatological Formulations for Local Effects

Children, adolescents, and parents must be aware of the need for and proper application of topical dermatologic drugs. Generally, these formulations are applied to clean skin surfaces from the inner to the outer aspect of the affected area, according to manufacturer recommendations. Strict sterile technique is required for burns, infections, or open skin lesions and, as with other types of drug therapy involving possible contact with body fluids, universal precautions also are required.

Drug absorption from topically applied dermatologic formulations is increased when the drug is applied to denuded or abraded skin or when application sites are covered with occlusive dressings or similarly acting materials (e.g., disposable diapers). Attention to absorption is important because of possible systemic toxicity and significant morbidity and mortality. For example, a 6-month-old infant with a pruritic rash associated with a varicella infection was treated at home with *Caladryl®* lotion (a combination topical product containing calamine, alcohol, diphenhydramine, and camphor). The lotion was applied to the infant's entire body for several days. Unfortunately, the diphenhydramine was systemically absorbed in amounts that resulted in toxicity. The infant developed progressive shock and subsequent fatal cardiorespiratory arrest. In 1993, *Caladryl* was reformulated in the United States, with pramoxine replacing diphenhydramine. Unfortunately, however, the original formulation continues to be available in Canada and the United States despite several additional reports of toxicity after topical application. Several topical antihistamine combination products (e.g., *Benadryl Itch Relief®*) also are available. Caution is warranted.

Although most skin conditions generally heal best if left uncovered, some require a dry or wet gauze dressing and possibly a plastic or occlusive dressing. Dry dressings may be used to protect affected areas from injury or to prevent a drug from being inadvertently removed (wiped off) after application. Wet dressings may be required to facilitate drug absorption. Plastic or occlusive dressings increase drug absorption at the site of application.

Children, adolescents, and parents should receive detailed instructions on what type of dressing to use and why. Parents also should be advised about the need to wear gloves to protect themselves from contact with dressings, infected skin lesions, and wounds. They also need to protect themselves from inadvertent contact with topically applied dermatologic drugs that they may be allergic to or that could produce expected effects if inadvertently absorbed systemically (e.g., corticosteroids). Parents also should protect clothing and bedding from permanent staining, which can occur with some topical formulations.

To promote healing and to prevent infection and injury of skin lesions, children and adolescents should not scratch pruritic areas, and their fingernails and toenails should be trimmed short and kept clean. Elbow cuff restraints or soft mitt restraints may be needed to prevent infants and small children from scratching affected areas, particularly when sleeping. Pediatric patients who have mental disorders (e.g., brain injury, cerebral palsy, mental retardation) also may require elbow cuff restraints or soft mitt restraints to protect treated skin sites. The provision of play and other diversional activities, particularly when children are isolated or require prolonged treatment, is important. Easily washed, age-appropriate toys with smooth edges should be provided to prevent trauma to and infection of the affected area. Oral antipruritic drugs (e.g., diphenhydramine *[Benadryl®]*) may be required to help relieve itching.

Disruptions in body image, emotional distress, and family dysfunction, which are often associated with dermatologic conditions in pediatric patients, also require attention from clinicians, particularly in cases involving long-term treatment or disfigurement. Referrals for individual psychotherapy or family counseling may be required. An individualized treatment plan and close, sustained communication usually are required between a family and its clinician and are important components for optimal topical dermatologic drug therapy.

Creams, gels, and ointments. Creams, gels, and ointments are usually thinly spread over affected skin sites or are gently rubbed onto the affected area with the fingertips or an applicator. Creams and gels should be applied sparingly to prevent overmoisturizing the affected skin area. They should be applied in the direction of hair growth to avoid associated folliculitis. Ointments should not be applied to hairy skin sites or intertriginous areas, as folliculitis and maceration can result.

Creams, gels, and ointments are usually supplied in tubes or jars and should be used carefully to avoid unnecessary waste and inadvertent contamination. Products in tubes should be squeezed onto the fingertips, a gauze, or an applicator. They should not be squeezed directly onto the treatment site because of the risks of injuring the site with the tip of the tube, particularly if the patient moves, and of contaminating the tube and its contents. Disposable applicators or tongue depressors should be used with dermatologic formulations supplied in jars.

Lotions. Lotions can be poured onto a clean gauze or cotton ball and gently patted onto the affected area. They should not be rubbed on, as irritation or injury to the treated site can result. Water- or alcohol-based lotions can be dripped directly onto the affected area and gently stroked into the skin. Some lotions require frequent reapplication because they tend to dry and flake off.

Powders. Medicated powders are applied topically for the treatment of various skin conditions (e.g., athlete's foot). Inhalation of medicated powders can result in respiratory tract irritation or injury, so care must be taken to ensure that the powder is not inhaled when it is applied. Unless specially formulated for use on moist skin, powders should be applied to clean, dry skin only. Applying powders to moist skin may result in clumping or caking at the site of application, which can result in local irritation, particularly in skin folds and creases.

Buccal, Sublingual, and Other Transmucosal Dosage Forms

The oral cavity is well perfused by the circulatory system, providing an important site for drug absorption. It also offers considerable advantages for drugs that are either unstable (i.e., degraded) in the GI tract or that undergo extensive first-pass hepatic metabolism. Drugs administered into the oral cavity but not swallowed include buccal tablets, which are placed in the cheek; sublingual tablets, which are placed under the tongue; and medicated chewing gums and oral sprays. Both buccal and sublingual tablets are retained at their sites of placement for rapid dissolution and absorption into the systemic circulation. The therapeutic action of drugs administered by these dosage forms generally occurs within minutes. Although buccal formulations are not generally available for pediatric use, some drugs commonly required by children and adolescents have been formulated in sublingual dosage forms (e.g., lorazepam *[Ativan®]*) and as medicated chewing gums (e.g., nicotine *[Nicorette®]*).

Although the oral cavity offers the benefits of convenience and rapid absorption, it provides a relatively small surface area for absorption, so only small amounts of drug can be administered at a time. The buccal mucosa (i.e., inner lips and cheeks) appears to be thicker than the floor of the mouth but shows considerable variation in thickness (100–900 micromillimeters). It is, however, more permeable than outer skin surfaces because it is not keratinized. Absorption depends on the physicochemical properties of the drugs, with small lipophilic molecules displaying an absorption advantage. Decreased saliva production (xerostomia), particularly among pediatric patients who are concurrently receiving drugs that produce a dry mouth (e.g., anticholinergics), can affect the absorption of drugs administered buccally or sublingually.[22] Therefore, patients should be assessed for xerostomia before buccal or sublingual drug

---

22. Dry mouth also is an ADR commonly associated with phenothiazines, tricyclic antidepressants, and other drugs that have anticholinergic actions. *See* Chapter 5 for additional discussion and examples on this subject.

therapy is initiated. If necessary, an alternative dosage form should be selected for those pediatric patients for whom xerostomia is problematic.

Buccally absorbed medicated chewing gums, oral sprays, and other products. Various products formulated for buccal absorption require different methods of administration based on their design and indication for use. The most common of these products and their administration are discussed here.

Nicotine chewable medicated gum. Nicotine has been formulated as a chewable gum (e.g., *Nicorette*) for the symptomatic management of smoking cessation. The drug is well absorbed from the oral mucosa. Generally, adolescents who require nicotine drug therapy should slowly chew one piece of nicotine gum over 30 minutes when the desire to smoke occurs. They should chew each piece of *Nicorette* slowly and stop chewing when they perceive a peppery taste or a slight tingling sensation in the mouth. They should then place the gum between the cheek and gums ("park" the gum) and resume chewing when the taste or tingling begins to disappear (approximately 1 minute). This procedure should be repeated over 30 minutes. For maximal nicotine absorption, adolescents should avoid swallowing while chewing the gum and should hold their saliva in their mouth as long as possible before swallowing. They also should be advised not to chew the gum formulation vigorously. Vigorous chewing increases the occurrence of ADRs (e.g., canker sores, excessive salivation, hiccups, jaw pain, throat irritation).

Sublingual tablets. Sublingual tablets are small, soft tablets formulated to dissolve over several minutes in order to rapidly provide therapeutic drug levels. For example, peak blood concentrations of sublingual lorazepam *(Ativan)* are obtained within 2–3 minutes as compared with 30 minutes for the oral tablet formulation. Older children and adolescents must understand that sublingual tablets should not be swallowed. After placement, they should be allowed to dissolve under the tongue. Children and adolescents also should be cautioned against swallowing their saliva for at least 2–3 minutes in order to allow sufficient time for sublingual absorption. In addition, they should be instructed to safely store their sublingual tablets in the original container (or a suitable supplemental one) in order to prevent loss of drug potency. It should be noted that the FDA and the HPB generally neither approve nor recommend sublingual tablets for pediatric patients.

Transdermal Dosage Forms

Transdermal drug delivery was first achieved with ointments, creams, and plasters. Drug absorption, however, was unpredictable and highly variable. Consequently, attention was given to the design of transdermal drug delivery systems (TDDSs) that provide a more accurate rate of drug delivery and a prolonged duration of drug absorption. TDDSs are thin, multilayered drug delivery patches that have a backing of drug-impermeable metallic plastic film. To ensure that drug bioavailability is independent of variations in skin permeability, the rate of drug delivery from the device to the skin surface is the rate-limiting step in transdermal absorption. Four-layer, three-layer, matrix diffusion, and microreservoir systems have been developed to control the rate and duration of transdermal drug delivery (Figure 1-2). The rate of drug release is usually set below the mean steady-state flux of drug across the skin to help ensure a controlled rate of drug delivery into the systemic circulation and to avoid drug "dumping" among patients who have increased skin permeability.

The principal rate-limiting barrier for transdermal drug absorption through intact skin is the dense, keratinized stratum corneum outer layer of the epidermis, which is avascular. Thus, drug absorption into the systemic circulation cannot occur until the drug reaches the dermis layer of the skin. The principal transport mechanism across the epidermis skin layer is passive diffusion. Several factors, including drug factors (e.g., pH, lipid solubility), dosage formulation variables (e.g., vehicle), and variation in skin condition (e.g., abrasions, age, disease), determine the rate

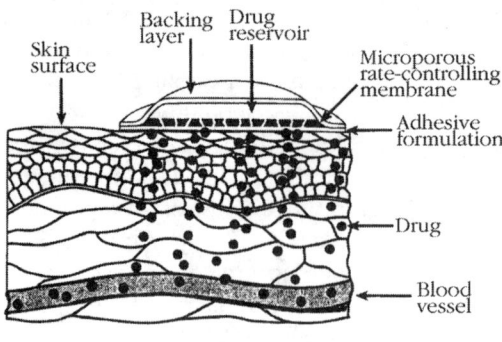

**FIGURE 1-2
Transdermal Drug Delivery System (TDDS)
Applied to the Skin Surface**

and extent of transdermal absorption. Regional variations in skin drug permeability are due primarily to differences in the structure and thickness of this layer. Drugs that penetrate the stratum corneum undergo systemic absorption because underlying tissues offer little resistance to the passive diffusion of drug molecules. Drug absorption through intact skin also can occur by the transfolicular route. Drugs, particularly those composed of large molecules (e.g., antibiotics, corticosteroids), penetrate by diffusion down hair follicles in the secretions of the eccrine and sebaceous glands.

TDDSs allow continuous drug delivery over relatively long periods, reduce fluctuations in drug blood concentrations, are convenient to use, and are generally highly accepted by patients because of their ease of application and care.

For a drug to be incorporated into a TDDS, several drug factors and the barrier properties and physicochemical characteristics of the skin must be considered. Generally, drugs that have both a low molecular weight (less than 1000 daltons) and adequate solubility in both oil and water should easily penetrate the skin. The drug also must be of sufficient concentration so that only a small surface area is required for adequate absorption. Drugs for which the daily injectable dose is below 5 mg and the therapeutic blood concentrations are within the microgram-per-liter range are likely candidates. In some cases, biotransformation of transdermally applied drugs can be facilitated by microorganisms present on the skin surface or by enzymes located within the epidermis. Drugs associated with topical irritation or hypersensitivity responses should be avoided. The most important requirement for incorporation into a TDDS is a drug's demonstrated need for controlled delivery (e.g., short half-life of elimination, ADRs associated with other methods of administration) or complex oral or intravenous dosing schedules. Although offering many advantages (e.g., accuracy of dose, avoidance of first-pass hepatic metabolism, minimal therapeutic failure and overdosage associated with the peaks and troughs of conventional drug therapy), TDDSs also have some disadvantages, including prolonged ADRs (although milder when compared to other routes of administration), local sensitivity reactions related to the drug or adhesive used, and variability in therapeutic drug response related to possible 10-fold variations in individual skin permeability, depending on individual patient factors.

Transdermal drug administration. Although the administration of various drugs formulated as TDDSs is relatively similar, certain differences exist among various products and different doses of the same product. The most commonly used TDDSs for adolescents are those for motion sickness (the scopolamine transdermal systems)[23] and tobacco smoking cessation (the nicotine transdermal systems).

Scopolamine transdermal systems. The scopolamine transdermal systems *(Transderm-Scop®, Transderm-V®)* contain 1.5 mg of scopolamine. The *Transderm-Scop,* however, is designed to deliver 0.5 mg of scopolamine at a constant rate over a 3-day period, whereas the *Transderm-V* is designed to deliver 1 mg over a 3-day period. These TDDSs

---

23. Scopolamine TDDSs are not generally used for infants and children because they are particularly susceptible to the ADRs associated with scopolamine, a naturally occurring belladonna alkaloid.

should be applied to a dry, hairless area behind the ear approximately 12 hours before the antiemetic effect is required. Only one TDDS should be worn at a time. If the system is inadvertently removed, it should be safely and appropriately discarded and replaced with a fresh system. Adolescents who require the use of these systems should be reminded to wash their hands thoroughly with soap and water and dry them before and after the application of these systems. Also, once the system has been applied, they should be instructed not to touch it until it is removed. When removed, the system should be safely discarded and the application site thoroughly washed with soap and water to prevent traces of scopolamine from coming into contact with the eyes. Contact with the eyes may result in blurring of vision and dilation of the pupils.

Nicotine transdermal systems. Nicotine TDDSs (e.g., *Nicoderm®, Nicotrol®, Prostep®*) are useful adjuncts to smoking cessation programs, particularly when used in combination with appropriate psychotherapy. These systems offer several advantages over nicotine chewing gum formulations because they do not require patients to learn proper chewing techniques and are not generally associated with ADRs such as hiccuping or nausea and vomiting. The dose is regulated, and slow absorption and relatively constant nicotine levels prevent the occurrence of signs and symptoms of nicotine withdrawal. The main ADR associated with the nicotine TDDSs is local skin irritation, such as erythema and pruritus. This ADR reportedly is associated with the pharmacologic action of nicotine on local blood flow and generally resolves when the application site is changed or when drug therapy with the TDDS is discontinued.

TDDSs generally can be applied to any clean, dry, hairless skin area. If a TDDS must be applied to a hairy skin site, hair should be clipped, not shaved, because shaving irritates the skin and increases drug absorption. Sites on the extremities below the knee or elbow are generally not recommended, and injured skin sites (e.g., skin areas that have abrasions or cuts) should be avoided. Effective adhesion of the TDDS to the skin surface is critical for maintaining the diffusion gradient. Adhesion cover patches may be used over the delivery system so that effective contact can be ensured during daily activities (e.g., showering, swimming) and for prolonged periods. Application sites should be rotated when fresh systems are applied.

The rate of drug release remains constant as long as the diffusion gradient between the system and the skin site is maintained. Drug diffusion begins immediately after the saturation of binding sites in the skin, and the drug is released constantly to establish therapeutic blood concentrations. After removal, blood concentrations decrease at a rate determined by the half-life of the drug (*see* Chapter 10). The quantity of drug in the reservoir determines the duration of action, since the size of the system determines the amount of drug absorbed per unit time. TDDSs thereby deliver the drug at a controlled rate per unit area. Most systems are available in more than one size so that drug dosage can be individualized. Attention to specific dosages among products is essential. Transdermal dosage should be checked carefully; dosing errors have occurred, particularly when one brand of a TDDS is replaced with another, perhaps for economic reasons.

As with other drug formulations, pediatric patients may require lower than usual adult dosages, depending on their age and body weight. Cutting the TDDS destroys the drug reservoir and directly affects the amount of drug delivered and systemically absorbed, so TDDSs should not be cut to obtain a desired dose. In some instances, cutting the TDDS may cause the release of the entire amount of drug stored in the reservoir and result in serious toxicity. Whenever possible, products with the most appropriate dosage for a particular patient should be selected. If such a product is not available, an alternative drug or method of administration is required.

Adolescents should be taught how to apply TDDSs correctly, how to care for them once applied, and how to store and dispose of them safely. Patients should be advised to store TDDSs in their individual unopened packages and to dispose of used systems so that they are inaccessible to younger siblings and to pets.[24]

Injectable Dosage Forms

Although infants, children, and adolescents may require epidermal, intra-arterial, intracardiac, intradermal, intradural, intralesional, intraperitoneal, or intrathecal injections, the most common routes are subcutaneous (SC), intramuscular (IM), and intravenous (IV). While still relatively uncommon, the intraosseous route also is an important alternative route for infants and young children who require emergency pediatric care. Injectable drugs are formulated as sterile pyrogen-free solutions, suspensions, emulsions (e.g., propofol *[Diprivan®]*), or powders (for reconstitution before use).

Injectable drugs are commonly formulated as solutions. Most solutions are aqueous, although nonaqueous solutions also are available (e.g., polyethylene glycol-based solutions). Some aqueous solutions (e.g., esmolol *[Brevibloc®]*, phenytoin *[Dilantin]*) may contain water-miscible liquids (e.g., propylene glycol, glycerol) to increase drug solubility or stability. Other solutions contain water-immiscible oils (e.g., corn, peanut, sesame) to enhance drug solubility or stability or to prolong the rate of drug release when sustained action is desired.[25] Although aqueous solutions (e.g., meperidine *[Demerol]*) can be injected subcutaneously, intramuscularly, or intravenously, other injectable formulations cannot because of their unique physical and chemical properties (e.g., lipid solubility, tissue-irritating qualities). For example, suspensions (e.g., isophane insulin suspension, NPH *[Iletin®]*) should not be injected intravenously because of the risk for capillary blockage by insoluble particles that are part of the suspension. And injectable formulations (e.g., chlorpromazine *[Largactil, Thorazine]*) formulated with benzyl alcohol[26] and sulfites for intramuscular use should not be injected subcutaneously; they are extremely irritating to subcutaneous tissues. Thus, in addition to individual patient factors, such as age, weight, disease state, and the condition of the injection site, consideration also must be given to the unique properties of the injectable formulation selected.[27] Ideal injectable formulations should provide a drug delivery vehicle that is nonirritating, nontoxic, nonsensitizing, and physiologically inert.

Drugs that are unstable in solution (e.g., ampicillin *[Omnipen-N®]*, cefoperazone *[Cefobid®]*, ticarcillin *[Ticar®]*) are formulated as dry powders for reconstitution as solutions or suspensions with an appropriate diluent (e.g., bacteriostatic water for injection, normal saline for injection, sterile water for injection) prior to their use. Some injectable formulations, such as chlordiazepoxide *(Librium®)*, are marketed with their own special diluent for intramuscular use only.

---

24. Discarded TDDSs may have sufficient amounts of drug remaining in the reservoir to pose significant risk of toxicity. Cases of poisoning involving small children and pets have been reported.

25. Some antipsychotic drugs (e.g., haloperidol *[Haldol]*), depending on the clinical indication for use (e.g., immediate control of acute psychotic symptomatology, simplified long-term adjunctive drug therapy for the management of schizophrenia or other psychotic disorders), have been specially formulated as various injectable salts (e.g., decanoate, enanthate, hydrochloride, lactate). The hydrochloride and lactate salts usually provide rapid action and may require additional dosing within a few hours. The decanoate and enanthate salts are generally used to provide prolonged action and can be dosed once a week or once a month, depending on the specific formulation.

26. Benzyl alcohol, which is used as a preservative for some injectable products, has been associated with a potentially fatal "gasping syndrome," particularly among some premature and low-birth-weight neonates and infants.

27. Note that propylene glycol, peanut oil, sesame oil, and other formulation ingredients (e.g., sulfites, tartrazine) are capable of causing severe hypersensitivity reactions among susceptible patients (*see* Chapter 5). A careful history that includes a detailed list of all known allergies and chronic medical disorders (e.g., asthma) is necessary to avoid prescribing or administering such formulations to susceptible patients.

Highly concentrated solutions of some injectable drugs (e.g., *Morphine HP®*) have been developed for patients who require high-dose, small-volume injections (e.g., patients who have chronic severe cancer pain and are tolerant to opiates). These highly concentrated solutions should not be confused with the standard injectable formulations that have lower dosage strengths. Fatal overdosage may result.[28]

Over the last decade, several liposome injectable products have been introduced, including the antifungal amphotericin B liposome *(AmBisome®)* and the antineoplastics aldesleukin (interleukin 2 [Biomira Corp]) and doxorubicin *(Caelyx®)*. Liposomes are microscopic vesicles composed of a phospholipid bilayer capable of encapsulating active drugs. The Stealth® liposomes of *Caelyx* are formulated with surface-bound methoxypolyethylene glycol (MPEG), a process often referred to as pegylation, to protect liposomes from detection by the mononuclear phagocyte system (MPS) and to increase blood circulation time. It is hypothesized that the doxorubicin pegylated liposomes are able to penetrate the altered and often compromised vasculature of tumors because of their small size (about 100 nm) and persistence in the circulation.

Injectable formulations usually produce a more rapid onset of action than oral dosage forms and generally have a higher absorption rate. The major disadvantage associated with their use, as compared with the other dosage forms, is the need to penetrate the protective skin layer. Such penetration can introduce pathogens into the body and cause injury to underlying blood vessels, bones, muscles, nerves, and subcutaneous tissues. Injections require a strict aseptic technique during all aspects of drug preparation (e.g., reconstitution; handling of needles, syringes, and intravenous tubing) and administration (e.g., intramuscular, intravenous, subcutaneous).[29] A sound knowledge of recommended injection sites and correct injection techniques also is required. In addition, an understanding of the principles of universal precautions (i.e., the use of gloves and the safe handling and disposal of injectable equipment) is needed because of the increased risk for contact with blood or other body fluids that may be infected with HIV.[30]

When an injection is required, it is imperative that, as appropriate, pediatric patients and their parents be advised of the benefits and associated risks. Nonhospitalized patients who require injections at home must have individual instruction about the appropriate use and disposal of injection supplies and equipment, aseptic techniques for drug preparation and administration, dose measurement, injection site selection and preparation for injection, monitoring of therapeutic

---

28. Highly concentrated solutions of morphine for injection (e.g., *Morphine HP*) may be used with or without dilution. These formulations are indicated for the relief of severe pain among patients who are opiate tolerant (e.g., patients who have terminal cancer and require long-term opiate analgesic pharmacotherapy) and who require intramuscular or subcutaneous opiate analgesia in dosages higher than those usually required by patients who are not opiate tolerant. These concentrated formulations allow smaller injection volumes and, thus, create less of the discomfort usually associated with the injection of larger volumes of drug. These formulations also may generally be diluted in large-volume intravenous solutions (e.g., dextrose 5% in water, sodium chloride injection) and injected by slow, continuous intravenous infusion.

29. Some injectable drugs, such as propofol *(Diprivan)* injectable emulsion (a single-use product for intravenous injection), have been formulated with disodium edetate to retard microbial growth in the event of accidental extrinsic contamination. However, strict aseptic technique must still be maintained during all aspects of their administration because they generally can still support microbial growth. The use of contaminated products has been associated with severe infections, sepsis, and death.

30. Postexposure prophylaxis (PEP), generally involving up to 4 weeks of antiretroviral therapy, is a well-established procedure for the management of occupational exposure to HIV among clinicians. However, the adverse effects associated with PEP are not yet well enough documented to state with certainty that it should be used in all cases of accidental exposure. Thus, although the administration of PEP after each accidental exposure would reduce risk rates for HIV infection, consideration must be given to the adverse effects associated with PEP, and clinicians should carefully consider whether or not to use this therapeutic modality.

effects, and the prevention of ADRs and other complications (e.g., overdosage) associated with their injectable drug therapy.

Developmental Considerations

The response of pediatric patients to injections depends largely on their developmental level and previous experience. Various techniques can be used to decrease the fear and pain associated with SC, IM, and IV injections. Specific techniques also can be used to prevent the needle from being withdrawn prematurely, breaking or scratching the skin, when injections are given and to prevent extravasation during intravenous drug therapy. A basic understanding of general developmental theory and its clinical application helps to provide optimal injectable drug therapy for infants, children, and adolescents.

Infants and toddlers. Neonates generally respond to the pain associated with an injection by crying and withdrawing the extremity in which the injection was made. A young infant who has not had injections previously usually will not protest. However, infants as young as 5 months who have had previous injections or venipunctures may protest when they see the equipment or even when they approach the hospital or clinic. The young toddler can associate the needle with a previous negative experience and may try to push it or the pediatric clinician away.

Older infants and toddlers should be approached confidently. The pediatric clinician should tell this age patient what is going to happen and then proceed with the injection. Most older infants and toddlers are strong enough to turn over, wriggle, and struggle. To prevent injury and to help to ensure that the patient does not perceive the procedure as punitive, a parent or another clinician should cuddle the child while the injection is administered or the venipuncture performed. For example, infants and toddlers can be cuddled in the parent's lap or held in a bear hug fashion against (and facing) the parent's chest. The bear hug position prevents the child from watching as the injection is administered and comfortably restrains her or him while allowing access to both the thigh and upper arm sites, which can be readily and gently stabilized.

Attention to site identification (i.e., landmarking) is essential to ensure that the injection is made safely when this and other approaches for gently restraining infants and toddlers are used. If necessary, patients this age also can be distracted during the procedure by being told to look at a bright picture on the wall or an interesting toy (e.g., squeak toy). Infants and toddlers should be gently cuddled and talked to in a soothing manner after the injection or venipuncture is completed. Allowing and encouraging parents to comfort their infant or toddler after the injection can help them to feel less guilty and helpless about the situation.

Preschoolers and young school-age children. If they are upset or frightened, preschoolers and young school-age children may require gentle manual restraint to prevent inadvertent injury. Parents can use a hand squeeze or hug as well as oral reassurance to help their young child remain still. With proper preparation, even young children can help position themselves and remain still, particularly if they are allowed to cry, close their eyes, blow through pursed lips, wriggle their toes, or count to 10 during the injection or venipuncture. Such activities effectively distract young children and help them increase their sense of control over the situation. A frightened or combative child in a clinical setting should not be manually restrained by several people; this approach is psychologically traumatic and causes increased fear, squirming, fighting, and loss of sense of control, which invariably causes greater problems the next time an injection, or any other potentially frightening procedure, is required.

If the injection or venipuncture has been upsetting to the preschooler or young child, time should be spent afterward reinforcing the reason for the procedure. Therapeutic needle play (e.g., simulating an injection with a doll or stuffed toy) can be used to help this age child cope with fears and anxieties. Physically aggressive play (e.g., throwing a ball, hammering on a pounding bench) also is helpful and provides the child with an acceptable means for releasing anger and tension. Children can maintain a sense of control and mastery if they receive individualized preparation before and support during and after an injection or venipuncture.

Preschool and young school-age children should be approached in a confident and understanding manner. It is often helpful if the clinician spends time with the young child before the procedure so that the clinician and the child can become familiar with each other. Pediatric clinicians should emphasize that the injection or venipuncture is necessary and, for example, will help the child to "get better faster" or "stay healthy and strong." Simple, honest explanations should be given, and young children should be assured that the injection is not punishment for a misdeed. Even preschool and young school-age children can be given choices (e.g., which hand for a venipuncture or which side for an injection), and their active participation should be encouraged, whenever possible.

Older school-age children and adolescents. Older school-age children and adolescents have difficulty with painful procedures such as injections and venipunctures because they feel they should be brave and adultlike. They may be concerned and embarrassed about regressing to younger behaviors (e.g., crying) during painful procedures and may redirect this concern as hostility or aggressiveness toward clinicians or parents. Adolescents should be supported and encouraged to talk about these normal and acceptable feelings. The reason for the procedure must be carefully explained, and privacy should be provided.

Parents. Parents should be involved, whenever possible, in their child's care—be the child an infant, toddler, preschooler, school-age child, or adolescent. However, some parents find injections and venipunctures (as well as other procedures) upsetting and may need someone to stand in for them. In such situations, parents should never be forced or coerced to assist with an injection or venipuncture nor should they ever be asked to hold the child down for an injection or venipuncture. Forcing a parent to participate in activities that are painful or perceived as threatening by their child can be damaging to the parent–child relationship by giving confusing messages to children, particularly infants, toddlers, and preschoolers, who generally view their parents as protectors. Parents may need assistance from pediatric clinicians with identifying age-appropriate ways to help and comfort their child and with helping him or her cope with unpleasant or painful procedures.

Dosage Forms and Related Equipment

Injectable drugs, including pediatric vaccines and toxoids, are generally supplied in sterile glass ampules, multiple-dose vials, or prefilled syringes or syringe cartridges (e.g., Carpuject®, Dosette®, Tel-E-Ject®, Tubex®).[31] Recommended guidelines for the preparation, storage, and disposal of injectable drugs, including reconstituted drugs, must be closely followed to ensure therapeutic benefit and prevent drug deterioration and contamination. In addition, all injectable drug products should be inspected for particulate

---

31. The Carpuject® unit-dose system is available for codeine, diazepam, fentanyl, hydromorphone, lorazepam, meperidine, morphine, naloxone, pentazocine *(Talwin®)*, phenytoin, and prochlorperazine. Dosette® syringes and cartridge–needle units are available for diazepam, dipyridamole, gentamicin, heparin, and sodium chloride. The drugs available in Tubex® closed injection systems include codeine, digoxin, dimenhydrinate, diphenhydramine, epinephrine, heparin, hydromorphone, lorazepam, meperidine, morphine, penicillin G procaine, pentobarbital, phenobarbital, promethazine, and sodium chloride. The Tubex® closed injection system delivers machine-measured doses of these drugs from sterile, clearly labeled, single-dose cartridge–needle units. These systems and similar cartridge systems help to reduce cross-contamination of injectable products and dosage errors.

matter and discoloration prior to use.[32] Clinicians also should be alert for drug product tampering, particularly drug products listed on the FDA narcotics schedule (e.g., amphetamines, barbiturates, benzodiazepines, opiate analgesics).

Ampules. Ampules, either glass or plastic (e.g., Polyamps®), hold a single dose of a liquid drug. Most glass ampules are prescored around their stems so that the stem snaps off easily. Plastic ampules come apart at the neck when the finger grip tab is twisted with the index finger and thumb. Before an ampule is opened, there must be assurance that all of the drug is in the ampule base. Any drug in the stem can be brought down into the base by gently "flicking" the stem with the fingertips. Assuring that the drug is in the base prevents inadvertent drug loss when the stem is snapped (or the neck twisted) off, ensuring that a sufficient volume of the drug is available for preparing an accurate dose when the drug is withdrawn.[33]

To withdraw the desired volume of drug from an ampule, a sterile needle is inserted toward the bottom of the ampule with the bevel of the needle facing up. The required volume of drug is then withdrawn into the syringe.[34] Filter needles (e.g., Monoject Filter Needle®, Monoject Filter Aspirator®) are recommended when using glass ampules to avoid withdrawing glass particles that might otherwise be tracked through or deposited in tissues. The drug also can be withdrawn with the ampule inverted. This technique is a matter of personal preference, but it is the preferred method when shorter needles are used. When withdrawing the drug, the needle must be kept in the solution to maintain capillary pressure and to prevent the drug from dribbling out of the ampule. Plastic ampules must be handled carefully, as any squeezing pressure from the fingertips may also result in drug loss. With either method, the drug should be withdrawn quickly to prevent airborne contamination. The needle should be replaced with a dry, sterile needle before the drug is injected. Replacing the needle prevents the drug from being tracked through sensitive skin layers.

Vials. Some injectable drugs are supplied in single- or multiple-dose vials (i.e., small sterilized glass bottles sealed with rubber stoppers). Drug vials are available in various sizes and usually hold 0.5–50 ml of solution or powdered drug ready for reconstitution. To protect the rubber stopper, vials are usually packaged with a plastic cap that can be snapped off with the thumb or a soft metal lid that can be lifted off with a small metal file. The rubber stopper should be cleansed with an antiseptic prior to drug withdrawal. The drug is removed from the vial, which is a closed system, by injecting an amount of air equal to the volume of drug to be withdrawn.[35] To ensure the accuracy of the dose,

---

32. Drug products that contain particulate matter or are outdated or discolored should not be used, because they may be contaminated or their potency affected. These products should be returned to the dispensing pharmacy or directly to the manufacturer for proper and safe disposal, not simply discarded in the trash. Several fatalities involving children and drug addicts who found and subsequently used discarded injectable drug products have been reported.

33. Glass ampules are opened by snapping the stem off. The base of the ampule is grasped with the fingers of the nondominant hand, and the stem is grasped with the thumb and index finger of the dominant hand. The tips of the thumbs should be facing each other. If desired, a foil-packaged sterile alcohol sponge can be placed over the stem under the thumbs for protection against inadvertent cuts when the stem is snapped. The ampule should be held away from the face to prevent glass particles or drug solution droplets from flying into the eyes, and the stem should be snapped off.

34. The needle bevel must be under solution when the drug is withdrawn. Unlike multidose vials, injecting air into the ampule to displace the volume of drug withdrawn is not required because it is an open system. To prevent contamination, the needle should not be allowed to touch the open edge of the ampule.

35. To decrease the possibility of introducing rubber cores from the stopper into the drug solution, it is recommended that the needle be inserted into the stopper with slight lateral pressure. The bevel of the needle should be facing up.

the drug should be withdrawn at eye level. To prevent the withdrawal of air, the needle bevel should be kept below the surface of the solution when the drug is withdrawn.

Sterile bacteriostatic water for injection and sterile normal saline are diluents commonly used to reconstitute powdered drug products supplied in vials. The manufacturer's directions on the label or package insert regarding the type and amount of diluent to use must be followed **exactly** (*see* Chapter 8). To facilitate dissolution of powders after a diluent is added, vials should be warmed in the hand and shaken gently or swirled. If shaking is contraindicated because of foaming or frothing, the vial can be gently rolled in the hands for a few minutes. Vials should be examined carefully for any undissolved drug before the dose is withdrawn.

After reconstitution, multiple-dose vials should be stored according to the manufacturer's directions. In hospital and residential care settings, they must be labeled with the date and time of reconstitution, type and amount of diluent used for reconstitution, and the name or initials of the person who performed the reconstitution. However, due to the large number of reported incidents of improper care and handling of multiple-dose vials (e.g., re-entering a vial with a contaminated needle, withdrawing excessive dosages) that have resulted in drug contamination, an incorrect dose, or a lethal overdosage, it is generally recommended that all multiple-dose vials be discarded after a single use. To avoid unnecessary waste and cost while helping to ensure patient safety, single-dose vials should be used whenever possible.[36]

Needles. Generally, injections are made with hyperchrome, stainless steel needles that are sterile, disposable, and individually packaged for convenience and to maintain sterility. Needles are designed to minimize the pain associated with insertion, penetrate skin and muscle without bending or breaking, and minimize tissue damage and the seepage of blood, lymph, and serum after withdrawal. Needles are withdrawn by making an incision that allows the close realignment of tissue edges. Needles are lubricated with a special medical grade silicone that reduces the force needed to penetrate the skin and prevents the adherence of tissues when the needle is withdrawn.

Needles consist of several parts, including the cannula lumen (channel), the hub, the primary and secondary bevels (i.e., the point tip and the heel of the bevel), and the sheath. The cannula determines the depth of drug delivery. The hub is the part of the needle that attaches to the syringe. The bevel of the needle provides both a sharp-cutting and nontearing, stretching action on the skin. The slant of the needle bevel varies, depending on its intended use, and is an important consideration for appropriate needle selection. The longer the bevel is, the sharper the needle. Needles with regular bevels are used for subcutaneous and intramuscular injections. Needles with short bevels are used for intradermal injections to facilitate correct needle placement and drug delivery. Short bevel needles also are used for intravenous injections because they minimize the possibility of piercing the opposite vein wall when the venipuncture or injection is made. The sheath protects the needle point.

Considerations in the selection of needles include the type, volume, and viscosity of the drug to be injected; the type of injection to be given (e.g., subcutaneous, intramuscular, intravenous); and the condition of the tissue to be injected (e.g., amount of subcutaneous fat, muscle size, health of veins). Needle gauge reflects the diameter of the needle. The lower the gauge number (e.g., 19 gauge), the larger the diameter. Conversely, the higher the gauge number (e.g., 25 gauge), the smaller the diameter. Generally, shorter needles with high gauge numbers (e.g., 0.5-inch, 27.5-gauge needles) are used for subcutaneous

---

36. In addition to ampules and vials, injectable drugs also are supplied in prefilled cartridges, such as the Tubex or Carpuject systems (see earlier discussion). These systems fit into reusable syringe holders designed to release their cartridges so that inadvertent contact with needles after injections (i.e., needle-stick injuries) is minimized.

injections. Longer needles with lower gauge numbers (e.g., 1.5-inch, 21-gauge needles) are used for intramuscular injections.[37]

Syringes. Sterile, disposable plastic syringes are generally used for the preparation and administration of injectable drugs. Such syringes are individually packaged for convenience and sterility. The syringe consists of a barrel or reservoir for holding the drug, a syringe tip for the attachment of the needle to the syringe, a plunger tip or pistonlike device for changing the volume in the barrel and preventing leakage of drug, calibrated markings for measuring the dose of a drug, a retainer ridge that prevents the plunger from being inadvertently withdrawn from the barrel, finger flanges for secure gripping during preparation and injection of the drug, and a thumb rest, which positions the thumb securely during the injection. Syringes are designed to meet the need for safety and accuracy of dose measurement. Several companies provide syringes with additional safety features, including positive stops to prevent the plunger from being accidentally withdrawn from the barrel during aspiration and easier-to-read markings to ensure accuracy. As with needle selection, syringe selection depends on the type and volume of drug solution to be injected and whether the injection is to be subcutaneous, intramuscular, or intravenous.

Equipment disposal. According to current Centers for Disease Control and Prevention (CDC) recommendations, all injectable equipment should be disposed of immediately after use in appropriate and accessible puncture-resistant receptacles (e.g., Sharps Collector®, Monoject High Volume Sharps Container®). The safe and ecologically appropriate disposal of injectable equipment from the home, clinic, and hospital is a concern for the community at large (e.g., garbage collectors, neighborhood children, pets), as well as for clinicians and their patients. Because of the risk for infection associated with the airborne transmission of microorganisms, needle-stick injuries, and inadvertent contact with infected blood, needles should not be clipped and syringes should not be destroyed before disposal.

Although disposable needles with shields (e.g., Needle-Pro®) protect clinicians from needle-stick injuries, their use does not obviate the need for appropriate care and technique. Because of the risk for needle-stick injuries, needles should not be recapped after use; all disposable injection equipment should be disposed of safely in appropriate puncture-resistant receptacles.

Injectable Site Preparation

To prevent infection, injection sites should be cleansed with an appropriate antiseptic prior to injection.[38] The two most common types of antiseptics are 70% isopropyl alcohol and iodophors such as povidone-iodine (*Betadine®*). Sensitivity to iodine (e.g., a previous hypersensitivity reaction to a specific iodine product or to shellfish) should be ascertained before iodophors are used. If an infant, child, or adolescent has an allergy to iodine, the site should be cleansed with 70% isopropyl alcohol.[39] If the skin site is dirty or covered with wound drainage or excrement, it first should be gently washed with a solution of warm

---

37. The gauge refers to the outer diameter of the needle. Needles are available in various gauges ranging from 18 to 27.5. To minimize tissue damage and pain, the highest gauge number (i.e., the smallest diameter needle) possible, considering drug and injection site factors, should be selected. Viscous drugs usually require needles with lower gauge numbers (i.e., larger diameters, such as a 19-gauge needle), while aqueous drugs can be administered with needles that have higher gauge numbers (i.e., smaller diameters such as a 25-gauge needle).

38. The site should be cleansed with the antiseptic in a circular fashion, moving from the center of the injection site outward approximately 2 inches (5 cm). The area should be allowed to dry before the injection is made so that the antiseptic is not tracked through the tissues, which can cause irritation and pain.

39. BD® disposable butterfly swabs are 70% isopropyl alcohol swabs commonly used for preparing injection sites. These swabs form a handle when opened so that the fingertips do not touch the swabbed skin.

water and soap, rinsed thoroughly, and then allowed to dry.

Subcutaneous Injections

Small volumes (less than 2 ml) of aqueous solutions or suspensions are commonly administered by subcutaneous injection. Drug formulations for subcutaneous injection (e.g., heparin, insulin, vaccines) should be isotonic to prevent irritation and pain at the injection site.[40] Concentrated or irritating drugs (e.g., chlorpromazine *[Largactil, Thorazine]*) should not be injected subcutaneously; they can cause sterile abscesses, pain, necrosis, and tissue sloughing at the injection site. However, the injection of certain other drugs (e.g., electrolyte solutions, opiate analgesics) by subcutaneous infusion (hypodermoclysis) has received renewed interest for managing fluid volume deficits and chronic severe pain (e.g., cancer pain).

Drug absorption from subcutaneous tissues is generally slow and complete. However, any factor that can affect blood flow to subcutaneous tissues (e.g., edema, exercise, shock) also can affect absorption rate. Significant differences in drug absorption also have been observed between upper arm, thigh, and abdominal sites. Variation in drug absorption depending on injection site is important when drugs such as insulin or heparin are injected subcutaneously.[41]

Equipment selection. To ensure that the drug is deposited in the subcutaneous tissue, a 25–27.5-gauge, 1/2–5/8-inch (1.27–1.59-cm) needle should be used, depending on the amount of subcutaneous tissue at the injection site (Figure 1-3). Obese children and adolescents may require a 1-inch or longer needle to ensure that the drug is deposited subcutaneously. A maximal volume of 0.5–1.5 ml may be injected at any one subcutaneous injection site, depending on the patient's size and the condition of the tissue. The injection of larger volumes may result in pain and irritation.

Subcutaneous injection sites. Subcutaneous injections deliver drug beneath the epidermal and dermal layers of the skin into the

---

40. Only insulin syringes (i.e., 0.5 ml [50 units] and 1 ml [100 units]) should be used for the dose measurement and subcutaneous injection of insulin. Multiple-dose vials of insulin should be stored according to manufacturer's guidelines and should be inspected before use. Insulin injection (regular) should be a clear solution. Insulin suspensions should be rolled gently between the hands to ensure uniform dispersion before the insulin dose is withdrawn. Shaking should be avoided because it may result in air bubbles or foam, which can affect accurate dose measurement. When two types of insulin are mixed, the clear regular insulin should be drawn into the syringe first. Each different type of insulin used must be of the same concentration (units per milliliter). NPH/regular mixtures of insulin are now available from the manufacturer in premixed formulations of 70% NPH and 30% regular. A 50/50 combination also is available. NPH/regular combinations of insulin are stable and are absorbed as if injected separately. In mixtures of regular and lente insulin, binding is detectable 5 minutes to 24 hours after mixing. If the regular/lente mixture is not administered within the first 5 minutes after mixing, the effect of the regular insulin is diminished. The excess zinc binds with the regular insulin and forms a lente-type insulin. Thus, it is critical that mixtures of regular with the lente insulins be mixed and injected immediately. These mixtures are stable for 1 month at room temperature or for 3 months when refrigerated. These mixtures also can be stored in prefilled plastic or glass syringes for 1 week to possibly 14 days when refrigerated. Filled syringes should be stored in a vertical position with the needle pointing upward to avoid plugging. Prior to injection, the plunger should be pulled back and the syringe tipped back and forth, to slightly agitate and remix the insulins. The mixture should be inspected for normal appearance before the injection is made. Semilente, ultralente, and lente insulins may be mixed in any ratio; they are chemically identical, differing only in size and structure of the insulin particles. These mixtures are stable for 1 month at room temperature or 3 months when refrigerated.

41. Note: To help prevent dosing errors frequently associated with the small amounts of drugs generally injected subcutaneously, such as heparin and insulin, pediatric clinicians are reminded to write out "units" and to avoid using the abbreviation "U" when prescribing, transcribing, or recording drug therapy. The "U" has been misread all too frequently as a "0," resulting in serious drug errors and related sequelae.

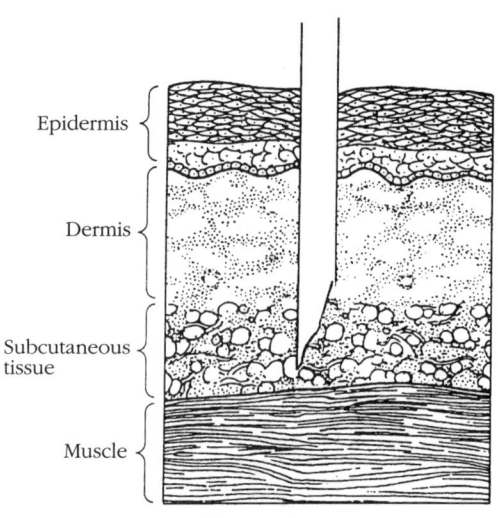

FIGURE 1-3
Subcutaneous Injection

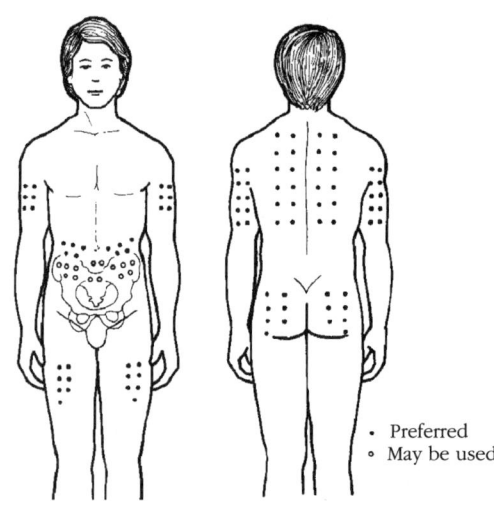

• Preferred
○ May be used

FIGURE 1-4
Subcutaneous Injection Sites

subcutaneous fat layer (Figure 1-3).[42] The preferred subcutaneous injection sites (Figure 1-4) are the upper arms, lower abdomen (from the belt line to the symphysis pubis and 2 inches [5 cm] from the umbilicus), anterior thighs, and buttocks. Fatty sites on the upper back above the scapulas also can be used. The site selected must be free from excoriations, hematomas, lesions, and moles. If injections are required frequently, injection sites should be rotated to prevent the occurrence of unabsorbed drug deposits, subcutaneous nodules, and sterile abscesses.

Performing the subcutaneous injection. After the cooperation of the pediatric patient has been obtained and he or she has been positioned comfortably and the site prepared, the needle should be inserted at a 90-degree angle to the skin surface (Figure 1-3).

Depending on the characteristics of the skin, the skin can be held taut for the insertion of the needle with the fingertips of the nondominant hand. If preferred, the subcutaneous tissue can be gently lifted away from the muscle with the fingertips and the needle inserted into the pocket that is formed. The use of the pocket technique is recommended for infants, children, and adolescents who are thin to avoid inadvertent intramuscular injection. To prevent undue pain and discomfort, the needle should be inserted quickly, bevel side up, with a darting motion. It should then be advanced smoothly into the tissue. To allow the drug to distribute easily into the tissues, skin held taut should be released after insertion of the needle and before injection of the drug. Releasing the skin also helps to minimize painful stimulation of subcutaneous nerve endings. When the pocket technique is used, the pocket should be maintained throughout the injection.

The syringe plunger should be gently pulled back before the drug is injected to ensure that the needle has not penetrated a blood vessel. If no blood is aspirated into the syringe, the drug should be slowly injected. If blood is aspirated into the syringe, the needle should be removed and gentle pressure applied to the site with a dry, sterile gauze. The needle and syringe should be disposed of appropriately and a fresh dose prepared and injected at a different subcutaneous site.

After the drug is injected, the needle should be quickly withdrawn at the same angle at which it was inserted. To prevent the needle

---

42. Subcutaneous injections should not be confused with intradermal injections, which are made into the vascular dermis layer and are used for the delivery of small volumes (less than 0.1 ml) of diagnostic, desensitizing, or immunizing products.

from clinging to and pulling on tissues, a dry, sterile gauze should be held at the site as the needle is withdrawn. To prevent bleeding at the site, after the needle is withdrawn, gentle pressure should be applied with sterile gauze. The site can then be gently massaged to increase drug absorption (unless contraindicated, such as when the anticoagulant heparin is injected). Tissue damage has been associated with frequent, repeated subcutaneous injections. These ADRs can be avoided or minimized by carefully rotating injection sites. It is generally recommended that any 1 inch (2.5 cm) in diameter area be used for subcutaneous injection no more than once every 3–4 weeks.

Heparin injections. Heparin should be administered subcutaneously by deep (intrafat) subcutaneous injection in healthy tissue sites above the iliac crest or at abdominal sites where there is an adequate fat layer, 2 inches (5 cm) from the umbilicus. To minimize tissue trauma and bleeding at the injection site, a 25–26-gauge needle usually is used. The tissue around the injection site should be grasped gently to form a roll and the needle should be inserted quickly at a 90-degree angle to the skin surface. The grasp should be relaxed slightly while the tissue roll is maintained and the heparin is injected. The needle should be withdrawn as the tissue roll is released. Pressure should be applied gently at the injection site for 5–10 seconds. The injection site should not be massaged before or after the injection. Although aspirating before the injection to assure that a blood vessel has not been entered does not appear to be necessary, there is no strong rationale to support that this not be done. (Note that, because of the risk for irritation, pain, and hematoma at the injection site, heparin should **not** be administered by intramuscular injection.)[43]

Insulin injections. Insulin is injected subcutaneously in healthy tissue sites in a pattern that depends on the pediatric patient's daily insulin requirements. Before the development of purified protein and human insulin formulations, injection site rotation was required to prevent hypertrophy and lipodystrophy. Although these ADRs are less problematic with currently available formulations, site rotation is still generally recommended. Attention to site rotation also has been recommended in regard to the variability of insulin absorption from different subcutaneous sites (e.g., abdomen, anterior thigh, upper arm).[44] Further research on site selection and rotation is required, particularly for the pediatric age group.

Insulin delivery devices. Insulin-dependent school-age children and adolescents can be taught to give themselves injections and to rotate injection sites. Several injection devices promote safe and accurate self-administration of insulin (e.g., Injectomatic®, Preci-Jet 50®); one popular device is the NovoPen® Insulin Delivery Device® or the Novolin-Pen® II or III. The Huma Pen Ergo® also is available. The NovoPen is a small, pen-shaped insulin delivery device that offers children and adolescents an easy and convenient method for managing their insulin therapy. The device is self-contained and allows the injection of insulin without the need for handling vials or syringes. The NovoPen can be adapted to various insulin regimens and can benefit many children and adolescents.

The NovoPen uses a replaceable 1.5-ml cartridge of *Novolin* human insulin (PenFill®) and a single-use, disposable 27-gauge needle. It delivers 2–36 units of insulin via a push-button mechanism.[45] This product is available in three forms—Novolin R PenFill® (short-acting

---

43. Whenever heparin is administered, clinicians should be reminded to monitor for heparin-induced thrombocytopenia (HIT), a potentially life-threatening ADR associated with heparin pharmacotherapy.

44. Generally, the rate of insulin absorption is more rapid when it is injected subcutaneously into abdominal sites (perhaps greater than 50% more rapid), followed by sites on the upper arms, thighs, and buttocks. Thus, it is generally recommended that sites be rotated within an area before moving to another area rather than rotating areas after each injection.

45. Because an accurate dose cannot be ensured, the NovoPen should **not** be used to deliver a single (one) unit of insulin.

regular human insulin injection), Novolin N PenFill® (intermediate-acting NPH human insulin isophane suspension), and Novolin 70/30 PenFill® (a mixture of 70% NPH human insulin isophane suspension and 30% regular human insulin injection)—so insulin regimens can be individualized. Cartridges with short-acting insulin can be stored unrefrigerated for up to 1 month; cartridges with other types of insulin can be kept unrefrigerated for up to 1 week.

For added convenience, the NovoPen can be stored in a case that includes space for three sterile disposable needles and one spare insulin cartridge. The dial-a-dose feature enables children and adolescents to select the amount of insulin required (within the 2–36-unit range). The NovoPen device ensures measurement accuracy. Thus, errors in measuring doses using traditional insulin syringes and inadvertent insulin loss caused by accidental movement of the plunger can be avoided. Some children need parental help in selecting the required dose, but they can be taught to inject the insulin, which requires only one hand.

To use the NovoPen device, the cap is removed and the device is turned end-to-end to mix the insulin. A sterile, disposable needle is attached and the dose selector set at the desired number of units. A locking ring is twisted into the locked position. The insulin is injected into the selected site by depressing the push button at the top end of the device. To prevent inadvertent insulin leakage, the needle should not be attached to the device until the child or adolescent is ready to inject the insulin. For the same reason, the needle should be removed and disposed of appropriately after each injection. For additional information on this and similar insulin devices, consult the patient education material available from the manufacturer.

Subcutaneous intermittent drug administration. Subcutaneous intermittent drug administration offers an alternative to intramuscular or intravenous analgesia for severe chronic pain (e.g., cancer pain) in both hospital and home settings. It avoids repeated injections, facilitates adequate pain control, promotes maintenance of activities of daily living (e.g., ambulation), and prevents unnecessary infusion of excess fluids, as is needed with intermittent or continuous intravenous infusions.

A subcutaneous injection site is selected (e.g., abdomen, lateral upper chest, lateral or anterior thigh) and gently pinched to form a bulge. Care must be taken that the needle is not inserted into breast tissue when chest sites are used. An intermittent infusion set (e.g., EZ® set) with a 25–27-gauge, 3/4-inch (1.75-cm) needle is used. The site is prepared according to protocol. The needle is inserted at a 30–45-degree angle, secured with tape or a transparent dressing, and appropriately labeled (i.e., "for subcutaneous use only"). The injection port is cleansed with an antiseptic and a maximum of 2 ml (i.e., the maximal volume of fluid that can be absorbed per hour from a subcutaneous site) of drug is slowly injected. Rapid injection causes burning or stinging and should be avoided. The site, usually maintained for 7 days, should be monitored carefully for irritation or infection daily.

Subcutaneous opiate analgesic infusion. Subcutaneous opiate infusion offers patients with advanced cancer and sustained pain a method of pain relief that can significantly reduce systemic ADRs. Unfortunately, a complication of therapy is the development of serious and painful subdermal plaques at needle-insertion sites. Plaque formation seems unrelated to needle size, site or angle of insertion, duration of placement, opiate dose or volume, or cancer diagnosis. There are no dermatologic warning signs of plaque formation, although induration is sometimes noted at the site before plaque formation occurs.

Although causes of plaque formation remain inconclusive, they appear to be related to hydraulic irritation, in which subdermal destruction may occur simply as a reaction to the hydraulic irritation (i.e., as a reaction to the infusion of a foreign substance into the subcutaneous tissue). Administered drug appears to be absorbed just as effectively from subcutaneous pockets with plaques as from those without. However, plaques do limit needle placement in the abdomen. In addition, the lesions are painful and disfiguring.

Continuous subcutaneous infusion. Terminally ill patients are increasingly choosing to die in their own homes with the assistance of family caregivers and the help of palliative care professionals. The use of continuous subcutaneous infusion (CSCI) of opiate analgesics has been important for promoting patient comfort in relation to pain management. Patients and their families require accurate and complete information regarding how to manage CSCI and other related aspects of palliative home care.

Continuous subcutaneous infusion benefits patients who have pain poorly controlled by orally ingested analgesics or who may be experiencing dysphagia or GI obstruction and cannot use oral analgesics. Continuous subcutaneous infusion also is indicated when prolonged use of the intravenous route for opiate analgesics is not feasible because of the need for close monitoring or because of activity limitations.

Continuous subcutaneous infusion involves the use of a portable, small, lightweight, battery-operated, refillable pump (e.g., Cormed®, Graesbyh MS26®, CADD-PCA®) that administers drug subcutaneously through a butterfly needle inserted into one of several subcutaneous injection sites, including the subclavian and anterior chest regions, outer aspects of the upper arms, abdomen, and thighs. Mobility is generally unaffected because the pump can be held in a holder bag or pajama pocket. This method provides continuous drug administration and replaces the need for repeated injections.

An interdisciplinary approach, such as palliative care services, is required, and proper support and teaching are essential. In addition to basic knowledge about the required opiate analgesics and how to obtain, store, and dispose of them safely and appropriately, patient instruction should include an overview of the basic parts and function of the infusion pump, general care of the pump during daily activities (e.g., ambulation, bathing, sleeping, traveling), specific ways to identify whether the pump is working properly, procedures for battery and drug cartridge changes, stopping and starting the pump, care of the tubing, and monitoring of alarm systems, including the meaning of various alarms and the what, when, and how in relation to appropriate action.

Monitoring and changing of CSCI sites also are important. Sites are usually changed every 3–7 days. Sites should be monitored for blockage, edema, pain, poor absorption, seepage of blood or other body fluid, redness, and other signs and symptoms that indicate the site should be changed.

Intramuscular Injections

Intramuscular injections should be made into healthy, well-vascularized muscle sites where drugs are generally absorbed rapidly and completely. Absorption rate can be affected by individual patient factors (e.g., blood profusion and general size and health of the muscle injected) and by the physicochemical properties of a drug formulation. For example, drugs formulated as aqueous solutions are readily absorbed after intramuscular injection into healthy tissue. Some drugs, however, are formulated as aqueous suspensions (e.g., penicillin G benzathine *[Bicillin L-A®, Permapen®]*) and solutions in oils (e.g., progesterone in peanut or sesame oil) so that intramuscular absorption will be slowed and the action will be sustained for an extended period. There also are gel formulations (e.g., corticotropin repository *[ACTH®, Acthar®]*) that are administered intramuscularly and are absorbed over 8–16 hours. In addition, the intramuscular route is used for long-acting depot drug formulations such as fluphenazine *(Modecate® Concentrate, Prolixin® Decanoate)* and haloperidol *(Haldol® Decanoate 50 or 100)*. These antipsychotic drugs are absorbed slowly so that their action is sustained, allowing once-a-month dosing as a means to promote patient compliance. These patient and drug factors also affect the volume of drug that can be safely injected into a particular muscle site.

The maximal recommended volume for an individual intramuscular injection at a specific site for infants is 0.5 ml. For children, it is 1–2 ml. Depending on the size and health of the muscle, a maximal volume of 1–5 ml is recommended for adolescents who have achieved adult height and weight. However, the volume tolerated varies among infants, children, and adolescents, depending on their physical size and general health. Careful assessment of pediatric patients and consideration of the proposed drug therapy are required before the volume of individual injections is determined.

Thus, as with other types of pediatric injections, intramuscular injection requires consideration of the age and general health of the infant, child, or adolescent; the indication for use; the type of drug formulation (e.g., aqueous solution, decanoate salt, emulsion, oleaginous solution, reconstituted powder, or suspension); the volume of drug needed; the equipment required (i.e., size of needle and syringe); the health of the skin and underlying muscle; and the number of injections required. Although most injectable products can be administered intramuscularly, this route is generally used for concentrated or irritating drugs that cannot be injected subcutaneously or intravenously. Intramuscular injection is also used for aqueous suspensions and drugs formulated with oils, which generally should not be administered intravenously because of the potential for emboli formation.

Drugs injected intramuscularly form a depot in the muscle tissue. Although absorption usually is complete, the absorption rate may vary widely because of the drug's physicochemical properties. Absorption also may be affected by physiological factors, including blood perfusion to the injection site. When drugs are injected intramuscularly, they generally produce a slower onset of action and longer duration of effect than when injected intravenously. Intramuscular absorption is generally more rapid than subcutaneous absorption because muscular tissue is more vascular than subcutaneous tissue. Absorption rates also may differ among the various intramuscular injection sites, depending on blood perfusion to the site (e.g., exercise of a group of muscles, muscle health).

Intramuscular injections are generally contraindicated for pediatric patients receiving anticoagulants (i.e., heparin *[Hepalean®]* or warfarin *[Coumadin®]*). They also are generally contraindicated for patients who have thrombocytopenia, because injections made deeply into the muscle can result in bleeding and severe tissue sloughing. Serum creatine phosphokinase (CPK) concentrations may rise after intramuscular injections, as a result of injury to muscle tissue, and may affect the interpretation of this laboratory test result.

Needles and syringes to be used for intramuscular injections must be selected to ensure that the drug is delivered deeply into healthy muscle sites where it can be absorbed and where therapeutic benefit can be obtained with minimal adverse reactions. Site accessibility and individual preference also must be considered. An infant's, child's, or adolescent's response to intramuscular injections depends on previous experience(s). The clinician needs to understand that children may have a fear of injections and may require emotional support. The clinician also needs to be aware of the various strategies that can be used to help pediatric patients. For example, toddlers and mentally challenged or confused pediatric patients may require gentle manual restraint during injection to prevent them from moving and inadvertently sustaining an injury (e.g., needle scratch). Young children may be concerned that "their insides might leak out" and may require the application of a plastic adhesive bandage to allay their fears. Other age-appropriate strategies are discussed in the following sections.

Equipment selection. Intramuscular injections for infants, children, and adolescents should be made with 5/8–3-inch (1.6–7.5-cm) needles. The length is determined by the amount of subcutaneous fat over the injection site (Figure 1-5). For young infants, a 5/8-inch needle is usually used. Children or thin, debilitated adolescents may require a 1-inch (2.5-cm) or smaller (5/8-inch) needle. For most children and adolescents, a 1- or 1.5-inch needle, respectively, is used.[46]

---

46. Needle length can affect the therapeutic efficacy of administered drugs. For example, when a too-short needle has been used for the intramuscular injection of vaccines (e.g., hepatitis B), decreased therapeutic effect has resulted because of inadvertent injection of the vaccine into the subcutaneous tissue.

CHAPTER 1: ADMINISTERING DRUGS TO INFANTS, CHILDREN, AND ADOLESCENTS

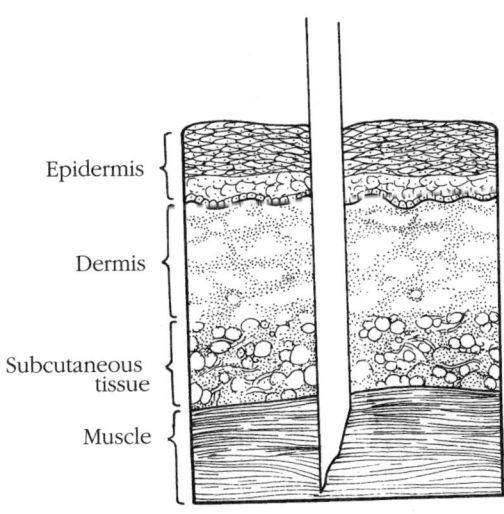

FIGURE 1-5
Intramuscular Injection

The needle gauge is determined by the viscosity of the drug formulation. A 19-gauge needle is usually indicated for viscous drug formulations (e.g., penicillin G procaine *[Wycillin®]*), whereas a 21–23-gauge needle may be used for an aqueous formulation (e.g., penicillin G *[Pfizerpen®]*). As a general rule, to avoid unnecessary tissue damage, the shortest length and highest gauge number needle possible for a particular drug and patient should be selected.[47]

Intramuscular injection sites. Intramuscular injection sites must be carefully identified to avoid injuring blood vessels, bones, and nerves.[48] Recommended intramuscular injection sites include the deltoid muscles of the upper arms, the gluteal muscles of the buttocks, and the rectus femoris and vastus lateralis muscles of the anterior and lateral thighs. The selection of a particular intramuscular injection site depends on accessibility (e.g., a cast or dressing may prevent access to a site); size and health of muscle (i.e., only large, healthy well-vascularized muscles should be selected); characteristics of the drug formulation to be injected (e.g., aqueous solution versus decanoate salt); number of injections required (e.g., one injection, such as an immunization, or four injections daily, which may be required for antibiotic therapy); and the patient's and clinician's personal preferences (e.g., nondominant arm).[49] Sites that pose infection risk should be avoided (e.g., diarrhea or urinary incontinence may increase the risk for infection of sites on the buttocks and thighs), as should sites that are sensitive,[50] are painful to touch, or that reveal hardened masses (e.g., sterile abscesses) upon palpation.

Deltoid site. The deltoid muscle is generally not recommended for the intramuscular

---

47. A two-needle technique (replacing the wet needle used to prepare the injection with a sterile dry needle) can be used to avoid tracking an irritating drug through the epidermis, dermis, and subcutaneous tissues when the injection is made. An airlock technique (withdrawing 0.2–0.5 ml of air into the syringe after replacing the needle) alone or in combination with the Z-track injection technique (see later discussion) can be used to prevent the drug from seeping out of the injection site along the needle track after injection.

48. Muscle contains more blood vessels and fewer sensory nerve endings than other tissues. Thus, the potential for puncturing blood vessels, which may result in bleeding or inadvertent intravenous injection, is great. Intramuscular injections also can cause nerve and bone damage, pain, and sometimes permanent disability, including paralysis and periostitis. Because of these dangers, landmarks and boundaries must be visualized in adequate light and palpated carefully. Although the child's or adolescent's privacy should be ensured, the site should be exposed sufficiently for accurate site identification. Children and adolescents who are concerned about the landmarking procedure can be told that the pediatric clinician is looking for the "special spot" or the "place where the drug will work best."

49. For example, the dorsogluteal muscle site is generally not recommended for the intramuscular injection of vaccines (e.g., hepatitis B, tetanus) because of the amount of subcutaneous fat over the injection site. Published literature has indicated that inadvertent injection into the subcutaneous tissue has resulted in diminished immune response of administered vaccines.

50. When a site has been selected, the muscle should be rolled between the fingertips and assessed for twitching. Highly sensitive areas twitch when the muscle is rolled between the fingertips. The intramuscular injection of a drug into a sensitive area can result in referred or sharp pain that feels as if a nerve has been "hit."

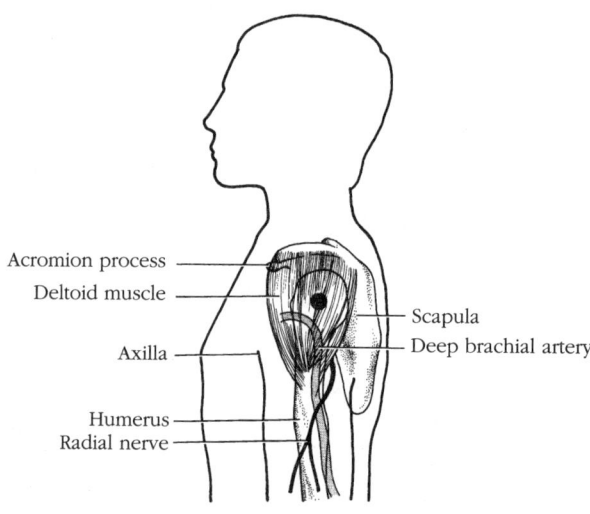

FIGURE 1-6
Deltoid Intramuscular Injection Site

injection of drugs for infants and toddlers younger than 18 months of age because of its small size and close proximity to the radial nerve and major blood vessels. However, the deltoid site may be the only site available for infants and toddlers in spica casts and generally can tolerate one or two small-volume (0.5 ml or less) injections of nonviscous, aqueous drug solutions (e.g., preoperative drug, analgesic drug following cast application). Although infants and toddlers can receive up to 0.5 ml and older children and adolescents generally can receive up to 2 ml of drug at this site if the muscle is healthy and well developed, it is generally recommended that the site be used only when necessary and only for small volumes (0.5 ml or less) of aqueous, nonirritating injectable drugs (e.g., immunizations). However, many nonambulatory children and adolescents who use nonmotorized wheelchairs may have deltoid muscles that are better developed than other muscle sites. For these children and adolescents, the deltoid site offers an important alternative site for intramuscular drug therapy.

To locate the densest area of the deltoid muscle and to avoid the radial nerve and major blood vessels, a point on the lateral aspect of the upper arm, about 1–2 inches (2.5–5 cm) inferior to the lower edge of the acromion process in line with the axilla, should be identified (Figure 1-6). The child or adolescent should be encouraged to relax the muscle by supporting the lower arm, and the needle should be inserted at a right angle to the skin or pointed slightly toward the acromion process.

Dorsogluteal site. The gluteal muscles are the most commonly used muscles for intramuscular injections for children and adolescents. However, the gluteal muscles have the slowest drug absorption rate of all muscles used for intramuscular drug therapy, and they also are likely to be degenerated in children and adolescents who are nonambulatory, inactive, or in poor general health.

Generally, children and adolescents should position themselves comfortably, lying face down (prone) on a flat surface with arms flexed toward the head. (Some children and adolescents may require help to assume this position.) To relax the gluteal muscles and reduce pain, children and adolescents should be asked to point their toes in ("toe-in"). The needle should be inserted at a right angle to the surface the child or adolescent is lying on. Although the prone position offers greater stability by restricting movement, the dorsogluteal site also can be injected when children or adolescents are lying on their side or standing. To relax the gluteal muscles when lying on the side, the child or adolescent should be positioned with the knee and hip of the upper leg flexed forward and the lower leg extended

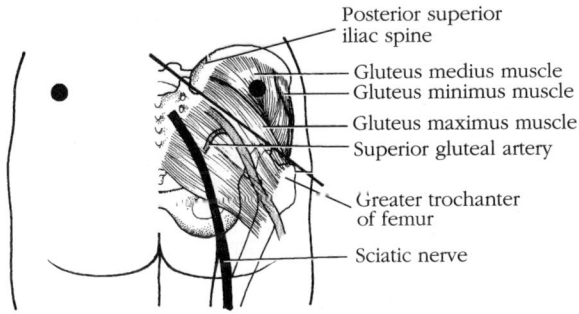

FIGURE 1-7
Dorsogluteal Intramuscular Injection Site

straight. To relax the gluteal muscles when standing, the child or adolescent should stand with the toes pointed in.

Accurate identification of bony prominences (i.e., "landmarks") is essential to avoid injuring the sciatic nerve and superior gluteal artery. To locate the dorsogluteal site, an imaginary diagonal line from the posterior superior iliac spine to the greater trochanter of the femur should be visualized. This imaginary line between the iliac spine and the greater trochanter is parallel and superior to the sciatic nerve. Thus, a site selected laterally and superiorly to this line will help to avoid the sciatic nerve and the major blood vessels (Figure 1-7). The dorsogluteal site is recommended for viscous or irritating drugs and drugs that can stain the skin (*see also* Z-Track injection).

The gluteal muscles are poorly developed among infants and toddlers younger than 18 months of age who have not started walking; among toddlers the dorsogluteal site can be used only for those who have been walking for at least 1 year. The gluteal muscles are likely to be degenerated among children and adolescents who are nonambulatory, frail, or emaciated. Thus, intramuscular injection into this site is contraindicated for these pediatric patients.

When large, healthy muscles are used, a maximum volume of 1 ml per injection can be injected into the dorsogluteal site for the 2.5–3-year-old child. The 3–6-year-old child can receive up to 1.5 ml per injection at the dorsogluteal site, and the 6–15-year-old can receive 1.5–2 ml. The older adolescent can comfortably receive up to 4 ml per injection at the dorsogluteal site.

Ventrogluteal site. The ventrogluteal site (Figure 1-8), comprising the gluteus medius and gluteus minimus muscles, has more muscle mass and less subcutaneous tissue than the dorsogluteal site. This site is accessible from prone, supine, side-lying, and standing positions. The ventrogluteal site is generally free of major nerves and blood vessels, which makes it a relatively safe site for intramuscular injections. However, care must be taken to avoid making the injection into a bone or joint. The ventrogluteal site generally is not recommended for infants and toddlers younger than 3 years of age, but it can be used to give up to 1 ml to toddlers older than 18

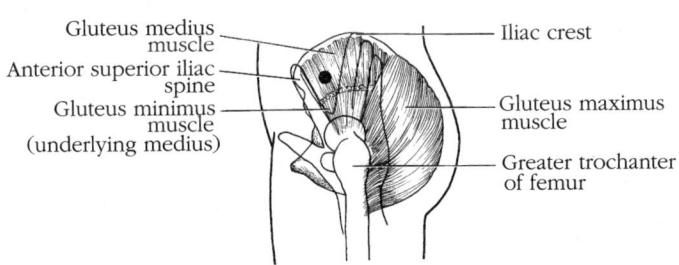

FIGURE 1-8
Ventrogluteal Intramuscular Injection Site

months if other recommended sites cannot be used. Preschoolers can receive up to 1.5 ml, and school-age children can receive up to 2 ml per injection at the ventrogluteal site. Adolescents can tolerate up to 5 ml. The ventrogluteal site also can be used for both ambulatory and nonambulatory pediatric patients, and it offers an alternative intramuscular injection site for patients whose muscle mass is likely to be degenerated at the dorsogluteal and vastus lateralis sites (e.g., children and adolescents with spina bifida).

This site can be located while the child or adolescent is standing or lying prone, supine, or on the side. The heel of the hand is placed over the greater trochanter of the femur, and the iliac crest is palpated with the fingertips, which are pointed toward the patient's head. The right hand is used for identifying the site on the left hip, and the left hand is used for identifying the site on the right hip. The index and middle fingers are spread to form a "V" with the tip of the index finger at the anterior superior iliac spine and the tip of the middle finger just below the iliac crest. Injections should be made at the center of the triangle formed between the index finger, middle finger, and iliac crest (Figure 1-8), with the needle perpendicular to the skin or directed slightly toward the iliac crest. The ventrogluteal muscle can be relaxed by the internal rotation of the femurs (i.e., "toeing-in") in the standing, prone, or supine position or by flexing the upper knee in front of the lower leg while in the side-lying position.

Vastus lateralis site. The vastus lateralis site is the preferred intramuscular injection site for infants and toddlers. It also is recommended for preschoolers, school-age children, and adolescents. The vastus lateralis muscle is well developed at birth and injections made into this site generally avoid major nerves and blood vessels. The vastus lateralis site has only a thin covering of subcutaneous tissue and, depending on the size and health of the muscle, can tolerate up to 4 ml of drug per injection and can be used for deep intramuscular and Z-track injections. However, the muscle is likely to be degenerated among nonambulatory and emaciated infants, children, and adolescents and should not be used for these pediatric patients.

The vastus lateralis is located on the anterolateral aspect of the thigh. For infants, toddlers, and preschoolers, the middle third of the muscle generally is used for injection. For school-age children and adolescents, the portion of the muscle body from a hand's breadth below the greater trochanter to a hand's breadth above the knee can be used (Figure 1-9A). Patients can be positioned in either a lying or sitting position. The needle should be inserted at a right angle to the muscle or directed slightly toward the knee. The injection should be made into the belly of the muscle by gently lifting the muscle away from the bone. Generally, infants and toddlers can tolerate a volume of up to 1 ml per injection comfortably, preschoolers can receive up to 1.5 ml, and school-age children can receive up to 2 ml. Older adolescents can receive injections of up to 4 ml per injection at this site. Needles should be selected in relation to the size of the muscle and the amount of subcutaneous tissue over the injection site. Generally, needles should not be inserted more than 1 inch for school-age children and adolescents.

An alternative technique for injecting the vastus lateralis muscle is recommended for infants, particularly those who require the injection of irritating drugs, such as long-acting penicillin (i.e., penicillin G procaine *[Wycillin]*). The needle should be inserted into the upper lateral quadrant of the thigh instead of the middle third of the anterior lateral thigh with the needle directed inferiorly and posteriorly at an angle of 45 degrees to the long axis of the leg. The muscle tissue should be compressed and lifted away from the bone with the nondominant hand to increase the penetrable muscle mass and stabilize the site during injection (Figure 1-9B). This technique decreases the risk for physical injury to tissues, nerves, or bones and resultant gangrene, paralysis, and other complications associated with the use of this site. (*See also* Rectus femoris site and quadriceps contracture.)

Rectus femoris site. The rectus femoris is smaller than the vastus lateralis; however, it is

CHAPTER 1: ADMINISTERING DRUGS TO INFANTS, CHILDREN, AND ADOLESCENTS

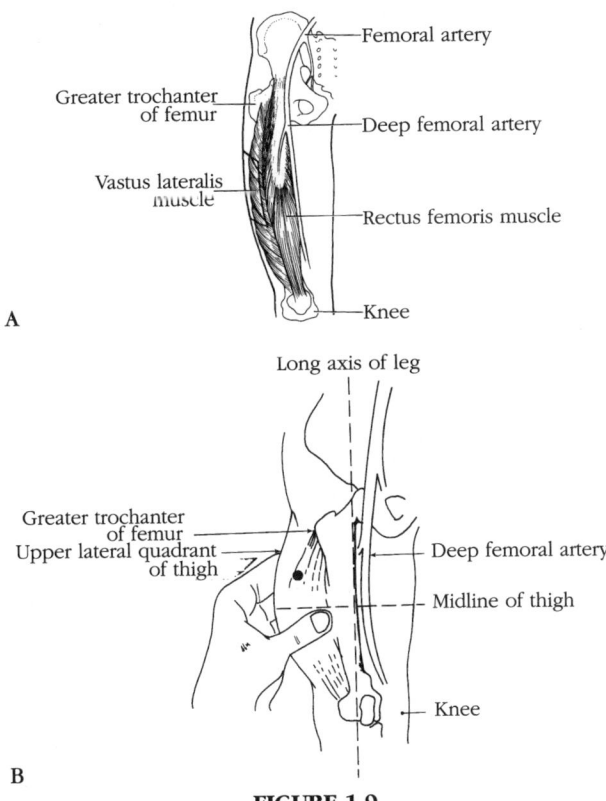

FIGURE 1-9
Vastus Lateralis Intramuscular Injection Site
(A) Middle third of anterior thigh. (B) Alternative site for young infants, upper lateral quadrant of thigh.

a recommended intramuscular injection site for infants and toddlers who have not started walking and for toddlers, preschoolers, school-age children, and adolescents. There are no major blood vessels or nerves in close proximity to the site, and it is readily accessible. The rectus femoris muscle is located on the anterior aspect of the thigh (Figure 1-10). Injections can be made into the midsection of this muscle while the infant, child, or adolescent is sitting or supine. Depending on the size and health of the muscle, infants, toddlers, and preschoolers can tolerate 0.5–1 ml per injection, and school-age children and adolescents can generally tolerate 1–3 ml. The site is identified in the same manner as the vastus lateralis site, but the anterior aspect of the thigh is used.

Quadriceps contracture. Quadriceps contracture is the loss of the ability to flex the knee associated with fibrosis and scarring of the thigh muscles caused by repeated intramuscular injections. This condition may not be noticed for a month or longer (for more than a year) after the associated intramuscular

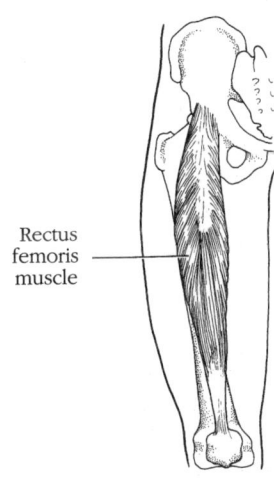

FIGURE 1-10
Rectus Femoris Intramuscular Injection Site

injection therapy. Although quadriceps contracture is associated primarily with frequent injections into the vastus lateralis or rectus femoris of newborns and young infants, it also has been noted among young infants for whom large volumes of drug were injected into a small muscle mass.

Therefore, to prevent quadriceps contracture, repeated intramuscular injections into the vastus lateralis and rectus femoris should be avoided whenever possible in newborns and infants. For example, infants who require more than one or two intramuscular injections should receive the required drug therapy by intravenous injection or infusion whenever possible to avoid muscle damage and the associated deformity. If intramuscular injection therapy cannot be avoided, warm compresses should be applied to the injection site after each injection. In addition, passive range of motion knee exercises and massage should be performed after each injection to disrupt and stretch immature scar tissue. Injection sites should be rotated after each injection and rotation site injection schedules should be posted to remind clinicians about the number and location of injections received.

Performing the intramuscular injection.

For intramuscular injections, children and adolescents should be encouraged to relax the muscle to decrease pain at the injection site and to facilitate drug dispersion. Emotional support, reassurance, and distraction during the injection are helpful. Infants and young children may require gentle manual restraint to prevent them from moving and inadvertently sustaining injury.

The site is prepared with an antiseptic, cleansing in a circular fashion from the center out for approximately 2 inches (5 cm). The syringe is held at a 90-degree angle to the skin surface, and the needle is quickly inserted in a darting manner to minimize the pain associated with the penetration of the skin and to facilitate penetration of the underlying tissue. The tissue is gently released, and the plunger is pulled back to determine whether the needle is in a blood vessel. If blood appears in the barrel of the syringe during aspiration, the needle should be withdrawn, gentle pressure applied to the site with a dry sterile gauze, and another dose prepared. If no blood is aspirated into the syringe, the dose is slowly injected to allow the drug to disperse into the muscle tissue. The needle is withdrawn quickly and smoothly in the direction in which it was inserted and a sterile gauze is held at the site.

Unless contraindicated because of the action or formulation of a particular drug, the site should be massaged after injection to distribute the drug in the tissues and increase its absorption. Massaging the site also decreases the pain associated with tissue stretching by the drug volume injected. Exercising the muscle also increases drug absorption and reduces pain. Applying a plastic adhesive bandage can help children maintain their feelings of body integrity and can be useful as a diversion or reward for "helping."

It is common for infants, children, and adolescents to experience pain and discomfort after intramuscular injections. The diluent or vehicle used in the drug formulation can be irritating to muscle tissues. For example, dextrose and saline solutions cause minimal damage, alcohol and propylene glycol solutions cause moderate damage, and severe muscle injury has been associated with diazepam *(Valium)* and phenytoin *(Dilantin)*. When several injections are required, rotation of injection sites is essential to prevent muscle injury and to ensure adequate drug absorption. (*See also* Quadriceps contracture.)

Monitoring of injection sites is essential for early recognition and care of complications related to injectable drug therapy. Site rotation must be carefully recorded. Critically ill infants and children are at particular risk for injury and infection because of the repeated use of a limited number of sites. Further research examining the use of intramuscular drug therapy for pediatric patients is required. Information on administration techniques, site selection, and the use of various injectable formulations is invaluable to those who make pediatric care decisions.

Topical anesthesia.
Some children and adolescents may have difficulty managing the pain associated with intramuscular injections.

Such patients may benefit from topical anesthesia provided by the *EMLA Patch®*, which consists of a single-dose, prepackaged dressing containing *EMLA 5%* emulsion (2.5% lidocaine and 2.5% prilocaine).[51] Coordinating outpatient intramuscular drug therapy with the child or adolescent is an important aspect of pediatric care and should be encouraged. The patch is available in Canada to pediatric patients at pharmacies without a prescription. The child, adolescent, or parent simply removes the aluminum backing and attaches the patch, as directed, to a clean, dry area of skin (i.e., the preplanned site for the intramuscular injection [or venipuncture]). The patch should remain in place for a minimum of 1 hour before the procedure. It is then removed, the area is cleaned, and the child or adolescent is prepared for the injection. Although an *EMLA* cream product also is available, the ease of patch administration appears to be a distinct advantage.

Z-Track injection. The Z-track method of intramuscular injection (Figure 1-11) prevents irritation and discoloration of the skin and subcutaneous tissues when viscous, irritating, or staining drugs (e.g., iron dextran *[INFeD®]*) are injected. A 19–20-gauge, 1–1.5-inch (2.5–3.75-cm) needle is used to withdraw the drug from the ampule or vial. The needle should be replaced with a dry, sterile needle to avoid tracking the drug through the skin and subcutaneous tissue, and 0.2–0.5 ml of air should be withdrawn into the syringe as an airlock before the dose is administered.

Although the Z-track technique can be used at other intramuscular injection sites, it is most commonly used at the dorsogluteal site. A 4-inch (10-cm) skin area is prepared with an antiseptic and allowed to dry. With the ulnar side (heel) of the nondominant hand, the skin and subcutaneous tissue at the injection site are retracted inferiorly (down) and medially (toward the center [median plane] of the body) at least 1 inch (2.5 cm) before the needle is inserted at a 90-degree angle. Although the skin and subcutaneous layers are retracted, the muscle remains in the original position. The needle should be inserted quickly and smoothly with a darting motion and the syringe plunger gently pulled back. If blood is not aspirated into the syringe, the drug should be slowly injected. The skin should be held in the retracted position for 10 seconds to allow dispersion into the muscle tissue. The needle should then be quickly and smoothly withdrawn and the skin and subcutaneous tissue allowed to return to their normal position. Pressure can be gently applied at the site; however, rubbing and massaging are contraindicated because of the potential for tissue irritation or staining. No more than 2 ml of irritating or staining drug should be injected into any one site. For courses of drug therapy that require more than one or two intramuscular injections, intravenous therapy using a suitable injectable formulation should be considered. The child or adolescent should be cautioned not to rub the site, exercise, or wear tight clothing immediately after the injection. Following these recommendations minimizes the chance of the drug seeping into the subcutaneous tissues and causing irritation or staining.

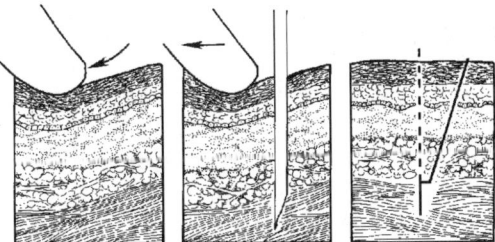

FIGURE 1-11
Z-Track Injection

Intravenous Injections and Infusions

Drug effects following intravenous injection or infusion are immediate and predictable, depending on the dose administered and the pharmacological properties of the drug, including its distribution and rate of elimination.

---

51. The *EMLA Patch* also has been used to decrease the pain associated with subcutaneous immunizations. Apparently, it has no adverse effect on antibody response to measles–mumps–rubella (MMR) vaccine and significantly reduces the pain associated with the subcutaneous injection of this vaccine. More research is needed.

Intravenous injections and infusions provide optimal drug delivery when used (1) to administer injectable drugs that have a short half-life (i.e., drugs that would otherwise require frequent intramuscular or subcutaneous injections); (2) to avoid the common complications associated with multiple intramuscular or subcutaneous injections (e.g., infection, pain, tissue damage); (3) to administer injectable antibiotic therapy to infants, children, and adolescents; and (4) to facilitate the concurrent administration of several different injectable drugs, particularly when the immediate action of a drug (e.g., analgesics, anticonvulsants, antidysrhythmics, antipsychotics, bronchodilators) is needed, such as in emergency situations.

Intravenous injections and infusions also are used when subcutaneous and intramuscular injections are contraindicated due to various patient factors (e.g., thrombocytopenia) or drug factors (e.g., the chemical characteristics or actions of a particular drug);[52] for patients who have compromised peripheral circulation (e.g., congestive heart failure, shock), because absorption is immediate and, unlike subcutaneous and intramuscular injections, is independent of blood flow to different tissues; and for maintaining fluid and electrolyte balance among infants, children, and adolescents who cannot tolerate liquids orally, and for replacing fluid and electrolytes lost through diarrhea, rapid respirations, suctioning, surgery, vomiting, or wound drainage.

Intravenous drug therapy at home, including in private homes and apartments, in residential care homes, and in rehabilitation care facilities, is increasingly common and can provide a safe and effective alternative to prolonged hospitalization for antimicrobial therapy, chronic cancer pain management, and other indications necessitating the prolonged administration of intramuscular or subcutaneous drugs. Intravenous drug therapy at home is expected to continue as patient demand and cost-effectiveness are increasingly demonstrated. With appropriate instruction and assistance from clinicians and other community resources (e.g., home healthcare assistants, palliative care team, community pharmacist), many children and adolescents and their caregivers can effectively manage home intravenous drug therapy. They can prepare intravenous admixtures, maintain peripheral and central venous access sites and devices (including Broviac/Hickman catheters and implantable devices), and operate electronic infusion pumps and controllers. Technological advances in intravenous infusion devices offer economy, flexibility, and convenience to patients who require in-home intravenous drug therapy.

Clinicians should be actively involved in the development of instructional materials that reflect current recommended administration procedures (e.g., written guidelines, demonstration videotapes) for promoting safe home intravenous maintenance, replacement, and drug therapy. Guidelines and instructions for the management of hazardous waste, including unused drug product, needles, and other equipment (e.g., plastic intravenous solution bags, plastic tubing) also must be developed. In addition, pediatric clinicians should participate in the development of comprehensive state or provincial regulations for intravenous drug therapy in the home setting.

Intravenous drug therapy has been affected by dramatic changes and developments over the last several decades, including requirements for universal precautions in response to HIV infection, and requirements for needleless drug delivery systems, portable infusion pumps, and liposomal drug delivery systems. Pediatric clinicians can expect further developments in intravenous drug delivery, including the application of microinfusion techniques and electrodiffusion principles and

---

52. For example, some injectable drugs (e.g., diazepam [*Valium*], nitroglycerin, phenytoin [*Dilantin*]) are formulated in combined propylene glycol and alcohol solvents. These solvents encourage rapid dilution by interstitial fluid and precipitation at subcutaneous and intramuscular injection sites. When injected intramuscularly or subcutaneously, these chemical characteristics of the drug formulation may result in slow and erratic drug absorption and irritation to subcutaneous and muscle tissue. Therefore, the intravenous route is preferred for these drugs when an injectable route is required.

the use of osmotic gradient devices and increased targeted drug delivery (e.g., magnetic microspheres, redox systems, monoclonal antibodies). Sustained-release intravenous dosage formulations (e.g., macromolecular drug carriers) also are being developed. These more recent advances in intravenous drug delivery are a response to the greater demands and acuity of care in a healthcare system increasingly operating under significant fiscal constraints. The complexity of clinical practice and the diversity of healthcare settings and approaches to costs and benefits of therapies are increasing, so it is incumbent upon all clinicians to become familiar with new, more cost-effective, and potentially safer methods of intravenous drug delivery.

Intravenous equipment. Intravenous drug therapy can be individualized to the specific needs of the infant, child, or adolescent by considering the types of intravenous solutions, venous access devices, intravenous tubing, and volume control devices, including electronic pumps and controllers, available for pediatric use. The equipment selected for intravenous injections and infusions depends on the patient's age and general health, the accessibility and number of healthy venipuncture sites, the specific drug to be injected or infused and its dosage and dosing interval, the duration of drug therapy, manufacturer guidelines for equipment use, cost of equipment, and amount of waste (e.g., drug, intravenous tubing, volume control devices).

Solutions and containers. A wide selection of intravenous solutions (e.g., sodium chloride 0.9% [normal saline]; dextrose 5% in water [D_5W]; Ringer's injection, lactated) are supplied in sterile vacuum-sealed glass bottles or, more commonly, polyvinyl chloride (PVC) bags[53] in various volumes (e.g., 50, 100, 250, 500, 1000 ml) for convenience and economy. The 500- and 1000-ml bags are used for fluid replacement and continuous intravenous infusions; 50-, 100-, and 250-ml bags are used for intravenous drug dilution and intermittent drug delivery.

PVC bags have generally replaced glass bottles for intravenous drug and fluid maintenance or replacement therapy because they offer several advantages (e.g., easier storage, lighter weight, less breakage). However, some disadvantages have been noted, including the greater propensity for many drugs in solution to adsorb to the inner plastic surface of PVC bags. For example, approximately 50% of diazepam *(Valium)* is adsorbed after 5 hours of contact with a PVC bag.[54] To avoid the potential significant adsorption of diazepam and other drugs (e.g., chlorpromazine [*Largactil, Thorazine*]), these drugs should be prepared in polyethylene bags (e.g., Stedim 6®) and administered with polyethylene infusion sets (*see* Tubing and drip chambers).

Solution bottles are fitted with rubber stoppers and sealed with metal caps or collars. They should be inspected carefully before use to ensure that seals are intact and the glass is not cracked. Solution bags should be inspected for puncture marks and leaks, particularly at the additive ports. All intravenous solution containers should be held up to the light and inspected for cloudiness and particulate matter. The expiration dates should be checked carefully, and labels should be read three times to avoid selecting and using the wrong solution.

Intravenous solution bottles have a vacuum and require that an equal volume of air be introduced through an integral airway (vent) to replace the volume of solution removed from the bottle during the infusion. Some intravenous solution bottles do not have integral airways and require vented tubing to permit filtered air to enter the bottle as the solution is infused and the bottle empties. Because solution bags compress as they empty, nonvented tubing can be used.

---

53. *See* Chapter 8 for additional details and discussion.

54. Insulin also may be adsorbed within 30–60 minutes when administered with plastic intravenous infusion sets (on average, approximately 25% and reportedly up to 80% of a dose may be adsorbed). The percent of insulin adsorbed is inversely proportional to the concentration of insulin infused. Careful patient monitoring is essential to ensure optimal intravenous insulin therapy.

Tubing and drip chambers. Specially designed intravenous tubing is supplied in sterile packages by various manufacturers for use with specific drug delivery systems and intravenous products. Intravenous tubing is available with drip chambers[55] that make it easy to see and count drops of solution so that the required amount can be administered accurately. Tubing also is available with in-chamber and in-line filter systems that decrease contaminants and particulate matter.

PVC tubing is commonly used and is adequate for most drugs and solutions but not for all drugs. For example, the vasodilator nitroglycerin *(Nitro-BID IV®, Tridil®)* is adsorbed by PVC intravenous tubing and, if used for infusion, underdosing can occur during the first 2 hours, until the tubing becomes saturated with nitroglycerin. Conversely, if the infusion rate is increased during this initial period to compensate for drug loss, toxicity can develop as the tubing becomes saturated. Polyethylene (PEL) tubing avoids this adsorption problem. However, the use of PEL tubing has been limited because of its opacity and inflexibility. To avoid these limitations, a PEL/PVC intravenous set has been developed; this set has been associated with significantly less loss of drug due to adsorption than the standard set, regardless of drug concentration or infusion rate.

Needleless and other delivery systems. Although small-volume intermittent infusions are commonly used for intravenous drug delivery, they have several limitations. These limitations include unpredictable infusion rates, which may result in inconsistent or incomplete drug delivery among pediatric patients who require intravenous drug therapy, or in fluid overload among pediatric patients who require fluid restriction; relatively high expense; and excessive waste of intravenous tubing and other equipment (e.g., needles and syringes). An increasing number of intravenous drug delivery systems (e.g., Add-Vantage®, Viaflex Plus®) have been designed to facilitate intravenous drug therapy, save time during preparation and administration of doses, and prevent dosing errors that can occur when reconstitution of drugs is required before intravenous administration. These drug delivery systems provide ready-to-use drugs and diluents or premixed drug solutions in easy-to-handle containers. Some drugs are available in frozen form.[56] The manufacturer's instructions for the storage, preparation, and use of these products should be followed.

Although recently developed intravenous drug delivery systems have many advantages, they also have been associated with several disadvantages, including serious errors related to incorrect use. Appropriate in-service education programs (e.g., seminars, newsletters, memoranda) should be provided to clinicians before intravenous drug delivery systems are introduced. Product manufacturers and pharmacy-based intravenous admixture services should assist with the development of instructional materials and should help improve labeling to prevent errors and adverse effects associated with the use of needleless intravenous devices. For example, reports of bacteremia associated with the use of these devices could be significantly reduced or entirely pre-

---

55. The drip chamber is calibrated so that a specified number of drops deliver a milliliter (1 ml) of solution. Thus, the infusion rate in milliliters per hour can be determined by counting drops for a short period (e.g., 15 seconds). Generally, drip chambers are supplied as macrodrip (e.g., 10, 12, 15 drops/ml) and microdrip (i.e., 60 drops/ml) systems. The number of drops per milliliter for macrodrip systems varies with the manufacturer, so it is important that the calibration on the package label is checked to ensure accurate calculation of the infusion rate. Microdrip systems have a small needle projection at the top of the inside of the drip chamber and, thus, can readily be visually differentiated from macrodrip systems. The microdrip systems are preferred because they decrease the risk of accidental drug overdosage and fluid overload by providing a more precise and controlled rate of drug and intravenous solution delivery. The infusion rate can be adjusted with a roller clamp on the tubing.

56. The manufacturer's specific instructions for thawing should be followed for all frozen products. Pediatric clinicians are cautioned not to thaw these products by microwave irradiation or immersion in a water bath (unless specifically directed by the manufacturer) because of the possible effect of heat on drug stability.

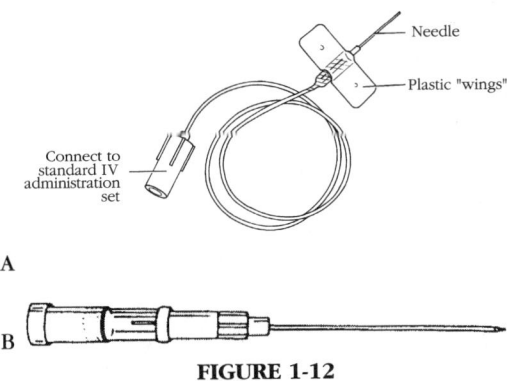

FIGURE 1-12
Peripheral Venous Access Devices for Infants, Children, and Adolescents
(A) Wing-tipped needle. (B) Over-the-needle catheter.

vented through implementation of the strict sterile technique used for needle devices.

Venous access devices. Veins can be accessed with peripheral, central, and implantable venous access devices. The selection and use of these devices are based on individual patient factors (e.g., age, general health, the size and condition of the patient's veins) and on factors related to the required intravenous drug therapy (e.g., vesicant effects of the drug, volume of drug to be administered, frequency of dosing, duration of therapy).

Peripheral venous access devices. Peripheral venous access devices include individually packaged, sterile, wing-tipped needles (e.g., Butterfly®) and over-the-needle catheters, which are available in a variety of gauges and lengths (Figure 1-12).[57] Needles and catheters should be carefully inspected for defects before use (e.g., broken needles or needles that have become detached from the hub, needle burrs). Generally, needles and catheters are coated with silicone to facilitate insertion and to decrease clotting at the bevel and tip. The wing-tipped needle is 0.5–1.25 inches (1.3–3.1 cm) long with tubing 3–12 inches (7.5–30 cm) in length. It is commonly used for one-time (i.e., slow or rapid intravenous injection) or short-term, intermittent intravenous drug therapy (i.e., 1–3 days). Over-the-needle catheters (e.g., Angiocath®) are radiopaque combination catheter and needle devices available in lengths of 1.25–2 inches (3.1–5 cm). An over-the-needle catheter has an inner needle and an outer catheter. After the combination is inserted into a vein, the needle is removed, leaving the catheter in the vein. Generally, over-the-needle catheters are used when an irritating drug (e.g., antibiotic) or long-term intravenous drug therapy (more than 3 days) is required.

Several peripheral venous access devices have been developed to protect against acci-

---

57. The selection of a peripheral venous access device often depends on the clinician's personal preference (i.e., some pediatric clinicians prefer wing-tipped needles, while others prefer catheters). Wing-tipped needles may be preferred because they are easily inserted. However, wing-tipped needles are not as stable as catheters after insertion because, being metal, they are rigid and can more easily damage or pierce the opposite vein wall, resulting in extravasation. Although wing-tipped needles can be used for long-term intravenous drug therapy, catheters may be preferred because they are more flexible and offer patients fewer activity restrictions. However, the catheter insertion site must be carefully assessed for signs of infection and phlebitis because these problems tend to occur more often with catheters than with wing-tipped needles, particularly when irritating drugs are infused (e.g., cephalothin *[Keflin®]*). Generally, the smallest possible diameter needle (i.e., the highest gauge number needle or catheter) should be used to maximize blood flow at the needle or catheter tip (see earlier discussion regarding needle selection); this size needle or catheter helps to rapidly dilute irritating drug solutions as they enter the bloodstream.

dental needle-stick injury and infection with the HIV, hepatitis B and C, or other blood-borne infectious microorganisms. For example, the PROTECTIV® IV catheter safety system offers needle-stick protection during and after venipuncture with an over-the-needle catheter. As the used (contaminated) needle is removed from within the catheter, a protective guard glides over it. A reassuring click indicates when the needle is locked safely inside the guard.

Peripheral venous access devices (either needles or catheters after they have been inserted) are often capped with intermittent infusion control (IIC) caps (e.g., intermittent heparin lock)[58] to promote freedom of movement and to prevent the necessity of repeated venipunctures. The IIC cap provides ready access for intravenous injections (i.e., "push" or "bolus" injections, which, depending on the drug and desired therapeutic action, are injected rapidly over 30 seconds or slowly over 1–5 minutes) and for intermittent intravenous drug infusions (i.e., when intravenous tubing is attached to the IIC cap for slow, intermittent infusion over 20–30 minutes, with a volume control device or small-volume infusion set).

The IIC cap is wiped with an alcohol swab, the site is checked for patency, and the drug is injected with a 1/2–1-inch (1.25–2.5-cm) needle. Previously, it was generally recommended that 1 ml of sterile normal saline (0.9% sodium chloride solution for injection) be injected into the IIC cap to flush the drug through the peripheral venous access device. The saline flush was then followed by a heparin flush (1 ml of heparin [100 units/ml]) to maintain the patency of the venous access device. In addition, heparin flushes generally were recommended every 8 hours and after each use of the venous access device for drug administration. However, irritation at the venipuncture site, phlebitis, and leakage of heparin around the venipuncture site have called into question these recommendations for maintaining the patency of venous access devices.

Although these recommendations have been examined, no conclusive guidelines have been provided because of conflicting results in the published literature. Normal saline flushes have been found to be as effective as heparin for maintaining patency of IIC capped devices with little association with phlebitis. However, research designed to determine cost-effectiveness has found that saline-flushed venous access devices require replacement twice as often as heparin–saline-flushed devices. Therefore, a heparin flush (alone, without saline) has been recommended for maintaining patency of venous access devices following the administration of drugs compatible with heparin. For drugs incompatible with heparin, the capped venous access device should be flushed first with 1 ml of normal saline and then with 1 ml of heparin solution. The use of other intravenous solutions (e.g., dextrose 5% in water for injection [D_5W]) also has been explored, with encouraging results. Further research, particularly involving pediatric patients, is needed.

An example of a potentially safer method for intravenous drug delivery is the needle-

---

58. To prevent clot formation in a heparin lock set, diluted heparin solution (Heparin Lock Flush Solution®) or 10–100 units/ml heparin solution should be injected into the injection hub to fill the entire set up to the needle or catheter tip. This solution must be replaced each time the heparin lock is used. Before any solution is administered through the heparin lock, aspiration should be performed to ensure patency of the venous access device and the location of the needle or catheter tip. If the drug is incompatible with heparin, the entire heparin lock set should be flushed with sterile water for injection or 0.9% sodium chloride injection before and after the drug is administered. After the second flush, the diluted heparin solution may be injected into the set. Because repeated injections of small doses of heparin can alter activated partial thromboplastin time (aPTT), a baseline aPTT should be obtained prior to the insertion of a heparin lock set. Another product is tinzaparin (*Innohep®*), a low-molecular-weight heparin that is indicated for the prevention of clotting in indwelling intravenous lines used for hemodialysis and extracorporeal circulation for patients who are not at high risk for bleeding. Tinzaparin should not be used interchangeably (unit for unit) with other low-molecular-weight heparins or with unfractionated heparin because of differences in anti-Xa and anti-IIa activities, dosages, manufacturing process, molecular weight, and units.

less InterLink® intravenous access system. This system uses a blunt plastic cannula in place of a needle for intravenous drug delivery applications, such as access to both single- and multiple-dose vials and intravenous tubing ports (i.e., Y-sites). Found to prevent accidental needle-stick injuries and infections, other similar needleless systems are under development. For example, the Blunt Point® sterile cartridge is used with the Tubex closed injection system and is compatible with other needleless systems.

Pediatric patients and their parents need to know what to do if the peripheral venous access device is inadvertently dislodged. They should be provided with a protocol for immediate management of the bleeding (i.e., apply pressure to the venipuncture site with a sterile gauze to stop the bleeding and immediately notify their clinician) and with procedures to follow for accessing emergency services or having a new venous access device inserted, if required. The site should be inspected for hemorrhage, discoloration, and other signs of prolonged clotting time. The IIC cap is generally changed when the peripheral venous access device (i.e., needle and catheter) is changed. Generally, they should be changed at least every 72 hours and more frequently if needed (e.g., if leaking occurs). More research is required examining how various drugs, needles, catheters, length of time the venipuncture site is used, and site dressing procedures affect rates of air embolism, extravasation, infection, and inflammation among pediatric patients.

Peripheral venous access devices are generally adequate for providing intravenous drug therapy for most pediatric patients. In some situations, however, other devices may be required, including central venous access devices (e.g., Broviac/Hickman catheters, multilumen central venous pressure catheters) and implantable venous access devices. These devices are usually reserved for pediatric patients who require intravenous opiate analgesics for severe acute or long-term pain associated with serious medical conditions (e.g., AIDS, burns, cancer, physical injury, surgery).

Central venous access devices. Broviac/Hickman catheters are central venous catheters made of silicone and designed for long-term infusion therapy. The Broviac catheter was introduced by Broviac in 1973 as a permanent indwelling right atrial catheter for delivering home nutritional support.[59] It was modified by Hickman and colleagues in 1979 to allow blood withdrawal, the infusion of intravenous drugs and solutions, and the delivery of blood products. These catheters can have one to three lumens, which are flushed after each use and every 24 hours (every 12 hours if not in use) with 2.5 ml of heparin (100 units /ml), or according to hospital or clinic protocol. Before a needle is inserted into the access port of the catheter, all tubing and needle connections should be vigorously scrubbed with povidone-iodine and allowed to dry. Alternatively, each connection can be vigorously scrubbed with isopropyl alcohol for 2 minutes.

Catheter insertion and removal is a minor surgical procedure completed medically under local or general anesthesia. Strict aseptic technique during insertion, drug administration, and site care is required because catheter-related infection, a major disadvantage associated with these devices, accounts for 10% of the time that pediatric patients who have central venous catheters spend in the hospital. In this regard, a review of the literature and clinical experience would indicate that infants and children younger than 2 years seem most susceptible to infection.

In addition to infection, central venous access devices are subject to other complica-

---

59. Concern regarding the possible contamination of total nutritional support formulas with aluminum and associated sequelae (e.g., encephalopathy, the inhibition of calcium uptake in the bones of premature infants, metabolic bone disease, and the induction of cholestasis) was raised by Popinska et al. (1999). In the absence of reliable labeling, these researchers recommend that clinicians use caution, particularly when pediatric patients require long-term use of nutritional products. Monitoring pediatric patients for excessive aluminum levels also seems prudent.

tions, including occlusion and dislodgement. If catheters become occluded or are dislodged, they must be replaced or an alternative device selected to maintain required drug, fluid, or other therapy (e.g., nutritional support). Occlusion or dislodgement presents a serious situation for pediatric patients who require central venous access devices for essential intravenous drug or other therapy. Fortunately, occlusion and dislodgement can be prevented by attention to recommended procedures for accessing and caring for the device; the application of protective dressings; and adequate instruction to children, adolescents, and parents regarding the care and management of the device. Unfortunately, occlusion can occur as a direct result of drug therapy or nutrition support.

Several techniques have been suggested for "salvaging" occluded central venous access devices. For example, irrigation of the device with a thrombolytic drug (e.g., streptokinase [Kabikinase®, Streptase®], urokinase [Abbokinase Open-Cath®]) has been suggested. These drugs have been successfully used to induce lysis of occlusions by activating the pediatric patient's fibrinolytic system.[60] However, because of their expected pharmacologic action, their use is contraindicated for infants, children, and adolescents who have active internal bleeding or who have had recent surgery.[61]

Occlusions associated with nutrition support have been successfully treated with a dilute hydrochloric acid solution. Occlusions associated with all-ion nutrient mixtures have been successfully treated with an alcohol solution. It is generally recommended that, if there is doubt about the nature of the occlusion, a thrombolytic drug probably should be used first. Regardless of the irrigation solution required, treatment should be implemented as soon as a sluggish flow rate is noted, **not** after total occlusion has occurred. It also is generally recommended that before a decision is made to remove an occluded catheter, which requires minor surgery, at least one attempt with each potentially successful irrigation solution should be made.

The multilumen central venous pressure (ML-CVP®) catheter is an alternative to the Broviac/Hickman catheter. It uses a single insertion site and provides three separate polyurethane lumens. It is suitable for pediatric patients who require intermediate-length courses of intravenous therapy and eliminates

---

60. If catheters are occluded by substances other than blood fibrin clots (e.g., drug precipitates), urokinase is generally not effective.

61. Note that excessive pressure must be avoided when urokinase is injected to restore the patency of intravenous catheters, including central venous catheters, because of the danger of either rupture of the catheter or expulsion of the clot into the systemic circulation. When urokinase is used for central venous catheter clearance, the patient should exhale and hold his or her breath while the catheter is not connected to the intravenous line or syringe to prevent air from entering the catheter. Generally, it is recommended that the intravenous tubing be disconnected from the central venous catheter hub and an empty 10-ml syringe attached. To determine occlusion of the catheter, an attempt to aspirate the clot with the 10-ml syringe should be made. If unsuccessful, the 10-ml syringe should be removed and a 1-ml tuberculin syringe filled with reconstituted urokinase attached. An amount of urokinase equivalent to the volume of the catheter should be injected slowly and gently. The tuberculin syringe should then be removed and a 5-ml syringe attached to the catheter. After approximately 5 minutes, an attempt should be made to aspirate the drug and residual clot with the 5-ml syringe. Aspiration attempts may be repeated every 5 minutes for up to 30 minutes (i.e., six times). If the catheter is not patent after 30 minutes, the catheter should be capped and the urokinase allowed to remain in the catheter for an additional 30–60 minutes. After this time, another attempt should be made to aspirate the clot. A second injection of urokinase may be necessary in resistant cases. When patency of the central venous catheter is restored, 4–5 ml of blood should be aspirated with the syringe to ensure complete removal of the drug and the residual clot and its fragments. The blood-filled syringe should be removed, appropriately discarded, and replaced with a 10-ml syringe filled with 0.9% sodium chloride injection. The catheter should then be gently irrigated with the 0.9% sodium chloride injection to ensure patency. Only then should the intravenous line be reattached to the catheter hub. To avoid infection, sterile technique must be used throughout this entire procedure.

the more traumatic insertion required with Broviac/Hickman catheters. The ML-CVP catheter can be used for both continuous and intermittent drug delivery and for administering incompatible drugs simultaneously. The locations of the exit points of the three lumens in the vein are staggered, and lumens can be rotated for drug administration to avoid mixing incompatible drugs. The device can be inserted percutaneously or by surgical cutdown into the internal or external jugular or subclavian veins.

Peripherally inserted central venous catheters. The peripherally inserted central venous catheter (PICVC) is an intermediate-term Silastic® long-line catheter. It is inserted peripherally, preferably at the antecubital region of the nondominant arm. The catheter is advanced so that the tip of the catheter is placed centrally in the superior vena cava. To allow maximal mobility of the elbow joint and extremity, the site of insertion should be at least two finger-breadths above or below the bend of the arm. Radiographic confirmation of the placement of the catheter tip ensures correct placement before drug therapy is initiated and also minimizes any complications associated with incorrect placement (e.g., extravasation, occlusion, thrombus).

The PICVC has gained wide acceptance as a comparatively low-risk and cost-effective alternative to ongoing venous access, particularly for pediatric patients who require intravenous drug therapy at home. The insertion of most PICVCs is performed by specially trained registered nurses. Fluoroscopically assisted insertion may facilitate the correct placement of the PICVC, particularly in patients with poor peripheral veins. Common complications associated with PICVCs, particularly with long-term use, include catheter and venous thrombosis, infection, occlusion, and phlebitis. Although the PICVC offers an alternative approach for intravenous drug therapy for many pediatric patients, because of the potential for severe tissue damage and resultant loss of limb associated with the accidental extravasation of vesicant drugs, the continuous infusion of vesicant drugs (e.g., antineoplastics) by PICVCs is not recommended. An alternative to the PICVC is the midline catheter.

Midline catheters. The midline catheter is inserted with aseptic technique in much the same manner as is the PICVC. However, the midline catheter is shorter and is only advanced into the vein of the upper arm below the axillary lateral line. The insertion of the midline catheter usually does not require radiographic verification of catheter tip placement. Complications associated with the use of midline catheters are essentially the same as those encountered with PICVCs.

The Landmark® midline catheters use a thrombo-resistant Aquavene® cannula that is relatively stiff during insertion, but softens after hydration within the vein. The cannula increases in length by approximately 0.5 inch (1.25 cm) and in gauge by two gauge sizes after full hydration within the vein (approximately 2 hours after insertion). **Thus, a catheter two gauge sizes smaller than normally required is selected for insertion,** and the arm is measured from the proposed insertion site to the desired placement site of the catheter tip (usually approximately 5–6 inches [13–15 cm] for older children and adolescents).

After insertion, the site is covered with a sterile, occlusive dressing, and the catheter is connected to intravenous luer-lock tubing or a heparin lock for intermittent use. The arm must be kept at rest in the extended position for 30 minutes after the catheter is inserted to allow adequate venous hydration of the catheter. Aquavene catheters should not be used for high-pressure injection (i.e., above 45 pounds per square inch), which may cause the catheter to rupture, nor, because the tonicity is too high for peripheral veins, should they be used for the infusion of hypertonic intravenous solutions (i.e., intravenous solutions exceeding 13% final glucose concentration). Hypertonic solutions are best infused with central venous catheters.

Implantable venous access devices. Implantable venous access devices include Infuse-a-Port®, Port-a-Cath®, and Mediport®. These devices provide central venous access for the delivery of intravenous drug therapy and solutions, systemic and intra-abdominal antineoplastic drug therapy (for intra-abdominal therapy, the catheter is inserted into the abdominal cavity rather than a central vein), nutrition support (including lipid emulsions), and administration of blood products. They also may be used for blood sample withdrawal.

Implantable vascular access devices eliminate the need for daily flushing and dressing changes. They should, however, be flushed with 5 ml of heparin (100 units/ml) every 5 days and after each use. If not accessed regularly, the devices should be flushed at least once a month with 10 ml of normal saline for injection followed by 3–5 ml of heparin (100 units/ml). Implantable devices require a Huber® needle, which should be supported with a 2 × 2-inch (5 × 5-cm) sterile gauze and SteriStrips® or a foam-padded Port-Gard® dressing during intravenous drug or solution infusion. The site should not be covered with a dressing when not in use. Insertion and removal of the device require minor surgery.

Although implantable vascular access devices offer many advantages, they also have several disadvantages. Strict aseptic technique and universal precautions are required to prevent infection, including septicemia. Other disadvantages include the need for the skin to be punctured each time the device is accessed and the possibility of thromboembolism, internal extravasation injury, catheter migration, and pain and inflammation at the access site. These adverse effects may require removal of the access device. Despite the disadvantages, however, the use of implantable vascular access devices is expected to increase because of their overall benefits. The selection of a particular manufacturer's device depends largely on the type of drug and other therapy required and on the surgeon's or oncologist's familiarity with or preference for a particular device.

Electronic infusion control devices. It is generally recommended that all infants and toddlers younger than 2 years receive intermittent or continuous intravenous drug therapy and intravenous maintenance or replacement therapy with an electronic infusion control device (EICD). The device delivers the exact amount of solution per unit of time and helps to prevent free-flow accidents and fluid volume overload, which are particularly dangerous for infants and toddlers, who have immature cardiovascular and renal systems and smaller total body volume than older children. Because the infusion rate can be controlled accurately, EICDs also are used for older children and adolescents when continuous intravenous drug therapy is required with drugs that have a narrow therapeutic index.

Although there are many brands and models of EICDs, there are only two main types: the gravity controller and the infusion pump. Both types are available in volumetric or nonvolumetric models. Volumetric EICDs are used when a specific volume of solution is required over a long period and the infusion rate is not critical. Nonvolumetric EICDs deliver solution at a constant drop rate and are used when the infusion rate must be measured with short-term accuracy. Cardiovascular drugs, such as dopamine *(Intropin)*, nitroglycerin *(Nitro-BID IV, Tridil)*, and sodium nitroprusside *(Nipride®)*, are best infused with nonvolumetric EICDs; nutrition support products (e.g., amino acids, dextrose, electrolytes, fat emulsions, minerals, vitamins) can be infused with volumetric EICDs.

Gravity controllers. Gravity provides the driving force for intravenous solution delivery with gravity controllers. The flow rate, however, may be regulated by mechanisms that electronically count the number of droplets.

Infusion pumps. Infusion pumps can be classified by mechanism of operation, including peristaltic, syringe, cassette, and reservoir pump. They may also be classified according to the timing of drug delivery (i.e., rapid or slow intravenous injection, intermittent infusion, continuous infusion), single- or multiple-solution delivery, or therapeutic application (e.g., patient-controlled analgesia).

Patient-controlled analgesia (PCA) is an increasingly common method of pain control.

Using a specially designed infusion pump programmed to prevent overdosage (e.g., Bard Harvard PCA®, Life Care PCA®), patients self-administer doses of an intravenous opiate analgesic when they need it. This method of pain control is generally well received by patients and is both safe and effective. In comparison with conventional intramuscular opiate analgesics, PCA is associated with fewer ADRs, better pulmonary recovery after abdominal surgery, less nursing time for drug administration tasks, lower total dose used, and improved individualization of drug dosing.

In the past, infusion pumps were designed for use in the acute hospital setting. Now portable infusion pumps (e.g., Bard Ambulatory PCA®) are used increasingly at home. Portable infusion pumps generally consist of a refillable drug reservoir with a large capacity that requires infrequent or no reservoir changes (so the risk of contamination and infection is low), a rate-controlling pump, an energy source, and a safety mechanism. As such infusion pumps become more cost-effective, their use is expected to increase because they offer the benefits of freedom of movement and the opportunity to stay at home.

Complications of EICDs. Unfortunately, EICDs also are subject to the common problems associated with intravenous drug or other therapy that uses nonelectronic infusion control devices. These problems include air in the tubing, disconnected tubing, empty solution chambers, inaccurate infusion rates, and occluded tubing. Thus, careful monitoring is required, particularly for pediatric patients and those who cannot self-monitor for and communicate about equipment malfunction or signs and symptoms of irritation or extravasation at the insertion site. Although various EICDs are equipped with alarm systems to indicate problems, EICDs continue to deliver drugs and solutions even when needles or catheters have become dislodged from the vein into interstitial tissue, which can result in irritation, pain at the insertion site, or severe tissue damage, particularly when irritating or vesicant drugs are being infused.

Regardless of these common problems, the use of EICDs has increased over the last several years, and advances in infusion therapy and computer technology have led to computerized infusion pumps with increasingly sophisticated drug delivery capabilities (e.g., multiple-rate and multiple-solution programming). Implantable pumps, pumps with chronobiological applications, osmotic-pressure devices, and open- and closed-loop systems also have been developed. The increasing complexity of EICD programming requires changes in the traditional roles of clinicians relative to the planning and delivery of intravenous drug and other therapy. Concerns also have been raised regarding the introduction of new models of EICDs without adequate training of clinicians.

It also has been argued that decisions regarding the selection and use of EICDs in pediatric settings should be based on clinical benefits (improved pediatric care) and cost-effectiveness (healthcare system efficiency). The cost of EICDs and reimbursement issues related to these costs also must be addressed to ensure that appropriate and beneficial therapy is not withheld from pediatric patients. It also has been emphasized that if other equally efficacious and more cost-effective methods of drug delivery are available, they should be used whenever possible. For example, a single-use disposable intravenous flow regulator (Sta-Set®, Controlled Flow Inc.) that allows accurate regulation of intravenous infusions without the additional cost of an EICD is available. This device and others may help to ensure safe intravenous drug and other therapy (e.g., nutritional therapy) while helping to improve the overall cost-effectiveness of therapy as hospital costs continue to escalate.

Performing venipuncture and intravenous injections. Intravenous drugs can be administered by three general methods, depending on their intended use and pharmacologic action: intravenous push, which can be rapid (less than 30 seconds) or slow (3–5 minutes); intermittent infusion (over 10 minutes to several hours); and continuous infusion (over 24 hours or longer). For example, diazepam *(Valium)* and meperidine *(Demerol)* are commercially available as injectable solutions for use (without further dilution) by slow intravenous push over 3–5 minutes. Dantrolene *(Dantrium®)*, flumazenil *(Anexate®, Romazicon®)*, and naloxone *(Narcan®)* can be injected by rapid intravenous push over 30 seconds. Other injectable drugs (e.g., amikacin *[Amikin®]*, gentamicin *[Garamycin®]*, miconazole *[Monistat IV®]*, penicillin G aqueous) may be diluted in small volumes of compatible intravenous solutions (less than 100 ml) in small-volume bags, bottles, and volume control devices (volumetric chambers [e.g., Buretrol®, Metriset®, Soluset®, Vol-U-Trol®]) and administered by intermittent intravenous infusion over a short period (30–60 minutes). Still other drugs (e.g., aminocaproic acid *[Amicar®]*, multivitamin infusion *[MVI Pediatric®]*) can be diluted in large volumes of intravenous solutions (500–1000 ml) and slowly administered as continuous infusions over long periods (24 hours or longer).

Factors such as recommended diluent and concentration, pH, incompatibilities with other drugs and solutions, stability, and infusion rate, as well as patient factors (e.g., cardiac and renal function) and the pharmacologic effect of the drug (i.e., desired action, protein binding, associated ADRs), must be considered when intravenous drug therapy is planned. *(See* Chapter 8 for additional guidance.)

Venipuncture. In many areas of clinical practice, venipuncture and the establishment of the intravenous site for drug and solution administration (Figure 1-13) is a responsibility shared by pediatric nurses and physicians.[62] Before intravenous therapy is initiated, chil-

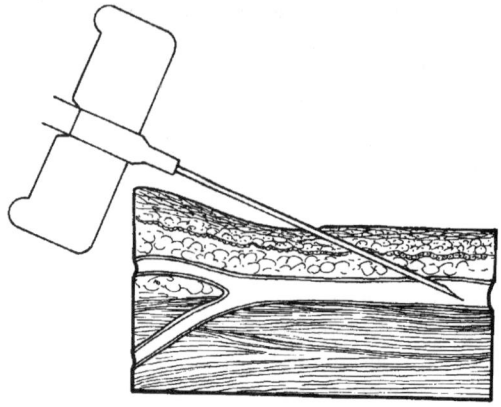

FIGURE 1-13
Intravenous Injection

dren, adolescents, and parents must understand the reasons for the required intravenous drug therapy, and they must know how and when it will be administered. They need to know how it will affect mobility and other activities. They also must learn to care for and monitor the venipuncture site. As is true with other forms of injectable drug therapy, pediatric patients must be carefully prepared for the venipuncture procedure according to their developmental level and previous experiences.

An important aspect of their preparation is to familiarize them with the equipment involved (Table 1-2). Although the preparation of patients and parents is often time consuming, ensuring appropriate preparation prevents undue fear and misunderstanding and promotes cooperation and willingness to participate.

The venipuncture site is selected in relation to the physicochemical properties of the

---

62. Pediatric clinicians are guided by state or provincial regulations, professional practice standards, and institutional policies in regard to their roles in the provision of intravenous drug therapy. There is significantly less margin for error with intravenous injection than with other methods of administration. Drugs injected intravenously act immediately and their effects are generally more difficult to reverse when an error is made. Hypersensitivity reactions and exaggerated or unusual pharmacologic effects can occur more readily. As a safeguard, intravenous drugs generally should be diluted in small volumes of appropriate intravenous solution and slowly infused over 30–60 minutes or longer, depending on the drug. The intravenous injection of drugs by rapid or slow intravenous push should be avoided whenever possible. Thus, if an undesired reaction occurs, the infusion can be discontinued before the entire dose is delivered. Additional training is required for the administration of some intravenous drugs, such as antineoplastics, because of the increased risk for severe tissue damage associated with the inadvertent extravasation of these drugs *(see* Chapter 12).

drug to be injected, the health of the veins and surrounding tissue, the frequency and duration of drug administration, and individual patient preference (i.e., nondominant hand). Prominent veins with adequate blood flow and elasticity should be selected when ever possible. Generally the smallest possible diameter (highest gauge number) needle and the largest possible vein should be used to optimize blood flow at the tip of the needle and dilution of the drug as it enters the vein, thus reducing vein irritation and avoiding the development of phlebitis. To avoid the need for frequent venipunctures, it is essential that venipunctures be made so that veins are not damaged and sites are maintained, particularly when patients have limited sites and require long-term therapy.[63]

Venipuncture is often difficult to perform on infants and toddlers because of the small size of their veins and because their veins are often covered by a thick layer of subcutaneous fat. The scalp veins are commonly used for intravenous drug therapy for infants because these veins are proportionately larger and more visible than the peripheral veins (Figure 1-14). When scalp veins are used, it is usually necessary to shave the hair. Shaving an infant's hair may distress some parents, who may worry that the hair will not grow back. Other parents may refuse to have their infant's hair shaved because of cultural, religious, or other reasons. As in many other areas, an individualized approach to the infant's care is required. Once the parents have consented, they may need to be reassured

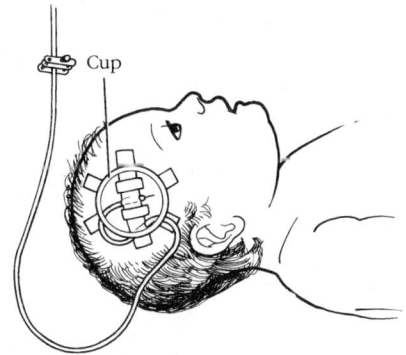

FIGURE 1-14
Scalp Vein Intravenous Injection Site

that care will be taken to shave only the hair necessary and that the hair will grow back.

Pediatric clinicians should explain that shaving the hair provides a clean area for the venipuncture, which helps to prevent infection. It also allows the venous access device to be securely taped in place and more easily removed (i.e., adhesive tape can be removed more easily and less painfully from a shaved site) when intravenous therapy is no longer required. Parents should know that, as long as the site is protected, use of the scalp site allows the infant more unrestricted movement of her/his hands and feet than when other venipuncture sites are used. It also facilitates infant care and cuddling. If necessary, sites on the dorsal aspect of the hands and feet also can be used for infants.

The basilic and cephalic veins on the dorsal aspect of the hands are commonly used for venipuncture for children and adolescents (Figure 1-15A).[64] Sites on the lower

---

63. Many of the procedures used in neonatal intensive care settings, including intravenous injections, damage the skin and cause needlemark scarring that may be embarrassing or cosmetically troublesome to children as they grow up. Attention to these concerns and the prevention of the disfigurement associated with intravenous injections should be encouraged.

64. If veins on the back of the hand are not readily visible, a warm compress can be applied to the site or it can be lowered below the rest of the body to enlarge the veins. Gentle tapping at the site with the fingertips and asking the patient to make a fist also are helpful. If these measures are ineffective, a rubber tourniquet can be applied above the venipuncture site between the elbow and wrist. Before the tourniquet is secured, a piece of gauze can be placed between it and the skin to prevent pinching. To enlarge scalp veins, a rubber band can be placed low on the infant's forehead above the eyebrows like a headband. To facilitate removal of the rubber band, a piece of tape should be folded over the rubber band to form a tab before it is applied. The tab can be used to pull the rubber band off or to remove it by pulling it way from the scalp so that it can be easily cut.

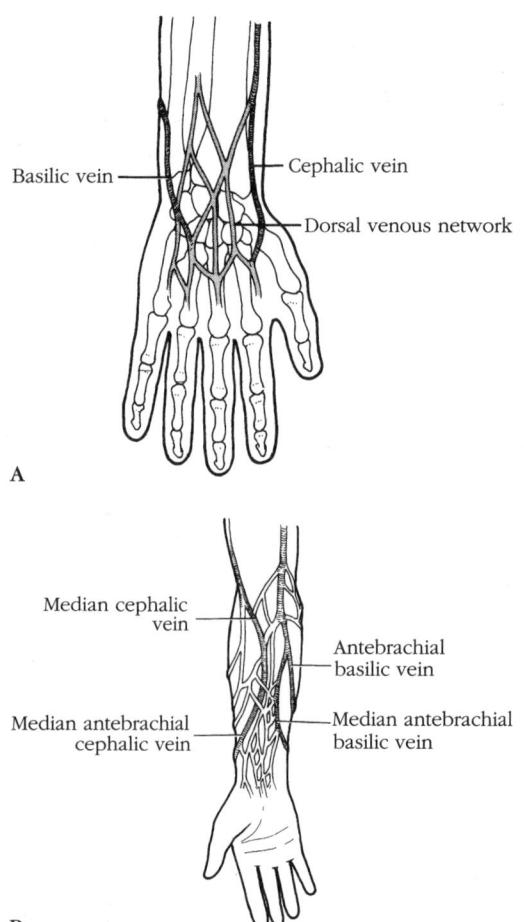

FIGURE 1-15
Intravenous Injection Sites for Children and Adolescents

(A) Basilic and cephalic veins on the dorsal aspect of the hand. (B) Superficial ventral basilic and cephalic veins of the forearm.

arm (Figure 1-15B) also may be used. When venipuncture sites are selected, distal sites should be selected first, and then more proximal sites should be used as needed. The needle or catheter should be inserted in a direction away from a movable joint to prevent inadvertent dislodgement and extravasation when the joint is moved. If required, a splint may be used to immobilize the joint. The antecubital fossa sites are usually reserved for rapid and slow intravenous injections (IV push injections) and blood withdrawal. These sites generally are not recommended for intermittent or continuous intravenous infusions because the elbow must be splinted to prevent dislodgement, resulting in stiffness and pain from immobility.

Infants and young children, as well as some older children and adolescents, may require gentle manual restraint of the extremity to stabilize the site. They should be positioned comfortably and the site prepared. It is often helpful to stabilize the extremity on a padded arm board. Any required equipment (e.g., intravenous solution, tubing, in-line filter, stand, controller or EICD) should be prepared prior to the venipuncture to prevent undue fear and so that it is ready for use once the venipuncture is completed. Parents should be encouraged to comfort and emotionally support their infant, child, or adolescent.

A 23–25-gauge wing-tipped or scalp vein needle (e.g., Butterfly) that is 0.5 inch (1.3 cm) in length or a 22–24-gauge over-the-needle catheter (e.g., Angiocath) that is 1 inch (2.5 cm) in length should be used for neonates and infants younger than 1 year. Scalp vein sites over the temporal areas and forehead are usually best for infants younger than 9 months. A 20–23-gauge wing-tipped needle or over-the-needle catheter that is 1–1.5 inches (2.5–3.75 cm) in length can be used for venipunctures on the dorsal aspect of the hand for older children and adolescents (Figure 1-15).

After the site has been cleansed with an appropriate antiseptic and a tourniquet (or rubber band) has been applied (if required), the skin should be pulled taut with the thumb of the nondominant hand below the venipuncture site, which helps to anchor the vein and prevent it from rolling. The needle should be inserted in the direction of blood flow to ensure that the injection or infusion is aimed in the same direction as the venous blood returning to the heart. Scalp vein blood generally flows from the top of the head down. To confirm the direction, a forefinger can be pressed gently on the vein at a site close to the infant's neck and the other forefinger gently pressed about 1 inch (2.5 cm) along the vein toward the head. The second forefinger should then be released and the vein should fill, indicating that the direction of flow is toward the occluding finger at the neck. When using scalp vein sites, the site may be stabilized by gently wrapping the infant with a blanket or "mummy" restraint and gently positioning and stabilizing the head manually on a firm surface (e.g., infant's crib mattress, examination table). When using veins in the hands or feet, it is often helpful to stabilize the extremity on a padded arm board.

It is particularly important to avoid arteries.[65] The needle should be inserted at a 20–30-degree angle to the skin with the bevel facing up. The skin should be entered just distal to the proposed site of vein entry (approximately 0.6–1.25 cm [¼–½ inch]). After the skin has been penetrated, the angle should be decreased to 15 degrees and the needle gently and slowly advanced into the vein (Figure 1-13). Blood should appear in the tubing. The needle of an over-the-needle catheter should be advanced a little farther and then removed, leaving the catheter in the vein.

Once the venipuncture is made, the tourniquet (if used) should be released, and the needle or catheter should be secured with tape or a transparent adhesive dressing so that the site can be observed easily. The needle or catheter should be flushed with normal saline solution before any drugs are administered to ensure patency of the site. If intravenous tubing is used, it should be secured with tape so it is free from kinks and does not pull on the needle or catheter. A padded arm board may be required to fully stabilize the site. When arm boards are used, the extremity should be kept in a natural anatomical position, and the fingers should be readily observable for monitoring circulation, voluntary movement, and sensation. All venous access devices should be labeled clearly with the dates and times inserted and the initials of the person who inserted the device. Needles and catheters that will remain in place can be flushed according to protocol and covered with a transparent dressing so that the site can be observed easily and monitored.[66]

Topical anesthesia. The fear and pain associated with venipunctures can be minimized with the application of a local topical anesthetic cream (i.e., *EMLA*® [eutectic mixture of local anesthetics]). This cream should be applied 1–2 hours before the venipuncture is performed. Successful local anesthesia of the intact skin layers at the venipuncture site has been reported for older infants (6–12 months), children, and adolescents. Although the use of *EMLA* is not feasible in all clinical situations (e.g., emergencies) because of the time required to achieve effective anesthesia, for selected pediatric patients it offers an effective means of reducing the pain perception and psychological trauma associated with venipunctures.

The major disadvantage associated with the use of *EMLA* is the required waiting period. But, given the benefits, this waiting time is generally acceptable.[67] *EMLA* cream should be applied only to intact skin (i.e., abraded or denuded skin areas should be avoided). Al-

---

65. The temporal arteries are the vessels most often inadvertently penetrated when scalp veins are used. Likewise, the brachial artery is close to the skin surface and adjacent to the cephalic vein. It can be inadvertently penetrated when sites above the wrist are used, including the antecubital fossa. If an artery is inadvertently punctured, the bright red blood will pulsate from the site. In contrast, blood from a vein is darker red and will not pulsate. If any artery is inadvertently punctured, firm pressure should be applied to the site for 10 minutes after the needle is withdrawn from the artery to stop bleeding and to prevent a hematoma from forming.

66. Some patients may require an arm-board splint to immobilize the site or soft restraints to prevent the needle from being removed. A plastic drug cup that has been cut in half lengthwise can be gently taped over the site to protect the needle from becoming dislodged. If necessary, roll gauze (e.g., Kling®) can be gently wrapped over the site, or stretchable netting (e.g., Tuberoll®) can be used for protection. Roll gauze must be unwrapped frequently to monitor for possible needle dislodgement and extravasation.

67. Patients and their parents can be taught to apply *EMLA* at home so that the site will be anesthetized upon their arrival at the clinic or office, where venipuncture can then be performed readily.

though generally well tolerated, its use is contraindicated for patients hypersensitive to amide-type local anesthetics (e.g., lidocaine [*Xylocaine®*]).[68]

A newer formulation (i.e., *EMLA Patch* [Canada]; *EMLA Disc* [United States]) consists of a single-dose, prepackaged occlusive dressing containing *EMLA* 5% emulsion (2.5% lidocaine and 2.5% prilocaine). The aluminum backing is removed and the patch is simply attached, as directed, to a clean, dry area of skin at the proposed venipuncture site. The patch should remain in place for a minimum of 1 hour. Then the patient is prepared, the patch is removed, the venipuncture site is cleansed, and the venipuncture is completed. Although the cream and patch formulations reportedly produce equivalent efficacy, the ease of applying the patch when compared to the cream appears to be a distinct advantage.

Slow and rapid intravenous injection (IV push). Some intravenous drugs are available commercially as ready-to-use products that require no further dilution. These intravenous drugs may be injected directly into the vein through a needle, catheter, IIC cap, or injection port in the tubing of a primary (fluid maintenance or replacement) intravenous infusion. The injection rate depends on the physicochemical nature of the drug and its pharmacologic action. For example, diazoxide *(Hyperstat®),* an antihypertensive, must be injected over 10–30 seconds because it is highly plasma protein bound; rapid administration overcomes the effect of protein binding so that a sufficient serum concentration and, thus, the desired effect are achieved. Other drugs, such as atropine, may be delivered over a minute to achieve an immediate effect. Other drugs generally should **not** be injected over less than 1 minute. The manufacturer's recommended rate of intravenous injection should be followed closely, as should individual patient response (*see also* Chapter 8). A red blood cell travels through the entire circulatory system in approximately 1 minute. If drugs are injected too rapidly, "speed shock" can occur, resulting in headache, tightness in the chest, shock, and cardiac arrest. Slow intravenous injection allows the drug to mix more thoroughly with the blood before delivery to the heart and brain, which can occur within 15 seconds.

Intravenous drugs can be injected into an injection port (sometimes called a Y-site) in the tubing of a compatible primary (fluid maintenance or replacement) continuous intravenous infusion. After the patency of the intravenous infusion site has been verified by visual inspection of blood return, the tubing above the injection port should be occluded with a roller clamp or hemostat. The injection port should be wiped with an antiseptic and allowed to dry. The needle should be inserted into the center of the port and the drug injected at the recommended rate. After the drug is injected, the roller clamp or hemostat is released, and the flow rate is readjusted. Pediatric patients should be observed closely for expected therapeutic benefit and any adverse reactions during injection and immediately afterward. The technique should be adapted accordingly when EICDs are being used.

Intermittent infusion. Intravenous additive sets, small-volume bags or bottles, and volume control devices (i.e., intermittent infusion control devices such as Burette®, Buretrol®, and Metriset®) are used for the intermittent infusion of intravenous drugs that require dilution before injection and infusion over 10 minutes to several hours. The intermittent infusion of selected drugs assures

---

68. Prilocaine, particularly when used concurrently with methemoglobin-inducing drugs (e.g., sulfonamides), may cause methemoglobinemia. Therefore, the use of *EMLA* formulations should also be avoided, or they should be used only with extreme caution, for neonates and infants, who may be at increased risk for methemoglobinemia because of immaturity of the methemoglobin reductase enzymatic pathway. For these same reasons, caution also is indicated when *EMLA* is used for pain associated with neonatal circumcision. Premature infants are particularly sensitive to methemoglobin-inducing drugs and tolerate methemoglobinemia less well.

maximal therapeutic benefit with minimal ADRs (e.g., toxicity, phlebitis at the infusion site). Intermittent infusion is used with IIC caps when pediatric patients require an intravenous drug several times a day and do not want the additional fluid or activity restrictions imposed by a continuous infusion. The use of various additive sets, small-volume bags and bottles, and small-volume control devices for intermittent infusion enables pediatric clinicians to avoid incompatibilities between drugs and between drugs and primary (maintenance or replacement) intravenous solutions.

When pediatric patients require continuous maintenance or replacement intravenous therapy, intermittent intravenous drug therapy can be infused into an injection port in the tubing of the primary infusion. Several additive sets and small-volume control devices for the intermittent infusion of intravenous drugs are available; equipment may differ among clinical facilities. As with other aspects of drug therapy, clinicians should be familiar both with the intravenous equipment used in their clinical practice settings and with all policies and procedures pertaining to it, thus ensuring patient safety and optimal drug therapy.

Generally, drugs can be infused simultaneously with compatible primary intravenous solutions. If the drug and primary intravenous solution are incompatible, they should be infused separately by occluding the tubing above the injection port with a roller clamp or hemostat or hanging the drug infusion container above the primary solution (gravity causes the solution in the higher position to infuse first). When drugs are administered through the same tubing as an incompatible primary intravenous solution, the tubing must be flushed with a compatible intravenous solution before the drug is infused. After drug infusion, the tubing must be flushed again before infusion of the incompatible primary intravenous solution is resumed.[69] The incompatibilities and associated diminished potency of antibiotics infused simultaneously with intravenous solutions containing multiple vitamins is a common example of the problems that result if intravenous tubing is not adequately flushed. The interaction between intravenous aminoglycosides and penicillins is another example of incompatibility that results in diminished therapeutic efficacy (see Chapters 6 and 8).

Continuous infusion. Various drugs can be added to large-volume primary (maintenance or replacement) intravenous solutions for slow continuous infusion (e.g., heparin).[70] Incompatibility with the solution and bioavailability are important considerations with this type of intravenous drug therapy. When drugs are added to primary solutions, an unexpected color change or cloudiness usually indicates an incompatibility. If more than one drug is added to a primary solution, the most concentrated drug should be added first and mixed thoroughly before other drugs are added. Drugs formulated with colored additives should be added last because they can mask precipitation and cloudiness. These same principles apply when drugs are prepared for intermittent infusion. Some drugs can be added directly to the primary solution, while other drugs can be added only after they have been reconstituted according to the manufacturer's recommendations (see also Chapter 8).[71]

---

69. For further discussion and examples of both compatible and incompatible intravenous drugs and solutions, see Chapter 8.

70. When heparin is added to a primary solution for continuous intravenous infusion, the primary container should be inverted six or more times to ensure that the heparin is mixed into the solution and does not pool. A slight discoloration does not affect potency.

71. A label specifying the drug added, its amount or concentration, the time and date it was added, and the initials of the person who added the drug must be attached to the primary solution container. A record of the infusion and any other pertinent observations must be documented appropriately. Because of the complexity of preparing such admixtures and the attendant risks for contamination and error, pharmacy departments at most hospitals are increasingly assuming primary responsibility for preparing intravenous admixtures.

Complications associated with intravenous injections and infusions. Although intravenous drug administration offers many advantages, some disadvantages include potentially serious complications such as overdosage and drug toxicity, air emboli and thrombus formation, extravasation, hypersensitivity reactions, infection, and phlebitis. Additional complications, such as fluid overload and drug toxicity, can arise with continuous intravenous infusions. These complications are associated with free-flow (uncontrolled infusion) accidents and can be particularly serious for neonates, small infants, and pediatric patients who have compromised body system function (e.g., cardiac, renal, hepatic). The activity restriction necessary for the maintenance of intravenous injection sites also is a concern, particularly for infants and young children, as well as for older children and adolescents if they are confused, mentally retarded, or have schizophrenia or other mental disorders. These pediatric patients may require constant supervision or the application of soft restraints to prevent the intravenous tubing from being pulled out and the venous access device displaced.

Careful attention must be paid to the guidelines for administering drugs intravenously; there is little room for error. When drugs are injected by rapid or slow intravenous injection (IV push), the drug is injected directly into the bloodstream and effects are virtually immediate. Emergency drugs, equipment, and personnel for the management of medical emergencies should be readily available. In addition, pediatric patients must be monitored carefully for untoward drug effects and the common complications associated with intravenous therapy.

Air embolism and thrombus. Air embolism (i.e., an air bubble in a vein, the right atrium or ventricle, or a capillary that may result in an infarct) is a concern for all clinicians who administer intravenous drug therapy. Although the amount of air required for fatal embolism has not been determined precisely, the inadvertent injection of air should be avoided whenever possible. The amount of air contained in intravenous tubing is approximately 10–15 ml. Fortunately, blood usually backs up into the tubing when a solution bag or volume control device has emptied and occludes the peripheral venous access device (e.g., needle or catheter) before air can enter the vein. However, thrombus formation may occur at the needle or catheter tip. Because of the risk of thrombus detachment and severe complications (e.g., pulmonary embolus), an occluded needle or catheter should not be irrigated with normal saline or heparin solution under any circumstances. Instead, the occluded needle or catheter should be removed, appropriately discarded and replaced with a new sterile needle or catheter at a new site.

Extravasation. One common local complication of intravenous drug therapy is extravasation, which occurs when the needle or catheter is improperly positioned outside of the vein and the drug or infusion solution is inadvertently injected or infused into the surrounding subcutaneous tissue. Tissue swelling around the venipuncture site may be observed, and the child or adolescent may complain of pain. In assessing swelling, the involved extremity should be compared with the opposite extremity. An early sign of extravasation is a slowed rate of infusion. However, this sign will be absent and intravenous solutions will continue to infuse if an EICD is being used.[72]

Fluid overload and drug toxicity. Infants, children, and adolescents who require drug

---

72. **Insertion of the needle or catheter near a movable joint should be avoided** to reduce the possibility of extravasation. An IIC cap should be used if the patient requires frequent intravenous therapy but does not require fluid maintenance or replacement therapy. Some drugs (e.g., vesicants) can be extremely irritating. For example, extreme care is required when antineoplastics and other drugs (e.g., highly alkaline drugs such as pentobarbital *[Nembutal®]* or secobarbital *[Seconal®]*) are injected. Extravasation of these drugs can result in pain and tissue necrosis. In addition, inadvertent intra-arterial injection has been associated with adverse effects ranging from transient pain along the course of the artery to gangrene of the limb, requiring amputation. To prevent extravasation, it is imperative that the patency of the needle or catheter be ensured before drugs are

therapy by continuous intravenous infusion (e.g., insulin) must be closely monitored, particularly because of the potential for fluid overload and drug toxicity. Although EICDs are increasingly used to control infusion rates, fluid overload and free-flow accidents continue to pose a serious problem for pediatric patients. For example, accidental uncontrolled free flow of an infusing drug (e.g., aminophylline, amphotericin B, dopamine, epinephrine, heparin, lidocaine, meperidine [Demerol], potassium chloride, sodium bicarbonate) after removal of administration sets from EICDs has resulted in serious injury and death. The use of devices that allow free flow should be avoided whenever continuous intravenous drug therapy is required. To promote patient safety, only trained personnel should be authorized to initiate, adjust, and remove intravenous equipment. All clinicians involved with intravenous drug therapy should receive adequate training regarding new equipment and procedures, and they should be retrained as needed, to maintain competency and avoid complications.

Hypersensitivity. Clinicians must be alert for hypersensitivity reactions when drugs are injected or infused intravenously. Monitoring is particularly important when drugs are injected by rapid or slow intravenous injection. Infants should be closely observed, and children and adolescents should be asked to report any unusual effects, including burning, chills, itching, local pain, or nausea. If these effects occur, the injection or infusion should be stopped immediately and appropriate intervention implemented. Emergency equipment and drugs (e.g., epinephrine) should be readily available in case of hypersensitivity reactions, particularly when a drug is used initially for a pediatric patient (see Chapter 5 for additional discussion). Test doses for drugs commonly associated with hypersensitivity reactions (e.g., penicillin) are recommended.

Infection. The intravenous administration of drugs poses a risk for infection because microorganisms can be introduced directly across the skin's protective barrier and into the systemic circulation. Pediatric clinicians should look for signs and symptoms of local (e.g., pain, redness, and swelling at the injection site) and systemic (e.g., fever) infection. Infection can result from contaminated drugs, equipment, or solutions; improper technique (e.g., lack of hand washing before preparing or administering injections); or poor injection or infusion site care. Approaches for minimizing infection among pediatric patients include stringent protocols for performing venipunctures and changing site dressings and infusion tubing. Collaboration among all involved with intravenous therapy is essential. Institutional venipuncture dressing procedures should be followed. In an increasing number of clinical facilities, pharmacists prepare intravenous admixtures in vertical laminar airflow hoods to maintain the sterility of intravenous products. Likewise, pharmaceutical manufacturers increasingly supply drugs in delivery systems ready for immediate intravenous use.

Phlebitis. Another common complication associated with intravenous drug therapy is phlebitis, which results from trauma to the vein caused by the needle, catheter, drug, or solution. Some drugs, such as cephalothin *(Keflin)* and potassium chloride for injection, are particularly irritating. When these drugs are used, the venipuncture site and surrounding skin at the site and over the vein should be observed closely for redness and increased warmth. A child's or adolescent's complaints of burning and pain along the vein should be heeded. If these signs and symptoms occur, the injection or infusion should be discontinued immediately and another site established. To prevent further damage to the vein, the affected site should not be used until it has healed adequately. Venipuncture sites should remain uncovered so they can be observed closely. Collodion dressings are recommended; they should be applied so that dress-

---

injected or infused. Pediatric clinicians are encouraged to develop treatment protocols for use in the event of extravasation associated with intravenous drug therapy and clinicians should be familiar with these protocols so they can be readily implemented (see Chapter 12).

ing changes will not result in the inadvertent displacement of the needle or catheter.

To monitor for phlebitis, the flash chamber or flash ball of the intravenous tubing can be gently compressed and the child or adolescent observed for pain or discomfort at the venipuncture site. This procedure dilates the vein at the entry site, which causes pain if the vein is inflamed. Pediatric patients receiving long-term intravenous therapy may require frequent site changes to avoid phlebitis and other complications (e.g., infection, scarring). Sites should be carefully cared for and alternated to allow healing between uses.

Preventing phlebitis can be difficult, particularly when irritating drugs are injected or infused and when long-term drug therapy is required. Frequent inspection of venipuncture sites and site changes at the earliest signs of tenderness, inflammation, or induration can reduce the incidence of phlebitis. Using small-volume bags or bottles or volume control devices to dilute irritating drugs and infusing them slowly whenever possible also can reduce the incidence of this complication. In addition, the use of in-line filters (0.22 or 0.45 µm) has been recommended. Their effectiveness has been questioned, however, particularly when drugs are infused in small volumes of intravenous solution or when they are infused slowly. Although these filters do not appear to affect accurate drug delivery, further pediatric research is required before definitive recommendations can be made.

Other recommendations for the prevention of phlebitis are changing intravenous tubing every 24 hours and changing intermittent infusion control devices (e.g., Buretrol devices) at least every 72 hours.[73] It also is recommended that the smallest diameter needle or catheter possible be used with the largest vein possible in order to reduce the risk for mechanical phlebitis and to optimize blood flow at the needle tip to dilute the drug, which decreases the risk for chemical phlebitis.

Activity restriction. When intravenous drug therapy is required, venipuncture sites should be selected to allow patients maximal activity. Parents should not be restricted from holding their infant or young child solely because of intravenous therapy. Pediatric clinicians should demonstrate how the infant or child who has a venous access device should be held and should show parents how to protect the device. Parents also need to manage intravenous stands and EICDs for out-of-bed activities. Children and adolescents, and their parents, should know how to protect the venipuncture site and how to monitor the intravenous flow rate, and they should report signs and symptoms of potential complications, particularly extravasation and phlebitis.

Even young children can learn to be careful with their venipuncture site and intravenous equipment. After they do learn, they generally do not require activity restrictions (i.e., bed rest) or the use of soft restraints. To prevent the tubing from being inadvertently pulled and the needle or catheter dislodged from its site, young infants and toddlers may require soft restraints when they are sleeping or are unattended.[74] Plastic drug cups that have been cut in half and commercially available protective devices can be used to protect venipuncture sites. Care must be taken to ensure that undo pressure is not applied to the vein when the cup or device is secured in place. All pediatric patients should be allowed as much normal activity as possible. They also should be taught, according to their developmental level, to promptly report any problems to their pediatric clinician or parent. Having such information can help

---

73. Phlebitis rates associated with leaving peripheral intravenous tubing in place for 72 versus 96 hours were not found to be significantly different among adult subjects; however, additional research is required. Although potential cost savings are a factor to be considered, leaving intravenous tubing in place for longer than 24 hours generally is not recommended for pediatric patients.

74. Although relatively uncommon, deaths by strangulation with intravenous tubing of unsupervised infants and toddlers while hospitalized have been reported. These needless tragedies could be prevented with adequate supervision, the appropriate use of soft restraints, and attention to the selection of intravenous equipment, including length of tubing and placement of infusion devices.

prevent or minimize serious complications associated with intravenous drug therapy. Patients' knowing that they have an important responsibility promotes their participation.

Intraosseous Infusions and Injections

The intraosseous route can be used to infuse intravenous fluids, blood, and drugs directly into the bone marrow cavity in emergency situations when peripheral and central venous access are not feasible because of circulatory collapse or severe dehydration.[75] It also is indicated when the endotracheal instillation of a drug is contraindicated (the endotracheal route can be used only for a select group of drugs) and when intravenous fluid and blood replacement is required (the endotracheal route cannot be used for intravenous fluid or blood replacement). Intraosseous infusion can be a life-saving alternative to the intravenous route for infants and young children who are critically ill or have serious burns or other injuries.

Intraosseous infusion, discovered by chance as a means for fluid and drug therapy just prior to World War II, was ignored for many years. More recently, it has become increasingly recognized as an important adjunct to the emergency care of neonates, infants, children, and adolescents. Intraosseous infusions currently are used by emergency nurses, physicians, and paramedics.

Generally, the intraosseous route is indicated for pediatric patients in extremis when two attempts at peripheral venous access have been unsuccessful. Contraindications to the intraosseous infusion of drugs include bone disorders (e.g., osteogenesis imperfecta, osteopetrosis) and the presence of infected burns or cellulitis at the injection site. Because of the increased risk for extravasation of the drug or solution into the subcutaneous tissues at the infusion site, the route also is contraindicated for patients who have recently fractured bones.

Intraosseous infusion involves the insertion of a rigid, large-bore needle through the bone cortex into the medullary cavity or spongy bone in an area with few or no overlying blood vessels, nerves, or major muscle groups (Figure 1-16).[76] Drugs and solutions are infused and rapidly absorbed by the extensive network of venous sinusoids in the bone and diffuse into the systemic circulation. Common intravenous solutions (e.g., dextrose 5% in water for injection; Ringer's injection, lactated; 4.5% normal saline for injection), blood products (e.g., packed red blood cells, plasma, whole blood), and drugs (e.g., adenosine, antibiotics, anticonvulsants, atropine, catecholamines, epinephrine, heparin, lidocaine, mannitol, methylene blue, morphine, phenytoin, sodium bicarbonate) can be administered by this route.

Potential administration sites include the sternum, iliac crest, femur, distal tibia, and proximal tibia. However, because it is flat, easily accessible, and avoids the epiphyseal growth plate, the anteromedial surface to the proximal tibia one to two finger-breadths below the tubercle is the site of choice. Access can be initiated without disrupting airway management during cardiopulmonary resuscitation. Although it is slightly more difficult to penetrate, the midanterior distal third of the femur offers an alternative site. However, the needle can slip off the bone (which is more rounded in this portion of the femur) and into the surrounding dense muscular and connective tissue.

Procedure. Although recommended techniques vary, the site is always prepared with an antiseptic. If the infant or child is conscious, a local anesthetic is required to prevent undue discomfort. The local anesthetic should be

---

75. For example, with children and adolescents, when atropine cannot be administered intravenously for advanced cardiac life support during cardiopulmonary resuscitation, it can be administered by endotracheal tube or by intraosseous infusion.

76. Several intraosseous administration devices have been used, including the Bone Injection Gun® and the Cook and Jamshidi intraosseous needles. Although some preliminary studies have examined the cost-effectiveness and ease of use of these devices, more research is needed. Until results are available, the selection and use of these devices depends on clinician familiarity and preference.

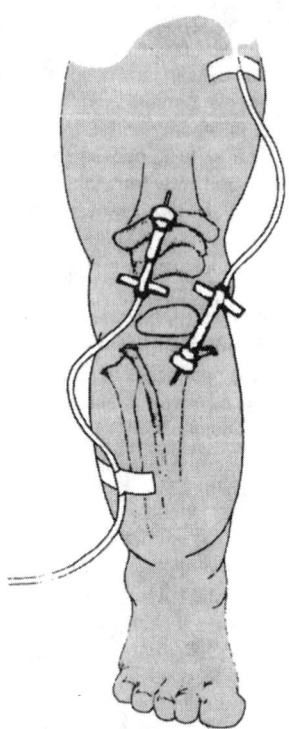

FIGURE 1-16
Intraosseous Infusion or Injection Sites

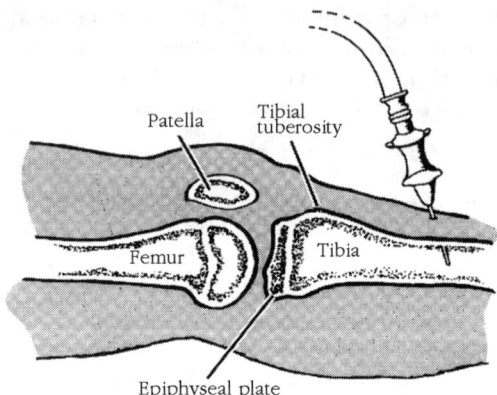

FIGURE 1-17
Intraosseous Infusion or Injection Needle Placement

infiltrated into the tissues from the skin surface down to the periosteum. The skin should be penetrated using strict aseptic technique and the needle should be firmly seated into the bone. Although needle preference varies, usually any rigid, large-bore needle with an inner stylet (a thin metal probe used to keep bone plugs from forming during insertion, which may occlude the needle), such as a disposable bone marrow aspiration needle, can be used. Although it is less rigid, a lumbar puncture needle is recommended for infants.

The needle is inserted at a 10–30-degree angle to the skin surface and directed toward the foot and away from the epiphyseal plate (Figure 1-17). With firm, downward pressure, a screwing or to-and-fro motion is used. A "pop" or sudden decrease in resistance signifies entrance into the medullary cavity. The inner stylet is removed and a syringe of normal saline is attached to the needle. Correct needle placement is confirmed if the syringe stands upright without support or if bone marrow contents are aspirated when the syringe plunger is pulled back. Alternatively, normal saline can be injected; the needle is positioned correctly if no evidence of extravasation is observed.[77] A free-flowing infusion without evidence of subcutaneous extravasation also verifies correct needle placement.

A conventional intravenous administration set can then be connected to the needle and used for subsequent therapy. The needle should be flushed with a heparin solution. Once anchored firmly into the bony cortex, the needle requires little intervention to secure it. The site should be observed for signs of extravasation of fluid into the subcutaneous tissues. Management of the site during infusion includes the application of a sterile dressing and the support or immobilization of the extremity. After venous access has been established, the intraosseous infusion can be discontinued and the site covered with a sterile dressing.

Complications. Although intraosseous infusion is an important adjunct to pediatric drug therapy in emergency situations, the technique has been associated with tibial fractures in young infants and other infrequent complications. These complications usually are associated with improper needle placement and extravasation of the drug or solution into the

---

77. Other methods have been suggested for confirming intraosseous needle placement, including the use of circumferential pressure at the intraosseous infusion site and the use of portable imaging devices.

subcutaneous tissues or leakage of body fluids from multiple puncture sites. Abscesses, local cellulitis, and pressure necrosis at the site of penetration also occur infrequently. However, severe tissue necrosis and resultant death after intraosseous placement have been reported. The complication causing the most concern is osteomyelitis, which appears to be related to long-term infusion of solutions or drugs into the bone marrow cavity. To prevent this complication, intraosseous infusions should be used for the briefest time possible (usually only an hour or two until intravenous access is established). There is no evidence of damage to the bone, bone marrow, or epiphyseal growth plate from the use of the intraosseous route. Studies of subsequent leg length after 1 year have failed to detect a difference in mean tibial length between the leg that received intraosseous infusion and the one that did not. Fat and bone emboli are a theoretical risk but have not been reported.

Training physicians, nurses, and paramedics to implement and manage intraosseous intravenous infusions and injections is increasingly common. In this regard, clear delineation of multidisciplinary responsibilities, including decisions for initiating intraosseous therapy and needle placement, are required. Attention to the pharmacokinetics of drugs administered by this route and other research also is required. The proper use of this administration route and technique can mean the difference between life and death for a severely ill infant or young child.

Summary

The responsibilities of clinicians are expanding as the complexity of providing drug therapy to infants, children, and adolescents increases. They must understand the use and effects of drugs in the pediatric patient and develop unique knowledge and skills in selecting and administering appropriate dosage forms. Whenever possible, clinicians also must promote the active participation of pediatric patients and their parents in required drug therapy. Recommended guidelines for the administration of oral, rectal, vaginal, ophthalmic, otic, intranasal, inhalation, topical, and injectable dosage forms have been provided, along with consideration of the general growth and development of infants, children, and adolescents. Pediatric clinicians must have a thorough knowledge and understanding of dosage forms available for pediatric use and correct methods of administration so they can provide appropriate and individualized drug therapy for their patients and work toward obtaining suitable pediatric drug formulations for both currently marketed and new drugs.

In in-patient settings, children, adolescents, and parents should be involved as much as possible in the various aspects of drug administration in order to improve their understanding and increase their ability to provide continued therapy at home. They should become active healthcare participants, which increases the efficacy of drug therapy and decreases errors in drug administration, ADRs, and overdosages or accidental pediatric poisonings in both hospital and home settings. Individual instruction of children and adolescents, as well as their parents, with attention to each pediatric patient's developmental abilities, is essential in this regard. With the information presented in this and subsequent chapters, clinicians will be better prepared to provide optimal drug therapy for their pediatric patients while promoting their developmental abilities in regard to their drug therapy.

References[78]

Abe, K. K., Blum, G. T., & Yamamoto, L. G. (2000). Intraosseous is faster and easier than umbilical

---

78. The approaches and techniques for administering drugs to infants, children, and adolescents, and related information contained in this chapter, have been derived from several sources, including the previous edition of *Problems in Pediatric Drug Therapy*, current product monographs, the listed references, and clinical experience. References listed are meant to provide the reader with some benchmarks only and do not constitute a comprehensive reference list. For additional references to original or earlier citations, please refer to the previous editions of this text.

venous catheterization in newborn emergency vascular access models. *American Journal of Emergency Medicine, 18,* 126–129.

Asai, T., Matsumoto, S., Matsumoto, H., et al. (1999). Prevention of needle-stick injury. Efficacy of a safeguarded intravenous cannula. *Anaesthesia, 54,* 258–261.

Barry, P. W., & O'Callaghan, C. (1998). Drug output from nebulizers is dependent on the method of measurement. *European Respiratory Journal, 12,* 463–466.

Burgt, J. A., Busse, W. W., Martin, R. J., et al. (2000). Efficacy and safety overview of a new inhaled corticosteroid, QVAR (hydrofluoroalkane-beclomethasone extrafine inhalation aerosol), in asthma. *Journal of Allergy and Clinical Immunology, 106,* 1209–1226.

Calkins, M. D., Fitzgerald, G., Bentley, T. B., et al. (2000). Intraosseous infusion devices: A comparison for potential use in special operations. *Journal of Trauma, 48,* 1068–1074.

Couper, R. T. (2000). Methaemoglobinaemia secondary to topical lignocaine/prilocaine in a circumcised neonate. *Journal of Paediatrics and Child Health, 36,* 406–407.

De Benedictis, F. M., Boner, A., Cavagni, G., et al. (2000). Treating asthma in children with beclomethasone dipropionate: Pulvinal versus Diskhaler. *Journal of Aerosol Medicine, 13*(1), 35–41.

Demedts, M., Cohen, R., & Hawkinson, R. (1999). Switch to non-CFC inhaled corticosteroids: A comparative efficacy study of HFA-BDP and CFC-BDP metered-dose inhalers. *International Journal of Clinical Practice, 53,* 331–338.

Dewar, A. L., Stewart, A., Cogswell, J. J., et al. (1999). A randomised controlled trial to assess the relative benefits of large volume spacers and nebulisers to treat acute asthma in hospital. *Archives of Disease in Childhood, 80,* 421–423.

Ellemunter, H., Simma, B., Trawoger, R., et al. (1999). Intraosseous lines in preterm and full term neonates. *Archives of Disease in Childhood Fetal and Neonatal Edition, 80,* F74–F75.

Erikson, E. H. (1950). *Childhood and society.* New York: Norton.

Erikson, E. H. (1963). *Childhood and society,* 2nd ed. New York: Norton.

Evans, R. J., Jewkes, F., Owen, G., et al. (1995). Intraosseous infusion–A technique available for intravascular administration of drugs and fluids in the child with burns. *Burns, 21,* 552–553.

Everard, M. L. (1996). Aerosol delivery in infants and young children. *Journal of Aerosol Medicine, 9,* 71–77.

Figgitt, D. P., & Plosker, G. L. (2000). Saquinavir soft-gel capsule: An updated review of its use in the management of HIV infection. *Drugs, 60*(2), 481–516.

Fiser, R. T., Walker, W. M., Seibert, J. J., et al. (1997). Tibial length following intraosseous infusion: A prospective, radiographic analysis. *Pediatric Emergency Care, 13,* 186–188.

Foex, B. A. (2000). Discovery of the intraosseous route for fluid administration. *Journal of Accident and Emergency Medicine, 17,* 136–137.

Fok, T. F., Monkman, S., Dolovich, M., et al. (1996). Efficiency of aerosol medication delivery from a metered dose inhaler versus jet nebulizer in infants with bronchopulmonary dysplasia. *Pediatric Pulmonology, 21,* 301–309.

Fox, P. E., & Rutter, N. (1998). The childhood scars of newborn intensive care. *Early Human Development, 51*(2), 171–177.

Freud, S. (1964a). *The standard edition of the complete psychological works of Sigmund Freud.* Vol. 19. J. Strachey (translator and editor) in collaboration with Anna Freud. London: Hogarth.

Freud, S. (1964b). *The standard edition of the complete psychological works of Sigmund Freud.* Vol. 20. J. Strachey (translator and editor) in collaboration with Anna Freud. London: Hogarth.

Frey, B., & Kehrer, B. (1999). Toxic methaemoglobin concentrations in premature infants after application of a prilocaine-containing cream and peridural prilocaine. *European Journal of Pediatrics, 158,* 785–788.

Friedman, F. D. (1996). Intraosseous adenosine for the termination of supraventricular tachycardia in an infant. *Annals of Emergency Medicine, 28,* 356–358.

Garcia, C. T., & Cohen, D. M. (1996). Intraosseous needle: Use of the miniature C-arm imaging device to confirm placement. *Pediatric Emergency Care, 12,* 94–97.

Goldberg, D., Johnston, J., Cameron, S., et al. (2000). Risk of HIV transmission from patients to surgeons in the era of post-exposure prophylaxis. *Journal of Hospital Infection, 44,* 99–105.

Halm, B., & Yamamoto, L. G. (1998). Comparing ease of intraosseous needle placement: Jamshidi versus Cook. *American Journal of Emergency Medicine, 16,* 420–421.

Halperin, S. A., McGrath, P., Smith, B., et al. (2000). Lidocaine-prilocaine patch decreases the pain associated with the subcutaneous administration of measles-mumps-rubella vaccine but does not adversely affect the antibody response. *The Journal of Pediatrics, 136,* 789–794.

Hannemann, L. A. (1999). What is new in asthma: New dry powder inhalers. *Journal of Pediatric Health Care, 13,* 159–165.

Herman, M. I., Chyka, P. A., Butler, A. Y., et al. (1999). *Annals of Emergency Medicine, 33,* 111–113.

Huchon, G., Hofbauer, P., Cannizzaro, B., et al. (2000). Comparison of the safety of drug delivery via HFA- and CFC-metered dose inhalers in CAO. *European Respiratory Journal, 15,* 663–669.

Hurren, J. S., & Dunn, K. W. (1995). Intraosseous

infusion for burns resuscitation. *Burns, 21,* 285–287.

Kelly, A. F., & Hewson, P. H. (2000). Factors associated with recurrent hospitalization in chronically ill children and adolescents. *Journal of Paediatric and Child Health, 36,* 13–18.

Kercsmar, C. M. (2000). Aerosol treatment of acute asthma: And the winner is ... *The Journal of Pediatrics, 136,* 428–431.

Koh, J. L., Fanurik, D., Stoner, P. D., et al. (1999). Efficacy of parental application of eutectic mixture of local anesthetics for intravenous insertion. *Pediatrics, 103,* 379.

Kunkel, G., Magnussen, H., Bergmann, K., et al. (2000). Respimat (a new soft mist inhaler) delivering fenoterol plus ipratropium bromide provides equivalent bronchodilation at half the cumulative dose compared with a conventional metered dose inhaler in asthmatic patients. *Respiration, 67,* 306–314.

Lai, K. K. (1998). Safety of prolonging peripheral cannula and i.v. tubing use from 72 to 96 hours. *American Journal of Infection Control, 26*(1), 66–70.

Leach, C. (1998). Targeting inhaled steroids. *International Journal of Clinical Practice, 96*(Suppl), 23–27.

Leach, C. (1999). Effect of formulation parameters on hydrofluoroalkane-beclomethasone dipropionate drug deposition in humans. *Journal of Allergy and Clinical Immunology, 104,* S250–S252.

Leonard, H. L. (2000). Clinical consult. *Child and Adolescent Psychopharmacology, 2,* 7.

Leversha, A. M., Campanella, S. G., Aickin, R. P., et al. (2000). Costs and effectiveness of spacer versus nebulizer in young children with moderate and severe acute asthma. *The Journal of Pediatrics, 136,* 497–502.

Lidocaine + prilocaine before 3 months of age: New indication. Correct use is crucial. *Prescrire International, 9,* 77–79.

Lindh, V., Wiklund, U., & Hakansson, S. (2000). Assessment of the effect of EMLA during venipuncture in the newborn by analysis of heart rate variability. *Pain, 86,* 247–254.

Mandelberg, A., Tsehori, S., Houri, S., et al. (2000). Is nebulized aerosol treatment necessary in the pediatric emergency department? *Chest, 117,* 1309–1313.

Nahata, M. C. (1999). Lack of pediatric drug formulations. *Pediatrics, 104*(3, Part 2), 607–609.

Nakanishi, A. K., Lamb, B. M., Foster, C., et al. (1997). Ultrasonic nebulization of albuterol is no more effective than jet nebulization for the treatment of acute asthma in children. *Chest, 111,* 1505–1508.

Newman, S. P. (1999). Use of gamma scintigraphy to evaluate the performance of new inhalers. *Journal of Aerosol Medicine, 12*(Suppl 1), S25–S31.

Nikander, K., Agertoft, L., & Pedersen, S. (2000). Breath-synchronized nebulization diminishes the impact of patient-device interfaces (face mask or mouthpiece) on the inhaled mass of nebulized budesonide. *Journal of Asthma, 37*(5), 451–459.

Nikander, K., Turpeinen, M., & Wollmer, P. (1999). The conventional ultrasonic nebulizer proved inefficient in nebulizing a suspension. *Journal of Aerosol Medicine, 12*(2), 47–53.

O'Dell, C., Maloney-Lutz, K., Shinnar, S., et al. (1995). Protocol for ACTH administration in refractory childhood seizures: Educational strategies. *Journal of Neuroscience Nursing, 27,* 363–369.

Pagliaro, A. M. (1995). Administering drugs to infants, children, and adolescents. In L. A. Pagliaro & A. M. Pagliaro, Eds., *Problems in pediatric drug therapy,* 3rd ed., pp. 3–101. Bethesda, MD: Drug Intelligence Publications.

Pagliaro, L. A., & Pagliaro, A. M. (1998). Administration of psychotropics. In L. A. Pagliaro & A. M. Pagliaro, *The pharmacologic basis of psychotherapeutics: An introduction for psychologists,* pp. 99–149. Philadelphia: Brunner/Mazel.

Pagliaro, L. A., & Pagliaro, A. M. (1999). *PNDR-Psychologists' neuropsychotropic drug reference.* Philadelphia: Brunner/Mazel.

Pagliaro, L. A., & Pagliaro, A. M. (1999). *PPDR-Psychologists' psychotropic drug reference.* Philadelphia: Brunner/Mazel.

Pavia, D., & Moonen, D. (1999). *Journal of Aerosol Medicine, 12*(Suppl 1), S33–S39.

Peden, D. B., Berger, W. E., Noonan, M. J., et al. (1998). Inhaled fluticasone propionate delivered by means of two different multidose powder inhalers is effective and safe in a large pediatric population with persistent asthma. *Journal of Allergy and Clinical Immunology, 102*(1), 32–38.

Piaget, J. (1950). *The psychology of intelligence.* London: Routledge & Kegan Paul.

Piaget, J. (1963). *The origins of intelligence in children,* 2nd ed. New York: Norton.

Piaget, J., & Inhelder, B. (1969). *The psychology of the child.* New York: Basic Books.

Ploin, D., Chapuis, F. R., Stamm, D., et al. (2000). High-dose albuterol by metered-dose inhaler plus a spacer device versus nebulization in preschool children with recurrent wheezing: A double-blind randomized equivalence trial. *Pediatrics, 106*(2, Part 1), 311–317.

Popinska, K., Kierkus, J., Lyszkowska, M., et al. (1999). Aluminum contamination of parenteral nutrition additives, amino acid solutions, and lipid emulsions. *Nutrition, 15,* 683–686.

Powell, C. V., & Everard, M. L. (1998). Treatment of childhood asthma. Options and rationale for inhaled therapy. *Drugs, 55,* 237–252.

Ranze, O., Ranze, P., Magnani, H. N., et al. (1999). Heparin-induced thrombocytopenia in paediatric patients—A review of the literature and a new case treated with danaparoid sodium. *European Journal of Pediatrics, 158*(Suppl 3), S130–S133.

Remple, G., & Coates, J. (1999). Special considerations for medication use in children with developmental disabilities. *Physical Medicine Rehabilitation Clinics of North America, 10,* 493–509.

Roberge, R. J., Krenzelok, E. P., & Mrvos, R. (2000). Transdermal drug delivery system exposure outcomes. *Journal of Emergency Medicine, 18,* 147–151.

Rosenfeld, M., Emerson, J., Astley, S., et al. (1998). Home nebulizer use among patients with cystic fibrosis. *The Journal of Pediatrics, 132,* 125–131.

Russo, P. L., Harrington, G. A., & Spelman, D. W. (1999). Needleless intravenous systems: A review. *American Journal of Infection Control, 27*(5), 431–434.

Shapiro, G., Mendelson, L., Kraemer, M. J., et al. (1998). Efficacy and safety of budesonide inhalation suspension (Pulmicort Respules) in young children with inhaled steroid-dependent, persistent asthma. *Journal of Allergy and Clinical Immunology, 102*(5), 789–796.

Shaver, K. (2001). Needle length and intramuscular vaccines. *Prescriber's Newsletter* [On-line]. Available: www.prescribersletter.com.

Simmons, C. M., Johnson, N. E., Perkin, R. M., et al. (1994). Intraosseous extravasation complication reports. *Annals of Emergency Medicine, 23,* 363–366.

Stein, S. W. (1999). Size distribution measurements of metered dose inhalers using Andersen Mark II cascade impactors. *International Journal of Pharmacy, 186,* 43–52.

Strausbaugh, S. D., Manley, L. K., Hickey, R. W., et al. (1995). Circumferential pressure as a rapid method to assess intraosseous needle placement. *Pediatric Emergency Care, 11,* 274–276.

Summary of drug market withdrawals, significant drug recalls, and changes in drug safety profiles in the United States: January 2000 to August 2000. (2000). Amprenavir *(Agenerase). DrugLink, 4*(10), 75.

Taddio, A., Pollock, N., Gilbert-MacLeod, C., et al. (2000). Combined analgesia and local anesthesia to minimize pain during circumcision. *Archives of Pediatrics and Adolescent Medicine, 154,* 620–623.

Turpeinen, M., Nikander, K., Malmberg, L. P., et al. (1999). Metered dose inhaler add-on devices: Is the inhaled mass of drug dependent on the size of the infant? *Journal of Aerosol Medicine, 12,* 171–176.

Update. Metformin HCl. *DrugLink, 4*(12), 1.

Walter-Sack, I., & Haefeli, W. E. (2000). Consideration of drug absorption in customizing drug therapy [article in German]. *Therapeutische Umschau. Revue therapeutique [sic], 57*(9), 557–562.

Wiebe, A. (2001). Couple seek answers: Parents of IV-strangled tot take Capital Health to court. *The Edmonton Sun,* February 13, p. News 3.

Wildhaber, J. H., Janssens, H. M., Pierart, F., et al. (2000). High-percentage lung delivery in children from detergent-treated spacers. *Pediatric Pulmonology, 29*(5), 389–393.

Zuckerman, J. N. (2000). The importance of injecting vaccines into muscle. *British Medical Journal, 321,* 1237–1238.

2

Drugs as Human Teratogens and Fetotoxins

Louis A. Pagliaro and Ann Marie Pagliaro

The word teratogenesis is derived from the Greek words "teratos" (monster) and "genesis" (generation, birth). It is generally used to denote the development of abnormal structures (i.e., birth defects, congenital anomalies, congenital malformations) in the embryo or fetus that result in prenatal death or a severely deformed neonate. A teratogen is broadly defined as any factor that causes teratogenesis. This chapter focuses on drugs as human teratogens.

Fetotoxins are drugs that, when used by women during pregnancy, are associated with fetal toxicities generally related to the expected pharmacologic actions of the particular drug. Fetal toxicity is defined as any adverse drug reaction (ADR) that may be displayed by the fetus/neonate as a consequence of maternal drug use, particularly during the last trimester of pregnancy or near term. For example, maternal nonsteroidal anti-inflammatory drug (NSAID) use near term may result in the premature closure of the ductus arteriosus in the exposed fetus; this defect is a result of the associated pharmacologic action of NSAIDs (i.e., suppression of prostaglandin synthesis). Another common example of fetotoxicity is the neonatal opiate analgesic-withdrawal syndrome. This syndrome occurs among neonates born to women who received long-term high-dose opiates, or to women who personally used opiates regularly (e.g., heroin addicts) during the last trimester.

This chapter focuses on published reports of human data that describe teratogenesis or fetotoxicity. Published reports of animal data have been generally excluded because of the physiologic and genetic differences between laboratory animals and humans. These differences severely confound findings of teratogenic susceptibility; also, equating dosage, stage of pregnancy, environmental conditions, age, and health status from experimental laboratory animals to humans is difficult, if not impossible. A classic example of the limitations associated with extrapolating animal data to humans is the thalidomide tragedy. Thalidomide, a sedative-hypnotic, was tested in several pregnant rodent species and no teratogenic effects were noted among offspring. When used by women during the first trimester, however, devastating teratogenic effects (e.g., phocomelia) were produced among fetuses/neonates (see Thalidomide monograph).

It has been estimated that a teratogenic effect can be found in 2%–3% of all neonates and that 20% of infant and early childhood deaths occurring during the first 5 years of life are related, at least in part, to teratogenic effects. Teratogenesis has been associated with many factors. These factors, and the rate of their occurrence (percentage), include unknown factor(s), 65%–70%; genetic factors, 20%; chromosomal aberrations, 5%–10%; and maternal/fetal environmental factors, 5%–10%. The factors comprising the last category can be further broken down into drugs, 2%–5%; infections, 2%–3% (e.g., cytomegalovirus infection; rubella [German measles]); disease, 1%–2% (e.g., epilepsy); and radiation, less than 1%. Although drugs account for less than 5% of all observed teratogenic effects, their associated effects can be severe and are largely preventable.

Maternal Pharmacotherapy and Other Drug Use during Pregnancy

It is estimated that pregnant women use, on average, 10 prescription and nonprescription drugs (range of 3–30 different drugs) during their pregnancies. The types of drugs most frequently used include antibiotics, antiemetics, CNS depressants (e.g., analgesics, sedative-hypnotics), diuretics, and vitamins and minerals, including iron supplements.

Pregnant women also use aspirin and other nonprescription drugs that may be associated with fetotoxic effects if used during the last trimester. These effects are generally related to the expected mechanisms of action of the drugs (e.g., bleeding tendency if aspirin is used during the last trimester). Thus, since 1983, the U. S. Food and Drug Administration (FDA) has required that all nonprescription drugs intended for systemic absorption be labeled with the following warning:[1]

As with any drug, if you are pregnant or nursing a baby, seek the advice of a health professional before using this product.

In addition, 10%–25% of women smoke one or more packages of cigarettes per day during pregnancy; 30% come in contact with pesticides or toxic chemicals that may be teratogenic; and 10%–45% consume more than two alcoholic drinks per day. Alcohol also is found in many cough and cold formulations. For example, *Vicks Formula 44D®* cough and decongestant liquid, *Vicks NyQuil Liquid®* nighttime cold/flu medicine, and *Cheracol Plus®* liquid each contain 10% alcohol.

Generally, drugs can be placed in three categories in relation to the safety of their use during pregnancy:

Category 1 = Dangerous for fetus
Category 2 = Relatively safe for fetus
Category 3 = Unknown

A detailed discussion of the available published evidence supporting the classification of a drug as a category 1 drug, dangerous for fetus, is presented in the monographs.

Category 2 drugs, those that are relatively safe for the fetus, are:

Analgesics: Acetaminophen
Antiasthmatics: Cromolyn, theophylline
Antibiotics: Cephalosporins, erythromycin, penicillins
Anticoagulants: Heparin
Antidepressants: Fluoxetine
Antidiabetics: Insulin
Antiemetics: Prochlorperazine
Antihypertensives: Hydrochlorothiazide
Antituberculars: Ethambutol, isoniazid
Cardiac glycosides: Digoxin
Sedative-hypnotics: Chloral hydrate
Vitamins and minerals: All

Category 3, unknown, would include about 80% of the drugs listed in the *Compendium of Pharmaceuticals and Specialties* (CPS) or the *Physicians' Desk Reference* (PDR). In these commonly used reference texts, either no statement is made regarding the use of category 3 drugs during pregnancy or one of the following general statements is found: "Safe use in pregnancy has *not* been established" or "There are no adequate and well controlled studies of (drug) use in pregnant women." Among the reasons that more information is not readily available are:

---

1. A majority of women reportedly do not know that they are pregnant until after the fourth week of pregnancy. Thus, this warning should be extended to all women of childbearing age, particularly if they are intending to become pregnant.

1. Human teratogenic experiments cannot be performed ethically.
2. Animal experiments designed to determine human teratogenic potential are not valid and reliable.
3. A drug that is nontoxic to the pregnant woman may be extremely toxic to the developing embryo or fetus because of differences in maternal and fetal metabolism, drug concentrations, and tissue sensitivity (*see* Monographs for examples and discussion).

Factors Affecting Teratogenesis

Clinicians should realize that there is usually no single direct cause–effect relationship between maternal use of a particular drug and the occurrence of a teratogenic insult. Usually the relationship is multivariate, depending upon the drug, dose, stage of pregnancy and fetal development, genetic predisposition of the mother and the fetus, concomitant maternal or fetal exposure to other potential teratogens, and the general health of the mother and the embryo/fetus.

For a drug to induce teratogenesis, it must reach the developing embryo or fetus by crossing from the maternal circulation to the embryonic tissues or fetal circulation. Such drug exposure occurs predominantly via the placenta (Figure 2-1). The rate and extent of placental drug exposure is governed by maternal factors, placental factors, embryo/fetal factors, environmental factors, and drug factors (Figure 2-2).

Maternal Factors

Maternal factors include age, stage of pregnancy, uterine blood flow, concomitant med-

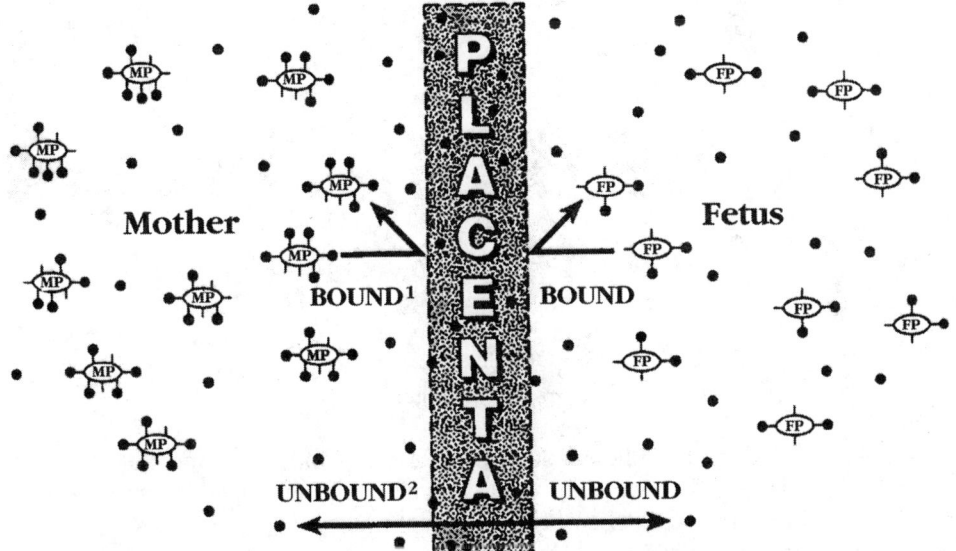

[1] The portion of drug bound to plasma protein or ionized that does not cross the placenta
[2] The portion of unionized or unbound drug that crosses the placenta

- unbound drug (note that the unbound drug concentration generally is in equilibrium across the placenta unless the drug is too large to cross)

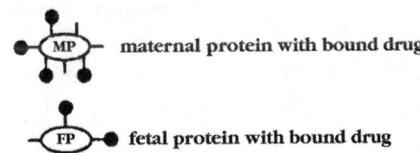

Note that the concentration of plasma protein as well as the protein-binding capacity may differ significantly between mother and fetus.

FIGURE 2-1

Drug Transfer across the Human Placenta

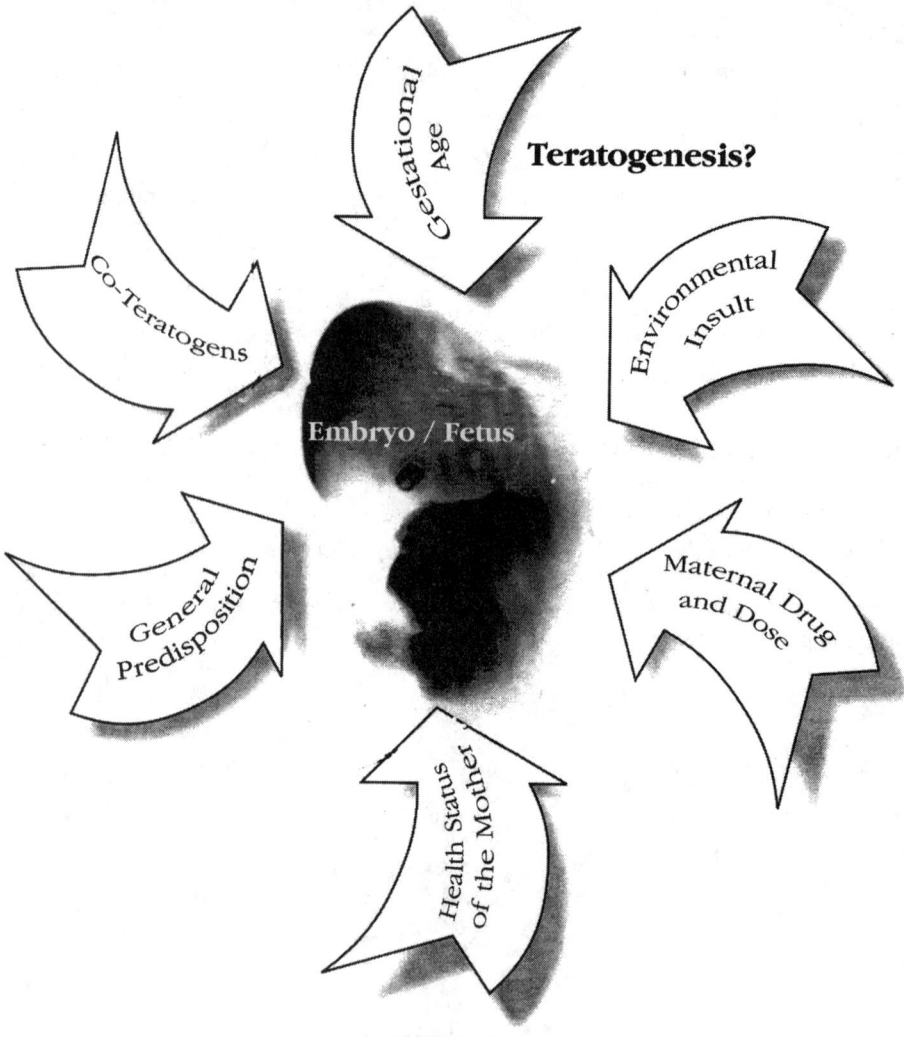

FIGURE 2-2
Factors in Teratogenesis

ical disorders (e.g., diabetes, phenylketonuria, thyroid disorders), and general health. Maternal factors also include diet; use of food additives (e.g., aspartame, nitrates); prescription and nonprescription drug use, including the use of alcohol and tobacco; the dose, time, and route of the drug administered; the distribution of the drug within the mother (concentration); and metabolism and elimination of the drug by the mother.

Placental Factors

Placental factors include placental age and health, the size and thickness of the placenta, placental blood flow, and the ability of the placenta to metabolize a drug to a teratogenic compound.

Embryo/Fetal Factors

Fetal factors include the age of the embryo/fetus, genetics, maturity of fetal hepatic drug-metabolizing systems, hepatic blood flow via the ductus venosus, and pH of fetal blood.

Environmental Factors

Environmental factors include pesticides (e.g., chlordane, DDT), pollutants (e.g., air and water pollutants), radiation, toxins (e.g., mercury, organic solvents), and infectious organisms.

Drug Factors

Drug factors include the drug's basic pharmacology and toxicology and physicochemical properties (e.g., lipid solubility [partition coefficient], ionization [pKa], protein binding). The molecular weight of a drug also is important.[2] During early pregnancy, drugs pass directly into the allantoic sac by passive diffusion. As pregnancy progresses, the placental membranes become progressively thinner, which decreases the diffusion distance.[3] Medical disorders, such as diabetes or toxemia of pregnancy, may also alter placental permeability.

Fetal serum levels are generally 30%–80% of maternal serum levels. There are, however, exceptions, such as diazepam, for which fetal serum concentration may be significantly higher than maternal serum concentration. (*See* Monographs for additional examples and related discussion.)

Once a drug crosses the placenta, it is in the fetal circulation, where it can produce expected pharmacologic as well as teratogenic effects. Whether the drug produces a teratogenic effect depends on several variables, the most important being timing. The critical period of greatest teratogenic risk for the embryo or fetus is generally the first trimester, the period during which the majority of organogenesis occurs. It is during this time, therefore, that major physical malformations are most likely to be induced. Timing also can serve to protect embryos and fetuses from certain teratogenic effects. For example, even if a drug is a known teratogen producing cleft palate, maternal use would not produce this defect if the palate had already fused. Thus, to evaluate the teratogenic potential of a drug, it is necessary to know not only whether it has been implicated in human teratogenesis, but also the critical period during which the embryo or fetus was exposed to it (Figure 2-3 and Table 2-1).

Summary

More data are needed to assure optimal maternal drug use with minimal embryonic and fetal risk for teratogenesis and fetotoxicity. Although there is extensive evidence implicating some drugs with teratogenic insult (e.g., barbiturates), published data for many other drugs often required by women during pregnancy (e.g., analgesics, anticonvulsants, immunizations) are inadequate. Unfortunately, a high percentage of women continue to be unnecessarily exposed to potentially dangerous drugs by their physicians and other prescribers during pregnancy. To decrease the likelihood of a teratogenic or fetotoxic drug insult, prescribers should first decide whether a drug is required during pregnancy and, if it is, should then determine which specific drug can be of therapeutic benefit to the mother, while offering the least likelihood of risk to the embryo or fetus. Prescribers must bear in mind, however, that the occurrence of teratogenesis is a **complex** process that depends **not only** on the drug, but also on many other factors. Thus, to minimize the occurrence of teratogenic and fetotoxic effects, prescribers need to:

1. Realize that **no drug** (prescription or nonprescription, including alcohol and other drugs and substances of abuse) can be considered completely safe for use during pregnancy.
2. Restrict drug use during pregnancy to "safe" drugs indicated for specific well-established indications. For example, although previously used for this pur-

(Continued on page 96)

---

2. Drugs that have a molecular weight of less than 500 cross the placenta easily; drugs that have a molecular weight of 500–1000 cross with some difficulty; and drugs that have a molecular weight exceeding 1000 generally are unable to cross the placenta. Most drugs have a molecular weight of 250–500.

3. Initially, these membranes are approximately 25 µm thick. At term, they decrease to approximately 2 µm. In addition, the placenta has thick and thin areas that create varying distances through which drugs may diffuse, and there may be shunting of blood away from the exchange area of the placenta.

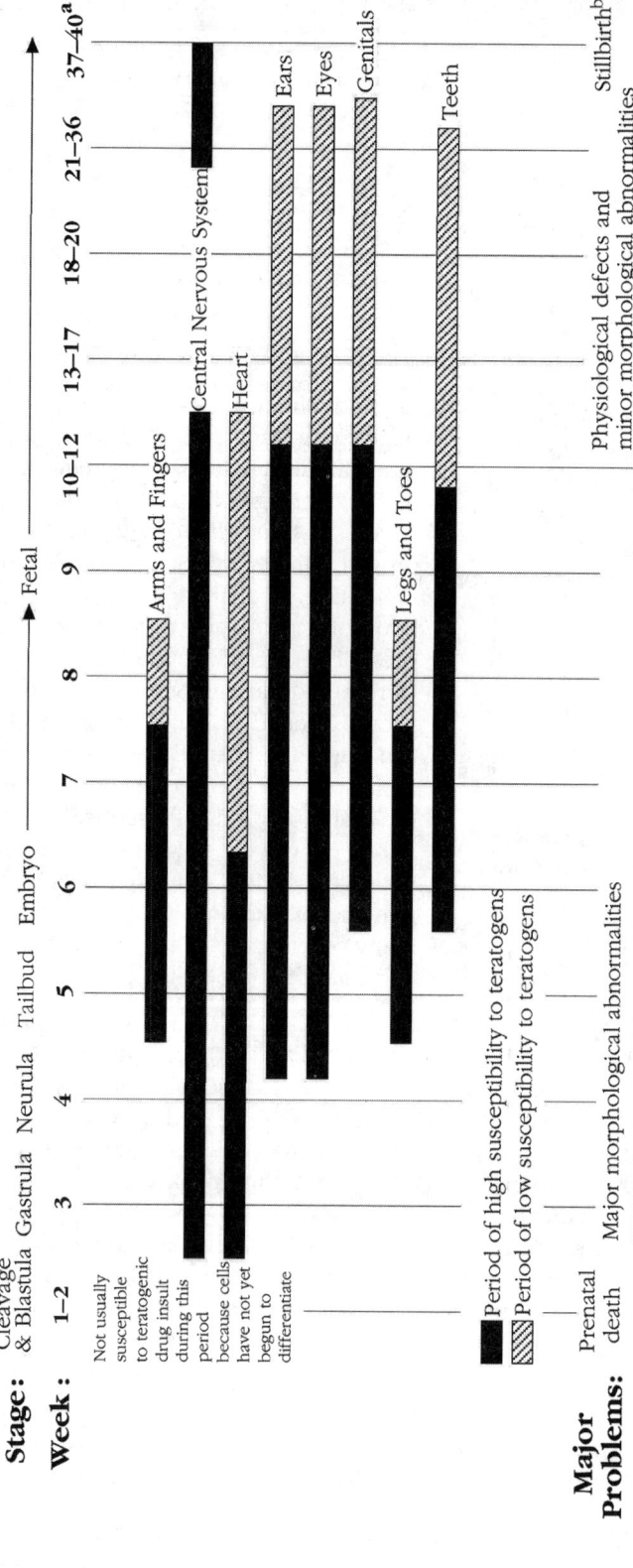

FIGURE 2-3

Variation in Tetratogenic Susceptibility of Organ Systems during Stages of Human Intrauterine Development

[a] Average time from fertilization to parturition is 38 weeks.
[b] Drugs administered during this period may cause neonatal depression at birth (or other effects directly related to the pharmacological effect of the administered drug).

TABLE 2-1
Human Gestational Development[a]

TIME AFTER FERTILIZATION	DEVELOPMENTAL STAGE AND ACTIVITY
First Month Postfertilization (Days 1–28)	
Days 1–3	**Cleavage Stage**
1	Fertilization and first cell division occur
2	Two cells appear and then four cells
3	Morula; 16 cells appear
Days 4–6	**Blastula Stage**
4	Early blastocyst (58 cells) forms
5	Free blastocyst (107 cells) forms
6	Attachment occurs
Days 7–13	**Gastrula Stage**
7	Implantation occurs
8	Bilaminar disc forms
9	External embryonic mesoderm forms
10	Primary yolk sac forms
11–13	Secondary yolk sac lined by endoderm forms
	Primitive streak begins
Days 14–19	**Primitive Streak Stage**
14–17	Primitive streak becomes half length
18	Intra-embryonic mesoderm forms
19	Primitive streak is completed
Days 20–28	**Neurula Stage**
20	Presomite neurula forms
	Yolk sac becomes visible
	Neural plate and neural groove form
21–22	Neural folds form
	Heart tube forms
	Intra-embryonic vessels start to form
	Head fold encloses foregut
	Cloacal membrane tail fold encloses hindgut
	Occipital somites (1–4) form
	Embryonic epidermis forms
23	Tail fold progresses
24–26	Cervical somites (5–12) form
	Rhombencephalic folds close
	Neural tube starts to form
27	Thoracic somites (13–20) form
	Thalamus starts to form
	Urachus starts to form
	Otic disc and vesicle start to form
	Optic vesicle starts to form
	Oral membranes start to form
	Heart tubes fuse and loop
	Laryngo-tracheal groove forms
	Pharyngeal pouches form
	Hepatic diverticulum forms
	Primary brain vesicles form
	Nephrogenic cord forms
	Nephric ducts form
28	Thoracic somites (21–24) form
	Tongue primordia develop
	Rathke's pouch (anterior pituitary gland) forms
	Thyroid rudiment forms
	Heart begins to beat
	Neural tube closes
	Crown-rump length 4–5 mm
Second Month Postfertilization (Days 29–56)	
Days 29–35	**Tailbud Stage**
29	Lumbar somites (25–27) form
	Appendicular ridges appear

TABLE 2-1 *continued*

TIME AFTER FERTILIZATION	DEVELOPMENTAL STAGE AND ACTIVITY
30	Lumbar somites (28–29) form
	Visceral arches become well separated
31	Sacral somites (30–32) form
	Limb buds start to form
	Optic cup appears
	Otic cup appears
	Pancreatic diverticula form
	Midbrain flexure forms
	Spinal nerve roots form
32	Sacral somites (33–34) form
33	Caudal somites (35–36) form
34	Caudal somites (37) form
	Greater curvature of stomach appears
35	Caudal somites (38–44) form
Days 36–56	**Embryo Stage**
36–39	Somite formation ends
	Tailbud regresses
	Aortico-pulmonary septation occurs
	Cardiac muscle begins to form
	Hemopoiesis begins in liver
	Dental laminae form
	Primitive nasal septum forms
	Pontine flexure forms
	Nerve plexus forms
	Cerebellum begins to form
	Intramembraneous ossification begins
	Chondrification begins
	Mullerian ducts begin to form
	Urethral plate begins to form
	Secondary bronchi begin to form
40	Hand plate appears
	Umbilical hernia begins to form
41–42	3rd and 4th visceral arches become covered by operculum
	Cervical flexure of head onto chest appears
	Pentadactyl rudiment appears
43–44	Cervical sinus closes
45–47	Urorectal septum appears
	Median processes of maxillaries begin to form
	Premaxillary processes start to form
	Sex differentiation begins
48	Primordial germ cells become visible
49	Testes begin to form (in male)
50–51	Facial clefts begin to close
52–53	Phalanges and first links appear
	Fingers and toes become visible
54–56	Origin of submandibular, parotid, and sublingual glands begins to develop
	External ear begins to form
	Large umbilical hernia becomes visible
	Smooth muscle begins to develop
	Mullerian ducts fuse to form utero-vaginal rudiment (in female)
	Primary follicles begin to develop (in female)
	Embryo assumes "human" appearance
	Crown-rump length ~24–34 mm, weight ~1 gram
Weeks 9–38	**Fetal Stage**
Third Month	
Weeks 9–12	
9	Finger- and toenail formation begins
	Testes start to descend (in male)
	Crown-rump length ~41 mm
10	Eyelids become fused
	Permanent tooth buds form
	Bones ossify
	Distinctive external genitalia appear
	Hematopoiesis begins in bone marrow
	Periderm plug forms in nostrils
	Periderm plug forms in ears

TABLE 2-1 *continued*

TIME AFTER FERTILIZATION	DEVELOPMENTAL STAGE AND ACTIVITY
	Islets of Langerhans form
	Epidermis formation becomes complete
	Thyroid gland formation becomes complete
	Lung formation becomes complete
	Gallbladder secretes bile
	Brain formation becomes essentially complete to the extent of neonate
11	"Respiratory" movement begins
12	Crown-rump length ~50–70 mm, weight ~15–20 grams
Fourth Month	
Weeks 13–16	
13	Gender becomes recognizable
14–15	Skeleton becomes visible on x-ray
	Vernix becomes visible
	Myelination occurs
	Mesenteries become well formed
	Metanephros formation becomes complete to the extent of neonate
	Heart formation becomes almost complete
	Hematopoiesis begins in spleen
16	Meconium collects
	Crown-rump length ~155 mm, weight ~165 grams
Fifth Month	Lanugo appears on body
Weeks 17–20	Hair forms on head
	Fetal movements begin to be detected by mother
	Crown-rump length ~185–210 mm, weight ~200–310 grams
Sixth Month	Fetal outline becomes palpable
Weeks 21–24	Dentine and enamel begin to form
	Eyebrows and lashes become well defined
	Pulmonary alveoli form
	Skin appears red and wrinkled
	Usually nonviable if born
	Crown-rump length ~220–240 mm, weight ~635–720 grams
Seventh Month	Cornification of epidermis surface layer occurs
Weeks 25–28	Eyelids open
	Periderm plugs in nostrils disappear
	Periderm plugs in ears disappear
	Testes approach scrotum (in male)
	Ovaries shift from dorsal to more caudal location within pelvis (in female)
	Viable if born (good chance to survive with proper care)
	Crown-rump length ~345 mm, weight ~1350 grams
Eighth Month	Calcium storage begins
Weeks 29–32	Fat becomes deposited subcutaneously
	Viable if born (good chance to survive with proper care)
	Crown-rump length ~395 mm, weight ~1800 grams
Ninth Month	Body rounds out
Weeks 33–36	Skin wrinkles smooth out
	Dull redness of skin fades
	Calcium storage continues
	Iron storage begins
	Viable if born
	Crown-rump length ~445 mm, weight ~2400 grams
Tenth Month	
Weeks 37–40	
(average time from fertilization to parturition is 38 weeks)	Body becomes plump
	Labia majora come in contact (in female)
	Nails extend to tips of fingers and toes
	Skin loses lanugo coat
	Vernix caseosa becomes deposited on skin surface
	Testes usually appear in scrotum (in male)
	Upper limbs become slightly longer than lower limbs
	Crown-rump length at term (~38 weeks) ~470 mm, weight ~3400 grams

[a] *See Problems in Pediatric Drug Therapy*, 3rd ed., L. A. Pagliaro and A. M. Pagliaro, Eds. 1995, pp. 105–243, for original references consulted for the preparation of this table.

pose, progestogens (e.g., hydroxyprogesterone, progesterone) are no longer recommended during the first trimester to prevent habitual or threatened abortion because of a lack of clearly demonstrated efficacy, the ability of these drugs to cause masculinization of the female fetus, and associated fetal heart and limb defects when used during the first 4 months of pregnancy.
3. Avoid the use of known teratogens during pregnancy (unless the perceived benefit outweighs the potential risk). For example, malaria prophylaxis with chloroquine[4] **during** pregnancy can help to prevent placental malaria infection associated with a high incidence of low birth weight among neonates and congenital infection.
4. Recognize that **many** drugs used near term can cause expected pharmacologic, including toxic, effects in the fetus or neonate. With proper recognition and care, these effects are generally reversible.

With these recommendations and using the information presented in this chapter, clinicians should be able to rationally prescribe drug therapy for women who are pregnant and decrease the occurrence of preventable drug-induced teratogenic and toxic effects among embryos/fetuses and neonates.

Teratogenesis Drug Monographs

The following monographs include three different evaluations of the human data derived from the published literature regarding the teratogenic risk of a particular drug when used by women during pregnancy. The first code is the FDA code for the drug, with the authors' modifications described later. The second code is the significance code, which is based on the authors' judgment of the probability that the drug might produce teratogenic or fetotoxic effects. The third code is the potency code, the authors' impression of the frequency with which the drug might produce the described effect.

For most monographs, sources of information for the FDA codes included the *Physicians' Desk Reference* (PDR), *Drug Facts and Comparisons,* and the *USP-DI (United States Pharmacopeia Dispensing Information).* Because all drugs have not been assigned a pregnancy category and do not include a code, the authors created additional codes.

In some instances, monographs have been included for drugs that have no assigned code. These are drugs for which there is no FDA code, or drugs that are not available for use in the United States. Such drugs are denoted by the NONE code to indicate that no assessment has been made.

Almost three hundred individual monographs[5] are presented for drugs in current use[6] in North America. These drugs are arranged in alphabetical order according to their nonproprietary United States Adopted Names (USAN). Each monograph contains, in addition to its evaluation code, a synopsis of the available published world literature concerning the particular drug in terms of its potential for human teratogenesis or fetotoxicity. Reference citations follow each individual monograph.

Maternal use of any drug during pregnancy involves some risk to the developing embryo, fetus, or neonate. Therefore, regardless of how safe a drug may be rated, it should **not** be used during pregnancy unless there is a clear indication for use and adequate attention has been given to these recommendations.

---

4. Chloroquine is not a known teratogen. However, it does readily cross the placenta and may achieve high concentrations in fetal ocular tissue.

5. Monographs are presented only for drugs for which human teratogenic data have been published. The absence of a drug from this series of monographs indicates only that teratogenic data have not been published or that available data were obtained from animal studies. The absence of a drug from this series of monographs should **not** be used to imply that the drug possesses no human teratogenic risk.

6. For teratogenic data regarding drugs that are no longer commonly available for use in North America (e.g., aminopterin), please see earlier editions of this text.

Teratogenesis Drug Monograph Codes

FDA Codes:

A: **Controlled Studies Show No Risk.** Adequate, well-controlled studies in pregnant women have failed to demonstrate a risk to the fetus in any trimester of pregnancy.

B: **No Evidence of Risk in Humans.** Adequate, well-controlled studies in pregnant women have not shown increased risk of fetal abnormalities despite adverse findings in animals, or, in the absence of adequate human studies, animal studies show no fetal risk. The chance of fetal harm is remote but remains a possibility.

C: **Risk Cannot Be Ruled Out.** Adequate, well-controlled human studies are lacking, and animal studies have shown a risk to the fetus or are lacking as well. There is a chance of fetal harm if the drug is administered during pregnancy but the potential benefits may outweigh the potential risk.

D: **Positive Evidence of Risk.** Studies in humans, or investigational or postmarketing data, have demonstrated fetal risk. Nevertheless, potential benefits from the use of the drug may outweigh the potential risk. For example, the drug may be acceptable if needed in a life-threatening situation or with serious disease for which safer drugs cannot be used or are ineffective.

X: **Contraindicated in Pregnancy.** Studies in animals or humans, or investigational or postmarketing reports, have demonstrated positive evidence of fetal abnormalities or risk that clearly outweighs any possible benefit to the patient.

Author Codes (used when no FDA code has been designated):

★: Indicates that statements in the literature recommend weighing the benefits versus risks, but no animal or human data are available.

●: Indicates that although statements in the literature recommend weighing the benefits versus the risks, animal and/or human data are available.

NONE: No assessment of teratogenic risk has been made.

Significance Codes:

1: Human teratogen
2: Probable human teratogen
3: Possible human teratogen
4: Improbable human teratogen
5: Not a human teratogen

Potency Codes:

1: Frequently produces effect
2: Occasionally produces effect
3: Rarely produces effect
4: Does not produce effect

Acetaminophen (Paracetamol)

FDA: **B**   SIGNIFICANCE: **5**   POTENCY: **4**

Although acetaminophen crosses the placenta in the unconjugated form, it has never been subjected to appropriate clinical teratogenic studies. One case report of the maternal use of acetaminophen during the tenth to twelfth week of pregnancy was associated with congenital cataracts and neonatal nephrotoxicity. Seven other cases involving acetaminophen and other drugs also have been published. One study of 226 infants born to women who had used acetaminophen during the first 4 months of pregnancy reported no increased incidence of congenital malformations. The wide use of acetaminophen during pregnancy, the scarcity of reported congenital malformations, and the one negative report make it highly unlikely that acetaminophen is a human teratogen.

Char, V. C., Chandra, R., Fletcher, A. B., et al. (1975). Polyhydramnios and neonatal renal failure—a possible association with maternal acetaminophen ingestion. *The Journal of Pediatrics, 86*, 638–639.

Collins, E. (1981). Maternal and fetal effects of acetaminophen and salicylates in pregnancy. *Obstetrics and Gynecology, 58*(Suppl 5), 57S–62S.

Harley, J. D., Farrar, J. F., Gray, J. B., et al. (1964). Aromatic drugs and congenital cataracts. *The Lancet, 1*, 472–473.

Heinonen, O. P., Slone, D., & Shapiro, S. (1977). *Birth defects and drugs in pregnancy*. Littleton, MA: Publishing Sciences Group.

Kurzel, R. B. (1990). Can acetaminophen excess result in maternal and fetal toxicity? *Southern Medical Journal, 83*(8), 953–955.

Levy, G., Garrettson, L. K., & Soda, D. M. (1975). Evidence of placental transfer of acetaminophen. *Pediatrics, 55*, 895.

Acetazolamide

FDA: C   SIGNIFICANCE: 3   POTENCY: 2–3

Unlike the case with many other anticonvulsants, extensive teratogenic studies of acetazolamide do not exist. However, teratogenic effects have been associated with its use during pregnancy. Reported congenital malformations include atrial septal defect, cerebellum abnormalities, cleft lip and palate, congenital hip dislocation, depressed nasal bridge, hypoplastic digits, limb defects, shortened extremities, and wide-set eyes. However, these reports must be tempered with the fact that the pregnant women in the report were also using other known teratogens. Further confounding these data is the argument that infants born to women who have epilepsy may have a higher incidence of congenital malformations. Regardless, acetazolamide should be used during pregnancy only if absolutely necessary.

Mallow, D. W., Herrick, H. K., & Gathman, G. (1980). Fetal exposure to anticonvulsant drugs. *Archives of Pathology and Laboratory Medicine, 104*, 215–218.

Nakane, Y., Okuma, T., Takahashi, R., et al. (1980). Multi-institutional study on the teratogenicity and fetal toxicity of antiepileptic drugs: A report of a collaborative study group in Japan. *Epilepsia, 21*, 663–680.

Acetohexamide

FDA: D   SIGNIFICANCE: 3–4   POTENCY: 3

No congenital malformations have been associated with acetohexamide use during pregnancy. However, teratogenic studies of acetohexamide have been limited because insulin and diet are the preferred treatment for managing diabetes among pregnant women and antihyperglycemics are not used widely for this group. However, fetotoxicity, particularly neonatal hypoglycemia, may be associated with acetohexamide when used to manage maternal diabetes during pregnancy. Appropriate assessment and monitoring of neonates born to mothers who received acetohexamide during pregnancy, especially during the last trimester, are indicated.

Kemball, M. L., McIver, C., Milner, R. D. G., et al. (1970). Neonatal hypoglycaemia in infants of diabetic mothers given sulphonylurea drugs in pregnancy. *Archives of Disease in Childhood, 45*, 696–701.

Malins, J. M., Cooke, A. M., Pyke, D. A., et al. (1964). Sulphonylurea drugs in pregnancy. *British Medical Journal, 2*, 187.

Acyclovir

FDA: B (systemic use)   C (topical use)
SIGNIFICANCE: 3   POTENCY: 3

One published study reported various congenital anomalies among nine of 168 infants born to women who had received acyclovir systemically during the first trimester. However, no congenital anomalies were reported for the offspring of women who received acyclovir systemically during the second or third trimester or used acyclovir topically throughout pregnancy. More data are needed, particularly data addressing systemic acyclovir use during the first trimester.

Andrews, E. B., Yankaskas, B. C., Cordero, J. F., et al. (1992). Acyclovir in pregnancy registry: Six years' experience. *Obstetrics and Gynecology Annual, 79*, 7–13.

Brown, Z. A., & Baker, D. A. (1989). Acyclovir therapy during pregnancy. *Obstetrics and Gynecology Annual, 73*(3), 526–531.

Brown, Z. A., & Watts, D. H. (1990). Antiviral therapy in pregnancy. *Clinica Obstetrica E Ginecologica, 33*, 276–289.

Frenkel, L. M., Brown, Z. A., Bryson, Y. J., et al. (1991). Pharmacokinetics of acyclovir in the human pregnancy and neonate. *American Journal of Obstetrics and Gynecology, 164*(2), 569–576.

Stray-Pedersen, B. (1990). Acyclovir in late pregnancy to prevent neonatal herpes simplex. *The Lancet, 336*, 756.

Alcohol (Ethanol)

AUTHOR: ●   SIGNIFICANCE: 1
POTENCY: 1 (dose dependent)

Alcohol is a recognized human neurotoxin and known human teratogen. As such, it ap-

TABLE 2-2
Congenital Malformations Associated with the Fetal Alcohol Syndrome[a]

MALFORMATION	INCIDENCE (%)
Postnatal growth failure	96.9
Prenatal growth failure	96.5
Microcephaly	92.8
Mental retardation	89.8
Short palpebral fissures	86.6
Hypoplastic maxilla	57.1
Midfacial hypoplasia	54.0
Abnormal palmar creases	52.0
Epicanthal folds	51.2
Skeletal/joint anomalies	47.3
Micrognathia	40.9
Cardiac defects	37.5
Genital anomalies	35.7
Cutaneous hemangioma	32.3
Pinnal anomaly	26.7
Other eye defects	6.0
Hypertelorism	4.0

[a] Based on data from four different studies involving 50 patients. Adapted from Hays, D. P. (1981). Teratogenesis: A review of the basic principles with a discussion of selected agents. (Part II). *Drug Intelligence and Clinical Pharmacy, 15,* 542–566; Pagliaro & Pagliaro (1996). *Substance use among children and adolescents.* New York: Wiley; and Pagliaro & Pagliaro (2000). *Substance use among women.* Philadelphia: Brunner/Mazel.

pears to affect specific brain structures, including the basal ganglia, the corpus callosum, and the cerebellum. This neurotoxicity appears to be mediated in the fetus by the microsomal alcohol-oxidizing system (i.e., cytochrome P-450 2E1) and the formation of alcohol's reactive metabolite, acetaldehyde. In 1968, Lemoine first reported the association between specific birth defects and maternal alcohol consumption during pregnancy. These birth defects were subsequently designated the fetal alcohol syndrome (FAS)[7] (Table 2-2 and Figure 2-4). Heavy drinking by women during pregnancy also has been related to significant impairments among their offspring, including impairments in executive functioning (e.g., concept formation and reasoning, cognitive flexibility, planning ability, selective inhibition) and in psychosocial functioning.

Although the FAS was first associated with heavy drinking during pregnancy, later studies found that it occurred with moderate drinking as well. More recently it has been suggested that even a small amount of alcohol consumption during pregnancy may be associated with subtle cognitive deficits or mild behavioral problems among offspring, including those with IQs within the normal range. For example, an increased incidence of learning disorders and behavioral (e.g., conduct disorder) and attentional disorders (e.g., attention-deficit/hyperactivity disorder [A-D/HD]) during childhood and adolescence have been associated with maternal alcohol consumption during pregnancy. Based on a review and risk analysis of all currently available published data, it is recommended that women abstain from all alcohol use during pregnancy.

Armant, D. R., & Saunders, D. E. (1996). Exposure of embryonic cells to alcohol: Contrasting ef-

---

7. Although some other classifications or descriptions may be used to designate various forms of alcohol-related teratogenic effects (e.g., alcohol-related birth defects [ARBD], fetal alcohol effects [FAE]), for scientific accuracy and parsimony, we argue that these simply be considered as less severe forms of FAS.

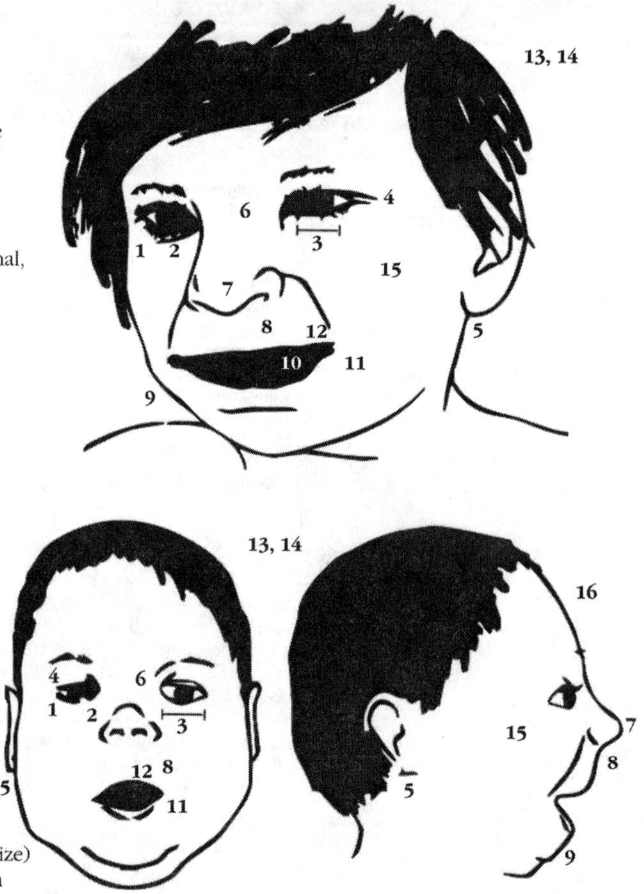

Eyes
1. ptosis (drooping lid)
2. strabismus (squint)
3. shortened palpebral fissure (opening between eyelids)
4. epicanthal fold

Ears
5. smaller or larger than normal, malformed, or low set

Nose
6. low nasal bridge
7. short with high or up-turned nasal tip

Mouth
8. philtrum (groove in upper lip): underdeveloped or absent
9. micrognathia (small jaw) or retrognathia (posteriorly displaced jaw)
10. teeth: absent enamel, malformed, or malocculded
11. wide mouth
12. thin vemilion border of upper lip

Head
13. microcephaly (small head size)
14. abnormally shaped cranium
15. midface hypoplasia (broad, flat face)
16. narrow receding forehead

FIGURE 2-4
Fetal Alcohol Syndrome

fects during preimplantation and postimplantation development. *Seminars in Perinatology, 20*(2), 127–139.

Becker, M., Warr-Leeper, G. A., & Leeper, H. A., Jr. (1990). Fetal alcohol syndrome: A description of oral, motor, articulatory, short-term memory, grammatical, and semantic abilities. *Journal of Communicative Disorders, 23*, 97–124.

Brown, R. T., Coles, C. D., Smith, I. E., et al. (1991). Effects of prenatal alcohol exposure at school age. II. Attention and behavior. *Neurotoxicology and Teratology, 13*, 369–376.

Brzezinski, M. R., Boutelet-Bochan, H., Person, R. E., et al. (1999). Catalytic activity and quantitation of cytochrome P–450 2E1 in the prenatal human brain. *Pharmacology and Experimental Therapeutics, 289*(3), 1648–1653.

Carney, L. J., & Chermak, G. D. (1991). Performance of American Indian children with fetal alcohol syndrome on the test of language development. *Journal of Communication Disorders, 24*, 123–134.

Casiro, O. G. (1991). Drinking and pregnancy. *Canadian Medical Association Journal, 145*, 1552–1554.

Coles, C. D., Brown, R. T., Smith, I. E., et al. (1991). Effects of prenatal alcohol exposure at school age. I. Physical and cognitive development. *Neurotoxicology and Teratology, 13*, 357–367.

Cramer, C., & Davidhizar, R. (1999). FAS/FAE: Impact on children. *Journal of Child Health Care, 3*(3), 31–34.

Floyd, R. L., Decoufle, P., & Hungerford, D. W. (1999). Alcohol use prior to pregnancy recognition. *American Journal of Preventive Medicine, 17*(2), 101–107.

Food & Drug Administration (1977). Fetal Alcohol Syndrome, *FDA Drug Bulletin*. Sept.-Oct.

Forbes, R. (1984). Alcohol-related birth defects. *Public Health (London), 98*, 238–241.

Government policies on alcohol and pregnancy. ICAP Report 6 (2000). *Journal of Substance Use, 4*(4), 216–219.

Hanson, J. W., Streissguth, A. P., & Smith, D. W.

(1978). The effects of moderate alcohol consumption during pregnancy on fetal growth and morphogenesis. *The Journal of Pediatrics, 92,* 457–460.

Idänpään-Heikkila, J., Jouppila, P., Akerblom, H. K., et al. (1972). Elimination and metabolic effects of ethanol in mother, fetus, and newborn infant. *American Journal of Obstetrics and Gynecology, 112,* 387–393.

Jacobson, S. W. (1998). Specificity of neurobehavioral outcomes associated with prenatal alcohol exposure. *Alcoholism: Clinical and Experimental Research, 22,* 313–320.

Jones, K. L., & Smith, D. W. (1973). Recognition of the fetal alcohol syndrome in early infancy. *The Lancet, 2,* 999–1001.

Jones, K. L., & Smith, D. W. (1977). Effects of alcohol on the fetus. *New England Journal of Medicine, 298,* 55–56.

Jones, K. L., Smith, D. W., Ulleland, C. N., et al. (1973). Pattern of malformation of offspring of chronic alcoholic mothers. *The Lancet, 1,* 1267–1271.

Lemoine, P., Harousseau, H., Borteyru, J. P., et al. (1968). Children of alcoholic parents. Observed anomalies (127 cases). *Ouest Medical, 21,* 476–478.

Little, R. E., Streissguth, A. P., Barr, H. M., et al. (1980). Decreased birth weight in infants of alcoholic women who abstained during pregnancy. *The Journal of Pediatrics, 96,* 974–977.

Mattson, S. N., Goodman, A. M., Caine, C., et al. (1999). Executive functioning in children with heavy prenatal alcohol exposure. *Alcoholism: Clinical and Experimental Research, 23*(11), 1808–1815.

Lopez, R., & Montoya, M. F. (1971). Abnormal bone marrow morphology in the premature infant associated with maternal alcohol infusion. *The Journal of Pediatrics, 79,* 1008–1010.

Nanson, J. L., & Hiscock, M. (1990). Attention deficits in children exposed to alcohol prenatally. *Alcoholism: Clinical and Experimental Research, 14,* 656–661.

Nichols, M. M. (1967). Acute alcohol withdrawal syndrome in a newborn. *American Journal of Diseases of Children, 113,* 714–715.

Oulette, E. M., Rosett, H. R., Rosman, N. P., et al. (1977). Adverse effects on offspring of maternal alcohol abuse during pregnancy. *New England Journal of Medicine, 297,* 528–530.

Pagliaro, A. M., & Pagliaro, L. A. (1996). *Substance use among children and adolescents.* New York: Wiley.

Pagliaro, A. M., & Pagliaro, L. A. (2000). *Substance use among women: A reference and resource guide.* Philadelphia: Brunner/Mazel.

Pagliaro, L. A. (1992). The straight dope: Focus on learning—Interpreting the interpretations. *Psynopsis, 14*(2), 8.

Pietrantoni, M., & Knuppel, R. A. (1990). Alcohol use in pregnancy. *Clinics in Perinatology, 18,* 93–111.

Roebuck, T. M., Mattson, S. N., & Riley, E. P. (1998). A review of the neuroanatomical findings in children with fetal alcohol syndrome or prenatal exposure to alcohol. *Alcoholism: Clinical and Experimental Research, 22,* 339–344.

Roebuck, T. M., Mattson, S. N., & Riley, E. P. (1999). Behavioral and psychosocial profiles of alcohol-exposed children. *Alcoholism: Clinical and Experimental Research, 23*(6), 1070–1076.

Schenker, S., Becker, H. C., Randall, C. L., et al. (1990). Fetal alcohol syndrome: Current status of pathogenesis. *Alcoholism: Clinical and Experimental Research, 14,* 635–647.

Shaywitz, S. E., Caparulo, B. K., & Hodgson, E. S. (1981). Developmental language disability as a consequence of prenatal exposure to ethanol. *Pediatrics, 68*(6), 850–855.

Shaywitz, S. E., Cohen, D. J., & Shaywitz, B. A. (1980). Behavior and learning difficulties in children of normal intelligence born to alcoholic mothers. *The Journal of Pediatrics, 96,* 978–982.

Sokol, R. J. (1981). Alcohol and abnormal outcomes of pregnancy. *Canadian Medical Association Journal, 125,* 143–148.

Streissguth, A. P., & Dehaene, P. (1993). Fetal alcohol syndrome in twins of alcoholic mothers: Concordance of diagnosis and IQ. *American Journal of Medical Genetics, 47*(6), 857–861.

Streissguth, A. P., Herman, C. S., & Smith, D. W. (1978). Intelligence, behavior, and dysmorphogenesis in the fetal alcohol syndrome. A report of 20 patients. *The Journal of Pediatrics, 92,* 363–367.

Walpole, I. R., & Hockey, H. (1980). Fetal alcohol syndrome: Implications to family and society in Australia. *Australian Paediatric Journal, 16,* 101–105.

Waltman, R., & Iniquez, E. S. (1972). Placental transfer of ethanol and its elimination at term. *Obstetrics and Gynecology, 40,* 180–185.

West, J. R., Black, A. C., Reimann, P. C., et al. (1981). Polydactyly and polysyndactyly induced by prenatal exposure to ethanol. *Teratology, 24,* 13–18.

Alglucerase

AUTHOR: **NONE** SIGNIFICANCE: **3–4**
POTENCY: **3–4**

A single case report noted no teratogenic effects for an infant delivered to a woman who had received alglucerase throughout her entire pregnancy. More data are needed.

Aporta Rodriguez, R., Escobar Vedia, J. L., Navarro Castro, A. M., et al. (1998). Alglucerase enzyme replacement therapy used safely and effectively throughout the whole pregnancy of a Gaucher disease patient. *Haematologica, 83*(9), 852–853.

Amantadine

FDA: C   SIGNIFICANCE: 3   POTENCY: 3

In a single published case report, a woman who took 100 mg of amantadine daily during the first trimester gave birth to an infant who had a single ventricle and pulmonary atresia. In another report, an infant was born with an inguinal hernia. Three normal births also have been reported among women who took amantadine at various stages during their pregnancies. More data are needed, particularly data addressing amantadine use during the first trimester.

Golbe, L. I. (1987). Parkinson's disease and pregnancy. *Neurology, 37,* 1245–1249.
Levy, M., Pastuszak, A., & Koren, G. (1991). Fetal outcome following intrauterine amantadine exposure. *Reproductive Toxicology, 5,* 79–81.
Nora, J. J., Nora, A. H., & Way, G. L. (1975). Cardiovascular maldevelopment associated with maternal exposure to amantadine. *The Lancet, 2,* 607.

Aminobenzoic Acid

FDA: C   SIGNIFICANCE: 3   POTENCY: 3

The Collaborative Perinatal Project reported congenital defects among five infants of 43 women who received aminobenzoic acid during the first trimester. More data are needed addressing maternal aminobenzoic acid use during pregnancy, particularly during the first trimester.

Heinonen, O. P., Slone D., & Shapiro, S. (1977). *Birth defects and drugs in pregnancy.* Littleton, MA: Publishing Sciences Group.

Aminoglutethimide

FDA: D   SIGNIFICANCE: 2   POTENCY: 1–2

Three cases have been reported involving the virilization of female external genitalia among neonates whose mothers received aminoglutethimide during pregnancy. These effects are consistent with the expected pharmacologic action of aminoglutethimide.

Iffy, L., Ansell, S., Bryant, J. S., et al. (1965). Nonadrenal female pseudohermaphroditism: An unusual case of fetal masculinization. *Obstetrics and Gynecology, 20,* 59–65.
LeMaire, W. J., Cleveland, W. W., Bejar, R. L., et al. (1972). Aminoglutethimide: A possible cause of pseudohermaphroditism in females. *American Journal of Diseases of Children, 124,* 421–423.

Aminophylline (Theophylline Ethylenediamine)

FDA: C   SIGNIFICANCE: 5   POTENCY: 4

No increase in congenital malformations was observed among the offspring of 76 women who received aminophylline during pregnancy and were followed as part of the Collaborative Perinatal Project. Treatment protocols for the management of acute asthmatic attacks during pregnancy have included aminophylline. With its frequent use during pregnancy, it is expected that birth defects, if they do occur, would have been noted. (*See* Theophylline monograph.)

Heinonen, O. P., Slone, D., & Shapiro, S. (1977). *Birth defects and drugs in pregnancy.* Littleton, MA: Publishing Sciences Group.
Pratt, W. R. (1981). Allergic diseases in pregnancy and breast feeding. *Annals of Allergy, 47,* 355–360.

Aminosalicylic Acid

FDA: C   SIGNIFICANCE: 4–5   POTENCY: 3–4

Although one study (123 patients) of aminosalicylic acid use during pregnancy reported an increased rate of congenital malformations for the treatment group, other larger studies (1619 patients) and a literature review have not supported this association. Although not discussed in the published clinical literature, the theoretical risk for neural-tube defects related to low folic acid concentrations associated with the use of aminosalicylic acid during pregnancy exists. Because of this theoretical risk, the use of a folic acid supplement may be indicated (*see* Folic Acid monograph). (*See also* Aspirin monograph.)

Marynowski, A., & Sianozecka, E. (1972). Porownanie czestosci wystepowania wad wrodzonych u noworodkow matek zdrowych i chorych, leczonych z powodu gruzlicy. *Ginekologia Polska, 43,* 713–715.
Snider, D. E., Layde, P. M., Johnson, M. W., et al. (1980). Treatment of tuberculosis during pregnancy. *American Review of Respiratory Disease, 122,* 65–79.
Warkany, J. (1979). Antituberculous Drugs. *Teratology, 20,* 133–138.

Amiodarone

FDA: D   SIGNIFICANCE: 2   POTENCY: 2

Neonatal goiter and abnormal thyroid function (i.e., hyperthyroidism and hypothyroidism) have been reported in several case studies of infants born to women who received amiodarone during pregnancy. These teratogenic effects are presumably due to the iodine content (37% by weight) of amiodarone.

de Wolf, D., De Schepper, J., Verhaaren, H., et al. (1988). Congenital hypothyroid goiter and amiodarone. *Acta Paediatrica Scandinavica, 77*, 616–618.

Foster, C. J., & Love, H. G. (1988). Amiodarone in pregnancy: Case report and review of the literature. *International Journal of Cardiology, 20*, 307–316.

Laurent, M., Betremieux, P., Biron, Y., et al. (1987). Neonatal hypothyroidism after treatment by amiodarone during pregnancy. *American Journal of Cardiology, 60*, 942.

Tubman, R., Jenkins, J., & Lim, J. (1988). Neonatal hyperthyroxinaemia associated with maternal amiodarone therapy: Case report. *Irish Journal of Medical Science, 157*, 243.

Amphotericin B

FDA: B   SIGNIFICANCE: 3   POTENCY: 3

Several reports have been published regarding the use of amphotericin B during pregnancy for systemic fungal infections. No teratogenic effects have been reported among offspring. More data are needed, particularly data addressing amphotericin B use during the first trimester.

Cohen, I. (1987). Absence of congenital infection and teratogenesis in three children born to mothers with blastomycosis and treated with amphotericin B during pregnancy. *Pediatric Infectious Disease, 6*, 76–77.

Ismail, M. A., & Lerner, S. A. (1982). Disseminated blastomycosis in a pregnant woman: Review of amphotericin B usage during pregnancy. *American Review of Respiratory Disease, 126*, 350–353.

Ampicillin

FDA: B   SIGNIFICANCE: 3–4   POTENCY: 3

Ampicillin use during pregnancy has been associated in two studies with an increased risk for congenital heart disease and transposition of the great arteries. However, several other studies and reports have failed to support these associations. Ampicillin does cross the placenta, but, based upon its long-standing use during pregnancy and the relative paucity of positive reports, teratogenic risk appears to be low. More data are needed, particularly data addressing ampicillin use during the first trimester.

Aselton, P., Jick, H., Milunsky, A., et al. (1985). First-trimester drug use and congenital disorders. *Obstetrics and Gynecology, 65*, 451–455.

Bachev, S., Petrova, L., Voicheva, V., et al. (1974). Experimental studies on the teratogenic effect, acute and chronic toxicity of ampicillin. *Savremenna Medicina, 25*, 29–32.

Bracken, M. B. (1986). Drug use in pregnancy and congenital heart disease in offspring. *New England Journal of Medicine, 314*, 1120.

Jick, H., Holmes, L. B., Hunter, J. R., et al. (1981). First-trimester drug use and congenital disorders. *Journal of the American Medical Association, 246*, 343–346.

Korzhova, V. V., Lisitsyna, N. T., & Mikhailova, E. G. (1981). Effect of ampicillin and oxacillin on fetal and neonatal development. *Bulletin of Experimental Biology and Medicine, 91*, 169–171.

Ancrod

AUTHOR: NONE   SIGNIFICANCE: 1   POTENCY: 1

Ancrod, the purified venom of the Malayan pit viper (agkistrodon rkodostoma), is used as a defibrinating agent. Because it is fetotoxic, ancrod use should be avoided during pregnancy. Its use has been associated with an increased risk for fetal death secondary to placental bleeding.

Bonnar, J. (1981). Venous thromboembolism and pregnancy. *Clinical Obstetrics and Gynecology, 8*, 455–473.

Anesthetics—Inhalation, Waste

AUTHOR: NONE   SIGNIFICANCE: 1–2   POTENCY: 1–2

Women who work in operating rooms appear to have a higher rate of spontaneous abortions (30% versus 10%) and congenital malformations among their offspring than control groups. Additionally, studies also indicate that there may be an increased rate of congenital malformations among infants whose fathers work in operating rooms and are exposed to anesthetic gases. On the basis of these data, anesthesiologists, anesthetists, dentists, dental assistants, operating room nurses, technicians, and other personnel who may be exposed to inhalation anesthetics and who are or who may become pregnant should work only in settings where effective scavenging systems for waste anesthetic gases are used. (*See* Halothane and Nitrous Oxide monographs.)

Cohen, E. N., Bellville, J. W., & Brown, B. W. (1971). Anesthesia, pregnancy, and miscarriage: A study of operating room nurses and anesthetists. *Anesthesiology, 35*, 343–347.

Committee on the Effects of Trace Anesthetics on the Health of Operating Room Personnel (1974). *Anesthesiology, 41*, 321–340.

Corbett, T. H. (1972). Anesthetics as a cause of abortion. *Fertility and Sterility, 23*, 866–869.

Corbett, T. H., Cornell, R. G., Endus, J. L., et al. (1974). Birth defects among children of nurse-anesthetists. *Anesthesiology, 41*, 341–344.

Fink, B. R. (1975). Fetal and environmental hazards. *Acta Anesthesiology Belgium, 26L*(Suppl), 182–189.

Fink, B. R., & Cullen, B. F. (1976). Anesthetic pollution: What's happening to us? *Anesthesiology, 45*, 79–83.

Joffe, J. M. (1979). Influence of drug exposure of the father on perinatal outcome. *Clinical Perinatology, 6*, 21–36.

Pedersen, H., & Finster, M. (1979). Anesthetic risk in the pregnant surgical patient. *Anesthesiology, 51*(5), 439–451.

Shnider, S. M. (1981). Choice of anesthesia for labor and delivery. *Obstetrics and Gynecology, 58*(5), 245–345.

Smith, B. E. (1975). Teratology in anesthesia. *Clinical Obstetrics and Gynecology, 17*, 145–163.

Spence, A. A., Cohen, E. M., Brown, B. W., et al. (1977). Occupational hazards for operating room-based physicians: Analysis to date from the United States and the United Kingdom. *Journal of the American Medical Association, 238*, 955–959.

Strobino, B. R., Kline, J., & Stein, Z. (1978). Chemical and physical exposures of parents: Effects on human reproduction and offspring. *Early Human Development, 1*, 371–399.

Tomlin, P. J. (1978). Teratogenic effects of waste anesthetic gases. *British Medical Journal, 1*, 108.

Vessey, M. P., & Nunn, J. F. (1980). Occupational hazards of anaesthesia. *British Medical Journal, 281*, 696–698.

Aspirin (Acetylsalicylic Acid)

FDA: **D**

SIGNIFICANCE: **1** (neonatal effects) **4** (malformations) POTENCY: **1** (neonatal effects) **3–4** (malformations)

Studies have shown that as many as 80% of women take aspirin sometime during pregnancy and that 10% of neonates may have a measurable salicylate serum level at birth. These findings are of some concern because most forms of salicylate are teratogenic in at least one animal species. In human pregnancies, retrospective case-matched controlled studies indicate an increased congenital malformation rate for the aspirin control group. One retrospective study of women who had rheumatic disorders and ingested an average of 3200 mg/day of aspirin during pregnancy found an association between aspirin use and increased length of gestation, postmaturity syndrome, and increased duration of labor. These findings were supported by an Australian study. However, two negative studies of 41,337 pregnancies found no increase in the rate of congenital malformations, perinatal mortality, or low birth weight. However, aspirin use late in pregnancy has been associated with such fetotoxic effects as neonatal bleeding, intracranial hemorrhage among premature neonates, and persistent pulmonary hypertension. Women who use aspirin close to delivery have increased blood loss. This effect has led some authors to recommend routine urine screening for salicylates in perinatal women.

Although the chance of aspirin being a teratogen is remote, it generally should not be used as an analgesic during pregnancy because of the availability of an acceptable alternative, acetaminophen. When aspirin is required during pregnancy, it should, whenever possible, be discontinued during the last trimester, particularly if the mother is at risk for premature delivery.

Benawra, R., Mangurten, H. H., & Duffell, D. R. (1980). Cyclopia and other anomalies following maternal ingestion of salicylates. *The Journal of Pediatrics, 96*(6), 1069–1071.

Blyer, W. A., & Breckenridge, R. T. (1970). Studies on the detection of adverse drug reactions in the newborn. II: The effect of prenatal aspirin on newborn hemostasis. *Journal of the American Medical Association, 3*, 2049–2053.

Collins, E. (1981). Maternal and fetal effects of acetaminophen and salicylates in pregnancy. *Obstetrics and Gynecology, 58*(Suppl 5), 57S–62S.

Collins, E., & Turner, G. (1975). Maternal effects of regular salicylate ingestion in pregnancy. *The Lancet, 2*, 335–337.

Corby, D. G., & Schulman, I. (1971). The effects of antenatal drug administration on aggregation of platelets of newborn infants. *The Journal of Pediatrics, 79*, 307–313.

Eriksson, M., Catz, C. S., & Yaffe, S. J. (1973). Drugs and pregnancy. *Clinical Obstetrics and Gynecology, 16*, 199–224.

Haslam, R. H. (1975). Neonatal purpura secondary to maternal salicylism. *The Journal of Pediatrics, 86*, 653.

Haslam, R. H., Ekert, H., & Gillman, G. L. (1974). Hemorrhage in a neonate possibly due to maternal ingestion of salicylate. *The Journal of Pediatrics, 84*, 556–557.

Levy, G., Procknal, J. A., & Garrettson, L. K. (1975). Distribution of salicylate between neonatal and maternal serum at diffusion equilibrium. *Clinical Pharmacology and Therapeutics, 18*, 210–214.

Lewis, R. B., & Shulman, J. D. (1973). Influence of acetylsalicylic acid, an inhibitor of prostaglandin synthesis, on the duration of human gestation and labour. *The Lancet, 2*, 1159–1161.

Nelson, M. M., & Forfar, J. O. (1971). Association between drugs administered during pregnancy and congenital abnormalities of the fetus. *British Medical Journal, 1*, 523–527.

Palmisano, P. A., & Cassady, G. (1969). Salicylate exposure in the perinate. *Journal of the American Medical Association, 209*, 556–558.

Perkin, R. M., Levin, D. L., & Clark, R. (1980). Serum salicylate levels and right-to-left ductus shunts in newborn infants with persistent pulmonary hypertension. *The Journal of Pediatrics, 96*, 721–726.

Richards, I. D. (1972). A retrospective inquiry into possible teratogenic effects of drugs in pregnancy. *Advances in Experimental Medicine and Biology, 27*, 441–455.

Rumack, C. M., Guggenheim, M. A., Rumack, B. H., et al. (1981). Neonatal intracranial hemorrhage and maternal use of aspirin. *Obstetrics and Gynecology, 58*(Suppl 5), 52S–56S.

Shapiro, S., Siskind, V., Monson, R. R., et al. (1976). Perinatal mortality and birth-weight relation to aspirin taken during pregnancy. *The Lancet, 1*, 1375–1376.

Slone, D., Siskind, V., Heinonen, O. P., et al. (1976). Aspirin and congenital malformations. *The Lancet, 1*, 1373–1375.

Turner, G., & Collins, E. (1975). Fetal effects of regular salicylate ingestion in pregnancy. *The Lancet, 2*, 338–339.

Atenolol

FDA: C   SIGNIFICANCE: 4–5   POTENCY: 4

Selective ß$_1$ blockers, including atenolol, have the theoretical advantage of not affecting uterine blood flow when used during pregnancy. In two studies of atenolol use during pregnancy, no effect on fetal intrauterine growth was observed. These studies involved 120 women who received atenolol 100–200 mg/day. In regard to fetotoxic effects, although fetal bradycardia was more frequent in the treatment than in the control group, no effects on fetal blood sugar or respiration were observed.

Fuerst, M. (1982). ß-blockers may have role in preeclampsia. *Journal of the American Medical Association, 248*, 516–518.

Lunell, N. O., Persson, B., Aragon, G., et al. (1979). Circulatory and metabolic effects of acute beta-1 blockade in severe pre-eclampsia. *Acta Obstetricia et Gynecologica Scandinavica, 58*, 443–445.

Wood, S. M., & Blainey, J. D. (1981). Hypertension and renal disease. *Clinical Obstetrics and Gynecology, 8*, 439–453.

Atropine

FDA: C   SIGNIFICANCE: 4   POTENCY: 4

Congenital malformations have not been associated with atropine use during pregnancy. Atropine does readily cross the placenta, however, and may produce expected pharmacologic effects in the fetus. When used by pregnant women in large doses near term, atropine has produced in neonates the usual signs and symptoms of atropine intoxication (e.g., abdominal distention, dry mucous membranes, CNS stimulation, drowsiness, fever, tachycardia).

Abboud, T., Raya, J., Sadri, S., et al. (1983). Fetal and maternal cardiovascular effects of atropine and glycopyrrolate. *Anesthesia and Analgesia, 62*, 426–430.

Avery, G. B. (1975). *Neonatology, pathophysiology, and management of the newborn*. Philadelphia: Lippincott.

Heinonen, O. P., Slone, D., & Shapiro, S. (1977). *Birth defects and drugs in pregnancy*. Littleton, MA: Publishing Sciences Group.

Hellman, L. M., Morton, G. W., Wallach, E. E., et al. (1963). An analysis of the atropine test for placental transfer in 28 normal gravidas. *American Journal of Obstetrics and Gynecology, 87*, 650–661.

John, A. H. (1965). Placental transfer of atropine and the effect on the foetal heart rate. *British Journal of Anaesthesia, 37*, 57.

Kanto, J., Virtanen, R., Iisalo, E., et al. (1981). Placental transfer and pharmacokinetics of atropine after a single maternal intravenous and intramuscular administration. *Acta Anaesthesiologica Scandinavica, 25*(2), 85–88.

Kivalo, I., & Saarikoski, S. (1977). Placental transmission of atropine at full-term pregnancy. *British Journal of Anaesthesia, 49*, 1017–1021.

Azathioprine

FDA: **D**   SIGNIFICANCE: **4**   POTENCY: **3**

Reports of the teratogenic potential of azathioprine have been obtained primarily from women who have undergone renal transplantation prior to pregnancy. However, findings may be confounded since azathioprine is frequently administered in combination with prednisone. Regardless, only three cases of congenital malformations among offspring have been reported: one with pulmonary stenosis, the second with polydactyly, and the third with growth retardation and facial dysmorphogenesis. Based on these limited data, it would appear unlikely that azathioprine is teratogenic at dosages used for renal transplant patients. However, fetotoxic effects have been noted among neonates of women who received azathioprine during pregnancy. These effects include adrenal insufficiency, intrauterine growth retardation, lymphopenia, and premature birth. In addition, thrombocytopenia, which is a known ADR associated with adult azathioprine use, has been reported among several infants born to women who received azathioprine during pregnancy.

Alstead, E. M., Ritchie, J. K., Lennard-Jones, J. E., et al. (1990). Safety of azathioprine in pregnancy in inflammatory bowel disease. *Gastroenterology, 99*, 443–446.

Barber, H. R. (1981). Fetal and neonatal effects of cytotoxic agents. *Obstetrics and Gynecology, 58*(Suppl 5), 41S–47S.

Brown, J. H., Maxwell, A. P., & McGeown, M. G. (1991). Outcome of pregnancy following renal transplantation. *Irish Journal of Medical Science, 160*(8), 255–256.

DeWitte, D. B., Buick, M. K., Cyran, S. E., et al. (1984). Neonatal pancytopenia and severe combined immunodeficiency associated with antenatal administration of azathioprine and prednisone. *The Journal of Pediatrics, 105*, 625–628.

Golbus, M. S. (1980). Teratology for the obstetrician: Current status. *Obstetrics and Gynecology, 55*, 269.

Golby, M. (1970). Fertility after renal transplantation. *Transplantation, 10*, 201.

Lower, G. D., Stevens, L. E., Najarian, J. S., et al. (1971). Problems from immunosuppressives during pregnancy. *American Journal of Obstetrics and Gynecology, 111*, 1120–1121.

Nolan, G. H., Sweet, R. L., Laros, R. K., et al. (1974). Renal cadaver transplantation followed by successful pregnancies. *Obstetrics and Gynecology, 43*, 732.

Ostrer, H., Stamberg, J., & Perinchief, P. (1984). Two chromosome aberrations in the child of a woman with systemic lupus erythematosus treated with azathioprine and prednisone. *American Journal of Medical Genetics, 17*, 627–632.

Penn, I., Makowski, E. L., & Harris, P. (1980). Parenthood following renal transplantation. *Kidney International, 18*, 221–233.

Price, H. V., Salaman, J. R., Laurence, K. M., et al. (1976). Immunosuppressive drugs and the foetus. *Transplantation, 21*, 294–298.

Registration Committee of the European Dialysis and Transplant Association. (1980). Successful pregnancies in women treated by dialysis and kidney transplantation. *British Journal of Obstetrics and Gynaecology, 87*, 839–845.

Rudolph, J. E., Schweizer, R. T., & Bartus, S. A. (1979). Pregnancy in renal transplant patients. *Transplantation, 27*, 26–29.

Sharon, E., Jones, J., Diamond, H., et al. (1974). Pregnancy and azathioprine in systemic lupus erythematosus. *American Journal of Obstetrics and Gynecology, 118*, 25.

Symington, G. R., Mackay, I. R., & Lambert, R. P. (1977). Cancer and teratogens: Infrequent occurrence after medical use of immunosuppressive drugs. *Australia and New Zealand Journal of Medicine, 7*, 368.

Tuchmann-Duplessis, H., & Mercier-Parot, L. (1968). Foetopathes therapeutiques: Production experimentale de malformations des members. *Union Medicale Canada, 97*, 283–288.

Williamson, R. A., & Karp, L. E. (1981). Azathioprine teratogenicity: Review of the literature and case report. *Obstetrics and Gynecology, 58*, 247–250.

BCG Vaccine

FDA: **C**   SIGNIFICANCE: **5**   POTENCY: **4**

BCG is a live bacterial vaccine. It has a history of safe use during pregnancy, but no controlled studies have been performed. More data are needed.

Hart, R. J. (1981). Immunizations. *Clinical Obstetrics and Gynecology, 8*, 421–430.

Belladonna

FDA: **C**   SIGNIFICANCE: **3**   POTENCY: **3**

Retrospective data have not shown an association between the use of belladonna during pregnancy and congenital malformations among offspring. However, a cohort study associated belladonna with an increased risk for congenital malformations, particularly eye and ear defects.

Heinonen, O. P., Slone, D., & Shapiro, S. (1977). *Birth defects and drugs in pregnancy.* Littleton, MA: Publishing Sciences Group.

Milkovich, L., & Van den Berg, B. J. (1976). An evaluation of the teratogenicity of certain antinauseant drugs. *American Journal of Obstetrics and Gynecology, 125,* 244.

Bendroflumethiazide

FDA: **C**   SIGNIFICANCE: **4–5**   POTENCY: **4**

No teratogenic effects have been associated with the use of bendroflumethiazide during pregnancy. However, only limited data are available for the first trimester. More data are needed.

Cuadros, A., & Tatum, H. J. (1964). The prophylactic and therapeutic use of bendroflumethiazide in pregnancy. *American Journal of Obstetrics and Gynecology, 89,* 891–897.

Heinonen, O. P., Slone, D., & Shapiro, S. (1977). *Birth defects and drugs in pregnancy.* Littleton, MA: Publishing Sciences Group.

Leather, H. M., Humphreys, D. M., Baker, P., et al. (1968). A controlled trial of hypotensive agents in hypertension in pregnancy. *The Lancet, 2,* 488–490.

Benzoyl Peroxide

FDA: **C**   SIGNIFICANCE: **4–5**   POTENCY: **4**

Benzoyl peroxide is commonly used in external topical formulations for skin conditions. It is usually used by adolescents for mild to moderate acne vulgaris. Benzoyl peroxide is absorbed into the skin, where it is metabolized to benzoic acid and excreted in the urine as benzoate. The extensive use of benzoyl peroxide among adolescents without reports of teratogenic effects would indicate that benzoyl peroxide is not a human teratogen or that, if it is, the incidence of teratogenicity is rare.

Benztropine

FDA: **C**   SIGNIFICANCE: **4**   POTENCY: **3**

There is a report of two infants born with birth defects whose mothers (n = 2) were receiving phenothiazine in combination with benztropine (2 mg/day). Both infants exposed in utero had the small left colon syndrome (i.e., abdominal distension, decreased intestinal motility, failure to pass meconium, vomiting). Whether this was a chance association, the action of coteratogens, or the result of benztropine alone can be determined only by the evaluation of additional data.

Falterman, G. G., & Richardson, C. J. (1980). Small left colon syndrome associated with maternal ingestion of psychotropic drugs. *The Journal of Pediatrics, 97,* 308–310.

Brompheniramine

FDA: **B**   SIGNIFICANCE: **4**   POTENCY: **3–4**

In one study, brompheniramine use during pregnancy was associated with an increased number of congenital malformations among offspring. Unfortunately, the defects were not specified. In another study, a slight increase in the frequency of congenital malformations was noted, but these were generally mild defects that occurred at widely varying rates among reporting institutions. Two other large studies in which women received brompheniramine during the first trimester (n = 270) or anytime while pregnant (n = 412) failed to support an increased incidence of congenital malformations. (*See* Chlorpheniramine monograph.)

Aselton, P., Jick, H., Milunsky, A., et al. (1984). First-trimester drug use and congenital disorders. *Obstetrics and Gynecology, 65,* 451–455.

Greenberger, P., & Patterson, R. (1978). Safety of therapy for allergic symptoms during pregnancy. *Annals of Internal Medicine, 89,* 234–237.

Heinonen, O. P., Slone, D., & Shapiro, S. (1977). *Birth defects and drugs in pregnancy.* Littleton, MA: Publishing Sciences Group.

Jick, H., Holmes, L. B., Hunter, J. R., et al. (1981). First-trimester drug use and congenital disorders. *Journal of the American Medical Association, 246,* 343–346.

Bupivacaine

FDA: **C**   SIGNIFICANCE: **2–3**   POTENCY: **1–2**

Several studies have supported the safety of bupivacaine epidural analgesia during labor. However, other studies have documented fetotoxic effects, including fetal bradycardia, when bupivacaine was administered by means of paracervical block. This effect, which occurred in up to 30% of patients, was generally transient. It is recommended that fetal heart rate be monitored during this procedure. Use of 0.75% bupivacaine for obstetrical anesthesia has been associated with maternal cardiac arrest and death.

Abboud, T. K., Khoo, S. S., Miller, F., et al. (1982). Maternal, fetal, and neonatal responses after epidural anesthesia with bupivacaine, 2-chloroprocaine, or lidocaine. *Anesthesia and Analgesia, 61,* 638–644.

Belfrage, P., Raabe, N., Thalme, B., et al. (1975). Lumbar epidural analgesia with bupivacaine in labor. *American Journal of Obstetrics and Gynecology, 121,* 360–365.

Cooper, L. V., Stephen, G. W., & Aggett, P. J. (1977). Elimination of pethidine and bupivacaine in the newborn. *Archives of Disease in Childhood, 52,* 638–641.

Lavin, J. P., Samuels, S. V., Miodovnik, M., et al. (1981). The effects of bupivacaine and chloroprocaine as local anesthetics for epidural anesthesia on fetal heart rate monitoring parameters. *American Journal of Obstetrics and Gynecology, 141*(6), 717–722.

Notarianni, L. J. (1981). Placental transfer of pethidine and bupivacaine. *Neuropharmacology, 20,* 1253–1258.

Puolakka, J., Jouppila, R., Jouppila, P., et al. (1984). Maternal and fetal effects of low-dosage bupivacaine paracervical block. *Journal of Perinatal Medicine, 12,* 75–84.

Scanlon, J. W., Ostheimer, G. W., Lurie, A. B., et al. (1976). Neurobehavioral responses and drug concentrations in newborns after maternal epidural anesthesia with bupivacaine. *Anesthesiology, 45,* 400–405.

Teramo, K. (1971). Effects of obstetrical paracervical blockade on the fetus. *Acta Obstetricia et Gynecologica Scandinavica, 16*(Suppl), 1–55.

Busulfan

FDA: D SIGNIFICANCE: 1–2 POTENCY: 2–3

There has been only one report of teratogenic effects when busulfan was used alone. Other reports primarily concern its use in combination with other antineoplastic drugs; such use resulted in several congenital defects (cleft palate, corneal opacities, cytomegaly, microphthalmia) and intrauterine and postnatal growth retardation. More data are needed.

Boros, S. J., & Reynolds, J. W. (1977). Intrauterine growth retardation following third-trimester exposure to busulfan. *American Journal of Obstetrics and Gynecology, 129,* 111–112.

Diamond, I. J., Anderson, M. M., & McCreadie, S. R. (1960). Transplacental transmission of busulfan (Myleran) in a mother with leukemia—Product of fetal malformation and cytomegaly. *Pediatrics, 25,* 85.

Golbus, M. S. (1980). Teratology for the obstetrician: Current status. *Obstetrics and Gynecology, 55,* 269–277.

Caffeine

FDA: C SIGNIFICANCE: 1 (reduced birth weight)
POTENCY: 1 (reduced birth weight)

Caffeine is a widely consumed drug, probably more so than alcohol. Some human studies have associated caffeine consumption with human teratogenic effects. One reference reported three cases in which maternal consumption of eight or more cups of coffee per day during pregnancy was associated with limb defects among offspring. However, more recent human studies have not supported teratogenic effects, although a fetotoxic effect has been conclusively associated with maternal caffeine use during pregnancy. Maternal ingestion of three or more cups of coffee per day has been associated with reduced birth weight. However, this effect may be confounded by concurrent tobacco use because of the high correlation between coffee consumption and smoking among women. (*See* Tobacco Smoking monograph.)

Bourlee, I., Lechat, M. F., Bouckaert, A., et al. (1978). Le cafe, facteur de risque pendant la grossesse? *Louvain Medicine, 97,* 279–284.

Infante-Rivard, C., Fernandez, A., Gauthier, R., et al. (1993). Fetal loss associated with caffeine intake before and during pregnancy. *Journal of the American Medical Association, 270,* 2940–2943.

Jacobson, M. F., Goldman, A. S., & Syme, R. H. (1981). Coffee and birth defects. *The Lancet, 1,* 1415–1416.

Kurppa, K., Holmberg, P. C., Kuosma, E., et al. (1982). Coffee consumption during pregnancy. *New England Journal of Medicine, 306,* 1548.

Lechat, M. F., Bourlée, I., Bouckaert, A., et al. (1980). Caffeine study. [Letter]. *Science, 207,* 1296–1297.

Linn, S., Schoenblum, S. C., Monson, R. R., et al. (1982). No association between coffee consumption and adverse outcomes of pregnancy. *New England Journal of Medicine, 306,* 141–145.

Martin, J. C. (1982). An overview: Maternal nicotine and caffeine consumption and offspring outcome. *Neurobehavioral Toxicology and Teratology, 4,* 421–428.

Martin, T., & Bracken, M. (1987). Maternal caffeine use and low birth weight. *American Journal of Epidemiology, 126,* 813–821.

Ritter, E. J., Scott, W. J., Wilson, J. G., et al. (1982). Potentiative interactions between caffeine and various teratogenic agents. *Teratology, 25,* 95–100.

Rossenberg, L., Mitchell, A. A., Shapiro, S., et al. (1982). Selected birth defects in relation to caffeine-containing beverages. *Journal of the American Medical Association, 247,* 1429–1432.

Weathersbee, D. S., Olsen, L. K., & Lodge, J. R. (1977). Topics in primary care—Caffeine and pregnancy. *Postgraduate Medicine, 62,* 64–69.

Calcium Salts

FDA: C   SIGNIFICANCE: 4–5   POTENCY: 4

The use of calcium salts in mineral supplements by women during pregnancy does not appear to present a significant teratogenic risk for the developing embryo or fetus.

Heinonen, O. P., Slone, D., & Shapiro, S. (1977). *Birth defects and drugs in pregnancy.* Littleton, MA: Publishing Sciences Group.

Captopril

FDA: C   SIGNIFICANCE: 2 (near term)
POTENCY: 2

No congenital anomalies were noted in 14 infants born to women who received captopril during the first trimester. Captopril does, however, appear to be fetotoxic. Near term, placental transfer of the drug results in expected pharmacologic effects among neonates (i.e., suppression of angiotensin-converting enzyme activity and increased renin plasma levels). Several cases of severe, but in one case reversible, neonatal renal failure have been reported and associated with captopril. In addition, use during the second or third trimester reportedly has been associated with fetal calvarial hypoplasia, fetal death, fetal hypotension, intrauterine growth retardation, oligohydramnios, pulmonary hypoplasia, and renal tubular dysplasia. The use of a different antihypertensive is recommended for pregnant women who require an antihypertensive during the last two trimesters. If this is not possible, the neonate should be monitored and treated appropriately. More data are needed in regard to maternal captopril use, particularly during the first and second trimesters.

Brent, R. L., & Beckman, D. A. (1991). Angiotensin-converting enzyme inhibitors, an embryopathic class of drugs with unique properties: Information for clinical teratology counsellors. *Teratology, 43,* 543–546.

Hanssens, M., Keirse, M. J. N. C., Vankelecom, F., et al. (1991). Fetal and neonatal effects of treatment with angiotensin-converting enzyme inhibitors in pregnancy. *Obstetrics and Gynecology, 78*(1), 128–135.

Kreft-Jais, C., & Boutroy, M. J. (1988). Angiotensin-converting enzyme inhibitors during pregnancy: A survey of 22 patients given captopril and nine given enalapril. *British Journal of Obstetrics and Gynaecology, 95,* 420–422.

Rosa, F. W., Bosco, L. A., Graham, C. F., et al. (1989). Neonatal anuria with maternal angiotensin-converting enzyme inhibition. *Obstetrics and Gynecology, 74,* 371–374.

Rothberg, A. D., & Lorenz, R. (1984). Can captopril cause fetal and neonatal renal failure? *Pediatric Pharmacology, 4,* 189–192.

Schubiger, G., Flury, G., & Nussberger, J. (1988). Enalapril for pregnancy-induced hypertension: Acute renal failure in a neonate. *Annals of Internal Medicine, 108,* 215–216.

Sedman, A. B., Kershaw, D. B., & Bunchman, T. E. (1995). Recognition and management of angiotensin converting enzyme inhibitor fetopathy. *Pediatric Nephrology, 9*(3), 382–385.

Carbamazepine

FDA: C   SIGNIFICANCE: 1   POTENCY: 1–2

Initial data regarding carbamazepine use during pregnancy were conflicting; fetotoxic effects were reported, although a possible protective effect also was identified. More recently, data indicate that carbamazepine is indeed a teratogen and produces similar effects as produced by other anticonvulsants when used during pregnancy: cardiac and CNS defects, cleft lip and/or palate, depressed nasal bridge, hypoplastic nails, intrauterine and postnatal growth retardation, and mental retardation. **In addition, because carbamazepine is a folic acid antagonist, its use during pregnancy results in an increased risk for neural-tube defects. Thus, the use of a folic acid supplement is generally recommended.** Of particular concern are data providing evidence that the combination of carbamazepine, valproate, and phenobarbital or phenytoin has a particularly high rate of teratogenicity. One study reported a 58% incidence. (*See* Folic Acid monograph.)

Hernandez–Diaz, S., Werler, M. M., Walker, A. M., et al. (2000). Folic acid antagonists during pregnancy and the risk of birth defects. *New England Journal of Medicine, 343*(22), 1608–1614.

Hilesmaa, V. K., Teramo, K., & Granstrom, M. L. (1981). Fetal head growth retardation associated with maternal antiepileptic drugs. *The Lancet, 2*, 165–167.

Jones, K. L., Lacro, R. V., Johnson, K. A., et al. (1989). Pattern of malformations in the children of women treated with carbamazepine during pregnancy. *New England Journal of Medicine, 320*, 1661–1666.

Kaneko, S., Otani, K., Kondo, T., et al. (1992). Malformation in infants of mothers with epilepsy receiving antiepileptic drugs. *Neurology, 42*(Suppl 5), 68–74.

Lindhout, D., Hoppener, R. J., & Minardi, H. (1984). Teratogenicity of antiepileptic drug combinations with special emphasis on epoxidation (of carbamazepine). *Epilepsia, 25*, 77–83.

Lindhout, D., Meinardi, H., & Barth, P. G. (1982). Hazards of fetal exposure to drug combinations. In D. Janz, L. Bossi, M. Dom, et al., Eds., *Epilepsy, pregnancy and the child*, pp. 275–280. New York: Raven.

Merlob, P., Mor, N., & Litwin, A. (1992). Transient hepatic dysfunction in an infant of an epileptic mother treated with carbamazepine during pregnancy and breast-feeding. *The Annals of Pharmacotherapy, 26*, 1563–1565.

Millar, J. H., & Nevin, N. C. (1973). Congenital malformations and anticonvulsant drugs. *The Lancet, 1*, 328.

Nakane, Y., Okuma, T., Takahashi, R., et al. (1980). Multi-institutional study of the teratogenicity and fetal toxicity of antiepileptic drugs: A report of a collaborative study group in Japan. *Epilepsia, 21*, 663–680.

Samren, E. B., van Duijn, C. M., Koch, S., et al. (1997). Maternal use of antiepileptic drugs and the risk of major congenital malformations: A joint European prospective study of human teratogenesis associated with maternal epilepsy. *Epilepsia, 38*(9), 981–990.

Shakir, R. A., & Abdulwahab, B. (1991). Congenital malformations before and after the onset of maternal epilepsy. *Acta Neurologica Scandinavica, 84*, 153–156.

Starrveld-Zimmerman, A. A., Van der Kolk, W. J., & Meinardi, H. (1973). Are anticonvulsants teratogenic? *The Lancet, 2*, 48–49.

Thomas, D., & Buchanan, N. (1981). Teratogenic effects of anticonvulsants. *The Journal of Pediatrics, 99*, 163.

Vestermark, V. (1983). Teratogenicity of carbamazepine: A review of the literature. *Developmental Brain Dysfunction, 6*, 266–278.

Cascara Sagrada
FDA: C   SIGNIFICANCE: 4–5   POTENCY: 4

Cascara sagrada use by pregnant women has not been associated with a significant teratogenic risk for the developing embryo or fetus.

Heinonen, O. P., Slone, D., & Shapiro, S. (1977). *Birth defects and drugs in pregnancy*. Littleton, MA: Publishing Sciences Group.

Casanthranol
FDA: C   SIGNIFICANCE: 3–4   POTENCY: 2–3

This anthraquinone-type laxative was associated with an increased risk for major congenital malformations in one small study involving several subjects. Another anthraquinone (i.e., dihydroxyanthraquinone) also has been shown to cross the placenta and to be detectable in amniotic fluid. It would seem prudent to avoid the use of the anthraquinone family of laxatives for constipation in pregnant women because of the availability of other laxatives with less teratogenic risk.

Blair, A. W., Burdon, M., Powell, J., et al. (1977). Fetal exposure to 1,8-dihydroxyanthraquinone. *Biological Neonate, 31*, 289.

Heinonen, O. P., Slone, D., & Shapiro, S. (1977). *Birth defects and drugs in pregnancy*. Littleton, MA: Publishing Sciences Group.

Cephalothin
FDA: B   SIGNIFICANCE: 5   POTENCY: 4

Several studies have examined the fetotoxic effects of cephalothin when administered to women during labor. Although cephalothin readily crosses the placenta, no adverse effects have been noted in the newborn. Within this clinical context, cephalothin may be considered to have a low potential for toxicity. However, more studies are needed to assess the teratogenic risk of long-term cephalothin use during the first and second trimesters.

Hirsch, H. A. (1971). The use of cephalothin antibiotics in pregnant women. *Postgraduate Medical Journal, 5*, 90–93.

MacAuley, M. A., & Charles, D. (1968). Placental transfer of cephalosporins. *American Journal of Obstetrics and Gynecology, 109*, 940–946.

Pruitt, A., & Dayton, P. (1971). A comparison of the

binding of drugs to adult and cord plasma. *European Journal of Clinical Pharmacology, 4*, 59–62.
Sheng, K. T., Huang, N. N., & Promadhattavedi, V. (1964). Serum concentrations of cephalothin in infants and children and placental transmission of the antibiotic. *Antimicrobial Agents and Chemotherapy, 1*, 200–206.

Chloral Hydrate

FDA: **C**   SIGNIFICANCE: **4–5** (congenital anomalies)

POTENCY: **4** (congenital anomalies)

Chloral hydrate use during pregnancy does not appear to present a significant teratogenic risk. However, chloral hydrate does cross the placenta and regular maternal use near term may result in fetotoxic effects associated with the expected pharmacology of chloral hydrate as a sedative-hypnotic (i.e., lethargy, poor suck). High-dose, long-term chloral hydrate use or regular personal use may result in the neonatal chloral hydrate-withdrawal syndrome.

Heinonen, O. P., Slone, D., & Shapiro, S. (1977). *Birth defects and drugs in pregnancy*. Littleton, MA: Publishing Sciences Group.

Chlorambucil

FDA: **D**   SIGNIFICANCE: **2–3**   POTENCY: **2–3**

Chlorambucil is an alkylating-type antineoplastic drug. There are three case reports of renal damage, including agenesis, among infants whose mothers had received chlorambucil during pregnancy. There also are some negative reports. More data are needed.

Golbus, M. S. (1980). Teratology for the obstetrician: Current status. *Obstetrics and Gynecology, 55*, 269–277.
Shotten, D., & Monie, I. W. (1963). Possible teratogenic effect of chlorambucil on a human fetus. *Journal of the American Medical Association, 186*, 74–75.
Steege, J. F., & Caldwell, D. S. (1980). Renal agenesis after first trimester exposure to chlorambucil. *Southern Medical Journal, 73*, 1414–1415.

Chloramphenicol

FDA: **C**   SIGNIFICANCE: **4**   POTENCY: **3**

Chloramphenicol use during pregnancy has been associated with cleft lip and/or palate among offspring. However, the reported incidence of teratogenic effects is not significantly increased above the incidence expected generally among pregnant women. No fetotoxic effects were noted when chloramphenicol was administered to women during labor. However, chloramphenicol does cross the placenta, and the potential for the gray baby syndrome (*see* Chapter 5) should be kept in mind, particularly when high doses are administered to the mother.

Heinonen, O. P., Slone, D., & Shapiro, S. (1977). *Birth defects and drugs in pregnancy*. Littleton, MA: Publishing Sciences Group.
Lischner, H., Seligman, S. J., Krammer, A., et al. (1961). An outbreak of neonatal deaths among term infants associated with administration of chloramphenicol. *The Journal of Pediatrics, 59*, 21–34.
Saxen, I. (1975). Associations between oral clefts and drugs taken during pregnancy. *International Journal of Epidemiology, 4*, 37–44.
Scott, W. C., & Warner, R. F. (1950). Placental transfer of chloramphenicol (Chloromycetin). *Journal of the American Medical Association, 142*, 1331–1332.
Stewart, K. S. (1981). Bacterial infections. *Clinical Obstetrics and Gynecology, 8*, 315–332.
Weiss, C. F., Glazko, A. J., & Weston, J. K. (1960). Chloramphenicol in the newborn infant, a physiologic explanation of its toxicity when given in excessive doses. *New England Journal of Medicine, 262*, 767–794.

Chlordiazepoxide

FDA: **D**   SIGNIFICANCE: **4**   POTENCY: **2–3**

Initial data indicated that an embryo exposed to chlordiazepoxide during the first 42 days after conception had a 4.5 times increased risk for severe congenital malformations and an increased risk for fetal death than nonexposed embryos. Subsequent studies failed to support this evidence. Because of the diversity of the anomalies initially reported, some researchers concluded that it was doubtful they were induced by chlordiazepoxide.

In regard to fetotoxic effects, neonates whose mothers receive long-term chlordiazepoxide during the last trimester may display the expected pharmacologic effects associated with chlordiazepoxide (e.g., convulsions, hyperexcitability, lethargy, respiratory depression, somnolence). A neonatal chlordiazepoxide-withdrawal syndrome (crying, insomnia, irritability, poor breast-feeding) may be observed, but it generally abates over several days, with complete recovery. (*See* Diazepam monograph.)

Crombie, D. L., Pinsent, R. J., Fleming, D. M., et al. (1975). Fetal effects of tranquilizers in pregnancy. *New England Journal of Medicine, 293,* 198–199.

Decancq, H. G., Bosco, J. R., & Townsend, E. H. (1965). Chlordiazepoxide in labor, its effect on the newborn infant. *The Journal of Pediatrics, 67,* 836–840.

Hartz, S. C., Heinonen, O. P., Shapiro, S., et al. (1975). Antenatal exposure to meprobamate and chlordiazepoxide in relation to malformations, mental development, and childhood mortality. *New England Journal of Medicine, 292,* 726–728.

Kullander, S., & Kallen, B. (1976). A prospective study of drugs and pregnancy. *Acta Obstetricia et Gynecologica Scandinavica, 55,* 24–33.

Lean, T. H., Ratnam, S. S., & Sivasamboo, R. (1968). The use of chlordiazepoxide in patients with severe pregnancy toxaemia (a preliminary study of effects on the newborn infants). *Journal of Obstetrics and Gynecology in the British Commonwealth, 75,* 853–855.

Milkovich, L., & Van den Berg, B. J. (1974). Effects of prenatal meprobamate and chlordiazepoxide hydrochloride on human embryonic and fetal development. *New England Journal of Medicine, 291,* 1268–1271.

Saxen, I., & Saxen, L. (1975). Association between maternal intake of diazepam and oral clefts. *The Lancet, 2,* 498.

Tuchmann-Duplesis, H. (1975). *Drug effects on the fetus.* Acton, MA: Publishing Sciences Group.

Tuchmann-Duplesis, H. (1983). The teratogenic risk. *American Journal of Industrial Medicine, 4,* 245–258.

Chloroform
AUTHOR: **NONE**   SIGNIFICANCE: **4**
POTENCY: **3**

No significant risk of congenital anomalies was noted among 128 women who were laboratory workers and had been exposed to chloroform during the first trimester. Another study examined the fetotoxic effects of chloroform when used as an inhalation anesthestic during labor. Of 526 neonates, 30 displayed some degree of apnea neonatorum. However, the incidence did not differ significantly from the control group. Signs and symptoms were reversible with proper recognition and care. Although chloroform is no longer used in North America as an anesthetic, it is still commonly available in many laboratories.

Axelsson, G., Lutz, C., & Rylander, R. (1984). Exposure to solvents and outcome of pregnancy in university laboratory employees. *British Journal of Industrial Medicine, 41,* 305–312.

Taylor, C. R. (1961). The effect of analgesia and anesthesia on the initial fetal respirations, with particular reference to the use of chloroform, levallorphan and halothane. *American Journal of Obstetrics and Gynecology, 81,* 1260–1265.

Chloroprocaine
FDA: **C**   SIGNIFICANCE: **4**   POTENCY: **3**

Chloroprocaine has been used for extradural analgesia during labor with little or no neurological depression or other fetotoxic effects (i.e., fetal heart rate deceleration). Studies during other phases of pregnancy have not been reported.

Abboud, T. K., Afrasiabi, A., Sarkis, F., et al. (1984). Continuous infusion epidural analgesia in parturients receiving bupivacaine, chloroprocaine, or lidocaine—Maternal, fetal, and neonatal effects. *Anesthesia and Analgesia, 63,* 421–428.

Hodgkinson, R., Marx, G. F., Kim, S. S., et al. (1977). Neonatal neurobehavioral tests following vaginal delivery under ketamine, thiopental and extradural anesthesia. *Anesthesia and Analgesia, 56,* 548–553.

Kuhnert, B. R., & Linn, P. L. The effect of chloroprocaine on neonatal neurobehavior. *Anesthesia and Analgesia, 64,* 1223–1224.

Scanlon, J. W., Brown, W. U., Weiss, J. B., et al. (1974). Neurobehavioral responses of newborn infants after maternal epidural anesthesia. *Anesthesiology, 40,* 121–126.

Chloroquine
FDA: **C**   SIGNIFICANCE: **3**   POTENCY: **3**

The data relating chloroquine use during pregnancy to teratogenesis are conflicting. Although both vestibular and cochlear otoxicity have been reported secondary to in utero exposure, negative reports also exist. If chloroquine is a teratogen, the incidence of teratogenicity is apparently low; it continues to be recommended for both the treatment and prophylaxis of malaria among pregnant women. Long-term use during pregnancy has been associated with neonatal chorioretinitis. Again, however, the risk appears to be minimal.

Beeley, L. (1981). Adverse effects of drugs in later pregnancy. *Clinical Obstetrics and Gynecology, 8*, 275–290.

Hart, C. W., & Naunton, R. F. (1964). The ototoxicity of chloroquine phosphate. *Archives of Otolaryngology, 80*, 407–412.

Klumpp, T. G. (1965). Safety of chloroquine in pregnancy. *Journal of the American Medical Association, 191*, 765.

Levy, M., Buskila, D., Gladman, D. D., et al. (1991). Pregnancy outcome following first trimester exposure to chloroquine. *American Journal of Perinatology, 8*(3), 174–178.

Parke, A. (1988). Antimalarial drugs and pregnancy. *American Journal of Medicine, 85*(Suppl 4A), 30–33.

Smith, D. W. (1966). Dysmorphology (teratology). *Journal of the American Medical Association, 69*, 1150–1169.

Trussell, R. R., & Beeley, L. (1981). Infestations. *Clinical Obstetrics and Gynecology, 8*, 333–340.

Wolfe, M. S., & Cordero, J. F. (1985). Safety of chloroquine in chemosuppression of malaria during pregnancy. *British Medical Journal, 290*, 1466–1467.

Chlorothiazide

FDA: **B**   SIGNIFICANCE: **4**   POTENCY: **3**

No teratogenic effects have been associated with chlorothiazide use during pregnancy. However, some authors recommend that chlorothiazide be avoided during pregnancy because its use has been associated with maternal cholestasis and pancreatitis. These authors also report decreased steroidogenesis by the placenta. Thrombocytopenia also is a rare complication. More data are needed.

Finnerty, F. A., & Assali, N. S. (1965). Thiazide and neonatal thrombocytopenia. *New England Journal of Medicine, 271*, 160–161.

Kraus, G. W., Marchese, J. R., & Yen, S. S. C. (1966). Prophylactic use of hydrochlorothiazide in pregnancy. *Journal of the American Medical Association, 198*, 1150–1154.

McBride, W. G. (1963). The teratogenic action of drugs. *Medical Journal of Australia, 2*, 689–693.

Rodriquez, S. U., Sanford, L. L., & Hiller, M. C. (1964). Neonatal thrombocytopenia associated with antepartum administration of thiazide drugs. *New England Journal of Medicine, 270*, 881–884.

Wesley, A. C., & Douglas, G. K. (1962). Continuous use of chlorothiazide for prevention of toxemia of pregnancy. *Obstetrics and Gynecology, 19*, 355–358.

Wood, S. M., & Blainey, J. D. (1981). Hypertension and renal disease. *Clinical Obstetrics and Gynecology, 8*, 439–453.

Chlorpheniramine

FDA: **B**   SIGNIFICANCE: **4**   POTENCY: **3–4**

Conflicting data concerning the teratogenic risk of chlorpheniramine have been reported. Among infants born to women (n = 1070) receiving chlorpheniramine during the first trimester a small, but significant, increase in risk for inguinal hernia or ear and eye anomalies was noted. However, this increased risk was not found in two similar sequential cohort studies (n = 275). In addition, the incidence of congenital anomalies was not increased among the offspring of women (n = 3931) who received chlorpheniramine at various times during their pregnancies. More data are needed. (See Brompheniramine monograph.)

Aselton, P., Jick, H., Milunsky, A., et al. (1985). First-trimester drug use and congenital disorders. *Obstetrics and Gynecology, 65*, 451–455.

Greenberger, P., & Patterson, R. (1978). Safety of therapy for allergic symptoms during pregnancy. *Annals of Internal Medicine, 89*, 234–237.

Heinonen, O. P., Slone, D., & Shapiro, S. (1977). *Birth defects and drugs in pregnancy*. Littleton, MA: Publishing Sciences Group.

Jick, H., Holmes, L. B., Hunter, J. R., et al. (1981). First-trimester drug use and congenital disorders. *Journal of the American Medical Association, 246*, 343–346.

Chlorpromazine

FDA: **C**   SIGNIFICANCE: **4**   POTENCY: **3**

Data regarding the teratogenic potential of chlorpromazine during pregnancy are conflicting. In one study of 315 infants exposed to phenothiazines in utero, the three-carbon side chain phenothiazines were associated with an increased rate of congenital malformations ($p < 0.01$). Observed defects included abdominal muscle aplasia, brachmesophalangy, cardiac malformations, cleft lip, clinodactyly, club hands and feet, hydrocephalus, hypospadias, microcephaly, and syndactyly. In another study, however, no such associations were found. If chlorpromazine is a teratogen, the overall incidence appears to be very low.

In regard to fetotoxicity, maternal use during labor has been associated with neonatal CNS depression and a neonatal extrapyramidal syndrome. Several case reports describe the occurrence of neurological dysfunction with extrapyramidal effects (hypertonia, muscle rigidity, tremor) among neonates whose mothers had received chlorpromazine during pregnancy. Although these effects were generally transient, they persisted for several months for some infants.

Ananth, J. (1976). Side effects on the fetus and infant of psychotropic drug use during pregnancy. *International Pharmacopsychiatry, 11*, 246–265.

Farkas, V. G., & Farkas, G. (1971). Teratogenic action of hyperemesis in pregnancy and of medication used to treat it. *Zentralblatt fur Gynakologie, 10*, 325–330.

Hammond, J. E., & Toseland, P. A. (1970). Placental transfer of chlorpromazine. A case report. *Archives of Disease in Childhood, 45*, 139.

Heinonen, O. P., Slone D., & Shapiro, S. (1977). *Birth defects and drugs in pregnancy.* Littleton, MA: Publishing Sciences Group.

Hill, R. M., Desmond, M. M., & Kay, J. L. (1966). Extrapyramidal dysfunction in an infant of a schizophrenic mother. *The Journal of Pediatrics, 69*, 589–595.

Levy, W., & Wiseniewski, K. (1974). Chlorpromazine causing extrapyramidal dysfunction in newborn infant of psychotic mother. *New York State Journal of Medicine, 74*, 684–685.

Rumeau-Rouquette, G., Goujard, J., & Huel, G. (1977). Possible teratogenic effects of phenothiazines in human beings. *Teratology, 15*, 57–64.

Slone, D., Siskind, V., Heinonen, O. P., et al. (1977). Antenatal exposure to the phenothiazines in relation to congenital malformations, perinatal mortality rate, birth weight, and intelligent quotient scores. *American Journal of Obstetrics and Gynecology, 128*, 468–488.

Sobel, D. E. (1960). Fetal damage due to ECT, insulin coma, chlorpromazine or reserpine. *American Medical Association Archives of General Psychiatry, 2*, 606–611.

Tamer, A., McKey, R., Arias, D., et al. (1969). Phenothiazine-induced extrapyramidal dysfunction in the neonate. *The Journal of Pediatrics, 75*, 479–480.

Chlorpropamide

FDA: **D**   SIGNIFICANCE: **2**   POTENCY: **2–3**

Initially, chlorpropamide was associated with a high rate of fetal mortality. Later studies demonstrated that 200–250 mg/day resulted in no effect on the fetus or neonate, whereas doses exceeding 500 mg/day increased the risk for perinatal mortality. Infants of diabetic mothers have an increased malformation rate associated with the disease. A single case report associated maternal chlorpropamide use with neonatal hypoglycemia and hypernatremia. Neonates of diabetic mothers should be routinely monitored for these effects.

Adashi, E. V., Piato, H., & Tyson, J. E. (1979). Impact of maternal euglycemia on fetal outcome in diabetic pregnancy. *American Journal of Obstetrics and Gynecology, 133*, 268–274.

Campbell, G. D. (1963). Chlorpropamide and foetal damage. *British Medical Journal, 1*, 59–60.

Douglas, C. P., & Richards, R. (1967). Use of chlorpropamide in the treatment of diabetes in pregnancy. *Diabetes, 16*, 60–61.

Jackson, W. P., Campbell, G. D., Notelovitz, M., et al. (1962). Tolbutamide and chlorpropamide during pregnancy in humans. *Diabetes, 11*(Suppl), 98–103.

Karlsson, K., & Kjellmer, I. (1972). The outcome of diabetic pregnancies in relation to the mothers' blood sugar level. *American Journal of Obstetrics and Gynecology, 112*, 213–220.

Landouer, W. (1972). Is insulin a teratogen? *Teratology, 5*, 129–136.

Malins, J. M., Cooke, A. M., Pyke, D. A., et al. (1964). Sulphonylurea drugs in pregnancy. *British Medical Journal, 2*, 187.

Notelovitz, M. (1975). Sulphonylurea therapy in the treatment of the pregnant diabetic. *South African Medical Journal, 45*, 226–229.

Passarge, E., & Lenz, W. (1966). Syndrome of caudal regression in infants of diabetic mothers: Observation of further cases. *Pediatrics, 37*, 672–675.

Piacquadio, K., Hollingsworth, D. R., & Murphy, H. (1991). Effects of in-utero exposure to oral hypoglycaemic drugs. *The Lancet, 338*, 866–869.

Sutherland, H. W., Bewsher, P. D., Cormack, J. D., et al. (1974). Effect of moderate dosage of chlorpropamide in pregnancy on fetal outcome. *Archives of Disease in Childhood, 49*, 283–291.

Sutherland, H. W., Stawers, J. M., Cormack, J. D., et al. (1973). Evaluation of chlorpropamide in chemical diabetes diagnosed during pregnancy. *British Medical Journal, 3*, 9–13.

Uhrig, J. D., & Hurley, R. M. (1983). Chlorpropamide in pregnancy and transient neonatal diabetes insipidus. *Journal of the Canadian Medical Association, 128*(4), 368, 370–371.

Zucker, P., & Gilbert, S. (1968). Prolonged symptomatic neonatal hypoglycemia associated with maternal chlorpropamide therapy. *Pediatrics, 42*, 824–825.

Chorionic Gonadotropin

FDA: **X**   SIGNIFICANCE: **2–3** (prior to pregnancy)

POTENCY: **1–2** (prior to pregnancy)

Use of human chorionic gonadotropin for the induction of ovulation has been associated with altered sex ratios (significantly increased proportion of female offspring), increased frequency of spontaneous abortion, and multifetal pregnancies (~1/3 of cases). The multifetal pregnancies are associated with an increased incidence of congenital anomalies, fetal death, perinatal death, and premature delivery. Human chorionic gonadotropin is contraindicated in pregnant women.

Cimetidine

FDA: B   SIGNIFICANCE: 4   POTENCY: 3–4

No congenital abnormalities were noted in two reports involving nine infants born to mothers who had received cimetidine during the first trimester. A large-scale retrospective cohort study investigating the effect on neonatal outcome of acid-suppressing drugs during pregnancy found no significant teratogenic risk associated with cimetidine. A field trial of cimetidine use in obstetric anesthesia prior to Caesarean section reported no neonatal complications. However, histamine plays a role in the fetal heart response to stress, and cimetidine can block this response. Until this latter effect is shown not to be a problem, a degree of caution is warranted. Additionally, there is one report of neonatal liver toxicity associated with cimetidine use during late pregnancy.

Glode, G., Saccar, C. L., & Pereira, G. R. (1980). Cimetidine in pregnancy: Apparent transient liver impairment in the newborn. *American Journal of Diseases of Children, 134*, 87–88.

Johnston, J. R., McCaughey, W., Moore, J., et al. (1982). A field trial of cimetidine as the sole oral antacid in obstetric anaesthesia. *Anaesthesia, 37*, 33–38.

Johnston, J. R., McCaughey, W., Moore, J., et al. (1982). Cimetidine as an oral antacid before elective Caesarean section. *Anaesthesia, 37*, 26–32.

Koren, G., & Zemlickis, M. (1991). Outcome of pregnancy after first trimester exposure to H2 receptor antagonists. *American Journal of Perinatology, 8*(1), 37–38.

Ruigomez, A., Garcia Rodriguez, L. A., Cattaruzzi, C., et al. (1999). Use of cimetidine, omeprazole, and ranitidine in pregnant women and pregnancy outcomes. *American Journal of Epidemiology, 150*, 476–481.

Wollerman, M., & Popp, J. G. (1979). Blockade by cimetidine of the effects of histamine on adenylate cyclase activity, spontaneous rate and contractibility in the developing prenatal heart. *Agents and Actions, 9*, 29.

Zuel, P., & DiNisia, O. (1978). Cimetidine treatment during pregnancy. *The Lancet, 2*, 945.

Citalopram

AUTHOR: NONE   SIGNIFICANCE: 3–4
POTENCY: 3–4

In a single case report, no adverse effects from maternal citalopram use were noted in a fetus aborted at 12 weeks. The mother had received 40 mg/day for the first 3 weeks after unrecognized conception and 60 mg/day for the following 3 weeks. The fetus had normal organ formation and a normal placenta. Neuropathological examination and chromosome analysis were also normal. Citalopram, a selective serotonin reuptake inhibitor, is pharmacologically related to fluoxetine and appears to share its same low potential for teratogenesis. More data are needed. (*See* Fluoxetine monograph.)

Seifritz, E., Holsboer-Trachsler, E., Haberthur, F., et al. (1993). Unrecognized pregnancy during citalopram treatment. *American Journal of Psychiatry, 150*, 1428–1429.

Clofazimine

FDA: C   SIGNIFICANCE: 4   POTENCY: 2–3
(skin discoloration)

In one report, two women who had Hansen's disease were treated with clofazimine during their entire pregnancy. Both infants were completely normal. However, some placental abnormalities were noted with the second birth. Two other references cite pigmented skin among offspring born to women who had received clofazimine during pregnancy. This recognized ADR associated with clofazimine is secondary to either prenatal exposure or ingestion in breast milk.

Browne, S. G., & Hogerzell, L. M. (1962). "B663" in the treatment of leprosy—Preliminary reports of a pilot trial. *Leprosy Review, 33*, 6.

Farb, H., West, D. P., & Pedvis-Leftick, A. (1982). Clofazimine in pregnancy complicated by leprosy. *Obstetrics and Gynecology, 59*, 122–123.

Holdiness, M. R. (1989). Clofazimine in pregnancy. [Letter]. *Early Human Development, 18*, 297–298.

Waters, M. F. (1968). Working party on B66: Symposium on B663 (Lamprene, Giegy) in the treatment of leprosy and leprosy reactions. *International Journal of Leprosy, 36,* 560.

Clomiphene

FDA: **X**   SIGNIFICANCE: **3**   POTENCY: **2**

The data regarding the teratogenic risk of clomiphene use during pregnancy are conflicting. In one study of women receiving either clomiphene or menotropins during pregnancy, a threefold greater incidence of Down's syndrome was noted. In other studies, an increased rate of neural-tube defects was observed. Both of these defects can be diagnosed by amniocentesis. However, several other studies found no significant increase in teratogenic risk associated with clomiphene. It would appear reasonable to advise women who have conceived with the help of this drug to seek diagnostic amniocentesis and/or high-resolution ultrasound examination. Clomiphene used for the induction of ovulation has been associated with multifetal gestation (usually twinning) in approximately 10% of pregnancies. Multifetal gestation is associated with a higher incidence of complications, including miscarriage and premature delivery.

Cornel, M. C., ten Kate L. P., & te Meerman, G. J. (1990). Association between ovulation stimulation, in vitro fertilisation, and neural tube defects? *Teratology, 42,* 201–203.
Creizel, A. (1989). Ovulation induction and neural tube defects. *The Lancet, 2,* 167.
Harlap, S. (1976). Ovulation induction and congenital malformations. *The Lancet, 2,* 2961.
James, W. H. (1977). Clomiphene, anencephaly and spina bifida. *The Lancet, 1,* 603.
Kurachi, K., Aono, T., Minagawa, J., et al. (1983). Congenital malformations of newborn infants after clomiphene-induced ovulation. *Fertility and Sterility, 40,* 187–189.
Mili, F., Lhoury, M. J., & Lu, X. (1991). Clomiphene citrate use and the risk of birth defects: A population-based case-control study. *Teratology, 43*(5), 422–423.
Mills, J. L. (1991). Clomiphene and neural-tube defects. *The Lancet, 337*(8745), 853.
Mills, J. L., Simpson, J. L., Rhoads, G. G., et al. (1990). Risk of neural tube defects in relation to maternal fertility and fertility drug use. *The Lancet, 336,* 103–104.
Nevin, N. C., & Harley, J. M. (1976). Clomiphene and neural tube defects. *Ulster Medical Journal, 45,* 59–64.
Oakley, G. P., & Flynt, J. W. (1972). Increased prevalence of Down's syndrome (mongolism) among the offspring of women treated with ovulation-inducing agents. *American Journal of Human Genetics, 24,* 20a.
Vollset, S. E. (1990). Ovulation induction and neural tube defects. *The Lancet, 335,* 178.

Clomipramine

FDA: **C**   SIGNIFICANCE: **3**   POTENCY: **2–3**
(withdrawal seizures)

No teratogenic data are available on clomipramine use during the first or second trimester. Several cases of neonatal-withdrawal seizures have been reported when clomipramine was used prior to delivery. More data are needed, particularly data on use during the first trimester.

Cowe, L., Lloyd, D. J., & Dawling, S. (1982). Neonatal convulsions caused by withdrawal from maternal clomipramine. *British Medical Journal, 284,* 1837–1838.
Musa, A. B. (1979). Neonatal effects of maternal clomipramine therapy. [Letter]. *Archives of Disease in Childhood, 54*(4), 405.
Ostergaard, G. Z., & Pedersen, S. E. (1982). Neonatal effects of maternal clomipramine treatment. *Pediatrics, 69*(2), 233–234.
Singh, S., Gulati, S., Narang, A., et al. (1990). Non-narcotic withdrawal syndrome in a neonate due to maternal clomipramine therapy. [Letter]. *Journal of Paediatric and Child Health, 26*(2), 110.

Clonazepam

FDA: **D**   SIGNIFICANCE: **3**   POTENCY: **3**

Data from a single population-based, case-controlled European study did not reveal an association between clonazepam use during pregnancy and a significant risk for congenital anomalies. More data are needed, particularly data on use during the first trimester.

Czeizel, A. E., Bod, M., & Halasz, P. (1992). Evaluation of anticonvulsant drugs during pregnancy in a population-based Hungarian study. *European Journal of Epidemiology, 8*(1), 122–127.

Clonidine

FDA: **C**   SIGNIFICANCE: **3–4**   POTENCY: **3**

One study conducted at birth and another conducted during childhood failed to find a significant risk for congenital anomalies among the offspring of women who had received clonidine during the second or third trimester. Transient neonatal hypertension was reported in one study in which clonidine was employed late during the third trimester. More data are needed, particularly data on use during the first trimester.

Boutroy, M. J., Gisonna, C. R., & Legagneur, M. (1988). Clonidine: Placental transfer and neonatal adaption. *Early Human Development, 17,* 275–286.

Horvath, J. S., Phippard, A., Korda, A., et al. (1985). Clonidine hydrochloride—A safe and effective antihypertensive agent in pregnancy. *Obstetrics and Gynecology, 66*(5), 634–638.

Huisjes, H. J., Hadders-Algra, M., & Touwen, B. C. L. (1986). Is clonidine a behavioral teratogen in the human? *Early Human Development, 17,* 399–407.

Clorazepate

FDA: **C**   SIGNIFICANCE: **3**   POTENCY: see monograph

A single case report of teratogenic effects associated with clorazepate use during the first trimester was found. The infant was born at 40 weeks gestation with multiple severe congenital malformations that resulted in death within 24 hours. More data are needed to determine whether these malformations were directly related to clorazepate and, if so, to determine their incidence (i.e., potency). (*See* Chlordiazepoxide and Diazepam monographs.) Another single report describes neurobehavioral depression (a noted pharmacologic effect of clorazepate) among neonates whose mothers received clorazepate near term.

Bavoux, F., Lanfranchi, C., Olive, G., et al. (1981). Adverse effects on newborns from intra uterine exposure to benzodiazepines and other psychotropic agents. *Therapie, 36,* 305–312.

Patel, D. A., & Patel, A. R. (1980). Clorazepate and congenital malformations. *Journal of the American Medical Association, 244,* 135–136.

Clotrimazole

FDA: **B**   SIGNIFICANCE: **4–5** (topical use)
POTENCY: **3–4** (topical use)

The topical (vaginal) application of clotrimazole during pregnancy was not associated with congenital anomalies in a single large-record linkage study. More data are needed in relation to maternal systemic (oral) clotrimazole use during pregnancy, particularly use during the first trimester.

Rosa, F. W., Baum, C., & Shaw, M. (1987). Pregnancy outcomes after first-trimester vaginitis drug therapy. *Obstetrics and Gynecology, 69,* 751–755.

Tettenborn, D. (1974). Toxicity of clotrimazole. *Postgraduate Medical Journal.* (July Supplement), 17–20.

Cocaine

FDA: **C**   SIGNIFICANCE: **2–3**   POTENCY: **2**

Use of cocaine during pregnancy has increased significantly during the last 20 years. It continues to be an illicit drug commonly abused by pregnant women. Cocaine use during pregnancy has been associated with cerebral infarction and other CNS anomalies, such as disruptive brain anomalies; intestinal atresia; intrauterine death, including spontaneous abortion; intrauterine growth retardation; limb reduction; low birth weight; necrotizing enterocolitis; neonatal seizures; neonatal tachycardia; and preterm delivery. In addition, various behavioral and learning disorders (attention-deficit/hyperactivity disorder) appear to have a significantly higher incidence among preschool and school-age children exposed to cocaine in utero. Autopsies performed on fetuses exposed in utero to cocaine have commonly revealed cerebral hemorrhages. However, the congenital anomalies and behavioral effects reportedly associated with maternal cocaine use during pregnancy have been attributed by some authors to confounding factors associated with the lifestyle of women who abuse cocaine (concomitant use of other abusable psychotropics, such as alcohol and nicotine [tobacco smoking], and inadequate prenatal care). Neonates also may display signs and symptoms of cocaine withdrawal if sufficient quantities were used by the mother near term.

Brown, E., Prager, J., Lee, H-Y., et al. (1992). CNS complications of cocaine abuse: Prevalence, pathophysiology, and neuroradiology. *American Journal of Roentgenology, 159,* 137–147.

Buehler, B. A., Conover, B., & Andres, R. L. (1996). Teratogenic potential of cocaine. *Seminars in Perinatology, 20*(2), 93–98.

Burg, F. D., & Schwartz, W. (1988). Neonatal drug withdrawal. *Drug Therapy, 48,* 82–87.

Chasnoff, I. J., Bussey, M. E., Savich, R., et al. (1986). Perinatal cerebral infarction and maternal cocaine use. *The Journal of Pediatrics, 108*, 456–459.

Czyrko, C., Del Pin, C. A., O'Neill, J. A., et al. (1991). Maternal cocaine abuse and necrotizing enterocolitis: Outcome and survival. *Journal of Pediatric Surgery, 26*(4), 414–421.

Dixon, S. D., & Bejar, R. (1989) Echoencephalographic findings in neonates associated with maternal cocaine and methamphetamine use: Incidence and clinical correlates. *The Journal of Pediatrics, 115*, 770–778.

Dominguez, R., Vila-Coro, A. A., Slopis, J. M., et al. (1991). Brain and ocular abnormalities in infants with in utero exposure to cocaine and other street drugs. *American Journal of Diseases of Children, 145*, 688–695.

Heier, L. A., Carpanzano, C. R., Mast, J., et al. (1991). Maternal cocaine abuse: The spectrum of radiologic abnormalities in the neonatal CNS. *American Journal of Neuroradiology, 12*(5), 951–956.

Hoyme, H. E., Jones, K. L., Dixon, S. D., et al. (1990). Prenatal cocaine exposure and fetal vascular disruption. *Pediatrics, 85*, 743–747.

Hutchings, D. E. (1993). The puzzle of cocaine's effects following maternal use during pregnancy: Are there reconcilable differences? *Neurotoxicology and Teratology, 15*, 281–286.

Jacobs, I. G., Roszler, M. H., Kelley, J. K., et al. (1989). Cocaine abuse: Neurovascular complications. *Radiology, 170*, 223–227.

Kapur, R. P., Cheng, M. S., & Shephard, T. H. (1991). Brain hemorrhages in cocaine-exposed human fetuses. *Teratology, 44*, 11–18.

Kosofsky, B. E. (1998). Cocaine-induced alterations in neuro-development. *Seminars in Speech and Language, 19*, 109–121.

Kramer, L. D., Locke, G. E., Ogunyemi, A., et al. (1990). Neonatal cocaine-related seizures. *Journal of Child Neurology, 5*, 60–64.

Little, B. B., Snell, L. M., Klein, V. R., et al. (1989). Cocaine abuse during pregnancy: Maternal and fetal implications. *Obstetrics and Gynecology, 73*, 157–160.

Lutiger, B., Graham, K., Einarson, T. R., et al. (1991). Relationship between gestational cocaine use and pregnancy outcome: A meta-analysis. *Teratology, 44*, 405–414.

Offidani, C., Pomini, F., Caruso, A., et al. (1995). Cocaine during pregnancy: A critical review of the literature. *Minerva Ginecologica, 47*(9), 381–390.

Pagliaro, L. A. (1992). The straight dope: Focus on learning—Interpreting the interpretations. *Psynopsis, 14*(2), 8.

Porat, R., & Brodsky, N. (1991). A risk factor for necrotizing enterocolitis. *Journal of Perinatology, 11*(1), 30–32.

Rizk, B., Atterbury, J. L., & Groome, L. J. (1996). Reproductive risks of cocaine. *Human Reproduction Update, 2*(1), 43–55.

Seghal, S., Ewing, C., Waring, P., et al. (1993). Morbidity of low-birthweight infants with intrauterine cocaine exposure. *Journal of the National Medical Association, 85*(1), 20–24.

Sheinbaum, K. A., & Badell, A. (1992). Physiatric management of two neonates with limb deficiencies and prenatal cocaine exposure. *Archives of Physical Medicine and Rehabilitation, 73*, 385–388.

Sims, M. E., & Walther, F. J. (1989). Neonatal ultrasound casebook. *Journal of Perinatology, 9*, 349–350.

Snodgrass, S. R. (1994). Cocaine babies: A result of multiple teratogenic influences. *Journal of Child Neurology, 9*(3), 227–233.

Spinazzola, R., Kenigsberg, K., Usmani, S. S., et al. (1992). Neonatal gastrointestinal complications of maternal cocaine abuse. *New York State Journal of Medicine, 92*(1), 22–23.

van den Anker, J. N., Cohen-Overbeek, T. E., Wladimiroff, J. W., et al. (1991). Prenatal diagnosis of limb-reduction defects due to maternal cocaine use. *The Lancet, 228*, 1332.

Van Dyke, D. C., & Fox, A. A. (1990). Fetal drug exposure and its possible implications for learning in the preschool and school-age population. *Journal of Learning Disabilities, 23*, 160–163.

Volpe, J. J. (1992). Effect of cocaine use on the fetus. *New England Journal of Medicine, 327*(6), 399–407.

Codeine

FDA: C   SIGNIFICANCE: 4–5 (congenital anomalies)

POTENCY: 3–4 (congenital anomalies)

Cleft lip/palate and congenital heart disease have been associated with codeine use during pregnancy. However, several large studies found no significant increase in congenital anomalies. Long-term, high-dose codeine use or regular personal use near term has been associated with the neonatal opiate-withdrawal syndrome.

Aselton, P., Jick, H., Milunsky, A., et al. (1985). First-trimester drug use and congenital disorders. *Obstetrics and Gynecology, 65*, 451–455.

Bracken, M. B. (1986). Drug use in pregnancy and congenital heart disease in offspring. *New England Journal of Medicine, 314*, 1120.

Bracken, M. B., & Holford, T. R. (1981). Exposure to prescribed drugs in pregnancy and association with congenital malformations. *Obstetrics and Gynecology, 58*, 336–344.

Heinonen, O. P., Slone, D., & Shapiro, S. (1977). *Birth defects and drugs in pregnancy*. Littleton, MA: Publishing Sciences Group.

Jick, H., Holmes, L. B., Hunter, J. R., et al. (1981). First-trimester drug use and congenital disor-

ders. *Journal of the American Medical Association, 246,* 343–346.

Mangurten, H. H., & Benawra, R. (1980). Neonatal codeine withdrawal in infants of nonaddicted mothers. *Pediatrics, 65,* 159–160.

Saxen, I. (1975). Association between oral clefts and drugs taken during pregnancy. *International Journal of Epidemiology, 4,* 37–44.

Van Leeuwen, G., Guthrie, R., & Stange, F. (1965). Narcotic withdrawal reaction in a newborn infant due to codeine. *Pediatrics, 36,* 635–636.

Colchicine

FDA: **C**   SIGNIFICANCE: **2**   POTENCY: **3**

In one report of 54 women who received colchicine during pregnancy, two infants had trisomy 21. Another report involving four women who discontinued the drug upon learning they were pregnant noted one spontaneous abortion. The birth of normal infants was reported for more than 50 women who took colchicine throughout their pregnancy and for three men who were taking the drug at the time of conception.

Ehrenfeld, M., Brzezinski, A., Levy, M., et al. (1987). Fertility and obstetric history in patients with familial Mediterranean fever on long-term colchicine therapy. *British Journal of Obstetrics and Gynaecology, 94,* 1186–1191.

Ferreira, N. R., & Frota-Pessoa, O. (1969). Trisomy after colchicine therapy. *The Lancet, 1,* 1160–1161.

Zemer, D., Pras, M., Sohar, E., et al. (1976). Colchicine in familial Mediterranean fever. *New England Journal of Medicine, 294,* 170–171.

Corticosteroids

FDA: **C**   SIGNIFICANCE: **4–5**   POTENCY: **3–4**

Long-term corticosteroid use during pregnancy may be indicated for women who: (1) have a minor degree of adrenal insufficiency and whose endogenous production may not meet the increased demands associated with pregnancy, (2) have adrenal insufficiency associated with Addison's disease or hypophysectomy, and (3) are receiving adrenosuppressive therapy for asthma, inflammatory bowel disease, rheumatoid arthritis, or other conditions. For the first two groups, drug therapy is aimed only at replacing normal physiologic amounts of the corticosteroids; such use should not be of concern from a teratogenic point of view. However, the dosages required by women in the third group are cause for concern. Any observed defects must, however, be considered in relation to the confounding effects of the underlying disease(s).

Although scattered case reports of human malformations have been associated with corticosteroid use during pregnancy, numerous reports, involving more than 1500 pregnancies, found no increase in congenital malformations. In addition, a 4-year follow-up of 318 children born to women who had received corticosteroids during pregnancy noted no developmental delays. However, a recent retrospective case-controlled study using a large sample reported a possible causal association between cleft lip and palate deformities among neonates born to mothers who used corticosteroids during the first trimester.

Neonatal adrenocortical suppression, a rare complication, occurred in one of 260 neonates in one study and two of 428 neonates in another. Thus, it appears improbable that corticosteroids are true teratogens. Rarely, they may produce neonatal adrenal insufficiency. Routine supplementation of neonates exposed in utero to corticosteroids does not seem appropriate. Instead, these neonates should be followed clinically for adrenal insufficiency and treated only when clinical signs or symptoms (dehydration, hypoglycemia, hyponatremia, vomiting) warrant intervention. (See Corticotropin and Dexamethasone monographs.)

Bongiovanni, A. M., & McPadden, A. J. (1960). Steroids during pregnancy and possible fetal consequences. *Fertility and Sterility, 11,* 181–186.

Carmichael, S. L., & Shaw, G. M. (1999). Maternal corticosteroid use and risk of selected congenital anomalies. *American Journal of Medical Genetics, 86*(3), 242–244.

DeCosta, E. J., & Abelman, M. A. (1953). Cortisone and pregnancy: An experimental and clinical study of the effects of cortisone on gestation. *American Journal of Obstetrics and Gynecology, 64,* 1062–1081.

Doig, R. K., & Coltman, O. M. (1956). Cleft palate following cortisone therapy in early pregnancy. *The Lancet, 2,* 730.

Fraser, F. C., & Sajoo, A. (1995). Teratogenic potential of corticosteroids in humans. *Teratology, 51*(1), 45–46.

Harris, J. W., & Ross, I. P. (1956). Cortisone therapy in early pregnancy: Relation to cleft palate. *The Lancet, 1,* 1045–1047.

Khudr, G., & Olding, L. (1973). Cyclopia. *American Journal of Diseases of Children, 125*, 120–122.

Merkatz, I. R., Schwartz, G. H., David, D. S., et al. (1971). Resumption of female reproductive function following renal transplantation. *Journal of the American Medical Association, 216*, 1749–1754.

Mogadam, M., Dobbins, W. O., Korelitz, B. I., et al. (1981). Pregnancy in inflammatory bowel disease: Effect of sulfasalazine and corticosteroids on fetal outcome. *Gastroenterology, 80*, 72–76.

Propert, A. J. (1962). Pregnancy and adrenocortical hormones. *The British Medical Journal, 1*, 967–972.

Reinish, J. M., Simon, N. G., Karon, W. G., et al. (1978). Prenatal exposure to prednisone in humans and animals retards intrauterine growth. *Science, 202*, 436–438.

Rolf, B. B. (1966). Corticosteroids and pregnancy. *American Journal of Obstetrics and Gynecology, 95*, 339.

Serment, H., Charpin, J., Tessier, G., et al. (1978). Corticotherapie et grossesse. *Bulletin de la Federation des Societes de Gynecologie et Obstetrique de Langue Francaise, 20*, 159–161.

Sidher, R., & Hawkins, D. F. (1981). Corticosteroids. *Clinical Obstetrics and Gynecology, 8*, 383–404.

Snyder, R. D., & Snyder, D. (1978). Corticosteroids for asthma during pregnancy. *Annals of Allergy, 41*, 340.

Warrell, D. W., & Taylor, R. (1968). Outcome for the fetus of mothers receiving prednisolone during pregnancy. *The Lancet, 1*, 117–118.

Wells, C. N. (1953). Treatment of hyperemesis gravidarum with cortisone. *American Journal of Obstetrics and Gynecology, 66*, 598–601.

Yackel, D. B., Kempers, R. D., & McConahey, W. W. (1966). Adrenocorticosteroid therapy in pregnancy. *American Journal of Obstetrics and Gynecology, 96*, 985–989.

Corticotropin (ACTH)

FDA: **C**   SIGNIFICANCE: **4–5**   POTENCY: **4**

A review of 688 fetuses exposed in utero to either corticotropin or corticosteroids showed no increase in the incidence of malformations. (*See* Corticosteroids monograph.)

Golbus, M. S. (1980). Teratology for the obstetrician: Current status. *Obstetrics and Gynecology, 55*, 269–277.

Cortisone

FDA: **D**   SIGNIFICANCE: **4**   POTENCY: **3**

Two early case reports suggested the potential for cortisone use during the first trimester to cause cleft palate. However, the lack of additional reports suggests a minimal risk. (*See* Corticosteroids and Corticotropin monographs.)

Doig, R. K., & Coltman, O. M. (1956). Cleft palate following cortisone therapy in early pregnancy. *The Lancet, 2*, 730.

Greene, R. M., & Kochhar, D. M. (1975). Some aspects of corticosteroid-induced cleft palate: A review. *Teratology, 11*, 47–56.

Harris, J. W., & Ross, I. P. (1956). Cortisone therapy in early pregnancy: Relation to cleft palate. *The Lancet, 1*, 1045–1047.

Co-Trimoxazole

FDA: **C**   SIGNIFICANCE: **4**   POTENCY: **4**

Three studies of pregnant women who received co-trimoxazole (a fixed ratio combination product containing trimethoprim and sulfamethoxazole) either during the first trimester (n = 141) or at various times during their pregnancies (n = 321) failed to find an increased risk for congenital anomalies. Use near term is not recommended because of the potential for the sulfonamide component (sulfamethoxazole) to cross the placenta and induce jaundice in the neonate. (*See* Sulfonamides monograph.)

Cromolyn Sodium (Sodium Cromoglycate)

FDA: **B**   SIGNIFICANCE: **4–5**   POTENCY: **3–4**

Large-scale studies of cromolyn sodium pharmacotherapy during pregnancy and possible teratogenic effects have not been completed. Available data do not indicate significant risk for congenital anomalies. These data are based on use of the inhaled powder. Other dosage forms of cromolyn have not been evaluated. More data are needed, especially data addressing cromolyn use during the first trimester.

Dyker, M. H. (1974). Evaluation of antiasthmatic agent cromolyn sodium. *Journal of the American Medical Association, 227*, 1061.

Wilson, J. (1982). Utilisation du cromoglycate de sodium au cours de la grossesse: Resultats sur 296 femmes asthmatiques. *Acta Therapeutica, 8*(Suppl), 45–51.

Cyclizine

FDA: **B**   SIGNIFICANCE: **4–5**   POTENCY: **3–4**

Cyclizine use during pregnancy has not been associated with human teratogenesis.

McBride, W. G. (1963). The teratogenic action of drugs. *Medical Journal of Australia, 2*, 689–693.

Milkovich, L., & Van den Berg, B. J. (1976). An evaluation of the teratogenicity of certain antinauseant drugs. *American Journal of Obstetrics and Gynecology, 125*, 244–248.

Cyclophosphamide

FDA: C **SIGNIFICANCE:** 1–2
POTENCY: 2–3

An increased incidence of congenital malformations was observed when cyclophosphamide was combined with radiation therapy during the first trimester. Possible teratogenic effects include digital defects (mainly affecting hands), flattened nasal bridge, palatal anomalies, and single coronary arteries. A more recent single case report suggested that cyclophosphamide is a human teratogen with a distinct phenotype. However, because of concurrent use of several other drugs, additional data are needed to support this suggestion.

Enns, G. M., Roeder, E., Chan, R. T., et al. (1999). Apparent cyclophosphamide (cytoxan) embryopathy: A distinct phenotype? *American Journal of Medical Genetics, 86*(3), 237–241.

Greenberg, L. H., Verdes, P., & Tanaka, K. R. (1964). Congenital anomalies probably induced by cyclophosphamide. *Journal of the American Medical Association, 188*, 423–426.

Nicholson, H. O. (1968). Cytotoxic drugs in pregnancy. *British Journal of Obstetrics and Gynecology, 75*, 307.

Cyclosporine

FDA: C **SIGNIFICANCE:** 3–4 **POTENCY:** 3

No malformations were found in more than 50 different pregnancies in which the mother received cyclosporine during all three trimesters, indicating that cyclosporine is not teratogenic. Several case reports noted various congenital anomalies, however, including fetal growth retardation and neonatal blood dyscrasias (neutropenia and thrombocytopenia), in offspring exposed to cyclosporine in utero. These effects could be due to the mother's underlying health condition (i.e., in relation to her need for an organ transplant) or to other drugs used concurrently. More data are needed regarding cyclosporine use during pregnancy, particularly data on use during the first trimester.

Al-Khader, A. A., Absy, M., Al-Hasani, M. K., et al. (1988). Successful pregnancy in renal transplant recipients treated with cyclosporine. *Transplantation, 45*(5), 987–988.

Burrows, D. A., O'Neil, T. J., & Sorrells, T. L. (1988). Successful twin pregnancy after renal transplant maintained on cyclosporine A immunosuppression. *Obstetrics and Gynecology, 72*(3), 459–461.

Kossoy, L. R., Herbert, C. M. III, & Wentz, A. C. (1988). Management of heart transplant recipients: Guidelines for the obstetrician-gynecologist. *American Journal of Obstetrics and Gynecology, 159*(2), 490–499.

Niesert, S., Gunter, H., & Grei, U. (1988). Pregnancy after renal transplantation. *British Medical Journal, 296*, 1736.

Pickrell, M. D., Sawer, R., & Michael, J. (1988). Pregnancy after renal transplantation: Severe intrauterine growth retardation during treatment with cyclosporin A. *British Medical Journal, 296*, 825.

Prieto, C., Errasti, P., Olaizola, J. I., et al. (1989). Successful twin pregnancies in renal transplant recipients taking cyclosporine. *Transplantation, 48*(6), 1065–1067.

Zeidan, B. S., Waltzer, W. C., Monheit, A. G., et al. (1991). Anemia associated with pregnancy in a cyclosporine-treated renal allograft recipient. *Transplantation Proceedings, 23*(4), 2301–2303.

Cyproheptadine

FDA: B **SIGNIFICANCE:** 5 **POTENCY:** 4

Cyproheptadine use during pregnancy has not been associated with human teratogenesis.

Sadovsky, E., Pfeiffer, Y., Polishuk, W. A., et al. (1972). The use of antiserotonin-cyproheptadine HCl in pregnancy: An experimental and clinical study. *Advances in Experimental Medicine and Biology, 27*, 399–405.

Cytarabine

FDA: C **SIGNIFICANCE:** 3 **POTENCY:** 2–3

Atresia of external auditory canals, microtia, and various limb abnormalities associated with cytarabine use during the first trimester have been reported in two case studies. Although these effects involve changes with the stage of fetal development that coincided with reported drug use, similar effects were not found in other similarly treated patients. More data are needed to determine whether these birth defects are directly related to cytarabine and, if so, their incidence (potency). Use near term has been associated with neutropenia, pancytopenia, and thrombocytopenia in exposed neonates.

Aviles, A., Diaz-Maqueo, J. C., Talavera, A., et al. (1991). Growth and development of children of mothers treated with chemotherapy during pregnancy: Current status of 43 children. *American Journal of Hematology, 36*, 243–248.

Colbert, N., Najman, A., Gorin, N. C., et al. (1980). Acute leukaemia during pregnancy: Favourable course of pregnancy in two patients treated with cytosine arabinoside and anthracyclines. *Nouvelle Presse Medicale, 12*, 175–178.

Gililland, J., & Weinstein, L. (1983). The effects of cancer chemotherapeutic agents on the developing fetus. *Obstetrical and Gynecological Survey, 38*(1), 6–12.

Morgenstern, G. (1980). Cytarabine in pregnancy. *The Lancet, 2*, 259.

Newcomb, M., Balducci, L., Thigpen, J. R., et al. (1978). Acute leukemia in pregnancy: Successful delivery after cytarabine and doxorubicin. *Journal of the American Medical Association, 239*, 2691–2692.

Pizzuto, J., Aviles, A., Noriega, L., et al. (1980). Treatment of acute leukemia during pregnancy: Presentation of nine cases. *Cancer Treatment Reports, 65*(4-5), 679–683.

Wagner, V. M., Hill, J. S., Weaver, D., et al. (1980). Congenital abnormalities in a baby born to cytarabine-treated mother. *The Lancet, 2*, 98–99.

Dactinomycin (Actinomycin D)

FDA: **C**   SIGNIFICANCE: **3**   POTENCY: **2**

A retrospective study of 306 women treated with various antineoplastics for childhood cancers found no overall significant difference in the outcome of their pregnancies when compared to the general population. However, the incidence of congenital heart defects found among children of women previously treated with dactinomycin was significantly greater than that found for the general population. More data are needed.

Green, D. M., Zevon, M. A., Lowrie, G., et al. (1991). Congenital anomalies in children of patients who received chemotherapy for cancer in childhood and adolescence. *New England Journal of Medicine, 325*, 141–146.

Danazol

FDA: **X**   SIGNIFICANCE: **1**   POTENCY: **1**

Several case reports substantiate the teratogenic potential of danazol used during the first trimester. Although male infants are morphologically normal, female infants frequently display pseudohermaphroditism (clitoral hypertrophy, labial fusion, and a urogenital opening at the base of the clitoris). Virilization of the female fetus appears likely when danazol doses exceed 200 mg/day. Reports suggest an increased incidence of spontaneous abortion and transient blockage of adrenocorticosteroid synthesis among exposed neonates.

Brunskill, P. J. (1992). The effects of fetal exposure to danazol. *British Journal of Obstetrics and Gynaecology, 99*, 212–215.

Castro-Magana, M., Cheruvanky, T., Collip, P. J., et al. (1981). Transient adrenogenital syndrome due to exposure to danazol in utero. *American Journal of Diseases of Children, 135*, 1032–1034.

Duck, S. C., & Katayama, K. P. (1981). Danazol may cause female pseudohermaphroditism. *Fertility and Sterility, 35*, 230–231.

Kingsbury, A. C. (1985). Danazol and fetal masculinization: A warning. *Medical Journal of Australia, 143*, 410–411.

Madanes, A., & Farber, M. (1982). Danazol. *Annals of Internal Medicine, 96*, 625–630.

Peress, M. R., Kreutner, A. K., Mathur, R. S., et al. (1982). Female pseudohermaphroditism with somatic chromosomal anomaly in association with in utero exposure to danazol. *American Journal of Obstetrics and Gynecology, 142*, 708–709.

Ross, F. W. (1984). Virilization of the female fetus with maternal danazol exposure. *American Journal of Obstetrics and Gynecology, 149*, 99–100.

Schwartz, R. P. (1982). Ambiguous genitalia in a term female infant due to exposure to danazol in utero. *American Journal of Diseases of Children, 136*, 474.

Shaw, R. W., & Farquhar, J. W. (1984). Female pseudohermaphroditism associated with danazol exposure in utero: Case report. *British Journal of Obstetrics and Gynecology, 91*, 386–389.

Wentz, A. (1982). Adverse effects of danazol in pregnancy. *Annals of Internal Medicine, 96*, 672–673.

Daunorubicin

FDA: **D**   SIGNIFICANCE: **3**   POTENCY: **2–3**

Several negative published case reports suggest that daunorubicin is not a teratogen. However, reports of an increased rate of fetal deaths and premature deliveries associated with the use of daunorubicin during pregnancy also exist. No large-scale studies have been published, and the interpretation of most reports is severely confounded by concurrent antineoplastics. More data are needed.

Colbert, N., Majman, A., Gorin, N. C., et al. (1980). Acute leukaemia during pregnancy: Favourable course of pregnancy in two patients treated with cytosine arabinoside and anthracyclines. *Nouvelle Presse Medicale, 9,* 175–178.

Doney, K. D., Kraemer, K. G., & Shepard, T. H. (1979). Combination chemotherapy for acute myelocytic leukemia during pregnancy: Three case reports. *Cancer Treatment Reports, 63,* 369–371.

Lowenthal, R. M., Marsden, K. A., Newman, N. M., et al. (1978). Normal infant after treatment of acute myeloid leukaemia in pregnancy with daunorubicin. *Australian and New Zealand Journal of Medicine, 8,* 431–432.

Reynoso, E. E., Shepherd F. A., Messner, H. A., et al. (1978). Acute leukemia during pregnancy: The Toronto leukemia study group experience with long-term follow-up of children exposed in utero to chemotherapeutic agents. *Journal of Clinical Oncology, 5,* 1098–1106.

Tobias, J. S., & Bloom, H. J. G. (1980). Doxorubicin in pregnancy. *The Lancet, 1,* 776.

Deferoxamine

FDA: C   SIGNIFICANCE: 4–5   POTENCY: 3–4

The lack of teratogenic effects in several case reports suggests that deferoxamine is not a teratogen. However, more data are needed regarding deferoxamine use during pregnancy.

Blanc, P., Hryhorczuk, D., & Danel, I. (1984). Deferoxamine treatment of acute iron intoxication in pregnancy. *Obstetrics and Gynecology, 64,* 12S–14S.

Olenmark, M., Biber, B., Dottori, O., et al. (1987). Fatal iron intoxication in late pregnancy. *Journal of Toxicology. Clinical Toxicology, 25,* 347–359.

Rayburn, W. F., Donn, S. M., & Wulf, M. E. (1983). Iron overdose during pregnancy: Successful therapy with deferoxamine. *American Journal of Obstetrics and Gynecology, 147,* 717–718.

Thomas, R. M., & Skalicka, A. E. (1980). Successful pregnancy in transfusion-dependent thalassaemia. *Archives of Disease in Childhood, 55,* 572–574.

Demeclocycline

AUTHOR: ●   SIGNIFICANCE: 1 (dental staining)   POTENCY: 1–2 (dental staining)

No increase in the incidence of congenital anomalies was noted in offspring of 90 women who received demeclocycline during the first trimester and 280 women who received demeclocycline at various times throughout their pregnancies. However, as noted in another study, use of demeclocycline during the third trimester may result in staining of the deciduous (baby) teeth.

Heinonen, O. P., Slone, D., & Shapiro, S. (1977). *Birth defects and drugs in pregnancy.* Littleton, MA: Publishing Sciences Group.

Macaulay, J. C., & Leistyna, J. A. (1964). Preliminary observations on the prenatal administration of demethylchlortetracycline HCl. *Pediatrics, 34,* 423–424.

Desipramine (Desmethylimipramine)

FDA: C   SIGNIFICANCE: 3–4   POTENCY: 2

Although probably not teratogenic, desipramine probably is fetotoxic. It has been implicated as a cause of neonatal urinary retention and a syndrome involving respiratory distress, peripheral cyanosis, hypertonia, tremor, clonus, and spasm among neonates exposed in utero. Urinary retention probably is a result of the anticholinergic effects of the drug; the remaining signs and symptoms probably are a result of adrenergic supersensitization.

Ananth, J. (1976). Side effects on fetus and infant of psychotropic drug use during pregnancy. *International Pharmacopsychiatry, 11,* 246–260.

Eggermont, E., Raveschot, V., Deneve, V., et al. (1972). The adverse influence of imipramine on the adaptation of the newborn infant to extrauterine life. *Acta Paediatrica Belgica, 26,* 197–204.

Webster, P. A. (1973). Withdrawal symptoms in neonates associated with maternal antidepressant therapy. *The Lancet, 2,* 318–319.

Dexamethasone

FDA: C   SIGNIFICANCE: 1 (leukocytosis)
POTENCY: 2 (leukocytosis)

Use of dexamethasone throughout pregnancy is indicated for congenital virilizing adrenal hyperplasia due to a genetic defect of 21-hydroxylase. It also is indicated to accelerate fetal lung maturation during the second and third trimesters to prevent or minimize respiratory distress syndrome among premature neonates. Case reports involving the use of dexamethasone in both of these clinical situations found no accompanying increased risk for congenital anomalies. However, dexamethasone use up to 10 days prior to delivery has been associated with transient neonatal leukocytosis. The leukocytosis apparently resolves within 1 week and is not directly associated with any morbidity. However, if neonatal leukocytosis is incorrectly ascribed to infection or leukemia, the neonate may be unnecessarily exposed to risk from related diagnostic procedures (bone marrow aspirates) or drugs (prophylactic administration of antibiotics). (*See* Corticosteroids monograph.)

Anday, E., & Harris, M. (1982). Leukemoid reaction associated with antenatal dexamethasone administration. *The Journal of Pediatrics, 101,* 614–616.
Collaborative Group on Antenatal Steroid Therapy: Effects of antenatal dexamethasone administration in the infant: Long-term follow-up. *The Journal of Pediatrics, 104*(2), 259–267.
Cosmi, E. V., & Di Renzo, G. C. (1989). Prevention and treatment of fetal lung immaturity. *Fetal Therapy, 4*(Suppl), 52–62.
David, M., & Forest, M. G. (1984). Prenatal treatment of congenital adrenal hyperplasia resulting from 21-hydroxylase deficiency. *The Journal of Pediatrics, 105*(5), 799–803.
Forest, M. G., Betuel, H., & David, M. (1989). Prenatal treatment in congenital adrenal hyperplasia due to 21-hydroxylase deficiency: Up-date 88 of the French Multicentric Study. *Endocrine Research, 15*(1&2), 277–301.
Otero, L., Conlon, C., Reynolds, P., et al. (1981). Neonatal leukocytosis associated with prenatal administration of dexamethasone. *Pediatrics, 68,* 778–780.
Pang, S., Pollack, M. S., Marshall, R. N., et al. Prenatal treatment of congenital adrenal hyperplasia due to 21-hydroxylase deficiency. *New England Journal of Medicine, 322*(2), 111–115.
Roberts, W. E., & Morrison, J. C. (1991). Pharmacologic induction of fetal lung maturity. *Clinica Obstetrica e Ginecologica, 34*(2), 319–327.

Dextroamphetamine

FDA: C   SIGNIFICANCE: 3   POTENCY: 2–3

Data associating dextroamphetamine use during pregnancy with teratogenic effects are both positive and negative. The use of dextroamphetamine during the first trimester has been associated with biliary atresia, cleft lip/palate, congenital heart disease, prematurity, and small size for gestational age. However, three cohort studies found no increase in congenital malformations among exposed neonates. More data are needed regarding dextroamphetamine use during pregnancy, particularly during the first trimester.

Briggs, G. G., Samson, J. H., & Crawford, D. J. (1975). Lack of abnormalities in a newborn exposed to amphetamine during gestation. *American Journal of Diseases in Children, 129,* 249–250.
Ericksson, M., Larson, G., Windbladh, B., et al. (1978). The influence of amphetamine addiction on pregnancy and the newborn infant. *Acta Paediatrica Scandinavica, 67,* 95–99.
Heinonen, O. P., Slone, D., & Shapiro, S. (1977). *Birth defects and drugs in pregnancy*. Littleton, MA: Publishing Sciences Group.
Levin, J. N. (1971). Amphetamine ingestion with biliary atresia. *The Journal of Pediatrics, 79,* 130–131.
Milkovich, L., & Van den Berg, B. J. (1977). Effects of antenatal exposure to anorectic drugs. *American Journal of Obstetrics and Gynecology, 129,* 637–642.
Nelson, M. M., & Forfar, J. O. (1971). Associations between drugs administered during pregnancy and congenital abnormalities of the fetus. *British Medical Journal, 1,* 523–527.
Nora, J. J., McNamara, D. G., & Fraser, F. C. (1967). Dexamphetamine sulfate and human malformations. *The Lancet, 1,* 570.
Nora, J. J., Vargo, T. A., Nora, A. H., et al. (1970). Dexamphetamine: A possible environmental trigger in cardiovascular malformations. [Letter]. *The Lancet, 1,* 1290.

Dextromethorphan

AUTHOR: NONE   SIGNIFICANCE: 4–5
POTENCY: 4

The negative data from two cohort studies, which included 359 women who took dextromethorphan during the third trimester and 580 women who took dextromethorphan at various times throughout pregnancy, provide evidence that dextromethorphan use does not pose a significant teratogenic risk.

Aselton, P., Jick, H., Milunsky, A., et al. (1985). First-trimester drug use and congenital disorders. *Obstetrics and Gynecology, 65,* 451–455.
Heinonen, O. P., Slone, D., & Shapiro, S. (1977). *Birth defects and drugs in pregnancy*. Littleton, MA: Publishing Sciences Group.

Dextrose (D-Glucose)

AUTHOR: NONE   SIGNIFICANCE: 1
(hyperbilirubinemia and hypoglycemia)
POTENCY: 2 (hyperbilirubinemia and hypoglycemia)

Two studies provide evidence that intravenous infusion of dextrose solutions at a rate exceeding 6 grams/hr during labor may result in neonatal hypoglycemia and hyperbilirubinemia. The glucose infusion raised maternal glucose levels, which correspondingly raised fetal glucose levels. The increased fetal glucose levels resulted in excess insulin being secreted, with resultant hypoglycemia in the neonate. These effects generally are reversible with proper recognition and care.

Kenepp, N., Kumar, S., Shelley, W. C., et al. (1982). Fetal and neonatal hazards or maternal hydration with 5% dextrose before caesarean section. *The Lancet, 1,* 1150–1152.

Singhi, S., Kang, E., & Hall, J. (1982). Hazards of maternal hydration with 5% dextrose. *The Lancet, 2,* 335–336.

Diazepam

FDA: D   SIGNIFICANCE: 3–4   POTENCY: 3

Early studies implicated diazepam use during pregnancy with cleft lip/palate and limb and digit malformations among offspring. More recent data indicate that diazepam is not teratogenic in usual therapeutic doses. Cleft lip/palate occurred when an acute overdose (580 mg) was taken during the first trimester. Diazepam use near term has been associated with hypothermia, hypotonia, low Apgar scores, and poor feeding. Any regular diazepam use during the last trimester may result in expected pharmacologic effects among neonates (lethargy, poor suck) and neonatal benzodiazepine-withdrawal syndrome.

Aarskog, D. (1975). Association between maternal intake of diazepam and oral clefts. *The Lancet, 2,* 921.

Aselton, P., Jick, H., Milunsky, A., et al. (1985). First-trimester drug use and congenital disorders. *Obstetrics and Gynecology, 65,* 451–455.

Backes, C. R., & Cordero, L. (1980). Withdrawal symptoms in the neonate from presumptive intrauterine exposure to diazepam: Report of a case. *Journal of American Osteopathology Association, 79,* 484–485.

Beeley, L. (1981). Adverse effects of drugs in later pregnancy. *Clinical Obstetrics and Gynecology, 8,* 275–290.

Bracken, M. B., & Holford, T. R. (1981). Exposure to prescribed drugs in pregnancy and association with congenital malformations. *Obstetrics and Gynecology, 58,* 336–344.

Cree, J. E., Meyer, J., & Hailey, D. M. (1973). Diazepam in labour: Its metabolism and effect on the clinical condition and thermogenesis of the newborn. *British Medical Journal, 4*(887), 251–255.

Czeizel, A. (1988). Lack of evidence of teratogenicity of benzodiazepine drugs in Hungary. *Reproductive Toxicology, 1,* 183–188.

Douglas-Ringrose, C. A. (1972). The hazards of neurotropic drugs in the fertile years. *Canadian Medical Association Journal, 106,* 1058.

Flowers, C. E., Rudolph, A. J., & Desmond, M. M. (1968). Diazepam (Valium) as an adjunct in obstetric analgesia. *Journal of Obstetrics and Gynecology, 34,* 68–81.

Idanpaa-Heikkila, J. E., Joupilla, P. I., Puolakka, J. O., et al. (1971). Placenta transfer and fetal metabolism of diazepam in early human pregnancy. *American Journal of Obstetrics and Gynecology, 109,* 1011–1016.

Istvan, E. J. (1970). Drug associated congenital abnormalities. *Canadian Medical Association Journal, 103,* 1394.

Jick, H., Holmes, L. B., Hunter, J. R., et al. (1981). First-trimester drug use and congenital disorders. *Journal of the American Medical Association, 246,* 343–346.

Laegreid, L., Hagberg, G., & Lundberg, A. (1992). Neurodevelopment in late infancy after prenatal exposure to benzodiazepines—A prospective study. *Neuropediatrics, 23,* 60–67.

Laegreid, L., Hagberg, G., & Lundberg, A. (1992). The effect of benzodiazepines on the fetus and the newborn. *Neuropediatrics, 23,* 18–23.

McCarthy, G. T., O'Connell, B., & Robinson, A. E. (1973). Blood levels of diazepam in infants of two mothers given large doses of diazepam during labor. *Journal of Obstetrics and Gynaecology of the British Commonwealth, 80,* 349–352.

Milkovich, L., & Van den Berg, B. J. (1975). Fetal effects of tranquillizers in pregnancy. *New England Journal of Medicine, 293,* 198–199.

Niswander, K. R. (1968). Effect of diazepam on meperidine requirements of patient during labor. *Journal of Obstetrics and Gynecology, 34*(1), 62–67.

Owen, J. R., Irani, S. F., & Blair, A. W. (1971). Effect of diazepam administered to mothers during labor on temperature regulation of neonate. *Archives of Disease in Childhood, 47,* 107–110.

Rementeria, J. L., & Bhatt, K. (1977). Withdrawal symptoms in neonates from intrauterine exposure to diazepam. *The Journal of Pediatrics, 90,* 123–126.

Rivas, F., Hernandez, A., & Cantu, J. (1984). Acentric craniofacial cleft in a newborn female prenatally exposed to a high dose of diazepam. *Teratology, 30,* 179–180.

Rosenberg, L., Mitchell, A. A., Parsells, J. L., et al. (1983). Lack of relation of oral clefts to diazepam use during pregnancy. *New England Journal of Medicine, 309,* 1282–1285.

Safra, M. J., & Oakley, O. P. (1975). Association between cleft lip with or without cleft palate and prenatal exposure to diazepam. *The Lancet, 2,* 478–479.

Saxen, I. (1975). Association between oral clefts and drugs taken during pregnancy. *International Journal of Epidemiology, 4,* 37–44.

Saxen, I., & Saxen, L. (1975). Association between maternal intake of diazepam and oral clefts. *The Lancet, 2,* 498.

Shiona, P. H., & Mills, J. L. (1984). Oral clefts and diazepam use during pregnancy. *New England Journal of Medicine, 311,* 919–920.

Tuchmann-Duplessis, H. (1983). The teratogenic risk. *American Journal of Industrial Medicine, 4,* 245–258.

Diazoxide

FDA: C   SIGNIFICANCE: 3   POTENCY: 2

Effects on hair growth, including both alopecia and hypertrichosis, were observed in four infants exposed to long-term diazoxide therapy during pregnancy. In other case reports, various fetotoxic effects, including bradycardia and hyperglycemia, were seen when diazoxide was administered to pregnant women near term. More data are needed regarding diazoxide use during pregnancy, particularly data on use during the first trimester.

Michael, C. A. (1986). Intravenous labetalol and intravenous diazoxide in severe hypertension complicating pregnancy. *Australian and New Zealand Journal of Obstetrics and Gynaecology, 26,* 26–29.

Milner, R. D., & Chouksey, S. K. (1972). Effects of fetal exposure to diazoxide in man. *Archives of Disease in Childhood, 47,* 537–543.

Morris, J. A., Arce, J. J., Hamilton, C. J., et al. (1977). The management of severe preeclampsia and eclampsia with intravenous diazoxide. *Obstetrics and Gynecology, 49*(6), 675–680.

Neuman, J., Weiss, B., Rabello, Y., et al. (1979). Diazoxide for the acute control of severe hypertension complicating pregnancy: A pilot study. *Obstetrics and Gynecology, 53*(Suppl 3), 50S–55S.

Nuroayhid, B., Brinkman, C. R., Katchen, B., et al. (1975). Maternal and fetal hemodynamic effects of diazoxide. *Obstetrics and Gynecology, 46,* 197–203.

Smith, M. J., Aynsley-Green, A., & Redman, C. W. G. (1982). Neonatal hyperglycaemia after prolonged maternal treatment with diazoxide. *British Medical Journal, 284,* 1234.

Diclofenac

FDA: B   SIGNIFICANCE: 2   POTENCY: 1–2

A single case report describes a term neonate with severe persistent pulmonary hypertension due to premature closure of the ductus arteriosus. The mother had received 5 days of diclofenac 2 weeks before delivery. Although this is the first reported case of persistent pulmonary hypertension of the newborn (PPHN) in association with use of diclofenac during pregnancy, PPHN has occurred with the use of other nonsteroidal anti-inflammatories (NSAIDs) and is consistent with their known pharmacology.

Zenker, M., Klinge, J., Kruger, C., et al. (1998). Severe pulmonary hypertension in a neonate caused by premature closure of the ductus arteriosus following maternal treatment with diclofenac: A case report. *Journal of Perinatal Medicine, 26,* 231–234.

Dicumarol

FDA: X   SIGNIFICANCE: 1   POTENCY: 1

Administration of dicumarol during pregnancy has been associated with cutaneous hematomas, fetal loss, hypoplasia of the nasal cartilage, intracranial hemorrhage, and stillbirth. Reportedly, these effects occurred in more than one-third of the pregnancies in which women received dicumarol. Although the total number of reported pregnancies (slightly more than 100) is small, these reports, together with similar reported observations for the closely related coumarin derivative warfarin (see Warfarin monograph), contraindicate dicumarol during pregnancy. Whenever possible, dicumarol should be replaced with heparin for women who require an anticoagulant during pregnancy. (See Heparin monograph.)

Fillmore, S. J., & McDevitt, E. (1970). Effects of coumarin compounds on the fetus. *Annals of Internal Medicine, 73,* 731–735.

Quaini, E., Vitali, E., Colombo, T., et al. (1986). Complicanze materne e fetali in 105 gravidanze di portatrici di protesi valvolari cardiache. *Minerva Ginecologica, 38,* 217–224.

Villasanta, U. (1965). Thromboembolic disease in pregnancy. *American Journal of Obstetrics and Gynecology, 93,* 142–160.

Dicyclomine

FDA: B   SIGNIFICANCE: 3–4   POTENCY: 3–4

A study involving approximately 100 women who received dicyclomine during the first trimester did not detect a significant increase in congenital anomalies among offspring when compared to pregnant women who did not receive dicyclomine. More data are needed regarding dicyclomine use during pregnancy, particularly data on use during the second and third trimesters and near term. (*See* Doxylamine monograph.)

Aselton, P., Jick, H., Milunsky, A., et al. (1985). First-trimester drug use and congenital disorders. *Obstetrics and Gynecology, 65,* 451–455.

Golbus, M. S. (1980). Teratology for the obstetrician: Current status. *Obstetrics and Gynecology, 55,* 269–277.

Heinonen, O. P., Slone, D., & Shapiro, S. (1977). *Birth defects and drugs in pregnancy.* Littleton, MA: Publishing Sciences Group.

Huff, P. S. (1980). Safety of drug therapy for nausea and vomiting of pregnancy. *Journal of Family Practice, 11,* 969–970.

McCredie, J., Kricker, A., Elliott, J., et al. (1984). The innocent bystander: Doxylamine/dicyclomine/pyridoxine and congenital limb defects. *The Medical Journal of Australia, 140,* 525–527.

Shiono, P. H., & Klebanoff, M. A. (1989). Bendectin and human congenital malformations. *Teratology, 40,* 151–155.

Wither, F. R., King, T. M., & Blake, D. A. (1981). The effects of chronic gastrointestinal medication on the fetus and neonate. *Obstetrics and Gynecology, 58*(5 Suppl), 79S–84S.

Dienestrol

FDA: X   SIGNIFICANCE: 2   POTENCY: 2–3

Dienestrol use during pregnancy has been associated with an increased risk for cardiovascular defects among offspring. More data are needed.

Heinonen, O. P., Slone, D., Monson, R. R., et al. (1977). Cardiovascular birth defects and antenatal exposure to female sex hormones. *New England Journal of Medicine, 296,* 67–70.

Diethylpropion

FDA: B   SIGNIFICANCE: 4–5   POTENCY: 4

The combined data from two large studies of pregnant women who received diethylpropion during pregnancy (n = 1500 [~300 during the first trimester]) failed to detect a significant increase in congenital anomalies among offspring.

Bunde, C. A., & Leyland, H. M. (1965). A controlled retrospective survey in evaluation of teratogenicity. *Journal of New Drugs, 5,* 193–198.

Heinonen, O. P., Slone, D., & Shapiro, S. (1977). *Birth defects and drugs in pregnancy.* Littleton, MA: Publishing Sciences Group.

Diethylstilbestrol

FDA: X   SIGNIFICANCE: 1   POTENCY: 1

Diethylstilbestrol (DES) was first synthesized in 1938. It came into widespread use after the publication of papers during the late 1940s that claimed efficacy for the management of threatened abortion or repeated spontaneous abortions. Later it was suggested that DES decreased the incidence of either pre- or postmature deliveries, stillbirth, and toxemia. In 1953, a double-blind, placebo-controlled trial by Dieckman et al. found DES not to be of benefit. Unfortunately, these results were generally ignored. More recent recalculation of the Dieckman et al. data showed that DES actually increased the rate of spontaneous abortions, neonatal deaths, and premature births.

By the mid-1960s, the use of DES had decreased significantly. However, it was not until 1971, when Herbst et al. linked in utero exposure to DES with clear cell adenocarcinoma of the vagina and cervix among young women, that the use of DES during pregnancy was discontinued.

During the 20+ years that DES was used during pregnancy, between 1,000,000 and 4,000,000 women were exposed to DES in utero. Most estimates place the exposed population for both women and men at 1,000,000–1,500,000. These data are for the United States only, not worldwide. More than 70% of females exposed to DES in utero developed genital tract lesions during early adulthood. The type of lesion depended on the timing of the exposure.

Lower genital tract anomalies included the following:

1. Vaginal adenosis has been observed in 73% of fetuses exposed prior to 8 weeks of age, 49% of fetuses exposed between 9 and 12 weeks, 29% of fetuses exposed between 13 and 16 weeks, and 7% of fetuses exposed at 17 weeks or more. Overall, 50%–75% of women exposed to DES in utero have this defect.

2. Clear cell adenocarcinoma of the vagina and cervix occurs at a rate of 1.4 per 1000 to 1.4 per 10,000 women exposed to DES in utero.
3. Cervical changes occur in 22%–58% of exposed fetuses. The incidence of cervical erosion has been observed at 100% for fetuses exposed before 8 weeks of gestation, 92% for fetuses exposed between 9 and 12 weeks, 81% for fetuses exposed between 13 and 16 weeks, and 70% for fetuses exposed at 17 weeks or more. Other noted changes include hoods, collars, septa, cockscombs, and stenosis.
4. Vaginal ridges occur in 23% of embryos and fetuses exposed before 8 weeks of gestation, 28% for fetuses exposed between 9 and 12 weeks, 19% for fetuses exposed between 13 and 16 weeks, and 13% for fetuses exceeding 17 weeks. Abnormal mucus also has been associated with in utero DES exposure.

Approximately 69% of exposed fetuses have upper genital tract anomalies. These anomalies include uterine defects such as T-shape, constriction bands, and hypoplasia. Withered appearance of fallopian tubes on radiograph also has been reported.

Reproductive difficulties include dysmenorrhea (40%–50%), infertility, menstrual irregularities (10%–40%), and adverse pregnancy outcome (40%). Women exposed to DES in utero have increased rates of spontaneous abortion (30%), ectopic pregnancy (57%), and premature delivery (16%). Premature delivery is frequently secondary to an incompetent cervix. In addition, women exposed to DES in utero may develop excessive scarring of their genital tracts from minor surgical procedures.

Both structural and reproduction abnormalities also have been noted in males. The structural abnormalities include urethral stenosis or hypospadias (4%); testicular abnormalities, such as hypotrophic testes, cryptorchidism, capsular induration, and absent testes (11%); epididymal cysts (17%); microphallus (1%); and seminoma (two cases). Reproductive abnormalities include oligospermia/azospermia, decreased sperm motility, altered sperm morphology, and decreased ability to penetrate an egg in vitro.

Adonian, R. W., & Kessler, R. (1979). Transplacental exposure to diethylstilbestrol in man. *Urology, 13,* 276–279.

Barnes, A. B., Colton, T., Gundersen, J., et al. (1980). Fertility and outcome of pregnancy in women exposed in utero to diethylstilbestrol. *New England Journal of Medicine, 302,* 609–613.

Berger, M. J., & Goldstein, D. P. (1980). Impaired reproductive performance in DES-exposed women. *Obstetrics and Gynecology, 55,* 25–27.

Conley, R. G., Sant, G. R., Ucci, A. A., et al. (1983). Seminoma and epididymal cysts in a young man with known diethylstilbestrol exposure in utero. *Journal of the American Medical Association, 249,* 1325–1326.

Cousins, L., Karp, W., Lacey, C., et al. (1980). Reproductive outcome of women exposed to diethylstilbestrol in utero. *Obstetrics and Gynecology, 56,* 70–76.

de Haas, I., Harlow, B. L., Cramer, D. W., et al. (1991). Spontaneous preterm birth: A case-control study. *American Journal of Obstetrics and Gynecology, 165,* 1290–1296.

Dieckman, W. J., Davis, M. E., Rynkiewicz, L. M., et al. (1953). Does the administration of diethylstilbestrol during pregnancy have therapeutic value. *American Journal of Obstetrics and Gynecology, 66,* 1062.

Driscoll, S. G., & Taylor, S. H. (1980). Effect of prenatal maternal estrogen on the male urogenital system. *Obstetrics and Gynecology, 56,* 537–542.

Farber, E., & Cameron, R. (1980). The sequential analysis of cancer development. *Advances in Cancer Research, 31,* 125–226.

Fetherston, W. C. (1975). Squamous neoplasia of vagina related to DES syndrome. *American Journal of Obstetrics and Gynecology, 122,* 176–181.

Fowler, W. C., Schmidt, C., Edelman, D. A., et al. (1981). Risks of cervical intraepithelial neoplasia among DES-exposed women. *Obstetrics and Gynecology, 58,* 720–724.

Fu, Y. S., Reagan, J. W., Richart, R. M., et al. (1979). Nuclear DNA and histologic studies of genital lesions in diethylstilbestrol-exposed progeny I. *American Journal of Clinical Pathology, 72,* 515–520.

Fu, Y. S., Reagan, J. W., Richart, R. M., et al. (1979). Nuclear DNA and histologic studies of genital lesions in diethylstilbestrol-exposed progeny II. *American Journal of Clinical Pathology, 72,* 521–526.

Gill, W. B., Schumacher, G. F. B., & Bibbo, M. (1977). Pathological semen and anatomical abnormalities of the genital tract in human male subjects exposed to diethylstilbestrol in utero. *Journal of Urology, 117,* 477–480.

Gill, W. B., Schumacher, G. F. B., Bibbo, M., et al. (1979). Association of diethylstilbestrol exposure in utero with cryptorchidism, testicular hypoplasia and semen abnormalities. *Journal of Urology, 122,* 36–39.

Henderson, B. E., Bemton, B., & Cosgrove, M. (1976). Urogenital tract abnormalities in sons of women treated with diethylstilbestrol. *Pediatrics, 58,* 505–507.

Herbst, A. L. (1981). Clear cell adenocarcinoma and the current status of DES-exposed females. *Cancer, 48,* 484–488.

Herbst, A. L. (1981). Diethylstilbestrol and other sex hormones during pregnancy. *Obstetrics and Gynecology, 58*(Suppl), 35–40.

Herbst, A. L., Cole, P., Colton, T., et al. (1977). Age-incidence and risk of diethylstilbestrol-related clear cell adenocarcinoma of the vagina and cervix. *American Journal of Obstetrics and Gynecology, 128,* 43.

Herbst, A. L., Hubby, M. M., Blough R. R., et al. (1980). A comparison of pregnancy experience in DES-exposed and DES-unexposed daughters. *Journal of Reproductive Medicine, 24,* 62–69.

Herbst, A. L., Kurman, R. J., & Scully, R. E. (1972). Vaginal and cervical abnormalities after exposure to stilbestrol in utero. *Obstetrics and Gynecology, 40,* 287–298.

Herbst, A. L., Poskanzer, D. C., Robboy, S. J., et al. (1975). Prenatal exposure to stilbestrol. *New England Journal of Medicine, 292,* 334–339.

Herbst, A. L., Ulfelder, H., & Poskanzer, D. C. (1971). Adenocarcinoma of the vagina. *New England Journal of Medicine, 284,* 878–881.

Hussey, H. H. (1974). Teratogenic effect of progestogen/estrogen. *Journal of the American Medical Association, 230,* 1019–1020.

Jeffries, J. A., Robboy, S. J., O'Brien, P. C., et al. (1984). Structural anomalies of the cervix and vagina in women enrolled in the diethylstilbestrol adenosis (DESAD) project. *American Journal of Obstetrics and Gynecology, 148,* 59–66.

Johnson, L. D., Driscoll, S. G., Hertig, A. T., et al. (1979). Vaginal adenosis in stillborns and neonates exposed to diethylstilbestrol and steroidal estrogens and progestins. *Obstetrics and Gynecology, 53,* 671–679.

Kaufman, R. H., Adam, E., Binder, G. L., et al. (1980). Upper genital tract changes and pregnancy outcome in offspring exposed in utero to diethylstilbestrol. *American Journal of Obstetrics and Gynecology, 137,* 299–308.

Kaufman, R. H., Adam, E., Grey, M. P., et al. (1980). Urinary tract changes associated with exposure in utero to diethylstilbestrol. *Obstetrics and Gynecology, 56,* 330–332.

Kaufman, R. H., Noller, K., Adam, E., et al. (1984). Upper genital tract abnormalities and pregnancy outcome in diethylstilbestrol-exposed progeny. *American Journal of Obstetrics and Gynecology, 148,* 973–984.

Kinch, R. A. (1979). Diethylstilbestrol: Risks of malignant disease and congenital malformations. *Canadian Medical Association Journal, 120,* 1483–1484.

Linn, S., Lieberman, E., Schoenbaum, S. C., et al. (1988). Adverse outcomes of pregnancy in women exposed to diethylstilbestrol in utero. *Journal of Reproductive Medicine, 33*(1), 3–7.

Mangan, C. E., Borow, L., Burnett-Rubin, M. M., et al. (1982). Pregnancy outcome in 98 women exposed to diethylstilbestrol in utero, their mothers, and unexposed siblings. *Obstetrics and Gynecology, 59,* 315–319.

Mangan, C. E., Guintoli, R. L., Sedlacek, T. V., et al. (1979). Six years' experience with screening of a diethylstilbestrol-exposed population. *American Journal of Obstetrics and Gynecology, 134,* 860–865.

Mattingly, R. F., & Stafl, A. (1976). Cancer risk in diethylstilbestrol exposed offspring. *American Journal of Obstetrics and Gynecology, 126,* 543–548.

Pillsbury, S. G. (1980). Reproductive significance of changes in the endometrial cavity associated with exposure in utero to diethylstilbestrol. *American Journal of Obstetrics and Gynecology, 137,* 178–182.

Professional and Public Relations Committee of the DESAD. (1976). Exposure in utero to diethylstilbestrol and related synthetic hormones. *Journal of the American Medical Association, 236,* 1107–1109.

Robboy, S. J., Noller, K. L., O'Brien, P., et al. (1984). Increased incidence of cervical and vaginal dysplasia in 3,980 diethylstilbestrol-exposed young women. Experience of the National Collaborative Diethylstilbestrol Adenosis Project. *Journal of the American Medical Association, 252,* 2979–2983.

Rosenfeld, D. L., & Bronson, R. A. (1980). Reproductive problems in the DES-exposed female. *Obstetrics and Gynecology, 55,* 453–456.

Sandberg, E. C. (1976). Benign cervical and vaginal changes associated with exposure to stilbestrol in utero. *American Journal of Obstetrics and Gynecology, 125,* 777–789.

Sandberg, E. C., Riffle, N. L., Higdon, J. V., et al. (1981). Pregnancy outcome in women exposed to diethylstilbestrol in utero. *American Journal of Obstetrics and Gynecology, 140,* 194–205.

Schmidt, G., Fowler, W. C., Talbert, W. M., et al. (1980). Reproductive history of women exposed to diethylstilbestrol in utero. *Fertility and Sterility, 33,* 21–24.

Seigler, A. M., Wong, C. F., & Friberg, J. (1979). Fertility of the diethylstilbestrol-exposed offspring. *Fertility and Sterility, 31,* 601–607.

Senekjian, E. K., Potkul, R. K., Frey, K., et al. (1988). Infertility among daughters either exposed or not exposed to diethylstilbestrol. *American Journal of Obstetrics and Gynecology, 158,* 493–498.

Stenchever, M. A., Williamson, R. A., Leonard, J., et al. (1981). Possible relationships between in utero diethylstilbestrol exposure and male fertility. *American Journal of Obstetrics and Gynecology, 140,* 186–193.

Stillman, R. J. (1982). In utero exposure to diethylstilbestrol: Adverse effects on the reproductive tract and reproductive performance in male and female offspring. *American Journal of Obstetrics and Gynecology, 142,* 905–921.

Ulfelder, H. (1976). DES-transplacental teratogen— and possibly also carcinogen. *Teratology, 131,* 101–104.

Vandrie, D. M., Puri, S., Upton, R. T., et al. (1983). Adenosquamous carcinoma of the cervix in a woman exposed to diethylstilbestrol in utero. *Obstetrics and Gynecology, 61*(Suppl), 845–875.

Digoxin

FDA: **C**   SIGNIFICANCE: **5**   POTENCY: **4**

Teratogenic studies of digoxin use throughout pregnancy failed to demonstrate a significant increase in congenital anomalies among offspring. In addition, digoxin has been used to treat fetal cardiac dysrhythmias and hydrops during the second and third trimesters without reports of teratogenic effects.

Aselton, P., Jick, H., Milunsky, A., et al. (1985). First-trimester drug use and congenital disorders. *Obstetrics and Gynecology, 65,* 451–455.

Heinonen, O. P., Slone, D., & Shapiro, S. (1977). *Birth defects and drugs in pregnancy.* Littleton, MA: Publishing Sciences Group.

Dimenhydrinate

FDA: **B**   SIGNIFICANCE: **5**   POTENCY: **4**

No association between dimenhydrinate use during pregnancy and teratogenesis was observed in two case-controlled studies and one prospective study. However, dimenhydrinate may have an oxytocic effect on the uterus at term and, thus, may shorten term or cause hyperstimulation and possible uterine rupture.

Collins, I. S. (1964). Hazards of drug therapy. *Medical Journal of Australia, 1,* 222.

Hara, G. S., Carter, R. P., & Krantz, K. E. (1980). Dramamine in labor: Potential boon or possible bomb? *Journal of the Kansas Medical Society, 81,* 134–136, 155.

Leathem, A. M. (1986). Safety and efficacy of antiemetics to treat nausea and vomiting in pregnancy. *Clinical Pharmacy, 5,* 660–668.

Milkovich, L., & Van den Berg, B. J. (1976). An evaluation of the teratogenicity of certain antinauseant drugs. *American Journal of Obstetrics and Gynecology, 125,* 244.

Nelson, M. M., & Forfar, J. O. (1971). Association between drugs administered during pregnancy and congenital abnormalities. *British Medical Journal, 1,* 523.

Diphenhydramine

FDA: **C**   SIGNIFICANCE: **4–5**   POTENCY: **3–4**

In one retrospective case-controlled study, diphenhydramine use during pregnancy was associated with an increased risk for cleft lip and/or palate among offspring. In three other large prospective studies, however, such use was safe.

Aselton, P., Jick, H., Milunsky, A., et al. (1985). First-trimester drug use and congenital disorders. *Obstetrics and Gynecology, 65,* 451–455.

Greenberger, P., & Patterson, R. (1978). Safety of therapy for allergic symptoms during pregnancy. *Annals of Internal Medicine, 89,* 234–237.

Heinonen, O. P., Slone, D., & Shapiro, S. (1977). *Birth defects and drugs in pregnancy.* Littleton, MA: Publishing Sciences Group.

Jick, H., Holmes, L. B., Hunter, J. R., et al. (1981). First-trimester drug use and congenital disorders. *Journal of the American Medical Association, 246,* 343–346.

Saxen, I. (1974). Cleft palate and maternal diphenhydramine intake. *The Lancet, 1,* 407–408.

Diphtheria Toxoid Vaccine

AUTHOR: **NONE**   SIGNIFICANCE: **5**
POTENCY: **4**

Most North American women were immunized for diphtheria as infants. However, if a woman's vaccination status is unknown and she is at risk for diphtheria exposure, a Schick test should be performed. Nonimmune (Schick-positive) women should receive low-dose immunization with an adsorbed vaccine.

Hart, R. J. (1981). Immunizations. *Clinical Obstetrics and Gynecology, 8,* 421–430.

Dipyridamole

FDA: **B**   SIGNIFICANCE: **4–5**   POTENCY: **3–4**

Various congenital anomalies have been associated with dipyridamole use during pregnancy. However, a consistent pattern has not been noted, the incidence rates are relatively low, and it has been argued that the reported teratogenic effects may be due to the maternal condition being treated (e.g., women with artificial heart valves tend to experience higher rates of fetal loss). These observations and the lack of observed risk for congenital anomalies in both prospective controlled studies and case reports of use of dipyridamole during pregnancy (i.e., to prevent fetal growth retardation and fetal death among women who have previously experienced these adverse outcomes of pregnancy) tend to support the contention that dipyridamole is not a teratogen.

Beaufils, M., Uzan, S., Donsimoni, R., et al. (1985). Prevention of pre-eclampsia by early antiplatelet therapy. *The Lancet, 1*, 840–842.

Beaufils, M., Uzan, S., Donsimoni, R., et al. (1986). Prospective controlled study of early antiplatelet therapy in prevention of preeclampsia. *Advances in Nephrology from the Necker Hospital, 15*, 87–94.

Chen, W. W. C., Chan, C. S., Lee, P. K., et al. (1982). Pregnancy in patients with prosthetic heart valves: An experience with 45 pregnancies. *Quarterly Journal of Medicine, 51*, 348–365.

Wallenburg, H. C. S., & Rotmans, N. (1987). Prevention of recurrent idiopathic fetal growth retardation by low-dose aspirin and dipyridamole. *American Journal of Obstetrics and Gynecology, 157*(5), 1230–1235.

Disopyramide

FDA: C   SIGNIFICANCE: 4   POTENCY: 3–4

As indicated in one report and in one case study, use of disopyramide during pregnancy did not affect the fetus. There was, however, one report of the stimulation of maternal uterine contractions associated with each maternal dose of the drug; these contractions abated when the drug was discontinued.

Barrillon, A., Grand, A., & Gerbaux, A. (1974). Treatment of the heart during pregnancy. *Annals de Medicine Interne (Paris), 125*, 437–445.

Leonard, R. F., Braun, T. E., & Levy, A. M. (1978). Initiation of uterine contractions by disopyramide during pregnancy. *New England Journal of Medicine, 299*, 84–85.

Sharted, E. J., & Milton, P. J. (1979). Disopyramide in pregnancy: A case report. *Current Medical Research and Opinion, 6*, 70–72.

Disulfiram

FDA: X   SIGNIFICANCE: 3   POTENCY: 2–3

Various congenital anomalies and effects (cleft palate, club feet, limb reduction, spontaneous abortion) have been associated with disulfiram use during pregnancy. Negative reports also have been published. These observations and the indication for disulfiram use (i.e., to assist alcoholic women in maintaining abstinence) confound the interpretation of accumulated data. More data are needed, particularly data on use during the first trimester.

Dehaene, P., Titran, M., & Dubois, D. (1984). Pierre Robin Syndrome and heart malformations in a newborn infant. The role of disulfiram during pregnancy. *Nouvelle Presse Medicale, 13*, 1394–1395.

Favre-Tissot, M., & Delatous, P. (1965). Psychopharmacologie et teratogenase a propos du sulfiram: Essai experimental. *Annals Medicopsychogigues (France), 1*, 735–740.

Gardner, R. J. M., & Clarkson, J. E. (1981). A malformed child whose previously alcoholic mother had taken disulfiram. *New Zealand Medical Journal, 93*, 184–186.

Jones, K. L., Chambers, C. C., & Johnson, K. A. (1991). The effect of disulfiram on the unborn baby. *Teratology, 43*(4), 438.

Nora, A. H., Nora, J. J., & Blu, J. (1977). Limb-reduction anomalies in infants born to disulfiram treated alcoholic mothers. *The Lancet, 2*, 6640.

Reitnauer, P. J., Callanan, N. P., Farber, R. A., et al. (1997). Prenatal exposure to disulfiram implicated in the cause of malformations in discordant monozygotic twins. *Teratology, 56*(6), 358–362.

Docusate

FDA: C   SIGNIFICANCE: 5   POTENCY: 4

Two large-scale teratogen studies involving ~1000 women who used docusate as a stool softener during pregnancy, primarily during the first trimester, indicated no significant increase in the risk for congenital anomalies.

Aselton, P., Jick, H., Milunsky, A., et al. (1985). First-trimester drug use and congenital disorders. *Obstetrics and Gynecology, 65*(4), 451–455.

Heinonen, O. P., Slone, D., & Shapiro, S. (1977). *Birth defects and drugs in pregnancy*. Littleton, MA: Publishing Sciences Group.

Jick, H., Holmes, L. B., Hunter, J. R., et al. (1981). First-trimester drug use and congenital disorders. *Journal of the American Medical Association, 246*(4), 343–346.

Doxorubicin

FDA: D   SIGNIFICANCE: 3–4   POTENCY: 2–3

Data from several case reports suggest that doxorubicin use during the last trimester poses no significant risk for the fetus. However, reports of teratogenesis associated with use during the first trimester are conflicting, with both normal deliveries and fetal loss. Because of the mechanism of action of this antineoplastic drug, caution is warranted until more data have been obtained, particularly if doxorubicin is used during the first and second trimesters.

Brusamolino, E., Lazzarino, M., Morra, E., et al. (1989). Combination chemotherapy with alternating MOPP-ABVD in advanced Hodgkin's disease. *Haematologica (Pavia), 74*(2), 173–179.

Dara, P., Slater, L. M., & Armentrout, S. A. (1981). Successful pregnancy during chemotherapy for acute leukemia. *Cancer, 47*, 845–846.

Garcia, V., San Miguel, J., & Borrasca, A. L. (1981). Doxorubicin in the first trimester of pregnancy. *Annals of Internal Medicine, 94*, 547.

Garg, A., & Kochupillai, V. (1985). Non-Hodgkin's lymphoma in pregnancy. *Southern Medical Journal, 78*(10), 1263–1264.

Karp, G. I., von Oeyen, P., Valone, F., et al. (1983). Doxorubicin in pregnancy: Possible transplacental passage. *Cancer Treatment Reports, 67*(9), 773–777.

Lowenthal, R., Funnell, C. F., Hope, D. M., et al. (1982). Normal infant after combination chemotherapy including teniposide for Burkitt's lymphoma in pregnancy. *Medical and Pediatric Oncology, 10*, 165–169.

Newcomb, M., Balducci, L., Thigpen, J. T., et al. (1978). Acute leukemia in pregnancy. Successful delivery after cytarabine and doxorubicin. *Journal of the American Medical Association, 239*(25), 2691–2692.

Pizzuto, J., Aviles, A., Noriega, L., et al. (1980). Treatment of acute leukemia during pregnancy: Presentation of nine cases. *Cancer Treatment Reports, 64*(4-5), 679–683.

Tobias, J. S., & Bloom, H. J. (1980). Doxorubicin in pregnancy. *The Lancet, 1*, 776.

Doxylamine

FDA: **B**   SIGNIFICANCE: **4**   POTENCY: **3–4**

Some controversy has been associated with the use of doxylamine in combination with dicyclomine and/or pyridoxine (i.e., *Bendectin®, Debendox®*). These combinations have been removed from the market because several reports denoted them as "low-grade" teratogens (i.e., affecting perhaps only 1–5 infants in every 1000 births) and because their use was associated with an increased risk for pyloric stenosis among offspring. However, most published reports and studies involving more than 3000 infants exposed in utero to doxylamine during the first trimester demonstrate **no** significant increase in congenital anomalies when compared to controls. (*See* Dicyclomine monograph.)

Bendectin and pyloric stenosis. (1983). *FDA Drug Bulletin, 13*, 14–15.

Clarke, M., & Clayton, D. G. (1981). Safety of Debendox. *The Lancet, 1*, 659–660.

Cordero, J. F., Oakley, G. P., Greenberg, F., et al. (1981). Is Bendectin a teratogen? *Journal of the American Medical Association, 245*, 2307–2310.

Fleming, D. M., Knox, J. D. E., & Crombie, D. L. (1981). Debendox in early pregnancy and fetal malformation. *British Medical Journal, 283*, 99–101.

Gibson, G. T., Calley, D. P., McMichael, A. J., et al. (1981). Congenital anomalies in relation to the use of doxylamine/dicyclomine and other antenatal factors. *The Medical Journal of Australia, 1*, 410–414.

Hall, J. B. (1981). Debendox in pregnancy. *The Lancet, 2*, 154–155.

Harron, D. W., Griffiths, K., & Shanks, R. G. (1980). Debendox and congenital malformations in Northern Ireland. *British Medical Journal, 281*, 1379–1381.

Hays, D. P. (1983). Bendectin: A case of morning sickness. *Drug Intelligence and Clinical Pharmacy, 17*, 826–827.

Heinonen, O. P., Slone, D., & Shapiro, S. (1977). *Birth defects and drugs in pregnancy*. Littleton, MA: Publishing Sciences Group.

Holmes, L. B. (1983). Teratogen update: Bendectin. *Teratology, 27*, 277–281.

Huff, P. S. (1980). Safety of drug therapy for nausea and vomiting of pregnancy. *The Journal of Family Practice, 11*, 969–970.

MacMahon, B. (1981). More on Bendectin. *Journal of the American Medical Association, 246*, 371–372.

McCredie, J., Kricker, A., Elliott, J., et al. (1984). The innocent bystander: Doxylamine/dicyclomine/pyridoxine and congenital limb defects. *The Medical Journal of Australia, 140*, 525–527.

Milkovich, L., & Van den Berg, B. J. (1976). An evaluation of the teratogenicity of certain antinauseant drugs. *American Journal of Obstetrics and Gynecology, 125*, 244–248.

Mitchell, A. A., Rosenberg, L., Shapiro, S., et al. (1981). Birth defects related to Bendectin use in pregnancy. *Journal of the American Medical Association, 245*, 2311–2314.

Morelock, S., Hingson, R., Kayne, H., et al. (1982). Bendectin and fetal development: A study at Boston City Hospital. *American Journal of Obstetrics and Gynecology, 142*, 209–213.

Shapiro, S., Heinonen, O. P., Siskind, V., et al.

(1977). Antenatal exposure to doxylamine succinate and dicyclomine hydrochloride (Bendectin) in relation to congenital malformations, perinatal mortality rate, birth weight, and intelligence quotient score. *American Journal of Obstetrics and Gynecology, 128,* 480–485.

Sheffield, L. J., & Batagol, R. (1985). The creation of therapeutic orphans—or, what have we learnt from the debendox fiasco? *Medical Journal of Australia, 143,* 143–147.

Shiono, P. H., & Klebanoff, M. A. (1989). Bendectin and human congenital malformations. *Teratology, 40,* 151–155.

Zierler, S., & Rothman, K. J. (1985). Congenital heart disease in relation to maternal use of Bendectin and other drugs in early pregnancy. *New England Journal of Medicine, 313,* 347–352.

Enalapril

FDA: **C**   SIGNIFICANCE: **2** (near term)
POTENCY: **2**

Several cases of severe, but in one case reversible, renal failure were reported among neonates exposed in utero to enalapril. Enalapril use near term also has been associated with placental transfer of the drug and resultant expected pharmacologic effects in the neonate (suppression of angiotensin-converting enzyme activity, increased renin plasma levels). In addition, enalapril use during the second or third trimester has been associated with the following teratogenic and fetotoxic effects: fetal anuria, fetal calvarial hypoplasia, fetal death, fetal hypotension, intrauterine growth retardation, oligohydramnios, pulmonary hypoplasia, and renal tubular dysplasia. For women who require antihypertensives during the last trimester, a different antihypertensive is recommended. If this is not feasible, the neonate should be monitored and treated appropriately. More data are needed to determine the teratogenic and fetotoxic effects of enalapril when used during the first and second trimesters.

Boutroy, M. J. (1989). Fetal effects of maternally administered clonidine and angiotensin-converting enzyme inhibitors. *Developmental Pharmacology and Therapeutics, 13,* 199–204.

Brent, R. L., & Beckman, D. A. (1991). Angiotensin-converting enzyme inhibitors, an embryopathic class of drugs with unique properties: Information for clinical teratology counsellors. *Teratology, 43,* 543–546.

Cunniff, C., Jones, K. L., Phillipson, J., et al. (1990). Oligohydramnios sequence and renal tubular malformation associated with maternal enalapril use. *American Journal of Obstetrics and Gynecology, 162,* 187–189.

Mehta, N., & Modi, N. (1989). Ace inhibitors in pregnancy. *The Lancet, 2,* 96.

Rosa, F. W., Bosco, L. A., Graham, C. F., et al. (1989). Neonatal anuria with maternal angiotensin-converting enzyme inhibition. *Obstetrics and Gynecology, 74,* 371–374.

Rothberg, A. D., & Lorenz, R. (1984). Can captopril cause fetal and neonatal renal failure? *Pediatric Pharmacology, 4,* 189–192.

Schubiger, G., Flury, G., & Nussberger, J. (1988). Enalapril for pregnancy-induced hypertension: Acute renal failure in a neonate. *Annals of Internal Medicine, 108*(2), 215–216.

Scott, A. A., & Purohib, D. M. (1989). Neonatal renal failure: A complication of maternal antihypertensive therapy. *American Journal of Obstetrics and Gynecology, 160,* 1223–1224.

Sedman, A. B., Kershaw, D. B., & Bunchman, T. E. (1995). Recognition and management of angiotensin converting enzyme inhibitor fetopathy. *Pediatric Nephrology, 9*(3), 382–385.

Ephedrine

FDA: **C**   SIGNIFICANCE: **4**   POTENCY: **3–4**

In a report of the Collaborative Perinatal Project, no significant increase in congenital malformations was observed among the offspring of 373 women who used ephedrine during the first trimester or of 873 women who used ephedrine at any time during their pregnancies. Near term, ephedrine has been administered to prevent or treat anaphylactic reactions and hypotension associated with epidural analgesia without producing fetotoxic effects.

Heinonen, O. P., Slone, D., & Shapiro, S. (1977). *Birth defects and drugs in pregnancy.* Littleton, MA: Publishing Sciences Group.

Hollmen, A. I., Jouppila, R., Albright, G. A., et al. (1984). Intervillous blood flow during caesarean section with prophylactic ephedrine and epidural anaesthesia. *Acta Anaesthesiologica Scandinavica, 28,* 396–400.

Epinephrine

FDA: **C**   SIGNIFICANCE: **3**   POTENCY: **3**

The use of epinephrine for the management of asthma among pregnant women has been associated with an increased risk for congenital malformations. However, the reported malformations could have been caused by a virus that precipitated the asthma attack or been from the hypoxia associated with the attack. Severe asthmatic attacks among women during pregnancy require immediate treatment. The continued use of epinephrine during pregnancy appears to be warranted.

Heinonen, O. P., Slone, D., & Shapiro, S. (1977). *Birth defects and drugs in pregnancy.* Littleton, MA: Publishing Sciences Group.

Pratt, W. R. (1981). Allergic diseases in pregnancy and breast feeding. *Annals of Allergy, 47,* 355–360.

Ergotamine

FDA: **X** SIGNIFICANCE: **4–5** POTENCY: **3–4**

In a large study of women (n = 900) with migraine headaches treated with ergotamine, no increase in congenital malformations was observed among their offspring. Ergot toxicity and resultant severe vasospasm would be expected to adversely affect the developing fetus. In fact, a case of fetal death associated with maternal ergotamine overdose has been reported. More data regarding ergotamine use during pregnancy are needed.

Au, K. L., Woo, J. S. K., & Wong, V. C. W. (1985). Intrauterine death from ergotamine overdosage. *European Journal of Obstetrics, Gynecology, and Reproductive Biology, 19,* 313–315.

Czeizel, A. (1989). Teratogenicity of ergotamine. *Journal of Medical Genetics, 26,* 69–71.

Heinonen, O. P., Slone, D., & Shapiro, S. (1977). *Birth defects and drugs in pregnancy.* Littleton, MA: Publishing Sciences Group.

Raymond, G. V. (1995). Teratogen update: Ergot and ergotamine. *Teratology, 51*(5), 344–347.

Wainscott, G., Sullivan, F. M., Volans, G. N., et al. (1978). The outcome of pregnancy in women suffering from migraine. *Postgraduate Medical Journal, 54,* 98.

Erythromycin

FDA: **B** SIGNIFICANCE: **5** POTENCY: **4**

Several large studies and numerous case reports involving more than 1000 women who received erythromycin during various trimesters failed to substantiate a significant teratogenic risk. There is, however, one report of a child with exencephalia associated with the administration of erythromycin during pregnancy. This child also had an obvious amniotic band deformity. Considering the extensive use of erythromycin, and only one case report, erythromycin use during pregnancy appears to be safe.

Aselton, P., Jick, H., Milunsky, A., et al. (1985). First-trimester drug use and congenital disorders. *Obstetrics and Gynecology, 65,* 451–455.

Cohen, I., Veille, J. C., & Calkins, B. M. (1990). Improved pregnancy outcome following successful treatment of chlamydia infection. *Journal of the American Medical Association, 263,* 3160–3163.

Eschenbach, D. A., Nugent, R. P., Rao, A. V., et al. (1991). A randomized placebo-controlled trial of erythromycin for the treatment of Ureaplasma urealyticum to prevent premature delivery. The Vaginal Infections and Prematurity Study Group. *American Journal of Obstetrics and Gynecology, 164,* 734–742.

Golbus, M. S. (1980). Teratology for the obstetrician: Current status. *Obstetrics and Gynecology, 55,* 269–277.

Heinonen, O. P., Slone, D., & Shapiro, S. (1977). *Birth defects and drugs in pregnancy.* Littleton, MA: Publishing Sciences Group.

Jick, H., Holmes, L. B., Hunter, J. R., et al. (1981). First-trimester drug use and congenital disorders. *Journal of the American Medical Association, 246,* 343–346.

Liban, E., & Abramovici, A. (1972). Fetal membrane adhesions and congenital malformations. *Advances in Experimental Medicine and Biology, 27,* 337–350.

McCormack, W. M., Rosner, B., Lee, Y. H., et al. (1987). Effect on birth weight of erythromycin treatment of pregnant women. *Obstetrics and Gynecology, 69,* 202–207.

McGregor, J. A., French, J. I., Richter, R., et al. (1990). Cervicovaginal microflora and pregnancy outcome: Results of a double-blind, placebo-controlled trial of erythromycin treatment. *American Journal of Obstetrics and Gynecology, 163,* 1580–1591.

Estradiol

FDA: **X** SIGNIFICANCE: **4–5** POTENCY: **3–4**

Use of estradiol during pregnancy, alone or in combination with a progesterone, has not been associated with teratogenic effects.

Michaelis, J., Michaelis, H., Gluck, E., et al. (1983). Prospective study of suspected associations between certain drugs administered during early pregnancy and congenital malformations. *Teratology, 27,* 57–64.

Spira, N., Goujard, J., Huel, G., et al. (1972). Investigation into the teratogenic action of sex hormones: First results of an epidemiologic survey involving 20,000 women. *Annual Review of Medicine, 41,* 2683–2694.

Tuchmann-Duplessis, H. (1983). The teratogenic risk. *American Journal of Industrial Medicine, 4,* 245–258.

Estrogens

FDA: **X**   SIGNIFICANCE: **2–3**   POTENCY: **2–3**

Although there are scattered reports associating estrogen use during pregnancy with various birth defects or associating the use of oral contraceptives with limb reduction defects, the only convincing data associated estrogens with an increased risk for cardiovascular abnormalities among offspring. However, these data do not include diethylstilbestrol. (*See* Diethylstilbestrol monograph and monographs for other individual estrogens.)

Greenwald, P., Barlow, J. J., Nasra, P. C., et al. (1971). Vaginal cancer after maternal treatment with synthetic estrogens. *New England Journal of Medicine, 285,* 390–392.

Heinonen, O. P., Slone, D., Monson, R. R., et al. (1977). Cardiovascular birth defects and antenatal exposure to female sex hormones. *New England Journal of Medicine, 296,* 67–70.

Herbst, A. L., Robboy, S. J., Scully, R. E., et al. (1974). Clear-cell adenocarcinoma of the vagina and cervix in girls: Analysis of 170 registry cases. *American Journal of Obstetrics and Gynecology, 119,* 713–724.

Janerich, D. T., Piper, J. M., Glebatis, D. M., et al. (1974). Oral contraceptives and congenital limb-reduction defects. *New England Journal of Medicine, 291,* 697–700.

Nelhaus, G. (1958). Artificially induced female pseudohermaphroditism. *New England Journal of Medicine, 258,* 935–938.

Noller, K. L., Decker, D. G., Lanier, D. P., et al. (1972). Clear-cell adenocarcinoma of the cervix after maternal treatment with synthetic estrogens. *Mayo Clinic Proceedings, 47,* 629–630.

Papp, Z., Garda, S., Dolhay, B., et al. (1976). Indirect effect of sex hormones on the fetus. *The Journal of Pediatrics, 88,* 524.

Tsukada, Y., Hewett, W. J., Barlow, J. J., et al. (1972). Clear-cell adenocarcinoma (mesonephroma) of the vagina, three cases associated with maternal synthetic nonsteroid therapy. *Cancer, 29,* 1208–1214.

Ethambutol

FDA: **B**   SIGNIFICANCE: **5**   POTENCY: **4**

Use of ethambutol during pregnancy has been studied extensively in hundreds of women. No increase in the malformation rate among offspring has been noted. Although ethambutol has been associated with ocular problems among infants and children, ocular toxicity has not been reported for infants exposed in utero.

Bobrowitz, I. D. (1974). Ethambutol in pregnancy. *Chest, 66,* 20–24.

Johnston, R. F., Harris, H. W., Knight, R. A., et al. (1966). Multiple retreatment drug programs for pulmonary tuberculosis. *Annals of the New York Academy of Sciences, 135,* 831–834.

Lewit, T., Nebel, L., Terracina, S., et al. (1974). Ethambutol in pregnancy: Observations on embryogenesis. *Chest, 66,* 25–26.

Place, V. A. (1964). Ethambutol administration during pregnancy. A case report. *Journal of New Drugs, 4,* 206–208.

Snider, D. E., Layde, P. M., Johnson, M. W., et al. (1980). Treatment of tuberculosis during pregnancy. *American Review of Respiratory Disease, 122,* 65–79.

Warkany, J. (1979). Antituberculous drugs. *Teratology, 20,* 133–137.

Ethinyl Estradiol

FDA: **X**   SIGNIFICANCE: **2**   POTENCY: **2**

Although one report associated the incidence of cardiovascular defects with in utero exposure to ethinyl estradiol, two other studies did not. More data regarding use of ethinyl estradiol during pregnancy are needed, particularly data on use during the first trimester.

Heinonen, O. P., Slone, D., & Monson, R. R., et al. (1977). Cardiovascular birth defects and antenatal exposure to female sex hormones. *New England Journal of Medicine, 296,* 67–70.

Kallander, S., & Kallen, B. (1976). A prospective study of drugs and pregnancy. *Acta Obstetricia and Gynecologica Scandinavica, 55,* 221–224.

Spira, N., Goujard, J., Huel, G., et al. (1972). Investigation into the teratogenic action of sex hormones: First results of an epidemiologic survey involving 20,000 women. *Annual Review of Medicine, 41,* 2683–2694.

Ethionamide

FDA: **D**   SIGNIFICANCE: **4**   POTENCY: **3**

The data on ethionamide are generally favorable. No association between its use during pregnancy and malformations among offspring was found in several studies. Only one study found an increased rate of malformations, although a specific pattern was not identified. Out of 23 infants, seven were affected. Noted defects included two cases of trisomy 21, heart defects, spina bifida, and GI atresia.

Potworowski, M., Sianozecka, E., & Szulfladowicz, R. (1966). Ethionamide treatment and pregnancy. *Polish Medical Journal, 5,* 1152–1158.

Schardein, J. L. (1976). *Drugs as teratogens.* Cleveland: CRC.

Warkany, J. (1979). Antituberculous drugs. *Teratology, 20,* 133–138.

Zierski, M. (1966). Effects of ethionamide on the development of the human fetus. *Gruzlica I Choroby Pluc, 34,* 349–352.

Ethisterone (17-α-Ethinyltestosterone)

FDA: **D**   SIGNIFICANCE: **2**   POTENCY: **2**

Ethisterone may cause masculinization of the female fetus exposed to it in utero. However, one report on its teratogenic effects failed to note any associated malformations.

Grumbach, M. M., Ducharme, J. R., & Moloshok, R. E. (1959). On the fetal masculinizing action of certain oral progestins. *Journal of Clinical Endocrinology and Metabolism, 19,* 1369–1380.

McBride, W. G. (1963). The teratogenic action of drugs. *Medical Journal of Australia, 2,* 689–693.

Wilkins, L. (1960). Masculinization of female fetus due to use of orally given progestins. *Journal of the American Medical Association, 172,* 1028–1032.

Ethosuximide

FDA: **C**   SIGNIFICANCE: **1–2**   POTENCY: **2–3**

Various congenital malformations have been observed among infants exposed to ethosuximide in utero. These malformations include accessory nipple; decreased scores for gross motor index, fine motor index, language index, and personal social index; mongoloid facies; short neck; simian crease; and pilonidal sinus. Approximately 6% of exposed infants were affected. However, negative reports also have been published.

Fabro, S., & Brown, N. A. (1979). The teratogenic potential of anticonvulsants. *New England Journal of Medicine, 300,* 1280–1281.

Hill, R. M., Vernlaud, W. M., Horning, M. G., et al. (1974). Infants exposed in utero to antiepileptic drugs. *American Journal of Diseases of Children, 127,* 645–653.

Millar, J. H., & Nevin, N. C. (1973). Congenital malformations and anticonvulsant drugs. *The Lancet, 1,* 328.

Nakane, Y., Okuma, T., Takahashi, R., et al. (1980). Multi-institutional study on the teratogenicity and fetal toxicity of antiepileptic drugs: A report of a collaborative study group in Japan. *Epilepsia, 21,* 663–680.

Speidel, B. D., & Meadow, S. R. (1972). Maternal epilepsy and abnormalities of the fetus and newborn. *The Lancet, 2,* 839–843.

Ethotoin

FDA: **C**   SIGNIFICANCE: **1**   POTENCY: **1–2**

Ethotoin is a less commonly used member of the hydantoin family. Three papers describe four infants who displayed signs and symptoms consistent with the fetal hydantoin syndrome. Observed defects include abnormal ears, abnormal facies, cleft lip/palate, depressed nasal bridge, developmental delay, growth retardation, hypertelorism, hypoplasia of distal phalanges/nails, hypospadias, metopic suture ridging, and strabismus. However, there also have been reports of normal infants (n = 4) exposed in utero. (*See* Phenytoin monograph.)

Finnell, R. H., & DiLiberti, J. H. (1983). Hydantoin-induced teratogenesis: Are arene oxide intermediates really responsible? *Helvetica Paediatrica Acta, 8,* 171–177.

Nakane, Y., Okuma, T., Takahashi, R., et al. (1980). Multi-institutional study on the teratogenicity and fetal toxicity of antiepileptic drugs: A report of a collaborative study group in Japan. *Epilepsia, 21,* 663–680.

Wallar, P. H., Genstler, D. E., & George, C. C. (1978). Multiple systemic and periocular malformations associated with the fetal hydantoin syndrome. *Annals of Ophthalmology, 10,* 1568–1572.

Zoblen, M., & Brand, N. (1977). Cleft lip and palate with the anticonvulsant ethotoin. *New England Journal of Medicine, 298,* 285.

Etretinate

FDA: **X**   SIGNIFICANCE: **2**   POTENCY: **1–2**

Several cases of congenital anomalies have been reported among infants born to women who received etretinate during pregnancy. These anomalies included craniofacial abnormalities (n = 3), neural-tube and other CNS defects (n = 4), and skeletal abnormalities (n = 3). Etretinate has a long half-life, which is related to its long-term storage in adipose tissue; it may be detected in serum 1 year or longer after its last use. A single case was reported of teratogenicity involving a complex of cardiac, craniofacial, and CNS malformations associated with etretinate use almost 1 year before conception. Because of the drug's prolonged half-life and possible teratogenic effects, it is recommended that women who have used etretinate to treat psoriasis employ effective methods of contraception for 2 years after they stop using it.

DiGiovanna, J. J., Zech, L. A., Ruddel, M. E., et al. (1984). Etretinate: Persistent serum levels of a potent teratogen. *Clinical Research, 32,* 579A.
Etretinate pregnancy caution. (1988). *The Pharmaceutical Journal,* November 12, 630.
Happle, R., Traupe, H., Bounameaux, Y., et al. (1984). Teratogenic effects of etretinate in humans. *Deutsche Medizinische Wochenschrift, 109,* 1476–1480.
Lammer, E. J. (1988). Embryopathy in infant conceived one year after termination of maternal etretinate. *The Lancet, 2,* 1080–1081.
Monga, M. (1997). Vitamin A and its congeners. *Seminars in Perinatology, 21*(2), 135–142.
Rinck, G., Gollnick, H., & Orfanos, C. E. (1989). Duration of contraception after etretinate. *The Lancet, 1*(8642), 845–846.
Rosa, F. W., Wilk, A. L., & Kelsey, F. O. (1986). Teratogen update: Vitamin A congeners. *Teratology, 33,* 355–364.

Fentanyl

FDA: **C** SIGNIFICANCE: **4** POTENCY: **3–4**

Fentanyl readily crosses the placenta. Although a single case of the neonatal opiate-withdrawal syndrome was associated with long-term fentanyl use during pregnancy, no teratogenic effects have been reported in the published literature. But, because of its expected pharmacologic effects on the fetus and neonate (CNS and respiratory depression), fentanyl is not recommended for use during labor and delivery.

Regan, J., Chambers, F., Gorman, W., et al. (2000). Neonatal abstinence syndrome due to prolonged administration of fentanyl in pregnancy. *British Journal of Obstetrics and Gynecology, 107*(4), 570–572.

Flecainide

FDA: **C** SIGNIFICANCE: **4–5** (third trimester use) POTENCY: **4** (third trimester use)

In a single case report, flecainide was reportedly administered throughout pregnancy without any observed teratogenic effect. Several reports cite the successful use of flecainide during the third trimester for the treatment of fetal supraventricular tachycardia without the occurrence of any teratogenic effects. More data are needed regarding flecainide use during pregnancy, particularly use during the first trimester.

Gembruch, U., Hansmann, M., & Bald, R. (1988). Direct intrauterine fetal treatment of fetal tachyarrhythmia with severe hydrops fetalis by antiarrhythmic drugs. *Fetal Therapy, 3,* 210–215.
MacPhail, S., & Walkinshaw, S. A. (1988). Fetal supraventricular tachycardia: Detection by routine auscultation and successful in-utero management. Case report. *British Journal of Obstetrics and Gynaecology, 95,* 1073–1076.
Perry, J. C., Ayres, N. A., & Carpenter, R. J., Jr. (1991). Fetal supraventricular tachycardia treated with flecainide acetate. *The Journal of Pediatrics, 118,* 303–305.
Wagner, X., Jouglard, J., Moulin, M., et al. (1990). Coadministration of flecainide acetate and sotalol during pregnancy: Lack of teratogenic effects, passage across the placenta, and excretion in human breast milk. *American Heart Journal, 119,* 700–702.
Wren, C., & Hunter, S. (1988). Maternal administration of flecainide to terminate and suppress fetal tachycardia. *British Medical Journal, 296,* 249.

Fluorouracil (5-Fluorouracil)

FDA: **D** SIGNIFICANCE: **2–3** POTENCY: **2–3**

In a single case report, an infant exposed in utero to fluorouracil was born with radial aplasia, imperforate anus, esophageal aplasia, and duodenal hypoplasia. In half a dozen other cases, however, normal infants were born to mothers who received fluorouracil, intravenously or topically, at various stages of their pregnancies. More data are needed regarding fluorouracil use during pregnancy, particularly use during the first trimester.

Kopelman, J. N., & Miyazawa, K. (1990). Inadvertent 5-fluorouracil treatment in early pregnancy: A report of three cases. *Reproductive Toxicology, 4,* 233–235.
Odom, L. D., Plouffe, L., Jr., & Butler, W. J. (1990). 5-Fluorouracil exposure during the period of conception: Report on two cases. *American Journal of Obstetrics and Gynecology, 163*(1), 76–77.
Stadler, H. E., & Knowles, J. (1971). Fluorouracil in pregnancy: Effect on the neonate. *Journal of the American Medical Association, 217*(2), 214–215.
Stephens, T. D., Golbus, M. S., Miller, J. R., et al.

(1980). Multiple congenital anomalies in a fetus exposed to 5-fluorouracil during the first trimester. *American Journal of Obstetrics and Gynecology, 137*, 747–749.

Turchi, J. J., & Villasis, C. (1988). Anthracyclines in the treatment of malignancy in pregnancy. *Cancer, 61*, 435–440.

Fluoxetine

FDA: **C**   SIGNIFICANCE: **4–5**   POTENCY: **4**

Fluoxetine crosses the placenta. Based on data from several studies (n = 250), however, it does not appear to be a human teratogen.

Baum, A. L., & Misri, S. (1996). Selective serotonin-reuptake inhibitors in pregnancy and lactation. *Harvard Review of Psychiatry, 4*(3), 117–125.

Goldstein, D. J. (1990). Outcome of fluoxetine-exposed pregnancies. *American Journal of Human Genetics, 47*, A136.

Pastuszak, A., Schick-Boschetto, B., Zuber, C., et al. (1993). Pregnancy outcome following first trimester exposure to fluoxetine (Prozac). *Journal of the American Medical Association, 269*, 2246–2248.

Shader, R. I. (1992). Does continuous use of fluoxetine during the first trimester of pregnancy present a high risk for malformation or abnormal development to the exposed fetus? *Journal of Clinical Psychopharmacology, 12*, 441.

Fluphenazine

FDA: **C**   SIGNIFICANCE: **4–5**   POTENCY: **3–4**

Although there is a report of an infant born with multiple congenital anomalies associated with fluphenazine use during pregnancy, there also is a negative report.

Donaldson, G. L., & Buz, R. G. (1983). Multiple congenital abnormalities in a newborn boy associated with maternal use of fluphenazine enanthate and other drugs during pregnancy. *Acta Paediatrica Scandinavica, 71*, 335–338.

Rumeau-Rouquette, C., Goujard, J., & Huel, G. (1977). Possible teratologic effects of phenothiazines in human beings. *Teratology, 15*, 57–64.

Folic Acid

FDA: **A**   SIGNIFICANCE: **5**
POTENCY: see monograph

Folic acid (4 mg/day) during the first half of the first trimester prevents neural-tube defects among the offspring of women who have had a previous affected pregnancy and are at high risk. Folic acid appears to provide significant (3.5-fold) protection against the recurrence of these defects in subsequent pregnancies. Folic acid supplementation also is recommended for epileptic women receiving anticonvulsant drugs (e.g., phenobarbital, phenytoin) and other drugs (e.g., triamterene, trimethoprim) that decrease folate serum levels.

Dansky, L. V., Rosenblatt, D. S., & Andermann, E. (1992). Mechanisms of teratogenesis: Folic acid and antiepileptic therapy. *Neurology, 42*(4, Suppl 5), 32–42.

Folic acid for prevention of neural tube defects. (1991). *Annals of Pharmacotherapy, 25*, 1158.

Glanville, N. T., & Cook, H. W. (1992). Folic acid and prevention of neural tube defects. *Canadian Medical Association Journal, 46*, 39.

Hernandez-Diaz, S., Werler, M. M., Walker, A. M., et al. (2000). Folic acid antagonists during pregnancy and the risk of birth defects. *New England Journal of Medicine, 343*(22), 1608–1614.

Lewis, D. P., Van Dyke, D. C., Stumbo, P. J., et al. (1998). Drug and environmental factors associated with adverse pregnancy outcomes. Part I: Antiepileptic drugs, contraceptives, smoking, and folate. *Annals of Pharmacotherapy, 32*(7-8), 802–817.

Use of folic acid for prevention of spina bifida and other neural tube defects: 1983–1991. (1991). *Journal of the American Medical Association, 266*, 1190–1191.

Furazolidone

AUTHOR: **NONE**   SIGNIFICANCE: **4–5**
POTENCY: **3–4**

No significant increase in the incidence of congenital anomalies was noted among the offspring of 132 women who took furazolidone during the first trimester. More data are needed.

Heinonen, O. P., Slone, D., & Shapiro, S. (1977). *Birth defects and drugs in pregnancy*. Littleton, MA: Publishing Sciences Group.

Furosemide (Frusemide)

FDA: **C**   SIGNIFICANCE: **2–3**   POTENCY: **2**

No teratogenic effects have been associated with furosemide administration during pregnancy. Furosemide use near term, however, may result in expected (diuretic) pharmacologic effects among neonates, specifically diuresis, hyperuricemia, hypokalemia, and hyponatremia. In addition, furosemide may decrease placental blood flow and may displace bilirubin from albumin. Therefore, it may pose an additional risk to neonates who are already at risk for jaundice. Some authors, however, consider it the diuretic of choice for use during pregnancy.

Barrillon, A., Grand, A., & Gerbaux, A. (1974). Treatment of the heart during pregnancy. *Annales Medecine Interne (Paris), 125,* 437–445.
Catz, C. A., & Abuelo, D. (1974). Drugs and pregnancy. *Drug Therapy, 4,* 79.
Corswell, W., & Semple, P. F. (1974). The effects of furosemide on uric acid levels in maternal blood, fetal blood, and amniotic fluid. *Obstetrics and Gynecology, 81,* 472.
Gnat, N. F., Madden, J. D., Shteri, P. K., et al. (1976). The metabolic clearance rate of dehydroisoandrosterone sulfate. IV. Acute effects of induced hypertension, and naturesis in normal and hypertensive pregnancies. *American Journal of Obstetrics and Gynecology, 124,* 143.
Jacobs, D. (1975). Maternal drug ingestion and congenital malformations. *South African Medical Journal, 49,* 2073.
Pecorari, D., Ragni, N., & Autera, C. (1969). Administration of furosemide to women during confinement, and its actions on newborn infants. *Acta Biomedica de' l Ateneo Parmense, 40,* 2.
Turmen, T., Thom, P., Louridas, A. T., et al. (1982). Protein binding and bilirubin displacing properties of bumetanide and furosemide. *Journal of Clinical Pharmacology, 22,* 551–556.
Witter, F. R., King, T. M., & Blake, D. A. (1981). Adverse effects of cardiovascular drug therapy on the fetus and neonate. *Obstetrics and Gynecology, 58*(Suppl 5), 100S–105S.

Gentamicin
FDA: **C**   SIGNIFICANCE: see monograph
POTENCY: see monograph

No studies in humans associate gentamicin use during pregnancy with teratogenic effects. It has been suggested that gentamicin may be ototoxic for the fetus, however; it should be used with caution during pregnancy.

Beeley, L. (1981). Adverse effects of drugs in later pregnancy. *Clinical Obstetrics and Gynecology, 8,* 275–290.
Tuchmann-Duplessis, H. (1975). *Drug effects on the fetus.* Acton, MA: Publishing Sciences Group.

Glutethimide
FDA: **C**   SIGNIFICANCE: **4–5**   POTENCY: **4**

The Collaborative Perinatal Project reported no significant increase in congenital malformations among the offspring of 67 women who received glutethimide during the first trimester or of the offspring of 640 women who received glutethimide at various times during their pregnancies.

Asnes, R. S., & Lamb, J. M. (1969). Neonatal respiratory depression secondary to maternal analgesics, treated by exchange transfusion. *Pediatrics, 43,* 94–96.
Heinonen, O. P., Slone, D., & Shapiro, S. (1977). *Birth defects and drugs in pregnancy.* Littleton, MA: Publishing Sciences Group.
Reveri, M., Pyati, S. P., & Pildes, R. S. (1977). Neonatal withdrawal symptoms associated with glutethimide (Doriden) addiction in the mother during pregnancy. *Clinical Pediatrics, 16,* 424–425.

Glyburide
FDA: **D**   SIGNIFICANCE: **4**   POTENCY: **2–3**

A prospective study involved more than 400 women who were between 11 and 33 weeks pregnant and randomly assigned to receive either glyburide or insulin for gestational diabetes mellitus. No significant differences in relation to teratogenic or fetotoxic effects were found. Effects specifically compared included incidence of fetal anomalies, hypoglycemia, largeness for gestational age, lung complications, macrosomia (i.e., birth weight above the 90th percentile on the intrauterine growth chart or greater than or equal to 4000 grams), and requirement for admission to a neonatal intensive care unit. Although these results are encouraging, more data are needed, particularly in relation to use of glyburide during the first trimester.

Langer, O., Conway, D. L., Berkus, M. D., et al. (2000). A comparison of glyburide and insulin in women with gestational diabetes mellitus. *New England Journal of Medicine, 343,* 1134–1138.

Gold Salts
FDA: **C**   SIGNIFICANCE: **4**   POTENCY: **3**

Gold crosses the placenta. In various reports involving more than 100 pregnant women, no teratogenic effects were associated with the use of gold salts. However, in one case in which gold was administered to a woman throughout the first trimester, the infant was born with cerebral degeneration, cleft lip and palate, and severe hypertelorism.

More data are needed regarding the use of gold salts during pregnancy, particularly data addressing use during the first trimester.

Needs, C. J., & Brooks, P. M. (1985). Antirheumatic medication in pregnancy. *British Journal of Rheumatology, 24*(3), 282–290.
Rocker, I., & Henderson, W. J. (1976). Transfer of gold from mother to fetus. *The Lancet, 2*, 1246.
Rogers, J. G., Anderson, R. M., Chow, C. W., et al. (1980). Possible teratogenic effects of gold. *Australian Paediatric Journal, 16*, 194–195.
Shepard, T. H. (1983). *Catalog of teratogenic agents*, 4th ed., pp. 212–213. Baltimore: Johns Hopkins.

Griseofulvin
FDA: **C**   SIGNIFICANCE: **4**   POTENCY: **3–4**

One report details two cases in which two mothers who received griseofulvin during the first trimester each gave birth to conjoined twins. Subsequent analyses of conjoined twin studies (n = 86) failed to support this association. More data are needed, particularly data addressing griseofulvin use during the first trimester.

Knudsen, L. B. (1987). No association between griseofulvin and conjoined twinning. [Letter]. *The Lancet, 2*, 1097.
Metneki, J., & Czeizel, A. (1987). Griseofulvin teratology. *The Lancet, 1*, 1042.
Rosa, F. W., Hernandez, C., & Carlo, W. A. (1987). Griseofulvin teratology, including two thoracopagus conjoined twins. *The Lancet, 1*, 171.

Guaifenesin
AUTHOR: **NONE**   SIGNIFICANCE: **5**
POTENCY: **4**

Two large studies in which women received guaifenesin during either the first trimester (n = 1123) or at various times during their pregnancies (n = 1336) failed to detect a significant risk for teratogenesis.

Aselton, P., Jick, H., Milunsky, A., et al. (1985). First-trimester drug use and congenital disorders. *Obstetrics and Gynecology, 65*, 451–455.
Heinonen, O. P., Slone, D., & Shapiro, S. (1977). *Birth defects and drugs in pregnancy*. Littleton, MA: Publishing Sciences Group.
Jick, H., Holmes, L. B., Hunter, J. R., et al. (1981). First-trimester drug use and congenital disorders. *Journal of the American Medical Association, 246*, 343–346.

Haloperidol
FDA: **C**   SIGNIFICANCE: **4–5**   POTENCY: **3–4**

Two case reports implicate haloperidol use during pregnancy with infant limb malformations (reduction defects). In other retrospective studies involving more than 100 pregnancies, negative results were reported.

Dieulangard, P., Coignet, J., & Vidal, J. C. (1966). On a case of phocomelia: Possibly caused by medication. *Bulletin de la Federation des Societes de Gynecologie et d'Obstetrique de Langue Francaise, 18*, 85–87.
Hanson, J. W., & Oakley, G. P. (1975). Haloperidol and limb deformities. *Journal of the American Medical Association, 231*, 26.
Kopelman, A. E., McCullar, F. W., & Heggeness, L. (1975). Limb malformations following maternal use of haloperidol. *Journal of the American Medical Association, 231*, 62–64.
Van Vaes, A., & Van de Velde, E. (1969). Safety evaluations of haloperidol in treatment of hyperemesis gravidarum. *Journal of Clinical Pharmacology, 9*, 224–227.

Halothane
AUTHOR: ★   SIGNIFICANCE: **3**
POTENCY: **2–3**

In addition to an increased risk for spontaneous abortions, as discussed under "Anesthetics–Inhalation, Waste," halothane, when used for obstetrical anesthesia, has been associated with an increased incidence of neonatal apnea. Another study (n = 25) found no significant increase in risk for congenital anomalies when halothane was used during the first trimester. More data are needed regarding the use of halothane during pregnancy. (*See* Anesthetics—Inhalation, Waste monograph.)

Heinonen, O. P., Slone, D., & Shapiro, S. (1977). *Birth defects and drugs in pregnancy*. Littleton, MA: Publishing Sciences Group.
Taylor, C. R. (1961). The effects of analgesia and anesthesia on the initial fetus respiration, with particular reference to the use of chloroform, levallorphan, and halothane. *American Journal of Obstetrics and Gynecology, 81*, 1260–1265.

Heparin
FDA: **C**   SIGNIFICANCE: **5**   POTENCY: **4**

Heparin is a large-molecular-weight compound and does not cross the placenta. Clinical trials have demonstrated no effects of maternal heparin use on the fetus. Heparin would appear to be the anticoagulant of choice for use during pregnancy. However, heparin has been associated with maternal vertebral fractures related to self-injection of the drug during pregnancy.

Bonar, J. (1981). Venous thromboembolism and pregnancy. *Clinical Obstetrics and Gynecology, 8*, 455–473.
Flessa, H. C., Kapstrom, A. B., Glueck, H. I., et al. (1965). Placental transport of heparin. *American Journal of Obstetrics and Gynecology, 93*, 570–573.
Ginsberg, J. S., & Hirsh, J. (1989). Anticoagulants during pregnancy. *Annual Review of Medicine, 40*, 79–86.
Ginsberg, J. S., Hirsh, J., Turner, C., et al. (1989). Risks to the fetus of anticoagulant therapy during pregnancy. *Thrombosis and Haemostasis, 61*(6), 197–203.
Ginsberg, J. S., Kowalchuk, G., Hirsh, J., et al. (1989). Heparin therapy during pregnancy. *Archives of Internal Medicine, 149*, 2233–2236.
Hill, R. M., & Stern, L. (1979). Drugs in pregnancy: Effects on the fetus and newborn. *Drugs, 17*, 182–197.
Hirsh, J., Cade, J. F., & Golbus, A. S. (1972). Anticoagulants in pregnancy. A review of indications and complications. *American Heart Journal, 83*, 301.
Merrill, L. K., & VerBurg, D. J. (1976). The choice of long-term anticoagulants for the pregnant patient. *Obstetrics and Gynecology, 47*, 711–714.
Squires, J. W., & Pinch, L. W. (1979). Heparin-induced spinal fracture. *Journal of the American Medical Association, 241*, 2417–2418.
Use of anticoagulants in pregnancy. (1987). *Drug and Therapeutics Bulletin, 25*(1), 1–4.
Wise, P. H., & Hall, A. J. (1980). Heparin-induced osteopenia in pregnancy. *British Medical Journal, 281*, 110–111.

Hepatitis B Vaccine

FDA: C SIGNIFICANCE: 4 POTENCY: 4

No birth defects were noted among infants whose mothers were vaccinated with hepatitis B vaccine during either the first trimester (n = 10) or the third trimester (n = 72). More data are needed, particularly data addressing hepatitis B vaccination during the second trimester.

Ayoola, E. A., & Johnson, A. O. K. (1987). Hepatitis B vaccine in pregnancy: Immunogenicity, safety and transfer of antibodies to infants. *International Journal of Gynaecology and Obstetrics, 25*, 297–301.
Levy, M., & Koren, G. (1991). Hepatitis B vaccine in pregnancy: Maternal and fetal safety. *American Journal of Perinatology, 8*(3), 227–232.

Heroin (Diacetylmorphine)

FDA: C SIGNIFICANCE: 1 (see monograph)
POTENCY: 1 (see monograph)

Although heroin and its metabolites readily cross the placenta, the use of heroin during pregnancy has not been associated with teratogenic effects. Its use during pregnancy has been associated with fetotoxic effects, however. A frequent finding among infants born to heroin-addicted mothers is intrauterine growth retardation; this finding has not been consistent, however. Although the growth retardation has been attributed to a decreased cell number, one study attributed it to several confounding variables (e.g., poor maternal nutrition, lack of prenatal care). Expected pharmacologic effects also may be observed among neonates. These effects include lethargy, poor suck, and neonatal opiate-withdrawal syndrome. Sudden infant death syndrome also is reported to be associated with maternal heroin addiction during pregnancy. A 13.5% first year mortality has been reported. These findings may be confounded, however, as women who are addicted to heroin also frequently abuse alcohol, cigarettes, and cocaine. They also generally have a higher incidence of sexually transmitted diseases, including human immunodeficiency virus (HIV) infection and acquired immunity deficiency syndrome (AIDS).

Claman, A. D., & Strong, R. I. (1962). Obstetric and gynecologic aspects of heroin addiction. *American Journal of Obstetrics, 83*, 252–257.
Connaughton, J. F., Reeser, D., Schut, J., et al. (1977). Perinatal addiction: Outcome and management. *American Journal of Obstetrics and Gynecology, 129*, 679–685.
Finnegan, L. P. (1979). In utero opiate dependence and sudden infant death syndrome. *Clinics in Perinatology, 6*, 163–180.
Harper, R. G., Solish, G. I., Parow, H. M., et al. (1974). The effect of a methadone treatment program upon pregnant heroin addicts and their newborn infants. *Pediatrics, 54*, 300–305.
Hill, R. M., & Desmond, M. M. (1963). Management of the narcotic withdrawal syndrome in

the neonate. *Pediatric Clinics of North America, 10*, 67–86.
Kahn, E. J., Neumann, L. L., & Polk, G. A. (1969). The course of the heroin withdrawal syndrome in newborn infants treated with phenobarbital or chlorpromazine. *The Journal of Pediatrics, 75*, 495–500.
Kandall, S. R., Albin, S., Gartner, L. M., et al. (1977). The narcotic dependent mother: Fetal and neonatal consequences. *Early Human Development, 1*, 159–169.
Lifschitz, M. H., Wilson, G. S., Smith, E., et al. (1983). Fetal and postnatal growth of children born to narcotic-dependent women. *The Journal of Pediatrics, 102*, 686–691.
Little, B. B., Snell, L. M., Klein, V. R., et al. (1990). Maternal and fetal effects of heroin addiction during pregnancy. *Journal of Reproductive Medicine, 35*(2), 159–162.
Naeye, R. L., Blanc, W., LeBlanc, W., et al. (1973). Fetal complications of maternal heroin addiction. *The Journal of Pediatrics, 83*, 1055–1061.
Newman, R. G., Bashkow, S., & Calko, D. (1975). Results of 313 consecutive live births of infants delivered to patients in the New York City methadone maintenance treatment program. *American Journal of Obstetrics and Gynecology, 121*, 233–237.
Ostrea, E. M., & Chavez, C. J. (1979). Perinatal problems (excluding neonatal withdrawal) in maternal drug addiction: A study of 830 cases. *The Journal of Pediatrics, 94*, 292–295.
Potsch, L., Skopp, G., Emmerich, T. P., et al. (1999). Report on intrauterine drug exposure during second trimester of pregnancy in a heroin-associated death. *Therapeutic Drug Monitoring, 21*(6), 593–597.
Reddy, A. M., Harper, R. G., & Stern, G. (1971). Observations on heroin and methadone withdrawal in the newborn. *Pediatrics, 48*, 353–358.
Schneck, H. (1958). Narcotic withdrawal symptoms in the newborn infant resulting from maternal addiction. *The Journal of Pediatrics, 52*, 584–587.
Stimmel, B., & Adamson, K. (1976). Narcotic dependency in pregnancy. Methadone maintenance compared to use of street drugs. *Journal of the American Medical Association, 235*, 1121–1124.
Stone, M. L., Salerno, L. J., Green, M., et al. (1971). Narcotic addiction in pregnancy. *American Journal of Obstetrics and Gynecology, 109*, 716–723.
Wilson, G. S., Desmond, M. M., & Verniaud, W. M. (1973). Early development of infants of heroin-addicted mothers. *American Journal of Diseases of Children, 126*, 457–462.
Zelson, C. (1973). Infant of the addicted mother. *Medical Intelligence, 288*, 1393–1396.
Zelson, C., Lee, S. J., & Casalino, M. (1973). Neonatal narcotic addiction—Comparative effects of maternal intake of heroin and methadone. *New England Journal of Medicine, 289*, 1216–1220.
Zelson, C., Rubio, E., & Wasserman, E. (1971). Neonatal narcotic addiction: 10 year observations. *Pediatrics, 48*, 178–189.

Hexachlorophene
AUTHOR: **NONE**   SIGNIFICANCE: **3–4**
POTENCY: **3–4**

A Swedish retrospective epidemiologic study raised concern over the teratogenic potential of the disinfectant hexachlorophene. The study found an increased malformation rate among the infants of women exposed frequently to hexachlorophene soap in hospitals. These data prompted a second study that found no association between hexachlorophene use and the malformation rate, except for a number of perinatal deaths during one year of the multiyear study. A third study that evaluated associations between hexachlorophene and oral clefts was negative. The teratogenic potential of hexachlorophene is unclear but appears to be low.

Baltzar, B., Ericson, A., & Kallen, B. (1979). Pregnancy outcome among women working in Swedish hospitals. *New England Journal of Medicine, 300*, 627–628.
Halling, H. (1979). Suspected link between exposure to hexachlorophene and malformed infants. *Annals of the New York Academy of Sciences, 320*, 426–435.
Hernberg, S., Holmberg, P., Rantala, K., et al. (1981). Relationship between congenital oral clefts and maternal chemical and physical exposures during pregnancy. *XX International Congress of Occupational Health*, Cairo, Egypt.
Hernberg, S., Kurppa, K., Ojajarvi, J., et al. (1983). Congenital malformations and occupational exposure to disinfectants: A case-referent study. *Scandinavian Journal of Work Environment and Health, 9*, 55.
Kallen, B. (1978). Hexachlorophene teratogenicity in humans disputed. *Journal of the American Medical Association, 240*(15), 1585–1586.

Hydralazine
FDA: **C**   SIGNIFICANCE: **4**   POTENCY: **3**

Hydralazine lowers maternal blood pressure without changing uterine blood flow. One report suggested that hydralazine use during pregnancy may be associated with an increased risk for teratogenesis. The data were not statistically significant, however, and the number of infants studied was small.

Heinonen, O. P., Slone, D., & Shapiro, S. (1977). *Birth defects and drugs in pregnancy*. Littleton, MA: Publishing Sciences Group.

Pitkin, R. M. (1980). Drugs in pregnancy. In F. J. Quilligan & N. Kretchmer, Eds., *Fetal and maternal medicine*, pp. 385–402. New York: Wiley.

Hydrochlorothiazide

FDA: **B**   SIGNIFICANCE: **5**   POTENCY: **4**

The only problem found from a review of the extensive use of hydrochlorothiazide during pregnancy has been one report of neonatal thrombocytopenia.

Arias, F., & Zamora, J. (1979). Antihypertensive treatment and pregnancy outcome in patients with mild chronic hypertension. *Obstetrics and Gynecology, 53*, 489–494.

Follis, N. E., Plauche, W. C., Mosey, L. M., et al. (1964). Thiazide versus placebo in prophylaxis of toxemia of pregnancy in primigravid patients. *American Journal of Obstetrics and Gynecology, 88*, 502–504.

Heinonen, O. P., Slone, D., & Shapiro, S. (1977). *Birth defects and drugs in pregnancy*. Littleton, MA: Publishing Sciences Group.

Jick, H., Holmes, L. B., Hunter, J. R., et al. (1981). First-trimester drug use and congenital disorders. *Journal of the American Medical Association, 246*, 343–346.

Kraus, G. W., Marchese, J. R., & Yen, S. S. C. (1966). Prophylactic use of hydrochlorothiazide in pregnancy. *Journal of the American Medical Association, 198*, 1150–1154.

Mackay, E. V., & Khoo, S. K. (1969). Clinical and laboratory study of a new diuretic agent (Vectren®) in pregnancy: A comparison with a diuretic agent in current use (Enduron®). *Medical Journal of Australia, 1*, 607–612.

McBride, W. G. (1963). The teratogenic action of drugs. *Medical Journal of Australia, 2*, 689–693.

Weseley, A. C., & Douglas, G. K. (1962). Continuous use of chlorothiazide for prevention of toxemia of pregnancy. *Obstetrics and Gynecology, 19*, 355–358.

Hydroflumethiazide

FDA: **B**   SIGNIFICANCE: **5**   POTENCY: **4**

Hydroflumethiazide use during pregnancy has not been associated with teratogenic or fetotoxic effects.

McBride, W. G. (1963). The teratogenic action of drugs. *Medical Journal of Australia, 2*, 689–693.

Schardein, J. (1976). *Drugs as teratogens*. Cleveland: CRC.

Hydroxyprogesterone

FDA: **X**   SIGNIFICANCE: **1–2**   POTENCY: **3**

Hydroxyprogesterone, a progestogen closely related to testosterone, has the potential to masculinize the female fetus. The observed incidence of this effect is, however, exceedingly rare. In one study of more than 1500 cases, only two cases of clitoral hypertrophy were reported.

Darling, M. R., & Hawkins, D. F. (1981). Sex hormones in pregnancy. *Clinical Obstetrics and Gynecology, 8*, 405–419.

Grumbach, M. M., Ducharme, J. R., & Moloshak, R. E. (1959). On the fetal masculinizing action of certain oral progestins. *Journal of Clinical Endocrinology and Metabolism, 19*, 1369–1380.

Istvan, E. J. (1970). Drug associated congenital abnormalities. *Canadian Medical Association Journal, 103*, 1394.

McBride, W. G. (1963). The teratogenic action of drugs. *Medical Journal of Australia, 2*, 689–693.

Serment, H., & Ruf, H. (1968). Therapeutiques hormonales. *Bulletin de la Federation des Societes de Gynecologie et d'Obstetrique de Langue Francaise, 20*, 69–76.

Hydroxyzine

FDA: **C**   SIGNIFICANCE: **4**   POTENCY: **3–4**

Two studies in which women received hydroxyzine either during the first trimester (n = 124) or at various times during pregnancy (n = 187) failed to detect a significant risk for congenital anomalies among offspring.

Erez, S., Schifrin, B. S., & Dirim, O. (1971). Double-blind evaluation of hydroxyzine as an antiemetic in pregnancy. *Journal of Reproductive Medicine, 7*, 35–37.

Heinonen, O. P., Slone, D., & Shapiro, S. (1977). *Birth defects and drugs in pregnancy*. Littleton, MA: Publishing Sciences Group.

Ibuprofen

FDA: **B**   SIGNIFICANCE: **2–3** (near term)
POTENCY: **2** (near term)

Results from two studies (one in which women received ibuprofen during the first trimester and one in which both overdoses and normal doses were taken at various times during pregnancy) failed to reveal an increased risk for congenital anomalies. However, the use of ibuprofen near term as a tocolytic for women with premature labor has been associated with oligohydramnios. In addition, inhibition of prostaglandin synthesis by ibuprofen may, theoretically, cause premature (i.e., in utero) closure of the ductus arteriosus in affected fetuses if the drug is administered near term. Use of ibuprofen during the third trimester, particularly near term, is not generally recommended.

Aselton, P., Jick, H., Milunsky, A., et al. (1985). First-trimester drug use and congenital disorders. *Obstetrics and Gynecology, 65,* 451–455.

Barry, W. S., Meinzinger, M. M., & Howse, C. R. (1984). Ibuprofen overdose and exposure in utero: Results from a postmarketing voluntary reporting system. *American Journal of Medicine, 77*(1a), 35–39.

Hendricks, S. K., Smith, J. R., Moore, D. E., et al. (1990). Oligohydramnios associated with prostaglandin synthetase inhibitors in preterm labour. *British Journal of Obstetrics and Gynaecology, 97,* 312–316.

Wiggins, D. A., & Elliott, J. P. (1990). Oligohydramnios in each sac of a triplet gestation caused by Motrin—Fulfilling Kock's postulates. *American Journal of Obstetrics and Gynecology, 162,* 460–461.

Imipramine

FDA: **D**   SIGNIFICANCE: **3–4**   POTENCY: **3–4**

Various teratogenic (adrenal hypoplasia, cleft palate, diaphragmatic hernias, exencephalia, limb defects, rib defects) and fetotoxic (cyanosis, irritability, neonatal dyspnea, profuse sweating, tachycardia, tachypnea) effects have been associated with imipramine use during pregnancy. Other studies have noted none of these effects.

However, a syndrome involving neonatal distress characterized by clonus, hypertonia, peripheral cyanosis, respiratory distress, spasm, tremor, and urinary retention secondary to the anticholinergic effects and to the sympathetic supersensitization of imipramine appears to be directly related to the use of imipramine near term. Neonates of mothers who receive imipramine during pregnancy should be monitored for these fetotoxic effects and treated appropriately. (*See* Nortriptyline monograph.)

Ananth, J. (1976). Side effects on fetus and infant of psychotropic drug use during pregnancy. *International Pharmacopsychiatry, 11,* 246–260.

Banister, P., DeFoe, C., Smith, E. S. O., et al. (1972). Possible teratogenicity of tricyclic antidepressants. *The Lancet, 1,* 838–839.

Barson, A. J. (1972). Malformed infant. *British Medical Journal, 2,* 45.

Crombie, D. L., Pinsent, R. J., & Fleming, D. (1972). Imipramine in pregnancy. *British Medical Journal, 1,* 745–755.

Eggermont, E., Roveschot, V., Deneue, V., et al. (1972). The adverse influence of imipramine on the adaptation of the newborn infant to extrauterine life. *Acta Pediatrica Belgica, 135,* 761–762.

Idanpaan-Heikkila, J., & Saxen, L. (1973). Possible teratogenicity of imipramine/chloropyramine. *The Lancet, 2,* 282–284.

Kuensberg, E. V., & Knox, J. D. (1972). Imipramine in pregnancy. *British Medical Journal, 2,* 292.

McBride, W. G. (1972). Limb deformities associated with iminodibenzyl hydrochloride. *Medical Journal of Australia, 1,* 492.

Morrow, A. W. (1972). Imipramine and congenital abnormalities. *New Zealand Medical Journal, 82,* 228–229.

Rachelefsky, G. S., Flynt, J. W., Ebbin, A. J., et al. (1972). Possible teratogenicity of tricyclic antidepressants. *The Lancet, 1,* 838–839.

Sim, M. (1972). Imipramine and pregnancy. *British Medical Journal, 2,* 45.

Tuchmann-Duplessis, H. (1975). *Drug effects on the fetus.* Acton, MA: Publishing Sciences Group.

Webster, P. A. (1973). Withdrawal symptoms in neonates associated with maternal antidepressant therapy. *The Lancet, 2,* 318–319.

Indomethacin

FDA: **D**   SIGNIFICANCE: **3** (early), **1** (late)   POTENCY: **2–3**

Indomethacin has been associated with oral cleft when used during early pregnancy. A more recent study, however, failed to demonstrate this teratogenic effect. Indomethacin has been used near term to arrest premature labor and to treat polyhydramnios. Indomethacin also is used to induce closure of the ductus arteriosus among premature infants and, when administered to pregnant women near term, can theoretically cause the same effect prenatally. Use of indomethacin during late pregnancy has been associated with hydrops fetalis, neonatal anuria, oligohydramnios, perinatal death, and persistent fetal circulation syndrome. Because of the potential for both therapeutic benefit and harmful effects, careful clinical evaluation and judgment must be used when indomethacin use near term is considered. The fetus and neonate must be closely monitored. Appropriate intervention, if required, must be readily available.

Aselton, P., Jick, H., Milunsky, A., et al. (1985). First trimester drug use and congenital disorders. *Obstetrics and Gynecology, 65*, 451–455.

Csaba, I. F., Sulyok, E., & Ertl, T. (1978). Relationship of maternal treatment with indomethacin to persistence of fetal circulation syndrome. *The Journal of Pediatrics, 92*, 484.

Douidar, S. M., Richardson, J., & Snodgrass, W. R. (1988). Role of indomethacin in ductus closure: An update evaluation. *Developmental Pharmacology and Therapeutics, 11*, 196–212.

Eronen, M., Pesonen, E., Kurki, T., et al. (1991). The effects of indomethacin and a beta-sympathomimetic agent on the fetal ductus arteriosus during treatment of premature labor: A randomized double-blind study. *American Journal of Obstetrics and Gynecology, 164*, 141–146.

Gal, P., Ransom, J. L., Schall, S., et al. (1990). Indomethacin for patent ductus arteriosus closure. Application of serum concentrations and pharmacodynamics to improve response. *Journal of Perinatology, 10*, 20–26.

Itskovitz, J., Abramovici, H., & Brandes, J. M. (1980). Oligohydramnios, meconium, and perinatal death concurrent with indomethacin treatment in human pregnancy. *Journal of Reproductive Medicine, 24*, 137–140.

Katz, Z., Lancet, H., Borenstein, R., et al. (1984). Absence of teratogenicity of indomethacin in ovarian hyperstimulation syndrome. *International Journal of Fertility, 29*, 186–188.

Kirshon, B., Mari, G., Moise, K. J., Jr., et al. (1990). Effect of indomethacin on the fetal ductus arteriosus during treatment of symptomatic polyhydramnios. *Journal of Reproductive Medicine, 35*, 529–532.

Kirshon, B., Moise, K. J., Jr., Mari, G., et al. (1991). Long-term indomethacin therapy decreases fetal urine output and results in oligohydramnios. *American Journal of Perinatology, 8*(2), 86–88.

Levin, D. L., Fixler, D. E., Morriss, F. C., et al. (1978). Morphologic analysis of the pulmonary vascular bed in infants exposed in utero to prostaglandin synthetase inhibitors. *The Journal of Pediatrics, 92*, 478–483.

Mari, G., Moise, K. J., Deter, R. L., et al. (1989). Doppler assessment of the pulsatility index of the middle cerebral artery during constriction of the fetal ductus arteriosus after indomethacin therapy. *American Journal of Obstetrics and Gynecology, 161*, 1528–1531.

Mogilner, B. M., Ashkenazy, M., Borenstein, R., et al. (1982). Hydrops fetalis caused by maternal indomethacin treatment. *Acta Obstetricia and Gynecologica Scandinavica, 61*, 183–185.

Moise, K. J., Jr. (1991). Indomethacin therapy in the treatment of symptomatic polyhydramnios. *Clinica Obstetrica e Ginecologica, 34*, 310–318.

Rubaltelli, F. F., Chiozza, M. L., Zanardo, V., et al. (1979). Effect on neonate of maternal treatment with indomethacin. *The Journal of Pediatrics, 94*, 161.

Saxen, I. (1975). Associations between oral clefts and drugs taken during pregnancy. *International Journal of Epidemiology, 4*, 37–44.

Influenza Virus Vaccine

FDA: C   SIGNIFICANCE: 5   POTENCY: 4

Maternal influenza vaccination during pregnancy using inactivated vaccine does not appear to increase the incidence of teratogenic effects among offspring. The composition of the influenza virus vaccine changes annually, however. New compositions thus have the theoretical risk of producing teratogenic effects.

Deinard, A. S., & Ogburn, P. (1981). A/NJ/8/76 influenza vaccination program: Effects on maternal health and pregnancy outcome. *American Journal of Obstetrics and Gynecology, 140*, 240–245.

Hart, R. J. (1981). Immunizations. *Clinical Obstetrics and Gynecology, 8*, 421–430.

Heinonen, O. P., Shapiro, S., Monson, R. R., et al. (1973). Immunizations during pregnancy against poliomyelitis and influenza in relation to childhood malignancy. *International Journal of Epidemiology, 2*, 229–235.

Heinonen, O. P., Slone, D., & Shapiro, S. (1977). *Birth defects and drugs in pregnancy*. Littleton, MA: Publishing Sciences Group.

Sumaya, C. V., & Gibbs, R. S. (1979). Immunization of pregnant women with influenza A/NEW Jersey/76 virus vaccine: Reactogenicity and immunogenicity in mother and infant. *Journal of Infectious Diseases, 140*, 141–146.

Insulin

FDA: B   SIGNIFICANCE: 5   POTENCY: 4

Insulin is a large molecule that does not cross the placenta. However, the effects of insulin on maternal blood glucose can cause shifts in glucose transfer across the placenta. Poor control of maternal blood sugar has been associated with an increased malformation rate among infants born to diabetic mothers. Insulin itself does not appear to have a direct teratogenic effect; the disease of diabetes mellitus with its associated hypoglycemia and hyperglycemia probably is responsible for the malformations. Therefore, it is generally recommended that insulin be used as indicated during pregnancy to maintain maternal blood glucose at levels as close to normal as possible.

Adashi, E. Y., Pinto, J., & Tyson, J. E. (1979). Impact of maternal euglycemia on fetal outcome in diabetic pregnancy. *American Journal of Obstetrics and Gynecology, 133*, 268–274.

Fuhrmann, K., Reiher, H., Semmler, K., et al. (1984). The effect of intensified conventional insulin therapy before and during pregnancy on the malformation rate in offspring of diabetic mothers. *Experimental and Clinical Endocrinology, 83*, 173–177.

Goldman, J. A., Dicker, D., Feldberg, D., et al. (1986). Pregnancy outcome in patients with insulin-dependent diabetes mellitus with preconceptional diabetic control: A comparative study. *American Journal of Obstetrics and Gynecology, 155*, 193–197.

Jackson, W. P., Campbell, J. D., Notelovitz, M., et al. (1962). Tolbutamide and chlorpropamide during pregnancy in human diabetes. *Diabetes, 11*(Suppl), 98–103.

Karlsson, K., & Kjellmer, I. (1972). The outcome of diabetic pregnancies in relation to the mother's blood sugar level. *American Journal of Obstetrics and Gynecology, 112*, 213–220.

Landauer, W. (1972). Is insulin a teratogen? *Teratology, 5*, 129–136.

Notelovitz, M. (1975). Sulphonylurea therapy in the treatment of the pregnant diabetic. *South African Medical Journal, 45*, 226–229.

Passarge, E., & Lenz, W. (1966). Syndrome of caudal regression in infants of diabetic mothers: Observation of further cases. *Pediatrics, 37*, 672–675.

Reece, E. A., Gabrielli, S., & Abdalla, M. (1988). The prevention of diabetes-associated birth defects. *Seminars in Perinatology, 12*(4), 292–301.

Iodide

AUTHOR: **NONE** SIGNIFICANCE: **1**
POTENCY: **1**

Iodide, a mucolytic, is found in many cough and cold formulations. Iodide may cross the placenta and inhibit the release of hormones from the fetal thyroid gland, which stimulates fetal thyroid-stimulating hormone (TSH) production and causes fetal thyroid hypertrophy and goiter. The hypertrophy can be quite severe, resulting in impaired respiration among neonates.

Anderson, G. S., & Bird, T. (1961). Congenital iodide goiter in twins. *The Lancet, 2*, 742–743.

Ayromlooi, J. (1972). Congenital goiter due to maternal ingestion of iodides. *Obstetrics and Gynecology, 39*, 818–822.

Carswell, F., Hutchison, J. H., & Kerr, M. M. (1970). Congenital goiter and hypothyroidism produced by maternal ingestion of iodides. *The Lancet, 1*, 1241–1243.

Galina, M. P., Avnet, N. L., & Einhorn, A. (1962). Iodides during pregnancy. *New England Journal of Medicine, 267*, 1124–1127.

Louw, J. H. (1963). Congenital goitre. A review with report of 3 cases of suffocative goitre in newborn. *South African Medical Journal, 37*, 976–983.

Senior, B., & Chernoff, H. L. (1971). Iodide goiter in the newborn. *Pediatrics, 47*, 510–515.

Iodoquinol (Diiodohydroxyquin)

FDA: **C** SIGNIFICANCE: **4–5** POTENCY: **4**

A study of 169 women who received oral iodoquinol during the first trimester and 172 women who received oral iodoquinol at various times during their pregnancies failed to detect an increased incidence of congenital anomalies. When applied topically for *Trichomonas vaginalis*, use of iodoquinol is considered acceptable, even during the first trimester.

Heinonen, O. P., Slone, D., & Shapiro, S. (1977). *Birth defects and drugs in pregnancy*. Littleton, MA: Publishing Sciences Group.

Trussell, R. R., & Beeley, L. (1981). Infestations. *Clinical Obstetrics and Gynecology, 8*, 333–340.

Iron Salts

FDA: **NONE**
SIGNIFICANCE: **3** (overdosage)
POTENCY: **2–3** (overdosage)

Several studies and case reports provide evidence that therapeutic dosages of the iron salts (e.g., ferrous gluconate, ferrous sulfate) during the various trimesters do not result in an increased risk for congenital anomalies. Although cases of spontaneous abortion have been reported in association with toxic iron overdosages, most case reports indicate that overdosages of iron do not result in increased risk for teratogenic effects.

Heinonen, O. P., Slone, D., & Shapiro, S. (1977). *Birth defects and drugs in pregnancy*. Littleton, MA: Publishing Sciences Group.

Hemminki, E., & Rimpela, U. (1991). A randomized comparison of routine versus selective iron supplementation during pregnancy. *Journal of the American College of Nutrition, 10*(1), 3–10.

Lacoste, H., Goyert, G. L., Goldman, L. S., et al. (1992). Acute iron intoxication in pregnancy: Case report and review of the literature. *Obstetrics and Gynecology, 80*, 500–501.

McElhatton, P. R., Roberts, J. C., & Sullivan, F. M. (1991). The consequences of iron overdose and its treatment with desferrioxamine in pregnancy. *Human and Experimental Toxicology, 10*, 251–259.

Olenmark, M., Biber, B., Dottori, O., et al. (1987). Fatal iron intoxication in late pregnancy. *Clinical Toxicology, 25*(4), 347–359.

Strom, R. L., Schiler, P., Seeds, A. E., et al. (1976). Fatal iron poisoning in a pregnant female: Case report. *Minnesota Medicine, 59*, 483–489.

Isoniazid (Isonicotinic Acid Hydrazide)

FDA: C   SIGNIFICANCE: 5   POTENCY: 4

Isoniazid has been used extensively during pregnancy. A single article presents data on five children with severe CNS damage who had been exposed to isoniazid in utero. A possible mechanism involving hypovitaminosis B_6 is described. However, as noted, if this association is valid, its incidence is quite rare. Because supplementation with vitamin B_6 is relatively easy and inexpensive, it would seem prudent that all pregnant women receiving isoniazid also take pyridoxine (50 mg/day orally).

American Thoracic Society. (1986). Treatment of tuberculosis and tuberculosis infection in adults and children. *American Review of Respiratory Disease, 134*, 355–363.

Lowe, C. R. (1964). Congenital defects among children born to women under supervision or treatment for pulmonary tuberculosis. *British Journal of Preventive Social Medicine, 18*, 14–16.

Marcus, J. C. (1967). Non-teratogenicity of antituberculosis drugs. *South African Medical Journal, 41*, 758–759.

Medchill, M. T., & Gillum, M. (1989). Diagnosis and management of tuberculosis during pregnancy. *Obstetrical and Gynecological Survey, 44*, 81–84.

Monet, P., Kalb, J. C., & Pujal, M. (1967). Doit-on craindre une influence teratogene eventuelle de l'isoniazide? *Revue Tuberculose (Paris), 31*, 845–848.

Varpela, E. (1964). On the effect exerted by first-line tuberculosis medicines on the foetus. *Acta Tuberculosea and Pneumologica Scandinavica, 35*, 53–69.

Warkany, J. (1979). Antituberculosis drugs. *Teratology, 20*, 133–138.

Isoproterenol

FDA: C   SIGNIFICANCE: 4   POTENCY: 3–4

Data from the Collaborative Perinatal Project involving women (n = 31) who received isoproterenol during the first trimester did not indicate any increase in the incidence of congenital anomalies. More data are needed.

Heinonen, O. P., Slone, D., & Shapiro, S. (1977). *Birth defects and drugs in pregnancy*. Littleton, MA: Publishing Sciences Group.

Isotretinoin

FDA: X   SIGNIFICANCE: 1   POTENCY: 1

Isotretinoin is a retinoic acid–vitamin A analog. Retinoic acid and its analogs are known for their teratogenicity. Isotretinoin is listed as a severe fetal hazard if used during pregnancy. Fetuses have been accidentally exposed to isotretinoin with the following results: anteverted nares, cleft palate, Dandy-Walker malformation, depressed nasal bridge, ear tag remnants, frontal bossing, heart defects, hydrocephalus, hypertelorism, limb reduction defects, low-set ears, mental retardation, microcephaly, micrognathia, microphthalmia, small ear canals, small ears, small mouth, small shoulder girdles, spontaneous abortion, trigonocephaly, and undifferentiated ears without antihelices. The risk for major physical defects after exposure during the first trimester has been reported to be approximately 20%. To avoid the possibility of accidental embryo/fetal exposure, implantable progesterone-type contraceptives (e.g., levonorgestrel implants *[Norplant System®]*) have been strongly recommended for women of childbearing age who require isotretinoin because of their greater efficacy over oral contraceptives for preventing pregnancy. Reportedly, approximately three out of 1000 women using isotretinoin get pregnant. Therefore, women not on an implantable contraceptive should use two other forms of contraception (e.g., condoms and an oral contraceptive). In addition, negative results should be obtained from two different pregnancy tests before isotretinoin is initiated. Pregnancy tests should also be readministered prior to each 30-day refill of isotretinoin. It also is recommended that contraceptive measures be used for at least 1 month following the discontinuation of isotretinoin.

Benke, P. J. (1984). The isotretinoin teratogen syndrome. *Journal of the American Medical Association, 251,* 3267–3269.
Braun, J. T., Franciosi, R. A., Mastri, A. R., et al. (1984). Isotretinoin dysmorphic syndrome. [Letter]. *The Lancet, 1,* 506–507.
De LaCruz, E., Sun, S., Vangvanichyakorn, K., et al. (1984). Multiple congenital malformations associated with maternal isotretinoin therapy. *Pediatrics, 74,* 428–430.
Doering, P. L., Araujo, O. E., Frohnapple, D. J., et al. (1992). Patterns of prescribing isotretinoin: Focus on women of childbearing potential. *Annals of Pharmacotherapy, 26,* 155–161.
FDA recommends additional requirements for Accutane pregnancy prevention program (1990). *American Journal of Hospital Pharmacy, 47,* 1912–1914.
Fernhoff, P. M., & Lammer, E. J. (1984). Craniofacial features of isotretinoin embryopathy. *The Journal of Pediatrics, 105,* 595–597.
Food and Drug Administration. (1983). Update on birth defects with isotretinoin. *FDA Drug Bulletin, 14,* 15–16.
Hill, R. M. (1984). Isotretinoin teratogenicity. *The Lancet, 1,* 1965.
Jellin, J. M. (2000). Dermatology. *Prescriber's Letter, 7*(10), 60.
Lammer, E. J., Chen, D. T., Hoar, R. M., et al. (1985). Retinoic acid embryopathy. *New England Journal of Medicine, 313,* 837–841.
Lynberg, M. C., Khoury, M. J., Lammer, E. J., et al. (1990). Sensitivity, specificity, and positive predictive value of multiple malformations in isotretinoin embryopathy surveillance. *Teratology, 42,* 513–519.
Monga, M. (1997). Vitamin A and its congeners. *Seminars in Perinatology, 21*(2), 135–142.
Rappaport, E. B., & Knapp, M. (1989). Isotretinoin embryopathy—A continuing problem. *Journal of Clinical Pharmacology, 29,* 463–465.
Recommendations for isotretinoin use in women of childbearing potential. (1991). *Teratology, 44,* 1–6.
Rizzo, R., Lammer, E. J., Parano, E., et al. (1991). Limb reduction defects in humans associated with prenatal isotretinoin exposure. *Teratology, 44,* 599–604.
Roche issues new warning on Accutane® and pregnancy. *APhA Weekly,* 1983. July 29, p. 119.
Roche strengthens Accutane pregnancy prevention program. (1990). *American Journal of Hospital Pharmacy, 47,* 2413–2414.
Rosa, F. W. (1983). Teratogenicity of isotretinoin. *The Lancet, 2,* 513.
Rosa, F. W., Wolk, A. L., & Kelsey, F. O. (1986). Vitamin A congeners. *Teratology, 33,* 355–364.
Strauss, J. S., Cunningham, W. J., Leyden, J. J., et al. (1988). Isotretinoin and teratogenicity. *Journal of the American Academy of Dermatology, 19,* 353–354.
Teratology Society. (1991). Recommendations for isotretinoin use in women of childbearing potential. *Teratology, 44,* 1–6.

Kanamycin

FDA: **D**   SIGNIFICANCE: **1**   POTENCY: **2–3**

Nine out of 391 infants exposed to kanamycin in utero had hearing impairment. Ototoxicity is a well-recognized kanamycin adverse drug reaction in both children and adults. Other individual cases of neonatal deafness associated with kanamycin use during pregnancy also have been reported.

Golbus, M. S. (1980). Teratology for the obstetrician: Current status. *Obstetrics and Gynecology, 55,* 269–277.
Jones, H. C. (1973). Intrauterine ototoxicity. A case report and review of literature. *Journal of the National Medical Association, 65*(3), 201–203.
Tuchmann-Duplessis, H. (1975). *Drug effects on the fetus.* Acton, MA: Publishing Sciences Group.

Kaolin

FDA: **C**   SIGNIFICANCE: **5**   POTENCY: **4**

There has been one retrospective study of kaolin use during pregnancy. No increase in the congenital malformation rate of offspring was detected.

Nelson, M. M., & Forfar, J. O. (1971). Association between drugs administered during pregnancy and congenital abnormalities. *British Medical Journal, 1,* 523.

Ketamine

FDA: **C**   SIGNIFICANCE: 2 (near term)
POTENCY: **2** (near term)

Ketamine may be fetotoxic. When used as an anesthetic during labor, moderate depression of neurobehavioral tests was observed among neonates for 2 days following delivery.

Hodgkinson, R., Bhatt, M., Kim, S. S., et al. (1978). Neonatal neurobehavioral tests following cesarean section under general and spinal anesthesia. *American Journal of Obstetrics and Gynecology, 132,* 670–674.

Labetalol

AUTHOR: **NONE** SIGNIFICANCE: **4–5**
POTENCY: **3–4**

In one report, no increase in congenital malformations was observed when labetalol was used by women during pregnancy. (*See* Metoprolol monograph.)

Lamming, G. D., Pipkin, F., & Symonds, E. M. (1980). Comparison of alpha and beta blocking drug, labetalol, and methyldopa in the treatment of moderate and severe pregnancy-induced hypertension. *Clinical Experiments in Hypertension, 2,* 865–895.

Levothyroxine

FDA: **A** SIGNIFICANCE: **5** POTENCY: **4**

A study of more than 2000 children born to women who took levothyroxine either during the first trimester (~25% of mothers) or at various times during their pregnancies (~75% of mothers) failed to find an increased risk for congenital anomalies. In several reports, levothyroxine taken during late pregnancy was beneficial (i.e., to treat hypothyroidism and goiter, to induce fetal lung maturity prior to premature delivery) without teratogenic effects. Levothyroxine and other thyroid hormones at therapeutic doses appear to be safe during pregnancy.

Heinonen, O. P., Slone, D., & Shapiro, S. (1977). *Birth defects and drugs in pregnancy.* Littleton, MA: Publishing Sciences Group.
Mashiach, S., Barkai, G., Sack, J., et al. (1978). Enhancement of fetal lung maturity by intra-amniotic administration of thyroid hormone. *American Journal of Obstetrics and Gynecology, 130*(3), 289–293.
van Herle, A. J., Young, R. T., Fisher, D. A., et al. (1975). Intra-uterine treatment of a hypothyroid fetus. *Journal of Clinical Endocrinology and Metabolism, 40,* 474–477.
Weiner, S., Scharf, J. I., Bolognese, R. J., et al. (1980). Antenatal diagnosis and treatment of a fetal goiter. *Journal of Reproductive Medicine, 24,* 39–42.

Lidocaine

FDA: **B** SIGNIFICANCE: **3** (during delivery)
POTENCY: **2–3** (during delivery)

Lidocaine anesthesia during labor and delivery has not been associated with congenital malformations among offspring. It may, however, be fetotoxic if administered in the presence of fetal acidosis. In this case, the usual CNS and cardiac toxicities may be observed among neonates secondary to ion trapping. In addition, several cases of alterations in brain stem auditory-evoked responses have been reported among neonates whose mothers received lidocaine regional anesthesia during delivery.

Abboud, T. K., Khoo, S. S., Miller, F., et al. (1982). Maternal, fetal, and neonatal responses after epidural anesthesia with bupivacaine, 2-chloroprocaine, or lidocaine. *Anesthesia and Analgesia, 61,* 638–644.
Bozynski, M. E. A., Schumacher, R. E., Deschner, L. S., et al. (1989). Effect of prenatal lignocaine on auditory brain stem evoked response. *Archives of Disease in Childhood, 64,* 934–938.
Brown, W. U., Bell, G. C., & Alper, M. H. (1976). Acidosis, local anesthesia and the newborn. *Obstetrics and Gynecology, 48,* 27–30.
Diaz, M., Graff, M., Hiatt, M., et al. (1988). Prenatal lidocaine and the auditory evoked responses in term infants. *American Journal of Diseases of Children, 142,* 160–161.
Heinonen, O. P., Slone, D., & Shapiro, S. (1977). *Birth defects and drugs in pregnancy.* Littleton, MA: Publishing Sciences Group.
Kileff, M., James, F. M., III, Dewan, D., et al. (1982). Neonatal neurobehavioral responses after epidural anesthesia for cesarean section with lidocaine and bupivacaine. *Anesthesiology, 57*(Suppl), A403.

Lincomycin

FDA: **B** SIGNIFICANCE: **5** POTENCY: **4**

In studies with seven-year follow-up data, use of lincomycin during pregnancy has not been shown to be teratogenic.

Mickal, A., Dildy, G. A., & Miller, H. J. (1966). Lincomycin in the treatment of cervicitis and vaginitis in pregnancy. *Southern Medical Journal, 59,* 567–570.
Mickal, A., & Panzer, J. D. (1975). The safety of lincomycin in pregnancy. *American Journal of Obstetrics and Gynecology, 121,* 1071–1074.

Lithium

FDA: **D** SIGNIFICANCE: **1** POTENCY: **1–2**

Lithium is a known human teratogen and is contraindicated during pregnancy. The data associating lithium with teratogenic effects initially came from the International Register of Lithium Babies. Data for 217 infants exposed to lithium in utero indicated that 183 were normal, seven were stillborn, two had trisomy 21, and 25 had congenital malformations. Of the 25 malformed infants, 18 had defects involving the heart and great vessels. These defects included coarctation of the aorta, mitral atresia, patent ductus arteriosus, single umbilical artery, tricuspid atresia, and ventricular septal defects. Six cases of Ebstein's malformation, which is characterized by distortion and downward displacement of the tricuspid valve along with anomalies of the right atrium and ventricle, also were reported.

A limitation of the Register data is the lack of a control group. In attempts to support the results of this study, a later study compared the ratio of cardiovascular defects in the Register study group with observed defects in the general population. This later study showed a total cardiovascular anomaly ratio of 1:1.3 in the study group versus 1:8 in the general population.

In another examination of the data, the ratio of Ebstein's malformation in the study group was 2.8% versus 0.005% in the general population. A Czechoslovakian study also found an increase in Ebstein's malformation among infants born to women who took lithium during pregnancy. In addition, a Scandinavian group, in a small study, found an increased perinatal death rate for lithium-exposed fetuses.

Fetotoxic effects associated with the use of lithium include congenital hypothyroidism and euthyroid goiters, which slowly subside over several months. Other neonatal fetotoxic effects include hypotonia, poor sucking, and poor respiratory effort. Infants normal at birth continue to develop normally.

Allan, L. D., Desai, G., & Tynan, J. J. (1982). Prenatal echocardiographic screening for Ebstein's anomaly for mothers on lithium therapy. *The Lancet, 2*, 875–876.
Ananth, J. (1993). Lithium during pregnancy and lactation. *Lithium, 4*, 231–237.
Arnon, R. G., Marin-Garcia, J., & Peeden, J. N. (1981). Tricuspid valve regurgitation and lithium carbonate toxicity in a newborn infant. *American Journal of Diseases of Children, 135*, 941–943.
Filtenborg, J. A. (1982). Persistent pulmonary hypertension after lithium intoxication in the newborn. *European Journal of Obstetrics, Gynecology, and Reproductive Biology, 138*, 321–323.
Fries, H. (1970). Lithium in pregnancy. *The Lancet, 1*, 123.
Goldfield, M. D., & Weinstein, M. R. (1973). Lithium carbonate in obstetrics: Guidelines for clinical use. *American Journal of Obstetrics and Gynecology, 116*, 15–22.
Kallen, B., & Tandberg, A. (1983). Lithium and pregnancy. *Acta Psychiatrica Scandinavica, 68*, 134–139.
Mizrahi, E. M., Hobbs, J. F., & Goldsmith, D. I. (1979). Nephrogenic diabetes insipidus in transplacental lithium intoxication. *The Journal of Pediatrics, 94*, 493–495.
Morrell, P., Sutherland, G. R., Buamah, P. K., et al. (1983). Lithium toxicity in a neonate. *Archives of Disease in Childhood, 58*, 439–541.
Nora, J. J., Nora, A. H., & Towes, H. (1974). Lithium, Ebstein's anomaly, and other congenital heart disease. [Letter]. *The Lancet, 2*, 594–595.
Park, J. M., Sridaromont, S., Ledbetter, E. O., et al. (1980). Ebstein's anomaly of the tricuspid valve associated with prenatal exposure to lithium carbonate. *American Journal of Diseases of Children, 134*, 703–704.
Robert, E., & Francannet, C. (1990). Comments on "teratogen update on lithium" by J. Warkany. [Letter]. *Teratology, 42*, 205.
Schou, M. (1976). What happened later to the lithium babies? A follow-up study of children born without malformations. *Acta Psychiatrica Scandinavica, 54*, 193–197.
Schou, M., Amdisen, A., Eskjaer, J., et al. (1968). Occurrence of goiter during lithium treatment. *British Medical Journal, 3*, 710–713.
Schou, M., & Weinstein, M. R. (1980). Problems of lithium maintenance treatment during pregnancy, delivery and lactation. *Aggressologie, 21* (a), 7–9.
Sedvall, G., Jonsson, B., & Petterson, U. (1969). Evidence of an altered thyroid function in man during treatment with lithium carbonate. *Acta Psychiatrica Scandinavica, 207*(Suppl), 59–67.
Sipek, A. (1989). Lithium and Ebstein's anomaly. *Cor Vasa, 31*, 149–156.
Stevens, D., Burman, D., & Midwinter, A. (1974). Transplacental lithium poisoning. *The Lancet, 2*, 595.
Stothers, J. K., Wilson, D. W., & Rayston, N. (1973). Lithium toxicity in newborn. *British Medical Journal, 3*, 233–234.
Tunnessen, W. W., & Hertz, C. G. (1972). Toxic effects of lithium in newborn infants: A commentary. *The Journal of Pediatrics, 81*, 804–807.
Warkany, J. (1988). Teratogen update: Lithium. *Teratology, 38*, 593–596.
Weinstein, M. R., & Goldfield, M. D. (1975). Cardiovascular malformations with lithium used during pregnancy. *American Journal of Psychiatry, 132*, 529–531.

Wilbanks, G. D., Bressler, B., Peete, C. H., et al. (1970). Toxic effects of lithium carbonate in a mother and newborn infant. *Journal of the American Medical Association, 213*, 865–867.

Woody, J. N., London, W. L., & Wilbanks, G. D., Jr. (1971). Lithium toxicity in a newborn. *Pediatrics, 47*, 94–96.

Loperamide

FDA: B   SIGNIFICANCE: 4   POTENCY: 2–3

A prospective, controlled multicenter study of loperamide use during pregnancy (n = 105) compared the outcomes of these pregnancies with a matched control group. No statistically significant differences were found in 89 women who used loperamide during the first trimester; it was concluded that loperamide use during pregnancy is not associated with an increased rate of major malformations. However, of the women who used loperamide at various times throughout their pregnancies, 20% (21 out of 105) delivered babies that were, on average, 200 grams smaller than the babies in the control group. More data are needed.

Einarson, A., Mastroiacovo, P., Arnon, J., et al. (2000). Prospective, controlled, multicentre study of loperamide in pregnancy. *Canadian Journal of Gastroenterology, 14*, 185–187.

Lorazepam

FDA: D   SIGNIFICANCE: 4 (congenital anomalies)

POTENCY: 3–4 (congenital anomalies)

Use of lorazepam near term has been associated with lethargy, poor muscle tone, and respiratory depression in the neonate. These fetotoxic effects appear to be particularly significant for premature neonates. They are, however, generally fully reversible with proper recognition and care. Long-term or regular personal use of lorazepam during pregnancy may result in the neonatal benzodiazepine-withdrawal syndrome. Teratogenic effects have not been reported.

McAuley, D. M., O'Neill, M. P., Moore, J., et al. (1982). Lorazepam premedication for labour. *British Journal of Obstetrics and Gynaecology, 89*, 149–154.

Sanchis, A., Rosique, D., & Catala, J. (1991). Adverse effects of maternal lorazepam on neonates. *Annals of Pharmacotherapy, 25*, 1137–1138.

Whitelaw, A. G. L., Cummings, A. J., & McFadyen, I. R. (1981). Effect of maternal lorazepam on the neonate. *British Medical Journal, 282*, 1106–1108.

Lysergic Acid Diethylamide (LSD)

AUTHOR: NONE   SIGNIFICANCE: 3–4

POTENCY: 4–5

Although there is no identifiable pattern, several reports associate various congenital anomalies with LSD use during pregnancy, including bladder exstrophy, CNS and eye defects, chromosomal breakage, inguinal hernias, and limb defects. The relatively few reports of anomalies in relation to use and the existence of several negative studies suggest that LSD is not a human teratogen. Of concern as use increases is a study linking LSD use with an increased incidence of spontaneous abortion.

Assemany, S. R., Neu, R. L., & Gardner, L. I. (1970). Deformities in a child whose mother took LSD. *The Lancet, 1*, 1290.

Bogdanoff, B., Rorke, L. B., & Yanoff, M. (1972). Brain and eye abnormalities, possible sequelae to prenatal use of multiple drugs including LSD. *American Journal of Diseases of Children, 123*, 145–148.

Dishotsky, N. I., Loughman, W. D., Mogar, R. E., et al. (1971). LSD and genetic damage. *Science, 172*, 431–441.

Eller, J. L., & Morton, J. M. (1970). Bizarre deformities in offspring of users of lysergic acid diethylamide. *New England Journal of Medicine, 283*, 395–397.

Gelehrter, T. D. (1976). Lysergic acid diethylamide (LSD) and exstrophy of the bladder. *The Journal of Pediatrics, 77*, 1065.

Hecht, F., Beals, R. K., Lees, M. H., et al. (1968). Lysergic-acid-diethylamide and cannabis as possible teratogens in man. *The Lancet, 2*, 1087.

Hsu, L. Y., Strauss, M., & Hirschhorn, K. (1970). Chromosome abnormality in offspring of LSD user. *Journal of the American Medical Association, 211*, 987–990.

Jacobson, C. B., & Berlin, C. M. (1972). Possible reproductive detriment in LSD users. *Journal of the American Medical Association, 222*, 1367–1373.

Long, S. Y. (1972). Does LSD induce chromosomal damage and malformations? A review of the literature. *Teratology, 6*, 75–90.

Loughman, W. D., Sargent, T. W., & Iraelstam, D. M. (1967). Leukocytes of humans exposed to lysergic acid diethylamide: Lack of chromosomal damage. *Science, 158*, 508–510.

McGlothlin, W. H., Sparkes, R. S., & Arnold, D. O.

(1970). Effect of LSD on human pregnancy. *Journal of the American Medical Association, 212,* 1483–1487.
Pagliaro, L. A. (1991). The straight dope: Cannibalism, birth defects, homosexuality, and other myths associated with drug and substance abuse. *Psynopsis, 13*(4), 8.
Tuchmann-Duplessis, H. (1983). The teratogenic risks. *American Journal of Industrial Medicine, 4,* 245–258.
Zwellweger, H., McDonalds, J. S., & Abbo, G. (1967). Is lysergic-acid diethylamide a teratogen? *The Lancet, 2,* 1066–1068.

Magnesium Sulfate

FDA: **B** SIGNIFICANCE: **2–3** (near term)
POTENCY: **1–2** (near term)

A study of the offspring of six women who received magnesium during the first trimester and 135 women who received magnesium at various times during their pregnancies failed to find an increased risk for congenital anomalies. Magnesium sulfate freely crosses the placenta, however, and may cause fetal bradycardia and neonatal neurological depression when administered intravenously to pregnant women for pre-eclampsia or eclampsia. These fetotoxic effects also are generally associated with neonatal hypermagnesemia and are usually transient. Continuous intravenous infusions of magnesium sulfate for several weeks prior to delivery for tocolysis have reportedly been associated with osseous lesions ostensibly due to the interaction between calcium and magnesium in the body.

Cumming, W. A., & Thomas, V. J. (1989). Hypermagnesemia: A cause of abnormal metaphyses in the neonate. *American Journal of Roentgenology, 152,* 1071–1072.
Foster, S. D. (1981). Magnesium sulfate: Eclampsia management; effects on neonates. *MCN, The American Journal of Maternal Child Nursing, 6,* 355.
Lamm, C. I., Noton, K. I., Murphy, R. J. C., et al. (1988). Congenital rickets associated with magnesium sulfate infusion for tocolysis. *The Journal of Pediatrics, 113*(6), 1078–1082.

Marijuana (Cannabis, Tetrahydrocannabinol)

AUTHOR: **NONE** SIGNIFICANCE: **4–5**
POTENCY: **3–4**

Scattered case reports relate marijuana use during pregnancy to fetotoxic effects. These effects appear to be limited to low-birth weight and other minor temporary neurological signs and symptoms (e.g., tremors) among neonates. Given the widespread use of marijuana by adolescent girls and young women of childbearing age and the relatively few reported teratogenic effects, the teratogenic potential of marijuana, if it exists at all, appears to be very low.

Conner, C. S. (1984). Marijuana and alcohol use in pregnancy. *Drug Intelligence and Clinical Pharmacy, 18,* 233–234.
Day, N., Sambamoorthi, U., Taylor, P., et al. (1991). Prenatal marijuana use and neonatal outcome. *Neurotoxicology and Teratology, 13*(3), 329–334.
Fried, P. (1982). Marijuana use by pregnant women and effects on offspring: An update. *Neurobehavioral Toxicity and Teratology, 4,* 451–454.
Fried, P. A., & O'Connell, C. M. (1987). A comparison of the effects of prenatal exposure to tobacco, alcohol, cannabis and caffeine on birth size and subsequent growth. *Neurotoxicology and Teratology, 9,* 79–85.
Fried, P. A., O'Connell, C. M., & Watkinson, B. (1992). 60- and 72-month follow-up of children prenatally exposed to marijuana, cigarettes, and alcohol: Cognitive and language assessment. *Journal of Developmental and Behavioral Pediatrics, 13,* 383–391.
Fried, P. A., & Watkinson, B. (1990). 36- and 48-month neurobehavioral follow-up of children prenatally exposed to marijuana, cigarettes, and alcohol. *Journal of Developmental and Behavioral Pediatrics, 11,* 49–58.
Fried, P. A., Watkinson, B., Dillon, R. F., et al. (1987). Neonatal neurological status in a low-risk population after prenatal exposure to cigarettes, marijuana, and alcohol. *Journal of Developmental and Behavioral Pediatrics, 8,* 318–326.
Gibson, G. T., Baghurst, P. A., & Colley, D. P. (1983). Maternal alcohol, tobacco and cannabis consumption and the outcome of pregnancy. *Australian and New Zealand Journal of Obstetrics and Gynaecology, 23,* 15–19.
Greenland, S., Richwald, G. A., & Honda, G. D. (1983). The effects of marijuana use during pregnancy. II. A study in a low-risk home-delivery population. *Drug and Alcohol Dependence, 11,* 359–366.
Hecht, F., Beals, R. K., Lees, M. H., et al. (1968). Lysergic-acid-diethylamide and cannabis as possible teratogens in man. *The Lancet, 2,* 1087.
Linn, S., Schoenbaum, S. C., Monson, R. R., et al. (1983). The association of marijuana use with outcome of pregnancy. *American Journal of Public Health, 73,* 1161–1164.
New, R. L. (1969). Cannabis and chromosomes. *The Lancet, 1,* 675.

O'Connell, C. M., & Fried, P. A. (1984). An investigation of prenatal cannabis exposure and minor physical anomalies in a low risk population. *Neurobehavioral Toxicology and Teratology, 6,* 345–350.

Qazi, Q. H., & Milman, D. H. (1983). Nontherapeutic use of psychoactive drugs. [Letter]. *New England Journal of Medicine, 309,* 797–798.

Tennes, K., Avitable, N., Blackard, C., et al. (1985). Marijuana: Prenatal and postnatal exposure in the human. *National Institute on Drug Abuse Research Monograph Series, 59,* 48–59.

Witter, F. R., & Niebyl, J. R. (1990). Marijuana use in pregnancy and pregnancy outcome. *American Journal of Perinatology, 7*(1), 36–38.

Zuckerman, B., Frank, D. A., Hingson, R., et al. (1989). Effects of maternal marijuana and cocaine use on fetal growth. *New England Journal of Medicine, 320,* 762–768.

Mebendazole

FDA: **C**   SIGNIFICANCE: **4–5**   POTENCY: **3–4**

Mebendazole is recommended for whipworm and mixed helminthic infestations. Of 112 women who received mebendazole during pregnancy, only one case of digit deformity was reported.

Shepard, T. H. (1983). *Catalog of teratogenic agents,* 4th ed. Baltimore: Johns Hopkins.

Trussell, R. R., & Beeley, L. (1981). Infestations. *Clinical Obstetrics and Gynecology, 8,* 333–340.

Mechlorethamine (Nitrogen Mustard)

FDA: **D**   SIGNIFICANCE: **3**   POTENCY: **2–3**

Adequate data regarding the teratogenic potential of mechlorethamine use during pregnancy are lacking. In one report of two women who received the drug during the first trimester, both had normal infants. In a second report, an infant was born with a small, malpositioned kidney. However, this report may have been confounded, as the nitrogen mustard had been administered as part of a combination antineoplastic regimen. In two other reported cases in which mechlorethamine was administered to treat Hodgkin's disease in pregnant women, one infant was born with oligodactyly and the other with an atrial septal defect. More data are needed.

Aviles, A., Diaz-Maqueo, J. C., Talavera, A., et al. (1991). Growth and development of children of mothers treated with chemotherapy during pregnancy. Current status of 43 children. *American Journal of Hematology, 36,* 243–248.

Deuschle, K. W., & Wiggins, W. S. (1953). Use of nitrogen mustard in management of two pregnant lymphoma patients. *Blood, 8,* 576.

Mennuti, M. T., Shepard, T. H., & Mellman, W. J. (1975). Fetal renal malformation following treatment of Hodgkin's disease during pregnancy. *Obstetrics and Gynecology, 46,* 194–196.

Thomas, L., & Andes, W. A. (1982). Fetal anomaly associated with successful chemotherapy for Hodgkin's disease during the first trimester of pregnancy. *Clinical Research, 30,* 424A.

Thomas, P. R. M., & Peckham, M. J. (1976). The investigation and management of Hodgkin's disease in the pregnant patient. *Cancer, 38,* 1443–1451.

Meclizine

FDA: **B**   SIGNIFICANCE: **4–5**   POTENCY: **4**

Large-scale human studies have failed to show any teratogenic effects associated with meclizine use during pregnancy. Meclizine has been recommended as the antiemetic of first choice for women during pregnancy.

Carter, M. P., & Wilson, F. W. (1962). "Ancoloxin" and foetal abnormalities. *British Medical Journal, 2,* 1609.

Collins, I. S. (1964). Hazards of drug therapy. *Medical Journal of Australia, 1,* 222.

Diggory, P. L., & Tomkinson, J. S. (1962). Meclizine and foetal abnormalities. *The Lancet, 2,* 1222–1223.

Leathem, A. M. (1986). Safety and efficacy of antiemetics used to treat nausea and vomiting in pregnancy. *Clinical Pharmacy, 5,* 660–668.

Lenz, W. (1966). Malformations caused by drugs in pregnancy. *American Journal of Diseases of Children, 112,* 99–106.

Mellin, G. W., & Katzenstein, M. (1963). Meclizine and fetal abnormalities. *The Lancet, 1,* 222–223.

Milkovich, L., & Van den Berg, B. J. (1976). An evaluation of the teratogenicity of certain antinauseant drugs. *American Journal of Obstetrics and Gynecology, 125,* 244–248.

Richards, I. D. (1972). A retrospective inquiry into possible teratogenic effect of meclizine in man. *Advances in Experimental Medicine and Biology, 27,* 441.

Smithells, R. W., & Chinn, E. R. (1964). Meclizine and foetal malformations: A prospective study. *British Medical Journal, 1,* 217–218.

Yerushalmy, J., & Milkovich, L. (1965). Evaluation of the teratogenic effect of meclizine in man. *American Journal of Obstetrics and Gynecology, 93,* 553–562.

Medroxyprogesterone

FDA: **X**   SIGNIFICANCE: **1–2**   POTENCY: **3**

The data relating medroxyprogesterone

use during pregnancy with teratogenic effects are conflicting. Medroxyprogesterone is an orally active progesterone closely related to testosterone. In one study, pseudohermaphroditism was reported in one of 172 infants. However, the studies on another defect, hypospadias, are both positive and negative. A large retrospective study from Thailand (n = 1229) suggested a strong association between in utero exposure to medroxyprogesterone and polysyndactyly. However, a smaller study (n = 366) that same year failed to find an increased risk for teratogenic effects. More data are needed.

Aarskog, D. (1979). Maternal progestins as a possible cause of hypospadias. *New England Journal of Medicine, 300*, 75–78.

Burstein, R., & Wasserman, H. C. (1964). The effect of Provera on the fetus. *Obstetrics and Gynecology, 23*, 931–934.

Darling, M. R., & Hawkins, D. F. (1981). Sex hormones in pregnancy. *Clinical Obstetrics and Gynecology, 8*, 405–419.

Mau, G. (1981). Progestins during early pregnancy and hypospadias. *Teratology, 24*, 285–287.

Pardthaisong, T., Gray, R. H., McDaniel, E. B., et al. (1988). Steroid contraceptive use and pregnancy outcome. *Teratology, 38*, 51–58.

Yovich, J. L., Turner, S. R., & Draper, R. (1988). Medroxyprogesterone acetate therapy in early pregnancy has no apparent fetal effects. *Teratology, 38*, 135–144.

Meperidine (Pethidine)

FDA: B   SIGNIFICANCE: 1 (near term)
POTENCY: 2 (near term)

No studies were found that relate meperidine use during early pregnancy to birth defects among offspring. When used as an analgesic during labor, meperidine can depress Apgar scores and cause transient respiratory depression among neonates. Although studies are not available, the authors' clinical experience indicates that long-term or regular personal use of meperidine during pregnancy, particularly near term, may result in expected pharmacologic effects (lethargy, poor suck) and the neonatal opiate analgesic-withdrawal syndrome (*see* Heroin and Methadone monographs). More data are needed, particularly data on use during the first trimester.

Busacca, M., Gementi, P., Gambini, E., et al. (1982). Neonatal effects of the administration of meperidine and promethazine to the mother in labor. Double blind study. *Journal of Perinatal Medicine, 10*, 48–53.

Cooper, L. V., Stephen, G. W., & Aggett, P. J. (1977). Elimination of pethidine and bupivacaine in the newborn. *Archives of Disease in Childhood, 52*, 638–641.

Hamza, J., Benlabed, M., Orhant, E., et al. (1992). Neonatal pattern of breathing during active and quiet sleep after maternal administration of meperidine. *Pediatric Research, 32*, 412–416.

Heinonen, O. P., Slone, D., & Shapiro, S. (1977). *Birth defects and drugs in pregnancy*. Littleton, MA: Publishing Sciences Group.

Hodgkinson, R., & Husain, F. J. (1982). The duration of effect of maternally administered meperidine on neonatal neurobehavior. *Anesthesiology, 56*(1), 51–52.

Jick, H., Holmes, L. B., Hunter, J. R., et al. (1981). First-trimester drug use and congenital disorders. *Journal of the American Medical Association, 246*, 343–346.

Koch, G., & Wendel, H. (1968). The effect of pethidine on the postnatal adjustment of respiration and acid base balance. *Acta Obstetricia et Gynecologica Scandinavica, 47*, 27–37.

Morrison, J. C., Wiser, W. L., Rosser, S. I., et al. (1973). Metabolites of meperidine related to fetal depression. *American Journal of Obstetrics and Gynecology, 115*, 1132–1137.

Shnider, S. M., & Moya, F. (1964). Effects of meperidine on the newborn infant. *American Journal of Obstetrics and Gynecology, 89*, 1009–1014.

Mephenytoin

FDA: C   SIGNIFICANCE: 1–2   POTENCY: 1–2

Several birth defects have been observed among neonates whose mothers received mephenytoin during pregnancy. These effects are similar to those seen with phenytoin and include anencephaly, congenital dislocated hips, developmental delay, diaphragmatic hernia, digit defects, genitourinary defects, hydrocephalus, ileal atresia, inguinal hernias, intrauterine and postnatal growth retardation, large fontanelles, microcephaly, nail hypoplasia, neonatal hemorrhage, talipes equinovarus, tracheoesophageal fistula, and various heart defects.

Hanson, J. W., Myrianthopoulos, N. C., Sedgwick, M. A., et al. (1976). Risk to the offspring of women treated with hydantoin anticonvulsants, with emphasis on the fetal hydantoin syndrome. *The Journal of Pediatrics, 89*, 662–668.

Hill, R. M., Verniaud, W. M., Horning, H. G., et al.

(1974). Infants exposed in utero to antiepileptic drugs. *American Journal of Diseases of Children, 127*, 645–653.

Schinzel, A. (1979). [Fetal hydantoin-syndrome in siblings.] *Schweizerische Medizinische Wochenschrift, 109*, 68–72.

Speidel, B. D., & Meadow, S. R. (1972). Maternal epilepsy and abnormalities of the fetus and newborn. *The Lancet, 2*, 839–843.

Mephobarbital

FDA: **D**   SIGNIFICANCE: **1–2**   POTENCY: **2–3**

Mephobarbital is a less commonly used anticonvulsant. In a Japanese study, a borderline statistically significant increase in congenital malformations was noted among neonates whose mothers received mephobarbital during pregnancy. Other studies also have associated mephobarbital with malformations, including anencephaly, atrial septal defects, broad alveolar ridge, broad nasal ridge, cleft lip/palate, congenital hip dislocation, developmental delay, digital thumb, inguinal hernias, large fontanelle, low hairline, nail hypoplasia, other heart anomalies, patent ductus arteriosus, talipes equinus, strabismus, and ventricular septal defects. However, whether these defects are due to mephobarbital, maternal epilepsy, or some other confounding factor remains unclear. More data are needed.

Annegers, J. F., Elveback, L. R., Hauser, W. A., et al. (1974). Do anticonvulsants have a teratogenic effect? *Archives of Neurology, 31*, 364–373.

Hill, R. M., Verniaud, W. M., Horning, M. G., et al. (1974). Infants exposed in utero to antiepileptic drugs. *American Journal of Diseases of Children, 127*, 645–653.

Nakane, Y., Okuma, T., Takahashi, R., et al. (1980). Multi-institutional study on the teratogenicity and fetal toxicity of antiepileptic drugs: A report of a collaborative study group in Japan. *Epilepsia, 21*, 663–680.

Speidel, B. D., & Meadow, S. R. (1972). Maternal epilepsy and abnormalities of the fetus and newborn. *The Lancet, 2*, 839–843.

Mepivacaine

FDA: **C**   SIGNIFICANCE: **1** (late)   POTENCY: **1** (late)

No published data associate mepivacaine use during early pregnancy with congenital malformations among offspring. When used as an analgesic during labor, mepivacaine has been associated with fetotoxic effects, including acidosis, fetal bradycardia, and neonatal depression.

Asling, J. H., Shnider, S. M., Margolis, A. J., et al. (1970). Paracervical block anesthesia in obstetrics. *American Journal of Obstetrics and Gynecology, 107*, 626–634.

Gordon, H. R. (1968). Fetal bradycardia after paracervical block. *New England Journal of Medicine, 279*, 910–914.

Morishima, H. O., Daniel, S. S., Finster, M., et al. (1966). Transmission of mepivacaine hydrochloride (Carbocaine®) across the human placenta. *Anesthesiology, 27*, 147–154.

Sinclair, J. C., Fox, H. A., Lentz, J. F., et al. (1965). Intoxication of the fetus by a local anesthetic. *New England Journal of Medicine, 273*, 1173–1177.

Meprobamate

FDA: **D**   SIGNIFICANCE: **3**   POTENCY: **2–3**

In a study of meprobamate use during the first 42 days of pregnancy (n = 66), a fourfold increase in severe congenital malformations, primarily cardiac defects, was found. Other studies during the first trimester revealed an increased incidence of either cleft palate or hypospadias among offspring. Two subsequent studies, however, did not support these associations. Some researchers agree that it is unlikely that meprobamate is a teratogen because of the heterogenicity of the observed defects. More data are needed.

Belafsky, H. A., Breslow, S., Hirsch, L. M., et al. (1969). Meprobamate during pregnancy. *Obstetrics and Gynecology, 34*, 378–386.

Hartz, S. C., Heinonen, O. P., Shapiro, S., et al. (1975). Antenatal exposure to meprobamate and chlordiazepoxide in relation to malformations, mental development, and childhood mortality. *New England Journal of Medicine, 292*, 726–728.

Heinonen, O. P., Slone, D., & Shapiro, S. (1977). *Birth defects and drugs in pregnancy*. Littleton, MA: Publishing Sciences Group.

Jick, H., Holmes, L. B., Hunter, J. R., et al. (1981). First trimester drug use and congenital defects. *Journal of the American Medical Association, 246*, 343–346.

Milkovich, L., & Van den Berg, B. J. (1974). Effects of prenatal meprobamate and chlordiazepoxide hydrochloride on human embryonic and fetal development. *New England Journal of Medicine, 291*, 1268–1271.

Milkovich, L., & Van den Berg, B. J. (1975). Fetal effects of tranquilizers in pregnancy. *New England Journal of Medicine, 293*, 198–199.

Tuchmann-Duplessis, H. (1975). *Drug effects on the fetus*. Acton, MA: Publishing Sciences Group.

Tuchmann-Duplessis, H. (1983). The teratogenic risk. *American Journal of Industrial Medicine, 4*, 245–258.

Mercaptopurine (6-Mercaptopurine)

FDA: D SIGNIFICANCE: 4 (malformations)
POTENCY: 4 (malformations)
1–2 (prematurity)

In an early review of the possible teratogenic effects of mercaptopurine, five women who received mercaptopurine during pregnancy produced three normal infants and two premature infants. In several other reports involving 50 different pregnant women who received mercaptopurine at various times during their pregnancies, prematurity and low-birth weight were common. No infant was born malformed. A recent case-controlled study of mercaptopurine use by **fathers** within 3 months of conception suggests a significant increase in the incidence of spontaneous abortions and various congenital anomalies. More data are needed.

Aviles, A., Diaz-Maqueo, J. C., Talavera, A., et al. (1991). Growth and development of children and mothers treated with chemotherapy during pregnancy: Current status of 43 children. *American Journal of Hematology, 36*, 243–248.

Catanzarite, V. A., & Ferguson, J. E., II. (1984). Acute leukemia and pregnancy: A review of management and outcome, 1972–1982. *Obstetrical and Gynecological Survey, 39*(11), 663–678.

Moloney, W. C. (1964). Management of leukemia in pregnancy. *Annals of the New York Academy of Sciences, 114*, 857–867.

Nicholson, H. O. (1968). Cytotoxic drugs in pregnancy. *British Journal of Obstetrics and Gynecology, 75*, 307.

Pizzuto, J., Aviles, A., Noriega, L., et al. (1980). Treatment of acute leukemia during pregnancy. Presentation of nine cases. *Cancer Treatment Reports, 64*, 679–683.

Rajapakse, R. O., Korelitz, B. I., Zlatanic, J., et al. (2000). Outcome of pregnancies when fathers are treated with 6-mercaptopurine for inflammatory bowel disease. *American Journal of Gastroenterology, 95*, 684–688.

Sokol, J. E., & Lessmann, E. M. (1960). Effects of cancer chemotherapeutic agents on the human fetus. *Journal of the American Medical Association, 172*, 1765–1771.

Methadone

FDA: C SIGNIFICANCE: 1 (addiction/withdrawal) **3** (intrauterine growth retardation) **5** (malformations)
POTENCY: 1 (addiction/withdrawal)
3 (intrauterine growth retardation)
4 (malformations)

Use of methadone during pregnancy has been associated with the birth of infants small for their gestational age. This growth deficit does not appear to persist into later childhood. Other fetotoxic effects include addiction. Approximately 80% of infants experience methadone withdrawal. Convulsions during treated withdrawal occur more frequently with methadone than with heroin. Methadone use during pregnancy also has been associated with sudden infant death syndrome. The data, however, are conflicting; if the association is valid, it might be explained by a study showing a decreased ventilatory response to carbon dioxide among neonates exposed to methadone in utero. These data must be interpreted in light of the observation that women who use methadone also are likely to abuse alcohol and smoke tobacco cigarettes. The use of methadone during pregnancy is not associated with the production of congenital malformations.

For women who want to discontinue methadone during pregnancy, methadone detoxification can be attempted under the appropriate conditions. Detoxification during the first trimester is associated with increased incidence of spontaneous abortions, and third trimester detoxification is associated with fetal distress. If methadone detoxification is to be tried, it should be attempted between the 14th and 28th weeks of gestation with very slow tapering of the dose.

Blinick, G., Jerez, E., & Wallach, R. C. (1973). Methadone maintenance, pregnancy, and progeny. *Journal of the American Medical Association, 225*, 477–479.

Chasnoff, I. J., Burns, K. A., Burns, W. J., et al. (1986). Prenatal drug exposure: Effects on neonatal and infant growth and development. *Neurobehavioral Toxicology and Teratology, 8*, 357–362.

Chavez, C. J., Ostrea, C. M., Stryker, J. D., et al. (1979). Sudden infant death syndrome among infants of drug dependent mothers. *The Journal of Pediatrics, 95*, 407.

Claman, A. D., & Strong, R. I. (1962). Obstetric and gynecologic aspects of heroin addiction. *American Journal of Obstetrics and Gynecology, 83*, 252–257.

Cohen, S. N., & Neumann, L. L. (1973). Methadone maintenance during pregnancy. *American Journal of Diseases of Children, 126*, 445–446.

Connaughton, J. F., Reeser, D., Schut, J., et al. (1977). Perinatal addiction: Outcome and management. *American Journal of Obstetrics and Gynecology. 129*, 679–685.

Finnegan, L. P. (1978). Management of pregnant drug-dependent women. *Annals of the New York Academy of Sciences, 311*, 135–146.

Harper, R. G., Solish, G. I., Parow, H. M., et al. (1974). The effect of a methadone treatment program upon pregnant heroin addicts and their newborn infants. *Pediatrics, 54*, 300–305.

Kandall, S. R., Albin, S., Gartner, L. M., et al. (1977). The narcotic-dependent mother: Fetal and neonatal consequences. *Early Human Development, 1*, 159–169.

Lifschitz, M. H., Wilson, G. S., Smith, E., et al. (1983). Fetal and postnatal growth of children born to narcotic-dependent women. *The Journal of Pediatrics, 102*, 686–691.

Lipsitz, P. J., & Blatman, S. (1973). The early neonatal period of 100 live-borns of mothers on methadone. *Pediatric Research, 7*, 404.

Newman, R. G., Bashkow, S., & Calko, D. (1975). Results of 313 consecutive live births of infants delivered to patients in the New York City methadone maintenance treatment program. *American Journal of Obstetrics and Gynecology, 121*, 233–237.

Olsen, G. D., & Leis, M. H. (1980). Ventilatory response to carbon dioxide of infants following chronic prenatal methadone exposure. *The Journal of Pediatrics, 96*, 983–989.

Pierson, P. S., Howard, P., & Kleber, H. D. (1972). Sudden death in infants born to methadone-maintained addicts. *Journal of the American Medical Association, 220*, 1733.

Rajegowda, B. K., Glass, L., Evans, H. E., et al. (1972). Methadone withdrawal in newborn infants. *The Journal of Pediatrics, 81*, 532–534.

Reddy, A. M., Harper, P. G., & Stern, G. (1971). Observations on heroin and methadone withdrawal in the newborn. *Pediatrics, 48*, 353–358.

Stimmel, B., & Adamsons, K. (1976). Narcotic dependency in pregnancy: Methadone maintenance compared to use of street drugs. *Journal of the American Medical Association, 235*, 1121–1124.

Stone, M. L., Salerno, L. J., Green, M., et al. (1971). Narcotic addiction in pregnancy. *American Journal of Obstetrics and Gynecology, 109*, 716–723.

Suffet, F., & Brotman, R. (1984). A comprehensive care program for pregnant addicts: Obstetrical, neonatal, and child development outcomes. *International Journal of the Addictions, 19*, 199–219.

Wilson, G. S., Desmond, M. M., & Wait, R. B. (1981). Follow-up of methadone-treated and untreated narcotic-dependent women and their infants: Health, developmental, and social implications. *The Journal of Pediatrics, 98*, 716–722.

Zelson, C., Rubio, E., & Wasserman, E. (1971). Neonatal narcotic addiction: 10 year observation. *Pediatrics, 48*, 178–189.

Zuspan, F. P., Gumpel, J. A., Mejia-Zelaya, A., et al. (1975). Fetal stress from methadone withdrawal. *American Journal of Obstetrics and Gynecology, 122*, 43–46.

Methamphetamine

FDA: C   SIGNIFICANCE: 3   POTENCY: 2–3

Three related studies associate methamphetamine use during pregnancy with fetal and neonatal effects. One study reported intracranial hemorrhages among nine of 24 infants whose mothers had used methamphetamine throughout their pregnancies. Another study found no significant risk for congenital anomalies among the infants of mothers who used methamphetamine either during the first trimester (n = 89) or at various times throughout their pregnancies (n = 320). The third study also failed to support an increased risk for congenital anomalies among infants of mothers who used methamphetamine throughout their pregnancies. Prenatal growth retardation (i.e., reduced head circumference, length, body weight) was noted, however. More data are needed, particularly in light of expectations for increased methamphetamine use among adolescent girls and women of childbearing age during the coming decade.

Dixon, S. D., & Bejar, R. (1989). Echoencephalographic findings in neonates associated with maternal cocaine and methamphetamine use: Incidence and clinical correlates. *The Journal of Pediatrics, 115*, 770–778.

Heinonen, O. P., Slone, D., & Shapiro, S. (1977). *Birth defects and drugs in pregnancy*. Littleton, MA: Publishing Sciences Group.

Little, B. B., Snell, L. M., & Gilstrap, L. C. (1988). Methamphetamine abuse during pregnancy: Outcome and fetal effects. *Obstetrics and Gynecology, 72*(4), 541–544.

Methenamine

FDA: C   SIGNIFICANCE: 4–5   POTENCY: 4

In the Collaborative Perinatal Project, 12 of 299 infants exposed to methenamine in utero during different periods of fetal development had congenital malformations. The incidence was not different from that of the general population, however, and 49 infants from the same study whose mothers had received methenamine during the first trimester did not experience an increased risk for congenital anomalies.

Heinonen, O. P., Slone, D., & Shapiro, S. (1977). *Birth defects and drugs in pregnancy.* Littleton, MA: Publishing Sciences Group.

Methimazole

FDA: **D**   SIGNIFICANCE: **1**   POTENCY: **1**

Methimazole use during pregnancy for hyperthyroidism has been associated with a small, nonobstructive goiter and an ulcerative midline scalp lesion in the neonate. Although neither of these defects presents a major problem, propylthiouracil appears to be the drug of choice for pregnant women since it does not produce the scalp lesion. Regardless, both drugs must be used with caution to prevent neonatal hypothyroidism and cretinism. Some investigators have suggested that when methimazole is required during pregnancy fetal heart rate monitoring should be used to adjust the dose.

Milham, S., & Elledge, W. (1972). Maternal methimazole and congenital defects in children. [Letter]. *Teratology, 5,* 125.
Mujtaba, O., & Barrow, G. N. (1975). Treatment of hyperthyroidism in pregnancy with propylthiouracil and methimazole. *Obstetrics and Gynecology, 46,* 282–286.
Refetoff, S., Ochi, Y., Selenkow, H. A., et al. (1974). Neonatal hypothyroidism and goiter in one infant of each of two sets of twins due to maternal therapy with antithyroid drugs. *The Journal of Pediatrics, 85,* 240–244.
Serup, J., & Petersen, S. (1977). Hyperthyroidism during pregnancy treated with propylthiouracil. *Acta Obstetricia and Gynecologica Scandinavica, 56,* 443–466.

Methotrexate (Amethopterin)

FDA: **D**   SIGNIFICANCE: **1**   POTENCY: **1**

Methotrexate, an analog of amethopterin, has been associated with teratogenic effects and spontaneous abortion when used by women during pregnancy. Identified anomalies include agenesis of the frontal bones, cranial synostosis, digital defects, hypertelorism, large fontanelle, oxycephaly, peculiar facies, postnatal growth retardation, and rib defects. As a folic acid antagonist, methotrexate may also induce neural-tube defects (*see* Folic Acid monograph). Methotrexate belongs to the group of antineoplastics called antimetabolites, which are associated with a 50% incidence of congenital malformations. Although negative reports have been published, it is recommended that women of childbearing age use effective contraceptive measures while receiving methotrexate and for 3 months following its discontinuation.

Diniz, E. M. A., Corradini, H. B., Ramos, J. L., et al. (1978). The effects of methotrexate on the developing fetus. *Revista do Hospital das Clinicas: Faculdade de Medicina da Universidade de Sao Paulo, 33,* 286–290.
Kozlowski, R. D., Steinbrunner, J. V., MacKenzie, H. H., et al. (1990). Outcome of first-trimester exposure to low-dose methotrexate in eight patients with rheumatic disease. *The American Journal of Medicine, 88,* 589–592.
Lambie, D. G., & Johnson, R. H. (1985). Drugs and folate metabolism. *Drugs, 30*(2), 145–155.
Milunsky, A., Graef, J. W., & Gaynor, M. F. (1968). Methotrexate-induced congenital malformations. *The Journal of Pediatrics, 72,* 790–795.
Powell, H. R., & Ekert, H. (1971). Methotrexate-induced congenital malformations. *Medical Journal of Australia, 2,* 1076–1077.
Tung, J. P., & Maibach, H. I. (1990). The practical use of methotrexate in psoriasis. *Drugs, 40,* 697–712.
Warkany, J. (1978). Aminopterin and methotrexate: Folic acid deficiency. *Teratology, 17,* 353–358.
Warkany, J., Beandy, P. H., & Hornstein, S. (1959). Attempted abortion with aminopterin (4-aminopteroylglutamic acid): Malformation of the child. *American Journal of Diseases of Children, 97,* 27.

Methotrimeprazine

FDA: **C**   SIGNIFICANCE: **2**   POTENCY: **1–2**

In a prospective study involving 315 women taking phenothiazine during pregnancy, the use of phenothiazine analogs with a three-carbon side chain, such as methotrimeprazine, was associated with an increased risk for congenital malformations among offspring, particularly cardiac defects.

Rumeau-Rouquette, C., Goujard, J., & Huel, G. (1977). Possible teratogenic effect of phenothiazines in human beings. *Teratology, 15,* 57–64.

Methsuximide

FDA: C SIGNIFICANCE: 1 POTENCY: 1

Methsuximide use during pregnancy has been associated with teratogenic and fetotoxic effects similar to those associated with other anticonvulsants (i.e., delayed development, hypoplasia of the nails and distal phalanges, neonatal hemorrhage). The observed incidence of these effects is ~6% for exposed infants, which is probably a lower rate than that observed for phenytoin and much lower than that observed with the oxazolidinediones.

Bleyer, W. A., & Skinner, A. L. (1976). Fatal neonatal hemorrhage after maternal anticonvulsant therapy. *Journal of the American Medical Association, 235,* 626–627.

Fabro, S., & Brown, N. A. (1979). The teratogenic potential of anticonvulsants. *New England Journal of Medicine, 300,* 1280–1281.

Hill, R. M., Verniaud, W. M., Horning, M. G., et al. (1974). Infants exposed in utero to antiepileptic drugs. *American Journal of Diseases of Children, 127,* 645–653.

Methyldopa (Methyldopate)

FDA: C SIGNIFICANCE: see monograph
POTENCY: see monograph

There is no significance or potency rating for methyldopa because this drug is beneficial during pregnancy under certain conditions and detrimental under others. When given to pregnant women, methyldopa crosses the placenta and achieves equal concentrations in fetal and maternal serum. In the clinical context of hypertension, methyldopa appears to decrease the incidence of spontaneous abortion without producing teratogenic effects among offspring. Infants of hypertensive mothers taking methyldopa during pregnancy had a lower incidence of motor retardation than those in the control group. For women who develop hypertensive crisis while receiving methyldopa, however, the fetal outcome is worse compared to that of untreated women. Methyldopa initiated between 16 and 20 weeks of gestation is associated with a smaller head size among neonates as compared to controls. By 6 years of age, however, there is catch-up head growth with no observed differences and no associated neurologic deficits. In hypertensive women who had proteinuria, methyldopa was associated with decreased birth weight among offspring and a shorter period of gestation. These data indicate that methyldopa has both positive and negative effects on the fetus/neonate. Some effects are temporary and the infant generally is able to compensate after birth. Use of methyldopa in hypertensive patients with proteinuria or patients with poor compliance who are subject to hypertensive crisis should be avoided if possible.

Arias, F., & Zamoro, J. (1979). Antihypertensive treatment and pregnancy outcome in patients with mild chronic hypertension. *Obstetrics and Gynecology, 53,* 489–494.

Jones, H. M., & Cummings, A. J. (1978). A study of the transfer of alpha-methyldopa to the human foetus and newborn infant. *British Journal of Clinical Pharmacology, 6,* 432.

Kincaid-Smith, P., & Bullen, M. (1966). Prolonged use of methyldopa in severe hypertension in pregnancy. *British Medical Journal, 1,* 274–276.

Leather, H. M., Humphreys, D. M., Baker, P., et al. (1968). A controlled trial of hypotensive agents in hypertension in pregnancy. *The Lancet, 2,* 488–490.

Moar, V. A., Jefferies, M. A., Mutch, L. M., et al. (1978). Neonatal head circumference and the treatment of maternal hypertension. *British Journal of Obstetrics and Gynecology, 85,* 933.

Mutch, L. M., Moar, V. A., Ounsted, M. K., et al. (1977). Hypertension during pregnancy, with and without specific hypotensive treatment. *Early Human Development, 1,* 59–67.

Ounsted, M. K., Moar, V. A., Good, F. J., et al. (1980). Hypertension during pregnancy with and without specific treatment; the development of the children at the age of four years. *British Journal of Obstetrics and Gynaecology, 87,* 19–24.

Redman, C. W., Beilin, L. J., Bonnar, J., et al. (1976). Fetal outcome in trial of antihypertensive treatment of pregnancy. *The Lancet, 2,* 753–756.

Methylene Blue

FDA: C SIGNIFICANCE: 3 (intra-amniotic near term)
POTENCY: 2 (intra-amniotic near term)

Intestinal atresia or stenosis was noted in several infants born to women who received an injection of methylene blue into the amniotic cavity during the second trimester. These reports involved multiple pregnancies (twins), which could be a confounding variable. Other studies of women who received methylene blue during the first trimester (n = 10) or at various times during their pregnancies (n = 35) failed to detect an increased risk for congenital anomalies. Intra-amniotic administration of methylene blue near term has resulted in neonatal hemolytic anemia and jaundice (adverse drug reactions associated with methylene blue use in neonates).

Cowett, R. M., Hakanson, D. O., Kocon, R. W., et al. (1976). Untoward neonatal effect of intra-amniotic administration of methylene blue. *Obstetrics and Gynecology, 48*(Suppl), 745–755.
Crooks, J. (1982). Haemolytic jaundice in a neonate after intra-amniotic injection of methylene blue. *Archives of Disease in Childhood, 57,* 872–886.
Dolk, H. (1991). Methylene blue and atresia or stenosis of ileum and jejunum. *The Lancet, 338,* 1021–1022.
Heinonen, O. P., Slone, D., & Shapiro, S. (1977). *Birth defects and drugs in pregnancy.* Littleton, MA: Publishing Sciences Group.
Katz, Z., & Lancet, M. (1981). Inadvertent intrauterine injection of methylene blue in early pregnancy. *New England Journal of Medicine, 304,* 1427.
McEnerney, J. K., & McEnerney, L. N. (1983). Unfavorable neonatal outcome after intraamniotic injection of methylene blue. *Obstetrics and Gynecology, 61,* 35S–37S.
Moorman-Voestermans, C. G. M., Heig, H. A., & Vos, A. (1990). Jejunal atresia in twins. *Journal of Pediatric Surgery, 25,* 638–639.
Nicolini, U., & Monni, G. (1990). Intestinal obstruction in babies exposed in utero to methylene blue. *The Lancet, 336,* 1258–1259.
Plunkett, G. D. (1973). Neonatal complications. *Obstetrics and Gynecology, 41,* 476–477.
Serota, F. T., Bernbaum, J. C., & Schwartz, E. (1979). The methylene blue baby. *The Lancet, 2,* 1142–1143.
Spahr, R. C., Salsburey, D. J., Kirssberg, A., et al. (1980). Intraamniotic injection of methylene blue leading to methemoglobinemia in one of twins. *International Journal of Gynaecology and Obstetrics, 17,* 477–478.
Vincer, M. J., Allen, A. C., Evans, J. R., et al. (1987). Methylene-blue-induced hemolytic anemia in a neonate. *Canadian Medical Association Journal, 136,* 503–504.

Methylenedioxy Methamphetamine (Ecstasy, MDMA)

AUTHOR: **NONE**   SIGNIFICANCE: **3–4**   POTENCY: **3–4**

A prospective study of children (n = 136) who were born to mothers who used methylenedioxy methamphetamine during pregnancy revealed an increased risk for congenital malformations, particularly malformations affecting the cardiac and musculoskeletal systems. More data are needed, particularly because, although methylenedioxy methamphetamine is widely used by adolescent girls and young women of childbearing age, there are no reports other than this study associating its use with teratogenic effects; and because adolescent girls and young women who use methylenedioxy methamphetamine generally use other drugs commonly used at Raves (*see* Chapter 7), including alcohol, tobacco, and ketamine, which may confound the interpretation of reported data.

McElhatton, P. R., Bateman, D. N., Evans, C., et al. (1999). Congenital anomalies after prenatal ecstasy exposure. *The Lancet, 354*(9188), 1441–1442.

Methylphenidate

FDA: **C**   SIGNIFICANCE: **4**   POTENCY: **3–4**

There was no significant increase in teratogenic effects among 11 neonates exposed to methylphenidate in utero. More data are needed regarding methylphenidate use during pregnancy, particularly on use during the first trimester.

Heinonen, O. P., Slone, D., & Shapiro, S. (1977). *Birth defects and drugs in pregnancy.* Littleton, MA: Publishing Sciences Group.

Methyltestosterone

FDA: **X**   SIGNIFICANCE: **1**   POTENCY: **1**

Methyltestosterone is a known teratogen that can masculinize the female fetus, even when taken late in pregnancy. If exposure occurs during the first trimester, complete labial fusion may occur.

Black, J. A., & Bentley, J. F. (1959). Effect on the foetus of androgens given during pregnancy. *The Lancet, 1,* 21.
Gold, A. P., & Michael, A. F. (1958). Testosterone-induced female pseudohermaphroditism. *The Journal of Pediatrics, 52,* 279–283.
Grumbach, M. M., & Ducharme, J. R. (1960). The effects of androgens on fetal sexual development: Androgen-induced female pseudohermaphroditism. *Fertility and Sterility, 11,* 157–180.
Grumwaldt, E., & Bates, T. (1957). Nonadrenal female pseudohermaphroditism after administration of testosterone to mother during pregnancy, report of case. *Pediatrics, 20,* 503.

Hayles, A. B., & Nolan, R. B. (1957). Female pseudohermaphroditism: Report of case in an infant born of a mother receiving methyltestosterone during pregnancy. *Proceedings of the Staff Meetings of the Mayo Clinic, 32*, 41.

Moncrieff, A. (1958). Nonadrenal female pseudohermaphroditism associated with hormone administration in pregnancy. *The Lancet, 2*, 267.

Nellhaus, G. (1958). Artificially-induced female pseudohermaphroditism. *New England Journal of Medicine, 258*, 935.

Tuchmann-Duplessis, H. (1975). *Drug effects on the fetus*. Acton, MA: Publishing Sciences Group.

Metoclopramide

FDA: **B**   SIGNIFICANCE: **3–4**   POTENCY: **3–4**

A single study of metoclopramide use during the first trimester (n = 25) found no teratogenic effects. More data are needed.

Sidhu, M. S., & Lean, T. H. (1970). The use of metoclopramide (Maxolon) in hyperemesis gravidarum. *Proceedings of the Obstetrics and Gynaecology Society of Singapore, 1*, 43–46.

Metoprolol

FDA: **B**   SIGNIFICANCE: **5**   POTENCY: **4**

Selective ß$_1$ blockers have the theoretical advantage in pregnancy of not affecting uterine blood flow. In studies of metoprolol use in 184 pregnant women, no effects on fetal growth, fetal heart rate, or neonatal blood glucose were observed.

Hogstedt, S., Lindeberg, S., Azelsson, O., et al. (1985). A prospective controlled trial of metoprolol-hydralazine treatment in hypertension during pregnancy. *Acta Obstetricia et Gynecologica Scandinavica, 64*, 505–510.

Sandstrom, B. (1978). Antihypertensive treatment with the adrenergic receptor blocker metoprolol during pregnancy. *Gynecologic and Obstetric Investigation, 9*, 195–204.

Sandstrom, B. (1982). Adrenergic beta-receptor blockers in hypertension of pregnancy. *Clinical and Experimental Hypertension, 1*, 127–141.

Wood, S. M., & Blainey, J. D. (1981). Hypertension and renal disease. *Clinical Obstetrics and Gynecology, 8*, 439–453.

Metronidazole

FDA: **B**   SIGNIFICANCE: **4–5**   POTENCY: **3–4**

There is no evidence that metronidazole is a human teratogen. In studies involving more than 2000 women of whom 25% received metronidazole during the first trimester, no increase in congenital malformations among offspring was observed with up to a 10-year follow-up. Metronidazole has been recommended for the treatment of amebiasis and *Trichomonas vaginalis* during pregnancy. However, these recommendations are not universal. (*See* Paromomycin monograph.)

Aselton, P., Jick, H., Milunsky, A., et al. (1985). First-trimester drug use and congenital disorders. *Obstetrics and Gynecology, 65*, 451–455.

Beard, C. M., Roller, K. L., O'Fallon, W. M., et al. (1979). Lack of evidence for cancer due to metronidazole. *New England Journal of Medicine, 301*, 519.

Berget, A., & Weber, T. (1972). Metronidazole in pregnancy. *Ubeskrift for Laeger, 134*, 2085.

Butler, C. D. (1990). Treatment of intestinal parasites during pregnancy. *Facts and Comparisons Drug Newsletter, 9*, 41–43.

Heinonen, O. P., Slone, D., & Shapiro, S. (1977). *Birth defects and drugs in pregnancy*. Littleton, MA: Publishing Sciences Group.

Jick, H., Holmes, L. B., Hunter, J. R., et al. (1981). First-trimester drug use and congenital disorders. *Journal of the American Medical Association, 246*, 343–346.

Morgan, I. (1985). Metronidazole treatment in pregnancy. *International Journal of Gynaecology and Obstetrics, 15*, 501–502.

Peterson, W. F., Stauch, J. E., & Ryder, C. D. (1966). Metronidazole in pregnancy. *American Journal of Obstetrics and Gynecology, 94*, 343.

Rosa, F. W., Bauman, C., & Shaw, M. (1987). Pregnancy outcomes after first-trimester vaginitis drug therapy. *Obstetrics and Gynecology, 69*, 751–755.

Trussell, R. R., & Beeley, L. (1981). Infestations. *Clinical Obstetrics and Gynecology, 8*, 333–340.

Miconazole

AUTHOR: **NONE**   SIGNIFICANCE: **4–5** (vaginal use)   POTENCY: **4** (vaginal use)

A retrospective, record linkage, case-controlled study of ~8000 infants with congenital anomalies and two other studies in which miconazole was administered vaginally either during the first trimester (n = 404) or at some time later during pregnancy (n = 248) failed to detect an increased risk for congenital anomalies. Unfortunately, no data are available for systemic miconazole use during pregnancy.

Jick, H., Holmes, L. B., Hunter, J. R., et al. (1981). First-trimester drug use and congenital disor-

ders. *Journal of the American Medical Association, 246,* 343–346.
McNellis, D., McLeod, M., Lawson, J., et al. (1977). Treatment of vulvovaginal candidiasis in pregnancy. *Obstetrics and Gynecology, 50,* 674–678.
Rosa, F. W., Baum, C., & Shaw, M. (1987). Pregnancy outcomes after first-trimester vaginitis drug therapy. *Obstetrics and Gynecology, 69*(5), 751–755.

Minoxidil

FDA: **C**   SIGNIFICANCE: **3**   POTENCY: **2**

Two reports of hypertrichosis involved infants whose mothers had received systemic minoxidil for hypertension during their pregnancies. The hypertrichosis, a recognized effect associated with minoxidil, resolved without intervention in a few months.

Kaler, S. G., Patrinos, M. E., Lambert, G. H., et al. (1987). Hypertrichosis and congenital anomalies associated with maternal use of minoxidil. *Pediatrics, 79*(3), 434–436.
Rosa, F. W., Idanpaan-Heikkila, J., & Asanti, R. (1987). Fetal minoxidil exposure. *Pediatrics, 80*(1), 120.

Misoprostol

FDA: **X**   SIGNIFICANCE: **1**   POTENCY: **1–2**

Misoprostol is contraindicated because of its abortifacient activity in pregnant women. Recent data from Brazil, where misoprostol is used both orally and vaginally as an abortifacient, strongly suggest that failed attempts at abortion with misoprostol may result in Moebius syndrome (i.e., a congenital maldevelopment of the cranial nerves resulting in unbalanced movements of the facial muscles and facial paralysis) among surviving neonates. Other congenital anomalies have been noted in conjunction with misoprostol use. Other reports, however, found no teratogenic effects among infants exposed to misoprostol in utero. More data are needed, particularly in regard to potentially confounding variables such as other drugs or activities that may have been used concurrently to end a pregnancy.

Genest, D. R., Di Salvo, D., Rosenblatt, M. J., et al. (1999). Terminal transverse limb defects with tethering and omphalocele in a 17 week fetus following first trimester misoprostol exposure. *Clinical Dysmorphology, 8,* 53–58.
Nunes, M. L., Friedrich, M. A., & Loch, L. F. (1999). Association of misoprostol, Moebius syndrome and congenital central alveolar hypoventilation. Case report. *Arquivos de Neuro-Psiquiatria, 57,* 88–91.
Orioli, I. M., & Castilla, E. E. (2000). Epidemiological assessment of misoprostol teratogenicity. *British Journal of Obstetrics and Gynaecology, 107,* 519–523.
Pastuszak, A. L., Schuler, L., Speck-Martins, C. E., et al. (1998). Use of misoprostol during pregnancy and Mobius syndrome in infants. *New England Journal of Medicine, 338,* 1881–1885.
Schuler, L., Pastuszak, A., Sanseverino, T. V., et al. (1999). Pregnancy outcome after exposure to misoprostol in Brazil: A prospective, controlled study. *Reproductive Toxicology, 13,* 147–151.

Morphine

FDA: **C**   SIGNIFICANCE: **5** (congenital anomalies)
POTENCY: **4** (congenital anomalies)

Congenital anomalies were not significantly increased among the offspring of women who received morphine during the first trimester (n = 70) or at various times during their pregnancies (n = 448). Neonatal lethargy, poor suck, and sedation have been associated with maternal morphine use near term. Long-term high dose or regular personal use of morphine during pregnancy has been associated with the neonatal opiate analgesic-withdrawal syndrome (diarrhea, irritability, sneezing, tremors, vomiting). (*See* Heroin and Meperidine monographs.)

Czeizel, A., Szentesi, I., Szekeres, I., et al. (1988). A study of adverse effects on the pregnancy after intoxication during pregnancy. *Archives of Toxicology, 61,* 1–7.
Heinonen, O. P., Slone, D., & Shapiro, S. (1977). *Birth defects and drugs in pregnancy.* Littleton, MA: Publishing Sciences Group.
Perlstein, M. A. (1974). Congenital morphinism. *Journal of the American Medical Association, 135,* 633.

Mumps Virus Vaccine

AUTHOR: ●   SIGNIFICANCE: **3–4**
POTENCY: **3–4**

Mumps virus is a live vaccine. It was administered to three women who were susceptible to mumps and were scheduled to have therapeutic abortions. The virus was cultured from the placenta but not from the fetus of two of these three women. The use of mumps virus vaccine during pregnancy has been questioned. However, maternal mumps infection during the first trimester is associated with a significant risk for miscarriage. Maternal mumps infection appears to have little risk of producing congenital anomalies. More data are needed.

Hill, A. B., Doll, R., Galloway, T. M., et al. (1958). Virus diseases in pregnancy and congenital defects. *British Journal of Preventive and Social Medicine, 12,* 1–7.
Korones, S. B., Todaro, J., Roane, J. A., et al. (1970). Maternal virus infection after the first trimester of pregnancy and status of offspring to 4 years of age in a predominantly Negro population. *The Journal of Pediatrics, 77,* 245–251.
Kurtz, J. B., Tomlinson, A. H., & Pearson, J. (1982). Mumps virus isolated from a fetus. *British Medical Journal, 284,* 471.
Siegel, M., & Fuerst, H. T. (1966). Low birth weight and maternal virus disease: A prospective study of rubella, measles, mumps, chickenpox, and hepatitis. *Journal of the American Medical Association, 197,* 680–684.
Yamanchi, T., Wilson, C., & St. Geme, J. W. (1974). Transmission of live attenuated mumps virus to the human placenta. *New England Journal of Medicine, 290,* 710–712.

Nalbuphine

FDA: **B** SIGNIFICANCE: **4** POTENCY: **4**

Use of nalbuphine near term has resulted in fetotoxic effects, including bradycardia, cyanosis, hypotonia, transient apnea, and neonatal respiratory depression. The placental transfer of nalbuphine is rapid and relatively complete. The effects reported are noted adverse drug reactions generally associated with nalbuphine. More data are needed, particularly data addressing nalbuphine use during the first trimester.

Guillonneau, M., Jacquz-Aigrain, E., de Crepy, A., et al. (1990). Perinatal adverse effects of nalbuphine given during parturition. *The Lancet, 335,* 1588.
Sgro, C., Escousse, A., Tennenbaum, D., et al. (1990). Perinatal adverse effects of nalbuphine given during labor. *The Lancet, 336,* 1070.

Nalidixic Acid

FDA: **C** SIGNIFICANCE: **4** POTENCY: **4**

One study of nalidixic acid use during various stages of pregnancy (first trimester, n = 6; second trimester, n = 26; third trimester, n = 31) failed to find a significant risk for congenital anomalies among offspring. More data are needed.

Murray, E. D. S. (1981). Nalidixic acid in pregnancy. *British Medical Journal, 282,* 224.

Naproxen

FDA: **B** SIGNIFICANCE: **3** (near term)
POTENCY: **1–2** (near term)

Three infants born to women who received naproxen during pregnancy had premature closure of the ductus arteriosus and persistent pulmonary hypertension. In the low oxygen levels of the fetal blood, prostaglandin E_2 (PGE_2) maintains the patency of the ductus arteriosus. Naproxen, a prostaglandin synthetase inhibitor, decreases PGE_2 production so that there is at least partial closure of the ductus in utero. This effect increases pulmonary artery pressure with secondary pulmonary vascular muscle hypertrophy and causes further pulmonary hypertension, resulting in difficulty with pulmonary circulation at birth.

Beeley, L. (1981). Adverse effects of drugs in later pregnancy. *Clinical Obstetrics and Gynecology, 8,* 275–290.
Wilkinson, A. R. (1980). Naproxen levels in preterm infants after maternal treatment. *The Lancet, 2,* 591–592.
Wilkinson, A. R., Aynsley-Green, A., & Mitchell, M. D. (1979). Persistent pulmonary hypertension and abnormal prostaglandin E levels in preterm infants after maternal treatment with naproxen. *Archives of Disease in Childhood, 54,* 942–945.

Niclosamide

FDA: **B** SIGNIFICANCE: **5** POTENCY: **4**

Niclosamide has been recommended for the treatment of tapeworm infestation during pregnancy. Data on its safety have not been substantiated, however. More data are needed.

Trussell, R. R., & Beeley, L. (1981). Infestations. *Clinical Obstetrics and Gynecology, 8,* 333–340.

Nifedipine

FDA: **C** SIGNIFICANCE: **4** POTENCY: **4**

In several studies on the second or third trimester use of nifedipine for preterm labor or pregnancy-induced hypertension, no teratogenic effects were noted. More data are needed, particularly data addressing use during the first trimester.

Bracero, L. A., Leikin, E., Kirshenbaum, N., et al. (1991). Comparison of nifedipine and ritodrine for the treatment of preterm labor. *American Journal of Perinatology, 8*(6), 365–369.

Fenakel, K., Fenakel, G., Appelman, Z. V. I., et al. (1991). Nifedipine in the treatment of severe preeclampsia. *Obstetrics and Gynecology, 77*, 331–337.

Ferguson, J. E., Dyson, D. C., Schutz, T., et al. (1990). A comparison of tocolysis with nifedipine or ritodrine: Analysis of efficacy and maternal, fetal, and neonatal outcome. *American Journal of Obstetrics and Gynecology, 163*, 105–111.

Meyer, W. R., Randall, H. W., & Graves, W. L. (1990). Nifedipine versus ritodrine for suppressing preterm labor. *Journal of Reproductive Medicine, 35*, 649–653.

Read, M. D., & Wellby, D. W. (1986). The use of a calcium antagonist (nifedipine) to suppress preterm labour. *British Journal of Obstetrics and Gynaecology, 93*, 933–937.

Nitrazepam

AUTHOR: **NONE**   SIGNIFICANCE: **2**
POTENCY: **3**

Use of nitrazepam during pregnancy has been associated with cleft lip and palate among offspring. It also has been associated with neonatal CNS depression and with the neonatal benzodiazepine-withdrawal syndrome, both of which are fully reversible with appropriate recognition and management.

Saxen, I., & Saxen, L. (1975). Association between maternal intake of diazepam and oral clefts. *The Lancet, 2*, 498.

Tuchmann-Duplessis, H. (1983). The teratogenic risk. *American Journal of Industrial Medicine, 4*, 245–258.

Nitrofurantoin

FDA: **B**   SIGNIFICANCE: **4–5** (first trimester effects)

POTENCY: **3–4** (first trimester effects)

The Collaborative Perinatal Project studied 83 women who received nitrofurantoin during the first trimester; congenital malformations were found in five infants. This rate of congenital malformations was not considered significant. However, the risk for hemolytic anemia in the newborn suggests a relative contraindication for the use of nitrofurantoin at or near term.

Heinonen, O. P., Slone, D., & Shapiro, S. (1977). *Birth defects and drugs in pregnancy.* Littleton, MA: Publishing Sciences Group.

Safety of antimicrobial drugs in pregnancy. (1987). *The Medical Letter, 29*, 61–63.

Nitrous Oxide

AUTHOR: ★   SIGNIFICANCE: **1–2**
POTENCY: **2**

Three studies of pregnant women who received nitrous oxide anesthesia either during the first trimester (n = 170) or at various times during their pregnancies (n = 580) found no significant risk for congenital anomalies among their offspring. In an occupational-exposure-related survey of dentists and dental assistants, a spontaneous abortion rate of 19% in the high user group versus 8% in a nonuser group was observed. For those pregnancies going to term, a malformation rate of 7.7% was observed in the high user group versus 3.6% in the nonuser group. However, this reported increased risk was not supported by later studies involving both dental assistants and veterinarians. (*See* Anesthetics—Inhalation, Waste monograph.)

Aldridge, L. M., & Tunstall, M. E. (1986). Nitrous oxide and the fetus. *British Journal of Anaesthesia, 58*, 1348–1356.

Cohen, E. N., Brown, B. W., Wu, M. L., et al. (1980). Occupational disease in dentistry and chronic exposure to trace anesthetic gases. *Journal of the American Dental Association, 101*, 21–31.

Crawford, J. S., & Lewis, M. (1986). Nitrous oxide in early human pregnancy. *Anaesthesia, 41*, 900–905.

Heidam, L. Z. (1984). Spontaneous abortions among dental assistants, factory workers, painters, and gardening workers: A follow up study. *Journal of Epidemiology and Community Health, 38*, 149–155.

Heinonen, O. P., Slone, D., & Shapiro, S. (1977). *Birth defects and drugs in pregnancy.* Littleton, MA: Publishing Sciences Group.

Johnson, J. A., Buchan, R. M., & Reif, J. S. (1987). Effect of waste anesthetic gas and vapor exposure on reproductive outcome in veterinary personnel. *American Industrial Hygiene Association Journal, 48*(1), 62–66.

Nonoxynol 9 (Nonoxinol 9)

AUTHOR: **NONE** SIGNIFICANCE: **5**
POTENCY: **4**

In an early study on the use of nonoxynol 9 by pregnant women, a 5.8% spontaneous abortion rate was recorded for the study group versus rates of 3.1% and 3.3% for two control groups. A higher incidence of congenital malformations also was observed among the study group's aborted fetuses. However, several authors rejected these findings on methodological grounds and because of the overwhelming majority of negative studies and case reports on nonoxynol 9. Spermicides in general are thought to be nonteratogenic.

Bracken, M. B. (1985). Spermicidal contraceptives and poor reproductive outcomes: The epidemiologic evidence against an association. *American Journal of Obstetrics and Gynecology, 151*(5), 552–556.
Cordero, J. F., & Layde, P. M. (1981). Vaginal spermicides, chromosome abnormalities and limb reduction defects. *American Journal of Human Genetics, 33*, 74A.
Einarson, T. R., Koren, G., Mattice, D., et al. (1990). Maternal spermicide use and adverse reproductive outcome: A meta-analysis. *American Journal of Obstetrics and Gynecology, 162*, 655–660.
Gibaldi, M. (1988). Spermicides and birth defects. *Perspectives in Clinical Pharmacy, 6*, 49–51.
Harlap, S., Shiono, P. H., & Ramcharan, S. (1985). Congenital abnormalities in the offspring of women who used oral and other contraceptives around the time of conception. *International Journal of Fertility, 30*(2), 39–47.
Huggins, G., Vessey, M., Flavel, R., et al. (1982). Vaginal spermicides and outcome of pregnancy: Findings in a large cohort study. *Contraception, 25*, 219–230.
Jick, H., Shiota, K., Shepard, T. H., et al. (1982). Vaginal spermicides and miscarriage seen primarily in the emergency room. *Teratogenesis, Carcinogenesis and Mutagenesis, 2*, 205–210.
Jick, H., Walker, A. M., Rothman, K. J., et al. (1981). Vaginal spermicides and congenital disorders. *Journal of the American Medical Association, 245*, 1329–1332.
Louik, C., Mitchell, A. A., Werler, M. M., et al. (1987). Maternal exposure to spermicides in relation to certain birth defects. *New England Journal of Medicine, 317*, 474–478.
Mills, J. L., Harley, E. E., Reed, G. F., et al. (1982). Are spermicides teratogenic? *Journal of the American Medical Association, 248*, 2148–2151.
Oakley, G. P. (1982). Spermicides and birth defects. [Editorial]. *Journal of the American Medical Association, 247*, 2405.
Polednak, A. P., Janerich, D. T., & Glebatis, D. M. (1982). Birth weight and birth defects in relation to maternal spermicide use. *Teratology, 26*, 27–38.
Shapiro, S., Slone, D., Heinonen, O. P., et al. (1982). Birth defects and vaginal spermicides. *Journal of the American Medical Association, 247*, 2381–2384.
Strobino, B., Kline, J., & Warburton, D. (1988). Spermicide use and pregnancy outcome. *American Journal of Public Health, 78*(3), 260–263.
Warburton, D., Neugut, R. H., Lustenberger, A., et al. (1987). Lack of association between spermicide use and trisomy. *New England Journal of Medicine, 317*(8), 478–482.
Watkins, R. N. (1986). Vaginal spermicides and congenital disorders. The validity of a study. *Journal of the American Medical Association, 256*(22), 3095.

Norethindrone (Norethisterone)

FDA: **X** SIGNIFICANCE: **1** POTENCY: **1–2**

Use of norethindrone during pregnancy is known to masculinize the female fetus, producing clitoral hypertrophy, labrosacral fusion, and pseudohermaphroditism. These effects appear to be dose related (note that generally lower therapeutic doses are used today than when these incidents were reported). The estimated incidence was ~18% for exposed female fetuses. Lack of association also has been reported, however. The degree of masculinization does not appear to be severe and usually can be treated with topical estrogens. No adverse effects on the male fetus have been noted.

Darling, M. R., & Hawkins, D. F. (1981). Sex hormones in pregnancy. *Clinical Obstetrics and Gynecology, 8*, 405–419.
Fine, E., Levin, H. M., & McConnell, E. L. (1963). Masculinization of female infants associated with norethindrone acetate. *Obstetrics and Gynecology, 22*, 210–212.
Golbus, M. S. (1980). Teratology for the obstetrician: Current status. *Obstetrics and Gynecology, 55*, 269–277.
Grumbach, M. M., Ducharme, J. R., & Moloshok, R. E. (1959). On the fetal masculinizing action of certain oral progestins. *Journal of Clinical Endocrinology and Metabolism, 19*, 1369–1380.
Hagler, S., et al. (1963). Fetal effects of steroid therapy during pregnancy. *American Journal of Diseases of Children, 106*, 589–590.
Ishizuka, N., Kawashima, Y., Nakanishi, T., et al. (1962). [Statistical observations on genital anomalies of newborns following the administration

of progestins to their mothers.] *Journal of the Japanese Obstetrical and Gynecological Society, 9,* 271.

Kullander, S., & Kallen, B. (1976). A prospective study of drugs and pregnancy. *Acta Obstetricia and Gynecologica Scandinavica, 55,* 221–224.

McBride, W. G. (1963). The teratogenic action of drugs. *Medical Journal of Australia, 2,* 689–693.

Schardein, J. L. (1980). Congenital abnormalities and hormones during pregnancy: A clinical review. *Teratology, 22,* 251–270.

Wilkins, L. (1960). Masculinization of female fetus due to use of orally given progestins. *Journal of the American Medical Association, 172,* 1028–1032.

Wilkins, L., Jones, H. W., Holman, G. H., et al. (1958). Masculinization of the female fetus associated with administration of progestins during gestation: Non adrenal female pseudo hermaphrodism. *Journal of Clinical Endocrinology and Metabolism, 18,* 559–585.

Nortriptyline

FDA: D   **SIGNIFICANCE: 5** (malformations) **1** (neonatal toxicity)
POTENCY: 4 (malformations) **1** (neonatal toxicity)

Large studies of the tricyclic antidepressants have shown them to be nonteratogenic but probably fetotoxic. Nortriptyline use during pregnancy has been implicated with neonatal urinary retention, a known adverse effect of the drug. It also has been associated with a neonatal distress syndrome involving respiratory distress, peripheral cyanosis, and hypertonia with tremor, spasm, or clonus. The nortriptyline neonatal distress syndrome is thought to be secondary to adrenergic supersensitization associated with the anticholinergic effects of the drug. As such, it might be called a neonatal nortriptyline-withdrawal syndrome. More data are needed. (*See* Imipramine monograph.)

Shearer, W. T., Schreiner, R. L., & Marshall, R. E. (1972). Urinary retention in a neonate secondary to maternal ingestion of nortriptyline. *The Journal of Pediatrics, 81,* 570–572.

Sjoqvist, F., Bergfors, P. G., Borga, O., et al. (1972). Plasma disappearance of nortriptyline in a newborn infant following placental transfer from an intoxicated mother: Evidence for drug metabolism. *The Journal of Pediatrics, 80,* 496–500.

Webster, P. A. (1973). Withdrawal symptoms in neonates associated with maternal antidepressant therapy. *The Lancet, 2,* 318–319.

Nystatin

FDA: C   **SIGNIFICANCE: 5**   **POTENCY: 4**

Four studies of women who used nystatin topically, primarily for the local treatment of candidiasis, during the first trimester (n = 543) or at various other times during their pregnancies (n = 230) found no increase in congenital anomalies among offspring.

Aselton, P., Jick, H., Milunsky, A., et al. (1985). First-trimester drug use and congenital disorders. *Obstetrics and Gynecology, 65,* 451–455.

Heinonen, O. P., Slone, D., & Shapiro, S. (1977). *Birth defects and drugs in pregnancy.* Littleton, MA: Publishing Sciences Group.

Jick, H., Holmes, L. B., Hunter, J. R., et al. (1981). First-trimester drug use and congenital disorders. *Journal of the American Medical Association, 246,* 343–346.

Rosa, F. W., Baum, C., & Shaw, M. (1987). Pregnancy outcomes after first-trimester vaginitis drug therapy. *Obstetrics and Gynecology, 69,* 751–755.

Ofloxacin

FDA: C   **SIGNIFICANCE: 3**   **POTENCY: 2–3**

A single case report examined ofloxacin use during the second trimester, and no teratogenic effects were found. More data on ofloxacin use during the first trimester are needed.

Peled, Y., Friedman, S., Hod, M., et al. (1991). Ofloxacin during the second trimester of pregnancy. *DICP, The Annals of Pharmacotherapy, 25,* 1181–1182.

Omeprazole

FDA: C   **SIGNIFICANCE: 3–4**   **POTENCY: 3–4**

A large-scale retrospective cohort study (n = 2236) investigating the effects of acid-suppressing drugs during the first trimester on neonatal outcome reported no significant teratogenic risk. More data are needed, particularly data on use during the later trimesters.

Ruigomez, A., Garcia Rodriguez, L. A., Cattaruzzi, C., et al. (1999). Use of cimetidine, omeprazole, and ranitidine in pregnant women and pregnancy outcomes. *American Journal of Epidemiology, 150,* 476–481.

Oral Contraceptives
Progestogen/Estrogen Combinations

FDA: X   **SIGNIFICANCE: 3**   **POTENCY: 2–3**

Studies examining use of progestogen/estrogen combination oral contraceptives in pregnancy have produced a great deal of conflicting and inconclusive data relative to possible teratogenic effects.

Use of the combination of norethindrone and mestranol in the second and third trimesters for threatened abortion has been associated with clitoral hypertrophy among female fetuses/neonates.

There also have been several studies associating neural-tube defects and the VACTERL syndrome (defects involving the vertebrae, anus, cardiovascular system, trachea, esophagus, renal tract, and limbs) with the use of various progestogen/estrogen combination products. A lack of association also has been reported, however.

The data on cardiac defects also are conflicting. Cardiac defects have been linked to use of progestogen and estrogen combination products during pregnancy. Other reports have found no such link.

The data provide no overwhelming evidence supporting teratogenic effects, but enough evidence has accumulated to warrant concern. There are several possible explanations for the conflicting evidence. Combination progesterone and estrogen use may be teratogenic only rarely (e.g., when the embryo/fetus is genetically susceptible or coteratogens also are present), or different products may differ in teratogenic effect. The use of oral contraceptives is associated with decreased maternal serum folate levels, which have been associated with teratogenic effects. Because evidence supporting the use of these combination oral contraceptives during pregnancy is lacking, it would seem prudent to avoid such use. More data are needed.

Cuckle, H. S., & Wald, N. J. (1982). Evidence against oral contraceptives as a cause of neural-tube defects. *British Journal of Obstetrics and Gynecology, 89*, 547–549.

Czeizel, A. (1980). Are contraceptive pills teratogenic? *Acta Morphologica Hungarica, 28*(1-2), 177–188.

Ferencz, C., & Wilson, P. D. (1980). Maternal hormone therapy and congenital heart disease. *Teratology, 21*, 225–239.

Gal, I., Kirman, B., & Stern, J. (1967). Hormonal pregnancy tests and congenital abnormalities. *Nature, 216*, 83–84.

Goujard, J., & Rumeau-Rouquette, C. (1977). First trimester exposure to progestogen oestrogen and congenital abnormalities. *The Lancet, 1*, 482–483.

Harlap, S., & Eldor, J. (1980). Births following oral contraceptive failures. *Obstetrics and Gynecology, 55*(4), 447–452.

Harlap, S., Prywes, R., & Davies, M. (1975). Birth defects and oestrogens and progesterones in pregnancy. *The Lancet, 1*, 682–683.

Heinonen, O. P., Slone, D., Monson, R. R., et al. (1976). Cardiovascular birth defects in antenatal exposure to female sex hormones. *New England Journal of Medicine, 296*, 67–70.

Janerich, D. T., Dugan, J. M., & Standfast, S. J. (1977). Congenital heart disease and prenatal exposure to exogenous sex hormones. *British Medical Journal, 1*, 1058–1060.

Janerich, D. T., Piper, J. M., & Glebatis, D. M. (1980). Oral contraceptives and birth defects. *American Journal of Epidemiology, 112*(1), 73–79.

Kasan, P. N., & Andrews, J. (1980). Oral contraception and congenital abnormalities. *British Journal of Obstetrics and Gynecology, 87*, 545–551.

Kelsey, F. O. (1980). The importance of epidemiology in identifying drugs which may cause malformations—With particular reference to drugs containing sex hormones. *Acta Morphologica Hungarica, 28*(1-2), 189–195.

Laurence, M., Miller, M., Vowles, M., et al. (1971). Hormonal pregnancy tests and neural tube malformation. *Nature, 233*, 495–496.

Lewis, D. P., Van Dyke, D. C., Stumbo, P. J., et al. (1998). Drug and environmental factors associated with adverse pregnancy outcomes. Part I: Antiepileptic drugs, contraceptives, smoking, and folate. *Annals of Pharmacotherapy, 32*(7-8), 802–817.

Matsunaga, E., & Shiota, K. (1979). Threatened abortion, hormone therapy and malformed embryos. *Teratology, 20*, 469–480.

Nora, J. J., & Nora, A. H. (1973). Birth defects and oral contraceptives. *The Lancet, 1*, 941–942.

Nora, J. J., & Nora, A. H. (1974). Can the pill cause birth defects? *New England Journal of Medicine, 291*, 731–732.

Nora, J. J., & Nora, A. H. (1978). Exogenous progestogens and estrogen implicated in birth defects. *Journal of the American Medical Association, 240*, 837–839.

Ortiz-Perez, H., Fuertes de la Haba, A., Bangdiwala, I. S., et al. (1979). Abnormalities among offspring of oral and nonoral contraceptive users. *American Journal of Obstetrics and Gynecology, 134*, 512–517.

Royal College of General Practice. (1976). The outcome of pregnancy in former contraceptive users. *British Journal of Obstetrics and Gynecology, 83*, 608–616.

Savolainen, E., Saksela, E., & Saxen, L. (1981). Teratogenic hazards of oral contraceptives analyzed in the national register. *American Journal of Obstetrics and Gynecology, 140,* 521–524.

Schardein, J. L. (1980). Congenital abnormalities and hormones during pregnancy. A clinical review. *Teratology, 22,* 251–270.

Voorhess, M. L. (1967). Masculinization of the female fetus associated with norethindrone-mestranol therapy during pregnancy. *The Journal of Pediatrics, 71,* 128–131.

Wilson, J. G., & Brent, R. L. (1981). Are female sex hormones teratogenic? *American Journal of Obstetrics and Gynecology, 141,* 567–580.

Oxazepam

FDA: **C**   SIGNIFICANCE: **3**   POTENCY: **2–3**

In one study, use of oxazepam during pregnancy was associated with cleft lip/palate. More data are needed. (*See* Diazepam monograph.)

Saxen, I., & Saxen, L. (1975). Association between maternal intake of diazepam and oral clefts. *The Lancet, 2,* 498.

Oxprenolol

AUTHOR: **NONE**   SIGNIFICANCE: **1–2**
POTENCY: **2**

In a single study, approximately 4% of infants exposed to oxprenolol in utero had intrauterine growth retardation. More data are needed. (*See* Propranolol monograph.)

Gallery, E. D., Saunders, D. M., Hunyor, S. N., et al. (1979). Randomized comparison of methyldopa and oxprenolol for treatment of hypertension in pregnancy. *British Medical Journal, 1,* 1591–1594.

Rotmensch, H. H., Elkayan, U., & Frishman, W. (1983). Antiarrhythmic drug therapy during pregnancy. *Annals of Internal Medicine, 98,* 487–497.

Oxymetazoline

FDA: **NONE**   SIGNIFICANCE: **4–5**
POTENCY: **4**

Congenital anomalies were not significantly increased among a sample of 250 infants whose mothers used oxymetazoline topical nasal spray during the first trimester.

Aselton, P., Jick, H., Milunsky, A., et al. (1985). First-trimester drug use and congenital disorders. *Obstetrics and Gynecology, 65,* 451–455.

Baxi, L. V., Gindoff, P. R., Pregenzer, G. J., et al. (1985). Fetal heart rate changes following maternal administration of a nasal decongestant. *American Journal of Obstetrics and Gynecology, 153,* 799–800.

Jick, H., Holmes, L. B., Hunter, J. R., et al. (1981). First-trimester drug use and congenital disorders. *Journal of the American Medical Association, 246,* 343–346.

Rayburn, W. F., Anderson, J. C., Smith, C. V., et al. (1990). Uterine and fetal doppler flow changes from a single dose of a long-acting intranasal decongestant. *Obstetrics and Gynecology, 76*(2), 180–182.

Oxytetracycline

AUTHOR: **NONE**   SIGNIFICANCE: **3–4**
POTENCY: **1–2** (tooth staining)

No significant risk for congenital anomalies was found in a study of 119 women who received oxytetracycline during the first trimester and 328 women who took it at various times during their pregnancies. Oxytetracycline does, however, cause staining of the deciduous teeth among infants exposed as fetuses during the second or third trimester.

Cohlan, S. Q. (1977). Tetracycline staining of teeth. *Teratology, 15,* 127–130.

Heinonen, O. P., Slone, D., & Shapiro, S. (1977). *Birth defects and drugs in pregnancy.* Littleton, MA: Publishing Sciences Group.

Toaff, R., & Ravid, R. (1966). Tetracyclines and the teeth. *The Lancet, 2,* 281–282.

Oxytocin

AUTHOR: ★   SIGNIFICANCE: **1** (neonatal jaundice)
POTENCY: **1–2** (neonatal jaundice)

Although two negative reports exist, other studies and case reports provide evidence that oxytocin may be fetotoxic when used near term. Oxytocin has been associated with generally reversible neonatal jaundice (hyperbilirubinemia) when used to induce or stimulate labor.

Beazley, J. M., & Alderman, B. (1975). Neonatal hyperbilirubinaemia following the use of oxytocin in labour. *British Journal of Obstetrics and Gynaecology, 82,* 265–271.

Chalmers, I., Campbell, H., & Turnbull, A. C. (1976). Oxytocin and neonatal jaundice. *British Medical Journal, 1,* 647–648.

Chew, W. C., & Swan, I. L. (1977). Influence of simultaneous low amniotomy and oxytocin infusion and other maternal factors on neonatal jaundice: A prospective study. *British Medical Journal, 1,* 72–73.

Davies, D. P., Gomersall, R., Robertson, R., et al. (1973). Neonatal jaundice and maternal oxytocin infusion. *British Medical Journal, 3,* 476–477.

Davis, G. H. (1984). Effects of oxytocin-induction of labor on neonatal hyperbilirubinemia. *Journal of the American Osteopathic Association, 84,* 365–367.

Lange, A. P., Secher, N. J., Westergaard, J. G., et al. (1982). Neonatal jaundice after labour induced or stimulated by prostaglandin E2 or oxytocin. *The Lancet, 1,* 991–994.

Liston, W. A., & Campbell, A. J. (1974). Dangers of oxytocin-induced labor to fetuses. *British Medical Journal, 3,* 606–607.

Sims, D. G., & Neligan, G. A. (1975). Factors affecting the increasing incidence of severe non-hemolytic neonatal jaundice. *British Journal of Obstetrics and Gynaecology, 82,* 863–867.

Paramethadione

FDA: **D** SIGNIFICANCE: **1** POTENCY: **1**

Paramethadione belongs to the oxazolidine-3,4-dione group of anticonvulsants, a group strongly associated with teratogenesis when used by pregnant women. Observed teratogenic effects include atrial and ventricular septal defects, cleft lip/palate, clinodactyly, developmental delay, epicanthal folds, inguinal hernias, intrauterine growth retardation, irregular teeth, malformed ears, microcephaly, patent ductus arteriosus, and V-shaped eyebrows. Women of childbearing age should be given a different anticonvulsant, if possible. (*See* Trimethadione monograph.)

Cohlan, S. Q. (1980). Drugs and pregnancy. *Progress in Clinical and Biological Research, 44,* 77–96.

Fabro, S., & Brown, N. A. (1979). Teratogenic potential of anticonvulsants. *New England Journal of Medicine, 300,* 1280–1281.

Feldman, G. L., Weaver, D. D., & Lavrien, E. W. (1977). The fetal trimethadione syndrome. *American Journal of Diseases of Children, 131,* 1389–1392.

German, J., Ehlers, K. H., Kowal, A., et al. (1970). Possible teratogenicity of trimethadione and paramethadione. *The Lancet, 2,* 261–262.

Goldman, A. S., & Yaffe, S. J. (1978). Fetal trimethadione syndrome. *Teratology, 17,* 103–106.

Rosen, R. C., & Lightner, E. S. (1979). Phenotypic malformations in association with maternal trimethadione therapy. *The Journal of Pediatrics, 92,* 240–244.

Zackai, E. H., Mellman, W. J., Neiderer, B., et al. (1975). The fetal trimethadione syndrome. *The Journal of Pediatrics, 87,* 280–284.

Paromomycin

FDA: **C** SIGNIFICANCE: **4–5** POTENCY: **3–4**

Three pregnant women with giardiasis were treated with paromomycin and had normal infants. Paromomycin has been recommended as the treatment of choice for giardiasis during pregnancy because it is poorly absorbed from the GI tract following oral administration. More data are needed.

Butler, C. D. (1990). Treatment of intestinal parasites during pregnancy. *Facts and Comparisons Drug Newsletter, 9,* 41–43.

Kreutner, A. K., Del Rene, V. E., & Anstey, M. S. (1981). Giardiasis in pregnancy. *American Journal of Obstetrics and Gynecology, 140,* 895–901.

Penicillamine (D-Penicillamine)

FDA: **D** SIGNIFICANCE: **3** POTENCY: **2–3**

There have been several reports of congenital malformations among neonates born to women who received penicillamine during pregnancy. Noted defects include a broad nasal bridge, bilateral inguinal hernias, flattened face, lax skin, loose joints, low-set ears, and small jaw. There also are many negative reports regarding the use of this drug during pregnancy. More data are needed.

Beck, R. B., Rosenbaum, K. N., Byers, P. H., et al. (1981). Ultrastructural findings in fetal penicillamine syndrome. Presentation and abstract. March of Dimes 14th Annual Birth Defects Conference, San Diego, California.

Crowhall, J. C., Scowen, E. F., Thompson, C. J., et al. (1967). Dissolution of cystine stones during d-penicillamine treatment of pregnant patients with cystinuria. *British Medical Journal, 2,* 216–218.

Endres, W. (1981). D-penicillamine in pregnancy—To ban or not to ban? *Klinische Wochenschrift, 59,* 535–537.

Harpey, J. P., Jaudon, M. C., Clavel, J. P., et al. (1983). Cutix laxa and low serum zinc after antenatal exposure to penicillamine. *The Lancet, 2,* 858.

Linares, A., Zarranz, J. J., Rodriguez-Alarcon, J., et al. (1979). Reversible cutix laxa due to maternal D-penicillamine treatment. *The Lancet, 2,* 43.

Lover, M., & Fairly, K. F. (1971). D-penicillamine treatment in pregnancy. *The Lancet, 1,* 1019–1020.

Lyle, W. H. (1968). Penicillamine in pregnancy. *The Lancet, 1,* 606.

Marecek, Z., & Graf, M. (1976). Pregnancy in penicillamine-treated patients with Wilson's disease. *New England Journal of Medicine, 295,* 841–842.

Mjolnerod, O. K., Rasmussen, K., Dommerud, S.

A., et al. (1971). Congenital connective-tissue defect probably due to d-penicillamine treatment in pregnancy. *The Lancet, 1,* 673–675.

Needs, C. J., & Brooks, P. M. (1985). Antirheumatic medication in pregnancy. *British Journal of Rheumatology, 24*(3), 282–290.

Rosa, F. W. (1986). Teratogen update: Penicillamine. *Teratology, 33,* 127–131.

Roubenoff, R., Hoyt, J., Petri, M., et al. (1988). Effects of antiinflammatory and immunosuppressive drugs on pregnancy and fertility. *Seminars in Arthritis and Rheumatism, 18*(2), 88–110.

Scheinberg, I. H., & Sternlieb, I. (1975). Pregnancy in penicillamine treated patients with Wilson's disease. *New England Journal of Medicine, 293,* 1300–1302.

Solomon, L., Abrams, G., Dinner, M., et al. (1977). Neonatal abnormalities associated with d-penicillamine treatment during pregnancy. [Letter]. *New England Journal of Medicine, 296,* 54–55.

Walshe, J. M. (1977). Copper chelation in patients with Wilson's disease. *Quarterly Journal of Medicine, 46,* 73.

Penicillin G

FDA: B   SIGNIFICANCE: 5   POTENCY: 4

Penicillin appears to have withstood the test of time. Penicillin at usual therapeutic doses during pregnancy has not been associated with teratogenic effects.

Aselton, P., Jick, H., Milunsky, A., et al. (1985). First-trimester drug use and congenital disorders. *Obstetrics and Gynecology, 65,* 451–455.

Golbus, M. S. (1980). Teratology for the obstetrician: Current status. *Obstetrics and Gynecology, 55,* 269–277.

Heinonen, O. P., Slone, D., & Shapiro, S. (1977). *Birth defects and drugs in pregnancy.* Littleton, MA: Publishing Sciences Group.

Jick, H., Holmes, L. B., Hunter, J. R., et al. (1981). First-trimester drug use and congenital disorders. *Journal of the American Medical Association, 246,* 343–346.

McLachlin, A. E., & Brown, D. D. (1947). Effects of penicillin-administration on menstrual and other sexual cycle functions. *British Journal of Venereal Diseases, 23,* 1–10.

Perin, L., Sissman, R., Detre, F., et al. (1950). La penicilline: A-t-elle une action abortive. *Bulletin de la Societe Francaise de Dermatologie et de Siphiligraphie, 57,* 534.

Pentazocine

FDA: C   SIGNIFICANCE: 4 (malformations) **1** (addiction)
POTENCY: 3–4 (malformations) **1–2** (addiction)

Several studies and case reports document that pentazocine use late in pregnancy is associated with fetal addiction and, subsequently, the neonatal opiate analgesic-withdrawal syndrome, characterized by a high-pitched cry, hyperactivity, irritability, and vomiting. Teratogenic effects have not been reported. (*See* Heroin monograph.)

Ananth, J. (1976). Side effects on fetus and infant of psychotropic drug use during pregnancy. *International Pharmacopsychiatry, 11,* 246–260.

Chasnoff, I. J., Hatcher, R., Burns, W. J., et al. (1983). Pentazocine and tripelennamine ("T's and Blue's"): Effects on the fetus and neonate. *Developmental Pharmacology and Therapeutics, 6,* 162–169.

Dunn, D. W., & Reynolds, J. (1982). Neonatal withdrawal symptoms associated with "T's and Blue's" (pentazocine and tripelennamine). *American Journal of Diseases of Children, 136,* 644–645.

Goetz, R. L., & Bain, R. V. (1974). Neonatal withdrawal symptoms associated with maternal use of pentazocine. *The Journal of Pediatrics, 84,* 887–888.

Kopelman, A. E. (1975). Fetal addiction to pentazocine. *Pediatrics, 55,* 888–889.

Little, B. B., Snell, L. M., Breckenridge, J. D., et al. (1990). Effects of T's and Blue's abuse on pregnancy outcome and infant health status. *American Journal of Perinatology, 7*(4), 359–362.

Scanlon, J. W. (1974). Pentazocine and neonatal withdrawal symptoms. *The Journal of Pediatrics, 85,* 735–736.

von Almen, W. F., & Miller, J. M. (1986). "T's and Blue's" in pregnancy. *Journal of Reproductive Medicine, 31,* 236–239.

Pentobarbital

FDA: D   SIGNIFICANCE: 4 (congenital anomalies) **2–3** (use near term)
POTENCY: 3–4 (congenital anomalies
2 (use near term)

Two studies of women who received pentobarbital either during the first trimester (n = 300) or at various times during their pregnancies (n = 1523) found no evidence of a significant risk for congenital anomalies. One early study indicated that pentobarbital is safe to use during labor. However, the known pharmacology of pentobarbital and reports of other barbiturate use during pregnancy and labor would indicate potential fetotoxic risk for respiratory depression, neonatal depression, and the neonatal barbiturate-withdrawal syndrome when used by women near term.

More studies are needed. (*See* Phenobarbital and Secobarbital monographs.)

Fealy, J. (1958). Placental transmission of pentobarbital sodium. *Obstetrics and Gynecology, 11*, 342–349.

Heinonen, O. P., Slone, D., & Shapiro, S. (1977). *Birth defects and drugs in pregnancy.* Littleton, MA: Publishing Sciences Group.

Jick, H., Holmes, L. B., Hunter, J. R., et al. (1981). First-trimester drug use and congenital disorders. *Journal of the American Medical Association, 246*, 343–346.

Perphenazine

FDA: **C**   SIGNIFICANCE: **5**   POTENCY: **4**

Perphenazine has not been associated with teratogenic effects. Use of phenothiazines during the last trimester has, however, been associated with a neonatal syndrome characterized by decreased reflexes, hypertonus, leukopenia, poor suck, tremors, and weakness. This syndrome may be dose related and may require a familial predisposition.

Ayd, F. J. (1964). Perphenazine: A reappraisal after eight years. *Diseases of the Nervous System, 71*, 311–317.

Ayd, F. J. (1968). Phenothiazine therapy during pregnancy. *International Drug Therapy Newsletter, 3*, 39.

Heinonen, O. P., Slone, D., & Shapiro, S. (1977). *Birth defects and drugs in pregnancy.* Littleton, MA: Publishing Sciences Group.

Hill, R. M., Desmond, M. M., & Kay, J. L. (1966). Extrapyramidal dysfunction in an infant of a schizophrenic mother. *The Journal of Pediatrics, 69*, 589–595.

Rumeau-Rouquette, C., Goujard, J., & Huel, G. (1977). Possible teratogenic effect of phenothiazines in human beings. *Teratology, 15*, 57–64.

Phenacemide

FDA: **D**   SIGNIFICANCE: **3–4**   POTENCY: **3–4**

One study of four mother/infant pairs reported no teratogenic effects when phenacemide was taken during pregnancy. More data are needed.

Nakane, Y., Okuma, R., Takahashi, R., et al. (1980). Multi-institutional study on the teratogenicity and fetal toxicity of antiepileptic drugs: A report of a collaborative study group in Japan. *Epilepsia, 21*, 663–680.

Phenazopyridine

FDA: **B**   SIGNIFICANCE: **4–5**   POTENCY: **4**

Three studies of women who received phenazopyridine either during the first trimester (n = 519) or at various times during their pregnancies (n = 1109) found no significant risk for teratogenic effects. More data are needed.

Aselton, P., Jick, H., Milunsky, A., et al. (1985). First-trimester drug use and congenital disorders. *Obstetrics and Gynecology, 65*, 451–455.

Heinonen, O. P., Slone, D., & Shapiro, S. (1977). *Birth defects and drugs in pregnancy.* Littleton, MA: Publishing Sciences Group.

Jick, H., Holmes, L. B., Hunter, J. R., et al. (1981). First-trimester drug use and congenital disorders. *Journal of the American Medical Association, 246*, 343–346.

Phencyclidine

FDA: **X**   SIGNIFICANCE: **3**   POTENCY: **3**

A single case of congenital malformation associated with phencyclidine (PCP) use during pregnancy has been reported. Fetotoxic effects attributed to phencyclidine also have been reported but are not clearly related to its use. These include abnormal suck, irritability, outbursts of agitation, and rapid changes in level of consciousness. Phencyclidine reportedly is used by 0.8% of women during pregnancy, frequently with other drugs.

Chasnoff, I. J., Burns, W. J., Hatcher, R. P., et al. (1983). Phencyclidine: Effects on the fetus and neonate. *Developmental Pharmacology and Therapeutics, 6*, 404–408.

Golden, N. L., Kuhnert, B. R., Sokol, R. J., et al. (1980). Angel dust: Effects on the fetus. *Pediatrics, 65*, 18–20.

Golden, N. L., Sokol, R. J., & Rubin, I. L. (1984). Phencyclidine use during pregnancy. *American Journal of Obstetrics and Gynecology, 148*, 254–259.

Harry, G. J., & Howard, J. (1992). Phencyclidine: Experimental studies in animals and long-term developmental effects on humans. In T. B. Sonderegger, Ed., *Perinatal substance abuse: Research findings and clinical implications.* Baltimore: The Johns Hopkins University Press, pp. 254–278.

Strauss, A. A., Modanlow, H. D., & Bosu, S. K. (1981). Neonatal manifestations of maternal phencyclidine (PCP) abuse. *Pediatrics, 68*, 550.

Tabor, B. L., Smith-Wallace, T., & Yonekura, M. L. (1990). Perinatal outcome associated with PCP versus cocaine use. *American Journal of Drug and Alcohol Abuse, 16*(3,4), 337–348.

Wachsman, L., Schuetz, S., Chan, L. S., et al. (1989). What happens to babies exposed to phencyclidine (PCP) in utero? *American Journal of Drug and Alcohol Abuse, 15*(10), 31–39.

Pheniramine

AUTHOR: **NONE**   SIGNIFICANCE: **5**
POTENCY: **4**

No significant risk for teratogenic effects was noted among the offspring of 831 women who used pheniramine during the first trimester or of 2442 women who used it at various times during their pregnancies. (*See* Brompheniramine monograph.)

Greenberger, P., & Patterson, R. (1978). Safety of therapy for allergic symptoms during pregnancy. *Annals of Internal Medicine, 89,* 234–237.

Heinonen, O. P., Slone, D., & Shapiro, S. (1977). *Birth defects and drugs in pregnancy.* Littleton, MA: Publishing Sciences Group.

Phenmetrazine

FDA: **C**   SIGNIFICANCE: **5**   POTENCY: **4**

In studies involving more than 450 pregnant women, no increase in congenital malformations was associated with the use of phenmetrazine.

Heinonen, O. P., Slone, D., & Shapiro, S. (1977). *Birth defects and drugs in pregnancy.* Littleton, MA: Publishing Sciences Group.

McBride, W. G. (1963). The teratogenic action of drugs. *Medical Journal of Australia, 2,* 639–643.

Milkovich, L., & Van den Berg, B. J. (1977). Effects of antenatal exposure to anorectic drugs. *American Journal of Obstetrics and Gynecology, 129,* 637–642.

Phenobarbital

FDA: **D**   SIGNIFICANCE: **1**   POTENCY: **1**

One published review recommended phenobarbital for women who require an anticonvulsant during pregnancy since it had an apparently safe record, with only one report of teratogenesis. The American Academy of Pediatrics has stated, however, that there is no reason to change a woman's anticonvulsant to phenobarbital during pregnancy. Several reports have associated the use of phenobarbital during pregnancy with various congenital malformations, and the Collaborative Study Group in Japan confirmed that phenobarbital is a teratogen. Observed defects include anencephaly, cleft lip/palate, congenital dislocated hip, developmental delay, hydrocephalus, hypoplastic phalanges, hypospadias, microcephaly, myelomeningocele, ocular agenesis, pre- and postnatal growth retardation, psychomotor retardation, short nose with low-set nasal bridge, talipes equinovarus, wide fontanelle, and various cardiac defects. In addition, because phenobarbital acts indirectly as a folic acid antagonist, maternal use during pregnancy results in increased risk for neural-tube defects among offspring. The use of a folic acid supplement is generally recommended. A neonatal barbiturate-withdrawal syndrome also has been reported. (*See* Phenytoin and other anticonvulsant monographs and the Folic Acid monograph.)

Bleyer, W. A., & Skinner, A. L. (1976). Fetal neonatal hemorrhage after maternal anticonvulsant therapy. *Journal of the American Medical Association, 235,* 626–627.

Committee on Drugs. (1979). Anticonvulsants and pregnancy. *Pediatrics, 63,* 331–333.

Dansky, L. V., & Finnell, R. H. (1991). Parental epilepsy, anticonvulsant drugs, and reproductive outcome: Epidemiologic and experimental findings spanning three decades. 2: Human studies. *Reproductive Toxicology, 5*(4), 301–335.

Desmond, M. M., Schwanecke, R. P., Wilson, G. S., et al. (1972). Maternal barbiturate utilization and neonatal withdrawal symptomatology. *The Journal of Pediatrics, 80,* 190–197.

Douglas-Ringrose, C. A. (1972). The hazards of neurotropic drugs in the fertile years. *Canadian Medical Association Journal, 106,* 1058.

Golbus, M. S. (1980). Teratology for the obstetrician: Current status. *Obstetrics and Gynecology, 55,* 269–277.

Heinonen, O. P., Slone, D., & Shapiro, S. (1977). *Birth defects and drugs in pregnancy.* Littleton, MA: Publishing Sciences Group.

Hernandez-Diaz, S., Werler, M. M., Walker, A. M., et al. (2000). Folic acid antagonists during pregnancy and the risk of birth defects. *New England Journal of Medicine, 343*(22), 1608–1614.

Hill, R. M., Verniaud, W. M., Horning, M. G., et al. (1974). Infants exposed in utero to antiepileptic drugs. *American Journal of Diseases of Children, 127,* 645–653.

Jones, K. L., Johnson, K. A., & Chamber, C. C. (1992). Pregnancy outcome in women treated with phenobarbital monotherapy. *Teratology, 45,* 452–453.

Koch, S., Goepfert-Geyer, I., Haeuser, I., et al. (1985). Neonatal behaviour disturbances in infants of epileptic women treated during pregnancy. *Progress in Clinical and Biological Research, 163*B, 453-461.

Koch, S., Losche, G., Jager-Roman, E., et al. (1992). Major and minor birth malformations and antiepileptic drugs. *Neurology, 42*(Suppl 5), 83–88.

Lowe, C. R. (1973). Congenital malformations among infants born to epileptic women. *The Lancet, 1*, 328.

Millar, J. H., & Nevin, N. C. (1973). Congenital malformations and anticonvulsant drugs. *The Lancet, 1*, 9–10.

Nakane, Y., Okuma, T., Takahashi, R., et al. (1980). Multi-institutional study on the teratogenicity and fetal toxicity of antiepileptic drugs: A report of a collaborative study group in Japan. *Epilepsia, 21*, 663–680.

Robert, E., Lofkvist, E., Manuguiere, F., et al. (1986). Evaluation of drug therapy and teratogenic risk in a Rhone-Alpes District population of pregnant epileptic women. *European Neurology, 25*, 436–443.

Rothman, K. J., Fyler, D. C., Goldblatt, A., et al. (1979). Exogenous hormones and other drug exposures of children with congenital heart disease. *American Journal of Epidemiology, 109*, 433–439.

Seip, M. (1976). Growth retardation, dysmorphic facies and minor malformations following massive exposure to phenobarbitone in utero. *Acta Pediatrica Scandinavica, 65*, 617–621.

Shapiro, S., Hartz, S. C., Siskind, V., et al. (1976). Anticonvulsants and parental epilepsy in the development of birth defects. *The Lancet, 1*, 272–275.

Speidel, B., & Meadow, S. R. (1972). Maternal epilepsy and abnormalities of the fetus and newborn. *The Lancet, 2*, 839–843.

Thakker, J. C., Kothari, S. S., Deshmukh, C. T., et al. (1991). Hypoplasia of nails and phalanges: A teratogenic manifestation of phenobarbitone. *Indian Pediatrics, 28*(1), 73–75.

Phenothiazines

AUTHOR: ●   SIGNIFICANCE: 3   POTENCY: 2

A French study of 12,764 women, 315 of whom received phenothiazine during the first trimester, found an increased rate of congenital malformations among the offspring of those who received phenothiazine analogs with a three-carbon side chain (e.g., acetylpromazine, chlorpromazine, methotrimeprazine, trimeprazine). Observed defects included abdominal muscular aplasia, brachymesophalangy, clinodactyly, club hands and feet, hydrocephalus, hypospadias, microcephaly, and syndactyly. In utero exposure to phenothiazines with a two-carbon side chain (e.g., promethazine, propiomazine) or piperazine and piperidine analogs did not increase the rate of malformations.

Other evidence is negative, including data from the Collaborative Perinatal Project in which no increase in congenital malformations was observed among the offspring of 1309 women who were receiving phenothiazines during pregnancy. In another study of 543 exposed pregnancies, again no increase in malformations was found. Both of these studies, however, had a skewed population in which most women received prochlorperazine. (*See* Prochlorperazine and other phenothiazine drug monographs.)

Heinonen, O. P., Slone, D., & Shapiro, S. (1977). *Birth defects and drugs in pregnancy*. Littleton, MA: Publishing Sciences Group.

Milkovich, L., & Van den Berg, B. J. (1976). An evaluation of the teratogenicity of certain antinauseant drugs. *American Journal of Obstetrics and Gynecology, 125*, 244–248.

Rumeau-Rouquette, C., Goujard, J., & Huel, G. (1977). Possible teratogenic effect of phenothiazines in human beings. *Teratology, 15*, 57–64.

Phenylephrine

FDA: C   SIGNIFICANCE: 4–5   POTENCY: 3–4

In three studies of 1499 women who received phenylephrine during the first trimester and 4194 women who received phenylephrine at various times during their pregnancies, no statistically significant increase in the rate of congenital malformations was observed. Another much smaller study found an increased risk for congenital heart disease among neonates whose mothers had used phenylephrine during the first trimester. A major confounding factor is the general use of phenylephrine as part of a multidrug regimen for the treatment of the common cold.

Aselton, P., Jick, H., Milunsky, A., et al. (1985). First-trimester drug use and congenital disorders. *Obstetrics and Gynecology, 65*, 451–455.

Heinonen, O. P., Slone, D., & Shapiro, S. (1977). *Birth defects and drugs in pregnancy*. Littleton, MA: Publishing Sciences Group.

Jick, H., Holmes, L. B., Hunter, J. R., et al. (1981). First-trimester drug use and congenital disor-

ders. *Journal of the American Medical Association, 246,* 343–346.

Pratt, W. R. (1981). Allergic diseases in pregnancy and breast feeding. *Annals of Allergy, 47,* 355–360.

Werler, M. M., Mitchell, A. A., & Shapiro, S. (1992). First trimester maternal medication use in relation to gastroschisis. *Teratology, 45,* 361–367.

Phenylpropanolamine
FDA: **C**   SIGNIFICANCE: **3**   POTENCY: **2–3**

One study of 726 women who took phenylpropanolamine during the first trimester found an increased rate of eye and ear defects and hypospadias among their neonates. In this same study, no significant increase in congenital anomalies was found when phenylpropanolamine was taken later in the pregnancy (n = 2489). Other later studies involving 426 women who took phenylpropanolamine during the first trimester failed to support a significant risk for congenital anomalies among offspring. More data are needed.

Heinonen, O. P., Slone, D., & Shapiro, S. (1977). *Birth defects and drugs in pregnancy.* Littleton, MA: Publishing Sciences Group.

Phenytoin (Diphenylhydantoin)
FDA: **D**   SIGNIFICANCE: **1**   POTENCY: **1**

Some studies have shown as high as a 24% incidence of congenital malformations among neonates exposed to anticonvulsants in utero. The Collaborative Perinatal Project reported that 11% of phenytoin-exposed neonates have the fetal hydantoin syndrome and 31% have congenital malformations associated with the syndrome. Observed defects are usually midline and include abnormal facies, ambiguous genitalia, anencephaly, cardiac malformations, CNS malformations, cleft lip/palate, club hands and feet, developmental delay, diaphragmatic hernias, dislocated hips, ear anomalies, genitourinary anomalies, hydrocephalus, hydronephrosis, hypoplastic digits and nails, hypospadias, ileal atresia, inguinal hernias, intrauterine and postnatal growth retardation, meningomyelocele, metopic suture ridging, microcephaly, neonatal hemorrhage, patent ductus arteriosus, skeletal defects, and ventricular septal defects. Other defects are seen less commonly. Although some authors have associated these defects with phenytoin generally, a similar pattern has been seen among neonates whose mothers received other anticonvulsants during pregnancy. It has been suggested that many of the teratogenic effects noted are directly related to the reduction in folic acid concentrations caused by these folic acid antagonists. (*See* other anticonvulsant monographs; *see also* Folic Acid monograph.)

Interestingly, the data from a Japanese collaborative study failed to associate congenital malformations with phenytoin use during pregnancy. The results of the Japanese study may be secondary to genetic predisposition. There also may have been a dose–effect relationship for the incidence of defects. Unfortunately, the only study on this possible relationship was small. Multiple births among mothers receiving phenytoin in which not all neonates were affected have been reported.

A single controlled study examined the effect of phenytoin use on intellectual functioning among school-age children (n = 20) and found a significant decrease in IQ scores. More data are needed. Most disturbing are reports of an even greater increased rate of congenital anomalies among the offspring of epileptic women who require several anticonvulsants during pregnancy. (*See* Phenobarbital and Folic Acid monographs.)

Adams, J., Vorhees, C. V., & Middaugh, L. D. (1990). Developmental neurotoxicity of anticonvulsants: Human and animal evidence on phenytoin. *Neurotoxicology and Teratology, 12,* 203–214.

Allen, R. W., Ogden, B., Bentley, F. L., et al. (1980). Fetal hydantoin syndrome, neuroblastoma, and hemorrhagic disease in a neonate. *Journal of the American Medical Association, 244*(13), 1464–1465.

Anticonvulsants found to have teratogenic potential. (1978). *Journal of the American Medical Association, 245,* 36.

Bracken, M. (1986). Drug use in pregnancy and congenital heart disease in offspring. *New England Journal of Medicine, 314,* 1120.

Bustamaute, S. A., & Stumpff, L. C. (1978). Fetal hydantoin syndrome in triplets: A unique experiment of nature. *American Journal of Diseases of Children, 132,* 978.

Dieterich, E., Steueling, A., Lukas, A., et al. (1980). Congenital anomalies in children of epileptic mothers and fathers. *Neuropediatrics, 11,* 274–283.

D'Souza, S. W., Robertson, I. G., Donnai, D., et al. (1990). Fetal phenytoin exposure, hypoplastic nails, and jitteriness. *Archives of Disease in Childhood, 65*, 320–324.

Ehrenbard, L. T., & Chaganti, R. S. (1981). Cancer in the fetal hydantoin syndrome. *The Lancet, 2*, 97.

Friis, M. L. (1989). Facial clefts and congenital heart defects in children of parents with epilepsy: Genetic and environmental etiologic factors. *Acta Neurologica Scandinavica, 79*, 433–459.

Gaily, E. (1990). Distal phalangeal hypoplasia in children with prenatal phenytoin exposure: Results of a controlled anthropometric study. *American Journal of Medical Genetics, 35*, 574–578.

Hanson, J. W., Myrianthopoulas, M. D., Harvey, M. A., et al. (1976). Risks to the offspring of women treated with hydantoin anticonvulsants with emphasis on the fetal hydantoin syndrome. *The Journal of Pediatrics, 89*, 662.

Hanson, J. W., & Smith, D. W. (1975). The fetal hydantoin syndrome. *The Journal of Pediatrics, 87*, 285–290.

Heinonen, O. P., Slone, D., & Shapiro, S. (1977). *Birth defects and drugs in pregnancy*. Littleton, MA: Publishing Sciences Group.

Hernandez-Diaz, S., Werler, M. M., Walker, A. M., et al. (2000). Folic acid antagonists during pregnancy and the risk of birth defects. *New England Journal of Medicine, 343*(22), 1608–1614.

Hill, R. M., Verniuad, W. M., Horning, M. G., et al. (1974). Infant exposed in utero to antiepileptic drugs. *American Journal of Diseases of Children, 127*, 645–653.

Howe, A. M., Lipson, A. H., Sheffield, L. J., et al. (1995). Prenatal exposure to phenytoin, facial development, and a possible role for vitamin K. *American Journal of Medical Genetics, 58*(3), 238–244.

Ishizaki, T., Yokochi, K., Chiba, K., et al. (1981). Placental transfer of anticonvulsants (phenobarbital, phenytoin, valproic acid) and the elimination from neonates. *Pediatric Pharmacology, 1*, 291–303.

Jimenez, J. F., Seibert, R. W., Char, F., et al. (1981). Melanotic neuroectodermal tumor of infancy and fetal hydantoin syndrome. *The American Journal of Pediatric Hematology/Oncology, 3*, 9–15.

Kelly, T. E., Edwards, P., Rein, M., et al. (1984). Teratogenicity of anticonvulsant drugs. II: A prospective study. *American Journal of Medical Genetics, 19*(3), 435–443.

Kelly, T. E., Rein, M., & Edwards, P. (1984). Teratogenicity of anticonvulsant drugs. IV: The association of clefting and epilepsy. *American Journal of Medical Genetics, 19*(3), 451–458.

Kogutt, M. S., & Young, L. W. (1984). Fetal hydantoin syndrome. *American Journal of Diseases of Children, 138*, 405–406.

Koren, G., Demitrakoudis, D., Weksberg, S., et al. (1989). Neuroblastoma after prenatal exposure to phenytoin: Cause and effect? *Teratology, 40*, 157–162.

Kousseff, B. G., Stein, M., Gellis, S. S., et al. (1981). Picture of the month: Fetal hydantoin syndrome. *American Journal of Diseases of Children, 135*, 371–372.

Loughnan, P. M., Gold, H., & Vance, J. C. (1973). Phenytoin teratogenicity in man. *The Lancet, 1*, 70.

Lowe, C. R. (1973). Congenital malformations among infants born to epileptic mothers. *The Lancet, 1*, 70.

Majewski, F., Raff, W., Fischer, P., et al. (1980). Zur teratogenitat von Antikonvulsiva. *Deutsche Medizinische Wochenschrift, 20*, 719–723.

Michalodimitrakis, M., Parchas, S., & Coutselinis, A. (1981). Fetal hydantoin syndrome: Congenital malformation of the urinary tract—A case report. *Clinical Toxicology, 18*, 1095–1097.

Millar, J. H., & Nevin, N. C. (1973). Congenital malformations and anticonvulsant drugs. *The Lancet, 1*, 328.

Mirkin, B. L. (1971). Diphenylhydantoin: Placental transport, fetal localization, neonatal metabolism, and possible teratogenic effects. *The Journal of Pediatrics, 78*, 329–337.

Mirkin, B. L. (1971). Placental transfer and neonatal elimination of diphenylhydantoin. *American Journal of Obstetrics and Gynecology, 109*, 930–933.

Monson, R. R., Rosenberg, L., Hartz, S. C., et al. (1973). Diphenylhydantoin and selected congenital malformations. *New England Journal of Medicine, 289*, 1049–1052.

Montgomery, B. J. (1979). Large study of teratogenic potential of anticonvulsants. *Journal of the American Medical Association, 242*, 321.

Nakane, Y., Okuma, T., Takahashi, R., et al. (1980). Multi-institutional study on the teratogenicity and fetal toxicity of antiepileptic drugs: A report of a collaborative study group in Japan. *Epilepsia, 21*, 663–680.

Pashayan, H., Pruzansky, D., & Pruzansky, S. (1971). Are anticonvulsants teratogenic? *The Lancet, 2*, 702–703.

Smith, D. W. (1977). Distal limb hypoplasia in the fetal hydantoin syndrome. *Birth Defects, 13*, 355–359.

Speidel, B. D., & Meadow, S. R. (1972). Maternal epilepsy and abnormalities of the fetus and newborn. *The Lancet, 2*, 839–843.

Stankler, C., & Campbell, A. G. (1980). Neonatal acne vulgaris: A possible feature of the fetal hydantoin syndrome. *British Journal of Dermatology, 103*, 453–455.

Swalman, K. F. (1980). Antiepileptic drugs, the developing nervous system, and the pregnant woman with epilepsy. *Journal of the American Medical Association, 244*, 1477.

Takashi, I. (1979). Evaluation of anticonvulsants. *Folia Psychiatrica et Neurologica Japanica, 33*, 372.

Taylor, W. F., Myers, M., & Taylor, W. R. (1980). Extrarenal Wilm's Tumor in an infant exposed to intrauterine phenytoin. *The Lancet, 2*, 481–482.

Truog, W. E., Feusner, J. H., & Baker, D. (1980). Association of hemorrhagic disease and the syndrome of persistent fetal circulation with the fetal hydantoin syndrome. *The Journal of Pediatrics, 96*, 112–114.

Van Dyke, D. C., Berg, M. J., & Olson, C. H. (1991). Differences in phenytoin biotransformation and susceptibility to congenital malformations: A review. *DICP, The Annals of Pharmacotherapy, 25*, 987–992.

Van Lang, Q. N., Tassinari, M. S., Keith, D. A., et al. (1984). Effect of in utero exposure to anticonvulsants on craniofacial development and growth. *Journal of Craniofacial Genetics and Developmental Biology, 4*, 115–133.

Vanoverloop, D., Schnell, R. R., Harvey, E. A., et al. (1992). The effects of prenatal exposure to phenytoin and other anticonvulsants on intellectual function at 4 to 8 years of age. *Neurotoxicology and Teratology, 14*, 329–335.

Pindolol

FDA: **B**   SIGNIFICANCE: **4–5**   POTENCY: **4**

Several studies examined the efficacy of pindolol for hypertension during pregnancy; no related teratogenic effects were identified.

Dubois, D., Petitcolas, J., Temperville, B., et al. (1982). Treatment of hypertension in pregnancy with beta-adrenoceptor antagonists. *British Journal of Clinical Pharmacology, 13*, 375S–378S.

Ellenbogen, A., Jaschevatzky, O., Davidson, A., et al. (1986). Management of pregnancy-induced hypertension with pindolol—Comparative study with methyldopa. *International Journal of Gynaecology and Obstetrics, 24*, 3–7.

Montan, S., Ingemarsson, I., Marsal, K., et al. (1992). Randomised controlled trial of atenolol and pindolol in human pregnancy: Effects on fetal haemodynamics. *British Medical Journal, 304*, 946–949.

Sukerman-Voldman, E. (1982). Pindolol therapy in pregnant hypertensive patients. *British Journal of Clinical Pharmacology, 13*, 379S.

Tuimala, R., & Hartikainen-Sorri, A-L. (1988). Randomized comparison of atenolol and pindolol for treatment of hypertension in pregnancy. *Current Therapeutic Research, Clinical and Experimental, 44*, 579–584.

Piperazine

FDA: **B**   SIGNIFICANCE: **4**   POTENCY: **3–4**

Piperazine has been recommended for the treatment of roundworm and threadworm infestations during pregnancy. However, there are no published data supporting the safe use of piperazine for this indication. More data are needed.

Data sheet changes for piperazine in pregnancy. (1988). *The Pharmaceutical Journal*, March 19, 367.

Trussell, R. R., & Beeley, L. (1981). Infestations. *Clinical Obstetrics and Gynecology, 8*, 333–340.

Pivampicillin

AUTHOR: ●   SIGNIFICANCE: **4–5**   POTENCY: **3–4**

A large retrospective analysis compared the birth outcomes of 791 women who took pivampicillin during their pregnancies to the birth outcomes of 7472 women who did not take it. No increase in risk for congenital malformations, preterm delivery, or low birth weight was noted. More data are needed.

Larsen, H., Nielsen, G. L., Sorensen, H. T., et al. (2000). A follow-up study of birth outcome in users of pivampicillin during pregnancy. *Acta Obstetricia et Gynecologica Scandinavica, 79*, 379–383.

Plague Vaccine

FDA: **C**   SIGNIFICANCE: see monograph   POTENCY: see monograph

Maternal infection with *Yersinia pestis* during pregnancy may result in spontaneous abortion. Plague vaccine is recommended for women who are traveling to areas of high risk of contact with the disease and for women who are working in laboratories where they may be exposed to the organism. More data are needed.

Hart, R. L. (1981). Immunizations. *Clinical Obstetrics and Gynecology, 8*, 421–430.

Mann, J. M., & Moskowitz, R. (1977). Plague and pregnancy. *Journal of the American Medical Association, 237*, 1854–1855.

Poliovirus Vaccine, Inactivated (Salk Vaccine)

FDA: **C**   SIGNIFICANCE: **5**   POTENCY: **4**

When a need is indicated, inactivated (killed) polio vaccine (IPV) may be safely administered to women during pregnancy. No teratogenic effects have been reported.

Hart, R. J. (1981). Immunizations. *Clinical Obstetrics and Gynecology, 8*, 421–430.

Heinonen, O. P., Shapiro, S., Monson, R., et al. (1973). Immunization during pregnancy against poliomyelitis and influenza in relation to childhood malignancy. *International Journal of Epidemiology, 2*, 229.

Heinonen, O. P., Slone, D., & Shapiro, S. (1977). *Birth defects and drugs in pregnancy.* Littleton, MA: Publishing Sciences Group.

Poliovirus Vaccine, Live Oral (Sabin Vaccine)

FDA: C   SIGNIFICANCE: 5   POTENCY: 4

Naturally occurring polio virus infections among pregnant women do not seem to have a harmful effect on the fetus. The use of the live oral polio vaccine (OPV) has been studied widely in pregnancy and has not been shown to cause spontaneous abortions or congenital malformations among offspring.

Harjulehto, T., Aro, T., Hovi, T., et al. (1989). Congenital malformations and oral poliovirus vaccination during pregnancy. *The Lancet, 1*, 771–772.

Heinonen, O. P., Slone, D., & Shapiro, S. (1977). *Birth defects and drugs in pregnancy.* Littleton, MA: Publishing Sciences Group.

Ornoy, A., Arnon, J., Feingold, M., et al. (1990). Spontaneous abortions following oral poliovirus vaccination in first trimester. *The Lancet, 335*, 800.

Siegel, M., & Greenberg, M. (1956). Poliomyelitis in pregnancy: Effect on fetus and newborn infants. *The Journal of Pediatrics, 49*, 280–288.

Special Advisory Committee on Oral Polio Vaccine. (1964). Oral poliomyelitis vaccines. *Journal of the American Medical Association, 190*, 49–51.

Prednisolone

FDA: C   SIGNIFICANCE: 3–4
POTENCY: 3 (dose dependent)

No increased risk for congenital anomalies among offspring is found in the literature on prednisolone use during pregnancy. However, dose-related fetal growth retardation has been reported. (*See* Prednisone and Corticosteroids monographs.)

Heinonen, O. P., Slone, D., & Shapiro, S. (1977). *Birth defects and drugs in pregnancy.* Littleton, MA: Publishing Sciences Group.

Nielsen, O. H., Andreasson, B., Bondesen, S., et al. (1983). Pregnancy in ulcerative colitis. *Scandinavian Journal of Gastroenterology, 18*(6), 735–742.

Nielsen, O. H., Andreasson, B., Bondesen, S., et al. (1984). Pregnancy in Crohn's disease. *Scandinavian Journal of Gastroenterology, 19*(6), 724–732.

O'Donnell, D., Sevitz, H., Seggie, J. L., et al. (1985). Pregnancy after renal transplantation. *Australian and New Zealand Journal of Medicine, 15*, 320–325.

Pirson, Y., van Lierde, M., Ghysen, J., et al. (1985). Retardation of fetal growth in patients receiving immunosuppressive therapy. *New England Journal of Medicine, 313*, 328.

Reinisch, J. M., Simon, N. G., Karow, W. G., et al. (1978). Prenatal exposure to prednisone in humans and animals retards intrauterine growth. *Science, 202*, 436–438.

Schatz, M., Patterson, R., Zeitz, S., et al. (1975). Corticosteroid therapy for the pregnant asthmatic patient. *Journal of the American Medical Association, 233*, 804–807.

Warrell, D. W., & Taylor, R. (1968). Outcome for the foetus of mothers receiving prednisone during pregnancy. *The Lancet, 1*, 117–118.

Prednisone

FDA: C   SIGNIFICANCE: 3–4
POTENCY: 3 (dose dependent)

No increased risk for congenital anomalies is found in the literature examining prednisone use during pregnancy. Dose-related fetal growth retardation has been reported, however. (*See* Prednisolone and Corticosteroids monographs.)

Heinonen, O. P., Slone, D., & Shapiro, S. (1977). *Birth defects and drugs in pregnancy.* Littleton, MA: Publishing Sciences Group.

Insley, B. M., & Imoto, R. M. (1986). Prednisone use in pregnancy. *Drug Intelligence and Clinical Pharmacy, 20*, 673–674.

Nielsen, O. H., Andreasson, B., Bondesen, S., et al. (1983). Pregnancy in ulcerative colitis. *Scandinavian Journal of Gastroenterology, 18*(6), 735–742.

Nielsen, O. H., Andreasson, B., Bondesen, S., et al. (1984). Pregnancy in Crohn's disease. *Scandinavian Journal of Gastroenterology, 19*(6), 724–732.

O'Donnell, D., Sevitz, H., Seggie, J. L., et al. (1985). Pregnancy after renal transplantation. *Australian and New Zealand Journal of Medicine, 15*, 320–325.

Schatz, M., Patterson, R., Zeitz, S., et al. (1975). Corticosteroid therapy for the pregnant asthmatic patient. *Journal of the American Medical Association, 233*, 804–807.

Primidone

FDA: D   SIGNIFICANCE: 1   POTENCY: 1

The use of primidone during pregnancy has been associated with various congenital malformations among offspring in a pattern similar to malformations associated with other anticonvulsants. Reported teratogenic effects include atrial septal defects, broad alveolar ridge, broad nasal bridge, cleft lip/palate, congenital hip dislocation, digital thumbs, fetal head growth retardation, hypertelorism, hypoplastic mandible, hypoplastic phalanges and nails, large fontanelle, low hairline, microcephaly, myelomeningocele, patent ductus arteriosus, pilonidal sinus, polydactyly, postnatal growth failure, tetralogy of Fallot, torticollis, and ventricular septal defects. As a folic acid antagonist, primidone may increase the risk for neural-tube defects. Use of a folic acid supplement may be indicated (see Folic Acid monograph). Primidone is metabolized significantly to phenobarbital. Fetotoxic effects are generally associated with the expected action of phenobarbital (e.g., lethargy, neonatal sedation, poor suck). (See Phenobarbital monograph.)

Fedrick, J. (1973). Epilepsy and pregnancy: A report from the Oxford Record Linkage Study. *British Medical Journal, 2*, 442–448.

Hernandez-Diaz, S., Werler, M. M., Walker, A. M., et al. (2000). Folic acid antagonists during pregnancy and the risk of birth defects. *New England Journal of Medicine, 343*(22), 1608–1614.

Hill, R. M., Verniaud, W. M., Horning, M. G., et al. (1974). Infants exposed in utero to antiepileptic drugs. *American Journal of Diseases of Children, 127*, 645–653.

Hoyme, H. E. (1990). Teratogenically induced fetal anomalies. *Clinics in Perinatology, 17*(3), 547–567.

Krauss, C. M., Holmes, L. B., Van Lang, Q., et al. (1984). Four siblings with similar malformations after exposure to phenytoin and primidone. *The Journal of Pediatrics, 105*, 750–755.

Majewski, F., & Steger, M. (1984). Fetal head growth retardation associated with maternal phenobarbitone/primidone and/or phenytoin therapy. *European Journal of Obstetrics, Gynecology, and Reproductive Biology, 141*, 188–189.

Myhre, S. A., & Williams, R. (1981). Teratogenic effects associated with maternal primidone therapy. *The Journal of Pediatrics, 99*, 160–162.

Nakane, Y., Okuma, T., Takahashi, R., et al. (1980). Multi-institutional study on the teratogenicity and fetal toxicity of antiepileptic drugs: A report of a collaborative study group in Japan. *Epilepsia, 21*, 663–680.

Rating, D., Nau, H., Jager-Roman, E., et al. (1982). Teratogenic and pharmacokinetic studies of primidone during pregnancy and in the offspring of epileptic women. *Acta Paediatrica Scandinavica, 71*, 301–317.

Rudd, N. L., & Freedom, R. M. (1979). A possible primidone embryopathy. [Letter]. *The Journal of Pediatrics, 94*, 835–837.

Thomas, D., & Buchanan, N. (1981). Teratogenic effects of anticonvulsants. [Letter]. *The Journal of Pediatrics, 99*, 163.

Procainamide

FDA: **C**   SIGNIFICANCE: **5**   POTENCY: **4**

No teratogenic effects have been associated with procainamide use during pregnancy. Procainamide has been used during the third trimester to treat fetal supraventricular tachycardia after digoxin and propranolol failed to restore normal rhythm. Some authors feel it is the preferred antidysrhythmic for use during pregnancy.

Barrillon, A., Grand, A., & Gerbaux, A. (1974). Treatment of the heart during pregnancy. *Annales de Medecine Interne (Paris), 125*, 437–445.

Dumesic, D. A., Silverman, N. H., Tobias, S., et al. (1982). Transplacental cardioversion of fetal supraventricular tachycardia with procainamide. *New England Journal of Medicine, 307*, 1128–1131.

Given, B. D., Phillippe, M., Sanders, S. P., et al. (1984). Procainamide cardioversion of fetal supraventricular tachyarrhythmia. *American Journal of Cardiology, 53*, 1460–1461.

Merx, W., Effert, S., & Heinrich, K. (1974). Heart disease in pregnancy, intra and postpartum. *Zeitschrift fur Geburtshilfe und Perinatologie (Stuttgart), 178*, 317–336.

Procaine

FDA: **C**   SIGNIFICANCE: **5**   POTENCY: **4**

A study of women who received procaine either during the first trimester (n = 1340) or at various times during their pregnancies (n = 3395) found no significant risk for teratogenic effects. In addition, when used for analgesia during labor, no fetotoxic effects were identified.

Heinonen, O. P., Slone, D., & Shapiro, S. (1977). *Birth defects and drugs in pregnancy*. Littleton, MA: Publishing Sciences Group.

Mellin, G. W. (1964). Drugs in the first trimester of pregnancy and the fetal life of Homo sapiens. *American Journal of Obstetrics and Gynecology, 90*, 1169–1180.

Usubiaga, J. E., Laluppa, M., Moya, F., et al. (1968). Passage of procaine hydrochloride and para-aminobenzoic acid across the human placenta.

American Journal of Obstetrics and Gynecology, 100, 918–923.

Procarbazine

FDA: **D**   SIGNIFICANCE: **3**   POTENCY: **2–3**

Of four infants exposed to procarbazine in utero, one was born with small pelvic kidneys and the other three were normal. More data are needed, particularly data addressing procarbazine use during the first trimester.

Dow, E. G. (1970). Procarbazine in pregnancy. [Letter]. *The Lancet, 2,* 984.
Mennuti, M. T., Shephard, T. H., & Mellman, W. J. (1975). Fetal renal malformation following treatment of Hodgkin's disease during pregnancy. *Obstetrics and Gynecology, 46,* 194–196.
Wells, J. H., Marshall, J. R., & Carbone, P. P. (1968). Procarbazine therapy for Hodgkin's disease in early pregnancy. *Journal of the American Medical Association, 205,* 935–937.

Prochlorperazine

FDA: **C**   SIGNIFICANCE: **5**   POTENCY: **4**

A few scattered published case reports associate prochlorperazine use during pregnancy with limb defects among offspring. In numerous studies involving ~3500 pregnant women who received prochlorperazine, however, no increase in the congenital malformation rate was observed. (*See* Phenothiazines monograph.)

Heinonen, O. P., Slone, D., & Shapiro, S. (1977). *Birth defects and drugs in pregnancy.* Littleton, MA: Publishing Sciences Group.
Jick, H., Holmes, L. B., Hunter, J. R., et al. (1981). First-trimester drug use and congenital disorders. *Journal of the American Medical Association, 246,* 343–346.
Kappelman, M. D. (1962). Prochlorperazine in labor and delivery. *Obstetrics and Gynecology, 19,* 118–120.
Kullander, S., & Kallen, B. (1976). A prospective study of drugs and pregnancy: II. Anti-emetic drugs. *Acta Obstetricia et Gynecologica Scandinavica, 55,* 105–111.
Mellin, G. W. (1975). A report of prochlorperazine utilization during pregnancy from fetal life study data bank. [Abstract]. *Teratology, 11,* 28a.
Milkovich, L., & Van den Berg, B. J. (1976). An evaluation of the teratogenicity of certain antinauseant drugs. *American Journal of Obstetrics and Gynecology, 125,* 244–248.
Rumeau-Rouquette, C., Goujard, J., & Huel, G. (1977). Possible teratogenic effect of phenothiazines in human beings. *Teratology, 15,* 57–64.

Progesterone

FDA: **X**   SIGNIFICANCE: **3–4**   POTENCY: **3–4**

Scattered case reports associate progesterone use during pregnancy with masculinization of the female fetus or hypospadias occurring in the male fetus. However, a German study of 648 pregnant women reported no increase in congenital malformations among offspring exposed to progesterone in utero. It is unlikely that progesterone is a teratogen.

Aarskoz, D. (1979). Maternal progestins as a possible cause of hypospadias. *New England Journal of Medicine, 300,* 75–78.
Hales, A. B., & Nolan, R. B. (1957). Masculinization of the female fetus, possibly related to administration of progesterone during pregnancy. *Mayo Clinic Proceedings, 32,* 200–203.
Michaelis, J., Michaelis, H., Gluck, E., et al. (1983). Prospective study of suspected associations between certain drugs administered during early pregnancy and congenital malformations. *Teratology, 27,* 57–64.
Tuchmann-Duplessis, H. (1983). The teratogenic risk. *American Journal of Industrial Medicine, 4,* 245–258.

Progestogens

FDA: **X**   SIGNIFICANCE: **1**   POTENCY: **2–3**

Use of progestogens during pregnancy has been associated with a modest degree of masculinization of the female fetus. Other reports associate progestogen use with cardiovascular anomalies, mainly affecting the great vessels. A syndrome involving vertebral, anal, cardiac, tracheal, esophageal, renal, and limb defects (VACTERL) also has been reported. In addition, one report of a positive correlation between prenatal progestin exposure and aggressive behavior was noted. Thus, it appears that progestogens are teratogenic and, perhaps, fetotoxic. The incidence, however, is not common. (*See* Oral Contraceptives monograph.)

Grumbach, M. M., Ducharme, J. R., & Moloshok, R. E. (1959). On the fetal masculinizing action of certain oral progestins. *Journal of Clinical Endocrinology and Metabolism, 19,* 1369–1380.
Harlap, S., Prywes, R., & Davies, A. M. (1975). Birth defects and oestrogens and progesterones in pregnancy. *The Lancet, 1,* 682.
Janerich, D. T., Dugan, J. M., Standfast, S. J., et al. (1977). Congenital heart disease and prenatal

exposure to exogenous sex hormones. *British Medical Journal, 1,* 1058.
Levy, E. P., Cohen, A., & Fraser, F. C. (1973). Hormone treatment during pregnancy and congenital heart defects. *The Lancet, 1,* 611.
Mau, G. (1981). Progestins during pregnancy and hypospadias. *Teratology, 24,* 285–287.
Nora, A. H., & Nora, J. J. (1975). A syndrome of multiple congenital anomalies associated with teratogenic exposure. *Archives of Environmental Health, 30,* 17–21.
Reinisch, J. M. (1981). Prenatal exposure to synthetic progestins increases potential for aggression in humans. *Science, 211,* 1171–1173.
Wilkins, L. (1960). Masculinization of female fetus due to use of orally given progestogens. *Journal of the American Medical Association, 172,* 1028–1030.

Promazine

FDA: **C**   SIGNIFICANCE: **4**   POTENCY: **3**

In one study, use of promazine during pregnancy was associated with congenital hip dislocation. The authors, however, felt that the association was coincidental. In another study, two-carbon side chain phenothiazines were not associated with an increased incidence of congenital malformations. Promazine belongs to this group of phenothiazine analogs but was not part of the study. (*See* Phenothiazines monograph.)

Kullander, S., & Kallen, B. (1976). A prospective study of drugs and pregnancy. II. Anti-emetic drugs. *Acta Obstetricia and Gynecologica Scandinavica, 55,* 105–111.
Rumeau-Rouquette, C., Goujard, J., & Huel, G. (1977). Possible teratogenic effect of phenothiazines in human beings. *Teratology, 15,* 57–64.

Promethazine

FDA: **C**   SIGNIFICANCE: **3**   POTENCY: **3**

Promethazine use during pregnancy has been associated with teratogenic effects. Negative reports also have been published. One study associates promethazine with brachymesophalangy, cleft palate, clindactyly, endocardial fibroelastosis, and microcephaly among offspring. Three other case-controlled studies found no teratogenic effects. More data are needed. (*See* Phenothiazines monograph.)

Aselton, P., Jick, H., Milunsky, A., et al. (1985). First-trimester drug use and congenital disorders. *Obstetrics and Gynecology, 65,* 451–455.
Farkas, V. G., & Farkas, G. (1971). Teratogenic action of hyperemesis in pregnancy and of medication used to treat it. *Zentralblatt Fur Gynakologie, 10,* 325–330.
General Practitioner Research Group. (1963). Drugs in pregnancy survey. *Practitioner, 191,* 775.
Heinonen, O. P., Slone, D., & Shapiro, S. (1977). *Birth defects and drugs in pregnancy.* Littleton, MA: Publishing Sciences Group.
Rumeau-Rouquette, C., Goujard, J., & Huel, G. (1977). Possible teratogenic effect of phenothiazines in human beings. *Teratology, 15,* 57–64.

Propoxyphene

FDA: **C**   SIGNIFICANCE: **3–4** (malformations)   **1** (neonatal symptoms)
POTENCY: **3** (malformations)   **2** (neonatal symptoms)

Propoxyphene use during pregnancy has been associated with such teratogenic effects among offspring as beaked nose, bifid uvula, congenital heart disease, congenital hip dislocation, defective abdominal wall, micrognathia, omphalocele, and widely spaced sutures. However, two cohort studies involving 3700 pregnant women who received propoxyphene at various times during their pregnancies failed to find a significant risk for teratogenic effects. Fetotoxic effects associated with propoxyphene use during pregnancy include the neonatal propoxyphene-withdrawal syndrome characterized by irritability, jitteriness, seizures, and tremors.

Ananth, J. (1976). Side effects on fetus and infant of psychotropic drug use during pregnancy. *International Pharmacopsychiatry, 11,* 246–260.
Boelter, W. (1980). Proposed fetal propoxyphene (Darvon®) syndrome. *Clinical Research, 28,* 115A.
Douglas-Ringrose, C. A. (1972). The hazards of neurotropic drugs in the fertile years. *Canadian Medical Association Journal, 106,* 1058.
Ente, G., & Mehra, M. C. (1978). Neonatal withdrawal from propoxyphene hydrochloride. *New York State Journal of Medicine, 78,* 2084–2085.
Golden, N. L., King, K. C., & Sokol, R. J. (1982). Propoxyphene and acetaminophen. Possible effects on the fetus. *Clinical Pediatrics, 21,* 752–754.
Klein, R. B., Blatman, S., & Little, G. A. (1975). Probable neonatal propoxyphene withdrawal: A case report. *Pediatrics, 55,* 882–884.
Quillian, W. W., & Dunn, C. A. (1976). Neonatal drug withdrawal from propoxyphene. *Journal of the American Medical Association, 235,* 2128.

Tyson, H. K. (1974). Neonatal withdrawal symptoms associated with maternal use of propoxyphene hydrochloride (Darvon). *The Journal of Pediatrics, 85,* 684–685.

Williams, D. A., Weiss, T., Wade, E., et al. (1983). Prune perineum syndrome: Report of a second case. *Teratology, 28,* 145–148.

Propranolol

FDA: **C**   SIGNIFICANCE: **1**   POTENCY: **2** (growth retardation)   **1** (neonatal effects)

Use of propranolol during pregnancy, particularly during the third trimester, has been associated with intrauterine growth retardation among neonates. Although one study reported more than a 90% incidence, most studies have placed the incidence at about 4%. In a small study, pregnant women were given propranolol 1 mg intravenously prior to caesarean section. All infants had a 5–6-minute delay in the onset of spontaneous respirations. Fetotoxic effects also have been associated with propranolol use during pregnancy; these effects include bradycardia, which usually is of no concern for the nonstressed fetus. For a delivery associated with fetal distress, however, propranolol prior to caesarean section may be deleterious to the neonate's adaptation to extrauterine life. Another fetotoxic effect is hypoglycemia. Propranolol alters pharmacokinetics in the neonate. The serum levels of propranolol double within the first 4 hours, secondary to redistribution. The exact role that this increase in propranolol serum levels, or its rapidity of change, has on the development of neonatal propranolol toxicity has not been thoroughly evaluated. More data are needed.

Bott-Kanner, G., Schwertzer, A., Reisner, S. H., et al. (1980). Propranolol and hydralazine in the management of essential hypertension in pregnancy. *British Journal of Obstetrics and Gynecology, 87,* 110–114.

Buechler, A. A., & Palmer, S. K. (1982). Intrapartum fetal death associated with propranolol: case report and review of physiology. *Wisconsin Medical Journal, 81,* 23–25.

Cottrill, C. M., McAllister, R. G., Gettes, L., et al. (1977). Propranolol therapy during pregnancy, labor, and delivery: Evidence for transplacental drug transfer and impaired neonatal drug disposition. *The Journal of Pediatrics, 91,* 812.

Ellahon, H. E., Silverberg, D. S., Reisin, E., et al. (1978). Propranolol for the treatment of hypertension in pregnancy. *British Journal of Obstetrics and Gynecology, 85,* 431–436.

Fiddler, G. I. (1974). Propranolol and pregnancy. *The Lancet, 2,* 722.

Gallery, E. D., Saunders, D. M., Hunyor, S. N., et al. (1979). Randomized comparison of methyldopa and oxprenolol for treatment of hypertension in pregnancy. *British Medical Journal, 1,* 1591–1594.

Habib, A., & McCarthy, V. S. (1977). Effects on the neonate of propranolol administered during pregnancy. *The Journal of Pediatrics, 91,* 808–811.

Joelsson, I., & Barton, M. D. (1969). The effect of blockade of the beta receptors on the sympathetic nervous system of the fetus. *Acta Obstetricia and Gynecologica Scandinavica, 48*(Suppl 3), 75–79.

Liberman, B. A., Stirrat, G. M., Cohen, S. L., et al. (1978). The possible adverse effect of propranolol on the fetus in pregnancies complicated by severe hypertension. *British Journal of Obstetrics and Gynaecology, 85,* 678–683.

Oakley, G. D., McGarry, K., Limb, D. G., et al. (1979). Management of pregnancy in patients with hypertrophic cardiomyopathy. *British Medical Journal, 1,* 1749–1750.

Pruyn, S. C., Phelan, J. P., & Buchanan, G. C. (1979). Long-term propranolol therapy in pregnancy: Maternal and fetal outcome. *American Journal of Obstetrics and Gynecology, 135,* 485–489.

Redmond, G. P. (1982). Propranolol and fetal growth retardation. *Seminars in Perinatology, 6*(2), 142–147.

Reed, R. L., Cheney, C. B., Fearon, R. B., et al. (1974). Propranolol therapy throughout pregnancy: A case report. *Anesthesia and Analgesia, 53,* 214.

Tcherdakoff, P. H., Colliard, M., Berrard, E., et al. (1978). Propranolol in hypertension during pregnancy. *British Medical Journal, 2,* 670.

Turnstall, M. B. (1969). The effect of propranolol on the onset of breathing at birth. [Abstract]. *British Journal of Anaesthesiology, 41,* 792.

Propylthiouracil

FDA: **D**   SIGNIFICANCE: **1**
POTENCY: **1** (goiter)

Although propylthiouracil crosses the placenta and has been associated with fetal hypothyroidism and, consequently, goiter, it is the drug of choice for hyperthyroidism (Graves' disease) in pregnant women. Approximately 10% of neonates born to women who receive propylthiouracil during pregnancy will have a goiter. However, these goiters are generally small and usually do not interfere with the neonate's respiratory function. Use of antithyroids during pregnancy requires caution because of their association with hypothyroidism and resulting cretinism. In this clinical situation, fetal thyroid function should be evaluated by monitoring fetal heart rate. It also is recommended that all neonates born to women who have Graves' disease managed with propylthiouracil during pregnancy be evaluated at birth in regard to thyroid function. (*See* Methimazole monograph.)

Aaron, H. H., Schneierson, S. J., & Siegel, E. (1955). Goiter in new born infant due to mother's ingestion of propylthiouracil. *Journal of the American Medical Association, 50*, 348–350.

Becks, G. P., & Burrow, G. N. (1991). Thyroid disease and pregnancy. *Medical Clinics of North America, 75*(1), 121–150.

Black, J. A. (1963). Neonatal goitre and mental deficiency. The role of iodides taken during pregnancy. *Archives of Disease in Childhood, 38*, 526–529.

Burrow, G. N. (1965). Neonatal goiter after maternal propylthiouracil therapy. *Journal of Clinical Endocrinology and Metabolism, 25*, 403–408.

Burrow, G. N. (1985). The management of thyrotoxicosis in pregnancy. *New England Journal of Medicine, 313*(9), 562–565.

Burrow, G. N., Bartsocas, C., Klatskin, E. H., et al. (1968). Children exposed in utero to propylthiouracil. Subsequent intellectual and physical development. *American Journal of Diseases of Children, 116*, 161–165.

Cheron, R. G., Kaplan, M. M., Larsen, P. R., et al. (1981). Neonatal thyroid function after propylthiouracil therapy for maternal Graves' disease. *New England Journal of Medicine, 304*(9), 525–528.

Davis, L. E., Lucas, M. J., Hankins, G. D. V., et al. (1989). Thyrotoxicosis complicating pregnancy. *American Journal of Obstetrics and Gynecology, 160*(1), 63–70.

Hayek, A., & Brooks, M. (1975). Neonatal hyperthyroidism following intrauterine hypothyroidism. *The Journal of Pediatrics, 87*(3), 446–448.

Hepner, W. R. (1952). Thiourea derivatives and the fetus, a review and report of a case. *American Journal of Obstetrics and Gynecology, 63*, 869–873.

Mujtaba, Q., & Burrow, G. N. (1975). Treatment of hyperthyroidism in pregnancy with propylthiouracil and methimazole. *Obstetrics and Gynecology, 46*, 282–286.

Serup, J., & Petersen, S. (1977). Hyperthyroidism during pregnancy treated with propylthiouracil. The significance of maternal and foetal parameters. *Acta Obstetricia and Gynecologica Scandinavica, 56*, 463–466.

Solomon, D. H. (1981). Pregnancy and PTU. *New England Journal of Medicine, 304*(9), 538–539.

Pseudoephedrine

FDA: B   SIGNIFICANCE: 4–5   POTENCY: 3–4

No increase in the rate of teratogenesis was observed in three studies in which women received pseudoephedrine during the first trimester (n = 941) or at various times during their pregnancies (n = 194). Because of its favorable toxicity profile, pseudoephedrine has been recommended as the preferred decongestant to use during pregnancy.

Aselton, P., Jick, H., Milunsky, A., et al. (1985). First-trimester drug use and congenital disorders. *Obstetrics and Gynecology, 65*, 451–455.

Heinonen, O. P., Slone, D., & Shapiro, S. (1977). *Birth defects and drugs in pregnancy*. Littleton, MA: Publishing Sciences Group.

Jick, H., Holmes, L. B., Hunter, J. R., et al. (1981). First-trimester drug use and congenital disorders. *Journal of the American Medical Association, 246*, 343–346.

Smith, C. V., Rayburn, W. F., Anderson, J. C., et al. (1990). Effect of a single dose of oral pseudoephedrine on uterine and fetal Doppler blood flow. *Obstetrics and Gynecology, 76*, 803–806.

Pyrantel Pamoate

FDA: C   SIGNIFICANCE: 4   POTENCY: 3–4

Reports of human teratogenic effects associated with pyrantel pamoate are lacking. This drug is poorly absorbed from the GI tract and has been recommended as the drug of choice for the treatment of ascariasis in pregnant women.

Butler, C. D. (1990). Treatment of intestinal parasites during pregnancy. *Facts and Comparisons Drug Newsletter, 9*, 41–43.

Pyrimethamine

FDA: C   SIGNIFICANCE: 3–4   POTENCY: 3

A European study of 64 women who received pyrimethamine during the first trimester did not find an increased risk for teratogenic effects. Pyrimethamine is recommended for chloroquine-resistant malaria. Because pyrimethamine is a folic acid antagonist, women who are malnourished or who have a folic acid deficiency should receive a folic acid supplement during the first trimester. (*See* Folic Acid monograph.) More data are needed, particularly data addressing pyrimethamine use during the first trimester.

Hengst, V. P. (1972). Investigations of the teratogenicity of daraprim (pyrimethamine) in humans. *Zentralblatt Fur Gynakologie, 94*, 551–555.
Lambie, D. G., & Johnson, R. H. (1985). Drugs and folate metabolism. *Drugs, 30*(2), 145–155.
Main, E. K., Main, D. M., & Krogstod, D. (1983). Treatment of chloroquine-resistant malaria during pregnancy. *Journal of the American Medical Association, 249*, 3207–3209.
Trussell, R. R., & Beeley, L. (1981). Infestations. *Clinical Obstetrics and Gynecology, 8*, 333–340.

Quinidine

FDA: **C**   SIGNIFICANCE: **4**   POTENCY: **3–4**

Quinidine has been given to pregnant women for more than 60 years, and it has been used successfully to treat fetal supraventricular tachycardia during the second and third trimesters. No teratogenic effects have been reported, although large doses may damage the eighth cranial nerve. Rarely, quinidine in usual recommended doses may induce premature labor. Toxic maternal doses have been associated with spontaneous abortions.

Conradsson, T. B., & Werko, L. (1974). Management of heart disease in pregnancy. *Progress in Cardiovascular Diseases, 16*, 407–419.
Guntheroth, W. G., Cyr, D. R., Mack, L. A., et al. (1985). Hydrops from reciprocating atrioventricular tachycardia in a 27-week fetus requiring quinidine for conversion. *Obstetrics and Gynecology, 66*(Suppl 3), 29S–33S.
Hill, L. M., & Malkasian, G. D. (1979). The use of quinidine sulfate throughout pregnancy. *Obstetrics and Gynecology, 54*, 366–368.
Lesch, M., Lewis, E., & Humphries, J. O. (1967). Paroxysmal ventricular tachycardia in the absence of organic heart disease: Report of a case and review of the literature. *Annals of Internal Medicine, 66*, 950–960.
McMillan, T. M., & Bellet, S. (1931). Ventricular paroxysmal tachycardia: Report of a case in a pregnant girl of sixteen years with an apparently normal heart. *American Heart Journal, 7*, 70–78.
Mendelson, C. L. (1956). Disorders of the heartbeat during pregnancy. *American Journal of Obstetrics and Gynecology, 72*, 1268–1301.
Merx, W. (1972). Heryrhythmuddtorungen in der schwangerschaft. *Deutsche Medizinische Wochenschrift, 97*, 1987–1988.
Meyer, J., Lackner, J. E., & Schochet, S. S. (1930). Paroxysmal tachycardia in pregnancy. *Journal of the American Medical Association, 94*, 1901–1904.

Spinnato, J. A., Shaver, D. C., Flinn, G. S., et al. (1984). Fetal supraventricular tachycardia: In utero therapy with digoxin and quinidine. *Obstetrics and Gynecology, 64*, 730–735.

Quinine

FDA: **X**   SIGNIFICANCE: **1**   POTENCY: **1–2**

Quinine is an abortifacient at high doses. Teratogenic effects have been associated with the use of quinine during pregnancy and include absence of external urethra, congenital glaucoma, corneal opacities, fetal death, flat nose, imperforate anus, intestinal atresia, low-set ears, mental retardation, optic nerve hypoplasia, ototoxicity, pseudohermaphroditism, and urogenital sinus. In addition, quinine near term has been associated with fetotoxic effects, including hemolytic anemia in glucose-6-phosphate dehydrogenase-deficient neonates and thrombocytopenia purpura. These fetotoxic effects resemble adverse drug reactions observed among children and adults who are taking quinine.

Barr, B. (1982). Teratogenic hearing loss. *Audiology, 21*, 111–127.
Dannenberg, A. L., Dorfman, S. F., & Johnson, J. (1983). Use of quinine for self-induced abortion. *Southern Medical Journal, 76*, 846–849.
Forbes, S. B. (1940). The etiology of nerve deafness with particular reference to quinine. *Southern Medical Journal, 33*, 613–621.
Glass, L., Rajegowda, B. K., Bowen, E., et al. (1973). Exposure to quinine and jaundice in a glucose-6-phosphate dehydrogenase-deficient newborn infant. *The Journal of Pediatrics, 82*, 734–735.
Mauer, A. M., DeVaux, W., & Lahey, M. E., (1957). Neonatal and maternal thrombocytopenic purpura due to quinine. *Pediatrics, 19*, 84–87.
McKinna, A. J. (1966). Quinine induced hypoplasia of the optic nerve. *Canadian Journal of Ophthalmology, 1*, 261–266.
Nishimura, H., & Tanimura, T. (1976). *Clinical aspects of the teratogenicity of drugs*. New York: Excerpta Medica, American Elsevier Publishing, pp. 140–143.
Reed, H., Briggs, J. N., & Martin, J. K. (1955). Congenital glaucoma, deafness, mental deficiency, and cardiac anomaly following attempted abortion. *The Journal of Pediatrics, 46*, 102–105.
Robinson, G. G., Brummitt, J. R., & Miller, J. R. (1963). Hearing loss in infants and preschool children. II. Etiological considerations. *Pediatrics, 32*, 115–124.
Taylor, H. M. (1937). Perinatal medication and its relation to the fetal ear. *Surgical Gynecology and Obstetrics, 64*, 542–546.

Tonimura, T., & Lee, S. (1972). Discussion on the suspected teratogenicity of quinine to humans. *Teratology, 6*, 122.

Winkel, C. F. (1948). Quinine and congenital injuries of ear and eye of foetus. *Journal of Tropical Medicine and Hygiene, 51*, 2–7.

Ranitidine

FDA: **B**   SIGNIFICANCE: **4**   POTENCY: **3–4**

A large-scale retrospective cohort study (n = 2236) on the effects of the use of acid-suppressing drugs during the first trimester on neonatal outcome reported no significant teratogenic risk associated with ranitidine. More data are needed, particularly data on use during the later trimesters.

Ruigomez, A., Garcia Rodriguez, L. A., Cattaruzzi, C., et al. (1999). Use of cimetidine, omeprazole, and ranitidine in pregnant women and pregnancy outcomes. *American Journal of Epidemiology, 150*, 476–481.

Reserpine

FDA: **D**   SIGNIFICANCE: **1** (near term)
POTENCY: **1** (near term)

A large-scale Hungarian case-control reporting system found no significant risk for teratogenic effects among the offspring of women who received reserpine during pregnancy for hypertension compared to a control group. However, fetotoxic effects have been associated with reserpine use. When administered within 48 hours of delivery, reserpine produces a neonatal syndrome characterized by hypothermia, lethargy, and nasal stuffiness/obstruction and discharge. Between 10% and 16% of neonates develop this syndrome, which may last up to 5 days. Because neonates are obligate nasal breathers, the nasal congestion may result in a fatal outcome. Neonatal deaths also have been related to the associated hypothermia.

Anagnostakis, D., & Matsanrotis, N. (1974). Neonatal cold injury and maternal reserpine administration. *The Lancet, 2*, 471.

Budnick, I. S., Leikin, S., & Hoeck, L. E. (1955). Effect in the newborn infant of reserpine administration antepartum. *American Journal of Diseases of Children, 90*, 286–289.

Czeizel, A. (1988). Reserpine is not a human teratogen. [Letter]. *Journal of Medical Genetics, 25*, 787.

Done, A. K. (1966). Perinatal pharmacology. *Annual Review of Pharmacology and Toxicology, 6*, 189.

Holman, G. H., & Lipsitz, P. J. (1966). Effect of toxemic pregnancy on the fetus and neonate. *Clinical Obstetrics and Gynecology, 9*, 922.

Sobel, D. E. (1960). Fetal damage due to ECT, insulin coma, chlorpromazine, or reserpine. *Archives of General Psychiatry, 2*, 606.

Sullivan, J. M. (1974). Blood pressure elevation in pregnancy. *Progress in Cardiovascular Diseases, 16*, 375–393.

Rifampin

FDA: **C**   SIGNIFICANCE: **3**   POTENCY: **3–4**

A study of 229 women who received rifampin during pregnancy reported 202 live births in which six infants had congenital malformations (three had skeletal reduction defects). This rate of congenital malformations is not significantly different from the rate for the general population. There also are negative reports. A review of 2787 women who received rifampin during pregnancy reported 2712 live births and a congenital malformation rate that does not suggest an increased risk. When the data for 446 women treated during the first trimester were examined, however, the rates of neural-tube defects (seven per 1000) and limb defects (195 per 1000) were unusually high. More data are needed, particularly data addressing use during the first trimester.

Antituberculosis drugs in pregnancy. (1980). *The Lancet, 2*, 1285–1286.

Jentgens, H. (1975). Antituberkulolische therapie mit ethambutol und rifampicin in der schwangerschaft. *Praxis der Pneumologie, 30*, 42–45.

Reimers, D. (1971). Missbildungen durch rifampicin? Bricht uber 2 faile von normaler fetales entwicklung nach rifampicin—therapie in der fruhschwangerschaft. *Muenchen Medizinische Wochenschrift, 113*, 1690–1691.

Snider, D. E., Layde, P. M., Johnson, M. W., et al. (1980). Treatment of tuberculosis during pregnancy. *American Review of Respiratory Diseases, 122*, 65–79.

Steen, J. S., & Stainton-Ellis, P. M. (1977). Rifampicin in pregnancy. *The Lancet, 2*, 604–605.

Rubella Virus Vaccine

FDA: **C**   SIGNIFICANCE: **3**   POTENCY: **3**

Pregnancy has been considered an absolute contraindication to rubella vaccination. This contraindication is being re-examined, however, because the risk appears to be minimal. Rubella vaccination results in viremia for up to 3 months after inoculation. Therefore, women who are not pregnant at the time of vaccination but become pregnant within 3 months have a theoretical risk of infecting the fetus. Rubella virus has been isolated from the placenta, from products of conception, and from the fetus. Fetal infections also have been confirmed by postnatal serologic testing of infants born to mothers who were vaccinated just prior to or during pregnancy. The critical question is whether fetal infections with the attenuated virus produce the congenital rubella syndrome characterized by neonatal cardiovascular disease, cataracts, deafness, glaucoma, growth retardation, retinopathy, and thrombocytopenia. To date, no exposed pregnancy that has gone to term has resulted in an affected neonate. However, cataract formation was observed histologically in an aborted fetus. Rubella vaccines are made with more than one strain of virus, so results for one strain may not apply to another. More data are needed.

Bolognese, R. J., Corson, S. L., Fuccillo, D. A., et al. (1973). Evaluation of possible transplacental infection with rubella vaccination during pregnancy. *American Journal of Obstetrics and Gynecology, 117*, 939–941.

Enders, G. (1985). Rubella antibody titers in vaccinated and nonvaccinated women and results of vaccination during pregnancy. *Review of Infectious Diseases, 7*(Suppl 1), S103–S107.

Fleet, W. F., Benz, E. W., Karzon, D. T., et al. (1974). Fetal consequences of maternal rubella immunization. *Journal of the American Medical Association, 227*, 621.

Hayden, G. F., Hermann, K. L., Bulmovici-Klein, E., et al. (1980). Subclinical congenital rubella infection associated with maternal rubella vaccination in early pregnancy. *The Journal of Pediatrics, 96*, 869–872.

Levine, M. M., Edsall, G., & Bruce-Chwatt, L. J. (1974). Live virus vaccines in pregnancy: Risks and recommendations. *The Lancet, 2*, 34–38.

Modlin, J. F., Herman, K., Brandling-Bennett, A. D., et al. (1976). Risk of congenital abnormality after inadvertent rubella vaccination of pregnant women. *New England Journal of Medicine, 294*, 972–974.

Preblud, S. R. (1985). Some current issues relating to rubella vaccine. *Journal of the American Medical Association, 254*, 253–256.

Preblud, S. R., Stetler, H. C., Frank, J. A., et al. (1981). Fetal risk associated with rubella vaccine. *Journal of the American Medical Association, 246*, 1413–1417.

Rubella vaccination during pregnancy—United States (1971–1988). *Morbidity and Mortality Weekly Report, 38*(17), 289–293.

Sheppard, S., Smithells, R. W., Dickson, A., et al. (1986). Rubella vaccination and pregnancy: Preliminary report of a national survey. *British Medical Journal (Clinical Research), 292*, 727.

Scopolamine (Hyoscine)
FDA: **C**   SIGNIFICANCE: **3–4**   POTENCY: **3**

A study of 388 infants born to women who received scopolamine during the first trimester and of 1053 infants born to mothers who received scopolamine at various times during their pregnancies found no significant risk for congenital anomalies. However, administration of scopolamine just prior to delivery may alter fetal cardiac rate and activity.

Ayromlooi, J., Tobias, M., & Berg, P. (1980). The effects of scopolamine and ancillary analgesics upon the fetal heart rate recording. *Journal of Reproductive Medicine, 25*, 323–326.

Heinonen, O. P., Slone, D., & Shapiro, S. (1977). *Birth defects and drugs in pregnancy.* Littleton, MA: Publishing Sciences Group.

Secobarbital
FDA: **C**   SIGNIFICANCE: **3–4** (neonatal effects)   POTENCY: **2–3** (neonatal effects)

A study of pregnant women who took secobarbital either during the first trimester (n = 378) or at various times during their pregnancies (n = 4248) found no significant risk for congenital anomalies. In a single case report, a woman who was addicted to secobarbital and used this drug regularly during pregnancy gave birth to an infant who displayed signs and symptoms of the neonatal barbiturate-withdrawal syndrome (e.g., hyperirritability, seizures). More data are needed regarding secobarbital use during pregnancy. (*See* Pentobarbital monograph.)

Bleyer, W. A., & Marshall, R. E. (1972). Barbiturate withdrawal syndrome in a passively addicted infant. *Journal of the American Medical Association, 221*, 185–186.

Heinonen, O. P., Slone, D., & Shapiro, S. (1977). *Birth defects and drugs in pregnancy.* Littleton, MA: Publishing Sciences Group.

Smallpox Vaccine

AUTHOR: ● **SIGNIFICANCE:** 1 **POTENCY:** 3

The World Health Organization presently recommends that only people who are working with the smallpox virus or with closely related viruses be immunized. For women who are pregnant, vaccination may result in fetal vaccinia and subsequent spontaneous abortion or perinatal death. Although a large study reported no effect on the teratogenic or spontaneous abortion rates of offspring born to women who were vaccinated during pregnancy and the incidence appears to be rare, smallpox vaccination should **not** be administered to pregnant women.

Adverse reactions to smallpox vaccination—1978. (1979). *Morbidity and Mortality Weekly Report, 28*, 265.
Epidemiology—unnecessary smallpox vaccination. (1979). *British Medical Journal, 2*, 1155.
Green, D. M., Reid, S. M., & Rhaney, K. (1966). Generalized vaccinia in the human fetus. *The Lancet, 1*, 1296–1298.
Hart, R. J. (1981). Immunizations. *Clinical Obstetrics and Gynecology, 8*, 421–430.
Levine, M. M., Edsall, G., & Bruce-Chwatt, L. J. (1974). Live virus vaccines in pregnancy: Risks and recommendations. *The Lancet, 2*, 34–38.
Saxen, L., Cantell, K., & Hakama, M. (1968). Relation between smallpox vaccination and outcome of pregnancy. *American Journal of Public Health, 58*, 1910–1921.

Sodium Iodide

FDA: X **SIGNIFICANCE:** 1 **POTENCY:** 1

The fetal thyroid gland begins to concentrate iodine at about 10 weeks of gestation. Use of sodium iodide I 131 after that time destroys this gland, resulting in cretinism. Several cases of neonatal hypothyroidism and hypoparathyroidism secondary to maternal iodide I 131 administration have been reported.

Bargmann, G. J., & Gardner, L. I. (1967). The cloistered thyroidologists. *The Lancet, 2*, 562.
Fisher, W. D., Voorhess, M. L., & Gardner, L. I. (1963). Congenital hypothyroidism in infant following maternal ^{131}I therapy. *Clinical Conference, 62*, 132–146.
Ibbertson, H. K., Seddon, R. J., & Croxson, H. S. (1975). Fetal hypothyroidism complicating medical treatment of thyrotoxicosis in pregnancy. *Clinical Endocrinology, 4*, 521–523.
Richards, G. E., Brewer, E. D., Conley, S. B., et al. (1981). Combined hypothyroidism and hypoparathyroidism in an infant after maternal ^{131}I administration. *The Journal of Pediatrics, 99*, 141–143.

Sodium Salicylate

FDA: C **SIGNIFICANCE:** 3 **POTENCY:** 2–3

A single study of 54 women who took sodium salicylate during the first trimester failed to detect an increased incidence of congenital anomalies. Salicylates readily cross the placenta, however, and may cause premature closure of the ductus arteriosus by inhibiting prostaglandin synthesis. More data are needed regarding sodium salicylate use during pregnancy. (*See* Aspirin monograph.)

Heinonen, O. P., Slone, D., & Shapiro, S. (1977). *Birth defects and drugs in pregnancy*. Littleton, MA: Publishing Sciences Group.

Streptokinase

FDA: C **SIGNIFICANCE:** 3–4 **POTENCY:** 3

Streptokinase use may cause severe hemorrhaging during the early puerperium and is usually contraindicated during this period. However, streptokinase is recommended during pregnancy for pulmonary embolus. Data on fetal toxicity are not available. More data are needed.

Bonner, J. (1981). Venous thromboembolism and pregnancy. *Clinical Obstetrics and Gynecology, 8*, 455–473.

Streptomycin

FDA: D **SIGNIFICANCE:** 1 **POTENCY:** 2

Streptomycin use during pregnancy has been associated with fetal ototoxicity. In a large review, one out of six exposed neonates was born with some degree of ototoxicity.

Conway, N., & Beit, B. D. (1965). Streptomycin in pregnancy: Effect on the foetal ear. *British Medical Journal, 2*, 260–263.
Donald, P. R., & Sellars, S. L. (1981). Streptomycin ototoxicity in the unborn child. *South African Medical Journal, 60*, 316.
Kern, V. G. (1962). Zur frage der intrauterinen streptomycin-schadigung. *Schweizerische Medizinische Wochenschrift, 92*, 77–79.
Lowe, C. R. (1964). Congenital defects among children born to women under supervision or treatment for pulmonary tuberculosis. *British Journal of Preventive Social Medicine, 18*, 14–16.
Marcus, J. C. (1967). Non-teratogenicity of anti-

tuberculosis drugs. *South African Medical Journal, 41*, 758–759.

Rasmussen, R. (1969). The ototoxic effect of streptomycin and dihydrostreptomycin on the foetus. *Scandinavian Journal of Respiratory Diseases, 50*, 61–67.

Robinson, C. G., & Cambon, K. G. (1964). Hearing loss in infants of tuberculosis mothers treated with streptomycin during pregnancy. *New England Journal of Medicine, 271*, 949–951.

Rubin, A., Winston, J., & Rutledge, M. L. (1951). Effects of streptomycin upon the human fetus. *American Journal of Diseases of Children, 82*, 14–16.

Snider, D. E., Layde, P. M., Johnson, M. W., et al. (1980). Treatment of tuberculosis during pregnancy. *American Review of Respiratory Disease, 122*, 65–79.

Varpela, E., Hietalahti, J., & Aro, M. J. (1969). Streptomycin and dihydrostreptomycin medication during pregnancy and their effect on the child's inner ear. *Scandinavian Journal of Respiratory Diseases, 50*, 101–109.

Watson, E. H., & Stow, R. M. (1948). Clinical notes, suggestions and new instruments, streptomycin therapy. *Journal of the American Medical Association, 137*, 1599–1600.

Sulfacetamide

FDA: C   SIGNIFICANCE: 3–4   POTENCY: 4

A single study of 93 women who used topical sulfacetamide during the first trimester found no increased risk for congenital anomalies. More data regarding sulfacetamide use during pregnancy are needed. (*See* Sulfonamides monograph.)

Heinonen, O. P., Slone, D., & Shapiro, S. (1977). *Birth defects and drugs in pregnancy.* Littleton, MA: Publishing Sciences Group.

Sulfamethoxazole

FDA: B   SIGNIFICANCE: 5   POTENCY: 4

Two different studies involving 166 women who received sulfamethoxazole during pregnancy found no increase in the rate of congenital malformations. (*See* Sulfonamides monograph.)

Heinonen, O. P., Slone, D., & Shapiro, S. (1977). *Birth defects and drugs in pregnancy.* Littleton, MA: Publishing Sciences Group.

Williams, J. D., Brumfitt, W., Condie, A. P., et al. (1969). The treatment of bacteriuria in pregnant women with sulphamethoxazole and trimethoprim. A microbiological, clinical, and toxicological study. *Postgraduate Medical Journal, 45*(Suppl), 71–76.

Sulfasalazine (Salicylazosulfapyridine)

FDA: B   SIGNIFICANCE: 4–5   POTENCY: 4

Four case reports associate sulfasalazine use during pregnancy with congenital malformations. Outweighing these reports are three studies of 60, 100, and 181 women who received sulfasalazine during pregnancy with no increase in malformations; 107 of these women received the drug during their entire pregnancy. Maternal sulfasalazine use during pregnancy may result in low folic acid serum concentrations and, theoretically, an increased risk for neural-tube defects among offspring. The use of a folic acid supplement may be indicated. (*See* Folic Acid and Sulfonamides monographs.)

Craxi, A., & Pagliarello, F. (1980). Possible embryotoxicity of sulfasalazine. [Letter]. *Archives of Internal Medicine, 140*, 1674.

Esbjorner, E., Jarnerot, G., & Wranne, L. (1987). Sulphasalazine and sulphapyridine serum levels in children to [sic] mothers treated with sulphasalazine during pregnancy and lactation. *Acta Paediatrica Scandinavica, 76*, 137–142.

Haxton, M. J., & Bell, J. (1983). Fetal anatomical abnormalities and other associated factors in middle-trimester abortion and their relevance to patient counselling. *British Journal of Obstetrics and Gynaecology, 90*, 501–506.

Hoo, J. J., Hadro, T. A., & von Behren, P. (1988). Possible teratogenicity of sulfasalazine. *New England Journal of Medicine, 318*, 1128.

Jarnerot, G., Into-Malmberg, M. B., & Esbjorner, E. (1981). Placental transfer of sulphasalazine and sulphapyridine and some of its metabolites. *Scandinavian Journal of Gastroenterology, 16*, 693–697.

Moyadam, M., Dobbins, W. O., Korelitz, B., et al. (1981). Pregnancy in inflammatory bowel disease: Effect of sulfasalazine and corticosteroids on fetal outcome. *Gastroenterology, 80*, 72–76.

Newman, N. M., & Correy, J. F. (1983). Possible teratogenicity of sulphasalazine. *Medical Journal of Australia, 1*, 528–529.

Nielsen, O. H., Andreasson, B., Bondesen, S., et al. (1983). Pregnancy in ulcerative colitis. *Scandinavian Journal of Gastroenterology, 18*, 735–742.

Willoughby, C. P., & Truelove, S. C. (1980). Ulcerative colitis and pregnancy. *Gut, 21*, 469–474.

Sulfisoxazole

FDA: B   SIGNIFICANCE: 5   POTENCY: 4

In three studies of women who received sulfisoxazole during the first trimester (n =

1121) or during various stages of pregnancy (n = 4287), no increase in the rate of congenital malformations was observed. (*See* Sulfonamides monograph.)

Aselton, P., Jick, H., Milunsky, A., et al. (1985). First-trimester drug use and congenital disorders. *Obstetrics and Gynecology, 65*, 451–455.

Heinonen, O. P., Slone, D., & Shapiro, S. (1977). *Birth defects and drugs in pregnancy*. Littleton, MA: Publishing Sciences Group.

Jick, H., Holmes, L. B., Hunter, J. R., et al. (1981). First-trimester drug use and congenital disorders. *Journal of the American Medical Association, 246*, 343–346.

Mellin, G. W. (1964). Drugs in the first trimester of pregnancy and the fetal life of Homo sapiens. *American Journal of Obstetrics and Gynecology, 90*, 1169–1180.

Sulfonamides

AUTHOR: NONE
SIGNIFICANCE: 4–5 (1st and 2nd trimester use)
POTENCY: 3–4 (1st and 2nd trimester use)

Sulfonamide use during the first and second trimesters does not appear to be associated with significant teratogenic risk. However, the known pharmacology of the sulfonamides suggests a risk for neonatal kernicterus. In addition, sulfonamide use near term may result in hemolysis among newborns who have glucose-6-phosphate dehydrogenase deficiency.

Safety of antimicrobial drugs in pregnancy. (1987). *The Medical Letter, 29*, 61–63.

Tacrolimus

FDA: C   SIGNIFICANCE: 3–4   POTENCY: 2–3

A retrospective study of 84 women who received immunosuppressant therapy with tacrolimus during their pregnancies (n = 100) did not report any significant congenital anomalies among offspring. However, several neonates reportedly experienced transient hyperkalemia, hypoxia, and renal dysfunction. More data are needed.

Kainz, A., Harabacz, I., Cowlrick, I. S., et al. (2000). Review of the course and outcome of 100 pregnancies in 84 women treated with tacrolimus. *Transplantation, 70*(12), 1718–1721.

Terbutaline

FDA: B   SIGNIFICANCE: 3–4   POTENCY: 3–4

Acute fetal distress has been successfully treated with maternal terbutaline during the intrapartum period. However, terbutaline use near term has been associated with fetotoxic effects, including fetal tachycardia and transient neonatal hypoglycemia. More data are needed, particularly data addressing terbutaline use during the first and second trimesters.

Epstein, M. G., Nicholls, E., & Stubblefield, P. G. (1979). Neonatal hypoglycemia after beta-sympathomimetic tocolytic therapy. *The Journal of Pediatrics, 94*, 449–453.

Ingemarsson, I., Arulkumaran, S., & Ratnam, S. S. (1985). Single injection of terbutaline in term labor. I. Effect on fetal pH in cases with prolonged bradycardia. *American Journal of Obstetrics and Gynecology, 153*(8), 859–864.

Mendez-Bauer, C., Shekarloo, A., Cook, V., et al. (1987). Treatment of acute intrapartum fetal distress by beta2-sympathomimetics. *American Journal of Obstetrics and Gynecology, 156*, 638–642.

Sharif, D. S., Huhta, J. C., Moise, K. J., et al. (1990). Changes in fetal hemodynamics with terbutaline treatment and premature labor. *Journal of Clinical Ultrasound, 18*, 85–89.

Shekarloo, A., Mendez-Bauer, C., Cook, V., et al. (1989). Terbutaline (intravenous bolus) for the treatment of acute intrapartum fetal distress. *American Journal of Obstetrics and Gynecology, 160*, 615–618.

Tejani, N. A., Verma, U. L., Chatterjee, S., et al. (1983). Terbutaline in the management of acute intrapartum fetal acidosis. *Journal of Reproductive Medicine, 28*, 857–861.

Wallace, R. L., Caldwell, D. L., Ansbacher, R., et al. (1978). Inhibition of premature labor by terbutaline. *Obstetrics and Gynecology, 51*, 387–393.

Terpin Hydrate

AUTHOR: NONE   SIGNIFICANCE: see monograph   POTENCY: see monograph

Three studies of women who used terpin hydrate during the first trimester (n = 390) or at various times during their pregnancies (n = 1762) found no significant risk for congenital anomalies. However, terpin hydrate requires cautious use during pregnancy because it is typically available only as an elixir containing ~40% alcohol. Long-term or high-dose use of terpin hydrate elixir may be associated with alcohol-related teratogenic or fetotoxic effects.

More data are needed. (*See* Alcohol monograph.)

Aselton, P., Jick, H., Milunsky, A., et al. (1985). First-trimester drug use and congenital disorders. *Obstetrics and Gynecology, 65*, 451–455.

Heinonen, O. P., Slone, D., & Shapiro, S. (1977). *Birth defects and drugs in pregnancy*. Littleton, MA: Publishing Sciences Group.

Testosterone

FDA: X   SIGNIFICANCE: 1   POTENCY: 1

Testosterone use during pregnancy has been associated with pseudohermaphroditism in the female fetus/neonate. When testosterone is used during the first 12 weeks of gestation, it may result in complete fusion of the labia. The most common teratogenic effect is clitoralmegaly with atrophy of the labia. Among affected infants, the ovaries, fallopian tubes, and uterus are normal, and normal female secondary sexual characteristics develop at puberty.

Gold, A. P., & Michael, A. F. (1958). Testosterone induced female pseudohermaphroditism. *The Journal of Pediatrics, 52*, 279–283.

Grumbach, M. M., & Ducharme, J. R. (1960). The effects of androgens on fetal sexual development. Androgen-induced female pseudohermaphrodism. *Fertility and Sterility, 11*, 157–180.

Reschini, E., Giustina, G., D'Alberton, A., et al. (1985). Female pseudohermaphroditism due to maternal androgen administration: 25-year follow-up. *The Lancet, 1*, 1226.

Tuchmann-Duplessis, H. (1983). The teratogenic risk. *American Journal of Industrial Medicine, 4*, 245–258.

Tetanus Toxoid Vaccine

AUTHOR: ●   SIGNIFICANCE: 5   POTENCY: 4

Maternal tetanus toxoid vaccination is not often required during pregnancy but may be indicated for some women. In developing areas of the world, maternal tetanus toxoid vaccination is recommended to provide neonates with passive maternal immunity.

Hart, R. J. (1981). Immunizations. *Clinical Obstetrics and Gynecology, 8*, 421–430.

Tetracycline

FDA: D   SIGNIFICANCE: 1 (dental staining)
POTENCY: 1 (dental staining)

Tetracycline is well known for its ability to stain the teeth of children exposed in utero during the second or third trimester. Tetracycline use during pregnancy also has been associated with enamel hypoplasia among offspring. In addition, tetracycline has been found in fetal bones obtained from therapeutic abortions. In one study, use of tetracycline was associated with decreased linear growth. Several cases of decreased growth also have been reported. Maternal tetracycline use during the first trimester will not affect the teeth of offspring because bone mineralization begins in the fourth month, and the effects of tetracycline involve complexing with calcium. Use of tetracycline during the second trimester stains the deciduous teeth and during the third trimester stains the crowns of permanent teeth. Case reports have associated tetracycline with digit defects, congenital cataracts, limb anomalies, and, in one case-controlled study, translocation of the great arteries. Negative studies also have been reported. In four studies involving more than 2000 pregnancies, tetracycline did not affect the malformation rate. Given these various effects, tetracycline should be avoided during pregnancy.

Aselton, P., Jick, H., Milunsky, A., et al. (1985). First-trimester drug use and congenital disorders. *Obstetrics and Gynecology, 65*, 451–455.

Carter, M. P., & Wilson, F. (1962). Tetracycline and congenital limb abnormalities. *British Medical Journal, 2*, 407–408.

Cohlan, S. Q. (1977). Tetracycline staining of teeth. *Teratology, 15*, 127–130.

Cohlan, S. Q., Bevelander, G., & Tiamsic, T. (1963). Growth inhibition of prematures receiving tetracycline. A clinical and laboratory investigation of tetracycline-induced bone fluorescence. *American Journal of Diseases of Children, 105*, 453–461.

Collins, I. S. (1964). Hazards of drug therapy. *Medical Journal of Australia, 1*, 122.

Coombes, B., Whalley, P. J., & Adams, R. H. (1972). Tetracycline and the liver. *Progress in Liver Diseases, 4*, 587.

Done, A. K. (1966). Perinatal pharmacology. *Annual Review of Pharmacology and Toxicology, 6*, 189.

Douglas, A. C. (1963). The deposition of tetracycline in human nails and teeth: A complication of long-term treatment. *British Journal of Diseases of the Chest, 57*, 43–46.

Elder, R. A., Santanariana, B. A., Smith, S. A., et al. (1967). Excess prematurity in tetracycline-treated bacteriuric patients whose infection persisted or returned. *Antimicrobial Agents and Chemotherapy, 7,* 101.

Harley, J. D., Farrar, J. F., Gray, J. B., et al. (1964). Aromatic drugs and congenital cataracts. *The Lancet, 1,* 472–473.

Heinonen, O. P., Slone, D., & Shapiro, S. (1977). *Birth defects and drugs in pregnancy.* Littleton, MA: Publishing Sciences Group.

Jick, H., Holmes, L. B., Hunter, J. R., et al. (1981). First-trimester drug use and congenital disorders. *Journal of the American Medical Association, 246,* 343–346.

Kline, A. H., Blattner, R. J., & Lunin, M. (1964). Transplacental effect of tetracycline on teeth. *Journal of the American Medical Association, 188,* 170–172.

Mull, M. M. (1966). The tetracyclines. *American Journal of Diseases of Children, 112,* 483–493.

Toaff, R., & Ravid, R. (1966). Tetracyclines and the teeth. *The Lancet, 2,* 281–282.

Totterman, L. E., & Saxen, L. (1969). Incorporation of tetracycline into human foetal bones after maternal drug administration. *Acta Obstetricia and Gynecologica Scandinavica, 48,* 542–549.

Thalidomide

FDA: **X**   SIGNIFICANCE: **1**   POTENCY: **1**

Thalidomide is regarded as a classic and potent human teratogen. Although widely used by pregnant women for its original indication (insomnia), thalidomide is no longer recommended for this indication in North America because of its associated teratogenic effects. Thalidomide was frequently used as a sedative-hypnotic by pregnant women during the 1950s and 1960s. The most striking of the teratogenic effects observed among offspring involved limb reduction defects, which included amelia and phocomelia of both the upper and lower extremities, congenital dislocated hip, deformities of the tibia and fibula, digital agenesis, femoral hypoplasia, foot deformities, and radial aplasia or hypoplasia. Other teratogenic effects included anophthalmos, anotia, coloboma, congenital heart disease, external ophthalmoplegia, facial palsy, genitourinary and GI tract anomalies, microphthalmos, microtia, and renal anomalies. The critical period for thalidomide-induced teratogenesis is from the 27th to the 40th day. Some authors claim that any pregnant woman taking the drug between the 3rd and 8th week postconception will have a malformed infant (implying a 100% rate of teratogenesis for this period), but this claim is **not** true. The mechanism for the teratogenic effects may involve a metabolite of thalidomide that causes neuropathy.

Thalidomide is available and is used in various countries for several indications, including graft-versus-host disease, leprosy, and multiple myeloma. Thalidomide is available for clinical use in North America for the cutaneous manifestations of erythema nodosum leprosum. To prevent or minimize inadvertent use by a pregnant woman, the FDA has established a special restricted distribution program called the System for Thalidomide Education and Prescribing Safety (S.T.E.P.S.®). The program restricts distribution to prescribers and pharmacists registered within the program. In addition, to receive thalidomide, all patients must be advised of, agree to, and comply with the requirements of S.T.E.P.S.® If the patient is an adolescent between 12 and 18 years of age, his or her parent or legal guardian must be apprised of the requirements and must agree to both monitor and ensure compliance.

Barr, B. (1982). Teratogenic hearing loss. *Audiology, 21,* 111–127.

Brent, R. L., & Holmes, L. B. (1988). Clinical and basic science lessons from the thalidomide tragedy: What have we learned about the causes of limb defects? *Teratology, 38,* 241–251.

Kajii, T. (1973). The effects of thalidomide intake during 113 human pregnancies. *Teratology, 8,* 163–166.

Knapp, K., Lenz, W., & Norwack, E. (1962). Multiple congenital abnormalities. *The Lancet, 2,* 725.

Lary, J. M., Daniel, K. L., Erickson, J. D., et al. (1999). The return of thalidomide: Can birth defects be prevented? *Drug Safety, 21,* 161–169.

Lenz, W. (1988). A short history of thalidomide embryopathy. *Teratology, 38,* 203–215.

Lenz, W., & Knapp, K. (1962). Thalidomide embryopathy. *Archives of Environmental Health, 5,* 100–105.

McBride, W. G. (1977). Thalidomide embryopathy. *Teratology, 16,* 79–82.

McBride, W. G. (1981). Another late thalidomide abnormality. *The Lancet, 2,* 368.

McCredie, J. (1973). Thalidomide and congenital Charcot's syndrome. *The Lancet, 2,* 1058–1061.

Mellin, G. W., & Katzenstein, M. (1962). The saga of thalidomide. *New England Journal of Medicine, 267,* 1184–1193.

Mellin, G. W., & Katzenstein, M. (1962). The saga

of thalidomide (concluded). *New England Journal of Medicine, 267,* 1238–1244.
Miller, M. T., & Stromland, K. (1999). Teratogen update: Thalidomide: A review, with a focus on ocular findings and new potential uses. *Teratology, 60,* 306–321.
Neubert, D. (1997). Never ending tales of the mode of the teratogenic action of thalidomide. *Teratogenesis, Carcinogenesis, and Mutagenesis, 17*(1), i–ii.
Newman, C. G. (1986). The thalidomide syndrome: Risks of exposure and spectrum of malformations. *Clinics of Perinatology, 13,* 555–572.
Nulsen, R. O. (1961). Trial of thalidomide in insomnia associated with the third trimester. *American Journal of Obstetrics and Gynecology, 81,* 1245–1248.
Pembrey, M. E., Clarke, C. A., & Frais, M. M. (1970). Normal child after maternal thalidomide ingestion in critical period of pregnancy. *The Lancet, 1,* 275–277.
Quibell, E. P. (1981). The thalidomide embryopathy: An analysis from the U.K. *Practitioner, 225,* 721–726.
Shull, G. E. (1984). Differential inhibition of protein synthesis: A possible biochemical mechanism of thalidomide teratogenesis. *Journal of Theoretical Biology, 110*(3), 461–486.
Smithells, R. W. (1973). Defects and disabilities of thalidomide children. *British Medical Journal, 1,* 269–272.
Stewart, A. (1963). Congenital defects due to thalidomide. *British Medical Journal, 1,* 123.
Terapane, J. F. (1970). Teratogenicity of phthalimidine derivative. *Teratology, 3,* 210.

Theophylline

FDA: **C**   SIGNIFICANCE: **4–5**   POTENCY: **3–4**

A study of 846 women who received theophylline as part of the Collaborative Perinatal Project found no increase in the rate of congenital malformations. A more recent report presented three cases of significant cardiovascular anomalies among neonates born to women who received theophylline throughout their pregnancies, but this finding was not supported by the results of a large-scale collaborative case-controlled study of congenital cardiovascular anomalies and disease. Currently, theophylline is generally regarded as the drug of choice for responsive chronic obstructive pulmonary disease among pregnant women. Theophylline, however, is a potential fetotoxin. It readily crosses the placenta and achieves serum concentrations in the fetus equal to, or greater than, maternal serum concentrations. Neonates exposed to theophylline near term have displayed signs and symptoms of theophylline toxicity, including jitteriness, tachycardia, and vomiting. (*See* Aminophylline monograph.)

Arwood, L. L., Dasta, J. F., & Friedman, C. (1979). Placental transfer of theophylline: Two case reports. *Pediatrics, 63,* 844–846.
Heinonen, O. P., Slone, D., & Shapiro, S. (1977). *Birth defects and drugs in pregnancy.* Littleton, MA: Publishing Sciences Group.
Horowitz, D. A., Jablonski, W. J., & Mehta, K. A. (1982). Apnea associated with theophylline withdrawal in a term neonate. *American Journal of Diseases of Children, 136,* 73–74.
Neff, R. K., & Leviton, A. (1990). Maternal theophylline consumption and the risk of stillbirth. *Chest, 97,* 1266–1267.
Park, J. M., Schmer, V., & Myers, T. L. (1990). Cardiovascular anomalies associated with prenatal exposure to theophylline. *Southern Medical Journal, 83,* 1487–1488.
Rubin, J. D., Loffredo, C., Correa-Villasenor, A., et al. (1991). Prenatal drug use and congenital cardiovascular malformations. *Teratology, 43,* 423.

Thiethylperazine

AUTHOR: ●   SIGNIFICANCE: **5**   POTENCY: **4**

Use of thiethylperazine during pregnancy has not been associated with teratogenic effects. However, it has been associated with fetotoxic effects, including extrapyramidal signs and symptoms. (*See* Phenothiazines monograph.)

Hill, R. M., Desmond, M. M., & Kay, J. L. (1966). Extrapyramidal dysfunction in an infant of a schizophrenic mother. *The Journal of Pediatrics, 69,* 589–595.
Rumeau-Rouquette, C., Goujard, J., & Huel, G. (1977). Possible teratogenic effect of phenothiazines in human beings. *Teratology, 15,* 57–64.

Thiopental

FDA: **C**   SIGNIFICANCE: **2–3** (neonatal effects)   POTENCY: **2** (neonatal effects)

In a single study of 152 women who received thiopental during the first trimester, no significant risk for congenital anomalies was noted. When administered during labor, thiopental produced neurobehavioral depression in the neonate for several days. (*See* Pentobarbital and Secobarbital monographs.)

Heinonen, O. P., Slone, D., & Shapiro, S. (1977). *Birth defects and drugs in pregnancy.* Littleton, MA: Publishing Sciences Group.

Hodgkinson, R., Marx, G. F., Kim, S. S., et al. (1977). Neonatal neurobehavioral tests following vaginal delivery under ketamine, thiopental, and extradural anesthesia. *Anesthetic and Analgesic Current Research, 56,* 548–553.

Jorgensen, N. P., & Marsal, K. (1988). Influence of thiopental anaesthesia on fetal motor behaviour in early pregnancy. *Early Human Development, 17,* 71–78.

Tobacco Smoking

AUTHOR: **NONE** SIGNIFICANCE: **1**
POTENCY: **1**

Although tobacco use during pregnancy has not been associated with major congenital anomalies among offspring, it is fetotoxic. In addition, tobacco smoke may function as a coteratogen. The incidence of club feet is significantly greater when women with a positive family history for club feet smoked tobacco during their pregnancies in comparison to the outcomes for pregnancies in which women either had a positive family history for club feet and did not smoke or smoked and did not have a positive family history for club feet. More data are needed.

The neonates of women who smoke tobacco show a dose-dependent (number of cigarettes smoked per day) relationship for decreased birth weight. These neonates weigh 100–400 grams less (average, 200 grams less) than those of nonsmokers and have a shorter body length. However, there appears to be a period of catch-up growth during the first year. Neonates of women who discontinue tobacco smoking during the first trimester are normal in size. Women who smoke have higher rates of premature deliveries, spontaneous abortions, abruptio placentae, and placenta previa than women who are nonsmokers. These effects are responsible, in part, for the higher perinatal mortality reported for neonates of women who smoke. The malformation rate for these neonates also may be increased. The risk for sudden infant death syndrome (SIDS) also is higher (4.4 times) for infants whose mothers are smokers. In addition, children whose mothers smoked during pregnancy do not score as well on tests for reading ability, mathematics, cognitive ability, IQ, vocabulary, or perceptual motor skills as children whose mothers did not. Obviously, women should be advised **not** to smoke during pregnancy.

Abel, E. L. (1980). Smoking during pregnancy: A review of effects on growth and development of offspring. *Human Biology, 52*(4), 593–625.

Abel, E. L. (1984). Smoking and pregnancy: *Journal of Psychoactive Drugs, 16*(4), 327–338.

Alberman, E., Creasy, M., & Elliot, M. (1976). Maternal factors associated with fetal chromosomal anomalies in spontaneous abortions. *British Journal of Obstetrics and Gynecology, 83,* 621–627.

Bracken, M. B., & Holford, T. R. (1981). Exposure to prescribed drugs in pregnancy and association with congenital malformations. *Obstetrics and Gynecology, 58*(3), 336–344.

Butler, N. R., & Goldstein, H. (1973). Smoking in pregnancy and subsequent child development. *British Medical Journal, 4,* 573–575.

Butler, N. R., Goldstein, H., & Ross, E. M. (1972). Cigarette smoking in pregnancy: Its influence on birth weight and perinatal mortality. *British Medical Journal, 2,* 127–130.

Cigarette smoking during the last 3 months of pregnancy among women who gave birth to live infants—Maine, 1988–1997. (1999). *Morbidity and Mortality Weekly Report, 48*(20), 421–425.

Comstock, G. W., Shah, F. K., Meyer, M. B., et al. (1971). Low birth weight and neonatal mortality rate related to maternal smoking and socioeconomic status. *American Journal of Obstetrics and Gynecology, 111,* 53–59.

Cope, L., Lancaster, P., & Stevens, L. (1973). Smoking in pregnancy. *Medical Journal of Australia, 1,* 673–677.

Davie, R., Butler, N., & Goldstein, H. (1972). *From birth to seven: A report of the National Child Development Study,* pp. 175–177. London: Longman and the National Children's Bureau.

Dunn, H. G., McBurney, A. K., Ingram, S., et al. (1976). Maternal cigarette smoking during pregnancy and the child's subsequent development. I. Physical growth to age 6½ years. *Canadian Journal of Public Health, 67,* 499–505.

Dunn, H. G., McBurney, A. K., Ingram, S., et al. (1977). Maternal cigarette smoking during pregnancy and the child's subsequent development. II. Neurological and intellectual maturation to the age of 6½ years. *Canadian Journal of Public Health, 68,* 43–50.

Frazier, T. M., Davis, G. H., Goldberg, H., et al. (1961). Cigarette smoking and prematurity: A prospective study. *American Journal of Obstetrics and Gynecology, 81,* 988–996.

Freid, P. A. (1989). Cigarettes and marijuana: Are there measurable long-term neurobehavioral teratogenic effects? *Neurotoxicology, 10*, 577–584.

Haustein, K. O. (1999). Cigarette smoking, nicotine and pregnancy. *International Journal of Clinical Pharmacology and Therapeutics, 37*, 417–427.

Honein, M. A., Paulozzi, L. J., & Moore, C. A. (2000). Family history, maternal smoking, and clubfoot: An indication of a gene–environment interaction. *American Journal of Epidemiology, 152*, 658–665.

King, J. C., & Fabro, S. (1983). Alcohol consumption and cigarette smoking: Effect on pregnancy. *Clinical Obstetrics and Gynecology, 26*, 437–448.

Kullander, S., & Kallen, B. (1971). A prospective study of smoking in pregnancy. *Acta Obstetricia and Gynecologica Scandinavica, 50*, 83–94.

Lowe, C. R. (1959). Effect of mothers' smoking habits on birth weight of their children. *British Medical Journal, 2*, 673–676.

McIntosh, I. D. (1984). Smoking and pregnancy: I. Maternal and placental risks. *Public Health Review, 12*, 1–28.

McMahon, B., Alpert, M., & Salber, E. J. (1966). Infant weight and parental smoking habits. *American Journal of Epidemiology, 82*, 247.

Miller, H. C., & Hassanein, K. (1964). Maternal smoking and growth of full term infants. *Pediatric Research, 8*, 960–963.

Miller, H. C., Hassanein, K., & Hensleigh, P. A. (1976). Fetal growth retardation in relation to maternal smoking and weight gain in pregnancy. *American Journal of Obstetrics and Gynecology, 125*, 55–60.

Moore, M. L., & Zaccaro, D. J. (2000). Cigarette smoking, low birth weight, and preterm births in low-income African American women. *Journal of Perinatology, 20*(3), 176–180.

Mulcahy, R., Murphy, J., & Martin, F. (1970). Placental changes and maternal weight in smoking and non-smoking mothers. *American Journal of Obstetrics and Gynecology, 106*, 703–704.

Murphy, J. F., & Mulcahy, R. (1971). The effect of age, parity, and cigarette smoking on baby weight. *American Journal of Obstetrics and Gynecology, 111*, 22–25.

Naeye, R. L. (1978). Effect of maternal cigarette smoking on the fetus and placenta. *British Journal of Obstetrics and Gynecology, 85*, 832–837.

Rush, D., & Callahan, K. R. (1989). Exposure to passive cigarette smoking and child development. A critical review. *Annals of the New York Academy of Science, 562*, 74–100.

Russell, C. S., Taylor, A., & Law, C. E. (1968). Smoking in pregnancy, maternal blood pressure, pregnancy outcome, baby weight and growth, and other related factors. *British Journal of Preventive and Social Medicine, 22*, 119–126.

Simpson, W. J. (1957). A preliminary report on cigarette smoking and the incidence of prematurity. *American Journal of Obstetrics and Gynecology, 73*, 808–815.

Sprauve, M. E., Lindsay, M. K., Drews-Botsch, C. D., et al. (1999). Racial patterns in the effects of tobacco use on fetal growth. *American Journal of Obstetrics and Gynecology, 181*(1), S22–S27.

Stillman, R. J., Rosenberg, M. J., & Sachs, B. P. (1986). Smoking and reproduction. *Fertility and Sterility, 46*(4), 545–566.

Underwood, P. B. (1967). Parental smoking empirically related to pregnancy outcome. *Obstetrics and Gynecology, 29*, 1–8.

Yerushalmy, J. (1964). Mother's cigarette smoking and survival of infant. *American Journal of Obstetrics and Gynecology, 88*, 505–518.

Tolbutamide

FDA: **D**   SIGNIFICANCE: **4**   POTENCY: **3–4**

Tolbutamide use has been associated with teratogenic effects in various case reports. However, retrospective studies have not demonstrated any pattern. More data are needed.

Campbell, G. D. (1961). Possible teratogenic effect of tolbutamide in pregnancy. *The Lancet, 1*, 891–892.

Coetzee, E. J., & Jackson, W. P. U. (1984). Oral hypoglycaemics in the first trimester and fetal outcome. *South African Medical Journal, 65*, 635–637.

Coopersmith, A., & Kerbel, N. C. (1962). Drugs and congenital anomalies. *Canadian Medical Association Journal, 87*, 193.

Dolger, H., Bookman, J. J., & Nechemias, C. (1967). The use of tolbutamide in the pregnant diabetic. *Diabetes, 16*, 522.

Dolger, H., Bookman, J. J., & Nechemias, C. (1969). Tolbutamide in pregnancy and diabetes. *Journal Mt. Sinai Hospital, NY, 36*, 471–474.

Endium, D. H., & Smith, G. J. (1961). Use of tolbutamide in pregnant diabetics. *Journal of Michigan State Medical Society, 60*, 1436–1438.

Ghanem, M. H. (1961). Possible teratogenic effects of tolbutamide in pregnant prediabetics. *The Lancet, 1*, 1227.

Heinonen, O. P., Slone, D., & Shapiro, S. (1977). *Birth defects and drugs in pregnancy*. Littleton, MA: Publishing Sciences Group.

Larsson, Y., & Sterky, G. (1960). Possible teratogenic effect of tolbutamide in a pregnant prediabetic. *The Lancet, 2*, 1424–1425.

Notelovitz, M. (1975). Sulphonylurea therapy in the treatment of the pregnant diabetic. *South African Medical Journal, 45*, 226–229.

Schiff, D., Aranada, J. V., & Stern, L. (1970). Neonatal thrombocytopenia and congenital malformations associated with administration of tolbutamide to the mother. *The Journal of Pediatrics, 77*, 457–458.

Sterne, J. (1973). Antidiabetic drugs and teratogenicity. *The Lancet, 1,* 1165.

Toluene

**AUTHOR: NONE   SIGNIFICANCE: 2
POTENCY: 1–2**

Toluene is a commercially available solvent. Maternal exposure to toluene may occur as a result of occupational hazard (e.g., painters) or deliberate abuse for its psychotropic effects. Reported cases involve the deliberate abuse of this solvent throughout pregnancy. Seven case reports and a prospective study involving 18 infants who had been exposed in utero to toluene provide support for a syndrome of toluene embryopathy, including cognitive and learning disorders (e.g., attention-deficit/hyperactivity disorder, mental retardation), developmental delay, microcephaly, minor craniofacial and limb anomalies, and variable growth deficiency. Possible concurrent use of other abusable drugs, notably alcohol and tobacco, confounds interpretation as does the lifestyle of solvent-abusing women, which may include low socioeconomic status, poor nutrition, and increased incidence of sexually transmitted diseases. More data are needed.

Arai, H., Yamada, M., Miyake, S., et al. (1997). Two cases of toluene embryopathy with severe motor and intellectual disabilities syndrome. *No To Hattatsu [Brain and Development], 29*(5), 361–366.
Hersh, J. H., Podruch, P. E., Rogers, G., et al. (1985). Toluene embryopathy. *The Journal of Pediatrics, 106,* 922–927.
Jones, H. E., & Balster, R. L. (1998). Inhalant abuse in pregnancy. *Obstetrics and Gynecology Clinics of North America, 25,* 153–167.
Lindemann, R. (1991). Congenital renal tubular dysfunction associated with maternal sniffing of organic solvents. *Acta Paediatrica Scandinavica, 80,* 882–884.
Pearson, M. A., Hoyme, H. E., Seaver, L. H., et al. (1994). Toluene embryopathy: Delineation of the phenotype and comparison with fetal alcohol syndrome. *Pediatrics, 93*(2), 211–215.
Seaver, L. H., Pearson, M. A., Rimsza, M. E., et al. (1991). Toluene embryopathy: Elucidation of phenotype and mechanism of teratogenesis in 12 patients. *American Journal of Human Genetics, 49*(Suppl 4), 237.
Wilkins-Haug, L., & Gabow, P. A. (1991). Toluene abuse during pregnancy: Obstetric complications and perinatal outcomes. *Obstetrics and Gynecology, 77,* 504–509.

Triamcinolone

FDA: C   SIGNIFICANCE: 4–5   POTENCY: 3–4

A single case report suggests an association between the use of very high doses of topical triamcinolone during the second trimester and severe intrauterine growth retardation. More data are needed. (*See* Corticosteroids monograph.)

Katz, V. L., Thorp, J. M., & Bowes, W. A. (1990). Severe symmetric intrauterine growth retardation associated with the topical use of triamcinolone. *American Journal of Obstetrics and Gynecology, 162,* 396–397.

Triamterene

FDA: B   SIGNIFICANCE: 4–5   POTENCY: 4

A study of 271 women who received triamterene at various times during their pregnancies (five during the first trimester) provided no evidence of a significant risk for congenital anomalies. However, because triamterene is a folic acid antagonist, its use during pregnancy may result in an increased risk for neural-tube defects. The use of a folic acid supplement may be indicated. (*See* Folic Acid monograph.) More data are needed.

Hernandez-Diaz, S., Werler, M. M., Walker, A. M., et al. (2000). Folic acid antagonists during pregnancy and the risk of birth defects. *New England Journal of Medicine, 343*(22), 1608–1614.
Lambie, D. G., & Johnson, R. H. (1985). Drugs and folate metabolism. *Drugs, 30*(2), 145–155.

Trifluoperazine

FDA: C   SIGNIFICANCE: 5   POTENCY: 4

In multiple studies of 1200 women who received trifluoperazine during pregnancy, no increase in the rate of congenital malformations was observed. However, cases of possible teratogenic effects have been reported. (*See* Phenothiazines monograph.)

General Practitioner Research Group: Drugs in pregnancy survey. (1963). *Practitioner, 191,* 775–780.
Hall, G. (1963). A case of phocomelia of the upper limbs. *Medical Journal of Australia, 1,* 449–450.
Heinonen, O. P., Slone, D., & Shapiro, S. (1977). *Birth defects and drugs in pregnancy.* Littleton, MA: Publishing Sciences Group.

McBride, W. G. (1963). The teratogenic action of drugs. *Medical Journal of Australia, 2*, 689–693.

Moriarty, A. J. (1963). Trifluoperazine and congenital malformations. *Canadian Medical Association Journal, 88*, 97.

Schire, I. (1963). Trifluoperazine and foetal anomalies. *The Lancet, 1*, 174.

Wheatley, D. (1964). Drugs and the embryo. *British Medical Journal, 1*, 630.

Trimeprazine

FDA: C   SIGNIFICANCE: 2   POTENCY: 2

In a prospective study, use of trimeprazine and other three-carbon side chain phenothiazines was associated with an increased risk for congenital malformations, including cardiac malformations, cleft lip, clinodactyly, club hands and feet, hydrocephalus, hypospadias, microcephaly, and syndactyly. (*See* Phenothiazines monograph.)

Rumeau-Rouquette, C., Goujard, J., & Huel, G. (1977). Possible teratogenic effect of phenothiazines in human pregnancy. *Teratology, 15*, 57–64.

Trimethadione

FDA: X   SIGNIFICANCE: 1   POTENCY: 1

Trimethadione use during pregnancy is associated with an unusually high rate of congenital malformations. In one study, 18 of 89 exposed infants were malformed. In another study of 53 women receiving trimethadione or paramethadione during pregnancy, there were 13 spontaneous abortions (24%) and 40 live births; 33 (88%) of the neonates had at least one major anomaly, including delayed mental development (50%), heart anomalies (50%) (patent ductus arteriosus, tetralogy of Fallot, transposition of the great vessels, ventricular septal defects), low-set ears (42%), urogenital malformations (30%), cleft lip/palate (28%), and skeletal malformations (25%). Other observed anomalies include clinodactyly, conductive hearing loss, growth retardation, inguinal hernia, irregular teeth, microcephaly, and ocular anomalies. Sixty-seven percent of these neonates later displayed speech impairment. They also have a characteristic facies with V-shaped eyebrows, a prominent forehead, epicanthal folds, and a broad nasal bridge similar to infants who have the Cornelia de Lange syndrome. Obviously, with this rate of malformations, trimethadione should be avoided during pregnancy. Women taking trimethadione and considering pregnancy should be switched to a different anticonvulsant before attempting to become pregnant. (*See* Paramethadione monograph.)

Feldman, G. L., Weaver, D., & Lovrien, F. W. (1977). The fetal trimethadione syndrome. *American Journal of Diseases of Children, 131*, 1389–1392.

German, J., Ehlus, K. H., Kowal, A., et al. (1970). Trimethadione and human teratogenesis. *Teratology, 3*, 349–362.

German, J., Kowal, A., & Ehlus, K. H. (1970). Possible teratogenicity of trimethadione and paramethadione. *The Lancet, 2*, 261–262.

Goldman, A. S., & Yaffe, S. J. (1991). Fetal trimethadione syndrome. *Teratology, 17*, 103–106.

Nakane, Y., Okuma, T., Takahashi, R., et al. (1980). Multi-institutional study on the teratogenicity and fetal toxicity of antiepileptic drugs: A report of a collaborative study group in Japan. *Epilepsia, 21*, 663–680.

Nichols, M. M. (1973). Fetal anomalies following maternal trimethadione ingestion. [Letter]. *The Journal of Pediatrics, 82*, 885–895.

Rosen, R. C., & Lightner, E. S. (1978). Phenotypic malformations in association with maternal trimethadione therapy. *The Journal of Pediatrics, 92*, 240–244.

Zackai, E. H., Mellman, W. J., Neiderer, B., et al. (1975). The fetal trimethadione syndrome. *American Journal of Diseases of Children, 87*, 280–284.

Trimethobenzamide

FDA: C   SIGNIFICANCE: 3–4   POTENCY: 2–3

A study of 192 women who took trimethobenzamide during the first trimester reported an increased incidence of severe congenital anomalies (type not specified) and an increased neonatal death rate secondary to the anomalies. However, three subsequent studies involving 1160 women who received trimethobenzamide at various times throughout their pregnancies (340 during the first trimester) failed to identify an increased risk for teratogenic effects.

Aselton, P., Jick, H., Milunsky, A., et al. (1985). First-trimester drug use and congenital disorders. *Obstetrics and Gynecology, 65*, 451–455.

Heinonen, O. P., Slone, D., & Shapiro, S. (1977). *Birth defects and drugs in pregnancy.* Littleton, MA: Publishing Sciences Group.

Jick, H., Holmes, L. B., Hunter, J. R., et al. (1981). First-trimester drug use and congenital disor-

ders. *Journal of the American Medical Association, 246,* 343–346.

Milkovich, L., & Van den Berg, B. J. (1976). An evaluation of the teratogenicity of certain antinauseant drugs. *American Journal of Obstetrics and Gynecology, 125,* 244–248.

Trimethoprim

FDA: C   SIGNIFICANCE: 4   POTENCY: 3–4

In a study of 120 women treated with sulfamethoxazole and trimethoprim during pregnancy (only 10 of whom received the drugs during the first trimester), no increase in the fetal malformation rate was noted. However, because trimethoprim is a folic acid antagonist, its use during pregnancy may result in an increased risk for neural-tube defects. Use of a folic acid supplement may be indicated. (*See* Folic Acid monograph.) More data are needed. (*See also* the Co-Trimoxazole [Trimethoprim and Sulfamethoxazole] monograph.)

Hernandez-Diaz, S., Werler, M. M., Walker, A. M., et al. (2000). Folic acid antagonists during pregnancy and the risk of birth defects. *New England Journal of Medicine, 343*(22), 1608–1614.

Lambie, D. G., & Johnson, R. H. (1985). Drugs and folate metabolism. *Drugs, 30*(2), 145–155.

Williams, J. D., Condie, A. P., Brumitt, W., et al. (1969). The treatment of bacteriuria in pregnant women with sulphamethoxazole and trimethoprim. *Postgraduate Medical Journal, 45*(Suppl), 71–76.

Tripelennamine

FDA: B   SIGNIFICANCE: 4   POTENCY: 3–4

In the only study of tripelennamine use during pregnancy, no increase in the rate of congenital malformations was observed. More data are needed.

Greenberger, P., & Patterson, R. (1978). Safety of therapy for allergic symptoms during pregnancy. *Annals of Internal Medicine, 89,* 234–237.

Triprolidine

AUTHOR: NONE   SIGNIFICANCE: 4   POTENCY: 4

Two studies of women who used triprolidine during the first trimester (n = 628) failed to find an increased risk for congenital anomalies. More data are needed.

Aselton, P., Jick, H., Milunsky, A., et al. (1985). First-trimester drug use and congenital disorders. *Obstetrics and Gynecology, 65,* 451–455.

Jick, H., Holmes, L. B., Hunter, J. R., et al. (1981). First-trimester drug use and congenital disorders. *Journal of the American Medical Association, 246,* 343–346.

Typhoid Vaccine

AUTHOR: ●   SIGNIFICANCE: 4–5   POTENCY: 3–4

No reports of teratogenic effects related to typhoid vaccine use during pregnancy were identified. Because typhoid vaccine is inactivated, pregnancy is not considered to be a contraindication to use, and this vaccine may be given to pregnant women. To minimize associated systemic reactions, the intradermal route is preferred. More data are needed.

Hart, R. J. (1981). Immunizations. *Clinical Obstetrics and Gynecology, 8,* 421–430.

Typhus Vaccine

AUTHOR: NONE   SIGNIFICANCE: 4–5   POTENCY: 3–4

Pregnancy is not considered a contraindication to the use of typhus vaccine. Although no data are available on the effects of maternal vaccination, the vaccine contains a killed Rickettsia and therefore should not cause a fetal infection. More data are needed.

Hart, R. J. (1981). Immunizations. *Clinical Obstetrics and Gynecology, 8,* 421–430.

Urokinase

FDA: B   SIGNIFICANCE: 3   POTENCY: 2–3

The use of thrombolytics in the early puerperium is usually contraindicated because of the possibility of massive maternal hemorrhage. However, the use of urokinase in the pregnant patient is recommended for massive pulmonary embolism. Data on fetal effects are not available. More data are needed.

Bonnar, J. (1981). Venous thromboembolism and pregnancy. *Clinical Obstetrics and Gynecology, 8,* 455–473.

Valproic Acid (Divalproex, Valproate Sodium)

FDA: D   SIGNIFICANCE: 1–2   POTENCY: 2

Valproate sodium crosses the placenta and achieves a fetal serum concentration that exceeds the maternal concentration. Although some studies have been negative, an increased rate of spina bifida has been observed among the offspring of women who received valproate sodium during pregnancy. One case of spina bifida was even noted in a negative report. In addition, the manufacturers of valproate sodium have acknowledged 98 unpublished cases of maternal valproate use during pregnancy that resulted in 19 abnormal pregnancies, including seven cases of spina bifida. Overall, the incidence of spina bifida among exposed fetuses appears to be between 1% and 2%. (Other congenital anomalies such as limb deficiencies have also been associated with valproic acid use in pregnancy.) For women who require valproate sodium during pregnancy and who are concerned about possible teratogenic effects, high-resolution ultrasound testing and the measurement of amniotic fluid or maternal serum alpha-fetoprotein concentrations may be used to detect fetal spina bifida prenatally. (*See* Folic Acid monograph.)

Anonymous. (1982). Valproate and malformations. [Editorial]. *The Lancet, 2*, 1313–1314.
Bantz, E. W. (1984). Valproic acid and congenital malformations. *Clinical Pediatrics, 23*, 352–355.
Bjerkedal, T., Czeizel, A., Goujard, J., et al. (1982). Valproic acid and spina bifida. *The Lancet, 2*, 1096, 1172.
Covanis, A., Gupta, A. K., & Jeavons, P. M. (1982). Sodium valproate: Monotherapy and polytherapy. *Epilepsia, 23*, 693–720.
Dickinson, R. G., Harland, R. C., Lynn, R. K., et al. (1979). Transmission of valproic acid (Depakene) across the placenta: Half-life of the drug in the mother and baby. *The Journal of Pediatrics, 94*, 832–835.
Jager-Roman, E., Deichl, A., Jakob, S., et al. (1986). Fetal growth, major malformations, and minor anomalies in infants born to women receiving valproic acid. *The Journal of Pediatrics, 108*, 997–1004.
Jeavons, P. M. (1982). Sodium valproate and neural tube defects. *The Lancet, 2*, 1282–1283.
Lammer, E. J., Sever, L. E., & Oakley, G. P. (1987). Teratogen update: Valproic acid. *Teratology, 35*, 465–473.
Lindhout, D., & Meinardi, H. (1984). Spina bifida and in-utero exposure to valproate. *The Lancet, 2*, 396.
Martinez-Frias, M. L. (1990). Clinical manifestation of prenatal exposure to valproic acid using case reports and epidemiologic information. *American Journal of Medical Genetics, 37*, 277–282.
Mastroiacovo, P., Bertollini, R., Morandini, S., et al. (1983). Maternal epilepsy, valproate exposure, and birth defects. *The Lancet, 2*, 1499.
Nakane, Y., Okuma, R., Takahashi, R., et al. (1980). Multi-institutional study on the teratogenicity and fetal toxicity of antiepileptic drugs: A report of a collaborative study group in Japan. *Epilepsia, 21*, 663–680.
Nau, H., & Hendrick, A. G. (1987). Valproic acid teratogenesis. *ISI Atlas of Science: Pharmacology, 49*, 52–56.
Omtzigt, J. G. C., Los, F. J., Grobbee, D. E., et al. (1992). The risk of spina bifida aperta after first-trimester exposure to valproate in a prenatal cohort. *Neurology, 42*(Suppl 5), 119–125.
Omtzigt, J. G. C., Nau, H., Los, F. J., et al. (1992). The disposition of valproate and its metabolites in the late first trimester and early second trimester of pregnancy in maternal serum, urine, and amniotic fluid: Effect of dose, co-medication, and the presence of spina bifida. *European Journal of Clinical Pharmacology, 43*, 381–388.
Robert, E., & Guibaud, P. (1982). Maternal valproic acid and congenital neural tube defect. *The Lancet, 2*, 937.
Robert, E., Lofkvist, E., & Mauguiere, F. (1984). Valproate and spina bifida. *The Lancet, 2*, 1392.
Rodriguez-Pinilla, E., Arroyo, I., Fondevilla, J., et al. (2000). *American Journal of Medical Genetics, 90*, 376–381.
Samren, E. B., van Duijn, C. M., Koch, S., et al. (1997). Maternal use of antiepileptic drugs and the risk of major congenital malformations: A joint European prospective study of human teratogenesis associated with maternal epilepsy. *Epilepsia, 38*(9), 981–990.
Serville, F., Carles, D., Guibaud, S., et al. (1989). Fetal valproate phenotype is recognisable by mid pregnancy. *Journal of Medical Genetics, 26*, 348–349.
Tein, I., & MacGregor, D. L. (1985). Possible valproate teratogenicity. *Archives of Neurology, 42*, 291–293.
Weinbaum, P. J., Cassidy, S. B., Ventzileos, A. M., et al. (1986). Prenatal detection of a neural tube defect after fetal exposure to valproic acid. *Obstetrics and Gynecology, 67*, 31S–33S.

Verapamil

FDA: **C** SIGNIFICANCE: **4** POTENCY: **3–4**

Verapamil has been used for acute and chronic management of maternal cardiac dysrhythmias during pregnancy. It also is used alone or in combination with other antidysrhythmics to treat fetal cardiac dysrhythmias during the second and third trimesters and has been used in combination with other tocolytics. Teratogenic effects have not been reported.

Barbillon, A., Grand, A., & Gerbaux, A. (1974). Treatment of the heart during pregnancy. *Annales de Medecine Interne (Paris), 125,* 437–445.

Carstensen, M. H., Bahnsen, J., & Sterzing, E. (1983). Tocolysis with beta-sympathomimetics alone or combined with the calcium antagonist verapamil. *Geburtshilfe und Frauenheilkunde, 43,* 481–485.

Gembruch, U., Hansmann, M., & Bald, R. (1988). Direct intrauterine fetal treatment of fetal tachyarrhythmia with severe hydrops fetalis by antiarrhythmic drugs. *Fetal Therapy, 3,* 210–215.

Gummerus, M. (1977). Treatment of premature labour and antagonization of the side effects of tocolytic therapy with verapamil. *Zeitschrift fur Geburtshilfe und Perinatologie, 181,* 334–340.

Klein, V., & Repke, J. T. (1984). Supraventricular tachycardia in pregnancy: Cardioversion with verapamil. *Obstetrics and Gynecology, 63*(Suppl), 16S–18S.

Marlettini, M. G., Crippa, S., Morselli-Labate, A. M., et al. (1990). Randomized comparison of calcium antagonists and beta-blockers in the treatment of pregnancy-induced hypertension. *Current Therapeutic Research, Clinical and Experimental, 48*(40), 684–692.

Orlandi, C., Marlettini, M. G., Cassani, A., et al. (1986). Treatment of hypertension during pregnancy with the calcium antagonist verapamil. *Current Therapeutic Research, 39*(6), 884–893.

Rotmensch, H. H., Elkayam, U., & Frischman, W. (1983). Antiarrhythmic drug therapy during pregnancy. *Annals of Internal Medicine, 98,* 487–497.

Wladimiroff, J. W., & Stewart, P. A. (1985). Treatment of fetal cardiac arrhythmias. *British Journal of Hospital Medicine, 34,* 134–140.

Wolff, F., Breuker, K. H., Schlencker, K. H., et al. (1980). Prenatal diagnosis and therapy of fetal heart rate anomalies: With a contribution on the placental transfer of verapamil. *Journal of Perinatal Medicine, 8,* 203–208.

Vinblastine

FDA: **D**   SIGNIFICANCE: **3–4**   POTENCY: **2–3**

There have been 21 reported cases of women receiving vinblastine during the first trimester (sometimes in combination with other antineoplastics), with no teratogenic effects. More data are needed.

Armstrong, J. G., Dyke, R. W., Fouts, P. J., et al. (1964). Delivery of a normal infant during the course of oral vinblastine sulfate therapy for Hodgkin's disease. *Annals of Internal Medicine, 61,* 106.

Aviles, A., Diaz-Maqueo, J. C., Talavera, A., et al. (1991). Growth and development of children of mothers treated with chemotherapy during pregnancy: Current status of 43 children. *American Journal of Hematology, 36,* 243–248.

Christman, J. E., Teng, N. N. H., Debovic, G. S., et al. (1990). Delivery of a normal infant following cisplatin, vinblastine, and bleomycin (PVB) chemotherapy for malignant teratoma of the ovary during pregnancy. *Gynecologic Oncology, 37,* 292–295.

Goguel, A. (1970). Hodgkin's disease and pregnancy. *La Presse Medicale, 78,* 1507–1510.

Lacher, M. J., & Geller, W. (1966). Cyclophosphamide and vinblastine sulfate in Hodgkin's disease during pregnancy. *Journal of the American Medical Association, 195*(6), 192–194.

Vincristine

FDA: **D**   SIGNIFICANCE: **3**   POTENCY: **3**

There is one case report of an infant with small malpositioned kidneys associated with in utero exposure to vincristine. More data are needed.

Mennuti, M. T., Shepard, R. H., & Mellman, W. J. (1974). Fetal renal malformation following treatment of Hodgkin's disease during pregnancy. *Obstetrics and Gynecology, 46,* 194–196.

Vitamin A

FDA: **C**   SIGNIFICANCE: **2–3**   POTENCY: **2–3**

Hypervitaminosis A is a known animal teratogen. The human data are far less clear, and associated teratogenic effects may be dependent on dose. The vitamin A analog, isotretinoin, is clearly a human teratogen (*see* Isotretinoin monograph). There are two cases of urinary tract anomalies associated with vitamin A intake. In another study, neonates with spina bifida were born to women who had elevated vitamin A serum levels. An increased risk for cranial neural crest defects and cardiac and craniofacial malformations also has been reported, but the role of vitamin A is unclear. More data are needed.

Bernhardt, I. B., & Dorsey, D. J. (1974). Hypervitaminosis A and congenital renal anomalies in a human infant. *Obstetrics and Gynecology, 43,* 750.

Collins, M. D., & Mao, G. E. (1999). Teratology of retinoids. *Annual Review of Pharmacology and Toxicology, 39,* 399–430.

Gal, L., Sharman, I. M., & Pryse-Davies, J. (1972). Vitamin A in relation to human congenital malformations. In *Advances in teratology, Vol. 5,* D. H. M. Woolman, Ed., New York: Academic.

Geelen, J. A. (1979). Hypervitaminosis A induced

teratogenesis. *CRC Critical Reviews in Toxicology, 6*(4), 351–375.

Miller, R. K., Hendrickx, A. G., Mills, J. L., et al. (1990). Periconceptional vitamin A use: How much is teratogenic? *Reproductive Toxicology, 12*(1), 75–88.

Monga, M. (1997). Vitamin A and its congeners. *Seminars in Perinatology, 21*(2), 135–142.

Pilotti, G. (1975). Hypervitaminosi A in gravidanzi e malformazioni neonatal dell'apparato urinario. *Minerva Ginecologica, 17*, 1103.

Vitamin A in pregnancy warning. (1990). *The Pharmaceutical Journal, 245*, 562.

Werler, M. M., Lammer, E. J., Rosenberg, L., et al. (1990). Maternal vitamin A supplementation in relation to selected birth defects. *Teratology, 42*, 497–503.

Vitamin D (Cholecalciferol)

AUTHOR: ● **SIGNIFICANCE:** 3–4
POTENCY: 3

In one study, excessive maternal vitamin D use was correlated with the incidence of neonate supravalvular aortic stenosis and neonatal hypercalcemia. However, in another study in which vitamin D was used to manage maternal hypoparathyroidism, no effect on the offspring was noted. More data are needed.

Friedman, W. F. (1968). Vitamin D and the supravalvular aortic stenosis syndrome. *Advances in Teratology, 3*, 85.

Goodenday, L. S., & Gordon, G. S. (1971). No risk from vitamin D in pregnancy. *Annals of Internal Medicine, 75*, 807–808.

Warfarin

FDA: D **SIGNIFICANCE:** 1 **POTENCY:** 1

The first report of teratogenesis involving an infant born to a woman who had received warfarin during pregnancy was in 1966, but it was not until 1976 that sufficient reports accumulated to define a fetal warfarin syndrome (warfarin embryopathy). Warfarin primarily produces midline defects and other defects that include absent nasal septum, bone stippling, cerebral agenesis, choana stenosis, delayed development, hydrocephalus, hypotonia, mental retardation, microphthalmia, midface hypoplasia, nasal hypoplasia, optic atrophy, punctuate skeletal lesions, seizures, short-broad hands, short femur and humerus, and simian creases. Exposure during the first trimester is associated with mental retardation, nasal hypoplasia, and the Conradi-Hunerman chondrodysplasia punctata syndrome. Second and third trimester exposure is associated with mental retardation, microcephaly, and optic atrophy. Maternal warfarin use during pregnancy also is associated with an increased risk for cerebral microbleeding and intraventricular hemorrhage, which may precede other signs and symptoms. Whenever possible, warfarin should be replaced by heparin in women who require an anticoagulant during pregnancy. (*See* Heparin monograph.)

Astedt, B. (1995). Antenatal drugs affecting vitamin K status of the fetus and the newborn. *Seminars in Thrombosis and Hemostasis, 21*(4), 364–370.

Baillie, M., Allen, E. D., & Elkington, A. R. (1980). The congenital warfarin syndrome: A case report. *British Journal of Ophthalmology, 64*, 633–635.

Bloomfield, D. K. (1970). Fetal deaths and malformations associated with the use of coumarin derivatives in pregnancy. *American Journal of Obstetrics and Gynecology, 107*, 883–888.

Buyse, E. G., Wermagoor, B. H., Bernard, J. T., et al. (1974). Anticoagulant therapy of patients with repeated placental infarction. *Obstetrics and Gynecology, 43*, 844.

DiSaia, P. J. (1966). Pregnancy and delivery of a patient with a Starr-Edwards mitral valve prosthesis. *Obstetrics and Gynecology, 28*, 469–472.

Golbus, M. S. (1980). Teratology for the obstetrician. Current status. *Obstetrics and Gynecology, 55*, 269–277.

Hall, J. G., Pauli, R. M., & Wilson, K. M. (1980). Maternal and fetal sequelae of anticoagulation during pregnancy. *American Journal of Medicine, 68*, 122–140.

Harrod, M. J., & Sherrod, P. S. (1981). Warfarin embryopathy in siblings. *Obstetrics and Gynecology, 57*(5), 673–676.

Hirsh, J., Cade, J. F., & O'Sullivan, E. F. (1970). Clinical experience with anticoagulant therapy during pregnancy. *British Medical Journal, 1*, 270.

Holzgreve, W., Carey, J. C., & Hall, B. P. (1976). Warfarin induced fetal abnormalities. *The Lancet, 2*, 914.

LaMontagne, J. M., LeClerc, J. E., Carrier, C., et al. (1984). Warfarin embryopathy–A case report. *The Journal of Otolaryngology, 13*, 127–129.

Pauli, R. M., Modden, J. D., Krangler, K. J., et al. (1976). Warfarin therapy initiated during pregnancy and phenotypic chondrodysplasia punctata. *The Journal of Pediatrics, 88*, 506–508.

Pettifor, J. M., & Benson, R. (1975). Congenital malformations associated with the administration of oral anticoagulants during pregnancy. *The Journal of Pediatrics, 86*, 459–462.

Richman, E. M., & Tahman, J. E. (1976). Fetal anomalies associated with warfarin therapy initiated shortly prior to conception. *The Journal of Pediatrics, 88*, 509–510.

Shaul, W. L., Emery, H., & Hall, J. G. (1975). Chondrodysplasia punctata and maternal warfarin use during pregnancy. *American Journal of Diseases of Children, 129*, 360–362.

Stevenson, R. E. (1980). Hazards of oral anticoagulants during pregnancy. *Journal of the American Medical Association, 243*(15), 1549–1551.

Use of anticoagulants in pregnancy. (1987). *Drug and Therapeutics Bulletin, 25*(1), 1–4.

Warkany, J. (1975). A warfarin embryopathy? *American Journal of Diseases of Children, 129*, 287–288.

Zakzouk, M. S. (1986). The congenital warfarin syndrome. *Journal of Laryngology and Otology, 100*, 215–219.

Yellow Fever Vaccine

FDA: C   SIGNIFICANCE: 4–5   POTENCY: 4

No teratogenic effects related to the administration of yellow fever vaccine during pregnancy have been reported. Yellow fever vaccine may be given to women at any time during pregnancy. Whenever possible, it is recommended that it be given after the first trimester to minimize any theoretical risk of teratogenesis. More data are needed.

Hart, R. J. (1981). Immunizations. *Clinical Obstetrics and Gynecology, 8*, 421–430.

Levine, M. M., Edsall, G., & Bruce-Chwatt, L. J. (1974). Live virus vaccines in pregnancy: Risks and recommendations. *The Lancet, 2*, 34–38.

Zidovudine

FDA: C   SIGNIFICANCE: 3–4   POTENCY: 2–3

More than 10,000 babies are born annually in North America to women who are HIV positive. The use of zidovudine and similar antiretroviral drugs can significantly reduce the rate of perinatal transmission (mother to neonate) of HIV. Published data on the potential teratogenic and fetotoxic effects of zidovudine are mixed. Two small retrospective studies (n <10) found risk for mitochondrial dysfunction to be greater among infants exposed to zidovudine in utero. Several other studies (n >250) failed to find a significant increase in congenital anomalies, premature birth, or fetotoxicity among neonates exposed in utero to zidovudine. Data implicating zidovudine as teratogenic or fetotoxic are difficult to interpret because of several confounding variables, including maternal multiple-drug therapy during pregnancy and the reported propensity for HIV-infected women to give birth to a greater number of infants with major congenital anomalies when compared to non-HIV-infected women.

Birth outcomes following zidovudine therapy in pregnant women. *Morbidity and Mortality Weekly Report, 43*(22), 409, 415–416.

Blanche, S., Tardieu, M., Rustin, P., et al. (1999). Persistent mitochondrial dysfunction and perinatal exposure to antiretroviral nucleoside analogues. *The Lancet, 354*(9184), 1084–1089.

Hernandez-Diaz, S., Werler, M. M., Walker, A. M., et al. (2000). Folic acid antagonists during pregnancy and the risk of birth defects. *New England Journal of Medicine, 343*(22), 1608–1614.

Kumar, R. M., Hughes, P. F., & Khurranna, A. (1994). Zidovudine use in pregnancy: A report on 104 cases and the occurrence of birth defects. *Journal of Acquired Immune Deficiency Syndrome, 7*(10), 1034–1039.

Lambie, D. G., & Johnson, R. H. (1985). Drugs and folate metabolism. *Drugs, 30*(2), 145–155.

Newschaffer, C. J., Cocroft, J., Anderson, C. E., et al. (2000). Prenatal zidovudine use and congenital anomalies in a Medicaid population. *Journal of Acquired Immune Deficiency Syndrome, 24*(3), 249–256.

Sperling, R. S., Stratton, P., O'Sullivan, M. J., et al. (1992). A survey of zidovudine use in pregnant women with human immunodeficiency virus infection. *New England Journal of Medicine, 326*(13), 857–861.

White, A., Eldridge, R., & Andrews, E. (1997). Birth outcomes following zidovudine exposure in pregnant women: The Antiretroviral Pregnancy Registry. *Acta Paediatrica Supplement, 421*, 86–88.

Zopiclone

AUTHOR: NONE   SIGNIFICANCE: 3–4   POTENCY: 2–3

A prospective Canadian matched-cohort study of 40 women who used zopiclone during the first trimester found no increase in the rate of major malformations. More data are needed, particularly data on use during the later trimesters.

Diav-Citrin, O., Okotore, B., Lucarelli, K., et al. (1999). Pregnancy outcome following first-trimester exposure to zopiclone: A prospective controlled cohort study. *American Journal of Perinatology, 16*, 157–160.

3

Drugs Excreted in Human Breast Milk

Neeta Bahal O'Mara and Milap C. Nahata

Breast milk generally is considered to be the best source of nutrition for infants during the first 4–6 months after birth. It is economical, safe, and an effective method for preventing illnesses through passive immunity; in fact, more than 60% of North American women breast feed (O'Mara & Nahata, 1995). However, many of these women require drug therapy for medical or psychological disorders. Other women may use various drugs and substances (e.g., alcoholic beverages, coffee or tea, natural health products). Unfortunately, these women may inadvertently expose their infants to the effects of these drugs and substances through their breast milk. In fact, it is estimated that women receive an average of seven drugs during labor and delivery, and that 90%–99% of mothers who choose to breast feed receive at least one drug during the first postpartum week (O'Mara & Nahata, 1995). While there is only limited information regarding the excretion of drugs in breast milk, there is even less information about the excretion of other substances in breast milk, particularly herbal and other natural health products. However, where available, data have been included in Table 3-1.

Not only may maternal drug or substance use affect breast-fed infants, lactation itself may be affected. For example, some drugs can inhibit lactation (e.g., bromocriptine), while others (e.g., metoclopramide, phenothiazines) can stimulate lactation. Thus, a number of questions must be considered by clinicians when discussing the use of drugs (e.g., whether to initiate therapy) or other substances (e.g., drinking alcoholic beverages, using herbal remedies) with women who are lactating. These questions include:

1. Is the drug or substance necessary?
2. Is there a safer alternative drug, substance, or therapy?
3. How does the drug or substance affect lactation?
4. How much of the dose of the drug or substance is excreted in breast milk?
5. How much of the drug or substance excreted in breast milk is absorbed by the breast-fed neonate or infant through breast feeding?
6. Once absorbed, can the neonate or infant eliminate the drug or substance efficiently?
7. What adverse drug reactions (ADRs) can be expected to occur among breast-fed neonates and infants?
8. What can be done to prevent or minimize a neonate's or infant's exposure to the drug or substance through breast feeding? For example, is the mother using the lowest effective dose? Can the timing of maternal drug use or breast

feeding be modified? Can breast feeding be discontinued temporarily, lactation maintained, and breast feeding resumed when the drug or substance is no longer required?

Knowledge of the pharmacokinetics of a particular drug or substance can assist clinicians to answer these questions and enable them to provide optimal drug therapy to women who are breast feeding. *See* Chapter 10 for additional discussion.

Absorption

During early infancy, an infant fed exclusively breast milk typically consumes approximately 150 ml/kg/day. As the infant matures and begins to receive supplemental food, the amount of breast milk consumed per kilogram of body weight decreases. Consequently, exposure to the drug or substance declines as the amount of breast milk ingested declines. The amount of a drug or substance that passes into the breast milk can be influenced by several factors, including its molecular weight, protein binding, pH and degree of ionization, and lipid solubility (O'Mara & Nahata, 1995). Drugs and substances that have large molecular weights (heparin, epinephrine, certain penicillins, cephalosporins) often are absorbed poorly from the GI tract. Thus, their absorption by a breast-fed infant is likely to be minimal.

Metabolism and Excretion

Careful consideration must be given to the metabolism and excretion of a drug or substance absorbed through breast feeding. Absorption by an infant of even small amounts of a drug or substance taken repeatedly by the mother can result in drug accumulation because of immature hepatic function (immature mechanisms of drug metabolism involving acetylation, oxidation, and glucuronidation) and renal function.

Unfortunately, availability of data on excretion of drugs and substances in breast milk is limited. Table 3-1 summarizes available data. Drugs and commonly used substances (alcohol, nicotine) are listed alphabetically by generic name. This table provides, when reported, the number of infants studied, the effect of the drug (**"not reported"** means that the article did not indicate whether there was an effect or that the infant was not breast fed, and **"none reported"** indicates that there was no detectable effect on the breast-fed infant), dose received by the mother and route of administration, the concentration of the drug or substance in the breast milk, the timing of the milk sample with respect to dosing, and original references.

The authors' evaluation of the data and the clinical significance of maternal drug or substance use for a breast-fed infant is provided **(0 = unlikely to be significant, + = possibly significant, ++ = probably significant, +++ = contraindicated)**. The distinction between "0" and "+" is somewhat arbitrary because, although the drug is often detected in breast milk, the clinical significance is unclear. For drugs or substances with a rating of ++, the risks and benefits of maternal drug or substance use to the mother and the breast-fed infant should be considered. Finally, for drugs with a rating of +++, breast feeding should be avoided or discontinued. For short-term use, lactation may be maintained and breast feeding resumed following the discontinuation of the drug. Lack of inclusion of a particular drug in the table does not indicate that the drug or substance is safe for breast-fed infants.

TABLE 3-1
Drugs Excreted in Human Breast Milk

DRUG[a]	NUMBER OF INFANTS	EFFECT ON INFANTS	MATERNAL DOSE	ROUTE	CONCENTRATION OF DRUG IN BREAST MILK	TIME AFTER MATERNAL DOSE	SIGNIFICANCE[b]	REFERENCE[c]
Acebutolol	3	Bradycardia, hypotension, tachypnea in one infant	200–1200 mg/day	PO	286–1545 ng/ml 4123 ng/ml	Before dose 1.5 hr after 400-mg dose	0	Boutroy 1986

- Concentration of metabolite (diacetolol) in milk is 2.3–24.7 times plasma concentration. Acebutol and diacetolol detectable up to 72 hr after discontinuation. Increased risk when dose exceeds 400 mg/day or when mother's renal function is diminished.

Acenocoumarol	20	None reported	4 mg as one-time dose, then 2 mg/day	PO	Not detected	1–10 hr	0	Houwert-de Jong 1981

- Drug not detectable in milk. Clotting times normal in breast-fed infants.

Acetaminophen	12	None reported	650 mg	PO	10–15 µg/ml	1–2 hr	0	Berlin 1980a
	3	None reported	500 mg	PO	4–4.4 µg/ml	2 hr		Bitzen 1981
	1	None reported	324 mg	PO	0.89 µg/ml	1–12 hr		Findlay 1981
	4	None reported	1000 mg	PO	2–14 µg/ml	1–3 hr		Notarianni 1987

- Maternal ingestion of usual doses unlikely to produce ADRs in breast-fed infants.

Acetazolamide	1	None reported	500 mg	PO	1.3–2.1 µg/ml	1–9 hr	0	Soderman 1984

- Small amounts excreted in milk. Unlikely to produce ADRs in breast-fed infants.

Acyclovir	1	None reported	200 mg every 3 hr	PO	0.43 µg/ml 1.31 µg/ml	0.5 hr 3.2 hr	0	Lau 1987
	1	None reported	200 mg five times a day	PO	0.78–1.26 µg/ml	4.25–5.5 hr		Meyer 1988
	1	None reported	800 mg five times a day	PO	4.16–5.81 µg/ml	1–9.5 hr		Taddio 1994

- Lag phase before peak concentration of acyclovir in milk occurs. Infants would receive 1–2 mg/day of acyclovir with typical oral maternal doses (Anderson, 1991). Still detectable in milk 48 hr after dose. Topical acyclovir applied to small areas of the mother's body should be safe (Anderson, 1991).

Alcohol (Ethanol)	1	Pseudo-Cushing syndrome	50 12-oz beers/week and other alcoholic beverages	PO	100 mg/dl	Not reported	++	Biniewicz 1978
	40	Dose-dependent inhibition of milk ejection reflex	0.1–2 grams/kg	PO	Not measured			Cobo 1973
	12	None when used in moderation by mother	0.6 gram/kg	PO	78 mg/dl	1 hr		Kesaniemi 1974
	8	None reported	0.75–1.5 grams/kg	PO	22–129 mg/dl	1–2 hr		Lawton 1985
	12	Lower than normal milk consumption	0.3 gram/kg	PO	0–32 mg/dl	0–3 hr		Mennella 1991

- Odor of milk altered and amount of milk ingested lower than normal after alcohol consumption (Mennella & Beauchamp, 1991). May affect motor development (Little et al., 1989). Maternal doses of alcohol exceeding 1 gram/kg may block the milk ejection reflex (Kacew, 1993).

Allopurinol	1	None reported	300 mg/day	PO	1.4 µg/ml	2–4 hr	+	Kamilli 1993

- Allopurinol and its active metabolite, oxypurinol, detected in milk. Oxypurinol detected in infant's plasma. No hypersensitivity signs and symptoms or changes in blood chemistry or hematology noted in infant.

Aloin	33	Increased bowel activity in 11 of 33 infants	15 mg aloin	PO	Detectable in small quantities	15-ml milk samples taken every 4 hr, collected, and pooled	++	Tyson 1937

- In usual doses, unlikely to produce ADRs in breast-fed infants, but higher doses may result in increased bowel activity.

---

[a] Drugs are listed in alphabetical order by generic name. Clinicians who use trade or brand names should consult the index.
[b] 0 = unlikely to be significant, + = possibly significant, ++ = probably significant, +++ = contraindicated.
[c] Only the first author and year of publication are provided. For complete reference citation, see the References that follow.

TABLE 3-1 continued

DRUG[a]	NUMBER OF INFANTS	EFFECT ON INFANTS	MATERNAL DOSE	ROUTE	CONCENTRATION OF DRUG IN BREAST MILK	TIME AFTER MATERNAL DOSE	SIGNIFI-CANCE[b]	REFERENCE[c]
Alprazolam	1	Restlessness, irritability, episodic screaming, crying, jerking, movements of extremities	0.5 mg bid or tid	PO	Not measured		++	Anderson 1989
	8	Not reported	0.5 mg	PO	3.7 ng/ml	1.1 hr		Oo 1995b

- Effects noted for 2–3 days following discontinuation of breast feeding; signs and symptoms thought to be associated with the alprazolam-withdrawal syndrome. Other benzodiazepines known to be excreted in milk. If a benzodiazepine is necessary, use of a short-acting one such as lorazepam or oxazepam is preferred.

| Aminosalicylic Acid (para-Aminosalicylic Acid) | 2 | None reported | 4 grams | PO | 1.1 mg/liter | 3 hr | 0 | Holdiness 1984 |

- Concentration in milk below therapeutic range. Probably safe for breast-fed infants.

Amiodarone	1	None reported	400 mg/day	PO	Amiodarone 2.8–16.4 mg/liter Desethylamiodarone 1.1–6.5 mg/liter	Various times	+++	McKenna 1983b
	1	None reported	Not reported	PO	Amiodarone 0.5–1.8 mg/liter Desethylamiodarone 0.4–0.8 mg/liter	Not reported		Pitcher 1983
	2	Not reported	200 mg/day	PO	1.7–3 mg/liter	Not reported		Plomp 1992

- Wide variation in amiodarone and desethylamiodarone concentrations in milk throughout the day. One infant had amiodarone serum concentrations of 0.1 μg/ml. After discontinuation of amiodarone, detectable concentrations noted 4 weeks later (Plomp et al., 1992). Estimated ingestion by the infant of 1.4–1.5 mg/kg/day is equivalent to low maintenance dosage for adult (McKenna et al., 1983b). Use of amiodarone for breast-feeding women should be avoided because of possible toxicity in breast-fed infants with long-term maternal use. Amiodarone 200 mg contains 75 mg iodine. The long half-life of amiodarone requires discontinuation for a considerable period to avoid exposure of infant during breast feeding.

Amitriptyline	1	None reported	100 mg	PO	135–151 ng/ml	14–16 hr	++	Bader 1980
	1	None reported	100 mg	PO	30–104 ng/ml	12–15 hr		Brixen-Rasmussen 1982
	1	None reported	175 mg/day	PO	42–71 ng/ml	Not reported		Breyer-Pfaff 1995

- Long-term effects unknown (American Academy of Pediatrics, 1994). Amitriptyline and its metabolite, E-10-hydroxynortriptyline, detected in breast milk, but not in infant's serum (Breyer-Pfaff et al., 1995).

| Amoxapine | 1 | None reported | 300 mg/day | PO | Amoxapine detectable (<20 ng/ml) 8-Hydroxyamoxapine 113–168 ng/ml | 0.75–11.5 hr | ++ | Gelenberg 1979 |

- Amoxapine and its active metabolite, 8-hydroxyamoxapine, detectable in milk. Long-term effects unknown (American Academy of Pediatrics, 1994).

| Amoxicillin | 6 | None reported | 1 gram | PO | 0.39–1.3 μg/ml | 4–5 hr | + | Kafetzis 1981 |

- Excreted in milk in low concentrations. Possibility of alteration in oropharyngeal flora and sensitization with subsequent hypersensitivity reaction. Monitor for candidiasis (e.g., oral thrush) and diarrhea.

| Amphetamine | 1 | None reported for up to 24 months | 5 mg qid | PO | 55–138 μg/ml | 4–16 hr | +++ | Steiner 1984 |

- Until effects on psychobehavioral development of breast-fed infants are known, amphetamine is contraindicated in breast-feeding women (American Academy of Pediatrics, 1994).

| Ampicillin | 14 | None reported | 350–700 mg tid | PO | 60–170 ng/ml | 1–5 hr | + | Branebjerg 1987 |

TABLE 3-1 continued

DRUG[a]	NUMBER OF INFANTS	EFFECT ON INFANTS	MATERNAL DOSE	ROUTE	CONCENTRATION OF DRUG IN BREAST MILK	TIME AFTER MATERNAL DOSE	SIGNIFI-CANCE[b]	REFERENCE[c]
Ampicillin continued	10	None reported	500 mg qid	PO	15–1670 ng/ml	2–6 hr		Campbell 1991
	2	None reported	500 mg every 6 hr	PO	14–1000 ng/ml	Not reported		Lohmeyer 1965
	6	None reported	270–540 mg tid or qid	PO	50–900 ng/ml	0.5–12 hr		Matheson 1988
	2	Not reported	500 mg	PO	0–200 ng/ml	1–6 hr		Matsuda 1984

- Considerable variation in reported concentrations in milk. Possibility of alteration in oropharyngeal flora and sensitization and subsequent hypersensitivity reaction. Monitor for candidiasis (e.g., oral thrush) and diarrhea.

DRUG	NUMBER OF INFANTS	EFFECT ON INFANTS	MATERNAL DOSE	ROUTE	CONCENTRATION	TIME	SIGNIF.	REFERENCE
Aspirin (Acetylsalicylic Acid)	10	None reported	650 mg	PO	17.3–48.3 mg/dl	5–8 hr	++	Berlin 1980a
	1	Metabolic acidosis	650 mg every 4 hr	PO	Not reported	Not reported		Clark 1981
	1	None reported	4000 mg/day	PO	18 mg/dl	Not reported		Erickson 1979
	2	None reported	450 mg	PO	0.11–0.17 mg/dl	3 hr		Findlay 1981
	6	None reported	500 mg / 1000 mg / 1500 mg	PO	0.58 mg/dl / 1.60 mg/dl / 3.87 mg/dl	2–4 hr		Jamali 1981
	8	None reported	300–1000 mg	PO	Less than plasma concentration	Peak at 3 hr		Putter 1975

- Variable amounts excreted in milk. In one case (Clark & Wilson, 1981), on third hospital day after exposure, infant's salicylate serum concentration was 24 mg/dl. Individual doses unlikely to cause ADRs in breast-fed infants. Chronic dosing may result in antiplatelet effect. Neonates eliminate salicylates slowly and have limited elimination capacity. May be contraindicated in mothers of infants with hematologic or clotting disorders. The risk of Reye's syndrome caused by salicylate in milk is unknown. Use with caution (American Academy of Pediatrics, 1994).

DRUG	N	EFFECT	DOSE	ROUTE	CONC	TIME	SIG	REF
Atenolol	4	None reported	100 mg	PO	293–2128 ng/ml	2–3 hr	++	Kulas 1984
	7	None reported	50–100 mg/day	PO	106–1676 ng/ml	Not reported		Liedholm 1981
	1	Cyanosis, bradycardia, poor perfusion	50 mg every 12 hr	PO	469 ng/ml	1.5 hr		Schmimmel 1989
	5	None reported	100 mg/day	PO	630 ng/ml	Not reported		Thorley 1983
	1	None reported	50 mg/day	PO	700–1600 ng/ml	4–12 hr		White 1984

- Concentration in milk variable. Infant atenolol serum concentration 2010 ng/ml 48 hr after breast feeding (Schmimmel et al., 1989). Others report negligible infant serum concentrations. Avoid breast feeding young infants when high maternal doses are necessary (Anderson, 1991).

DRUG	N	EFFECT	DOSE	ROUTE	CONC	TIME	SIG	REF
Atropine		May inhibit lactation or cause anticholinergic effects in breast-fed infants					++	O'Brien 1974; Rivera-Calimlim 1977; Wilson 1981

- There are conflicting reports without adequate documentation.

DRUG	N	EFFECT	DOSE	ROUTE	CONC	TIME	SIG	REF
Azithromycin	1	Not reported	500 mg/day	PO	1.3–2.8 µg/ml	1–30 hr	+	Kelsey 1994
Aztreonam	12	None reported	1 gram	IM or IV	0.2–0.3 µg/ml	2.4–6 hr	0	Fleiss 1985

- Concentrations in milk are low, and GI absorption is poor; unlikely to cause ADRs in breast-fed infants.

DRUG	N	EFFECT	DOSE	ROUTE	CONC	TIME	SIG	REF
Baclofen	1	Not reported	20 mg	PO	0.61 µmol/liter	4 hr	0	Eriksson 1981

- Only 1/1000 of dose excreted in milk in 24 hr.

DRUG	N	EFFECT	DOSE	ROUTE	CONC	TIME	SIG	REF
Bendroflume-thiazide	40	None reported	5 mg bid for 5 days	PO	Not measured		++	Reiher 1963

- Lactation suppressed in all subjects, most likely as a result of dehydration. Large maternal doses should be avoided. Unlikely to have an effect on breast-fed infant when mother does not experience dehydration (Drugs . . . , 1974; Healy, 1961).

DRUG	N	EFFECT	DOSE	ROUTE	CONC	TIME	SIG	REF
Bretylium	1	None reported	400 mg every 8 hr	PO	Not measured		+	Gutgesell 1990

- Limited data available. Excretion in milk and effects on breast-fed infants unknown.

DRUG	N	EFFECT	DOSE	ROUTE	CONC	TIME	SIG	REF
Bromocriptine	Not reported	None reported	2.5 mg bid or tid	PO	Not measured		+++	del Re 1973

- Contraindicated in breast-feeding women (American Academy of Pediatrics, 1994). Inhibits lactation. Used to suppress lactation during the postpartum period.

Footnotes are on page 203.

TABLE 3-1 continued

DRUG[a]	NUMBER OF INFANTS	EFFECT ON INFANTS	MATERNAL DOSE	ROUTE	CONCENTRATION OF DRUG IN BREAST MILK	TIME AFTER MATERNAL DOSE	SIGNIFI- CANCE[b]	REFERENCE[c]
Bupropion	1	None reported	100 mg	PO	0.189 µg/ml	2 hr	+	Briggs 1993

• Bupropion and its metabolite, threo-hydrobupropion, are not detected in infant's plasma.

Butabarbital	1	None reported	8 mg bid for seven doses	PO	370 ng/ml	1.5 hr	+	Horning 1975

• Small amounts excreted in milk. Unlikely to produce ADRs in breast-fed infants when taken daily by mother in small divided doses rather than as a single daily dose.

Butorphanol	12	Not reported	2 mg	IM	0.7–1.5 ng/ml	1–3 hr	0	Pittman 1980
			8 mg	PO	1.8–3.6 ng/ml	1–3 hr		

• Unlikely to cause ADRs in breast-fed infants because of low concentration in milk.

Caffeine	9	None reported	750 mg	PO	1.9–28.6 µg/ml	24-hr collection period	+	Ryu 1985
	6	None reported	100 mg	PO	1.2–4.3 µg/ml	0.75–2 hr		Stavchansky 1988
	5	Irritability	150–300 mg	PO	1.1–2.5 µg/ml	0.5–1 hr		Tyrala 1979

• Excreted in milk in trace amounts. Coffee consumption (>3 cups/day) may decrease iron concentrations in milk (Nehlig & Debry, 1994). Caffeine accumulation and prolonged half-life of caffeine in premature and term neonates possible.

Captopril	12	None reported	100 mg tid	PO	4.7 ng/ml	3.8 hr	0	Devlin 1981b

• Minute amounts (0.002% of maternal dose) excreted in milk.

Carbamazepine	1	Cholestatic hepatitis	600 mg/day	PO	Not measured		++	Frey 1990
	19	Poor sucking in one of 19 infants	7.1–24.6 mg/kg/day	PO	2.0–3.1 µg/ml	Not reported		Froescher 1984
	9	None reported	Not reported	PO	1.9 µg/ml	Not reported		Kaneko 1979
	11	None reported	11 mg/kg/day	PO	1.8 µg/ml	Not reported		Kuhnz 1983

• Metabolite (carbamazepine-epoxide) also detected in milk (Froescher et al., 1984). Infant steady-state carbamazepine serum concentration 1.0–4.7 µg/ml (Kuhnz et al., 1983). If poor sucking, sedation, or lethargy occurs in infant, milk intake should be reduced or breast feeding should be discontinued.

Carbimazole	1	Not reported	40 mg/day	PO	Methimazole 83–182 ng/ml	1–8 hr	++	Johansen 1982
	11	None reported	5–15 mg/day	PO	Not measured			Lamberg 1984
	1	None reported	30 mg/day	PO	Methimazole 0–92 ng/ml	Not reported		Rylance 1987

• See Methimazole entry in this table. Propylthiouracil should be used instead, if possible.

Carisoprodol	1	None reported	700 mg tid	PO	0.9 µg/ml carisoprodol and 11.6 µg/ml meprobamate	Before morning dose	++	Nordeng 2001

• Carisoprodol and its active metabolite, meprobamate, detected in breast milk. An exclusively breast-fed infant could receive ~1.9 mg/kg/day of carisoprodol.

Cascara	22	Increased bowel activity in 10 of 22 infants	4 ml fluidextract	PO	Five of 10 milk samples tested had detectable concentrations	24-hr pooled milk samples	+++	Tyson 1937

• May cause increased infant bowel activity with usual maternal doses. Use of cascara should be avoided in breast-feeding women.

Cefadroxil	6	Not reported	1 gram	PO	1.2–2.4 µg/ml	6–7 hr	+	Kafetzis 1981

• Unlikely to produce detectable serum concentrations in infants. Possibility of alteration in oropharyngeal flora and sensitization and subsequent hypersensitivity reaction. Monitor for candidiasis (e.g., oral thrush) and diarrhea.

Cefazolin	20	Not reported	2 grams	IV	1.16–1.51 µg/ml	2–4 hr	+	Yoshioka 1979

• Unlikely to produce detectable serum concentrations in breast-fed infants. Possibility of alteration in oropharyngeal flora and sensitization and subsequent hypersensitivity reaction. Monitor for candidiasis (e.g., oral thrush) and diarrhea.

Cefonicid	10	Not reported	1 gram	IM	Trace amounts–0.3 µg/ml	1 hr	+	Lou 1984

• Unlikely to produce detectable serum concentrations in breast-fed infants. Possibility of alteration in oropharyngeal flora and sensitization and subsequent hypersensitivity reaction. Monitor for candidiasis (e.g., oral thrush) and diarrhea.

TABLE 3-1 continued

DRUG[a]	NUMBER OF INFANTS	EFFECT ON INFANTS	MATERNAL DOSE	ROUTE	CONCENTRATION OF DRUG IN BREAST MILK	TIME AFTER MATERNAL DOSE	SIGNIFI- CANCE[b]	REFERENCE[c]
Cefotaxime	12	Not reported	1 gram	IV	0.25–0.52 µg/ml	2–3 hr	+	Kafetzis 1980
	2	Not reported	1 gram	IV	0 trace amounts	1–6 hr		Matsuda 1984

• Unlikely to produce detectable serum concentrations in infants. Possibility of alteration in oropharyngeal flora and sensitization and subsequent hypersensitivity reaction. Monitor for candidiasis (e.g., oral thrush) and diarrhea.

Cefprozil	9	Not reported	1000-mg single dose	PO	0.3–3.4 µg/ml	2–24 hr	+	Shyu 1992

• Peak occurs at about 6 hr, but cefprozil detectable in milk throughout 24-hr interval. Possibility of alteration in oropharyngeal flora and sensitization and subsequent hypersensitivity reaction. Monitor for candidiasis (e.g., oral thrush) and diarrhea.

Ceftazidime	11	Not reported	2 grams every 8 hr for 5 days	IV	5.2 µg/ml 3.8 µg/ml	1 hr 8 hr (trough)	+	Blanco 1983

• Unlikely to produce detectable serum concentrations in infants. Possibility of alteration in oropharyngeal flora and sensitization and subsequent hypersensitivity reaction. Monitor for candidiasis (e.g., oral thrush) and diarrhea.

Ceftriaxone	20	Not reported	1 gram	IM or IV	0.2–0.6 µg/ml	4–24 hr	+	Kafetzis 1983
	1	None reported	2 grams/day	IV	1.61–7.89 µg/ml	1–24 hr (on day 7)	+	Bourget 1993

• Unlikely to produce detectable serum concentrations in infants. Possibility of alteration in oropharyngeal flora and sensitization and subsequent hypersensitivity reaction. Monitor for candidiasis (e.g., oral thrush) and diarrhea.

Cephalexin	6	Not reported	1 gram	PO	0.24–0.85 µg/ml	4–5 hr	+	Kafetzis 1981
	2	Not reported	500 mg	PO	Trace amounts– 0.8 µg/ml	1–6 hr		Matsuda 1984

• Unlikely to produce detectable serum concentrations in infants. Possibility of alteration in oropharyngeal flora and sensitization and subsequent hypersensitivity reaction. Monitor for candidiasis (e.g., oral thrush) and diarrhea.

Cephalothin	6	Not reported	1 gram	IV	0.36–0.62 µg/ml	1–2 hr	+	Kafetzis 1981

• Unlikely to produce detectable serum concentrations in infants. Possibility of alteration in oropharyngeal flora and sensitization and subsequent hypersensitivity reaction. Monitor for candidiasis (e.g., oral thrush) and diarrhea.

Cephradine	12	Not reported	500 mg every 6 hr for 2 days	PO	0.68 µg/ml	1 hr	+	Mischler 1978

• Unlikely to produce detectable serum concentrations in infants. Possibility of alteration in oropharyngeal flora and sensitization and subsequent hypersensitivity reaction. Monitor for candidiasis (e.g., oral thrush) and diarrhea.

Chloral Hydrate	50	None reported	1.33 grams	Rectal	100 µg/ml (50%– 100% of blood concentration)	Not reported	+++	Bernstine 1956
	1	Drowsiness	Hypnotic dose	PO	Not measured			Lacey 1971

• Both chloral hydrate and its active metabolite, trichloroethanol, are detectable in milk for up to 24 hr after an individual dose. Infant may receive sedative dose if breast fed when milk concentration is at its peak.

Chlor- amphenicol	1	Refusal of breast, falling asleep during feeding, vomiting after feeding	Not reported	PO	16 and 25 µg/ml (50% of maternal serum concentration)	Not reported	+++	Havelka 1968
	10	None reported	250–500 mg every 6 hr for 7–10 days	PO	0.26–3.5 µg/ml	During second day		Havelka 1972

• Measured milk concentrations may be twice the actual chloramphenicol concentration because some assays measure chloramphenicol and its inactive metabolite. Milk concentrations are not sufficient to cause gray baby syndrome, but there is a theoretical risk of bone marrow suppression (American Academy of Pediatrics, 1994). Avoid breast feeding during chloramphenicol therapy.

Chloroquine	1	Not reported	600 mg	PO	Not reported	Not reported	+	Edstein 1986
	5	Not reported	300 mg	PO	3.97 µg/ml	3.1 hr		Ette 1987
	11	None reported	600 mg	PO	4.4 µg/ml	14.4 hr		Ogunbona 1987

• Chloroquine milk concentrations are greater than maternal plasma concentrations (Edstein et al., 1986). Small amounts of chloroquine and even smaller amounts of its metabolite, desethylchloroquine, may be ingested by breast-fed infants. Unlikely to produce ADRs. Low plasma concentrations in infants may promote development of drug-resistant strains of malaria.

Chlorothiazide	11	Not reported	500 mg	PO	<1 µg/ml	1–3 hr	+	Werthmann 1972

• Small quantities excreted in milk. Unlikely to produce ADRs in breast-fed infants unless mother becomes dehydrated.

Footnotes are on page 203.

TABLE 3-1 continued

DRUG[a]	NUMBER OF INFANTS	EFFECT ON INFANTS	MATERNAL DOSE	ROUTE	CONCENTRATION OF DRUG IN BREAST MILK	TIME AFTER MATERNAL DOSE	SIGNIFI-CANCE[b]	REFERENCE[c]
Chlor-promazine	1	Not reported	1200 mg	PO	290 ng/ml	2 hr	++	Ayd 1973
	4	Lethargy, drowsiness in one of two breast-fed infants	Not reported	PO	7–98 ng/ml	Not reported		Wiles 1978

- Chlorpromazine and its metabolites detected in milk samples. Monitor for drowsiness and lethargy. Long-term effects unknown (American Academy of Pediatrics, 1994).

| Chlorthalidone | 9 | Not reported | 50 mg/day | PO | 0.09–0.86 µg/ml | Not reported | ++ | Mulley 1978 |

- Half-life in adults is ~60 hr. Elimination in breast-fed infants may be delayed, resulting in accumulation. Discontinuation is recommended prior to the initiation of breast feeding.

Cimetidine	1	Not reported	400 mg as one-time dose or three 200-mg doses	PO	4.8–6.0 µg/ml	Not reported	++	Somogyi 1979
	12	Not reported	100 mg	PO	Average 0.7 µg/ml	Not reported		Oo 1995a
			600 mg	PO	Average 4.2 µg/ml	Not reported		
			1200 mg	PO	Average 9.6 µg/ml	Not reported		

- Milk concentrations remain elevated with chronic dosing. Caution during breast feeding is advised. Peak cimetidine concentration occurs at about 3 hr (Oo et al., 1995a). Alternative drugs (e.g., famotidine, nizatidine, sucralfate) should be considered.

Ciprofloxacin	1	Not reported	500 mg	PO	2.0–3.0 µg/ml	4–16 hr	++	Cover 1990
	10	Not reported	750 mg every 12 hr for three doses	PO	2.26–3.79 µg/ml	2–4 hr		Giamarellou 1989
	1	None reported	500 mg/day	PO	0.98 µg/ml	10.5 hr		Gardner 1992

- Highly concentrated in milk. Bioavailability of ciprofloxacin in infant may be reduced due to concomitant milk ingestion (i.e., calcium–ciprofloxacin binding drug interaction) (Fleiss, 1992). Clinical significance unknown.

| Cisplatin | 1 | Not reported | 100 mg/m² over 26 hr | IV | Not detected | 0.25–71.25 hr | + | Egan 1985 |

- Limited data available.

| Citalopram | 1 | Uneasy sleep | 40 mg/day | PO | 205 ng/ml | Not reported | ++ | Schmidt 2000 |

- Citalopram detected in infant's serum. Infant's sleep normalized after citalopram dose reduction in mother and decreased breast milk ingestion. Long-term effects unknown.

| Clemastine | 1 | Drowsiness, irritability, refusal to feed, high-pitched cry, neck stiffness | 1 mg bid | PO | 5–10 µg/liter | 20 hr | ++ | Kok 1982 |

- Mother also received chronic phenytoin and carbamazepine. Signs and symptoms developed in infant after initiation of clemastine. Clemastine detected in initial milk sample, but not after effects in infant resolved. Use with caution (American Academy of Pediatrics, 1994).

Clindamycin	1	Bloody diarrhea	600 mg every 8 hr	IV	Not measured		++	Mann 1980
	2	Not reported	600 mg every 6 hr	IV	2.1–3.8 µg/ml	2–4 hr (peak)		Smith 1975
	2	Not reported	300 mg every 6 hr	PO	0.8–1.8 µg/ml	Not reported		
	5	Not reported	150 mg tid	PO	<0.5–3.1 µg/ml	Not reported		Steen 1982a

- Small amounts excreted in milk. Bloody diarrhea resolved upon discontinuation of breast feeding (Mann, 1980). Cause–effect relationship uncertain.

| Clofazimine | 8 | Not reported | 50 mg/day or 100 mg every other day | PO | 0.8–1.7 µg/ml | 4–6 hr | + | Venkatesan 1997 |

- Milk concentrations higher than maternal blood concentrations. Infant may ingest 13.5%–30% of maternal dose.

Clomipramine	1	None reported	125 mg/day	PO	215.8–342.7 ng/ml	4–6 days after birth	++	Schimmell 1991
			150 mg/day	PO	269.8–624.2 ng/ml	10–35 days after birth		
	4	None reported	75–125 mg/day	PO	Not measured			Wisner 1995

- Based on milk concentrations, infant would receive about 0.4% of maternal dose (Schimmell et al., 1991). No clomipramine or its metabolite detected in blood of infants (Wisner et al., 1995). Long-term effects unknown.

TABLE 3-1 continued

DRUG[a]	NUMBER OF INFANTS	EFFECT ON INFANTS	MATERNAL DOSE	ROUTE	CONCENTRATION OF DRUG IN BREAST MILK	TIME AFTER MATERNAL DOSE	SIGNIFI-CANCE[b]	REFERENCE[c]
Clonazepam	1	Apnea, periodic breathing episodes	Not reported	PO	11–13 ng/ml	Not reported	+	Fisher 1985
	1	None reported	2 mg tid	PO	10 ng/ml	4 hr		Soderman 1987

- Infant serum concentration 4.7 μg/liter (Soderman & Matheson, 1987). Based on milk concentration, the maximum intake by infant is 2.5% of maternal dose.

Clonidine	9	Hypoglycemia, hypotension, hyperexcitability	Average of 241–391 μg/day	PO	>2 ng/ml	Not reported	+	Hartikainen-Sorri 1987
	1	None reported	37.5 μg tid	PO	0.6 ng/ml	2.5 hr		Bunjes 1993

- Clonidine milk concentration is twice the concurrent maternal serum concentration. Infant serum concentration is approximately 50% of maternal serum concentration. Effects in infants are similar to those seen in infants born to untreated mothers with pre-eclampsia.

Clorazepate	7	Not reported	20 mg	IM	7.5–11.5 ng/ml (of nordiazepam and clorazepate)	2–4 days	++	Rey 1979

- Nordiazepam concentrations detected in blood of infants. Elimination of nordiazepam in infant is prolonged due to immature hepatic enzymes.

Clozapine	1	Not reported	500 mg/day	PO	63.5 ng/ml	Not reported	++	Barnas 1994
			100 mg/day	PO	115.6 ng/ml	Not reported		

- Milk concentrations relatively high due to lipophilic properties of clozapine.

Cocaine	1	Apnea, seizures	Topical cocaine powder (used as a nipple anesthetic)	Topical	Not detected	1 day	+++	Chaney 1988
	1	Irritability, vomiting, diarrhea, tremulousness, dilated pupils	0.5 gram	Intranasal	Detectable	Up to ~36 hr		Chasnoff 1987

- Cocaine is contraindicated in breast-feeding mothers (American Academy of Pediatrics, 1994).

Codeine	4	Apnea, bradycardia	60 mg every 4–6 hr for 4–6 days	PO	Not measured		++	Davis 1985
	5	None reported	65 mg as one-time dose, or 65 mg for two doses, or 32 mg for six doses at unspecified intervals	PO	Not detected	2–4 hr after last dose		Kwit 1935
	2	None reported	60 mg	PO	Codeine 33.8–314 ng/ml Morphine 1.9–20.5 ng/ml	0.33–4 hr		Meny 1993

- Although low concentrations are detected in milk, accumulation can occur over 4–5 days and result in respiratory depression in breast-fed infants.

Colchicine	4	None reported	1 mg/day	PO	3.6–6.46 ng/ml	1 hr	+	Ben-Chetrit 1996
	1	None reported	1 mg/day	PO	10–31 ng/ml	2–7 hr		Guillonneau 1995
	1	None reported	0.6 mg tid	PO	<0.5–2.5 ng/ml	0.33–1 hr		Milunsky 1991

- To minimize infant exposure, give colchicine as bedtime dose and breast feed at least 8 hr later (Guillonneau et al., 1995).

Cyanocobalamin (Vitamin B_{12})	5	None reported	Normal dietary intake (in United States)	PO	0.03–0.05 ng/ml	Not reported	0	Collins 1951
	Not reported	None reported	Normal dietary intake (in Russia)	PO	0.25–0.52 ng/ml	Not reported		Knowles 1972

- Differences in milk concentrations probably caused by variations in dietary intake. Cyanocobalamin (vitamin B_{12}) is a normal constituent of breast milk.

Footnotes are on page 203.

TABLE 3-1 continued

DRUG[a]	NUMBER OF INFANTS	EFFECT ON INFANTS	MATERNAL DOSE	ROUTE	CONCENTRATION OF DRUG IN BREAST MILK	TIME AFTER MATERNAL DOSE	SIGNIFI-CANCE[b]	REFERENCE[c]
Cyclo-phosphamide	1	Neutropenia	800 mg/week	IV	Not measured		+++	Amato 1977
	1	Reduction in leukocyte and platelet counts	300 mg/day	IV	Not measured			Durodola 1979
	1	Not reported	500 mg	IV	Detectable, but not quantified	1–6 hr		Wiernik 1971

- Contraindicated in breast-feeding mothers because it is detected in milk (American Academy of Pediatrics, 1994). Mother of infant who developed neutropenia received vincristine and prednisolone concurrently with cyclophosphamide (Amato & Niblett, 1977).

| Cycloserine | 5 | None reported | 250 mg qid | PO | 6–19 µg/ml (31%–118% of maternal blood concentration) | Not reported | + | Morton 1955–1956 |

- May be highly concentrated in milk. At a maternal dose of 1 gram/day, infant could receive 11.3% of the therapeutic dose (Snider & Powell, 1984). Clinical significance unknown.

Cyclosporine	1	None reported	325 mg/day	PO	16 ng/ml	22 hr	+++	Flechner 1985
	7	None reported	Not reported	PO	50–227 ng/ml	Not reported		Nyberg 1998
	1	None reported	300 mg/day	PO	79–286 ng/ml	Not reported		Munoz-Flores-Thiagarajan 2001

- Detectable in infant's serum in one study (Flechner et al., 1985), but not in others (Nyberg et al., 1998; Munoz-Flores-Thiagarajan et al., 2001). Contraindicated in breast-feeding mothers because of possible immune suppression, uncertain effects on growth, and possible association with carcinogenesis (American Academy of Pediatrics, 1994).

| Cyproheptadine (See comment) | | | | | | | ++ | Wortsman 1979 |

- Used to treat galactorrhea. May reduce milk production due to antiserotonergic properties.

| Dapsone | 3 | None reported | 100 mg | PO | Not reported | | + | Edstein 1986 |
| | 1 | Hemolytic anemia | 50 mg/day | PO | 1092 ng/ml | Not reported | | Sanders 1982 |

- About 5%–10% of maternal dose excreted in milk over 9-day study period (Edstein et al., 1986). Infant serum concentration of dapsone 439 ng/ml (Sanders et al., 1982). Low serum concentration in infants may promote development of drug-resistant malaria strains. Avoid in breast-feeding mothers of infants with glucose-6-phosphate dehydrogenase deficiency.

| Demeclocycline | 45 | None reported | 300–2700 mg/day | PO | 0.06–1.4 µg/ml (average of 70% of maternal serum concentration) | Detectable for up to 3 days after last dose | ++ | Von Kobyletzki 1964 |

- Individual doses greater than 600 mg resulted in detectable milk concentrations. Theoretical possibility of tooth staining and inhibition of bone growth. Limit demeclocycline therapy to 10 days in breast-feeding mothers.

| Desipramine | 1 | None reported | 300 mg | PO | Desipramine 316–328 ng/ml 2-Hydroxydesipramine 327–381 ng/ml | 9–10 hr | ++ | Stancer 1986 |

- Milk concentrations of desipramine and metabolite 30% higher than maternal serum concentration. Infant serum concentrations substantially lower than maternal serum concentration. Prolonged exposure to low concentrations may adversely affect the developing catecholaminergic and serotonergic neuronal systems (Buist et al., 1990). Long-term effects unknown (American Academy of Pediatrics, 1994).

| Desmopressin (DDAVP) | 1 | Not reported | 10 µg | Intra-nasal | <1.5 ng/liter | 0–4 hr | 0 | Burrow 1981 |

- Limited data available. Unlikely to produce ADRs in breast-fed infants because of low concentrations in milk.

Diazepam	1	None reported	Up to 80 mg/day	PO	Up to 307 ng/ml	1.1–2.6 hr	++	Dusci 1990
	3	Neonatal jaundice possibly caused by inhibition of bilirubin metabolism	10 mg tid for 6 days	PO	51 ng/ml 78 ng/ml	4 days 6 days		Erkkola 1972
	1	None reported	5 mg for three doses over a 4-hr period	IV	100 ng/ml	25 hr after last dose		Horning 1975

TABLE 3-1 continued

DRUG[a]	NUMBER OF INFANTS	EFFECT ON INFANTS	MATERNAL DOSE	ROUTE	CONCENTRATION OF DRUG IN BREAST MILK	TIME AFTER MATERNAL DOSE	SIGNIFI-CANCE[b]	REFERENCE[c]
Diazepam *continued*	1	After 3rd day, lethargy and weight loss; EEG consistent with sedation; symptoms resolved upon discontinuation of diazepam	10 mg tid for 3 days	PO	Not measured			Patrick 1972
	1	Sedation if nursed soon after dose; no sedation if >8 hr after dose	6–10 mg/day	PO	Diazepam 7.5–87 ng/ml Desmethyldiazepam 19.2–77 ng/ml	1.5–10 hr		Wesson 1985

- Accumulation of diazepam and metabolite, desmethyldiazepam, is possible because of immature metabolism in infants. Sufficient amounts are excreted in milk to cause infant sedation, so avoid maternal oral doses >30 mg/day (Kanto, 1982). Long-term effects unknown (American Academy of Pediatrics, 1994).

Dicumarol	125	Normal prothrombin times in most infants	200 mg as one-time dose; then dosage titrated to prothrombin time	PO	Not measured		+	Brambel 1950

- Monitor infant prothrombin times. May give phytonadione to infants as prophylaxis for hemorrhage when large maternal doses are necessary.

Digoxin	11	Not reported	0.25 mg/day	PO	0.6 ng/ml	Not reported	0	Chan 1978
	1	None reported	0.75 mg/day	PO	1.9 ng/ml	Not reported		Finley 1979
	11	Not reported	500 μg	IV	1–4 ng/ml	0.5–24 hr		Reinhardt 1982

- Infant serum concentrations 0.2–0.6 ng/ml (Finley et al., 1979). Caution should be used when interpreting infant's serum concentrations; they may be overestimated due to the presence of digoxinlike immunoreactive substances.

Diltiazem	1	Not reported	60 mg qid	PO	200 ng/ml	2 hr	+	Okada 1985

- Maternal serum and milk concentrations are similar. Until the effect of calcium channel blockers on infants is known, caution should be used when breast feeding.

Diphtheria Vaccine	Not reported	Not reported	0.5 ml	IM	<0.3% of administered dose	Not reported	0	Valquist 1949

- Breast feeding is not a contraindication to the administration of diphtheria vaccine to the mother (Immunization Practices Advisory Committee, 1989).

Disopyramide	1	None reported	200 mg tid	PO	Disopyramide 2.6–5.7 mg/liter N-Monodesalkyl disopyramide 1.8–4.4 mg/liter	4–8 hr	+	Barnett 1982
	1	None reported	450 mg tid (chronic therapy)	PO	2.6–4.4 mg/liter	2–8 hr		Ellsworth 1989
	1	Crying, restlessness	200 mg bid	PO	0.58 mg/liter 0.98 mg/liter	Before dose 3.5 hr after dose		Hoppu 1986
	1	None reported	100 mg five times a day	PO	1.7 mg/liter	2 hr		MacKintosh 1985

- Breast-fed infants may receive relatively large doses of disopyramide and its metabolite, N-monodesalkyl disopyramide. Use with caution in breast-feeding mothers, only if no suitable alternative exists. Monitor for evidence of anticholinergic effects.

Doxepin	1	None reported	150 mg/day	PO	Doxepin 60 μg/liter Desmethyldoxepin 111 μg/liter	17.2–17.7 hr	++	Kemp 1985
	1	Shallow respirations, limpness, drowsiness, pallor	25 mg tid	PO	Doxepin 27–29 μg/liter Desmethyldoxepin 7–11 μg/liter	4–5 hr		Matheson 1985

(Continued)

Footnotes are on page 203.

PROBLEMS IN PEDIATRIC DRUG THERAPY

TABLE 3-1 continued

DRUG[a]	NUMBER OF INFANTS	EFFECT ON INFANTS	MATERNAL DOSE	ROUTE	CONCENTRATION OF DRUG IN BREAST MILK	TIME AFTER MATERNAL DOSE	SIGNIFICANCE[b]	REFERENCE[c]
Doxepin *continued*	1	Muscle hypotonia, vomiting, weight loss	35 mg/day	PO	Doxepin + desmethyldoxepin 60–100 µg/liter	13–15 hr		Frey 1999

- Despite low desmethyldoxepin milk concentrations, an 8-week-old infant had a high metabolite serum concentration (58–66 µg/liter) with a very low doxepin serum concentration (3 µg/liter) (Matheson et al., 1985). Accumulation of desmethyldoxepin may be the result of immature hepatic function (hydroxylation and conjugation) in infant. Doxepin should be used cautiously in breast-feeding women. Long-term effects unknown (American Academy of Pediatrics, 1994).

DRUG	N	EFFECT	MATERNAL DOSE	ROUTE	CONC IN MILK	TIME	SIG	REF
Doxorubicin	1	Not reported	70 mg/m^2	IV	Doxorubicin 128 ng/ml Doxorubicinol 111 ng/ml	24 hr	+++	Egan 1985

- Contraindicated in breast-feeding women because effects on growth and carcinogenesis potential in infants are unknown (American Academy of Pediatrics, 1994). Large amounts of doxorubicin and its metabolite, doxorubicinol, are excreted into milk.

| **Doxycycline** | 15 | None reported | 200 mg, then 100 mg 24 hr later | PO | >70 ng/ml and 380 ng/ml (30%–40% of maternal serum concentration) | 3 and 24 hr after second dose | ++ | Morganti 1968 |

- Doxycycline concentrations in milk may progressively increase with continued therapy. Theoretical possibility of tooth staining and inhibition of bone growth (Tokuda et al., 1969). Limit doxycycline therapy to 10 days in breast-feeding women.

Enalapril	3	Not reported	5 mg	PO	Enalaprilat <0.2 ng/ml	Not reported	+	Huttunen 1989
			10 mg	PO	Enalaprilat <0.2 ng/ml	Not reported		
	5	None reported	20 mg	PO	Enalapril 0–5.9 ng/ml	4–6 hr		Redman 1990
					Enalaprilat 0–2.3 ng/ml	4–6 hr		
	1	Not reported	10 mg/day	PO	Enalapril 0.82–2.05 ng/ml	4–24 hr		Rush 1991
					Enalaprilat 0.55–0.75 ng/ml			

- Unlikely to produce ADRs in breast-fed infants because of small amounts excreted in milk. In lactating women with even slight renal impairment, high serum concentrations of enalaprilat (active metabolite) may result in high enalaprilat concentrations in milk.

| **Epinephrine** | | None reported | | | | | 0 | Riordan 1987 |

- Unlikely to produce ADRs in breast-fed infants because epinephrine is destroyed in the GI tract. Sympathomimetics inhibit milk flow in animals by inhibition of secretion and release of oxytocin and by peripheral vasoconstriction. Use of epinephrine by breast-feeding mothers may reduce milk production.

| **Ergonovine** | 12 | None reported | 200 µg | PO | Not measured | | ++ | Shane 1974 |

- May reduce prolactin serum concentrations. Large doses may result in sufficient prolactin inhibition to decrease lactation.

| **Ergot Alkaloids** | 16 | Ergotism (vomiting, diarrhea, weak pulse, unstable blood pressure, convulsions) in 14 of 16 infants | Unspecified dose of liquid extract of ergot | PO | Detectable, but not quantified | Not reported | +++ | Fomina 1934 |

- Other ergot alkaloids may suppress lactation and cause ergotism (Floss, 1973). Ergot alkaloids should be avoided in breast-feeding women (American Academy of Pediatrics, 1994). (*See* Bromocriptine and Ergonovine entries in this table.)

| **Erythromycin** | 2 | Not reported | 500 mg | PO | 0.8–1.4 µg/ml | 2–6 hr | + | Matsuda 1984 |
| | 1 | Pyloric stenosis | 250 mg tid | PO | Not measured | | | Stang 1986 |

- Reported concentrations of erythromycin in milk greater than in maternal serum. In single case report of pyloric stenosis, infant had a history of birth asphyxia and was receiving phenobarbital (Stang, 1986). Possibility of alteration of oropharyngeal flora. Monitor for candidiasis (e.g., oral thrush) and diarrhea.

| **Ethambutol** | 1 | Not reported | 15 mg/kg | PO | 1.5–4.6 mg/liter | 3 hr | + | Snider 1984 |

- Limited information available. Similar concentrations in maternal serum and milk. Use cautiously in breast-feeding women. Clinical significance unknown.

CHAPTER 3: DRUGS EXCRETED IN HUMAN BREAST MILK

TABLE 3-1 continued

DRUG[a]	NUMBER OF INFANTS	EFFECT ON INFANTS	MATERNAL DOSE	ROUTE	CONCENTRATION OF DRUG IN BREAST MILK	TIME AFTER MATERNAL DOSE	SIGNIFI-CANCE[b]	REFERENCE[c]
Ether	2	None reported	170 and 250 grams	Inhalation	Similar to maternal blood concentration	8–10 hr	++	Gramen 1922

- Avoid in breast-feeding women because general anesthetics can cause severe respiratory depression in breast-fed infants.

Ethosuximide	9	Not reported	Not reported	PO	21.3 µg/ml	Not reported	++	Kaneko 1979
	5	None reported	9.3–23.6 mg/kg/day	PO	27–77.5 µg/ml	Not reported		Kuhnz 1984
	1	None reported	250 mg bid	PO	426–1136 µg/ml	Not reported		Rane 1981
	2	Not reported	750–1000 mg/day	PO	34–52 µg/ml	Not reported		Tomson 1994

- Ethosuximide serum concentration of 15–40 µg/ml in breast-fed infants (Kuhnz et al., 1984). Consider using an alternative anticonvulsant because milk concentration is ~80% of concurrent maternal serum concentration. Ethosuximide serum concentration of infant was 17 µg/ml (Tomson & Villen, 1994).

Etoposide	1	None reported	80 mg/m² on days 1–3	IV	120 ng/ml	Day 3	++	Azuno 1995

- Patient began to breast feed infant 3 weeks after antineoplastic therapy. Etoposide not detected in milk by 24 hr after last dose.

Famotidine	8	Not reported	40 mg	PO	72 ng/ml	6 hr	+	Courtney 1988

- Appears to be less extensively secreted into milk than other H_2-antagonists. Famotidine concentrations in milk lag behind measured maternal serum concentrations. Peak milk concentration occurs 6 hr after a dose (versus peak serum concentration 2 hr after dose).

Fentanyl	10	Not reported	50–400 µg	IV	<0.05–0.15 µg/ml	4 hr	+	Leuschen 1990
					<0.05–0.14 µg/ml	24 hr		

- Single doses unlikely to produce ADRs in breast-fed infants because of limited excretion in milk and short half-life in maternal serum.

Flecainide	11	None reported	100 mg every 12 hr	PO	134–1529 ng/ml	12 hr	+	McQuinn 1990

- Metabolites have some activity but were not measured. In general, milk concentration is 2.5 times corresponding plasma concentration. In adults, plasma concentrations >1000 ng/ml are associated with toxic effects. It is unlikely that infant plasma concentrations will approach this value based on the amount excreted in milk.

Fluconazole	1	Not reported	150 mg	PO	0.98–2.93 µg/ml	2–48 hr	+	Force 1995

- Due to long half-life, single dose of fluconazole may result in detectable milk concentrations for 48 hr or longer.

Fluoride	Not reported	Not reported	Variable (average of 1.13 ppm)	PO	Average 0.25 ppm	Not reported	0	Bercovici 1960; Ekstrand 1981; Ericsson 1969, 1972

- Poorly secreted into milk. Most clinicians recommend fluoride supplementation for infants to prevent dental caries (American Academy of Pediatrics, 1986; Berlin, 1990).

Fluoxetine	1	Possible increase in irritability	20 mg/day	PO	Fluoxetine 28.8 ng/ml Norfluoxetine 41.6 ng/ml	Not reported	++	Isenberg 1990
	1	None reported	20 mg/day	PO	Fluoxetine 17–67 ng/ml Norfluoxetine 13–52 ng/ml	4–8 hr		Burch 1992
	1	Crying, decreased sleep, vomiting, watery stools	20 mg/day	PO	Fluoxetine 69 ng/ml Norfluoxetine 90 ng/ml	Not reported		Lester 1993
	10	None reported	0.17–0.85 mg/kg/day	PO	Fluoxetine 17.4–293 ng/ml Norfluoxetine 23.4–379.1 ng/ml	2–24 hr		Taddio 1996

- Fluoxetine and a metabolite, norfluoxetine, detectable in milk and infant's plasma. In one infant, when changed to formula, symptoms of colic subsided. When rechallenged with breast milk 3 weeks later, colic recurred (Lester et al., 1993). Cognitive and psychomotor development normal in four infants at 12 months (Yoshida et al., 1998). One retrospective study of 64 women suggests reduced growth in offspring that may be clinically important for infants for whom weight gain is already a concern (Chambers et al., 1999). Long-term effects unknown.

Footnotes are on page 203.

TABLE 3-1 continued

DRUG[a]	NUMBER OF INFANTS	EFFECT ON INFANTS	MATERNAL DOSE	ROUTE	CONCENTRATION OF DRUG IN BREAST MILK	TIME AFTER MATERNAL DOSE	SIGNIFI-CANCE[b]	REFERENCE[c]
Flurbiprofen	10	Not reported	100 mg	PO	0.09 µg/ml	1–20 hr	0	Cox 1987
	12	Not reported	50 mg qid for nine doses	PO	0–0.07 µg/ml	2 hr		Smith 1989

• Minimal amounts are excreted in milk. Unlikely to produce ADRs in breast-fed infants.

Fluvoxamine	1	Not reported	100 mg bid	PO	750–1200 nmol/liter	1–12 hr	++	Hagg 2000

• Small amounts excreted in milk. Long-term effects unknown.

Folic Acid	2	None reported	100–200 µg/day	PO	40–70 ng/ml	10 days	0	Metz 1968
	42	None reported	Normal dietary intake (in India)	PO	16.5 ng/ml			Ramasastri 1965

• Amounts excreted in milk are sufficient to prevent megaloblastic anemia in infant.

Furosemide	Not reported	Not reported	Not reported	PO	Not reported		+	O'Brien 1974
								Takyi 1970

• Not readily excreted in milk. May cause dehydration in mother, resulting in reduced lactation.

Gallium Citrate Ga 67	1	Not reported	3 mCi	IV	70 nCi/ml	96–120 hr	+++	Larson 1971

• Significant amounts are excreted in milk. Interrupt breast feeding for at least 2 weeks after receiving gallium citrate Ga 67 (American Academy of Pediatrics, 1994).

Gentamicin	10	None reported	80 mg/day	IM	<0.27–0.74 µg/ml	1–7 hr	+	Celiloglu 1994

• Five to 10 infants had detectable gentamicin serum concentrations (mean 0.41 ± 0.05 µg/ml). Monitor for candidiasis (e.g., oral thrush) and diarrhea.

Ginseng	1	Neonatal androgenization (increased hair growth, enlarged testes)	650 mg bid	PO	Not measured		++	Koren 1990

• Similar effects reported in animal studies. Ginseng should not be used by breast-feeding women.

Gold	1	Gold detected in infant serum (51 mg/liter)	10 mg (gold sodium thiomalate)	IM	15–93 µg/liter	Variable	++	Bennett 1990
	1	Trace amounts found in serum and red blood cells; skin rash	135 mg	IM	8600 µg/liter 10,000 µg/liter	Not reported Not reported		Blau 1973
	2	None reported	70 mg	IM	<1–153 µg/liter	Variable		Ostensen 1986
			50 mg (gold sodium thiomalate)	IM	<1–185 µg/liter	Variable		
	1	None reported	50 mg (aurothioglucose)	IM	40 µg/liter	Variable		Rooney 1987

• Limited amounts of gold are secreted into milk. However, concentrations detected in infants' serum (Bennett et al., 1990) indicate that GI absorption occurs. Avoid breast feeding because of small amounts detected in serum and red blood cells of breast-fed infants.

Growth Hormone
(*See* comment)

• Preliminary studies suggest that growth hormone may increase milk production (Milsom et al., 1992, 1998).

Haloperidol	1	None reported	29 mg/day for 6 days	PO	5 ng/ml	11 hr	++	Stewart 1980
	1	None reported	5 mg bid	PO	23.5 ng/ml	Not reported		Whalley 1981

• Small amounts found in milk. Long-term effects unknown (American Academy of Pediatrics, 1994).

Heparin		None reported					0	

• Not excreted into milk or absorbed orally because of its high molecular weight (Anderson, 1991; Wilson, 1981).

TABLE 3-1 continued

DRUG[a]	NUMBER OF INFANTS	EFFECT ON INFANTS	MATERNAL DOSE	ROUTE	CONCENTRATION OF DRUG IN BREAST MILK	TIME AFTER MATERNAL DOSE	SIGNIFI-CANCE[b]	REFERENCE[c]
Heroin	22	Signs and symptoms of opiate-withdrawal syndrome observed in 13 of 22 infants	2–45 mg/day	IV	Detectable, but not quantified	Not reported	+++	Cobrinik 1959

- Contraindicated in breast-feeding women (American Academy of Pediatrics, 1994). Appears in milk and may prolong addiction developed in utero in breast-fed infants of mothers addicted to opiates. Maternal opiate use should be discontinued prior to initiation of breast feeding.

Hydralazine	1	None reported	50 mg tid	PO	127 ng/ml	2 hr	+	Liedholm 1982

- Small amount ingested by breast-fed infant.

Hydrochloro-thiazide	1	None reported	50 mg	PO	50–110 ng/ml (mean 80 ng/ml)	24 hr	+	Miller 1982

- Negligible amount excreted in milk. May cause dehydration in mother, resulting in reduced lactation.

Hydroxy-chloroquine	1	None reported	310 mg/day hs	PO	0.85–1.46 ng/ml	2–17.7 hr	+	Nation 1984
	1	Not reported	200 mg bid	PO	10.6 ng/ml	After 48 hr of therapy		Ostensen 1985

- Distributes extensively into blood cells. Milk concentration is up to 5.5 times that of concurrent maternal plasma concentration. Accumulation can occur in breast-fed infants because of long half-life.

Hydroxyurea	1	Not reported	5000 mg tid	PO	3.8–8.4 mg/liter	2 hr	++	Sylvester 1987

- The amount of hydroxyurea ingested by infant is low, but its effects are unknown.

Ibuprofen	12	Not reported	400 mg every 6 hr	PO	<1.0 µg/ml	2–6 hr	0	Townsend 1984
	1	None reported	400 mg	PO	<0.5 µg/ml	1–8 hr		Weibert 1982

- Minimal amounts excreted in milk. No ibuprofen metabolites detected in milk.

Imipramine	1	None reported	200 mg/day	PO	Imipramine 4–29 ng/ml Desipramine (metabolite) 17–35 ng/ml	1–23 hr	++	Sovner 1979

- Infant would receive ~0.04 mg/kg/day at usual maternal doses; recommended initial therapeutic dose for children is 1–1.5 mg/kg/day. Milk and maternal plasma concentrations are similar. Infant plasma concentration well below therapeutic concentrations. Accumulation can occur in infants because of immaturity of drug-metabolizing enzymes. Long-term effects unknown (American Academy of Pediatrics, 1994).

Indomethacin	1	Generalized seizures	200 mg/day	PO	Not measured		+	Eeg-Olofsson 1978
	16	None reported	75–300 mg (0.94–4.29 mg/kg/day)	PO/Rectal	<20–115 µg/liter	0.7–22.6 hr		Lebedevs 1991

- According to manufacturer, milk concentrations are similar to maternal plasma concentrations. Indomethacin detected in plasma in one of seven infants (Lebedevs et al., 1991).

Insulin		None reported		SC			0	Davies 1989

- Not excreted into milk because of its high molecular weight. If insulin passed into milk, it would be destroyed in infant's GI tract. Mothers who breast feed may require reduction of insulin to about 75% of prepregnancy requirements and may need to supplement carbohydrate intake.

Iodine	1	Hypothyroidism	Topical povidone-iodine during pregnancy and lactation	Topical	Not reported		++	Danzinger 1987
	1	Hypothyroidism	Douching twice a day	Vaginal	Not reported	Not reported		Delange 1988
	1	Normal T$_4$ and TSH levels, elevated serum and urine iodine levels	50 mg/day	Vaginal	25 times maternal serum concentration	Not reported		Postellon 1982

- Readily absorbed by mother topically and orally and concentrated in milk. May cause thyroid suppression and hypersensitivity reactions in breast-fed infants.

Footnotes are on page 203.

TABLE 3-1 continued

DRUG[a]	NUMBER OF INFANTS	EFFECT ON INFANTS	MATERNAL DOSE	ROUTE	CONCENTRATION OF DRUG IN BREAST MILK	TIME AFTER MATERNAL DOSE	SIGNIFI-CANCE[b]	REFERENCE[c]
Iron	7	None reported	Normal dietary intake (in Denmark)	PO	181–220 ng/ml	Not reported	0	Saarinen 1977

• Small amount of iron (0.5–1.5 mg/liter) in milk is adequate to prevent iron-deficiency anemia in infants because iron in breast milk is better utilized than oral iron supplements. Maternal use of supplemental iron unlikely to appreciably affect iron concentration in milk.

Isoniazid	1	Not reported	300 mg	PO	Isoniazid 16.6 µg/ml Acetylisoniazid 3.76 µg/ml	3 hr 5 hr	+	Berlin 1979b
	1	None reported	5–10 mg/kg	PO	6–12 µg/ml	1–10 hr		Ricci 1954–1955

• Isoniazid and a metabolite, acetylisoniazid, concentrate in milk. Risk of liver toxicity (isoniazid- or acetylisoniazid-induced hepatitis). Concurrent use of isoniazid with aminosalicylic acid may increase serum half-life of isoniazid, which may increase its concentration in milk (Holdiness, 1984).

Ivermectin	4	Not reported	150 µg/kg	PO	4.2–20.6 ng/ml	1–24 hr	+	Ogbuokiri 1994

• Amount the infant is exposed to is considerably less than therapeutic doses.

Kanamycin	4	None reported	2 grams	PO	1.1–1.6 µg/ml	Not reported	+	Chyo 1962
	4	None reported	1 gram	IM	12–19 µg/ml	0.5–1 hr		

• Peak serum concentration in mother occurred 3 hr after oral administration and two of four mothers had a measurable milk concentration. Peak milk concentration in mother occurred 1 hr after IM administration. Not well-absorbed orally, so unlikely to produce ADRs in breast-fed infants.

Ketoconazole	1	None reported	200 mg/day	PO	0.22 µg/ml Not detected	3.25 hr 24 hr	+	Moretti 1995

• Low concentrations excreted into milk. Monitor for nausea, vomiting, and skin rash.

Ketorolac Tromethamine	10	Not reported	10 mg qid for 2 days	PO	0–7.9 ng/ml	2 hr	0	Wischnik 1989

• Low concentrations excreted into milk.

Labetalol	3	Not reported	600–1200 mg/day	PO	129–662 µg/ml	1–3 hr	++	Lunell 1985

• One infant had labetalol plasma concentrations similar to mother's. Milk concentrations exceeded maternal plasma concentration throughout most of the 8-hr dosing interval.

Lamivudine	20	Not reported	150 mg bid	PO	<0.5–8.2 µg/ml	Not reported	+	Moodley 1998
			300 mg bid	PO	<0.5–6.09 µg/ml	Not reported		

• Limited information available.

Lead	29	Not reported	Amount in normal diet (in United States)	PO	6–58 ng/ml	Not reported	++	Knowles 1974
	100	Not reported	Amount in normal diet (in United States)	PO	17 ng/ml (mean)	Not reported		Rabinowitz 1985

• Samples taken from white middle-class American women who may have lower levels than the general population (Knowles, 1974). Lead levels are similar in breast milk and canned milk and formulas (Rabinowitz et al., 1985). Lead ointment should not be used on breasts (Dillon, 1974), and all dietary sources of lead should be avoided by breast-feeding women.

Levodopa/ Carbidopa	1	None reported	50/200 levodopa/carbidopa sustained-release qid	PO	0.19–0.32 µg/ml	4–6 hr	+	Thulin 1998
			50/200 levodopa/carbidopa single dose	PO	0.85 µg/ml	3 hr		

• Amount of levodopa ingested by breast-fed infant is small and subtherapeutic.

Levonorgestrel	100	Reduced weight gain in female infants during 4th month postpartum	Norplant® (delivers ~100 µg/day from day 1 to 100, then gradually decreases to 30 µg/day during years 2–7)	Subdermal	23–311 pg/ml	During first 40 days after implantation	+	Diaz 1985

TABLE 3-1 continued

DRUG[a]	NUMBER OF INFANTS	EFFECT ON INFANTS	MATERNAL DOSE	ROUTE	CONCENTRATION OF DRUG IN BREAST MILK	TIME AFTER MATERNAL DOSE	SIGNIFI-CANCE[b]	REFERENCE[c]
Levonorgestrel *continued*	250	None reported	0.03 mg/day	PO	Not measured			McCann 1989

- Unlikely to produce ADRs in breast fed infants because amounts excreted in breast milk are small. *See* Oral Contraceptives entry in this table.

Lidocaine	1	Not reported	Bolus, then 2 mg/min	IV	2 µg/ml 0.8 µg/ml	5 hr 7 hr	+	Zeisler 1986
	1	Not reported	20 mg	Dental injection	Lidocaine 44–66 µg/liter Monoethylglycinexylidide 35–41 µg/liter	2–6.5 hr		Lebedevs 1993

- Milk concentrations about 40% of maternal serum concentrations. Lidocaine and metabolite, monoethylglycinexylidide detected in milk (Lebedevs et al., 1993). Unlikely to produce ADRs in breast-fed infants because of poor oral bioavailability and immature hepatic enzymes. Possibility of idiosyncratic or hypersensitivity reaction.

Lincomycin	9	None reported	500 mg every 6 hr for 3 days	PO	50%–122% of maternal serum concentration	6 hr	++	Medina 1963

- May achieve higher concentrations in milk than in maternal serum, so lincomycin should be avoided in breast-feeding women.

Lindane (Gamma Benzene Hexachloride)	Not reported	None reported	Amount in normal diet	PO	480 µg/kg of milk fat	Not reported	++	Luquet 1975

- Measured in pooled milk. May pass into milk after topical application of lindane lotion to mother's skin. Milk concentrations may remain elevated for more than 7 days following topical exposure. Alternative drugs (e.g., permethrin, pyrethrins) preferred for women who are breast feeding (Anderson, 1991).

Lithium	8	None reported	Not reported	PO	0.16–0.56 mEq/liter; 35%–50% of maternal serum concentration	Not reported	+++	Schou 1973
	1	Hypotonia, hypothermia, cyanosis, lethargy, T-wave inversion on ECG	600–1200 mg	PO	0.6 mEq/liter	Not reported		Tunnessen 1972

- May be contraindicated in breast-feeding women (American Academy of Pediatrics, 1994). Monitor infant's fluid status and sodium and lithium serum concentrations. A breast-fed infant of a mother receiving lithium exhibited restlessness and muscle twitches (infant serum concentration 1.4 mEq/liter) (Skausig & Schou, 1977). Controversy over safety of lithium therapy for women who are breast feeding remains unresolved (Ananth, 1978; Linden & Rich, 1983; Schou, 1990; Sykes et al., 1976). However, in the interest of pediatric health and safety, it is recommended that breast feeding be avoided.

Loperamide	6	Not reported	4 mg every 12 hr for two doses	PO	0.27 ng/ml 0.19 ng/ml	6 hr after 2nd dose 24 hr after 2nd dose	+	Nikodem 1992

- Low concentrations of loperamide and a metabolite, loperamide oxide, detected in milk. During long-term loperamide therapy, monitor breast-fed infants for constipation.

Loratadine	6	Not reported	40 mg	PO	Maximum concentration 20.4–30 ng/ml	0–2-hr pooled sample	+	Hilbert 1988

- Low amounts excreted in milk.

Lorazepam	4	Not reported	3.5 mg	PO	8–9 ng/ml	4 hr	++	Summerfield 1985
	1	None reported	2.5 mg bid	PO	12 ng/ml	Not reported		Whitelaw 1981

- Unlikely to have a significant effect on breast-fed infants. Neonates, especially premature infants, conjugate lorazepam slowly and may be at increased risk for toxicity. Long-term effects unknown (American Academy of Pediatrics, 1994).

Footnotes are on page 203.

TABLE 3-1 continued

DRUG[a]	NUMBER OF INFANTS	EFFECT ON INFANTS	MATERNAL DOSE	ROUTE	CONCENTRATION OF DRUG IN BREAST MILK	TIME AFTER MATERNAL DOSE	SIGNIFI- CANCE[b]	REFERENCE[c]
Magnesium Sulfate	10	None reported	4 grams as one-time dose, then 1 gram/hr for 24 hr	IV	64 µg/ml	Immediately after discontinuation of infusion	0	Cruikshank 1982
					38 µg/ml	24 hr after discontinuation of infusion		

- Administered antepartum. Maternal magnesium serum concentrations fall to normal values 24 hr after birth. Some mothers have difficulty establishing milk supply after magnesium administration (Anderson, 1991). Breast-fed infant would receive an estimated 1.5 mg/day of additional magnesium compared to breast-fed infant of untreated mother.

Medroxy-progesterone
(See comment)

- No adverse long-term effects on growth or development reported in 1215 children exposed to medroxyprogesterone during breast feeding (Pardthaisong et al., 1992).

Mefloquine	2	Not reported	250-mg single dose	PO	32–53 ng/ml	4 hr–56 days	+	Edstein 1988

- Small amounts excreted in milk. More data needed to determine infant exposure in mothers who receive multiple doses for prophylaxis or treatment.

Meperidine (Pethidine)	9	None reported	50 mg	IV	130 µg/ml	2 hr	+	Peiker 1980
	2	None reported	75 mg	IV	209 ng/ml	Not reported		Quinn 1986
			150 mg	IV	275 ng/ml	Not reported		

- Meperidine and its active metabolite, normeperidine, detectable in milk. Does not reach significant levels with single doses. Repeated doses can cause high concentrations of meperidine and normeperidine in milk (Anderson, 1991).

Mesalamine (5-Amino-salicylic Acid)	1	Diarrhea	500 mg bid	Rectal	Not measured		++	Nelis 1989
	1	Not reported	1 gram tid	PO	0.1 µg/ml	5 hr		Klotz 1993

- Upon rechallenge on four occasions, diarrhea recurred within 8–12 hr after administration (Nelis, 1989).

Mestranol	4	Not reported	150 µg/day	PO	0.3–0.6 ng/ml (calculated)	Not reported	+	Wijmenga 1969

- Wijmenga and van der Molen (1969) used radioactive-labeled drug and measured active and metabolized products but did not distinguish between them. (See Oral Contraceptives entry in this table.)

Methadone	10	None reported	50–80 mg/day	PO	230–570 ng/ml; average of 83% of maternal serum concentration	Not reported	++	Blinick 1975
	2	None reported	60–73 mg/day	PO	110–250 ng/ml	1–22.5 hr		Geraghty 1997
	4	May minimize signs and symptoms of heroin-withdrawal syndrome in neonate	10–40 mg/day	PO	50–170 ng/ml	3–5 days after delivery		Ostrea 1978
	1	Death	Not reported	PO	Not measured			Smialek 1977
	12	None reported	20–80 mg/day	PO	39–232 ng/ml	1.7–3.9 hr		Wojnar-Horton 1997

- In the single case of infant death, infant's methadone serum concentration at autopsy was 40 ng/ml (Smialek et al., 1977). If mother is heroin free and receiving low-dose methadone (<20–40 mg/day) as part of an opiate maintenance program, breast feeding may be continued. Avoid breast feeding for 2–6 hr after each dose when peak milk concentrations occur (Kreek et al., 1974).

Methimazole	1	None reported	2.5 mg bid	PO	20–70 µg/liter	0–12 hr	++	Tegler 1980

- Enters milk freely. May interfere with infant's thyroid function, so serum thyroxine and TSH should be monitored in breast-fed infant every 2–4 weeks (Cooper, 1987). Propylthiouracil should be used, if possible.

TABLE 3-1 continued

DRUG[a]	NUMBER OF INFANTS	EFFECT ON INFANTS	MATERNAL DOSE	ROUTE	CONCENTRATION OF DRUG IN BREAST MILK	TIME AFTER MATERNAL DOSE	SIGNIFI-CANCE[b]	REFERENCE[c]
Methotrexate (Amethopterin)	1	Not reported	22.5 mg/day	PO	2.6 ng/ml; 8% of maternal plasma concentration	10 hr (peak)	+++	Johns 1972

- Contraindicated in breast-feeding women because effects on growth and carcinogenesis potential in breast-fed infants are unknown (American Academy of Pediatrics, 1994). Low weekly doses for arthritis may be safe in breast-feeding women.

Methyldopa	1–3	None reported	250 mg bid	PO	1.4 µg/ml	3 hr	+	Hauser 1985
		None reported	500 mg	PO	0.2–1.14 µg/ml	3–6 hr		White 1985

- Although methyldopa was detected in infant's serum and urine, no ADRs were reported. Monitor respiration, blood pressure, and alertness in breast-fed infants (especially premature infants).

Methylergonovine	10	Not reported	200 µg tid for 7 days	PO	Not measured		++	del Pozo 1975
	8	Not reported	125 µg tid	PO	<0.5–1.3 ng/ml 0–1.2 ng/ml	1 hr 8 hr		Erkkola 1978

- No decrease in maternal prolactin serum concentration has been reported, but suppression of lactation has occurred with other ergot derivatives. (See Ergot Alkaloids entry in this table.)

Metoclopramide	5	None reported	10 mg bid	PO	52–156 ng/ml	1–2 hr	++	Kauppila 1983
	10	None reported	10 mg	PO	125.7 ng/ml	2 hr		Lewis 1980
	5	Not reported	10 mg tid for 7–10 days	PO	Not measured			Sousa 1975

- Used to stimulate lactation (Ehrenkranz & Ackerman, 1986; Ertl et al., 1991; Kauppila et al., 1983). Infant prolactin serum concentrations elevated (Kauppila et al., 1983). Potential to cause CNS effects (Gupta & Gupta, 1985). Concern because of defects in neural development in newborn animals exposed to dopamine receptor antagonists (Anderson, 1991). Avoid breast feeding for 3–4 hr after each dose and limit duration of therapy to 10–14 days (Anderson, 1991).

Metoprolol	3	None reported	50–100 mg	PO	507 ng/ml	1.5 hr	++	Kulas 1984
	3	None reported	50 mg bid for 1 day, then 100 mg bid for 4 days	PO	260–1767 ng/ml	Not reported		Liedholm 1981
	9	Not reported	50–100 mg	PO	78–1158 ng/ml	1.5–6 hr		Sandstrom 1980

- Concentration in milk is approximately 2.5–3 times higher than maternal serum concentration. Infant serum concentration negligible. Avoid breast feeding for 3–4 hr after each dose.

Metronidazole	3	Not reported	2 grams as a one-time dose	PO	46 µg/ml 19 µg/ml 3.5 µg/ml	2 hr 12 hr 24–48 hr	+++	Erickson 1981
	10	None reported	200 mg	PO	1–7.7 µg/ml; 45%–180% of maternal serum concentration	4–12 hr		Gray 1961
	15	None reported	400–600 mg	PO	1.6–12.9 µg/ml	0.5–6.5 hr		Heisterberg 1983
	12	None reported	1200 mg/day	PO	15.5 µg/ml	2 hr		Passmore 1988

- Use cautiously in breast-feeding women because metronidazole is an in vitro mutagen (American Academy of Pediatrics, 1994). Discard milk produced in 24-hr period after 2-gram dose (Erickson et al., 1981).

Mexiletine	1	Not reported	200 mg every 8 hr	PO	959 ng/ml	Not reported	+	Lewis 1981
	1	Poor feeding	250 mg tid	PO	Not measured			Lownes 1987

- Milk concentrations generally greater than maternal plasma concentrations. Higher plasma concentrations required to produce therapeutic effects in infants compared to adults. Unlikely to affect breast-fed infants.

Midazolam	12	None reported	15 mg	PO	<3.3 ng/ml	7 hr	+	Matheson 1990

- Detectable in milk after oral dose. Rapidly declines to undetectable concentrations within 4 hr. Long-term effects unknown (American Academy of Pediatrics, 1994).

Milk of Magnesia (Magnesium Hydroxide)	Not reported	None reported	Not reported	PO	Not measured		0	Baldwin 1963

- Poorly absorbed saline laxatives, such as magnesium salts, do not appear to cause problems in breast-fed infants. It is unlikely that there are measurable concentrations in milk.

Footnotes are on page 203.

TABLE 3-1 continued

DRUG[a]	NUMBER OF INFANTS	EFFECT ON INFANTS	MATERNAL DOSE	ROUTE	CONCENTRATION OF DRUG IN BREAST MILK	TIME AFTER MATERNAL DOSE	SIGNIFI-CANCE[b]	REFERENCE[c]
Mineral Oil	Not reported	None reported	15 ml	PO	Not measured		0	Baldwin 1963
• Not absorbed in mother's GI tract, so unlikely to achieve significant concentration in milk.								
Minocycline	1	None reported	200 mg	PO	800 ng/ml	8 hr	++	Brogden 1975
• Two reports of black discoloration of milk with minocycline therapy (Basler & Lynch, 1985; Hunt et al., 1996). Milk had an increased amount of iron. Small amount (18 µg) excreted in milk in 12 hr (Brogden, 1975). Limit therapy to 10 days in breast-feeding women.								
Minoxidil	1	Increased blood pressure	7.5 mg	PO	41.7–55 ng/ml 2.9–3.1 ng/ml	1 hr 6 hr	+	Valdivieso 1985
• Mother also received propranolol and furosemide. Lack of hypertrichosis and normal blood chemistries in infant suggest lack of effect from minoxidil.								
Mitoxantrone	1	None reported	6 mg/m² on days 1–5	IV	0.6 µg/ml	Day 3	++	Azuno 1995
• Patient began to breast feed infant 3 weeks after antineoplastic therapy. Mitoxantrone detectable 28 days after administration.								
Morphine	5	Not reported	5–15 mg	IV or IM	500 ng/ml (peak)	1 hr	++	Feilberg 1989
	1	None reported	5 mg	PO	10–100 ng/ml	0–1 hr		Robieux 1990
• Milk concentration generally higher than maternal plasma concentration. Infant serum concentration 4 ng/ml, which provides analgesic effect (Robieux et al., 1990).								
Moxalactam	8	Not reported	2 grams every 8 hr	IV	1.56–3.24 mg/ml	Not reported	+	Miller 1984
• Theoretically, could cause suppression of normal gut flora, overgrowth of other organisms, and enterocolitis in breast-fed infant.								
Nadolol	12	Not reported	80 mg/day for 5 days	PO	442.9 ng/ml	6 hr	++	Devlin 1981a
• Nadolol concentrations in milk are higher than those of some other antihypertensive drugs. Use with caution in breast-feeding women.								
Nalidixic Acid	1	Hemolytic anemia	1 gram qid	PO	Not measured		+	Belton 1965
	13	Not reported	2 grams	PO	0.3–1.1 µg/ml	24-hr pooled sample		Traeger 1980
• Mother also received amobarbital; no enzyme deficiencies found in the infant, who improved with bottle feeding (Belton & Jones, 1965). Avoid use in breast-feeding mothers of glucose-6-phosphate dehydrogenase-deficient infants to minimize risk of hemolysis.								
Naproxen	1	None reported	375 mg bid	PO	1.2 µg/ml	4 hr	0	Jamali 1983
• Amount of naproxen dose received by infant is minimal and unlikely to cause significant consequences.								
Nefazodone	1	Drowsiness, lethargy, poor feeding, unable to maintain body temperature	300 mg/day	PO	358 µg/liter	3 hr	++	Yapp 2000
• Nefazodone and metabolites detected in milk. ADRs noted in premature infant which resolved upon cessation of breast feeding. Safety unknown in full-term infants. Long-term effects unknown.								
Nicotine	20	None reported	1 cigarette		Nicotine (N) 55 µg/ml Cotinine (C) 136 µg/ml	0.5 hr	++	Dahlstrom 1990
	34	Shock, vomiting, diarrhea, increased heart rate, restlessness, decreased maternal serum prolactin concentrations (decreased milk production)	1–10 cigarettes/day 11–20 cigarettes/day 21–40 cigarettes/day		N 18 ng/ml C 76 ng/ml N 28 ng/ml C 125 ng/ml N 48 ng/ml C 230 ng/ml			Luck 1987
• Breast-feeding women should refrain from smoking. Milk exposure to nicotine and its metabolite cotinine varies with the number of cigarettes smoked per day and the time between smoking and breast feeding. Nicotine and cotinine concentrations are higher in maternal milk than maternal plasma (Dahlstrom et al., 1990). Nicotine and cotinine have been detected in infants' urine (Dahlstrom et al., 1990).								

TABLE 3-1 continued

DRUG[a]	NUMBER OF INFANTS	EFFECT ON INFANTS	MATERNAL DOSE	ROUTE	CONCENTRATION OF DRUG IN BREAST MILK	TIME AFTER MATERNAL DOSE	SIGNIFI-CANCE[b]	REFERENCE[c]
Nifedipine	1	Not reported	10 mg	PO	12.85 ng/ml	0.5 hr	+	Ehrenkranz 1989
			20 mg	PO	16.35 ng/ml	1 hr		
			30 mg	PO	53.35 ng/ml	0.5 hr		
	1	Not reported	10 mg every 8 hr	PO	12.89 ng/ml	0.5 hr		
			20 mg every 8 hr	PO	16.35 ng/ml	1 hr		
			30 mg every 8 hr	PO	53.35 ng/ml	0.5 hr		
	1	Not reported	20 mg	PO	15 ng/ml	1 hr		Penny 1989
			20 mg	PO	46 ng/ml	2 hr		
	6	Not reported	10 mg tid	PO	<1–10.3 ng/ml	1–8 hr		Manninen 1991

- Small amounts excreted in milk. Unlikely to pose risk to breast-fed infant. To reduce infant exposure, delay breast feeding for 3–4 hr after immediate-release nifedipine administration.

Nimodipine	1	Not reported	1 mg/hr for 2 hr, then 2 mg/hr for 22 hr	IV	0.42–4.7 ng/ml	During infusion and 2 hr after infusion	+	Carcas 1996
	1	Not reported	60 mg every 4 hr	PO	0–3 ng/ml	0–4 hr		Tonks 1995

- Milk concentrations fluctuate widely within the dosing interval and throughout the day. Unlikely to produce ADRs in breast-fed infant (Carcas et al., 1996).

Nitrofurantoin	3	Not reported	50 mg tid	PO	0.49 µg/ml	3 hr	+	Pons 1990
	3	Not reported	100 mg tid	PO	1.19 µg/ml	3 hr		
	9	Not reported	200 mg	PO	0.3–0.5 µg/ml	2 hr		Varsano 1973

- Concentration in milk greater than concentration in maternal plasma 3 hr after a dose. Avoid use in mothers of breast-fed infants with glucose-6-phosphate dehydrogenase deficiency.

Nizatidine	6	None reported	150 mg	PO	0.52 µg/ml	12 hr	+	Obermeyer 1990
	3	Not reported	150 mg every 12 hr	PO	0.3–0.7 µg/ml	12-hr pooled sample		

- Unlikely to produce ADRs in breast-fed infants.

Norethynodrel	6	Not reported	5 mg	PO	Trace amounts detectable	Not reported	++	Laumas 1967
	9	Not reported	5 mg/day for 3 days	PO	Detectable	Not reported		Laumas 1970

- Both studies used radioactive-labeled drug and found trace amounts of active and metabolized drug in milk but were unable to distinguish between them. Estrogenic activity also tested in milk and found in some milk samples. (*See also* Oral Contraceptives entry in this table.)

Nortriptyline	7	None reported	50–80 mg/day	PO	Not measured		+	Wisner 1991

- Although infant nortriptyline serum levels were undetectable, low serum concentrations of a less active metabolite, 10-hydroxynortriptyline, were found in two of four breast-fed infants in whom blood samples were evaluated.

Ofloxacin	10	Not reported	400 mg	PO	2.41 µg/ml	2 hr	++	Giamarellou 1989
					1.91 µg/ml	4 hr		

- Concentration in milk generally exceeds concurrent maternal serum concentration. Clinical significance unknown.

Olsalazine	1	None reported	500 mg	PO	0.28–0.43 µg/ml	10–24 hr	+	Miller 1993

- Not detected in milk. Concentrations of the resulting 5-aminosalicylic acid in breast milk are low and are likely safe for breast-fed infant.

Oral Contraceptives		Reduction in milk volume, changes in protein and nitrogen composition of breast milk, decreased infant weight gain, feminization of male infants	1 tablet/day	PO	Detectable	Not reported	+	Croxatto 1983 Curtis 1964 Diaz 1983 Koetsawang 1982, 1987 Liewellyn-Jones 1975 Lonnerdal 1980 Pincus 1966 World Health Organization, 1988

- Although changes in nutritional content of milk are minimal, they should be considered before recommending oral contraceptives for malnourished mothers. Extent of milk volume suppression is less with progestin-only contraceptives.

Footnotes are on page 203.

TABLE 3-1 continued

DRUG[a]	NUMBER OF INFANTS	EFFECT ON INFANTS	MATERNAL DOSE	ROUTE	CONCENTRATION OF DRUG IN BREAST MILK	TIME AFTER MATERNAL DOSE	SIGNIFI-CANCE[b]	REFERENCE[c]
Oxazepam	1	None reported	10 mg tid	PO	11–26 µg/ml	Not reported	+	Wretlind 1987

• Small amounts excreted in milk because of low lipid solubility. Unlikely to cause ADRs in breast-fed infants more than 1–3 days old. Half-life of oxazepam significantly prolonged during first 1–3 days of life (Kanto, 1982).

Oxycodone	6	None reported	5–10 mg every 4–7 hr	PO	<5–226 ng/ml	0.25–12 hr	+	Marx 1986

• Maximum concentration in milk occurs 1.5–2 hr after each dose. Concentration in milk is greater than concentration in maternal plasma.

Oxytocin	113	None reported	40 units/ml as nasal spray prior to each feeding	Intra-nasal	Not measured		0	Luhman 1963

• Used to facilitate lactation. Oxytocin appears to increase volume of milk excreted without altering composition of milk (when compared with untreated mothers) (Ruis et al., 1981).

Paroxetine	1	None reported	20 mg/day	PO	7.6 µg/liter	4 hr	++	Spigset 1996
	6	None reported	10–30 mg/day	PO	26–81 µg/liter	2–12 hr		Begg 1999

• Less than 1% of maternal dose is ingested by breast-fed infant. Long-term effects unknown (American Academy of Pediatrics, 1994).

Pefloxacin	10	Not reported	400 mg	PO	2.93–3.54 µg/ml	2–6 hr	++	Giamarellou 1989

• Concentrations in milk are similar to maternal serum concentrations. Clinical significance unknown.

Penicillin G	11	None reported	100,000 units (benzathine)	IM	0.01–0.06 unit/ml (3%–13% of maternal plasma concentration)	1–2 hr	+	Greene 1946
	2	Not reported	360 mg	IM	0.1–0.4 µg/ml	1–2 hr		Matsuda 1984
	13	None reported	200,000–600,000 units (benzathine)	IM	0.06–0.96 unit/ml	4 hr		Rozansky 1949

• Insufficient quantities in milk to treat infection in infant but could cause a hypersensitivity reaction or alter GI flora. Monitor breast-fed infants for rash, diarrhea, and candidiasis (e.g., oral thrush).

Penicillin V	Not reported	None reported	125–250 mg	PO	0.05–0.3 unit/ml	Not reported	+	Knowles 1972

• Concentrations in milk higher than those achieved with penicillin G, but ADRs are similar to those caused by penicillin G. Monitor breast-fed infants for rash, diarrhea, and candidiasis (e.g., oral thrush).

Pentobarbital	1	Sedation with hypnotic maternal doses	100 mg/day for 3 days	PO	170 ng/ml	19 hr after last dose	++	Horning 1975

• Sedative doses in the mother would not affect breast-fed infant. Large single doses may have greater potential for causing drowsiness in infants than multiple small doses. If barbiturate use is unavoidable, use of a short-acting barbiturate in small, divided daily doses is preferred to a single daily dose.

Pentoxifylline	5	Not reported	400 mg	PO	≤163 ng/ml	2–4 hr	+	Witter 1985

• Clinical significance is unknown. Unlikely to produce ADRs in breast-fed infants.

Phencyclidine (PCP)	1	Not reported	Not reported	Inhalation	3.9 ng/ml	Not reported	+++	Kaufman 1983

• PCP is a potent hallucinogen that is contraindicated in breast-feeding women (American Academy of Pediatrics, 1994). Reported to cause behavioral problems, lethargy, irritability, and coma in breast-fed infants (Nicholas et al., 1982).

Phenobarbital	8	Not reported	Quantity to achieve maternal serum concentration 19.3 µg/ml	PO	10.4 µg/ml	Not reported	++	Kaneko 1979
	13	None reported	Not reported	PO	36% of maternal serum concentration	Not reported		Kuhnz 1988

• May cause sedation in breast-fed infants. Use with caution in breast-feeding women (American Academy of Pediatrics, 1994). Sufficient amounts of barbiturates may be absorbed by breast-fed infants to stimulate liver enzymes and alter the metabolism of other drugs or bilirubin. Monitor serum concentrations (Nau et al., 1982).

Phenolphthalein	39	Increased bowel activity in 16 of 39 infants	65 mg	PO	<300 ng/ml	24-hr pooled samples	+	Tyson 1937

• Small amounts excreted in milk.

TABLE 3-1 continued

DRUG[a]	NUMBER OF INFANTS	EFFECT ON INFANTS	MATERNAL DOSE	ROUTE	CONCENTRATION OF DRUG IN BREAST MILK	TIME AFTER MATERNAL DOSE	SIGNIFI-CANCE[b]	REFERENCE[c]
Phenytoin	?	None reported	300 mg/day	PO	1.0–3.2 µg/ml	Not reported	+	Mirkin 1971
(Diphenyl-	1	None reported	200 mg bid	PO	1.8–2.0 µg/ml	3–7 hr		Soderman 1987
hydantoin)								
	6	None reported	200–400 mg	PO	0.2–3.0 µg/ml	Not reported		Steen 1982b
	1	None reported	100 mg tid	PO	4.2 µg/ml (peak) 1–2 µg/ml	3 hr Rest of dosing interval		Svensmark 1960

- Small amounts excreted into milk. In one study, two of six breast-fed infants had detectable blood concentrations (Steen et al., 1982b). Rarely, idiosyncratic reactions may occur in breast-fed infants. One case report was of cyanosis and methemoglobinemia in a breast-fed infant whose mother was taking both phenytoin and phenobarbital (Finch & Lorber, 1954).

DRUG[a]	NUMBER OF INFANTS	EFFECT ON INFANTS	MATERNAL DOSE	ROUTE	CONCENTRATION OF DRUG IN BREAST MILK	TIME AFTER MATERNAL DOSE	SIGNIFI-CANCE[b]	REFERENCE[c]
Phytonadione (Vitamin K$_1$)	120	Prothrombin times not affected until 3rd day after dose	40 mg	PO	Not measured		+	Dyggve 1956
	1	None reported	100 µg (similar to amount in normal meal)	PO	100% higher than maternal serum concentration	Not reported		Kries 1987

- At usual maternal doses, unlikely to produce ADRs in normal breast-fed infants. Exogenous vitamin K$_1$ use by mother results in an increase in vitamin K$_1$ concentration in milk (Kries et al., 1987). Maternal vitamin K$_1$ supplementation with 5 mg/day increases vitamin K$_1$ concentrations in milk to levels comparable with that in infant formula (Greer et al., 1997). Monitor infant prothrombin times if mother receives exogenous vitamin K$_1$.

DRUG[a]	NUMBER OF INFANTS	EFFECT ON INFANTS	MATERNAL DOSE	ROUTE	CONCENTRATION OF DRUG IN BREAST MILK	TIME AFTER MATERNAL DOSE	SIGNIFI-CANCE[b]	REFERENCE[c]
Piroxicam	2	None reported	20 mg 40 mg	PO PO	0.17 µg/ml 0.22 µg/ml	15.5 hr 2.2 hr	0	Ostensen 1983
	4	None reported	20 mg	PO	0.07–0.1 µg/ml			Ostensen 1988

- About 1%–3% of maternal dose excreted in milk (Ostensen et al., 1988). Unlikely to produce ADRs in breast-fed infants.

DRUG[a]	NUMBER OF INFANTS	EFFECT ON INFANTS	MATERNAL DOSE	ROUTE	CONCENTRATION OF DRUG IN BREAST MILK	TIME AFTER MATERNAL DOSE	SIGNIFI-CANCE[b]	REFERENCE[c]
Polio Virus Vaccine, Oral (OPV)		None reported					0	Deforest 1973 Greenberger 1993 Immunization Practices Advisory Committee 1989 John 1976 Kim-Farley 1982

- The Centers for Disease Control Immunization Practices Advisory Committee recommends routine immunization of infants with OPV regardless of breast feeding. After 6 weeks of age, neutralizing antibodies in milk have little effect on successful immunization.

DRUG[a]	NUMBER OF INFANTS	EFFECT ON INFANTS	MATERNAL DOSE	ROUTE	CONCENTRATION OF DRUG IN BREAST MILK	TIME AFTER MATERNAL DOSE	SIGNIFI-CANCE[b]	REFERENCE[c]
Prednisolone	7	None reported	5 mg	PO	Average of 0.07%–0.23% of dose per liter of milk	48-hr pooled samples	++	McKenzie 1975
	6	Not reported	10–80 mg	PO	30–317 ng/ml	1 hr		Ost 1985
	3	Not reported	50 mg	IV	40–400 ng/ml	0–6 hr		Greenberger 1993

- Exposure of breast-fed infant minimal, especially in mothers receiving 20 mg once or twice daily. At higher doses, avoidance of breast feeding for 3–4 hr after each dose may minimize breast milk exposure to infant (Anderson, 1987b). The more predictable and earlier peak concentrations with prednisolone compared to prednisone may be advantageous.

DRUG[a]	NUMBER OF INFANTS	EFFECT ON INFANTS	MATERNAL DOSE	ROUTE	CONCENTRATION OF DRUG IN BREAST MILK	TIME AFTER MATERNAL DOSE	SIGNIFI-CANCE[b]	REFERENCE[c]
Prednisone	1	Not reported	120 mg	PO	627 ng/ml*	Not reported	++	Berlin 1979a
	1	Not reported	10 mg	PO	28.3 ng/ml*	2 hr		Katz 1975
	1	Not reported	20 mg	PO	102 ng/ml*	Not reported		Sagraves 1981

- Milk concentrations here (*) reflect prednisone + prednisolone. When dosages >20 mg/day or long-term therapy is required, consider using prednisolone and avoiding breast feeding for 3–4 hr following each dose to minimize exposure of infant (Anderson, 1987b).

DRUG[a]	NUMBER OF INFANTS	EFFECT ON INFANTS	MATERNAL DOSE	ROUTE	CONCENTRATION OF DRUG IN BREAST MILK	TIME AFTER MATERNAL DOSE	SIGNIFI-CANCE[b]	REFERENCE[c]
Primidone	4	Lethargy, hypotonia, poor feeding, drug-withdrawal signs and symptoms	7.4–8.5 mg/kg	PO	Primidone 0.4–8.2 µg/ml Phenylethyl-malonamide 0.94–2.6 µg/ml Phenobarbital 0.84–5.2 µg/ml	Not reported	++	Nau 1980

Continued

Footnotes are on page 203.

TABLE 3-1 continued

DRUG[a]	NUMBER OF INFANTS	EFFECT ON INFANTS	MATERNAL DOSE	ROUTE	CONCENTRATION OF DRUG IN BREAST MILK	TIME AFTER MATERNAL DOSE	SIGNIFI-CANCE[b]	REFERENCE[c]
Primidone continued	12	Not reported	Quantity to achieve maternal serum concentration of 0.8–15.7 μg/ml	PO	2.8 μg/ml	Not reported		Kaneko 1979

- Use with caution in breast-feeding women (American Academy of Pediatrics, 1994). Primidone and its active metabolites, phenylethylmalonamide and phenobarbital, appear in milk. Monitor for sedative effects (Kuhnz et al., 1988).

Procainamide	1	Not reported	500 mg	PO	Procainamide 10.2 mg/liter N-Acetylprocainamide 3.4 mg/liter	6 hr	+	Pittard 1983

- Procainamide and a metabolite, N-acetylprocainamide, appear in milk. However, minimal amounts are excreted into milk with long-term use.

Propafenone	1	Not reported	300 mg tid	PO	32 ng/ml	Not reported	+	Libardoni 1991

- Small amounts excreted in milk. Clinical significance unknown.

Propoxyphene	6	Not reported	65 mg	PO	Propoxyphene 24.2–210 ng/ml Norpropoxyphene (active metabolite) 54.1–606 ng/ml	2 hr	0	Kunka 1984

- Unlikely to produce ADRs in breast-fed infants because only small amounts are excreted in milk.

Propranolol	1	None reported	40 mg as one-time dose	PO	2–9 ng/ml	2–5 hr	0	Bauer 1979
			40 mg qid	PO	64 ng/ml	3 hr		
	3	Not reported	1.2–2.6 mg/kg/day	PO	13.5–74.9 ng/ml	2.75–8.17 hr		Smith 1983
	1	None reported	20 mg bid	PO	20 ng/ml	1–2 hr		Taylor 1981
	10	None reported	80–100 mg/day	PO	27 ng/ml	2 hr		Thorley 1983

- Only small amounts are excreted into milk, even with relatively large maternal doses. Unlikely to produce ADRs in breast-fed infants.

Propyl-thiouracil	9	None reported	400 mg	PO	0.7 μg/ml	Not reported	+	Kampmann 1980
	1	None reported	125 mg	PO	Not measured			Lamberg 1984

- Not concentrated in milk. Recommended maternal doses of up to 300 mg/day result in transfer of minimal and clinically insignificant amounts (0.025% of maternal dose) to the breast-fed infant. Drug of choice for mothers who are breast feeding because of greater risks associated with other antithyroid drugs (Cooper, 1987). Monitor circulating thyroid hormone levels of breast-fed infants.

Pseudo-ephedrine	3	None reported	60 mg	PO	~1000 ng/ml	1–1.5 hr	0	Findlay 1984

- Amount excreted in milk in 24-hr period is 0.4%–6% of maternal dose. Concentration in milk higher than in maternal plasma. Unlikely to produce ADRs in breast-fed infants because of small amounts excreted in milk.

Pyrazinamide	1	Not reported	1 gram	PO	1.5 mg/liter	3 hr	+	Holdiness 1984

- Unlikely to produce ADRs in breast-fed infants because of low concentrations in milk. Monitor liver function periodically for hepatotoxicity in breast-fed infants.

Pyridostigmine	2	None reported	60 mg	PO	13–25 ng/ml	2–8 hr	+	Hardell 1982

- Unlikely to produce ADRs in breast-fed infants unless infant renal function is impaired.

Pyridoxine (Vitamin B_6)		May suppress lactation		PO			++	Andon 1985 Canales 1976 Foukas 1973 Macdonald 1976 Marcus 1975

- Some studies show a suppression of lactation with maternal use of high doses (600 mg/day) of pyridoxine (Foukas, 1973; Marcus, 1975), but other studies show no effect on lactation (Canales et al., 1976; Macdonald, 1976). Usual amounts of pyridoxine in diet unlikely to have an effect on lactation.

TABLE 3-1 continued

DRUG[a]	NUMBER OF INFANTS	EFFECT ON INFANTS	MATERNAL DOSE	ROUTE	CONCENTRATION OF DRUG IN BREAST MILK	TIME AFTER MATERNAL DOSE	SIGNIFI-CANCE[b]	REFERENCE[c]
Pyrimethamine	18	Not reported	50–75 mg as one-time dose	PO	3.1–3.3 µg/ml	6 hr	++	Clyde 1956, 1960
	3	Not reported	12.5 mg	PO	Not reported	Not reported		Edstein 1986

- Enough excreted in milk over 2-day period to treat malaria in 6-month-old infants. Detectable in milk 48 hr after dose. Up to 45.6% of maternal dose excreted in milk. Although sufficient amounts are excreted in milk, prophylaxis of breast-fed infants with a single drug is not recommended because resistant malaria strains may develop. Exposure to low concentrations of antimalarial drugs on a long-term basis may promote development of drug resistance.

| Quinidine | 1 | Not reported | 600 mg (quinidine sulfate) | PO | 6.4–8.2 mg/ml | 3 hr | ++ | Hill 1979 |

- Concentrations in milk similar to maternal serum concentrations. There is a potential for accumulation in breast-fed infants because of their immature liver function. Effects on breast-fed infants unknown.

| Quinine | 6 | None reported | 600–1300 mg | PO | 0.4–1.6 µg/ml | 1.5–6 hr | 0 | Terwilliger 1934 |

- Only small quantities are excreted in milk, even with high maternal doses. Unlikely to produce ADRs in breast-fed infants.

| Ranitidine | 1 | None reported | 150 mg | PO | 309 ng/ml | 5.5 hr | + | Kearns 1985 |

- There is a lag between the ranitidine concentration profiles in milk compared to maternal plasma. Highest milk to maternal plasma ratio seen at 12 hr after dose. Lowest ratio at 1.5–5.5 hr after dose. To minimize exposure of breast-fed infant, feed at least 1–2 hr after each dose. Alternative drugs (famotidine, nizatidine, sucralfate) should be considered (Anderson, 1991).

| Rifampin | 1 | None reported | 450 mg | PO | 21.3 mg/liter | 12 hr | + | Lenzi 1969 |

- Small amounts (0.05% maternal dose) excreted in milk. Unlikely to produce ADRs in breast-fed infants (Snider & Powell, 1984).

Rubella Virus Vaccine	1	None reported	HPV-77 DE$_5$ strain	SC	Virus detectable	12 days	0	Bulmovici-Klein 1977
	9	None reported	0.5–0.7 ml Cendehill strain	SC	Not reported			Farquhar 1972
	16	No clinical symptoms of rubella	Live, attenuated rubella virus vaccine	SC	Not reported			Losonsky 1982

- Rubella virus observed in milk of more than 69% of vaccinated women (Losonsky et al., 1982). Transient seroconversion to rubella virus in 25% of breast-fed infants (Losonsky et al., 1982). No transfer of live virus with Cendehill strain (Farquhar, 1972). No evidence that milk from women immunized with rubella is harmful to breast-fed infants (Immunization Practices Advisory Committee, 1989). Approximately 50% of breast-fed infants exhibit an immune response (Anderson, 1991).

Senna	25	None reported	100 mg (Senokot®)	PO	<0.34 µg/ml	Not reported	+	Baldwin 1963
	10	Increased stools in six of 10 infants	4-ml fluidextract	PO	<2.8 µg/ml	24-hr pooled samples		Tyson 1937
	50	None reported	1 teaspoonful (Senokot® granules)	PO	Not measured			Werthmann 1973

- Senna formulations commonly used previously (e.g., fluidextract) contained larger amounts of senna. Larger than usual maternal doses of senna may cause an increase in bowel activity in breast-fed infants. Usual maternal doses probably are safe.

Sertraline	1	None reported	100 mg/day	PO	8.8–43 ng/ml	1–22 hr	++	Altshuler 1995
	8	None reported	50–200 mg/day	PO	12–20 µg/liter (in one patient)	0–24 hr		Kristensen 1998
	12	None reported	25–200 mg/day	PO	17–173 ng/ml	0–24 hr		Stowe 1997
	9	None reported	50–200 mg/day	PO	Not measured			Wisner 1998

- Peak sertraline milk concentration occurs at 6–8 hr. In four infants, no sertraline or a major metabolite, N-desmethylsertraline, was detected in plasma (Kristensen et al., 1998). In another study, seven of nine infants had undetectable sertraline concentrations but one infant had unusually high concentrations (50% of mother's plasma concentration) (Wisner et al., 1998). Long-term effects unknown (American Academy of Pediatrics, 1994).

| Sodium Iodide I 125 | 1 | Not reported | 100 µCi | IV | 4 nCi/ml
0.3 nCi/ml | 20 hr
300 hr | +++ | Palmer 1979 |

- May cause thyroid suppression in breast-fed infants. Radioactivity in milk detectable for 12 days.

Footnotes are on page 203.

TABLE 3-1 continued

DRUG[a]	NUMBER OF INFANTS	EFFECT ON INFANTS	MATERNAL DOSE	ROUTE	CONCENTRATION OF DRUG IN BREAST MILK	TIME AFTER MATERNAL DOSE	SIGNIFI-CANCE[b]	REFERENCE[c]
Sodium Iodide I 131	2	Not reported	100 µCi	PO	39 nCi/ml 1.3–2 nCi/ml	6 hr (peak) 24 hr	+++	Nurenberger 1952
	6	Not reported	10 µCi, then 30 µCi	PO	0.3%–26.8% of dose	48-hr pooled serum		Weaver 1960
	1	Not reported	200 MBq 4000 MBq	PO	10⁶ Bq/ml 10 Bq/ml	Day 0 >Day 30		Robinson 1994

- May cause thyroid suppression and, with high doses, destruction of the thyroid gland of the infant. May increase the risk of thyroid cancer in breast-fed infant. Use T_3 and T_4 tests instead of radioactive testing, when possible.

Sotalol	1	None reported	80 mg tid 80 mg bid	PO	3.6–4.1 mg/liter 2.4–3.2 mg/liter	6.3–7 hr 2.8–3.3 hr	+	Hackett 1990
	5	None reported	200–800 mg/day	PO	4.8–20.2 mg/liter	Not reported		O'Hare 1980

- Monitor breast-fed infants for bradycardia, hypotension, respiratory distress, and hypoglycemia (Hackett et al., 1990).

Spironolactone	1	None reported	25 mg qid	PO	104 ng/ml (canrenone) 47 ng/ml (canrenone)	2 hr 14.5 hr	0	Phelps 1977

- Small quantities of canrenone (a metabolite of spironolactone) excreted in milk.

Streptomycin	8	None reported	1 gram	IM	1.1–1.3 mg/liter 0.6 mg/liter	6 hr 24 hr	+	Fujimori 1960

- May alter intestinal flora in breast-fed infants. Monitor for diarrhea and candidiasis (e.g., oral thrush).

Sulfasalazine (Salicylazo-sulfapyridine)	1	None reported	500 mg qid	PO	Not detectable	Not reported	++	Berlin 1980b
	1	Bloody diarrhea	3 grams/day	PO	Not reported	Not reported		Branski 1986
	8	None reported	Average of 2.6 grams/day	PO	Sulfasalazine 4.1 µg/ml Sulfapyridine 6–30 µg/ml	Not reported		Esbjorner 1987
	12	Not reported	1–3 grams/day	PO	<5 µg/ml in five of 31 milk samples	Not reported		Jarnerot 1979

- In one study (Branski et al., 1986), a breast-fed infant's sulfapyridine plasma concentration was 5.3 µg/ml (therapeutic range 20–50 µg/ml), whereas the mother's plasma concentration was 42 µg/ml. The infant's diarrhea resolved within 48–72 hr after the mother discontinued her sulfasalazine use. Use with caution (American Academy of Pediatrics, 1994).

Sumatriptan	5	Not reported	6 mg	SC	Average 87.2 µg/liter	2.5 hr	+	Wojnar-Horton 1996

- Low concentrations excreted in milk. If desired, to avoid even minor exposure to breast-fed infant, express and discard milk for 8 hr after dose.

Technetium Tc 99m	1	None reported	10 mCi	IV	5.8 µCi/ml 0.02 µCi/ml 0.001 µCi/ml	3.25 hr 24 hr 45 hr	+++	Maisels 1983
	2	Not reported	4 mCi	IV	3 and 5.2 times maternal serum concentration	17.2 hr		Spencer 1970
	2	Not reported	12 mCi	IV	610 nCi/ml 100 nCi/ml Detectable	2 hr 10 hr 24 hr		Wyburn 1973
	1	Not reported	10 mCi	IV	10 nCi/ml 3 nCi/ml Not detectable	22 hr 46 hr 70 hr		Vagenakis 1971

- Concentrates in milk. Do not breast feed for 72 hr after Tc 99m administration (American Academy of Pediatrics, 1994).

Technetium Tc 99m Albumin Aggregated	1	None reported	2 mCi	IV	0.45 µCi activity/ 15 ml milk 0.014 µCi activity/ 15 ml milk	4 hr 18 hr	+++	Berke 1973
	1	None reported	4 mCi	IV	1.1 µCi activity/ 15 ml milk 0.02 µCi activity/ 15 ml milk	3 hr 24 hr		Pittard 1982

- Concentrates in milk. Do not breast feed for 72 hr after Tc 99m albumin aggregated administration (American Academy of Pediatrics, 1994).

TABLE 3-1 continued

DRUG[a]	NUMBER OF INFANTS	EFFECT ON INFANTS	MATERNAL DOSE	ROUTE	CONCENTRATION OF DRUG IN BREAST MILK	TIME AFTER MATERNAL DOSE	SIGNIFI- CANCE[b]	REFERENCE[c]
Temazepam	10	None reported	10–20 mg/day	PO	26–28 ng/ml (in one patient)	Not reported	++	Lebedevs 1992

• Detected in milk in one of 10 subjects. Oxazepam (a metabolite) not detected in any sample (Lebedevs et al., 1992). Long-term effects unknown (American Academy of Pediatrics, 1994).

Terbutaline	2	None reported	2.5 mg tid	PO	2.5–4.6 ng/ml	1.2–7.8 hr	0	Boreus 1982
	2	None reported	5 mg tid	PO	3.2–3.8 ng/ml	3–8 hr		Lonnerholm 1982
	4	None reported	2.5–5 mg tid	PO	2.5–4.8 ng/ml	0–8 hr		Lindberg 1984

• Only small amounts of terbutaline excreted into milk, not detectable in infant plasma. Unlikely to produce ADRs in breast-fed infants because of small amounts.

Tetracycline	2	Not reported	150 mg	PO	0.3–1.2 µg/ml	Not reported	++	Matsuda 1984
	5	None reported	500 mg qid for 3 days	PO	0.43–2.53 µg/ml	2–4 hr		Posner 1955

• Tooth staining and inhibition of bone growth theoretically possible but not reported. Calcium in breast milk may inhibit GI absorption by infants of the small amounts of tetracycline in breast milk. Infant serum concentrations less than milk concentrations (Posner, 1955). Limit tetracycline therapy to 7–10 days in breast-feeding women (Anderson, 1991).

Tetrahydro- cannabinol (Cannabis, Marijuana, THC)	68	Decreased motor development at 1 year	Not reported	Not reported	Not reported		+++	Astley 1990
	1	Drowsiness	Smoked once a day	Inhalation	105 ng/ml	Not reported		Perez-Reyes 1982
	1	Drowsiness	Smoked seven times/day	Inhalation	340 ng/ml	Not reported		

• Excreted in milk. Concentration can occur (Perez-Reyes & Wall, 1982), and tetrahydrocannabinol may then be absorbed and metabolized by breast-fed infants.

Theobromine	10	None reported	1.2-oz chocolate bar	PO	1.5–3.7 µg/ml	3–5 hr	+	Berlin 1981
	6	None reported	113-gram Hershey's milk chocolate (240 mg theobromine)	PO	3.7–7.5 mg/liter (peak)	2.1–3.3 hr		Resman 1977

• If a mother consumed a 4-oz chocolate bar every 6 hr, and a 5–10-kg infant ingested 1 liter of milk in a 24-hr period, infant could receive 10 mg of theobromine (1–2 mg/kg/day) and experience adverse effects because of the long half-life of theobromine.

Theophylline	3	Not reported	3.2–5.3 mg/kg	IV	0.9–3.6 µg/ml	1–3 hr	++	Stec 1980
	1	Agitation, irritability	4.25 mg/kg	PO	4 µg/ml	Not reported		Yurchak 1976

• Less than 1% of maternal theophylline dose is excreted in milk (Stec et al., 1980). Slow elimination and low plasma protein binding in breast-fed infants may result in accumulation. Avoid high maternal theophylline serum concentrations. Caffeine and theobromine intake should be restricted to avoid cumulative effects. Monitor infant's serum concentration if signs and symptoms occur (Anderson, 1991).

Thiamine (Vitamin B$_1$)	175	None reported	Normal dietary intake (in India)	PO	99–130 ng/ml	Not reported	0	Fehily 1944

• Women with severe thiamine deficiency should avoid breast feeding to prevent thiamine deficiency in their breast-fed infants.

Thiopental	16	Not reported	3.8–6.3 mg/kg	IV	9 µg/ml	2 hr	0	Andersen 1987
	1	None reported	125 mg over 35 min	IV	7.5–20 µg/ml	14 min after end of infusion		Mayo 1942

• Small quantities excreted in milk.

Thiouracil	2	Not reported	1 gram	PO	90–120 mg/ml; 300% higher than maternal serum concentration	2 hr	+++	Kay 1944

• Significant milk concentrations can occur and suppress thyroid function in breast-fed infants, resulting in goiter. Breast feeding generally should be avoided while taking thiouracil.

Footnotes are on page 203.

TABLE 3-1 continued

DRUG[a]	NUMBER OF INFANTS	EFFECT ON INFANTS	MATERNAL DOSE	ROUTE	CONCENTRATION OF DRUG IN BREAST MILK	TIME AFTER MATERNAL DOSE	SIGNIFI-CANCE[b]	REFERENCE[c]
Timolol	9	None reported	5 mg tid	PO	15.9 ng/ml	Not reported	++	Fidler 1983
	1	None reported	0.5% ophthalmic solution bid	OD	5.6 ng/ml	1.5 hr		Lustgarten 1983

• Concentrates in milk. Monitor breast-fed infants for bradycardia and hypotension. Use of timolol should be avoided when high maternal oral doses are necessary (Anderson, 1991).

Tobramycin	1	Not reported	80 mg	IM	0.6 µg/ml	1 hr	+	Uwaydah 1975
					0.58 µg/ml	8 hr		

• Unlikely to achieve significant plasma concentrations in breast-fed infants because of poor GI absorption. Monitor for candidiasis (e.g., oral thrush) and diarrhea.

Tocainide	1	Not reported	400 mg every 8 hr	PO	28 µg/ml	2 hr	+	Wilson 1988

• Milk concentration is twice concurrent maternal serum concentration. Use with caution in breast-feeding women.

Tolbutamide	2	Not reported	500 mg	PO	3–18 µg/ml; 9%–40% of maternal serum concentration	4 hr	+	Moiel 1967

• Unlikely to produce ADRs in breast-fed infants. However, risk of hypoglycemia must be considered. Insulin may be preferred in breast-feeding women.

Tolmetin	1	Not reported	400 mg	PO	0.18 µg/ml	0.67 hr	0	Sagraves 1985

• Small amounts excreted in milk. Unlikely to produce ADRs in breast-fed infants.

Trazodone	6	Not reported	50 mg	PO	100 ng/ml	2 hr	++	Verbeeck 1986

• Small amounts excreted in milk. Amount of active metabolite, 1-m-chlorophenyl piperazine, in milk not measured. Long-term effects unknown (American Academy of Pediatrics, 1994).

Trimethoprim	20	None reported	160 mg bid-tid	PO	1.2–2.4 µg/ml	Not reported	+	Arnauld 1972

• Present in milk in low concentrations. Unlikely to produce ADRs in breast-fed infants.

Tuberculin Test (TB Test)	13	Eight of 13 infants born to skin test tuberculin-positive mothers developed reactive lymphocytes to tuberculin after 4 weeks of breast feeding	PPD	ID	Reactive-lymphocytes detectable	4 weeks	+	Schlesinger 1977
	9	None of nine infants of skin test tuberculin-negative mothers had any reactive lymphocytes to tuberculin after 4 weeks of breast feeding	PPD	ID	Reactive-lymphocytes not detectable	4 weeks		

• No infant developed tuberculin-positive skin test at 4 weeks. However, breast-fed infants may acquire T cell responsiveness to a specific antigen (e.g., tuberculin) by ingestion of milk from tuberculin-positive mothers.

Valproic Acid	1	None reported	1600 mg/day	PO	3–7 µg/ml	Not reported	+	Alexander 1979
	11	None reported	Not reported	PO	<0.5 µg/ml	Not reported		Nau 1981
	16	Not reported	300–2400 mg/day	PO	0.4–3.9 µg/ml (~5% of maternal serum concentration)	Not reported		von Unruh 1984

• Valproic acid concentration in milk is low (5%–10% of maternal serum concentration) (Philbert et al., 1985). Unlikely to produce ADRs in breast-fed infants. However, monitor for rare idiosyncratic reactions (e.g., hepatotoxicity).

Vancomycin	10	Not reported	Not reported	IV	12.7 µg/ml in one of 10 mothers	4 hr	0	Reyes 1989

• Unlikely to produce ADRs in breast-fed infants because of poor oral bioavailability.

TABLE 3-1 continued

DRUG[a]	NUMBER OF INFANTS	EFFECT ON INFANTS	MATERNAL DOSE	ROUTE	CONCENTRATION OF DRUG IN BREAST MILK	TIME AFTER MATERNAL DOSE	SIGNIFI-CANCE[b]	REFERENCE[c]
Venlafaxine	3	Not reported	3.04–8.18 mg/kg/day	PO	400–4200 µg/liter	0–12 hr	++	Ilett 1998

- None detected in infants' plasma, but all infants had detectable plasma concentrations of metabolite, O-desmethylvenlafaxine. Monitor for agitation, insomnia, poor feeding, and failure to thrive. Long-term effects unknown.

Verapamil	1	None reported	240 mg	PO	8–40 ng/ml	1 hr	+	Anderson 1983
	1	None reported	80 mg tid	PO	Verapamil 25.8 ng/ml Norverapamil 8.8 ng/ml	Not reported		Anderson 1987a
	1	None reported	120 mg tid	PO	Verapamil 133–205 ng/ml Norverapamil 50–65 ng/ml	4 hr		Miller 1986

- Infant's verapamil and norverapamil (active metabolite) serum concentrations not detectable (Anderson et al., 1987a; Miller et al., 1986).

Vigabatrin	2	Not reported	1000 mg bid	PO	1.82–3.96 mg/liter 2.94–5.08 mg/liter	3 hr 6 hr	+	Tran 1998

- Up to 4% of maternal dose ingested by breast-fed infant.

Vitamin D	1	None reported	50,000 units/day	PO	Not measured		+	Goldberg 1972
	1	None reported	10,000 units/day	PO	6700–7660 units/liter	Not reported		Greer 1984

- Normal vitamin D concentration in breast milk <20 units/liter. In mothers receiving large vitamin D doses, monitor infant's calcium serum concentration. Vitamin D supplementation is recommended for breast-fed infants of women with vitamin D deficiency (Rothberg et al., 1982).

Warfarin	1	None reported; normal prothrombin times (10.7 sec)	10 mg/day	PO	Not measured		+	Baty 1976
	13	Slightly elevated prothrombin times in three of seven breast-fed infants	30–40-mg loading dose, then maintenance dose of 5–11 mg/day (six patients) or 2–12 mg/day (seven patients)	PO	<25 mg/ml	3 days after maintenance dose started and 4 hr after last dose		Orme 1977
	2	None reported; normal prothrombin times	Not reported	PO	Not detectable	Not reported		McKenna 1983a

- Small quantities appear in milk. Maternal doses <12 mg/day unlikely to produce ADRs in breast-fed infants (Anderson, 1991). Monitor infant's prothrombin time with maternal doses >12 mg/day, if infant is at risk for vitamin K deficiency, or if there is evidence of bleeding (Clark et al., 2000).

Zolpidem	5	Not reported	20 mg	PO	0.76–3.88 µg (volume not specified)	3 hr	+	Pons 1989

- Not detected in milk 13–16 hr after maternal dose.

Footnotes are on page 203.

References

Alexander, F. W. (1979). Sodium valproate and pregnancy. *Archives of Disease in Childhood, 54,* 240–245.

Altshuler, L. L., Burt, V. K., McMullen, M., et al. (1995). Breastfeeding and sertraline: A 24-hour analysis. *Journal of Clinical Psychiatry, 56,* 243–245.

Amato, D., & Niblett, J. S. (1977). Neutropenia from cyclophosphamide in breast milk. *Medical Journal of Australia, 1,* 383–384.

American Academy of Pediatrics. Committee on Drugs. (1982). Psychotropic drugs in pregnancy and lactation. *Pediatrics, 69,* 241–244.

American Academy of Pediatrics. Committee on Drugs. (1994). Transfer of drugs and other chemicals into human milk. *Pediatrics, 93,* 137–150.

American Academy of Pediatrics. Committee on Nutrition. (1985). *Pediatric nutrition handbook,* 2nd ed. Elk Grove Village, IL: American Academy of Pediatrics.

American Academy of Pediatrics. Committee on Nutrition. (1986). Fluoride supplementation. *Pediatrics, 77,* 758–761.

American Academy of Pediatrics. Committee on Nutrition. (1992). The use of whole cow's milk in infancy. *Pediatrics, 89,* 1105–1109.

Ananth, J. (1978). Side effects in the neonate from psychotropic agents excreted through breast-feeding. *American Journal of Psychiatry, 135,* 801–805.

Andersen, L. W., Qvist, T., Hertz, J., et al. (1987). Concentration of thiopentone in mature breast milk and colostrum following an induction dose. *Acta Anaesthesiologica Scandinavica, 31,* 30–32.

Anderson, H. J. (1983). Excretion of verapamil in human milk. *European Journal of Clinical Pharmacology, 25,* 279–280.

Anderson, P., Bondesson, U., Mattiasson, I., et al. (1987a). Verapamil and norverapamil in plasma and breast milk during breast feeding. *European Journal of Clinical Pharmacology, 31,* 625–627.

Anderson, P. O. (1987b). Corticosteroid use by breast-feeding mothers. *Clinical Pharmacy, 6,* 445.

Anderson, P. O. (1991). Drug use during breast feeding. *Clinical Pharmacy, 10,* 594–624.

Anderson, P. O., & Mcguire, G. C. (1989). Neonatal alprazolam withdrawal: Possible effects of breast feeding. *Annals of Pharmacotherapy, 23,* 614.

Andon, M. B., Howard, M. P., Moser, P. B., et al. (1985). Nutritionally relevant supplementation of vitamin B_6 in lactating women: Effect on plasma prolactin. *Pediatrics, 76,* 769–773.

Arnauld, R. (1972). Étude du passage de la triméthoprime dans le lait maternel. *Ouest Medicine, 25,* 959–964.

Astley, S. J., & Little, R. E. (1990). Maternal marijuana use during lactation and infant development at one year. *Neurotoxicology and Teratology, 12,* 161–168.

Atkinson, H. C., & Beggs, E. J. (1990). Prediction of drug distribution into human milk from physiochemical characteristics. *Clinical Pharmacokinetics, 18,* 151–167.

Atkinson, H. C., Beggs, E. J., & Darlow, B. A. (1988). Drugs in human milk. Clinical pharmacokinetic considerations. *Clinical Pharmacokinetics, 14,* 217–240.

Ayd, F. J. (1973). Excretion of psychotropic drugs in human breast milk. *International Drug Therapy Newsletter, 8,* 33–40.

Azuno, Y., Kaku, K., Fujita, N., et al. (1995). Mitoxantrone and etoposide in breast milk. *American Journal of Hematology, 48,* 131–132.

Bader, T. F., & Newman, K. (1980). Amitriptyline in human breast milk and the nursing infant's serum. *American Journal of Psychiatry, 137,* 855–856.

Baldwin, W. F. (1963). Clinical study of senna administration to nursing mothers—Assessment of effects on bowel habits. *Canadian Medical Association Journal, 89,* 566–568.

Barnas, C., Bergant, A., Hummer, M., et al. (1994). Clozapine concentrations in maternal and fetal plasma, amniotic fluid, and breast milk. *American Journal of Psychiatry, 151,* 945.

Barnett, D. B., Hudson, S. A., & McBurney, A. (1982). Disopyramide and its N-monodesalkyl metabolite in breast milk. *British Journal of Clinical Pharmacology, 14,* 310–312.

Basler, R. S. W., & Lynch, P. J. (1985). Black galactorrhoea as a consequence of minocycline and phenothiazine therapy. *Archives of Dermatology, 121,* 417–418.

Baty, J. D. (1976). May mothers taking warfarin breast feed their infants? *British Journal of Clinical Pharmacology, 3,* 969.

Bauer, J. H., Pape, B., Zajicek, J., et al. (1979). Propranolol in human plasma and breast milk. *American Journal of Cardiology, 43,* 860–862.

Begg, E. J., Duffull, S. B., Saunders, D. A., et al. (1999). Paroxetine in human milk. *British Journal of Clinical Pharmacology, 48,* 142–147.

Belton, E. M., & Jones, R. V. (1965). Hemolytic anemia due to nalidixic acid. *The Lancet, 2,* 691.

Ben-Baruch, G., Menezer, J., Goshen, R., et al. (1992). Cisplatin excretion in human milk. *Journal of the National Cancer Institute, 84,* 451–452.

Ben-Chetrit, E., Scherrmann, J. M., & Levy, M. (1996). Colchicine in breast milk of patients with familial Mediterranean fever. *Arthritis and Rheumatism, 39,* 1213–1217.

Bennett, P. N., Humphries, S. J., Osborne, J. P., et al. (1990). Use of sodium aurothiomalate during lactation. *British Journal of Clinical Pharmacology, 29,* 777–779.

Bercovici, B., Gedalia, I., & Brzezinski, A. (1960). Fluorine in human milk. Its relation to urinary fluorine levels. *Obstetrics and Gynecology, 16,* 319–321.

Berke, R. A., Hoops, E. C., Kereiakes, J. C., et al. (1973). Radiation dose to breast-feeding child after mother has ^{99m}Tc-MAA lung scan. *Journal of Nuclear Medicine, 14,* 51–52.

Berlin, C. M., Jr. (1981). Excretion of the methylxanthines in human milk. *Seminars in Perinatology, 5,* 389–394.

Berlin, C. M., Jr. (1990). Fluoride supplementation for breast-fed infants. *Journal of the American Medical Association, 263,* 2371.

Berlin, C. M., Jr., & Lee, C. (1979b). Isoniazid and acetylisoniazid disposition in human milk, saliva and plasma. *Federation Proceedings, 38,* 426.

Berlin, C. M., Jr., & Yaffe, S. J. (1980b). Disposition of sulfasalazine and metabolites in human breast milk. *Developmental Pharmacology and Therapeutics, 1,* 31–39.

Berlin, C. M., Jr., Kaiser, D. G., & Demers, L. (1979a). Excretion of prednisone and prednisolone in human milk. *Pharmacologist, 21,* 264.

Berlin, C. M., Jr., Pascuzzi, M. J., & Yaffe, S. J. (1980a). Excretion of salicylate in human milk. *Clinical Pharmacology and Therapeutics, 27,* 245–246.

Berlin, C. M., Jr., Yaffe, J. Y., & Ragni, M. (1980c). Disposition of acetaminophen in milk, saliva, and plasma of lactating women. *Pediatric Pharmacology, 1,* 135–141.

Bernstine, J. B. (1956). Maternal blood and breast milk estimation following the administration of chloral hydrate during the puerperium. *Journal of Obstetrics and Gynaecology of the British Empire, 63,* 228–231.

Biniewicz, A., Robinson, M. J., & Senior, B. (1978). Pseudo-Cushing syndrome caused by alcohol in breast milk. *The Journal of Pediatrics, 93,* 965–967.

Bitzen, P. O., Gustafsson, B., Jostell, K. G., et al. (1981). Excretion of paracetamol in human breast milk. *European Journal of Clinical Pharmacology, 20,* 123–125.

Blanco, J. D., Jorgensen, J. H., Castaneda, Y. S., et al. (1983). Ceftazidime levels in human breast milk. *Antimicrobial Agents and Chemotherapy, 23,* 479–480.

Blau, S. P. (1973). Metabolism of gold during lactation. [Letter]. *Arthritis and Rheumatism, 16,* 777–778.

Blinick, G. (1975). Methadone assays in pregnant women progeny. *American Journal of Obstetrics and Gynecology, 121,* 617–621.

Boreus, L. O., de Chateau, P., Lindberg, C., et al. (1982). Terbutaline in breast milk. *British Journal of Clinical Pharmacology, 13,* 731–732.

Bourget, P., Quinquis-Desmaris, V., & Fernandez, H. (1993). Ceftriaxone distribution and protein binding between maternal blood and milk postpartum. *Annals of Pharmacotherapy, 27,* 294–297.

Boutroy, M. J., Bianchetti, G., Dubruc, C., et al. (1986). To nurse when receiving acebutolol: Is it dangerous for the neonate? *European Journal of Clinical Pharmacology, 3,* 737–739.

Bowes, W. A., Jr. (1980). The effect of medications on the lactating mother and her infant. *Clinical Obstetrics and Gynecology, 23,* 1073–1080.

Brambel, C. E., & Hunter, R. E. (1950). Effect of dicumarol on the nursing infant. *American Journal of Obstetrics and Gynecology, 59,* 1153–1159.

Branebjerg, P. E., & Heisterberg, L. (1987). Blood and milk concentrations of ampicillin. *Journal of Perinatal Medicine, 15,* 555–558.

Branski, D., Kerem, E., Gross-Kieselstein, E., et al. (1986). Bloody diarrhea—A possible complication of sulfasalazine transferred through human breast milk. *Journal of Pediatric Gastroenterology and Nutrition, 5,* 316–317.

Breyer-Pfaff, U., Nill, K., Entenmann, A., et al. (1995). Secretion of amitriptyline and metabolites into breast milk. *American Journal of Psychiatry, 152,* 812–813.

Briggs, G. G., Samson, J. H., Ambrose, P. J., et al. (1993). Excretion of bupropion in breast milk. *Annals of Pharmacotherapy, 27,* 431–433.

Brixen-Rasmussen, L., Halgrener, J., & Jorgenson, A. (1982). Amitriptyline and nortriptyline excretion in human breast milk. *Psychopharmacology, 76,* 94–95.

Brogden, R. N. (1975). Minocycline—A review. *Drugs, 9,* 251–291.

Buist, A., Norman, T. R., & Dennerstein, L. (1990). Breastfeeding and the use of psychotropic medication: A review. *Journal of Affective Disorders, 19,* 197–206.

Bulmovici-Klein, E., Hite, R. L., Byrne, T., et al. (1977). Isolation of rubella virus in milk after post-partum immunization. *The Journal of Pediatrics, 91,* 939–941.

Bunjes, R., Schaefer, C., & Holzinger, D. (1993). Clonidine and breast-feeding. *Clinical Pharmacy, 12,* 178–179.

Burch, K. J., & Wells, B. G. (1992). Fluoxetine/norfluoxetine concentrations in human milk. *Pediatrics, 89,* 676–677.

Burrow, G. N., Wassenaar, W., Robertson, G. L., et al. (1981). DDAVP treatment of diabetes insipidus during pregnancy and the post-partum period. *Acta Endocrinologica, 97,* 23–25.

Campbell, A. C., McElnay, J. C., & Passmore, C. M. (1991). The excretion of ampicillin in breast milk and its effect on the suckling infant. *British Journal of Clinical Pharmacology, 31,* 230.

Canales, E. S., Soria, J., Zarate, A., et al. (1976). The influence of pyridoxine on prolactin secretion and milk production in women. *British Journal of Obstetrics and Gynaecology, 83,* 387.

Carcas, A. J., Abad-Santos, F., deRosendo, J. M., et al. (1996). Nimodipine transfer into human breast milk and cerebrospinal fluid. *Annals of Pharmacotherapy, 30,* 148–150.

Celiloglu, M., Celiker, S., Guven, H., et al. (1994). Gentamicin excretion and uptake from breast milk by nursing infants. *Obstetrics and Gynecology, 84,* 263–265.

Chambers, C. D., Anderson, P. O., Thomas, R. G., et al. (1999). Weight gain in infants breastfed by mothers who take fluoxetine. *Pediatrics, 104,* e61.

Chan, V., Tse, T. F., & Wong, V. (1978). Transfer of digoxin across the placenta and into breast milk. *British Journal of Obstetrics and Gynaecology, 85,* 605–609.

Chaney, N. E., Franke, J., & Wadlington, W. B. (1988). Cocaine convulsions in a breast-feeding baby. *The Journal of Pediatrics, 112,* 134–135.

Chasnoff, I. J., Lewis, D. E., & Squires, L. (1987). Cocaine intoxication in a breast-fed infant. *Pediatrics, 80,* 836–838.

Chyo, N. (1962). Clinical studies of kanamycin applied in the field of obstetrics and gynecology. *Asian Medical Journal, 5,* 265–275.

Clark, J. H., & Wilson, W. G. (1981). A 16-day-old breast-fed infant with metabolic acidosis caused by salicylate. *Clinical Pediatrics, 20,* 53–54.

Clark, S. L., Porter, T. F., & West, F. G. (2000). Coumarin derivatives and breast-feeding. *Obstetrics and Gynecology, 95*(6 part 1), 938–940.

Clyde, D. F. (1956). Transfer of pyrimethamine in human milk. *Journal of Tropical Medicine and Hygiene, 59,* 277–284.

Clyde, D. F. (1960). Prolonged malaria prophylaxis through pyrimethamine in mother's milk. *East African Medical Journal, 37,* 659–660.

Cobo, E. (1973). Effect of different doses of ethanol on the milk-ejecting reflex in lactating women. *American Journal of Obstetrics and Gynecology, 115,* 817–821.

Cobrinik, R. W. (1959). The effect of maternal narcotic addiction on the newborn infant. *Pediatrics, 24,* 288–304.

Collins, R. A. (1951). The folic acid and vitamin B_{12} content of milk of various species. *Journal of Nutrition, 43,* 313–321.

Cooper, D. S. (1987). Anti-thyroid drugs: To breast feed or not to breast feed. *American Journal of Obstetrics and Gynecology, 157,* 234–235.

Courtney, T. P., Shaw, R. W., Cedar, E., et al. (1988). Excretion of famotidine in breast milk. *British Journal of Clinical Pharmacology, 26,* 639.

Cover, D. L., & Mueller, B. A. (1990). Ciprofloxacin penetration into human breast milk: A case report. *Annals of Pharmacotherapy, 24,* 703–704.

Cox, S. R., & Forbes, K. K. (1987). Excretion of flurbiprofen into breast milk. *Pharmacotherapy, 7,* 211–215.

Croxatto, H. (1983). Fertility regulation in nursing women: IV. Long-term influence of a low-dose combined oral contraceptive initiated at day 30 postpartum upon lactation and infant growth. *Contraception, 27,* 13–25.

Cruikshank, D. P., Varner, M. W., & Pitkin, R. M. (1982). Breast milk magnesium and calcium concentrations following magnesium sulfate treatment. *American Journal of Obstetrics and Gynecology, 143,* 685–688.

Curtis, E. M. (1964). Oral-contraceptive feminization of a normal male infant. *Obstetrics and Gynecology, 23,* 295–296.

Dahlstrom, A., Lundell, B., Curvall, M., et al. (1990). Nicotine and cotinine concentrations in the nursing mother and her infant. *Acta Paediatrica Scandinavica, 79,* 142–147.

Danzinger, Y., Pertzelan, A., & Mimouni, M. (1987). Transient congenital hypothyroidism after topical iodine in pregnancy and lactation. *Archives of Disease in Childhood, 62,* 295–296.

Davies, H. A., Clark, J. D. A., Dalton, K. J., et al. (1989). Insulin requirements of diabetic women who breast feed. *British Medical Journal, 298,* 1357–1358.

Davis, J. M., & Bhutani, V. K. (1985). Neonatal apnea and maternal codeine use. *Pediatric Research, 19,* 170A.

Deforest, A., Parker, P. B., DiLiberti, J. H., et al. (1973). The effect of breast-feeding on the antibody response of infants to trivalent oral poliovirus vaccine. *The Journal of Pediatrics, 83,* 93–95.

del Pozo, E. (1975). Lack of effect of methylergonovine on postpartum lactation. *American Journal of Obstetrics and Gynecology, 123,* 845–846.

del Re, R. B. (1973). Prolactin inhibition and suppression of puerperal lactation by bromergocryptine (CB 154). *Obstetrics and Gynecology, 41,* 884–890.

Delange, F., Chandine, J. P., Abrassart, C., et al. (1988). Topical iodine, breast feeding, and neonatal hypothyroidism. *Archives of Disease in Childhood, 63,* 106–107.

Devlin, R. G., Duchin, K. L., & Fleiss, P. M. (1981a). Nadolol in human serum and breast milk. *British Journal of Clinical Pharmacology, 12,* 393–396.

Devlin, R. G., & Fleiss, P. M. (1981b). Captopril in human blood and breast milk. *Journal of Clinical Pharmacology, 21,* 110–113.

Diaz, S. (1983). Fertility regulation in nursing women: III. Short-term influence of a low-dose combined oral contraceptive upon lactation and infant growth. *Contraception, 27,* 1–11.

Diaz, S., Herreros, C., Juez, G., et al. (1985). Fertility in nursing women: VII. Influence of Norplant® levonorgestrel implants upon lactation and infant growth. *Contraception, 32,* 53–74.

Dillon, H. K. (1974). Lead concentration in human milk. *American Journal of Diseases of Children, 128,* 491–492.

Drugs and human lactation. (1988). P. N. Bennett, I. Matheson, N. M. G. Duke, et al., Eds. Amsterdam: Elsevier.

Drugs in breast milk. (1974). *The Medical Letter on Drugs and Therapeutics, 16,* 25–27.

Drugs in pregnancy and lactation, 5th ed. (1998). G. G. Briggs, R. K. Freeman, & S. J. Yaffee, Eds. Baltimore, MD: Williams and Wilkins.

Durodola, J. I. (1979). Administration of cyclophosphamide during late pregnancy and early lactation: A case report. *Journal of the National Medical Association, 71,* 165–166.

Dusci, L. J., Good, S. M., Hall, R. W., et al. (1990). Excretion of diazepam and its metabolite in human milk during withdrawal from combination high-dose diazepam and oxazepam. *British Journal of Clinical Pharmacology, 29,* 123–126.

Dyggve, H. V. (1956). Influence on the prothrombin time of breast fed newborn babies of one single dose of vitamin K, or Synkavite® given to the mother within two hours after birth. *Acta Obstetricia et Gynecologica Scandinavica, 35,* 440–444.

Edstein, M. D., Veenendaal, J. R., & Hyslop, R. (1988). Excretion of mefoquine in human breast milk. *Chemotherapy, 34,* 165–169.

Edstein, M. D., Veenendaal, J. R., Newman, K., et al. (1986). Excretion of chloroquine, dapsone and pyrimethamine in human milk. *British Journal of Clinical Pharmacology, 22,* 733–735.

Eeg-Olofsson, O., Malmros, I., Elwin, C. E., et al. (1978). Convulsions in a breast-fed infant after maternal indomethacin. *The Lancet, 2,* 215.

Egan, P. C., Costanza, M. E., Dodion, P., et al. (1985). Doxorubicin and cisplatin excretion into human milk. *Cancer Treatment Reports, 69,* 1387–1389.

Ehrenkranz, R. A., & Ackerman, B. A. (1986). Metoclopramide effect on faltering milk production by mothers of premature infants. *Pediatrics, 78,* 614–620.

Ehrenkranz, R. A., Ackerman, B. A., & Hulse, J. D. (1989). Nifedipine transfer into human milk. *The Journal of Pediatrics, 114,* 478–480.

Ekstrand, J., Boreus, L. O., & de Chateau, P. (1981). No evidence of transfer of fluoride from plasma to breast milk. *British Medical Journal, 283,* 761–762.

Ellsworth, A. J., Horn, J. R, Raisys, V. A., et al. (1989). Disopyramide and N-monodesalkyl disopyramide in serum and breast milk. *Annals of Pharmacotherapy, 23,* 56–57.

Erickson, S. H., & Oppenheim, G. L. (1979). Aspirin in breast milk. *Journal of Family Practice, 8,* 189–190.

Erickson, S. H., Oppenheim, G. L., & Smith, G. H. (1981). Metronidazole in breast milk. *Obstetrics and Gynecology, 57,* 48–50.

Ericsson, Y. (1969). Fluoride excretion in human saliva and milk. *Caries Research, 3,* 159–166.

Ericsson, Y. (1972). Pilot studies on the fluoride metabolism in infants on different feedings. *Acta Paediatrica Scandinavica, 61,* 459–464.

Eriksson, G., & Swahn, C. (1981). Concentrations of baclofen in serum and breast milk from a lactating woman. *Scandinavian Journal of Clinical Investigation, 41,* 185–187.

Erkkola, R., & Kanto, J. (1972). Diazepam and breast feeding. *The Lancet, 1,* 125–126.

Erkkola, R., Kanto, J., Allonen, H., et al. (1978). Excretion of methylergometrine (methylergonovine) into the human breast milk. *International Journal of Clinical Pharmacology, 16,* 579–580.

Ertl, T., Sulyok, E., Ezer, E., et al. (1991). The influence of metoclopramide on the composition of human breast milk. *Acta Paediatrica Hungarica, 31,* 415–422.

Esbjorner, E., Jarnerot, G., & Wranne, L. (1987). Sulphasalazine and sulphapyridine serum levels in children of mothers treated with sulphasalazine during pregnancy and lactation. *Acta Paediatrica Scandinavica, 76,* 137–142.

Ette, E. I., Essien, E. E., Ogonor, J. I., et al. (1987). Chloroquine in human milk. *Journal of Clinical Pharmacology, 27,* 499–502.

Farquhar, J. D. (1972). Follow-up on rubella vaccinations and experience with subclinical reinfection. *The Journal of Pediatrics, 81,* 460–465.

Fehily, L. (1944). Human milk intoxication due to B_1 avitaminosis. *British Medical Journal, 2,* 590–592.

Feilberg, V. L., Rosenborg, D., Christensen, C. B., et al. (1989). Excretion of morphine in human breast milk. *Acta Anaesthesiologica Scandinavica, 33,* 426–428.

Fidler, J., Smith, V., & de Swiet, M. (1983). Excretion of oxprenolol and timolol in breast milk. *British Journal of Obstetrics and Gynaecology, 90*(10), 961–965.

Finch, E., & Lorber, J. (1954). Methemoglobinemia in the newborn probably due to phenytoin excreted in human milk. *Journal of Obstetrics and Gynaecology of the British Empire, 61,* 833–834.

Findlay, J. W. A., Butz, R. F., Sailstad, J. M., et al. (1984). Pseudoephedrine and triprolidine in plasma and breast milk of nursing mothers. *British Journal of Clinical Pharmacology, 18,* 901–906.

Findlay, J. W. A., DeAngelis, R. L., Kearney, M. F., et al. (1981). Analgesic drugs in breast milk and plasma. *Clinical Pharmacology and Therapeutics, 29,* 625–633.

Finley, J. P., Waxman, M. B., Wong, P. Y., et al. (1979). Digoxin excretion in human milk. *The Journal of Pediatrics, 94,* 339–340.

Fisher, J. B., Edgren, B. E., Mammel, M. C., et al. (1985). Neonatal apnea associated with maternal clonazepam therapy: A case report. *Obstetrics and Gynecology, 66*(Suppl), 34S–35S.

Flechner, S. M., Katz, A. R., Rogers, A. J., et al. (1985). The presence of cyclosporine in body tissues and fluids during pregnancy. *American Journal of Kidney Diseases, 5,* 60–63.

Fleiss, P. M. (1992). The effect of maternal medications on breast feeding infants. *Journal of Human Lactation, 8,* 7.

Fleiss, P. M., Richwald, G. A., & Gordin, J. (1985). Aztreonam in human serum and breast milk. *British Journal of Clinical Pharmacology, 19*, 509–511.

Floss, H. G. (1973). Influence of ergot alkaloids on pituitary prolactin and prolactin-dependent processes. *Journal of Pharmaceutical Sciences, 62*, 699–715.

Fomina, P. I. (1934). Untersuchungen über den übergang des aktiven agens des mutterkorns in die milch stillender mütter. *Archiv für Gynäkologie, 157*, 275–285.

Force, R. W. (1995). Fluconazole concentrations in breast milk. *Pediatric Infectious Disease Journal, 14*, 235–236.

Ford, K., & Labbok, M. (1990). Who is breast feeding? Implications of associated social and biomedical variables for research on the consequences of method of infant feeding. *American Journal of Clinical Nutrition, 52*, 451–456.

Foukas, M. D. (1973). An antilactogenic effect of pyridoxine. *Journal of Obstetrics and Gynaecology of the British Commonwealth, 19*, 718–720.

Frey, B., Schubiger, G., & Musy, J. P. (1990). Transient cholestatic hepatitis in a neonate associated with carbamazepine exposure during pregnancy and breastfeeding. *European Journal of Pediatrics, 150*, 136–138.

Frey, O. R., Scheidt, P., & vanBrenndorff, A. I. (1999). Adverse effects in a newborn infant breast-fed by a mother treated with doxepin. *Annals of Pharmacotherapy, 33*, 690–693.

Froescher, W., Eichelbaum, M., Niesen, M., et al. (1984). Carbamazepine levels in breast milk. *Therapeutic Drug Monitoring, 6*, 266–271.

Fujimori, S. (1960). International Abstract Surgery. *Surgery Gynecology and Obstetrics, 111*, 289.

Gardner, D. K. (1987). Drug passage into breast milk: Principles and concerns. *Journal of Pediatric and Perinatal Nutrition, 1*, 27–37.

Gardner, D. K., Gabbe, S. G., & Harter, C. (1992). Simultaneous concentrations of ciprofloxacin in breast milk and serum in mother and breast-fed infant. *Clinical Pharmacy, 11*, 352–354.

Gelenberg, A. J. (1979). Amoxapine, a new antidepressant, appears in human milk. *Journal of Nervous and Mental Disease, 167*, 635–636.

Geraghty, B., Graham, E. A., Logan, B., et al. (1997). Methadone levels in breast milk. *Journal of Human Lactation, 13*, 227–230.

Giamarellou, H., Kolokythas, E., Petrikkos, G., et al. (1989). Pharmacokinetics of three newer quinolones in pregnancy and lactating women. *American Journal of Medicine, 87*(Suppl 5A), 49S–51S.

Goldberg, L. D. (1972). Transmission of a vitamin-D metabolite in breast milk. *The Lancet, 2*, 1258–1259.

Gramen, K. (1922). Bestimmungen über den übergang des athers in die muttermilch. *Acta Chirurgica Scandinavica*, (Suppl 1), 83.

Gray, M. S. (1961). Further observations on metronidazole (Flagyl®). *British Journal of Venereal Diseases, 37*, 278–279.

Greenberger, P. A., Odeh, Y. K., Frederiksen, M. C., et al. (1993). Pharmacokinetics of prednisolone transfer to breast milk. *Clinical Pharmacology and Therapeutics, 53*, 324–328.

Greene, H. J. (1946). Excretion of penicillin in human milk following parturition. *American Journal of Obstetrics and Gynecology, 51*, 732–733.

Greer, F. R., Hollis, B. W., & Napoli, J. L. (1984). High concentrations of vitamin D_2 in human milk associated with pharmacologic doses of vitamin D_2. *The Journal of Pediatrics, 105*, 61–64.

Greer, F. R., Marshall, S. P., Foley, A. L., et al. (1997). Improving the vitamin K status of breast feeding infants with maternal vitamin K supplements. *Pediatrics, 99*, 88–92.

Guillonneau, M., Aigrain, E. J., Galliot, M., et al. (1995). Colchicine is excreted at high concentrations in human breast milk. *European Journal of Obstetrics and Gynecology, 61*, 177–178.

Gupta, A. P., & Gupta, P. K. (1985). Metoclopramide as a lactagogue. *Clinical Pediatrics, 24*, 269–272.

Gutgesell, M., Overholt, E., & Boyle, R. (1990). Oral bretylium tosylate use during pregnancy and subsequent breastfeeding: A case report. *American Journal of Perinatology, 7*, 144–145.

Hackett, L. P., Wojnar-Horton, R. E., Dusci, L. J., et al. (1990). Excretion of sotalol in breast milk. *British Journal of Clinical Pharmacology, 29*, 277–278.

Hagg, S., Graunberg, K., & Carleborg, L. (2000). Excretion of fluvoxamine into breast milk. *British Journal of Clinical Pharmacology, 49*, 286–288.

Hardell, L. I., Lindstrom, B., Lonnerholm, G., et al. (1982). Pyridostigmine in human breast milk. *British Journal of Clinical Pharmacology, 14*, 565–567.

Hartikainen-Sorri, A. L., Heikkinen, J. E., & Koivisto, M. (1987). Pharmacokinetics of clonidine during pregnancy and nursing. *Obstetrics and Gynecology, 69*, 598–600.

Hauser, G. J., Almog, S., Tirosh, M., et al. (1985). Effect of alpha-methyldopa excreted in human milk on the breast-fed infant. *Helvetica Paediatrica Acta, 40*, 83–86.

Havelka, J. (1968). Excretion of chloramphenicol in human milk. *Chemotherapy, 13*, 204–211.

Havelka, J., & Frankova, A. (1972). Study of side effects of maternal chloramphenicol therapy in newborns. *Ceskoslovenska Pediatrie, 21*, 31–33.

Healy, M. (1961). Suppressing lactation with oral diuretics. *The Lancet, 1*, 1353–1354.

Heisterberg, L., & Branebjerg, P. E. (1983). Blood and milk concentrations of metronidazole in mothers and infants. *Journal of Perinatal Medicine, 11*, 114–120.

Hilbert, J., Radwanski, E., Affrime, M. B., et al. (1988). Excretion of loratadine in human breast milk. *Journal of Clinical Pharmacology, 28*, 234–239.

Hill, L. M., & Malkasian, G. D., Jr. (1979). The use of quinidine sulfate throughout pregnancy. *Obstetrics and Gynecology, 54*, 366–368.

Holdiness, M. R. (1984). Antituberculosis drugs and breast feeding. *Archives of Internal Medicine, 144*, 1888.

Hoppu, K., Neuvonen, P. J., & Korte, T. (1986). Disopyramide and breast feeding. *British Journal of Clinical Pharmacology, 21*, 553.

Horning, M. G. (1975). Identification and quantification of drugs and drug metabolites in human breast milk using GC-MS-COM methods. *Modern Problems in Pediatrics, 15*, 73–79.

Houwert-de Jong, M., Gerards, L. J., Tetteroo-Tempelman, C. A. M., et al. (1981). May mothers taking acenocoumarol breast feed their infants? *European Journal of Clinical Pharmacology, 21*, 61–64.

Hunt, M. J., Salisbury, E. L., Grace, J., et al. (1996). Black breast milk due to minocycline therapy. *British Journal of Dermatology, 134*, 943–944.

Huttunen, K., Grunhagen-Riska, C., & Fuhrquist, F. (1989). Enalapril treatment of a nursing mother with slightly impaired renal function. *Clinical Nephrology, 31*, 278.

Ilett, K. F., Hackett, L. P., Dusci, L. J., et al. (1998). Distribution and excretion of venlafaxine and O-desmethylvenlafaxine in human milk. *British Journal of Clinical Pharmacology, 45*, 459–462.

Immunization Practices Advisory Committee. (1989). General recommendations on immunization. *Morbidity and Mortality Weekly Reports, 38*, 205–227.

Isenberg, K. E. (1990). Excretion of fluoxetine in human breast milk. *Journal of Clinical Psychiatry, 51*, 169.

Jamali, F., & Keshavarz, E. (1981). Salicylate excretion in breast milk. *International Journal of Pharmacy, 8*, 285–290.

Jamali, F., & Stevens, D. (1983). Naproxen excreted in milk and its uptake by the infant. *Drug Intelligence and Clinical Pharmacy, 17*, 910–911.

Jarnerot, G., & Into-Malmberg, M. B. (1979). Sulphasalazine treatment during breast feeding. *Scandinavian Journal of Gastroenterology, 14*, 869–871.

Johansen, K., Nyboe, A., Kampmann, J. P., et al. (1982). Excretion of methimazole in human milk. *European Journal of Clinical Pharmacology, 23*, 339–341.

John, T. J., Devarajan, L. V., Luther, L., et al. (1976). Effect of breast-feeding on seroresponse of infants to oral poliovirus vaccination. *Pediatrics, 57*, 47–53.

Johns, D. G. (1972). Secretion of methotrexate into human milk. *American Journal of Obstetrics and Gynecology, 112*, 978–980.

Kacew, S. (1993). Adverse effects of drugs and chemicals in breast milk on the nursing infant. *Journal of Clinical Pharmacology, 33*, 213–221.

Kafetzis, D. A., Brater, D. C., Fanourgakis, J. E., et al. (1983). Ceftriaxone distribution between maternal blood and fetal blood and tissues at parturition and between blood and milk postpartum. *Antimicrobial Agents and Chemotherapy, 23*, 870–873.

Kafetzis, D. A., Lazarides, C. V., Siafas, C. A., et al. (1980). Transfer of cefotaxime in human milk and from mother to foetus. *Journal of Antimicrobials and Chemotherapy, 6*(Suppl A), 135–141.

Kafetzis, D. A., Siafas, C. A., Georgakopoulos, P. A., et al. (1981). Passage of cephalosporins and amoxicillin into the breast milk. *Acta Paediatrica Scandinavica, 70*, 285–288.

Kamilli, J., & Gresser, U. (1993). Allopurinol and oxypurinol in human breast milk. *Clinical Investigator, 71*, 161–164.

Kampmann, J. P., Hansen, J., Johansen, K., et al. (1980). Propylthiouracil in human milk, revision of a dogma. *The Lancet, 1*, 736.

Kaneko, S., Sato, T., & Suzuki, K. (1979). The levels of anticonvulsant in breast milk. *British Journal of Clinical Pharmacology, 7*, 624–627.

Kanto, J. H. (1982). Use of benzodiazepines during pregnancy, labor and lactation, with particular reference to pharmacokinetic considerations. *Drugs, 23*, 354–380.

Katz, F. H., & Duncan, B. R. (1975). Entry of prednisolone into human milk. [Letter]. *New England Journal of Medicine, 293*, 1154.

Kaufman, K. R., Petrucha, R. A., Pitts, F. N., et al. (1983). PCP in amniotic fluid and breast milk: Case report. *Journal of Clinical Psychiatry, 44*, 269–270.

Kauppila, A., Arvela, P., Koivisto, M., et al. (1983). Metoclopramide and breast feeding: Transfer into milk and the newborn. *European Journal of Clinical Pharmacology, 25*, 819–823.

Kay, G. A., & Jandorf, B. J. (1944). Thiouracil: Its absorption, distribution and excretion. *Journal of Clinical Investigation, 23*, 613–627.

Kearns, G. L., McConnell, R. F., Trang, J. M., et al. (1985). Appearance of ranitidine in breast milk following multiple dosing. *Clinical Pharmacy, 4*, 322–324.

Kelsey, J. J., Moser, L. R., Jennings, J. C., et al. (1994). Presence of azithromycin breast milk concentrations: A case report. *American Journal of Obstetrics and Gynecology, 170*, 1375–1376.

Kemp, J., Ilfett, K. F., Booth, J., et al. (1985). Excretion of doxepin and N-desmethyldoxepin in human milk. *British Journal of Clinical Pharmacology, 20*, 497–499.

Kesaniemi, Y. (1974). Ethanol and acetaldehyde in the milk and peripheral blood of lactating women after ethanol administration. *Journal of Obstetrics and Gynaecology of the British Commonwealth, 81*, 84–86.

Kim-Farley, R., Brink, E., Orestein, W., et al. (1982). Vaccination and breast feeding. *Journal of the American Medical Association, 248*, 2451–2452.

Klotz, U., & Harings-Kaim, A. (1993). Negligible excretion of 5-aminosalicylic acid in breast milk. *The Lancet, 342*, 618–619.

Knowles, J. A. (1972). Drugs in milk. *Pediatric Currents, 21*, 28–32.

Knowles, J. A. (1974). Breast milk: A source of more than nutrition for the neonate. *Clinical Toxicology, 7*, 69–82.

Koetsawang, S. (1982). Transfer of contraceptive steroids in milk of women using long-acting gestagens. *Contraception, 25*, 321–331.

Koetsawang, S. (1987). The effects of contraceptive methods on the quality and quantity of breast milk. *International Journal of Gynecology and Obstetrics, 25*(Suppl), 115–127.

Kok, T. H. H. G., Taitz, L. S., & Bennett, M. J. (1982). Drowsiness due to clemastine transmitted in breast milk. *The Lancet, 1*, 914.

Koren, G., Radnor, S., Martin, S., et al. (1990). Maternal ginseng use associated with neonatal androgenization. *Journal of the American Medical Association, 264*, 2866.

Kreek, M. J., Schecter, A., Gutjahr, C. L., et al. (1974). Analyses of methadone and other drugs in maternal and neonatal body fluids: Use in evaluation of symptoms in a neonate of a mother maintained on methadone. *American Journal of Drug and Alcohol Abuse, 1*, 409–419.

Kries, R. V., Shearer, M., McCarthy, P. T., et al. (1987). Vitamin K_1 content of maternal milk: Influence of the stage of lactation, lipid composition, and vitamin K_1 supplements given to the mother. *Pediatric Research, 22*, 513–517.

Kristensen, J. H., Ilett, K. F., Dusci, L. J., et al. (1998). Distribution and excretion of sertraline and N-desmethylsertraline in human milk. *British Journal of Clinical Pharmacology, 45*, 453–457.

Kuhnz, W., Jager-Roman, E., Rating, D., et al. (1983). Carbamazepine and carbamazepine-10,11-epoxide during pregnancy and postnatal period in epileptic mothers and their nursed infants: Pharmacokinetics and clinical effects. *Pediatric Pharmacology, 3*, 199–208.

Kuhnz, W., Koch, S., Helge, H., et al. (1988). Primidone and phenobarbital during lactation period in epileptic women: Total and free serum levels in the nursed infant and their effects on neonatal behavior. *Developmental Pharmacology and Therapeutics, 11*, 147–154.

Kuhnz, W., Koch, S., Jakob, S., et al. (1984). Ethosuximide in epileptic women during pregnancy and lactation period. Placental transfer, serum concentrations in nursed infants and clinical status. *British Journal of Clinical Pharmacology, 18*, 671–677.

Kulas, J., Lunell, N. O., Rosing, U., et al. (1984). Atenolol and metoprolol. A comparison of their excretion into human breast milk. *Acta Obstetricia et Gynecologica Scandinavica, 118* (Suppl), 65–69.

Kunka, R. L., Venkateramanan, R., Stern, R. M., et al. (1984). Excretion of propoxyphene and norpropoxyphene in breast milk. *Clinical Pharmacology and Therapeutics, 35*, 675–680.

Kwit, N. T., & Hatcher, R. A. (1935). Excretion of drugs in milk. *American Journal of Diseases in Children, 49*, 900–904.

Lacey, J. H. (1971). Dichloralphenazone and breast milk. *British Medical Journal, 4*, 684.

Lamberg, B. A., Ikonen, E., Osterlund, K., et al. (1984). Anti-thyroid treatment of maternal hyperthyroidism during lactation. *Clinical Endocrinology, 21*, 81–87.

Larson, S. M., & Schall, G. L. (1971). Gallium 67 concentrations in human breast milk. *Journal of the American Medical Association, 218*, 257.

Lau, R. J., Emery, M. G., & Galinsky, R. E. (1987). Unexpected accumulation of acyclovir in breast milk with estimation of infant exposure. *Obstetrics and Gynecology, 69*, 468–471.

Laumas, K. R. (1967). Radioactivity in breast milk of lactating women after oral administration of ^{3}H-norethynodrel. *American Journal of Obstetrics and Gynecology, 98*, 411–413.

Laumas, V. (1970). The possibility of estrogenic activity in the human and goat milk after administration of oral gestagens. *Contraception, 2*, 331–338.

Lawton, M. E. (1985). Alcohol in breast milk. *Australian and New Zealand Journal of Obstetrics and Gynecology, 25*, 71–73.

Lebedevs, T. H., Wojnar-Hortan, R. E., Yapp, P., et al. (1991). Excretion of indomethacin in breast milk. *British Journal of Clinical Pharmacology, 32*, 751–754.

Lebedevs, T. H., Wojnar-Hortan, R. E., Yapp, P., et al. (1993). Excretion of lignocaine and its metabolite monoethylglycinexylidide in breast milk following its use in a dental procedure. *Journal of Clinical Periodontology, 20*, 606–608.

Lebedevs, T. H., Wojnar-Hortan, R. E., Yapp, P., et al. (1992). Excretion of temazepam in breast milk. *British Journal of Clinical Pharmacology, 33*, 204–206.

Lenzi, E., & Santuari, S. (1969). Preliminary observations on the use of a new semi-synthetic rifamycin derivative in gynecology and obstetrics. *Atti Accademia Lancisiana Roma, 13*, (Suppl 1), 87–94.

Lester, B. M., Cucca, J., Andreozzi, L., et al. (1993). Possible association between fluoxetine hydrochloride and colic in an infant. *Journal of the American Academy of Child and Adolescent Psychiatry, 32*, 1253–1255.

Leuschen, M. P., Wolf, L. J., & Rayburn, W. F. (1990). Fentanyl excretion in breast milk. *Clinical Pharmacy, 9*, 336–337.

Lewis, A. M., Patel, L., Johnston, A., et al. (1981). Mexiletine in human blood and breast milk. *Postgraduate Medical Journal, 57*, 546–547.

Lewis, P. J., Devenish, C., & Kahn, C. (1980). Controlled trial of metoclopramide in the initiation of breast feeding. [Letter]. *British Journal of Clinical Pharmacology, 9*, 217–219.

Libardoni, M., Piovan, D., Busato, F., et al. (1991). Transfer of propafenone and 5-OH-propafenone to foetal plasma and maternal milk. *British Journal of Clinical Pharmacology, 32*, 527–528.

Liedholm, H. (1981). Accumulation of atenolol and metoprolol in human breast milk. *European Journal of Clinical Pharmacology, 20*, 229–231.

Liedholm, H., Wahlin-Boll, E., Ingemarsson, I., et al. (1982). Transplacental passage and breast milk concentrations of hydralazine. *European Journal of Clinical Pharmacology, 21*, 417–419.

Liewellyn-Jones, D. (1975). Inhibition of lactation. *Drugs, 10*, 121–129.

Lindberg, C., Boreus, L. O., deChateau, P., et al. (1984). Transfer of terbutaline into breast milk. *European Journal of Respiratory Diseases, 65* (Suppl 134), 87–91.

Linden, S., & Rich, C. L. (1983). The use of lithium during pregnancy and lactation. *Journal of Clinical Psychiatry, 44*, 358–361.

Little, R. E., Anderson, K. W., Ervin, C. H., et al. (1989). Maternal alcohol use during breast feeding and infant mental and motor development at one year. *New England Journal of Medicine, 321*, 425–430.

Lohmeyer, H., & Halfpap, E. (1965). Pharmakokinetische untersuchungen und klinische erfahrungen mit ampicillin bei der behandlung von infektionen des urogenitaltrakts der frau. *Zeitschrift für Geburtshilfe und Gynäkologie, 164*, 184–202.

Lonnerdal, B., Forsum, E., & Hambraeus, L. (1980). Effect of oral contraceptives on composition and volume of breast milk. *American Journal of Clinical Nutrition, 33*, 816–824.

Lonnerholm, G., & Lindstrom, B. (1982). Terbutaline excretion into breast milk. *British Journal of Clinical Pharmacology, 13*, 729–730.

Losonsky, G., Fishaut, J., Strussenberg, J., et al. (1982). Effect of immunization against rubella on lactation products: II. Maternal–neonatal interactions. *Journal of Infectious Diseases, 145*, 661–666.

Lou, M. A., Wu, Y. H., & Jacob, L. S. (1984). Penetration of cefonicid into human breast milk and various body fluids and tissues. *Reviews of Infectious Diseases, 6*(Suppl 4), S816–S820.

Lownes, H. E., & Ives, T. J. (1987). Mexiletine use in pregnancy and lactation. *American Journal of Obstetrics and Gynecology, 157*, 446–447.

Luck, W., & Nau, H. (1987). Nicotine and cotinine concentrations in the milk of smoking mothers: Influence of cigarette consumption and diurnal variation. *European Journal of Pediatrics, 146*, 21–26.

Luhman, L. A. (1963). The effect of intranasal oxytocin on lactation. *Obstetrics and Gynecology, 83*, 54–55.

Lunell, N. O., Kulas, J., & Rane, A. (1985). Transfer of labetalol into amniotic fluid and breast milk in lactating women. *European Journal of Clinical Pharmacology, 28*, 597–599.

Luquet, F. M. (1975). Pollution of human milk in France with organochlorine insecticide residues. *Pathologie et Biologie, 23*, 45–49.

Lustgarten, J. S., & Posos, S. M. (1983). Topical timolol and the nursing mother. *Archives of Ophthalmology, 101*, 1381–1382.

Macdonald, H. N. (1976). The failure of pyridoxine in suppression of puerperal lactation. *British Journal of Obstetrics and Gynaecology, 83*, 54–55.

MacKintosh, D., & Buchanan, N. (1985). Excretion of disopyramide in human breast milk. *British Journal of Clinical Pharmacology, 19*, 856–857.

Maisels, M. J., & Gilcher, R. O. (1983). Excretion of technicium in human milk. *Pediatrics, 71*, 841–842.

Mann, C. F. (1980). Clindamycin and breast-feeding. *Pediatrics, 66*, 1030–1031.

Manninen, A. K., & Juhakoski, A. (1991). Nifedipine concentrations in maternal and umbilical serum, amniotic fluid, breast milk and urine of mothers and offspring. *International Journal of Clinical Pharmacology Research, 11*, 231–236.

Marcus, R. G. (1975). Suppression of lactation with high doses of pyridoxine. *South African Medical Journal, 49*, 2155–2156.

Marx, C. M., Pucino, F., Carlson, J. D., et al. (1986). Oxycodone excretion in human milk in the puerperium. *Drug Intelligence and Clinical Pharmacy, 20*, 474.

Matheson, I., Lunde, P. K. M., & Bredesen, J. E. (1990). Midazolam and nitrazepam in the maternity ward: Milk concentrations and clinical effects. *British Journal of Clinical Pharmacology, 30*, 787–793.

Matheson, I., Pande, H., & Alertsen, A. R. (1985). Respiratory depression caused by N-desmethyldoxepin in breast milk. *The Lancet, 2*, 1124.

Matheson, I., Samseth, M., & Sande, H. A. (1988). Ampicillin in breast milk during puerperal infection. *European Journal of Clinical Pharmacology, 34*, 657–659.

Matsuda, S. (1984). Transfer of antibiotics into maternal milk. *Biological Research in Pregnancy, 5*, 57–60.

Mayo, C. C., & Schlicke, C. P. (1942). Appearance of a barbiturate in human milk. *Proceedings of the Staff Meetings of the Mayo Clinic, 17*, 87–88.

McCann, M. F., Moggia, A. V., Higgins, J. E., et al. (1989). The effects of a progestin-only oral contraceptive (levonorgestrel 0.03 mg) on breast feeding. *Contraception, 40*, 635–648.

McKenna, R., Cole, E. R., & Vasan, U. (1983a). Is warfarin contraindicated in the lactating mother? *The Journal of Pediatrics, 103,* 325–327.

McKenna, W. J., Harris, L., Rowland, E., et al. (1983b). Amiodarone therapy during pregnancy. *American Journal of Cardiology, 51,* 1231–1233.

McKenzie, S. A. (1975). Secretion of prednisolone into breast milk. *Archives of Disease in Childhood, 50,* 894–896.

McQuinn, R. L., Pisani, A., & Wafa, S. (1990). Flecanide excretion in human breast milk. *Clinical Pharmacology and Therapeutics, 48,* 262–268.

Medina, A., Fiske, N., Hjeh-Harvey, I., et al. (1963). Absorption, diffusion and excretion of a new antibiotic, lincomycin. *Antimicrobial Agents and Chemotherapy, 3,* 189–196.

Mennella, J. A., & Beauchamp, G. K. (1991). The transfer of alcohol to breast milk. Effects on flavor and the infant's behavior. *New England Journal of Medicine, 325,* 981–985.

Meny, R. G., Naumburg, E. G., Alger, L. S., et al. (1993). Codeine and the breast-fed neonate. *Journal of Human Lactation, 9,* 237–240.

Metz, J. (1968). Folic acid binding by serum and milk. *American Journal of Clinical Nutrition, 21,* 289–297.

Meyer, L. J., de Miranda, P., Sheth, N., et al. (1988). Acyclovir in human breast milk. *American Journal of Obstetrics and Gynecology, 158,* 586–588.

Miller, L. G., Hopkinson, J. M., Motil, K. J., et al. (1993). Disposition of olsalazine and metabolites in breast milk. *Journal of Clinical Pharmacology, 33,* 703–706.

Miller, M. E., Cohn, R. D., & Burghart, M. S. (1982). Hydrochlorothiazide disposition in a mother and her breast-fed infant. *The Journal of Pediatrics, 101,* 789–791.

Miller, M. R., Withers, R., Bhamra, R., et al. (1986). Verapamil and breast-feeding. *European Journal of Clinical Pharmacology, 30,* 125–126.

Miller, R. D., Keegan, K. A., Thrupp, L. D., et al. (1984). Human breast milk concentration of moxalactam. *American Journal of Obstetrics and Gynecology, 148,* 348–349.

Milsom, S. R., Breier, B. H., Gallaher, B. W., et al. (1992). Growth hormone stimulates galactopoiesis in healthy lactating women. *Acta Endocrinologica, 127,* 337–343.

Milsom, S. R., Rabone, D. L., Gunn, A. J., et al. (1998). Potential role for growth hormone in human lactation insufficiency. *Hormone Research, 50,* 147–150.

Milunsky, J. M., & Milunsky, A. (1991). Breast-feeding during colchicine therapy for familial Mediterranean fever. *The Journal of Pediatrics, 119,* 164.

Mirkin, B. L. (1971). Diphenylhydantoin: Placental transport, fetal localization, neonatal metabolism, and possible teratogenic effects. *The Journal of Pediatrics, 78,* 329–337.

Mischler, T. W., Corson, S. L., Larranaga, A., et al. (1978). Cephradine and epicillin in body fluids of lactating and pregnant women. *Journal of Reproductive Medicine, 21,* 130–135.

Moiel, R. H., & Ryan, J. R. (1967). Tolbutamide (Orinase) in human breast milk. *Clinical Pediatrics, 6,* 480.

Moodley, J., Moodley, D., Pillay, K., et al. (1998). Pharmacokinetics and antiretroviral activity of lamivudine alone or when coadministered with zidovudine in human immunodeficiency virus type-1-infected pregnant women and their offspring. *Journal of Infectious Diseases, 178,* 1327–1333.

Moretti, M. E., Ito, S., & Koren, G. (1995). Disposition of maternal ketoconazole in breast milk. *American Journal of Obstetrics and Gynecology, 173,* 1625–1626.

Morganti, G. (1968). Comparative concentrations of a tetracycline antibiotic in serum and maternal milk. *Antibiotica, 6,* 216–223.

Mortola, J. F. (1989). The use of psychotropic agents in pregnancy and lactation. *Psychiatric Clinics of North America, 12,* 69–87.

Morton, R. F. (1955–1956). Studies on the absorption, diffusion, and excretion of cycloserine. *Antibiotics Annual, 3,* 169–172.

Mountford, P. J., & Coakley, A. J. (1989). A review of the secretion of radioactivity in human breast milk: Data, quantitative analysis and recommendations. *Nuclear Medicine Communications, 10,* 15–22.

Mulley, B. A., Parr, G. D., Pau, W. K., et al. (1978). Placental transfer of chlorthalidone and its elimination in maternal milk. *European Journal of Clinical Pharmacology, 13,* 129–131.

Munoz-Flores-Thiagarajan, K. D., Easterling, T., Davis, C., et al. (2001). Breast-feeding by a cyclosporine-treated mother. *Obstetrics and Gynecology, 97*(5 part 2), 816–818.

Nation, R. L., Hackett, L. P., Dusci, L. J., et al. (1984). Excretion of hydroxychloroquine in human milk. *British Journal of Clinical Pharmacology, 17,* 368–369.

Nau, H., Kuhnz, W., Egger, H. J., et al. (1982). Anticonvulsants during pregnancy and lactation. Transplacental, maternal and neonatal pharmacokinetics. *Clinical Pharmacokinetics, 7,* 508–543.

Nau, H., Rating, D., Hauser, I., et al. (1980). Placental transfer and pharmacokinetics of primidone and its metabolites, phenobarbital, PEMA and hydroxyphenobarbital in neonates and infants of epileptic mothers. *European Journal of Clinical Pharmacology, 18,* 31–42.

Nau, H., Rating, D., Koch, S., et al. (1981). Valproic acid and its metabolites: Placental transfer, neonatal pharmacokinetics, transfer via mother's milk and clinical status in neonates of epileptic mothers. *Journal of Pharmacology and Experimental Therapeutics, 219,* 768–777.

Nehlig, A., & Debry, G. (1994). Consequences on the newborn of chronic maternal consumption of coffee during gestation and lactation: A review. *Journal of the American College of Nutrition, 13*, 6–21.

Nelis, G. F. (1989). Diarrhea due to 5-aminosalicylic acid in breast milk. *The Lancet, 1*, 383.

Nice, F. J. (1995). OTC medications and breastfeeding: An update. *Pharmacy Times, 61*, 29–31.

Nicholas, J. M., Lipshitz, J., & Schreiber, E. C. (1982). Phencyclidine: Its transfer across the placenta as well as into breast milk. *American Journal of Obstetrics and Gynecology, 143*, 143–146.

Nikodem, V. C., & Hofmeyr, G. J. (1992). Secretion of the antidiarrheal agent loperamide oxide in breast milk. *European Journal of Clinical Pharmacology, 42*, 695–696.

Nordeng, H., Zahlsen, K., & Spigset, O. (2001). Transfer of carisoprodol to breast milk. *Therapeutic Drug Monitoring, 23*, 298–300.

Notarianni, L. J., Oldham, H. G., & Bennett, P. N. (1987). Passage of paracetamol into breast milk and its subsequent metabolism by the neonate. *British Journal of Clinical Pharmacology, 24*, 63–67.

Nurenburger, C. E., & Lipscomb, A. (1952). Transmission of radioiodine (^{131}I) to infants through human maternal milk. *Journal of the American Medical Association, 150*, 1398–1400.

Nyberg, G., Haljamac, U., Frisenette-Fich, C., et al. (1998). Breast-feeding during treatment with cyclosporine. *Transplantation, 65*, 253–255.

Obermeyer, B. D., Bergstrom, R. F., Callaghan, J. T., et al. (1990). Secretion of nizatidine into human breast milk after single and multiple doses. *Clinical Pharmacology and Therapeutics, 47*, 724–730.

O'Brien, T. E. (1974). Excretion of drugs in human milk. *American Journal of Hospital Pharmacy, 31*, 844–854.

Ogbuokiri, J. F., Ozumba, B. C., & Okonkwo, P. O. (1994). Ivermectin levels in human breast milk. *European Journal of Clinical Pharmacology, 46*, 89–90.

Ogunbona, F. A., Onyeji, C. O., Bolaji, O. O., et al. (1987). Excretion of chloroquine and desethylchloroquine in human milk. *British Journal of Clinical Pharmacology, 23*, 473–476.

O'Hare, M. F., Murnaghan, G. A., Russell, C. J., et al. (1980). Sotalol as a hypotensive agent in pregnancy. *British Journal of Obstetrics and Gynaecology, 87*, 814–820.

Okada, M., Inoue, H., Nakamura, Y., et al. (1985). Excretion of diltiazem in human milk. *New England Journal of Medicine, 312*, 992–993.

O'Mara, N. B., & Nahata, M. C. (1995). Drugs excreted in human breast milk. In L. A. Pagliaro & A. M. Pagliaro, Eds., *Problems in Pediatric Drug Therapy*, 3rd ed., pp. 247–335, Hamilton, IL: Drug Intelligence Publications.

Oo, C. Y., Kuhn, R. J., Desai, N., et al. (1995a). Active transport of cimetidine into human milk. *Clinical Pharmacology and Therapeutics, 58*, 548–555.

Oo, C. Y., Kuhn, R. J., Desai, N., et al. (1995b). Pharmacokinetics in lactating women: Prediction of alprazolam transfer into milk. *British Journal of Clinical Pharmacology, 40*, 231–236.

Orme, M. L'E, Lewis, P. J., de Swiet, M., et al. (1977). May mothers given warfarin breast-feed their infants? *British Medical Journal, 1*, 1564–1565.

Ost, L., Wettrell, G., Bjorkhem, I., et al. (1985). Prednisolone excretion in human milk. *The Journal of Pediatrics, 106*, 1008–1011.

Ostensen, M. (1983). Piroxicam in human breast milk. *European Journal of Clinical Pharmacology, 25*, 829–830.

Ostensen, M., Brown, N. D., Chiang, P. K., et al. (1985). Hydroxychloroquine in human breast milk. *European Journal of Clinical Pharmacology, 28*, 357.

Ostensen, M., Matheson, I., & Laufen, H. (1988). Piroxicam in breast milk after long-term treatment. *European Journal of Clinical Pharmacology, 35*, 567–569.

Ostensen, M., Skavdal, K., Myklebust, G., et al. (1986). Excretion of gold into human breast milk. *European Journal of Clinical Pharmacology, 31*, 251–252.

Ostrea, E. M., Chavez, C. J., & Stryker, J. C. (1978). In *The care of the drug dependent woman and her infant*, p. 18. Lansing, MI: Michigan Department of Public Health.

Palmer, K. E. (1979). Excretion of ^{125}I in breast milk following administration of labelled fibrinogen. *British Journal of Radiology, 52*, 672–673.

Pardthaisong, T., Yenchit, C., & Gray, R. (1992). The long-term growth and development of children exposed to Depo-Provera during pregnancy or lactation. *Contraception, 45*, 313–324.

Passmore, C. M., McElnay, J. C., Rainey, E. A., et al. (1988). Metronidazole excretion in human milk and its effect on the suckling neonate. *British Journal of Clinical Pharmacology, 26*, 46–51.

Patrick, M. J. (1972). Diazepam and breast feeding. *The Lancet, 1*, 542–543.

Peiker, G., Muller, B., Ihn, W., et al. (1980). Excretion of pethidine in mother's milk. *Zentralblatt für Gynäkologie, 102*, 537–541.

Penny, W. J., & Lewis, M. J. (1989). Nifedipine is excreted in human milk. *European Journal of Clinical Pharmacology, 36*, 427–428.

Perez-Reyes, M., & Wall, M. E. (1982). Presence of delta 9-tetrahydrocannabinol in human milk. *New England Journal of Medicine, 307*, 819–820.

Phelps, D. L., & Karim, A. (1977). Spironolactone: Relationship between concentration of dethioacetylated metabolite in human serum and milk. *Journal of Pharmaceutical Sciences, 66*, 1203.

Philbert, A., Pedersen, B., & Dam, M. (1985). Concentration of valproate during pregnancy, in the newborn and in breast milk. *Acta Neurologica Scandinavica, 72,* 460–463.

Pincus, G. (1966). Radioactivity in the milk of subjects receiving radioactive 19-norsteroids. *Nature, 212,* 924–925.

Pitcher, D., Leather, H. M., Storey, G. C. A., et al. (1983). Amiodarone in pregnancy. *The Lancet, 1,* 597–598.

Pittard, W. B., & Glazier, H. (1983). Procainamide excretion in human milk. *The Journal of Pediatrics, 102,* 631–632.

Pittard, W. B., Merkatz, R., & Fletcher, B. D. (1982). Radioactive excretion in milk following administration of technicium Tc 99 macroaggregated albumin. *Pediatrics, 70,* 231–234.

Pittman, K. A., Smyth, R. D., Losada, M., et al. (1980). Human perinatal distribution of butorphanol. *American Journal of Obstetrics and Gynecology, 138,* 797–800.

Plomp, T. A., Vulsma, T., deVijlder, J. J. M., et al. (1992). Use of amiodarone during pregnancy. *European Journal of Obstetrics and Gynecology and Reproductive Biology, 43,* 201–207.

Pons, G., Francoual, C., Guillet, P., et al. (1989). Zolpidem excretion in breast milk. *European Journal of Clinical Pharmacology, 37,* 245–248.

Pons, G., Rey, E., Richard, M. O., et al. (1990). Nitrofurantoin excretion in human milk. *Developmental Pharmacology and Therapeutics, 14,* 148–152.

Posner, A. C. (1955). Further observations on the use of tetracycline hydrochloride in prophylaxis and treatment of obstetric infections. *Antibiotics Annual,* 594–598.

Postellon, D., & Aronow, R. (1982). Iodine in mother's milk. [Letter]. *Journal of the American Medical Association, 247,* 463.

Putter, J. (1975). Quantitative analysis of the main metabolites of acetylsalicylic acid. Comparative analysis in the blood and milk of lactating women. *Zeitschrift für Geburtshilfe und Perinatologie, 178,* 135–138.

Quinn, P. G., Kuhnert, B. R., Kaine, C. J., et al. (1986). Measurement of meperidine and normeperidine in human breast milk. *Biomedical and Environmental Mass Spectrophotometry, 13,* 133–135.

Rabinowitz, M., Leviton, A., & Needleman, H. (1985). Lead in milk and infant blood: A dose-response model. *Archives of Environmental Health, 40,* 283–286.

Ramasastri, B. V. (1965). Folate activity in human milk. *British Journal of Nutrition, 19,* 581–586.

Rane, A., & Tunell, R. (1981). Ethosuximide in human milk and in plasma of a mother and her nursed infant. *British Journal of Clinical Pharmacology, 12,* 855–858.

Redman, C. W. G., Kelly, J. G., & Cooper, W. D. (1990). The excretion of enalapril and enalaprilat in human breast milk. *European Journal of Clinical Pharmacology, 38,* 99.

Reiher, K. M. (1963). Unterdrückung der laktation durch anregung dur diurese. *Zentralblatt für Gynäkologie, 85,* 188–190.

Reinhardt, D., Richter, O., Genz, T., et al. (1982). Kinetics of the translactal passage of digoxin from breast feeding mothers to their infants. *European Journal of Pediatrics, 138,* 49–52.

Resman, B. M., Blumenthal, H. P., & Jusko, W. J. (1977). Breast milk distribution of theobromine and chocolate. *The Journal of Pediatrics, 91,* 477–480.

Rey, E., Giraux, P., d'Athis, P., et al. (1979). Pharmacokinetics of the placental transfer and distribution of clorazepate and its metabolite, nordiazepam, in the feto-placental unit and in the neonate. *European Journal of Clinical Pharmacology, 15,* 181–185.

Reyes, M. P., Ostrea, E. M., Cabinian, A. E., et al. (1989). Vancomycin during pregnancy: Does it cause hearing loss or nephrotoxicity in the infant? *American Journal of Obstetrics and Gynecology, 161,* 977–981.

Ricci, G., & Copaitich, T. (1954–1955). Modalita di eliminazione dell'isoniazide somministrata per via orals attraverso il latte di donna. *Rassegna di Clinica Terapia a Scienza Affini, 53,* 209–214.

Riordan, J. (1987). Drugs secreted in human breast milk. In L. A. Pagliaro & A. M. Pagliaro, Eds. *Problems in Pediatric Drug Therapy,* 2nd ed., pp. 193–258. Hamilton, IL: Drug Intelligence Publications.

Rivera-Calimlim, L. (1977). Drugs in breast milk. *Drug Therapy, 2,* 20.

Robieux, I., Koren, G., Vandenbergh, H., et al. (1990). Morphine excretion in breast milk and resultant exposure of a nursing infant. *Clinical Toxicology, 28,* 365–370.

Robinson, P. S., Barker, P., Campbell, A., et al. (1994). Iodine-131 in breast milk following therapy for thyroid carcinoma. *Journal of Nuclear Medicine, 35,* 1797–1801.

Romney, B. M., Nickoloff, E. L., Esser, P. D., et al. (1986). Radionuclide administration to nursing mothers: Mathematically derived guidelines. *Radiology, 160,* 549–554.

Rooney, T. W., Lorber, A., Veng-Pedersen, P., et al. (1987). Gold pharmacokinetics in breast milk and serum of a lactating woman. *Journal of Rheumatology, 14,* 1120–1122.

Rothberg, A. D., Pettifor, J. M., Cohen, D. F., et al. (1982). Maternal–infant vitamin D relationship during breast feeding. *The Journal of Pediatrics, 101,* 500–503.

Rozansky, R., & Bre, A. (1949). The excretion of penicillin in human milk. *Journal of Laboratory and Clinical Medicine, 34,* 497–500.

Ruis, H., Rolland, W., Broeders, G., et al. (1981). Oxytocin enhances onset of lactation among mothers delivering prematurely. *British Medical Journal, 283,* 340–343.

Rush, J. E., Snyder, D. L., Barrish, A., et al. (1991).

Comment on Huttunen, K., Gronhagen-Riska, C., and Fryhrquist, F. (1989). Enalapril treatment of a nursing mother with slightly impaired renal function. *Clinical Nephrology, 35,* 234.

Rylance, G. W., Woods, C. G., Donnelly, M. C., et al. (1987). Carbimazole and breastfeeding. *The Lancet, 1,* 928.

Ryu, J. E. (1985). Caffeine in human milk and in serum of breast-fed infants. *Developmental Pharmacology and Therapeutics, 8,* 329–337.

Saarinen, U. M., Siimes, M. A., & Dallman, P. R. (1977). Iron absorption in infants—High bioavailability of breastmilk iron as indicated by the extrinsic tag method of iron absorption and by the concentration of serum ferritin. *The Journal of Pediatrics, 91,* 36–39.

Sagraves, R., Kaiser, D., & Sharpe, G. L. (1981). Prednisone and prednisolone concentration in the milk of lactating mother. *Drug Intelligence and Clinical Pharmacy, 15,* 484.

Sagraves, R., Waller, E. S., & Goehrs, H. R. (1985). Tolmetin in breast milk. *Drug Intelligence and Clinical Pharmacy, 19,* 55–56.

Sanders, S. W., Zone, J. J., Foltz, R. L., et al. (1982). Hemolytic anemia induced by dapsone transmitted through breast milk. *Annals of Internal Medicine, 96,* 465–466.

Sandstrom, B., & Regardh, C. G. (1980). Metoprolol excretion into breast milk. *British Journal of Clinical Pharmacology, 9,* 518–519.

Schimmell, M. S., Katz, E. Z., Shaag, Y., et al. (1991). Toxic neonatal effects following maternal clomipramine therapy. *Clinical Toxicology, 29,* 479–484.

Schlesinger, J. J., & Covelli, H. D. (1977). Evidence for transmission of lymphocyte responses to tuberculin by breast feeding. *The Lancet, 2,* 529–532.

Schmidt, K., Olesen, O. V., & Jensen, P. N. (2000). Citalopram and breast-feeding: Serum concentration and side effects in the infant. *Biological Psychiatry, 47,* 164–165.

Schmimmel, M. S., Eidelman, A. J., Wilschanski, M. A., et al. (1989). Toxic effects of atenolol consumed during breast feeding. *The Journal of Pediatrics, 114,* 476–478.

Schou, M. (1990). Lithium treatment during pregnancy, delivery, and lactation: An update. *Journal of Clinical Psychiatry, 10,* 410–413.

Schou, M., & Amdisen, A. (1973). Lithium and pregnancy: III. Lithium ingestion by children breast-fed by women on lithium treatment. *British Medical Journal, 2,* 138.

Shane, J. M., & Naftolin, F. (1974). Effects of ergonovine maleate on puerperal lactation. *American Journal of Obstetrics and Gynecology, 120,* 129–131.

Shyu, W. C., Shah, V. R., Campbell, D. A., et al. (1992). Excretion of cefprozil into human breast milk. *Antimicrobial Agents and Chemotherapy, 36,* 938–941.

Skausig, O. B., & Schou, M. (1977). Diegivning under lithiumbehandling. *Ugeskrift for Laeger, 139,* 400–401.

Smialek, J. E., Montoforte, J. R., Aronow, R., et al. (1977). Methadone deaths in children. *Journal of the American Medical Association, 238,* 2516–2517.

Smith, I. J., Hinson, J. L., Johnson, V. A., et al. (1989). Flurbiprofen in post-partum women: Plasma and breast milk disposition. *Journal of Clinical Pharmacology, 29,* 174–184.

Smith, J. A. (1975). Clindamycin in human breast milk. *Canadian Medical Association Journal, 112,* 806.

Smith, M. T., Livingstone, I., Hooper, W. D., et al. (1983). Propranolol, propranolol glucuronide, and naphthoxylactic acid in breast milk and plasma. *Therapeutic Drug Monitoring, 5,* 87–93.

Snider, D. E., & Powell, K. E. (1984). Should women taking antituberculosis drugs breast-feed? *Archives of Internal Medicine, 144,* 589–590.

Soderman, P., Hartvig, P., & Fagerlund, C. (1984). Acetazolamide excretion into human breast milk. *British Journal of Clinical Pharmacology, 17,* 599–600.

Soderman, P., & Matheson, I. (1987). Clonazepam in breast milk. *European Journal of Pediatrics, 147,* 212–213.

Somogyi, A., & Gugler, R. (1979). Cimetidine excretion into breast milk. *British Journal of Clinical Pharmacology, 7,* 627–629.

Sousa, P. L. R. (1975). Metoclopramide and breast feeding. *British Medical Journal, 1,* 512.

Sovner, R., & Orsulak, P. J. (1979). Excretion of imipramine and desipramine in human breast milk. *American Journal of Psychiatry, 136,* 1483.

Spencer, R. P. (1970). Breast secretion of ^{99m}Tc administration. *Journal of Nuclear Medicine, 12,* 188.

Spigset, O., Carleborg, L., Norstrom, A., et al. (1996). Paroxetine level in breast milk. *Journal of Clinical Psychiatry, 57,* 39.

Stancer, H. C., & Reed, K. L. (1986). Desipramine and 2-hydroxydesipramine in human breast milk and the nursing infant's serum. *American Journal of Psychiatry, 143,* 1597–1600.

Stang, H. (1986). Pyloric stenosis associated with erythromycin ingested through breastmilk. *Minnesota Medicine, 69,* 669–670, 682.

Stavchansky, S., Combs, A., Sagraves, R., et al. (1988). Pharmacokinetics of caffeine in breast milk and plasma after single oral administration of caffeine to lactating mothers. *Biopharmaceutics and Drug Disposition, 9,* 285–299.

Stec, G. P., Greenberger, P., Ruo, T. I., et al. (1980). Kinetics of theophylline transfer to breast milk. *Clinical Pharmacology and Therapeutics, 28,* 404–408.

Steen, B., & Rane, A. (1982a). Clindamycin passage into human milk. *British Journal of Clinical Pharmacy, 13,* 661–664.

Steen, B., Rane, A., Lonnerholm, G., et al. (1982b). Phenytoin excretion in human breast milk and plasma levels in nursed infants. *Therapeutic Drug Monitoring, 4,* 331–334.

Steiner, E., Villen, T., Hallberg, M., et al. (1984). Amphetamine secretion in breast milk. *European Journal of Clinical Pharmacology, 27,* 123–124.

Stewart, R. B., Karas, B., & Springer, P. C. (1980). Haloperidol excretion in human milk. *American Journal of Psychiatry, 137,* 849–850.

Stowe, Z. N., Owens, M. J., Landry, J. C., et al. (1997). Sertraline and desmethylsertraline in human breast milk and nursing infants. *American Journal of Psychiatry, 154,* 1255–1260.

Summerfield, R. J., & Nielsen, M. G. (1985). Excretion of lorazepam into breast milk. *British Journal of Anaesthesia, 57,* 1042–1043.

Svensmark, O. (1960). 5,5-diphenylhydantoin [Dilantin®] blood levels after oral or intravenous dosage in man. *Acta Pharmacologica et Toxicologica, 16,* 331–346.

Sykes, P. A., Quarrie, J., & Alexander, F. W. (1976). Lithium carbonate and breast feeding. *British Medical Journal, 2,* 1299.

Sylvester, R. K., Lobell, M., Teresi, M., et al. (1987). Excretion of hydroxyurea into milk. *Cancer, 60,* 2177–2178.

Taddio, A., Ito, S., & Koren, G. (1996). Excretion of fluoxetine and its metabolite, norfluoxetine, in human breast milk. *Journal of Clinical Pharmacology, 36,* 42–47.

Taddio, A., Klein, J., & Koren, G. (1994). Acyclovir excretion in human breast milk. *Annals of Pharmacology, 28,* 585–586.

Takyi, B. E. (1970). Excretion of drugs in human milk. *Journal of Hospital Pharmacy, 28,* 317–326.

Taylor, E. A., & Turner, P. (1981). Anti-hypertensive therapy with propranolol during pregnancy and lactation. *Postgraduate Medical Journal, 57,* 427–430.

Tegler, L., & Lindstrom, B. (1980). Antithyroid drugs in milk. [Letter]. *The Lancet, 2,* 591.

Terwilliger, W. G., & Hatcher, R. A. (1934). The elimination of morphine and quinine in human milk. *Surgical Gynecology and Obstetrics, 58,* 823–826.

Thorley, K. J., & McAinsh, J. (1983). Levels of beta-blockers atenolol and propranolol in the breast milk of women treated for hypertension in pregnancy. *Biopharmaceutics and Drug Disposition, 4,* 299–301.

Thulin, P. C., Woodward, W. R., Carter, J. H., et al. (1998). Levodopa in human breast milk: Clinical implications. *Neurology, 50,* 1920–1921.

Tokuda, G., Yuasa, M., Mihara, S., et al. (1969). Clinical studies of doxycycline in obstetrical and gynecological fields. *Chemotherapy* (Tokyo), *17,* 339–344.

Tomson, T., & Villen, T. (1994). Ethosuximide enantiomers in pregnancy and lactation. *Therapeutic Drug Monitoring, 16,* 621–623.

Tonks, A. M. (1995). Nimodipine levels in breast milk. *Australia and New Zealand Journal of Surgery, 65,* 693–694.

Townsend, R. J., Benedetti, T. J., Erickson, S. H., et al. (1984). Excretion of ibuprofen into breast milk. *American Journal of Obstetrics and Gynecology, 149,* 184–186.

Traeger, A., & Peiker, G. (1980). Excretion of nalidixic acid via mother's milk. *Archives of Toxicology* (Suppl 4), 388–390.

Tran, A., O'Mahoney, T., Rey, E., et al. (1998). Vigabatrin: Placental transfer in vivo and excretion into breast milk of the enantiomers. *British Journal of Clinical Pharmacology, 45,* 409–411.

Tunnessen, W. M., & Hertz, C. G. (1972). Toxic effects of lithium in newborn infants: A commentary. *The Journal of Pediatrics, 81,* 804–807.

Tyrala, E. A., & Dodson, W. E. (1979). Caffeine secretion into breast milk. *Archives of Disease in Childhood, 54,* 787–800.

Tyson, R. M., Shrader, E. A., & Perlman, H. H. (1937). Drugs transmitted through breast milk: I. Laxatives. *The Journal of Pediatrics, 11,* 824–832.

UNICEF, WHO, & UNESCO. (1989). *Facts for life. A communication challenge.* New York: UNICEF.

Uwaydah, M., Bibi, S., & Salaman, S. (1975). Therapeutic efficacy of tobramycin—A clinical and laboratory evaluation. *Journal of Antimicrobial Chemotherapy, 1,* 429–437.

Vagenakis, A. G. (1971). Duration of radioactivity in the milk of a nursing mother following ^{99m}Tc administration. *Journal of Nuclear Medicine, 12,* 188.

Valdivieso, A., Valdes, G., Spiro, T. E., et al. (1985). Minoxidil in breast milk. *Annals of Internal Medicine, 102,* 135.

Valquist, B., & Hogstedt, C. (1949). Minute absorption of diphtheric antibodies from the gastrointestinal tract in infant. *Pediatrics, 4,* 410.

Varsano, I., Fischl, J., & Shochet, S. B. (1973). The excretion of PO ingested nitrofurantoin in human milk. *The Journal of Pediatrics, 82,* 886–887.

Venkatesan, K., Mathur, A., Girdhar, A., et al. (1997). Excretion of clofazimine in human milk in leprosy patients. *Leprosy Review, 68,* 242–246.

Verbeeck, R. K., Ross, S. G., & McKenna, E. A. (1986). Excretion of trazodone in breast milk. *British Journal of Clinical Pharmacology, 22,* 367–370.

Von Kobyletzki, D., & Strauch, D. (1964). Experimentelle untersuchungen zur frage der diaplazentaren passage und der ausscheidung mit der muttermilch von demethylchlorotetracyclin. *Zeitschrift für Geburtshilfe und Gynäkology, 161,* 292–305.

von Unruh, G. E., Froescher, W., Hoffman, F., et al. (1984). Valproic acid in breast milk: How much is really there? *Therapeutic Drug Monitoring, 6,* 272–276.

Weaver, J. C. (1960). Excretion of radioiodine in

human milk. *Journal of the American Medical Association, 173,* 872–875.

Weibert, R. T., Townsend, R. J., Kaiser, D. G., et al. (1982). Lack of ibuprofen secretion into human milk. *Clinical Pharmacy, 1,* 457–458.

Werthmann, M. W., & Krees, S. V. (1972). Excretion of chlorothiazide in human breast milk. *The Journal of Pediatrics, 81,* 781–783.

Werthmann, M. W., & Krees, S. V. (1973). Quantitative excretion of Senekot® in human breast milk. *Medical Annals of the District of Columbia, 42,* 4–5.

Wesson, D. R., Camber, S., Harkey, M., et al. (1985). Diazepam and desmethyldiazepam in breast milk. *Journal of Psychoactive Drugs, 17,* 55–56.

Whalley, L. J., Blain, P. G., & Prime, J. K. (1981). Haloperidol secreted in breast milk. *British Medical Journal, 282,* 1746–1747.

White, W. B., Andreoli, J. W., & Cohn, R. D. (1985). Alpha-methyldopa disposition in mothers with hypertension and in their breast fed infants. *Clinical Pharmacology and Therapeutics, 37,* 387–390.

White, W. B., Andreoli, J. W., Wong, S. H., et al. (1984). Atenolol in human plasma and breast milk. *Obstetrics and Gynecology, 63*(Suppl), 42S–44S.

Whitelaw, A. G. L., Cummings, A. J., & McFadyen, I. R. (1981). Effect of maternal lorazepam on the neonate. *British Medical Journal, 282,* 1106–1108.

Wiernik, P. H., & Duncan, J. H. (1971). Cyclophosphamide in human milk. *The Lancet, 1,* 912.

Wijmenga, H. G., & van der Molen, H. J. (1969). Studies with 4-^{14}C-mestranol in lactating women. *Acta Endocrinologica, 61,* 665–677.

Wiles, D. H., Orr, M. W., & Kolakowska, T. (1978). Chlorpromazine levels in plasma and milk of nursing mothers. *British Journal of Clinical Pharmacology, 5,* 272–273.

Wilson, J. H. (1988). Breast milk tocainide levels. *Journal of Cardiovascular Pharmacology, 12,* 497.

Wilson, J. T. (1981). *Drugs in breast milk.* Baltimore, MD: Williams and Wilkins.

Wischnik, A., Manth, S. M., Lloyd, J., et al. (1989). The excretion of ketorolac tromethamine into breast milk after multiple oral dosing. *European Journal of Clinical Pharmacology, 36,* 521–524.

Wisner, K. L., & Perel, J. M. (1991). Serum nortriptyline levels in nursing mothers and their infants. *American Journal of Psychiatry, 148,* 1234–1236.

Wisner, K. L., Perel, J. M., & Blummer, J. (1998). Serum sertraline and N-desmethylsertraline levels in breast-feeding mother–infant pairs. *American Journal of Psychiatry, 155,* 690–692.

Wisner, K. L., Perel, J. M., & Fuglia, J. P. (1995). Serum clomipramine and metabolite levels in four nursing mother–infant pairs. *Journal of Clinical Psychiatry, 56,* 17–20.

Witter, F. R., & Smith, R. V. (1985). The excretion of pentoxifylline and its metabolites in human breast milk. *American Journal of Obstetrics and Gynecology, 151,* 1094–1097.

Wojnar-Horton, R. E., Hackett, L. P., Yapp, P., et al. (1996). Distribution and excretion of sumatriptan in human milk. *British Journal of Clinical Pharmacology, 41,* 217–221.

Wojnar-Horton, R. E., Kristensen, J. H., Yapp, P., et al. (1997). Methadone distribution and excretion into breast milk of clients in a methadone maintenance programme. *British Journal of Clinical Pharmacology, 44,* 543–547.

World Health Organization Task Force on Oral Contraceptives. (1988). Effects of hormonal contraceptives on breast milk composition and infant growth. *Studies in Family Planning, 19,* 361–369.

Wortsman, J., Soler, N. G., & Hirschowitz, J. (1979). Cyproheptadine in the management of galactorrhea-amenorrhea syndrome. *Annals of Internal Medicine, 90,* 923–925.

Wretlind, M. (1987). Excretion of oxazepam in breast milk. *European Journal of Clinical Pharmacology, 33,* 209–210.

Wyburn, J. R. (1973). Human breast milk excretion of radionuclides following administration of radiopharmaceutical. *Journal of Nuclear Medicine, 14,* 115–117.

Yapp, P. Ilett, K. F., Kristensen, J. H., et al. (2000). Drowsiness and poor feeding in a breast-fed infant: Association with nefazodone and its metabolites. *Annals of Pharmacotherapy, 34,* 1269–1272.

Yoshida, K., Smith, B., Craggs, M., et al. (1998). Fluoxetine in breast-milk and developmental outcomes in breast-fed infants. *British Journal of Psychiatry, 172,* 175–179.

Yoshioka, H., Cho, K., Takimato, M., et al. (1979). Transfer of cefazolin into human milk. *The Journal of Pediatrics, 94,* 151–152.

Yurchak, A. M., & Jusko, W. J. (1976). Theophylline secretion into breast milk. *Pediatrics, 57,* 518–525.

Zeisler, J. A., Gaarder, T. D., & DeMesquita, S. A. (1986). Lidocaine excretion in breast milk. *Drug Intelligence and Clinical Pharmacy, 20,* 691–693.

4

Pediatric Poisoning

Wendy Klein-Schwartz and Gary M. Oderda

Unintentional poisoning is one of the leading causes of injury in children in North America today. In 2000, poison centers reported 2,168,248 poison exposures to the American Association of Poison Control Centers (AAPCC) Toxic Exposure Surveillance System (TESS). Of these exposures, 52.7% involved children younger than 6 years (Litovitz et al., 2001). Table 4-1 shows the age distribution of these exposures.

Fortunately, the effects of most of these exposures were not severe. The majority (86.7%) of children younger than 6 years experienced no toxic effects or were not followed clinically after ingesting a nontoxic or minimally toxic drug or substance or a subtoxic dose of a toxic drug or substance because toxic effects were not anticipated. The outcomes for these children were mild in 9.4%, moderate or severe in 0.9%, unknown in 1.4%, and unrelated to the exposure in 1.6%. There were 20 deaths.

The number of deaths from poisonings involving young children has declined dramatically during the past 30 years. In 1968, 284 children younger than 5 years died from unintentional poisoning from toxic solids and liquids. The number of fatalities dropped to 114 in 1975, 73 in 1980, and 25 in 1998 (Update: Childhood Poisonings . . . , 1985; Vital Statistics of the United States . . . , 2001). Table 4-2 compares U.S. 1979 and 1998 national mortality data for children and adolescents. Both the number of reported deaths and the death rate have decreased in all age groups. Several factors have played a role in this decrease, including the use of child-resistant closures, increased public awareness about poisoning, the establishment of regional poison control centers, and improved medical management of poisoning.

Nonpharmaceutical and pharmaceutical drugs and substances may be implicated in childhood poisonings. The nonpharmaceutical substances most frequently implicated in pediatric poisonings include cosmetic and personal care products, cleaning products, foreign bodies, plants, pesticides, arts/crafts/office supplies, and hydrocarbons (Litovitz et al., 2001). The most frequently involved pharmaceuticals include analgesics, topical formulations, cough and cold products, vitamins, GI preparations, antimicrobials, antihistamines, and hormones and hormone antagonists. Many of these drugs and substances are readily accessible to children but are not highly toxic. Young children can come in contact with hazardous nonpharmaceutical substances such as hydrocarbons and pesticides (Litovitz & Manoguerra, 1992). Pharmaceuticals that are considered to be particularly hazardous, based on potency and/or clinical cases of pediatric exposure, include camphor,

TABLE 4-1
Age Distribution of Poison Exposure Based on AAPCC TESS Data, 2000

AGE (YEARS)	EXPOSURES	EXPOSURES, %	DEATHS	DEATH RATE PER 1000 EXPOSURES
<6	1,142,796	52.7	20	0.02
6–12	151,221	7.0	6	0.04
13–19	160,505	7.4	66	0.41
>19	696,171	32.1	826	1.19
Unknown	17,555	0.8	2	0.11
Total	2,168,248	100	920	0.42

cardiovascular drugs, diphenoxylate–atropine, salicylates (especially methyl salicylate), theophylline, and tricyclic antidepressants (Koren, 1993; Liebelt & Shannon, 1993; Litovitz & Manoguerra, 1992).

In addition to morbidity and mortality, pediatric poisonings contribute to increased healthcare costs. A study of the cost at an urban hospital over a 4-year period of 638 hospitalizations due to poisoning found that the length of stay decreased from 1992 to 1995 which resulted in a decrease in the charges per case (Woolf et al., 1997). However, charges of almost $1 million resulted from poison-related admissions in 1995. The most common and most costly hospitalizations involved poisonings with acetaminophen, antidepressants, and lead.

Unintentional poisoning exposures occur among infants as young as 6 months. Even at this young age, infants can crawl, pick up items such as a tablet dropped on the floor, and grab leaves from plants. It is important that parents be made aware of poison prevention techniques and of the location and telephone number of their regional poison control center. As more parents use day-care services for their infants and children, attention to these precautions by day-care staff also is required.

Regional poison control centers provide information on poisoning to both healthcare professionals and to the general public. Poison control centers save healthcare dollars by enabling parents to manage many reported cases of poisoning at home and prevent unnecessary visits to healthcare facilities (Miller & Lestina, 1997). These centers are staffed by pharmacists and/or nurses specially trained in poison information and the use of resources in clinical toxicology. In addition to providing consultations on specific actions to take in regard to suspected or known poisoning cases, regional poison control centers collect data on poisonings and provide education to healthcare professionals and poison prevention education to the general public. Pediatric healthcare professionals should be familiar with the regional poison center in their area and consult the center for help in managing poisonings when they occur. **In the United States, a national number**

TABLE 4-2
U.S. Mortality Data for Poisoning, 1979 and 1998[a]

AGE (YEARS)	1979		1998	
	DEATHS	DEATH RATE[b]	DEATHS	DEATH RATE[b]
<1	30	0.85	13	0.33
1–4	96	0.78	31	0.20
5–9	31	0.18	12	0.06
10–14	69	0.37	31	0.16
15–19	657	3.07	360	1.84

[a] U.S. Vital Statistics; includes poisonings classified as accident, suicide, homicide, non-dependent drug abuse, and undetermined intent.
[b] Deaths per 100,000 population.

(1-800-222-1222) connects callers to the poison control center in their area.

General Considerations

Poisoning can occur by virtually any route of exposure, including oral, inhalation, injectable, rectal, and topical routes. In cases of pediatric poisoning, the most common route is the oral route. Regardless of the route of exposure, a thorough assessment is essential.

Assessment

Obtaining an accurate history from the child, parent, or caregiver is crucial. The information required to analyze a poison case includes identification of the poisonous drug or substance (name of commercial product); amount involved with the exposure; route of exposure; time elapsed after the exposure; the patient's age, weight, symptomatology, physical findings, pre-existing medical conditions, and current drug therapy or other drug and substance use; and any emergency treatment (e.g., home remedies) that may have been administered prior to seeking medical or other professional assistance.

If the name of a commercial product and the amount ingested are known, the potential for toxicity can be determined based on the ingredients and their concentrations. The pediatric patient's age and weight are important for assessing the toxicity potential of an exposure and for determining appropriate therapy, particularly for proper dosing of antidotes. The time elapsed since exposure may indicate when maximal toxicity can be expected and what treatment (e.g., induction of vomiting versus ingestion of activated charcoal) is appropriate. Symptomatology and physical findings are the most important information available for assessing a poisoned pediatric patient. It is not unusual for poison control centers to encounter symptomatic patients who inaccurately report ingesting nontoxic drugs or substances or subtoxic doses of potentially toxic drugs or substances. Thus, patients need to be carefully assessed regardless of the information provided in their histories.

Pre-existing medical conditions and current drug therapy (prescription or nonprescription drugs) or the use of other drugs and substances (e.g., abusable psychotropics, herbal remedies) may affect the degree of toxicity or the appropriate treatment. A parent or other caregiver may have administered a home remedy before calling the poison control center or seeking medical care. In some instances, the use of home remedies is helpful, and, in many other situations, it makes no difference. However, in some cases, it complicates patient management. For example, the administration of salt water as an emetic often does not produce vomiting and can produce significant toxicity and death from hypernatremia (Barer et al., 1973).

Management

The management of pediatric poisoning generally includes supportive medical care to ensure vital organ function and the following three interventions: prevention of further absorption of the poison, promotion of elimination of the poison, and the administration of appropriate antidotes. These aspects of patient management are discussed in more detail in the following section.

Supportive Medical Care

Providing supportive medical care is the most important component of the treatment of pediatric poisoning. Fortunately, most pediatric patients who receive adequate supportive medical care detoxify the poison and recover on their own. It is essential that vital organ functions be maintained during the acute phase of the poisoning exposure so that recovery can occur. Thus, the initial assessment of patients with suspected poisoning should focus on vital organ functions. Because many poisons can affect the respiratory system, the CNS, the cardiovascular system, and body temperature regulation systems, specific areas of concern include coma, respiratory depression or airway obstruction, seizures, hypotension and shock or hypertension, cardiac dysrhythmias, hypothermia or hyperthermia, cerebral or pulmonary edema, acid–base disturbances, and long-term complications of coma such as pneumonia and decubitus ulcers.

Prevention of GI Absorption

The time frame for considering GI decontamination varies, depending on the poison involved. A general guideline is that GI decontamination should be performed within 1–2 hours of the ingestion of the poison. However, rapidly absorbed poisons (e.g., alcohols) are usually absorbed within 1 hour of ingestion. Poorly absorbed poisons (e.g., aspirin) or poisons that decrease GI motility (e.g., anticholinergics) may remain in the GI tract longer. Absorption from the GI tract can be minimized by inducing vomiting, performing gastric lavage, administering activated charcoal, or performing whole bowel irrigation. **Although ipecac syrup is sometimes used in the home setting, activated charcoal is the primary means of GI decontamination in healthcare settings.**

The role of ipecac syrup, lavage, and activated charcoal in GI decontamination has changed markedly over the past 15 years. Decontamination trends show that ipecac use has dropped from 13.4% of exposures in 1983 to 0.8% of exposures managed by poison control centers in 2000. During the same time period, the use of activated charcoal increased from 4.0% to 6.7% of exposures (Litovitz et al., 2001). Numerous studies of volunteers and poisoned patients comparing the efficacy of ipecac syrup, lavage, and/or activated charcoal have led to the following conclusions.

- Activated charcoal is either as effective or superior to ipecac syrup or lavage with or without activated charcoal (Albertson et al., 1989; Bosse et al., 1995; Curtis et al., 1984; Kornberg & Dolgin, 1991; Kulig et al., 1985; Neuvonen et al., 1983; Pond et al., 1995; Tenenbein et al., 1987a).
- Early administration of ipecac syrup is more effective than lavage for small children (Boxer et al., 1969), particularly if the poison is a solid (e.g., tablet) because of the small diameter of lavage tubes.
- When large-bore lavage tubes are used, lavage is more effective than ipecac syrup for adults (and presumably adolescents) (Auerbach, 1986; Tandberg et al., 1986).
- Ipecac syrup administration delays the administration of activated charcoal, prolongs time in the emergency department, and increases the risk for aspiration (Albertson et al., 1989; Kornberg & Dolgin, 1991).

Ipecac syrup and gastric lavage are no longer utilized routinely for most overdoses that are managed in the emergency department. However, although supportive clinical data are lacking, lavage is still sometimes considered for potentially life-threatening overdoses if the procedure can be undertaken within 60 minutes of the ingestion of the poison (American Academy of Clinical Toxicology . . . , Ipecac syrup, 1997; American Academy of Clinical Toxicology . . . , Gastric lavage, 1997). Activated charcoal may be considered if the ingestion has occurred within 1 hour. However, there are insufficient data to support or exclude its use after 1 hour (American Academy of Clinical Toxicology . . . , Single dose activated charcoal, 1997). Because data on the use of cathartics with activated charcoal are conflicting, their routine use is not endorsed (American Academy of Clinical Toxicology . . . , Cathartics, 1997). However, when a cathartic is used, a single dose of the cathartic minimizes associated adverse drug reactions (ADRs) (e.g., diarrhea).

Many studies of GI decontamination have been performed in adults; however, there are few studies involving children. A study of children 12–20 months of age with salicylate overdoses in whom both emesis and lavage were performed in random order found ipecac-induced emesis to be superior to lavage (Boxer et al., 1969). In 455 children with acetaminophen poisoning, emesis (spontaneous or induced) within 30 minutes of ingestion reduced acetaminophen plasma concentrations by approximately 50% when compared to a control group without GI decontamination (Bond et al., 1993). However, by 90 minutes after ingestion, the emesis had no demonstrable effect. A prospective randomized trial of 70 children younger than 6 years presenting with mild-to-moderate acute oral overdoses who received either ipecac syrup and activated charcoal or only activated charcoal found that ipecac syrup delays the administration of activated charcoal and prolongs the time required in the emergency department (Kornberg & Dolgin, 1991). Patients who received ipecac syrup were more likely to vomit the activated charcoal than those who received activated charcoal alone (56% compared to 16%). Activated charcoal alone was recommended as the GI decontamination method of choice.

Ipecac syrup. Ipecac syrup and other emetics are used to induce vomiting. **Absolute contraindications to the use of emetics include significant CNS depression, the presence of seizures, the ingestion of caustic poisons, or the ingestion of a poison that could produce rapid onset of CNS depression or seizures.** There is a high risk for aspiration if vomiting occurs in a patient who has CNS depression or seizures. Induction of emesis following the ingestion of a caustic poison exposes the esophagus to the caustic poison for a second time, thus producing additional esophageal damage, and increases the risk for esophageal perforation. Emetics are usually avoided in cases of hydrocarbon ingestions because of the possible increased risk for aspiration.

Although its use is declining, ipecac syrup can be given to induce vomiting in the home or day-care setting. While no longer routinely recommended for use in hospitals, ipecac syrup can be administered early after the ingestion of drugs or substances that are not adsorbed by activated charcoal (e.g., iron). Although ipecac syrup-induced vomiting has been shown to reduce serum concentrations of the ingested poison, data demonstrating that ipecac syrup alters clinical outcomes are lacking (Bond et al., 1993). Ipecac syrup is available without prescription in 15- and 30-ml quantities and 30 ml should be kept in all homes that have children younger than 5 years. Ipecac syrup acts both locally on the GI mucosa and centrally by stimulating the chemoreceptor trigger zone and the vomiting center to produce emesis. Studies have demonstrated that ipecac syrup is both effective for inducing vomiting and safe for infants as young as 6 months and children (Litovitz et al., 1985; McCray et al., 1984). However, the quantity of the poison removed with vomiting is variable. Ipecac syrup is not recommended for infants younger than 6 months. Recommended initial doses are 10 ml for infants who are 6–12 months, 15 ml for children, and 15–30 ml for adolescents. Clear liquids should be administered in amounts of 120–180 ml (4–6 ounces) for young children and 360–480 ml (12–16 ounces) for adolescents. Studies have demonstrated that ipecac syrup is 90%–100% effective for inducing vomiting, with an onset of action of approximately 20 minutes. If vomiting does not occur within 15–20 minutes, more clear liquids should be administered and the initial dose of ipecac syrup should be repeated.

Common ADRs following therapeutic doses of ipecac syrup include sedation and diarrhea. Chronic abuse of ipecac syrup by adolescents with eating disorders may cause severe GI effects, tachycardia, hypotension, ECG changes, skeletal muscle weakness, tremors, and convulsions (Manno & Manno, 1972). Fatalities were reported for a 26-year-old patient who had anorexia nervosa and who ingested three or four 30-ml bottles of ipecac syrup daily for 3 months to lose weight and for a 14-month-old toddler who received a therapeutic dose of ipecac syrup (Adler et al., 1980; Robertson, 1979). The toddler's death was attributed to an anatomic defect.

Gastric lavage. Gastric lavage is an alternate method for removing poisons from the stomach. **It is contraindicated after ingestion of caustic poisons, for patients who are convulsing (unless the convulsions are controlled), and for patients who are comatose or who do not have an adequate gag reflex (unless a cuffed endotracheal tube is in place to protect the airway).** The most appropriate patient position for lavage is lying on the left side with the head down (Ellenhorn, 1997). A lavage tube is inserted into the patient's mouth and guided through the esophagus to the stomach. The tube position is checked by aspiration of the gastric contents and by forcing air through the tube and auscultating the stomach. After aspirating the stomach contents, lavage solution is instilled, allowed to mix with gastric contents, and removed. The initial gastric aspirate may be saved for laboratory analysis if the identity of the ingested poison is uncertain. Lavage is continued until gastric returns are clear. The use of water as a lavage solution should be avoided for infants because of the associated risk for water intoxication. Suitable lavage solutions for infants and children include 0.9% sodium chloride (normal saline), 0.45% sodium chloride (half normal saline), or 5%–6% polyethylene glycol (PEG) lavage solutions.

The utility of lavage for the management of pediatric poisonings is somewhat limited because of the small diameter of the lavage tubes that must be used. For young children, lavage may be considered within 1 hour after ingestion of a life-threatening amount of a liquid poison or for poisons that are not adsorbed by activated charcoal (e.g., alcohols, iron, lithium). For adolescents, lavage may be considered for the management of life-threatening poisonings if the procedure can be performed within 1 hour of the ingestion of the poison.

Activated charcoal. Activated charcoal is a fine black powder that has a large surface area. It effectively adsorbs many drugs and chemicals. The dose is 1 gram/kg of body weight or 15–30 grams for children and 60–100 grams for adolescents. Activated charcoal is mixed with water to form a slurry that can be drunk or poured down a gastric lavage tube. It is allowed to pass through the GI tract. Activated charcoal tablets are not effective for the adsorption of poisons.

Several preweighed and prepackaged charcoals are commercially available. Some consist of activated charcoal and water. Others are mixed with either 70% sorbitol or carboxymethylcellulose to increase their palatability. The formulation with sorbitol also acts as a cathartic. These prepackaged activated charcoal products offer convenience because additional weighing and mixing in the clinical setting are not required.

Activated charcoal is considered most effective when administered within 1 hour of the ingestion of a poison. More studies are needed to assess its efficacy for longer time periods after the ingestion of a poison. Activated charcoal is **ineffective** for alcohols (including ethanol, isopropyl alcohol, and methanol), glycols (such as ethylene glycol), mineral acids and alkalis, hydrocarbons, cyanide, iron, and lithium. Adverse effects associated with activated charcoal include vomiting, aspiration in CNS-depressed patients who do not have airway protection, and GI obstruction in patients who have decreased GI motility.

For some drugs, two doses of activated charcoal may be warranted to prevent delayed absorption. These drugs are slowly absorbed from the GI tract and exhibit marked delays in peak blood concentrations in cases of overdoses. A second dose of activated charcoal may be indicated approximately 4 hours after the first dose for carbamazepine, salicylates, valproic acid, and sustained-release products.

The role of activated charcoal for the management of poisonings outside a healthcare facility is unclear. Parents have difficulty getting children to drink the entire dose of activated charcoal slurry (Grbcich & Lacouture, 1987). Activated charcoal is administered sooner after the ingestion when used at home rather than waiting for administration at the emergency department, but the amount ingested varies greatly (average of 11.8 grams with a standard deviation of 7.9) (Spiller & Rodgers, 1997).

Cathartics. Cathartics are used to speed the transit of the activated charcoal–poison complex through the GI tract. Although data regarding the effect of cathartics on clinical outcome are lacking, cathartics are often administered with the first dose of activated charcoal. Saline cathartics (e.g., magnesium sulfate and magnesium citrate) or sorbitol are most commonly recommended. However, sorbitol may enhance the transit of activated charcoal to a greater extent than magnesium citrate or magnesium sulfate (Krenzelok et al., 1985). The concentration and dosage of magnesium sulfate should be no greater than 10% and 250 mg/kg, respectively. The appropriate dose of magnesium citrate is 200 ml for adolescents or 5 ml/kg for children. The appropriate dose of sorbitol is 1–3 grams/kg as a 35%–70% solution for adolescents and 1–1.5 grams/kg as a 35% solution for children.

Fluid and electrolyte disturbances are a significant concern when cathartics are used for pediatric patients because cathartics cause loss of fluids and electrolytes from the GI tract. These problems are even more likely to develop when multiple-dose activated charcoal and cathartic regimens are used to enhance GI clearance of a poison because the patient is more likely to loose significant quantities of fluids and electrolytes. A 3-month-old infant who had chronic theophylline poisoning developed severe hypernatremia, dehydration, and shock following approximately 150 ml of a charcoal–sorbitol suspension containing 70% sorbitol (110–120 grams of sorbitol) that was administered over 3–4 hours (Farley, 1986).

Whole bowel irrigation. Whole bowel irrigation involves rapid enteral administration of large volumes of polyethylene glycol lavage solutions over several hours. The procedure mechanically cleanses the bowel and has been used for years as a routine bowel preparation for colonoscopy and large bowel surgery. Whole bowel irrigation also is used for GI decontamination in cases of acute oral drug overdosages. The procedure involves the administration of a polyethylene glycol electrolyte lavage solution such as *Golytely®* or *Colyte®* by nasogastric tube at 2 liters/hr for adolescents and 0.5 liter/hr for children for up to 6 hours. The end point for the irrigation is reached when the rectal effluent has the same appearance as the infusate. A study in human volunteers using the ampicillin "overdose" model found that whole bowel irrigation resulted in a 67% decrease in ampicillin bioavailability when compared to the control group (Tenenbein et al., 1987b).

In addition to decreasing drug absorption by mechanical cleansing, whole bowel irrigation may increase enteroenteric and enterohepatic elimination in a similar manner to multiple-dose activated charcoal because of the large volume of fluid in the GI tract. **Potential indications for whole bowel irrigation include oral overdoses with iron and other drugs and substances that are not adsorbed by activated charcoal and possibly oral overdoses with sustained-release products.** Whole bowel irrigation was used successfully for the management of six children who had iron poisoning, three of whom still had a large number of iron tablets in the stomach (identified by abdominal roentgenogram) following ipecac and/or lavage (Tenenbein, 1987).

Promotion of Elimination

After a poison is absorbed into the systemic circulation and distributed throughout the body, several procedures can be used to promote its elimination and help to prevent or minimize its toxic effects. These procedures are generally indicated only in severe poisonings and often play a secondary role to supportive care, prevention of absorption, and the administration of antidotes.

Multiple doses of activated charcoal. Multiple doses of activated charcoal are used to prevent reabsorption and enhance the clearance of poisons that are transferred from the bloodstream into the stomach or that undergo enteroenteric or enterohepatic recirculation. Activated charcoal is usually administered at 4-hour intervals until the serum concentration of the poison is no longer in the toxic range or the signs and symptoms associated with the poisoning have resolved. Alternatively, lower doses could be administered at more frequent intervals (Ilkhanipour et al., 1992). Multiple doses of activated charcoal dramatically reduce the elimination half-life for a limited number of drugs. Greatest benefit has been demonstrated in cases of theophylline overdosages or poisonings in which multiple-dose charcoal administered to patients with life-threatening toxicities has resulted in complete resolution of associated signs and symptoms

(Paloucek & Rodvold, 1988). Multiple-dose activated charcoal is recommended for acute or chronic overdosages or poisonings with dapsone, phenobarbital, and phenytoin. However, improved outcome has not been demonstrated conclusively. A randomized trial of patients who were identified as having a phenobarbital overdose demonstrated a reduction in the phenobarbital half-life from 90 to 36 hours in the treated versus control group (Pond et al., 1984). No differences were seen between the two groups, however, in time course or outcome.

Although some sources suggest that multiple-dose activated charcoal will decrease the half-life of drugs with high volumes of distribution, such as tricyclic antidepressants and digoxin (Campbell & Chyka, 1992), it is unlikely that this procedure will remove significant quantities of these drugs via the GI tract. In addition, the administration of multiple doses of activated charcoal to patients who have tricyclic antidepressant overdoses and who are experiencing CNS depression and/or seizures increases the risk for aspiration. Potential complications of multiple-dose activated charcoal include bowel obstruction and charcoal aspiration (Pond, 1986; Tenenbein, 1991). A cathartic can be administered with the first dose of a multiple-dose activated charcoal regimen, but not with subsequent doses of activated charcoal. Multiple doses of cathartics can result in fluid and electrolyte disturbances (e.g., hypermagnesemia). Hypernatremia developed in a 2-year-old child when multiple doses of a charcoal–sorbitol suspension were administered (McCord, 1987).

Alteration of urine pH. Alteration of the urinary pH is used primarily for poisons for which the urinary excretion of the active component is the predominant pathway of elimination. The goal is to maximize the amount of the poison that is in the ionized state in the renal tubules because ionized substances are not reabsorbed. Although alkalinization enhances the elimination of weak acids, no controlled trials demonstrate an effect on clinical outcome. **Acidification of the urine is not clinically indicated because it increases the risk for acute renal failure secondary to rhabdomyolysis and myoglobinuria.**

Urinary alkalinization can be considered for poisonings and overdoses involving phenobarbital, salicylates, chlorpropamide, and 2,4-dichlorophenoxyacetic acid (2,4-D). Alkalinization of the urine is not possible if hypokalemia is present because hydrogen ion is excreted into the renal tubules instead of potassium in an attempt to conserve potassium. Because metabolic acidosis and hypokalemia are common in severe salicylate poisonings involving children, alkalinization of the urine may be difficult, or impossible, to achieve until potassium serum concentrations are replenished.

Sodium bicarbonate is the only acceptable drug for urinary alkalinization. For pediatric patients, 2 mEq/kg of sodium bicarbonate for injection is added to the intravenous solution (e.g., 5% dextrose in water for infusion or 5% dextrose and 2.5% normal saline for infusion) and infused over 1–2 hours. Additional 1–2-mEq/kg doses should be administered to maintain the urinary pH at 7.0 or higher. Urinary and serum pH and sodium and potassium serum concentrations must be monitored carefully. If the patient is hypokalemic, oral or intravenous potassium should be administered after renal function is evaluated and determined to be sufficient (i.e., potassium supplementation is contraindicated for patients who are anuric).

Hemodialysis and hemoperfusion. Hemodialysis and hemoperfusion effectively enhance the elimination of some poisons. For hemodialysis to be effective, the following criteria must be met (Schreiner, 1977):

- The poison should diffuse through the dialyzing membrane at a reasonably rapid rate.
- The poison must be distributed in plasma water or rapidly equilibrated with plasma water.
- There should be a relationship between serum concentration and duration of exposure and clinical toxicity.
- The amount dialyzed should constitute a

significant addition to the normal body mechanisms for elimination.

In severe poisonings with alcohols (particularly methanol and ethylene glycol), lithium, and salicylates, hemodialysis should be considered. Used concurrently with the administration of ethanol or fomepizole to block metabolism to more toxic metabolites, hemodialysis removes methanol and ethylene glycol from the body.

Hemoperfusion is a procedure that involves passing blood through an adsorbent material, usually a coated charcoal or a resin. The efficacy of hemoperfusion is related primarily to the affinity of the adsorbent for the poison, the rate of blood flow through the adsorbent column, and the rate of equilibration of the poison in peripheral tissues with that in the blood. The factors that influence the effectiveness of dialysis, such as high molecular weight, poor water solubility, and plasma protein binding, do not influence hemoperfusion (Koffler et al., 1978; Pond et al., 1979; Vale et al., 1975; Winchester et al., 1977). The drugs phenobarbital and theophylline are removed by both hemodialysis and hemoperfusion, but hemoperfusion is more effective. Phenobarbital overdoses can usually be managed with supportive medical care alone.

Antidotes

Systemic antidotes are available for only a few drugs and other substances commonly involved in pediatric poisoning. In some instances, the antidote can save lives. In most instances, antidotes are an adjunct to, not a substitute for, supportive medical care. If an antidote is available, it is important to consider whether it is indicated for a particular patient. For example, the opiate antagonist naloxone *(Narcan®)* would not be indicated for an asymptomatic 2-year-old child who accidently drank a small amount of her older sister's cough syrup, which contained codeine, although it would do no harm (if the pediatrician were in doubt) because it is a pure opiate antagonist. Conversely, an antidote such as physostigmine can produce serious life-threatening toxicity and is rarely used. Table 4-3 provides a description of clinically useful antidotes.

Treatment of Common Pediatric Poisonings

Several drugs and substances are involved in the majority of pediatric poisonings, including aspirin and other salicylates, acetaminophen, nonsteroidal anti-inflammatory drugs (NSAIDs [excluding the salicylates]), iron, antihistamines, caustics, hydrocarbons, and alcohols and ethylene glycol. A detailed discussion of the treatment for overdoses with each of these drugs and substances follows.

Aspirin and Other Salicylates

Aspirin and other salicylates are involved in both acute and chronic poisonings. Acute salicylate poisonings, which at one time were the leading cause of poisoning in children younger than 5 years, have decreased markedly as a result of the Poison Prevention Packaging Act of 1970. This act mandated the child-resistant packaging now required for many drugs and household products, including aspirin. However, children and adolescents younger than 20 years accounted for 67% of salicylate exposures reported to the American Association of Poison Control Centers Toxic Exposure Surveillance System in 2000 (Litovitz et al., 2001). There were 14,177 exposures involving salicylates in children younger than 6 years and 8967 salicylate exposures among children and adolescents 6–19 years of age. There were four aspirin-related fatalities, all of which involved adolescents committing suicide.

Chronic overdoses of salicylates, usually related to long-term high dosage salicylate therapy, are associated with greater morbidity and mortality than acute overdoses (Gaudreault et al., 1982; Yip et al., 1994). On presentation, these children and adolescents are usually more severely ill and exhibit the following signs and symptoms: hyperventilation, fever, dehydration, acidosis, and CNS effects. Misdiagnosis (e.g., as an infection) may

(Continued on page 256)

TABLE 4-3
Antidotes for Pediatric Poisoning

INDICATION	ANTIDOTE (TRADE NAME)	USUAL PEDIATRIC DOSAGE AND ADMINISTRATION[a]	COMMENTS
Acetaminophen poisoning	Acetylcysteine (Mucomyst®)	In United States, 140 mg/kg PO loading dose followed by 70 mg/kg PO every 4 hr for 17 doses.	IV administration of acetylcysteine is not approved in the United States. See Chapter 14 for details regarding IV use.
Arsenic, gold, lead, or mercury poisoning	Dimercaprol (BAL in Oil®)	Dosage varies according to indication; generally 4 mg/kg IM every 4 hr.	Used in combination with other chelators for severe lead poisoning.
Atropine and other pure anticholinergic drug poisoning	Physostigmine salicylate (Antilirium® [United States only])	**Children:** 0.02 mg/kg IM or slow IV, **not** to exceed 0.5 mg/min; repeat as needed up to total dose of 2 mg. Repeat lowest effective dose if signs and symptoms recur.	Indicated for seizures, severe hypertension, supraventricular tachydysrhythmias, severe hallucinations and delirium related to anticholinergic poisoning. Potential toxicity often outweighs potential benefits. May cause cholinergic crisis, including bradycardia and convulsions. Avoid use in cases involving cyclic antidepressant overdosage. Patient should be on a cardiac monitor.
Benzodiazepine poisoning	Flumazenil (Anexate®, Romazicon®)	**Children:** No standardized dose; initial dose of approximately 0.01 mg/kg IV followed by 0.005 mg/kg/min has been reported in children (Jones et al., 1991; Kelly et al., 1988). **Adolescents:** 0.2–0.3 mg IV over 30 sec initially; repeat at 60-sec intervals, as indicated, up to total dose of 3 mg; some patients who respond only partially to 3 mg may need up to 5 mg for complete response.	Contraindicated if poisoning includes tricyclic antidepressants or other drugs with potential to induce seizures or cardiac dysrhythmias. Currently not approved by the FDA or HPB for use in infants or children.
Beta-adrenergic blocker poisoning	Glucagon	Initially, 50–150 μg/kg as an IV bolus, then 1–5 mg/hr as indicated.	Increases myocardial contractility. Use as an antidote is not FDA or HPB approved.
Calcium-channel blocker poisoning	Calcium chloride injectable, 10% (contains 27.2 mg of elemental calcium per milliliter)	5–7 mg/kg of elemental calcium by slow IV administration.	Monitor calcium serum concentrations if more than one dose is required; produces positive inotropic effect; less effective for AV block or hypotension; less useful in cases of severe intoxication.
Copper, lead, mercury, or arsenic poisoning	Penicillamine (Cuprimine®)	**Children:** 20–40 mg/kg/day PO as a single dose or in divided doses (maximum 2 grams/day)	Avoid use in children with penicillin allergy.
Cyclic antidepressant poisoning	Sodium bicarbonate	Initially, 1–2 mEq/kg by IV bolus, then IV infusion to maintain blood pH of 7.5.	Indicated for the treatment of poisoning-related cardiac dysrhythmias, conduction disturbances, and hypotension.
Cyanide poisoning	Amyl nitrite inhalant, sodium nitrite IV, sodium thiosulfate IV (Cyanide Antidote Kit®)	Administer amyl nitrite inhalant for 30 sec of each minute until sodium nitrite can be administered IV. **Children >25 kg:** Administer sodium nitrite 300 mg IV, then immediately administer sodium thiosulfate 12.5 grams IV. **Children ≤25 kg:** Administer doses according to hemoglobin concentration: HEMOGLOBIN (grams/dl) / 3% SODIUM NITRITE (ml/kg) 8 / 0.22 10 / 0.27 12 / 0.33 14 / 0.39 HEMOGLOBIN (grams/dl) / 25% SODIUM THIOSULFATE (ml/kg) 8 / 1.10 10 / 1.35 12 / 1.65 14 / 1.95	Follow manufacturer's instructions in kit carefully; inappropriate sodium nitrate dosing can produce severe methemoglobinemia and death.

[a] See Chapters 13 and 14 for additional information regarding dosage and administration.

TABLE 4-3 continued

INDICATION	ANTIDOTE (TRADE NAME)	USUAL PEDIATRIC DOSAGE AND ADMINISTRATION[a]	COMMENTS
Digoxin poisoning	Digoxin immune Fab (Digibind®)	Dose of digoxin immune Fab (in number of 38-mg vials) = total body load of digoxin (mg)/0.5. **Approximate *Digibind* dose for reversal of a single large digoxin overdose** | NUMBER OF DIGOXIN TABLETS* OR CAPSULES	*DIGIBIND* DOSE, NUMBER OF VIALS | |---|---| | 25 | 10 | | 50 | 20 | | 75 | 30 | | 100 | 40 | | 150 | 60 | | 200 | 80 | *0.25-mg tablets with 80% bioavailability (e.g., Lanoxin®) or 0.2-mg capsules with 100% bioavailability (e.g., Lanoxicaps®).	For acute intoxication, use table provided as a guide. For chronic intoxication, use glycoside serum concentrations to guide treatment. *See* Chapter 14 for additional information.
Ethylene glycol or methanol poisoning	Alcohol (ethanol)	Loading dose: 7.6 ml/kg of alcohol 10% IV over 30–60 min followed by 1.4 ml/kg/hr oral maintenance dose; increase dosage during hemodialysis.	Maintain alcohol blood concentration of 100 mg/dl. Simultaneous glucose administration usually is required.
	Fomepizole (Antizol®)	Administer as a slow IV infusion over 30 min. Loading dose: 15 mg/kg; then 10 mg/kg every 12 hr for four doses, followed by 15 mg/kg every 12 hr until ethylene glycol or methanol blood concentration is less than 20 mg/dl.	Change dosing interval to every 4 hr during dialysis. Approved in United States for ethylene glycol poisoning but probably effective for methanol poisoning also.
Iron poisoning	Deferoxamine mesylate (Desferal®)	Initially, 1000 mg IM; then 500 mg every 4 hr as indicated (maximum 6 grams/day). If the patient is in a state of cardiovascular collapse, then desferoxamine can be administered IV at a maximum rate of 15 mg/kg/hr for the first 1000 mg administered. Subsequent IV dosing, if required, should be at a reduced rate not to exceed 125 mg/hr (maximum 6 grams/day).	Indicated for patients with positive GI radiograph, iron serum concentration greater than 350 µg/dl, and/or signs or symptoms of iron poisoning.
Isoniazid poisoning	Pyridoxine	Administer 1 gram of pyridoxine by slow IV infusion for each gram of isoniazid ingested (to a maximum pyridoxine dose of 70 mg/kg). Repeat dose as required for treatment of persistent or recurrent seizures.	Indicated for treatment of seizures and acidosis related to isoniazid poisoning.
Lead poisoning	Edetate calcium disodium (calcium disodium edetate, calcium EDTA) (used alone or in conjunction with dimercaprol) (*Calcium Disodium Versenate®*)	50–75 mg/kg/day IM in three to six equally divided doses for 5 days (maximum dosage 500 mg/kg over 5 days); wait 2 days and repeat 5-day course of therapy, if necessary.	Generally indicated for lead blood concentrations ≥45 µg/dl. May consider for use among patients with 35–44 µg/dl concentration.
	Succimer (DMSA) (*Chemet®*)	Initially, 10 mg/kg or 350 mg/m^2 PO every 8 hr for 5 days and then every 12 hr for 14 days.	
Methemoglobinemia (poisoning with nitrates, nitrites, and others)	Methylene blue	0.2 ml/kg IV over 5–10 min.	Use 10-mg/ml solution. The dose is equivalent to 2 mg/kg. Use methylene blue very cautiously, if at all, to treat methemoglobinemia in patients with glucose-6-phosphate dehydrogenase deficiency because it is ineffective in some of these patients and may induce an acute hemolytic episode.

TABLE 4-3 continued

INDICATION	ANTIDOTE (TRADE NAME)	USUAL PEDIATRIC DOSAGE AND ADMINISTRATION[a]	COMMENTS
Opiate poisoning	Naloxone (*Narcan®*)	**Children:** Initially, 0.1 mg/kg IV push; repeat at 2–3-min intervals as needed to reverse respiratory depression. **Adolescents:** Initially, 2–4 mg IV push; repeat at 2–3-min intervals as needed to reverse respiratory depression.	Duration of action is short, so repeated doses every 1–2 hr usually are necessary. An IV infusion (2/3 of total required IV push dose/hr) may be useful, particularly in cases of poisoning with long-acting opiates (e.g., methadone and propoxyphene). Infusion rate and concentration should be individualized according to response. Patients should be monitored closely.
Organo-phosphate (e.g., organic phosphorus insecticides) poisoning	Pralidoxime chloride (*Protopam®*)	**Children:** Initially, 25–50 mg/kg (up to 1 gram) IM or IV; repeat every 8–12 hr as indicated if muscle weakness persists.	Use in conjunction with atropine; of little benefit greater than 36 hr after exposure.
Organo-phosphate or carbamate poisoning	Atropine sulfate	Initially, 0.05 mg/kg IV, not to exceed 2 mg; repeat every 10–30 min as indicated.	Administer atropine until excessive pulmonary secretions associated with the poisoning are effectively controlled or signs and symptoms of atropine intoxication appear.

[a] See Chapters 13 and 14 for additional information regarding dosage and administration.

delay appropriate assessment and management of the overdose. Fortunately, chronic salicylate overdose is an infrequent problem among children because of the declining use of aspirin in this age group related to concerns about Reye's syndrome.

The factors that increase the severity of salicylate overdoses include impaired renal function, pre-existing fever or dehydration, and age. Children younger than 4 years are more susceptible to the toxic effects of salicylates. Although an uncommon route of exposure, topically applied salicylates also can cause toxicity. Two neonates and three children 6–12 years old developed clinical features of salicylate toxicity and elevated salicylate serum concentrations following the topical application of 1%–10% salicylic acid for 1–5 days (Brubacher & Hoffman, 1996).

Clinical manifestations of mild-to-moderate salicylate toxicity or poisoning include confusion, difficulty hearing, dizziness, drowsiness, headache, hyperventilation, nausea, tinnitus, and vomiting with resulting respiratory alkalosis. Metabolic acidosis usually develops over the first 12 hours and is universal for young children by 20 hours after the overdose (Done, 1968). Metabolic acidosis results from the stimulation of catabolism, which leads to an increased production of metabolic intermediate acids including lactate, pyruvate, and the ketoacids. Hypoglycemia is more common among children than adults because children have decreased glycogen stores and gluconeogenesis is impaired. More severe salicylate poisoning produces coma, dehydration, delirium, fever, hemorrhage, pulmonary edema, restlessness, and seizures. Delayed CNS depression, including coma, may occur 24–48 hours after aspirin is discontinued in chronic salicylate poisoning among children (Dove & Jones, 1982). Dehydration is secondary to vomiting, decreased ingestion of oral liquids, increased water loss due to hyperventilation and sweating, and increased urine output associated with the excretion of salicylate. In cases of moderate salicylate poisonings, water losses are estimated at 2–3 liters/m^2 while deficits of 4–6 liters/m^2 may occur in cases of severe salicylate poisoning.

Elevated temperature is a serious complication of salicylate poisoning, particularly among children, and is caused by increased heat production at the tissue level as a result of uncoupling of oxidative phosphorylation. Noncardiogenic pulmonary edema, though rare, is a potentially life-threatening manifestation of salicylate poisoning and is probably related to a salicylate-induced increase in pulmonary vascular permeability to protein (Fisher et al., 1985; Kahn & Blum, 1979). In a series of 20 children who had salicylate poisoning, two children developed pulmonary edema and both died (Fisher et al., 1985). There is disagreement as to whether the pulmonary edema was from acute lung injury or cardiogenic (Wald et al., 1985). Cardiovascular effects include conduction disturbances, dysrhythmias, hypotension, and, in cases of severe salicylate poisonings, cardiovascular collapse (Mukerji et al., 1986; Pei & Thompson, 1987). Terminal events include cerebral edema and cardiovascular failure.

Ingestions of less than 150 mg/kg of aspirin generally require no specific treatment except the administration of a demulcent such as milk. Ipecac syrup or activated charcoal can be administered at home for an ingestion of 150–300 mg/kg of aspirin. If 300 mg/kg or more or an unknown amount of aspirin has been ingested, the patient should be treated in a medical facility. If a nonaspirin salicylate is ingested, the dose is converted to aspirin-equivalents by multiplying by the aspirin conversion factor (ACF). Table 4-4 provides the ACFs for some common nonaspirin salicylates.

GI decontamination with activated charcoal can be attempted up to 12 hours after the salicylate poisoning exposure because salicylate overdoses produce pylorospasm, which delays gastric emptying and can produce a mass of drug that serves as a reservoir for continued absorption. A second dose of activated charcoal may be administered 4 hours after the first dose to adsorb the drug remaining in the GI tract. Neither multiple-dose activated charcoal nor whole bowel irrigation increases the clearance of salicylate and, therefore, neither is recommended (Campbell & Chyka, 1992; Kirshenbaum et al., 1990; Mayer et al., 1992).

Laboratory evaluation of acute salicylate poisoning should include a salicylate serum concentration at 6 hours or longer after the ingestion. Salicylate serum concentrations should be determined every 2 hours until the concentrations decline. The **Done nomogram,** which predicts the prognosis of an acute poisoning, **is no longer used** to guide patient management. When used for adolescents and adults who have acute salicylate overdoses, the nomogram overestimates toxicity, especially when serum concentrations are obtained more than 12 hours after the ingestion (Dugandzic et al., 1989). It also has no role in the assessment of chronic salicylate poisonings. Other laboratory evaluation should include blood glucose, serum electrolytes (particularly potassium), arterial blood gases, bicarbonate, and prothrombin time.

Alkalinization plays an important role in the treatment of salicylate poisoning. Sodium bicarbonate should be administered to correct the metabolic acidosis and to "ion trap" salicylate out of the brain and into the plasma (Done, 1978). Sodium bicarbonate should be administered (1–2 mEq/kg every 1–2 hours as needed) to achieve a plasma pH of 7.5. Alkalinization of the urine enhances the renal elimination of salicylate but may be difficult to achieve for the child who has severe salicylate poisoning; it has not been proved to positively affect outcome for these patients. Therefore, aggressive attempts at urine alkalinization are not warranted. However, with the correction of hypokalemia and the base deficit by the administration of sodium bicarbonate for injection in intravenous solutions, urine alkalinization may result in some patients.

Intravenous replacement therapy should aim to correct dehydration, acid–base and electrolyte imbalances, and hypoglycemia. Hyperthermia is managed by external means

TABLE 4-4
Aspirin Conversion Factors (ACF)

NONASPIRIN COMPOUND	ACF
Bismuth Subsalicylate	0.59
Choline Salicylate	0.75
Magnesium Salicylate	1.21
Methyl Salicylate	1.40
Phenyl Salicylate	0.84
Potassium Salicylate	1.02
Salicylic Acid	1.30
Sodium Salicylate	1.12
Triethanolamine Salicylate	0.63

including sponging with tepid water or using cooling blankets. Coagulation abnormalities and hemorrhage are rare and are related to impaired formation of vitamin K-dependent clotting factors that should respond to phytonadione.

Patients who have severe salicylate poisoning may require more effective means for removing the drug from the body. Hemodialysis is indicated for patients who have a 6-hour salicylate serum concentration of ≥100 mg% in acute overdose, refractory acidosis, persistent CNS signs and symptoms, or progressive clinical deterioration despite appropriate intravenous therapy. Hemodialysis also is indicated for patients who have severe salicylate poisoning with renal failure. Although hemoperfusion removes salicylate from the blood, it cannot be used to correct the acid–base and electrolyte disturbances that can be corrected by hemodialysis.

Acetaminophen

Acetaminophen has almost completely replaced aspirin as an analgesic and antipyretic for pediatric patients. Although acetaminophen is safe and relatively devoid of ADRs with therapeutic doses, **overdoses produce serious liver damage**. As acetaminophen availability and use have increased, there has been a concomitant increase in the number of overdoses. Acetaminophen (alone or in combination with other drugs) accounted for 5.0% of exposures in the AAPCC Toxic Exposure Surveillance System for 2000, with children and adolescents younger than 20 years of age accounting for 56% of these exposures (Litovitz et al., 2001). There were 34,401 exposures involving children younger than 6 years and 25,609 involving children and adolescents 6–19 years old. Acetaminophen alone or in combination with diphenhydramine or hydrocodone was the primary drug responsible for seven fatalities of which six involved intentional ingestions by adolescents.

The clinical course of an acetaminophen overdose has been described in four phases (Prescott, 1983; Rumack, 1983; Rumack & Matthew, 1975). The **first phase** develops within a few hours of the ingestion and consists of nausea, vomiting, anorexia, diaphoresis, malaise, and drowsiness. These initial signs and symptoms are relatively nonspecific and often mild. Thus, medical care generally is not sought until later during the course of the acetaminophen poisoning or overdose, which decreases the effectiveness of antidotal therapy. This delay tends to occur more commonly among adolescents who attempt to commit suicide with an overdose of acetaminophen than among children, for whom medical advice is usually sought as soon as the acetaminophen poisoning is discovered.

The **second phase** occurs up to 48 hours after the overdose or poisoning. The initial signs and symptoms resolve, but liver enlargement and tenderness and right upper quadrant pain develop. Laboratory evidence of liver damage includes hepatic enzyme elevation, increases in bilirubin levels, and prolongation of prothrombin time. Urine output may decrease as a result of dehydration from vomiting and decreased ingestion of oral liquids or the development of inappropriate antidiuretic hormone secretion.

The **third phase** occurs on days 3–5 postingestion and is characterized by severe liver damage manifested as jaundice, coagulation defects, hypoglycemia, metabolic acidosis, and hepatic encephalopathy. Acetaminophen produces centrilobular necrosis with sparing of the periportal areas (Black, 1984; Mitchell et al., 1974; Piperno et al., 1978). Acute renal tubular necrosis 5–7-days postingestion has been reported to occur in as high as 10%–40% of patients, but it is seen less frequently since the advent of specific antidotal therapy. Renal failure may be secondary to hepatic failure or may be a direct nephrotoxic effect (Curry et al., 1982; Kleinman et al., 1980; Wilkinson et al., 1977). Death, although not common, is related to hepatic failure. If the patient survives the acute injury to the liver, hepatic function gradually returns to normal during the **fourth phase,** which occurs over 1–2 weeks. Increased fibrous tissue on follow-up liver biopsies is the only residual evidence of acetaminophen's toxicity.

Acetaminophen produces hepatic toxicity through the formation of a toxic metabolite (Black, 1984; Piperno et al., 1978). In therapeutic doses, acetaminophen is primarily metabolized to glucuronide and sulfate conjugates that account for 80%–90% of the dose. Less than 2% of the dose is excreted renally unchanged. The remainder is metabolized by the cytochrome P-450 mixed function oxidase system to a toxic substance that is probably a highly reactive arylating agent. Normally, the reactive metabolite is detoxified by conjugation with glutathione and is further conjugated and excreted renally as the cysteine and mercapturic acid conjugates. In an overdose or poisoning, the sulfate and glucuronide pathways become saturated. A large proportion of the dose is metabolized via the cytochrome P-450 system and glutathione is rapidly utilized and depleted. When glutathione stores in the liver drop to 20%–30% of normal, the amount of glutathione is insufficient to detoxify the reactive metabolite that becomes available to bind covalently to liver macromolecules, producing hepatocellular damage.

The generally accepted hepatotoxic dose for adolescents and adults is 10–15 grams, although there are case reports of mild elevations of liver enzymes following ingestion of 5–7.5 grams (Fernandez & Fernandez-Brito, 1977; Prescott, 1983). Age-related differences in sensitivity to acetaminophen toxicity have been proposed (Peterson & Rumack, 1981; Rumack, 1983). Children may be more resistant than adolescents and adults to the hepatotoxic effects of acetaminophen as a result of differences in metabolic disposition (increased formation of the sulfate conjugate relative to the glucuronide conjugate may occur) (Lieh-Lai et al., 1984; Miller et al., 1976). The rate of glutathione synthesis is higher among young animals when compared to older animals, which may partly explain the decreased susceptibility of children to acetaminophen hepatotoxicity (Lauterburg et al., 1980). Only three pediatric deaths from single acute ingestions have been reported and, in two of these deaths, the exact amount of acetaminophen involved in the ingestion is not specified (Penna & Buchanan, 1991; Rumack & Matthew, 1975; Weber & Cutz, 1980).

Chronic acetaminophen toxicity has been reported in children from repeated "therapeutic" administration of dosages exceeding recommended dosages. Although death due to an acute overdose of acetaminophen among young children is rare, fatalities have been reported with chronic overdosages (Heubi et al., 1998; Penna & Buchanan, 1991). Chronic acetaminophen overdosages are often the result of the administration of adult formulations to children. In one report, the threshold for hepatotoxicity was 150 mg/kg/day or more for more than 2–4 days (Henretig et al., 1989). A compilation of 47 reports of acetaminophen toxicity involving infants and children 5 weeks to 10 years old found that 24 of 43 children died and three additional children survived following liver transplantation (Heubi et al., 1998). Doses of acetaminophen ranged from 60 to 420 mg/kg/day for 1–42 days.

A retrospective review of the outcome of acetaminophen overdose in a selected pediatric population at liver transplant centers found that 28 patients had severe liver toxicity and six of these patients required a liver transplant (Rivera-Penera et al., 1997). Ten of 14 children younger than 10 years had severe liver toxicity and, in all of these cases, the toxicity was caused by multiple toxic doses administered by parents. Acetaminophen doses ranged from 75 to 750 mg/kg/day for 1–5 days and suggest a therapeutic index as low as 1.7 (Heubi & Bien, 1997). An 18-month-old child who died of acetaminophen toxicity after 120 mg/kg/day for 4 days was considered at increased risk because of diminished hepatic reserve resulting from prolonged total parenteral nutrition as an infant (Pershad et al., 1999).

Children ingesting less than 200 mg/kg of acetaminophen generally can be managed at home (Bond et al., 1994). At the Maryland Poison Center, children ingesting less than 200 mg/kg are managed with observation only. Children ingesting 200 mg/kg or more and adolescents who ingest more than 140 mg/kg or 7.5 grams are managed in a medical facility with activated charcoal, assessment of acetaminophen plasma concentrations, and oral acetylcysteine therapy. Although some in vitro and human volunteer studies have found that activated charcoal adsorbs acetylcysteine (Ekins et al., 1987; Klein-Schwartz &

Oderda, 1981), the dose of acetylcysteine is large enough that this interaction is clinically insignificant. Therefore, activated charcoal can be administered to patients who will be receiving oral acetylcysteine.

Acetylcysteine therapy should be initiated as soon as possible after an acetaminophen overdose. It is most effective if initiated within 8 hours of the overdose but has an effect on liver enzyme elevations for up to 24 hours following the overdose (and possibly longer) (Harrison et al., 1990; Smilkstein et al., 1988). Late administration of acetylcysteine to patients who have acetaminophen-induced hepatic failure improves the survival rate and lowers the incidence of complications (Keays et al., 1991).

The initiation of acetylcysteine therapy should take into consideration the history of acetaminophen exposure and the potential toxicity of the amount ingested. The decision to complete the full course of therapy is based on the acetaminophen plasma concentration obtained later. An acetaminophen plasma concentration should be obtained at 4 hours or more after the exposure and interpreted utilizing a modified Matthew–Rumack nomogram (Figure 4-1) (Rumack & Matthew, 1975; Rumack et al., 1981). If the acetaminophen plasma concentration is below the lower line on the nomogram, acetylcysteine therapy should be discontinued because the concentration is nontoxic. If the concentration is at or above the lower line, a full course of acetylcysteine therapy should be administered because hepatotoxicity can be expected without treatment. Following ingestions involving acetaminophen tablets or capsules, acetaminophen plasma concentrations obtained earlier than 4 hours postingestion may not accurately reflect the potential for hepatotoxicity because absorption may not be complete. However, recent evidence suggests that absorption occurs more rapidly if acetaminophen elixir (or solution) is ingested and that the acetaminophen plasma concentration should be measured at 2 hours after ingestion rather than 4 hours (Anderson et al., 1999). A 2-hour acetaminophen plasma concentration of 225 mg/liter or greater has been proposed as the concentration at which antidotal therapy with acetylcysteine would be indicated (Anderson et al., 1999; Rumack, 1999).

Acetylcysteine protects against acetaminophen hepatotoxicity either by acting as a glutathione precursor or substitute or by enhancing the activity of the sulfate conjugation pathway. Acetylcysteine's potent antioxidant activity may also prevent or reverse secondary microcirculatory changes and restore microcirculatory blood flow (Mitchell, 1988). The oral dosing regimen is a loading dose of 140 mg/kg followed by 17 maintenance doses of 70 mg/kg. Acetylcysteine is available as a 10% or 20% solution and should be diluted to a 5% solution before it is administered.

In Great Britain and Canada, acetylcysteine is routinely administered intravenously at a total dose of 300 mg/kg over 20 hours. A 48-hour intravenous regimen (140 mg/kg load followed by 12 maintenance doses of 70 mg/kg every 4 hours; total dose 980 mg/kg) was investigated in the United States and compared with the published data on the 20-hour intravenous and 72-hour oral regimens (Smilkstein et al., 1991). If acetylcysteine therapy was initiated within 10 hours of the acetaminophen ingestion, efficacy was similar for all three regimens. If therapy was initiated 10–24 hours after the ingestion, the 48-hour regimen was superior to the 20-hour intravenous regimen (Smilkstein et al., 1991). For 25 pediatric patients who had acetaminophen poisoning, the 52-hour intravenous regimen was as effective as the 72-hour oral regimen in a comparison using historical control pediatric subjects (Perry & Shannon, 1998). Hepatotoxicity did not occur among children treated within 10 hours and occurred in only 9.8% of those treated between 10 and 24 hours.

There are several disadvantages to the use of oral and intravenous acetylcysteine. Major ADRs associated with oral acetylcysteine, which is usually administered by nasogastric tube, include nausea and vomiting. Chilling each dose of the oral acetylcysteine formulation or administering each dose slowly (by nasogastric drip) is sometimes helpful. Administration of antiemetics may be necessary.

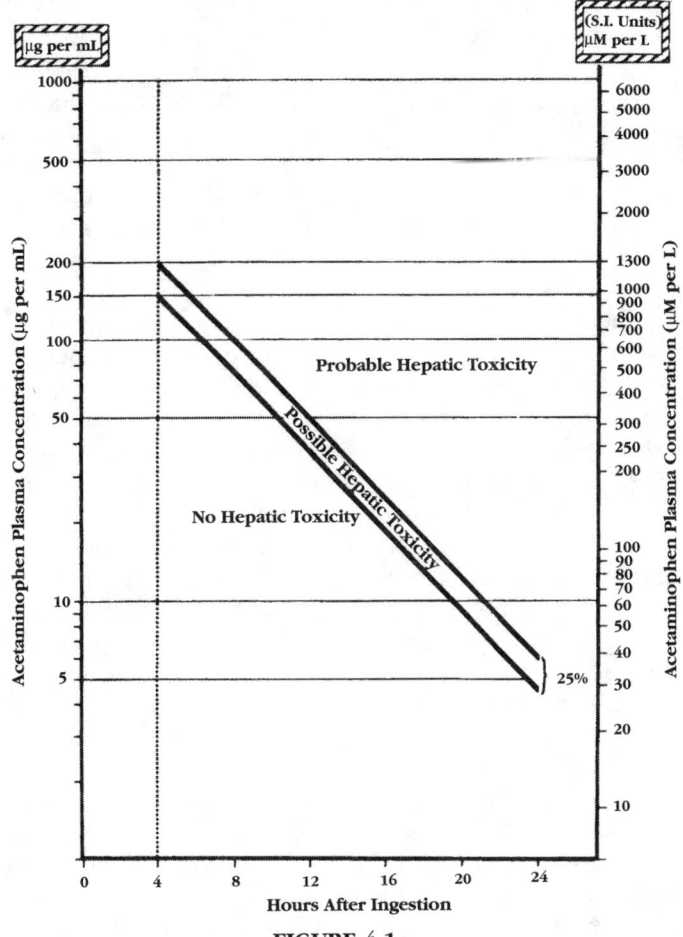

FIGURE 4-1

Rumack–Matthew Nomogram for Acetaminophen Poisoning

This graph should be used only in relation to a single acute ingestion. The time coordinates refer to time of ingestion. Serum levels drawn before 4 hours may not represent peak levels. The lower solid line 25% below the standard nomogram is included to allow for possible errors in acetaminophen plasma assays and estimated time from ingestion of an overdose. (Adapted from Rumack–Matthew Nomogram for Acetaminophen Poisoning, *Pediatrics*, 55(6), 1975. (Reprinted with permission.)

If the patient vomits within 1 hour of receiving the dose, it should be re-administered.

ADRs that are associated with the acetylcysteine intravenous formulation include hypersensitivity reactions (e.g., erythema, urticaria, bronchospasm) and, rarely, anaphylaxis and death. The fatalities are associated with the administration of excessive dosages of acetylcysteine (Penna & Buchanan, 1991). In a retrospective evaluation of 76 patients, including 35 children younger than 18 years, only four patients developed ADRs, none of which were life threatening (Yip et al., 1998).

The laboratory evaluation of a patient who had an acute acetaminophen overdose should include baseline liver function tests (aspartate aminotransferase, alanine aminotransferase, bilirubin serum levels, prothrombin time). These tests should be performed on admission (to establish a baseline) and repeated daily for patients who have severe toxicity. The creatinine serum concentration also should be monitored. Patients who develop hepatotoxicity should receive supportive medical care.

Nonsteroidal Anti-Inflammatory Drugs (NSAIDs) Other Than Aspirin and Other Salicylates

In 2000, poison control centers reported 81,036 nonsalicylate NSAID exposures. Of these poisoning exposures, 57,876 (71.4%) were exposures to ibuprofen (Litovitz et al., 2001). Children younger than 6 years accounted for 32,987 ibuprofen exposures while 12,459 occurred in children between 6 and 19 years old.

Nonsalicylate NSAIDs have complex mechanisms of action, but all appear to be related to the inhibition of cyclo-oxygenase, which results in the decreased production of prostaglandin precursors and thromboxanes from arachidonic acid. Inhibition of oxidative phosphorylation and inhibition of cyclo-oxygenase-1 appear to be related to many of the toxic effects including those affecting the GI tract (Hayllar & Bjarnason, 1995).

The ADRs associated with chronic administration of nonsalicylate NSAIDs should be distinguished from those observed with acute overdose or poisoning. Chronic administration of nonsalicylate NSAIDs is more common in adults but can occur in pediatric patients (e.g., in cases of juvenile rheumatoid arthritis). Up to 30% of patients who are receiving chronic nonsalicylate NSAID therapy will have gastric ulceration and/or bleeding (Roth, 1988).

The other major ADR associated with the chronic use of nonsalicylate NSAIDs is renal toxicity, including interstitial nephritis, tubular necrosis, papillary necrosis, and decreased renal blood flow. Experience with nonsalicylate NSAIDs during early pregnancy varies, depending on the drug, but all nonsalicylate NSAIDs should be avoided late in pregnancy because they may cause premature closure of the patent ductus arteriosus, neonatal pulmonary hypertension, inhibition of labor, and prolonged pregnancy.

Overdoses and poisonings associated with nonsalicylate NSAIDs are rarely life threatening for children or adults. For most nonsalicylate NSAIDs, serious toxicity is not seen until at least 5–10 times the therapeutic dose is ingested. For children, ibuprofen doses of 100 mg/kg or more are associated with toxicity. Lower doses may produce serious toxicity for mefenamic acid and phenylbutazone. **The following discussion of clinical effects and treatment is specific for ibuprofen, the most commonly ingested nonsalicylate NSAID.**

Most ibuprofen overdoses and poisonings produce GI effects, including nausea, vomiting, and epigastric pain, and mild CNS effects, predominantly lethargy. Although there were no pediatric fatalities associated with ibuprofen overdoses or poisonings reported to the American Association of Poison Control Centers (AAPCC) in 2000, a review of nonsalicylate NSAID overdoses suggests that most fatalities involve children (Halpern et al., 1993).

Overdoses and poisonings involving large amounts of ibuprofen produce ADRs affecting several body systems, including the GI, CNS, metabolic, cardiovascular, and renal. ADRs affecting the GI system include nausea, vomiting, epigastric pain, esophagitis, GI bleeding, ulcerations, perforations, and intestinal strictures. Metabolic acidosis is seen in some cases. ADRs affecting the cardiovascular system generally are uncommon but can include hypertension, hypotension, bradycardia, tachycardia, and atrial fibrillation. In regard to the CNS, lethargy is common in mild-to-moderate exposures. Other ADRs involving the CNS may be observed in more serious cases of overdose or poisoning and include delirium, dizziness, disorientation, tinnitus, headache, hallucinations, and coma. ADRs affecting the renal system include acute renal failure, which has been reported following NSAID ingestion and also has been reported in an ibuprofen overdose involving a child (Kim et al., 1995). In most cases it has been transient.

Determination of serum concentrations of ibuprofen or other nonsalicylate NSAIDs is of little value for the evaluation and management of overdoses and poisonings. There is a poor correlation between ibuprofen serum concentrations and clinical effects. Considering the poor predictive value of the ibuprofen nomogram and the absence of a specific antidote or specific treatment, serum concentrations should not be determined for the management of these overdoses and poisonings (Hall et al., 1992).

The mainstay of treatment for nonsalicylate NSAID overdoses and poisonings is GI decontamination and supportive medical care. There is a role for ipecac syrup at home for children who have ingested 100–200 mg/kg of ibuprofen recently and are asymptomatic. Ipecac syrup should not be administered after very large overdoses or poisonings because seizures, CNS depression, and apnea have been reported among children who have ingested 400 mg/kg or more of ibuprofen (Smolinske et al., 1990).

If a large amount of ibuprofen has been ingested, children should be referred to an acute care facility and be given activated charcoal. In the event of seizures, they should be treated with intravenous diazepam (0.2–0.5 mg/kg; repeat every 5 minutes as needed) or lorazepam (0.05–0.1 mg/kg). Children whose seizures are uncontrolled with either benzodiazepine may be given phenobarbital, phenytoin, or fosphenytoin. They should be monitored and also treated for hypotension, dysrhythmias, and respiratory depression. Methods to enhance the excretion of ibuprofen are generally not useful. Ibuprofen is greater than 99% protein bound. Most other nonsalicylate NSAIDs have protein binding of 90% or more. Although it has been suggested that cholestyramine will enhance the excretion of ibuprofen in severely overdosed or poisoned patients, there are no controlled studies, and only limited data, to support this treatment.

Iron

Unintentional ingestion of products containing iron is relatively common in children and was the most frequent cause of pediatric poisoning fatalities between 1883 and 1990 (Litovitz & Manoguerra, 1992). Many iron products look and taste like candy. Ingestion of iron and vitamins with iron accounted for 3648 and 26,560, respectively, potentially toxic exposures reported to the AAPCC Toxic Exposure Surveillance System in 2000 (Litovitz et al., 2001). Children younger than 6 years were involved in 61% of exposures to iron products and 83% of vitamin with iron exposures.

The clinical manifestations of iron poisoning can be divided into five phases. The **first phase** occurs 30 minutes–2 hours after the poisoning and is characterized by vomiting, hematemesis, diarrhea, and abdominal pain. These effects are caused by a direct effect of the iron on the GI mucosa to produce ulceration and necrosis. Shock may occur during this phase because of fluid, blood, and electrolyte losses. Other signs and symptoms of phase one include irritability, seizures, lethargy, and coma. Of 172 children who had acute iron poisoning, the most common presenting sign was vomiting (80%), followed by drowsiness or lethargy (52%), diarrhea (48%), and shock and coma (17%) (Westlin, 1966). Patients also may develop tachypnea, tachycardia, and hypotension. Leukocytosis and hyperglycemia have been reported for patients who had iron serum concentrations higher than 300 µg% (Lacouture et al., 1981). However, other studies have questioned the value of these parameters as screening tests for iron poisoning (Knasel & Collins-Barrow, 1986).

The **second phase** is a period of apparent recovery when phase one signs and symptoms decrease or resolve and an improvement in the patient's clinical condition occurs. However, approximately 2–12 hours after the first phase, some patients proceed to the **third phase,** which is characterized by marked shock and refractory metabolic acidosis. Shock is believed to be caused by vasodilation and increased capillary permeability as the result of increased concentrations of free iron, ferritin, and possibly serotonin and histamine. Venous return decreases, leading to a decrease in cardiac output, hypotension, and shock (Lacouture et al., 1981; Robotham & Lietman, 1980). Metabolic acidosis develops as a result of tissue hypoperfusion, inhibition of the Kreb's cycle by iron with accumulation of intermediate acids, and oxidation of iron-forming ferric hydroxides and the release of hydrogen ions.

The **fourth phase** occurs at 2–4 days after

the iron ingestion and is characterized by hepatic necrosis as a result of the disruption of liver cell mitochondrial function either by lipid peroxidation or shunting electrons away from the electron transport system (Robotham & Lietman, 1980). A very small number of patients proceed to the **fifth phase** and develop pyloric scarring and stenosis with obstruction at 2–4 weeks after the ingestion.

The first step in assessing the potential for toxicity after iron ingestion is to determine the milligram-per-kilogram dose of elemental iron ingested. The most common iron salts available are the fumarate, sulfate (hydrated), and gluconate salts, which contain 33%, 20%, and 12% elemental iron, respectively. The minimal toxic dose is 20–60 mg/kg of elemental iron (Stein et al., 1976). Although the usual lethal dose of iron is probably greater than 180 mg/kg, the minimal lethal dose reported for a 21-month-old child was 300–600 mg total (Greenblatt et al., 1976). The concentration of iron in the product may affect the degree of toxicity associated with an iron ingestion. Although fatalities have been reported with high concentration adult products (usually over 60 mg of elemental iron per tablet), low concentration children's iron products have not been reported to cause serious toxicity or deaths. According to the Maryland Poison Center triage guidelines, an iron ingestion of less than 20 mg/kg is managed with milk and observation only, 20–60 mg/kg without signs and symptoms is treated with ipecac syrup at home, while patients ingesting 60 mg/kg or more are sent to a medical care facility for assessment and treatment (Klein-Schwartz et al., 1990).

The management of iron poisoning includes supportive medical care, GI decontamination, and the administration of the antidote, deferoxamine. Supportive medical care usually involves intravenous therapy to correct hypotension, acidosis, and electrolyte disturbances. Laboratory evaluation should include iron serum concentration, complete blood counts, blood glucose, blood pH, liver function tests, and electrolyte serum concentrations. Stool and gastric contents should be tested for occult blood, which indicates GI injury.

Iron serum concentrations are obtained 2–4 hours after ingestion of immediate-release iron products and 4–6 hours after ingestion of sustained-release products. Iron serum concentrations that are obtained late after the ingestion do not always accurately reflect the seriousness of the exposure because free iron is rapidly cleared from the plasma. James (1970) reported the development of moderate-to-severe toxicity in 14 of 22 patients who had iron serum concentrations of 300–500 µg%, concluding that iron serum concentrations that are less than 500 µg% do not always signify mild poisoning if the sample is obtained late after the ingestion. In contrast, Westlin (1966) found shock or coma in nine of 112 children who had initial iron serum concentrations that were less than 500 µg%, compared with 17 of 46 children who had iron serum concentrations of 500 µg% or more.

Ipecac syrup is administered for the management of pediatric iron ingestions unless vomiting, hematemesis, abdominal pain, or bloody diarrhea is present. Lavage can be performed if a serious poisoning is suspected or, after ipecac-induced emesis, an incomplete emptying of the stomach is demonstrated by an abdominal roentgenogram. Sodium bicarbonate, diluted sodium phosphate/biphosphate, or deferoxamine lavage solutions were advocated in the past, but they are no longer recommended because of both a lack of demonstrated efficacy and potential toxicity (Bachrach et al., 1979; Czajka et al., 1981; Geffner & Opas, 1980; Whitten et al., 1966). Studies of adult volunteers suggest that magnesium hydroxide decreases iron absorption, but there is no experience regarding its use with children (Wallace et al., 1998). Activated charcoal does not bind iron well and, thus, is not recommended.

Iron is radiopaque, thus, as already noted, an abdominal roentgenogram can be obtained to evaluate the extent of iron removal after emesis is obtained with ipecac syrup or the stomach contents are emptied with gastric lavage. However, the usefulness of the roentgenogram is limited when the ingestion involves multiple-vitamin products because these products generally contain smaller amounts of elemental iron than other iron products. Thus, they produce briefer, less dense radio-opacity when compared to products that contain a higher concentration of iron (Ng et al., 1979). If the roentgenogram is positive, whole bowel irrigation should be performed. Whole bowel irrigation was performed in six patients ranging in age from 2 to 19 years; three patients who had been treated with ipecac and/or lavage had positive radiographic findings prior to whole bowel irrigation (Tenenbein et al., 1987b).

The clinical use of ipecac and lavage in cases of iron poisoning can sometimes fail because of the adherence of iron to GI mucosa. For example, an abdominal radiograph showed at least 16 whole iron tablets in the stomach following GI decontamination (i.e., emesis and lavage) of an 11-month-old infant (Everson et al., 1991). The radiograph was negative for tablets in the stomach within 4 hours after initiating whole bowel irrigation. A 33-month-old boy who ingested at least 160 mg/kg of elemental iron received whole bowel irrigation for 5 days because of persistence of iron in the GI tract (Kaczorowski & Wax, 1996). In rare cases, emergency gastrotomy may be required to remove iron embedded in the gastric mucosa (Peterson & Fifield, 1980).

Deferoxamine mesylate is indicated for all patients who have more than transient minor signs and symptoms, patients who have a positive abdominal radiograph demonstrating multiple radiopacities, patients who have an iron serum concentration greater than 500 µg%, or any symptomatic patient who has an iron serum concentration of 350 µg% or greater (Mills & Curry, 1994; Stein et al., 1976). Deferoxamine complexes with iron to form ferrioxamine, which is excreted renally, producing red-orange urine. Deferoxamine also may exert a protective effect at the cellular level (Robotham & Lietman, 1980). Deferoxamine does not remove iron from essential forms such as hemoglobin, myoglobin, or iron-containing enzymes in the body.

Deferoxamine mesylate is available as a sterile powder for reconstitution in 500-mg ampules. It is administered by intravenous infusion at 15 mg/kg/hr. Faster rates may cause hypotension, tachycardia, and flushing. ADRs associated with deferoxamine are uncommon. Four patients who received deferoxamine continuously for 30 hours or more developed adult respiratory distress syndrome (ARDS), but it is unclear if deferoxamine was responsible (Mills & Curry, 1994; Tenenbein et al., 1992).

In most cases of iron poisoning, clinical improvement occurs with 6–12 hours of deferoxamine therapy. However, therapy may need to be continued for 2–3 days for the treatment of severe iron poisonings. Urine color change should not be used as a monitoring parameter during deferoxamine therapy because urine color may not change in some patients, despite high iron serum concentrations. Deferoxamine therapy can be discontinued when signs and symptoms of systemic iron poisoning have resolved, iron serum concentrations are normal or low (less than 300 µg%), and previously positive abdominal radiographs are negative (Mills & Curry, 1994).

Antihistamines

Prescription and nonprescription antihistamines (H_1-receptor antagonists) are commonly found in most homes and are often inadvertently available to infants and children. Antihistamines primarily are used to treat allergies, motion sickness, and itching. They also are used to provide palliation for symptoms of the common cold. H_1-receptor antagonists were involved in 23,273 poison exposures in children younger than 6 years and 11,152 exposures in children and adolescents 6–19 years of age as reported to poison centers in 2000 (Litovitz et al., 2001). Diphenhydramine was the primary drug responsible for two pediatric deaths. One death was associated with the intentional misuse of diphenhydramine by the parent of a 2-month-old infant and the other was related to the suicide of an 18-year-old adolescent.

All antihistamines, except for those that are nonsedating, produce similar ADRs related to their CNS depressant and anticholinergic effects. The CNS depressant effects range from sedation to coma. The anticholinergic effects include dilated pupils, flushed dry skin, tachycardia, delirium, hallucinations, seizures, hyperthermia, decreased bowel motility, and urinary retention. A newborn was very sedated at birth as the result of diphenhydramine ingestion by the mother just before delivery (Miller, 2000).

For the treatment of antihistamine poisonings, GI decontamination with activated charcoal is recommended. Physostigmine is usually not needed but can be considered for antihistamine overdoses that produce significant anticholinergic effects. Physostigmine will reverse central and peripheral anticholinergic effects including delirium, hallucinations, seizures, coma, and tachycardia. Bradycardia and possibly seizures may occur if physostigmine is administered too rapidly. Physostigmine can produce cholinergic toxicity including bradycardia, diarrhea, increased secretions, and vomiting if too large a dose is administered.

The earlier nonsedating antihistamines were structurally related to the tricyclic antidepressants and overdoses produced life-threatening ventricular dysrhythmias. Terfenadine *(Seldane®)*, a nonsedating antihistamine, was voluntarily withdrawn from the U. S. market in 1998 because of its potential to produce the ventricular dysrhythmia torsades de pointes. Terfenadine's metabolism by the cytochrome P-450 isoenzyme CYP3A4 is inhibited by other drugs, such as ketoconazole and erythromycin and other macrolide antibiotics, resulting in the accumulation of terfenadine and toxicity. Cardiotoxicity with QT prolongation associated with torsades de pointes also has been reported with acute terfenadine overdoses. Similar cardiotoxic effects have been reported with astemizole among young children and adolescents (Clark & Love, 1991; Wiley et al, 1992). Astemizole was withdrawn from the U. S. market in 1998.

Fexofenadine *(Allegra®)*, the active metabolite of terfenadine, produces similar therapeutic effects but reportedly does not exhibit toxicity from this type of drug interaction. (*See* Chapter 6 for further discussion of these drug interactions.)

Newer nonsedating antihistamines, such as loratadine *(Claritin®)* and cetirizine *(Zyrtec®)*, are safer than astemizole and terfenadine because they do not cause clinically significant cytochrome P-450-related drug interactions or QT prolongation (Eick et al., 2001). Ingestion of large doses may result in sedation. Unless very large doses are ingested, children usually can be managed at home with observation.

Caustic Poisonings

The oral ingestion of caustic poisons produces injuries ranging from superficial to severe burns and necrosis of the oropharynx, esophagus, and stomach. The caustic poisons commonly found in the home include drain cleaners, oven cleaners, industrial and nonindustrial strength cleaners, toilet bowl cleaners, rust removers, and tile cleaners. Corrosive injury among children also can result from exposure to methacrylic acid in artificial nail primers (Woolf & Shaw, 1998).

Exposure to caustic poisons accounted for 5.1% of cases reported to the American Association of Poison Control Centers Data Collection System in 2000 (Litovitz et al., 2001). Of these cases, 49% involved children and adolescents younger than 20 years. There were 41,643 exposures to potentially caustic poisons among children younger than 6 years and 12,523 exposures among children and adolescents 6–19 years of age. Adolescents who ingest large volumes of a caustic poison in an attempt to commit suicide generally have more extensive injuries than do young children involved in accidental caustic poison exposures who generally swallow smaller volumes (Hawkins et al., 1980; Mansson, 1978). Mortality rates of 3.4% for alkaline corrosives and as high as 11.8%–18% for acids have been reported (Hawkins et al., 1980; Tucker et al., 1974).

Alkalis and acids produce injury by different mechanisms. **Alkalis produce injury by liquefaction necrosis that allows them to penetrate deeply into tissues by direct extension** (Muhlendahl et al., 1978). In an alkaline corrosive ingestion, the oropharynx and esophagus are the most common sites of injury, resulting in esophageal strictures. Corrosive gastric injury causing gastric outlet obstruction is another consequence of alkali ingestion (Ciftci et al., 1999). **Acids produce** coagulation necrosis that usually results in the destruction of the surface epithelium and submucosa (Haller et al., 1971; Tucker et al., 1974). The stomach is most frequently injured by acids, which may result in pyloric stenosis. The critical pH for alkaline corrosive injury is 12, while for acids it is 2. For alkalis, titratable alkaline reserve may more accurately predict esophageal injury than pH (Hoffman et al., 1989). Other important factors include the volume ingested, the contact time, stomach contents, and tonicity of the pyloric sphincter (Muhlendahl et al., 1978).

Solid alkaline corrosives adhere to mucous membranes, limiting the damage to the oropharynx and upper esophagus (Kirsh & Ritter, 1976). Liquids produce diffuse damage to the esophagus and stomach, resulting in circumferential or near circumferential burns that can progress to extensive stricture formation (Cello et al., 1980; Leape et al., 1971). The incidence of strictures with liquid alkaline corrosives is as high as 100% compared to 10%–25% for solids (Kirsh & Ritter, 1976; Leape et al., 1971). Esophageal burns can occur in the absence of oral injury, especially after the ingestion of a liquid alkaline corrosive (Kirsh & Ritter, 1976). However, one study found that the extent of the initial oropharyngeal injury predicted esophageal injury (Ferguson et al., 1989). Overall, esophageal injury occurs in 6%–20% of acid ingestions, while approximately 20% of patients who have esophageal injury following an alkali ingestion will also have gastric injury (Penner, 1980).

Ammonia and bleach products can produce mucosal edema and burns when ingested. However, the injury is generally superficial and stricture formation is extremely rare because these products rarely penetrate deeply enough to injure the submucosa or muscularis propria.

Children may swallow smaller amounts of acids because they are bitter tasting and cause immediate pain upon ingestion (Rothstein, 1986). Alkaline poisons are often tasteless and odorless and may result in children swallowing larger amounts before protective reflexes are involved (Rothstein, 1986). Fifteen of 22 pediatric patients who ingested lye (an alkali) developed significant strictures and 11 of these patients eventually required colon intraposition (Moazam et al., 1987).

Clinical manifestations of a corrosive ingestion include pain; dysphagia; profuse salivation and drooling; inflammatory edema of the lips, tongue, and palate; and hematemesis (Cello et al., 1980; Tewfik & Schloss, 1980). Fever, tachypnea, tachycardia, and hypotension secondary to the extensive mucosal damage may occur. Involvement of the epiglottis and vocal cords is evidenced by dyspnea, hoarseness, or stridor. Substernal, back, or abdominal pain are indicative of mediastinal or peritoneal extension. Aspiration pneumonia, laryngeal obstruction, shock, mediastinitis, esophageal perforation, gastric perforation, and peritonitis are initial complications of the ingestion of a corrosive poison. The late complications, primarily esophageal strictures, are usually evident within 2 months after the ingestion.

There is considerable controversy regarding the relationship between the signs and symptoms of a caustic ingestion and the degree of esophageal injury. A study of 378 children who ingested a caustic poison found that 55 (18%) of 298 symptomatic patients had grade two lesions and five (2%) developed strictures; of 80 asymptomatic patients, 10 (12%) had grade two lesions and one (1%) developed a stricture (Gaudreault et al., 1983). On the basis of these findings, the researchers concluded that signs and symptoms do not predict the presence or severity of an esophageal lesion following a caustic poison ingestion.

In contrast, Crain et al. (1984) found that signs and symptoms predicted esophageal injury at endoscopy after finding serious esophageal injury in seven of 14 patients who had two or more serious signs and symptoms (vomiting, drooling, stridor) and no injury in 65 patients with none or only one of these findings. In a multicenter study of 336 alkaline corrosive ingestions, no single or group of initially reported signs and symptoms identified all patients who had second- or third-degree esophageal burns (Gorman et al., 1992). The investigators recommended that endoscopy not be used for asymptomatic patients because all patients with serious burns were symptomatic.

The **treatment of ingestions** involving caustic poisons includes immediate treatment and treatment of resultant injuries and related complications. These aspects of treatment are now discussed.

Immediate treatment. Immediate treatment following the ingestion of a caustic poison involves the dilution of the ingested poison with 4–8 ounces of milk or water to decrease contact time. There is controversy over the role that dilution has in the management of ingestions involving strong caustic poisons. Opponents of the practice argue that dilution is ineffective because the damage is instantaneous, heat of dilution will increase injury, and the administration of oral liquids will increase the chance of spontaneous vomiting. Although injury may be immediate for concentrated caustics, the exact pH (and thus the likelihood that intervention will be effective) is rarely known at the time of exposure. The administration of oral liquids will wash off a solid caustic that is adhering to mucous membranes. Because dilution is only effective within a relatively short time after exposure, it should be performed immediately before taking the patient to an emergency department. Damage is complete by the time the patient arrives in the emergency department, so dilution is not indicated in this setting.

Emesis, lavage, charcoal, cathartics, and neutralization are contraindicated in a caustic poison exposure. Vomiting exposes the esophagus and oropharynx to the caustic poison for a second time, resulting in additional injury as well as increasing the risk of perforation and aspiration. Although cautious gastric lavage with a soft rubber tube has been performed successfully, this procedure generally should be avoided because of the risk for esophageal and gastric perforation as well as the worsening of respiratory distress among patients who have laryngeal edema. Activated charcoal poorly adsorbs caustic poisons and can promote granulation formation if it becomes embedded in ulcerated areas. Neutralization is contraindicated because the reaction is exothermic and will increase the degree of damage.

Esophagoscopy and treatment of esophageal injury. Esophagoscopy is performed within the first 24–48 hours after the ingestion of a caustic poison to evaluate the extent of injury and to identify patients who require further treatment for their injuries. Because the absence of oral burns does not rule out esophageal or gastric injury, esophagoscopy will identify patients who require close observation and further treatment (Gaudreault et al., 1983).

The extent of esophageal injury is classified as a first-, second-, or third-degree burn. Some controversy exists over which patients require esophagoscopy. While some investigators recommend that an esophagoscopy be performed for all patients who have a history of a corrosive ingestion, others recommend that it be performed for symptomatic patients only (Crain et al., 1984; Gaudreault et al., 1983; Gorman et al., 1992; Knopp, 1979; Muhlendahl et al., 1978).

Corticosteroid therapy. Corticosteroids have been recommended to decrease inflammation and prevent stricture formation among patients who have esophageal burns after ingestion of caustic poisons. However, their efficacy in regard to the treatment of esophageal burns is unclear. The role of corticosteroids is poorly defined because of conflicting reports, uncontrolled studies, inconsistency in esophageal burn classification schemes, lack of consistency in patient selection criteria for esophagoscopy, lack of identification of the nature of the caustic poison (i.e., acid or alkali), and inconsistent corticosteroid dosage regimens.

A controlled study of 60 patients treated for ingestion of caustic poisons at a single pediatric hospital over an 18-year period demonstrated a lack of corticosteroid efficacy (Anderson et al., 1990). None of the 19 patients with first-degree burns, in either the steroid or control group, developed strictures or required esophageal replacement. For patients with third-degree burns, 90% of the steroid group developed strictures, and one-third of those patients required esophageal replacement. All of the children in the control group developed strictures, and 64% of them required esophageal replacement. One of 14 patients receiving corticosteroids with second-degree burns developed strictures and required esophageal replacement, but no strictures were observed in the control group. Overall there were no statistically significant differences in stricture development between the two groups. However, statistical power, which was not addressed by the investigators, is an important concern because of the small number of patients studied.

In a retrospective study of 41 patients with a caustic ingestion who received either no treatment or treatment with antibiotics and corticosteroids, the incidence of esophageal strictures in the treatment group (seven of 31 patients) was comparable to that in the group that did not receive treatment (two of 10 patients) (Ferguson et al., 1989). However, data comparing the initial depth of injury in the two groups are not provided and the size of individual subgroups is small.

In contrast, corticosteroids reportedly decreased esophageal strictures in a meta-analysis of 361 patients from 13 published studies with esophageal injury following ingestion of caustic poisons. Strictures developed in 54 of 228 (24%) patients with either second- or third-degree burns treated with corticosteroids and antibiotics compared with 13 of 25 (52%) patients with second- or third-degree burns without treatment (Howell et al., 1992). These differences were statistically significant.

Corticosteroids are not indicated in first-degree burns because these burns generally heal without strictures. Corticosteroids are probably ineffective in third-degree burns because the injury is so severe. In addition, their use may be dangerous because they impair wound healing and inhibit scar formation, making the esophagus more vulnerable to perforation. Corticosteroids also mask the signs and symptoms of infection while making the person more susceptible to infection. However, some clinicians still recommend that corticosteroid therapy may be considered for children who have second-degree burns, but it must be initiated early (Hawkins et al., 1980; Rothstein, 1986). Children usually receive 2 mg/kg/day of prednisone orally for 3 weeks, followed by gradual tapering of the dosage over several weeks.

Antibiotics. Antibiotics are indicated for patients who have evidence of infection or prophylactically for patients who are treated with corticosteroids. Supportive medical care, including airway and respiratory support, intravenous therapy, and pain management, may be required.

Esophagrams. Esophagrams taken shortly after exposure to a caustic poison are considered unreliable because they may appear normal despite injury (Mansson, 1978; Stannard, 1978; Sugawa et al., 1981). Esophagrams are of value later and are generally performed several weeks after the ingestion to identify and evaluate strictures.

Esophageal dilations and surgery. If strictures occur, esophageal dilations should be performed in an attempt to achieve an adequately functioning esophagus (Campbell et al., 1977; Ferguson et al., 1989; Stiff et al., 1996). Dilations may be effective after only one or two procedures or may be needed for months or years. In general, deep, circumferential, multiple, and long strictures are resistant to dilations, while short smooth strictures are more likely to respond to dilations. If dilations are ineffective, surgical replacement of the esophagus with segments of the stomach, jejunum, or colon may be attempted. Surgical management of alkali or acid injury to the stomach can include gastrectomy, gastrostomy, and pyloroplasty (Ciftci et al., 1999; Stiff et al., 1996).

Complications. A potential long-term complication of esophageal burns is squamous cell carcinoma of the esophagus that is 1000 times more likely to occur in people who sustained an esophageal burn between 40 and 56 years earlier than for other people in the same age group (Applequist & Salno, 1980).

The morbidity associated with a corrosive ingestion depends largely on the extent of the initial injury and is often significant. Extended hospitalizations and multiple procedures including esophagoscopies, esophagrams, dilations, and surgery are often necessary. Thus, the prevention of caustic poison exposures in children through the use of safety closures and keeping caustic poisons out of the reach of children is extremely important.

Hydrocarbons

Many household products, including furniture polishes, waxes, spot removers, and lighter fluids, contain hydrocarbons and are pleasantly scented, making them attractive to children. Hydrocarbons accounted for 2.8% of exposures for all age groups reported to the American Association of Poison Control Centers Toxic Exposure Surveillance System in 2000 (Litovitz et al., 2001). Children and adolescents accounted for 53% of these exposures. There were 23,418 exposures among children younger than 6 years and 8389 among children and adolescents 6–19 years of age. The abuse of hydrocarbons by inhalation was responsible for five deaths involving adolescents. Hydrocarbon aspiration caused the death of a 12-month-old toddler. Clinical or radiographic evidence of pneumonitis was reported in 12% of 950 patients following hydrocarbon ingestion, with progressive pulmonary toxicity in less than 1% (Anas et al., 1981). Overall mortality rates of 0.2% and 0.5% as well as mortality rates as high as 1.3% and 1.5% have been reported in patients who were initially symptomatic (Anas et al., 1981; Machado et al., 1988).

There are several types of hydrocarbons, including aliphatics, such as kerosene, gasoline, and mineral seal oil; aromatics, such as toluene, xylene, and benzene; and halogenated hydrocarbons, such as fluorinated and chlorinated hydrocarbon insecticides. Turpentine and pine oil also are hydrocarbons. The following discussion will concentrate on the manifestations and treatment of aliphatic hydrocarbon ingestions, including turpentine and pine oil.

The primary toxicity associated with aliphatic hydrocarbon ingestions is aspiration pneumonia. Aspiration risk is greatest for hydrocarbons that have low viscosities, such as gasoline, kerosene, mineral seal oil, naphtha, stoddard solvent, and turpentine. Hydrocarbons that have high viscosities, such as motor oil, are considered relatively free from aspiration hazard. Hydrocarbons with low surface tension will spread rapidly over the lung surface. Hydrocarbons with high volatility increase injury by replacing alveolar air with vaporized hydrocarbon.

The risk for aspiration following hydrocarbon ingestion was characterized in a retrospective review of 950 children brought to an outpatient clinic or emergency department (Anas et al., 1981). Of 950 children, 800 were asymptomatic with a normal chest roentgenogram and were discharged after a 6–8-hour observation period. Of the 150 children who were admitted to the hospital, 136 (91%) had uncomplicated hospitalizations. Although progressive respiratory signs and symptoms developed in 14 patients, respiratory signs and symptoms resolved in seven patients within 24 hours. Only seven patients experienced additional pulmonary complications and two of these patients died. These data indicate that the majority of children do not require hospitalization and that hospitalization is necessary only for children who are symptomatic within 6–8 hours following hydrocarbon ingestion.

When hydrocarbons are aspirated, they produce bronchospasm that contributes to ventilation-perfusion abnormalities and hypoxia (Eade et al., 1974). Hydrocarbons produce direct destruction of the airways and pulmonary capillaries. On autopsy, the following have been described: hyperemia; interstitial inflammation; necrosis of bronchial, bronchiolar, and alveolar tissues; hemorrhagic pulmonary edema; vascular thromboses; and necrotizing bronchopneumonia. Hydrocarbons may alter surface tension in the lungs, resulting in atelectasis and early distal airway closure.

The clinical manifestations of hydrocarbon aspiration include gagging, choking, and coughing (Eade et al., 1974). A hydrocarbon odor on the child's breath is usually noted. Patients develop dyspnea, a persistent cough, and grunting respirations. On physical examination, increases in respiratory rate and heart rate, intercostal retractions, diminished breath sounds, dullness of percussion, rales, and rhonchi are noted. Signs and symptoms of respiratory involvement usually progress during the first 24 hours and begin to subside between days 2 and 5. Patients who have mild pulmonary manifestations often recover in 24–48 hours.

Chest roentgenogram abnormalities may be present within 30 minutes after ingestion of hydrocarbons, but they often take longer to develop. By 12 hours, almost all patients with lung involvement have roentgenogram findings consistent with chemical pneumonia. Findings range from fine perihilar densities, which may extend into the mid-lung fields, to basal infiltrates. Basal pneumonitis and atelectasis can occur. Lobar consolidation, pleural effusions, pneumothoraces, and pneumatoceles have all been encountered but are less common. Clinical signs and symptoms and roentgenographic findings do not always correlate. Anas et al. (1981) found that 36 of 71 asymptomatic patients had abnormal initial chest roentgenograms and only two patients developed signs and symptoms and progression of the roentgenogram abnormalities. In contrast, 76 of 79 symptomatic patients had abnormal chest roentgenograms by 6 hours after the hydrocarbon ingestion.

In addition to the pulmonary findings, patients may experience GI symptomatology, including vomiting and diarrhea, as a result of the local irritation. Irritability, drowsiness, lethargy, coma, and seizures have been described in moderate-to-severe cases and are most likely the result of hypoxia, not a direct effect of the hydrocarbon on the CNS. Fever and leukocytosis have been reported among patients who have radiographic evidence of pneumonia (Anas et al., 1981; Beamon et al., 1976). These effects are caused by extensive tissue necrosis and inflammation, not infection.

Bacterial pneumonia is rare after hydrocarbon aspiration. Children who have severe aspiration pneumonia may develop complications of intravascular hemolysis and disseminated intravascular coagulation (Algren & Rogers, 1992; Banner & Walson, 1983). Severe, reversible left ventricular dysfunction requiring inotropic support developed in a 19-month-old toddler after the ingestion of a paint thinner (Anene & Castello, 1994). Rarely, ingestion of massive amounts of hydrocarbons may overwhelm the capacity of the liver to remove the hydrocarbons that have been absorbed, resulting in systemic toxicity, including renal failure (Janssen et al., 1988).

Treatment depends on the type of hydrocarbon ingested and the initial signs and symptoms of hydrocarbon poisoning. The majority of patients who ingest aliphatic hydrocarbons are asymptomatic initially and can be observed safely at home for cough, dyspnea, and fever (Anas et al., 1981; Arena, 1987). If initial signs and symptoms include coughing, choking, or dyspnea, pediatric patients should be referred to a medical facility for evaluation. If patients are asymptomatic on arrival at the medical facility and the chest roentgenogram is negative, they may be discharged home after an observation period of 6 hours. Regardless of the results of the chest roentgenogram, symptomatic patients should be admitted to the medical facility or hospital for observation. The more difficult triage decision involves the asymptomatic patient who has a positive roentgenogram. The conservative approach would be to admit the patient overnight for observation, although observation in the emergency department for 6 hours is probably sufficient.

Treatment of hydrocarbon pneumonitis consists of supportive medical care. Interventions are directed primarily to the respiratory system and include maintaining adequate ventilation and oxygenation with the administration of oxygen, mechanical ventilation, and positive and expiratory pressure (PEEP), as needed, according to the patient's response (Zucker et al., 1986).

If conventional therapy is inadequate, alternative options for severe pneumonitis include extracorporeal membrane oxygenation (ECMO) or high-frequency jet ventilation (Bysani et al., 1994). ECMO was used successfully for two infants who had hydrocarbon aspiration (mineral oil, mineral seal oil) unresponsive to conventional therapy (Scalzo et al., 1990). Antipyretics may be required for fever and anticonvulsants may be indicated for seizures not controlled by correcting hypoxia. Corticosteroids should not be administered because their efficacy for the treatment of hydrocarbon pneumonitis is lacking (Brown et al., 1974; Marks et al., 1972; Steele et al., 1972).

GI emptying is not recommended when aliphatic hydrocarbons are ingested alone, regardless of the amount ingested. If a toxic amount of an aromatic or halogenated hydrocarbon or dangerous additive in an aliphatic hydrocarbon base is ingested, activated charcoal should be administered.

The overall prognosis in regard to hydrocarbon pneumonitis is favorable with aggressive respiratory support. A follow-up study conducted 8–14 years after hydrocarbon exposure revealed residual pulmonary function abnormalities consistent with small airway obstruction and loss of elastic recoil in 14 of 17 children despite the fact that the signs and symptoms of respiratory abnormalities completely resolved after the initial exposure (Gurwitz et al., 1978). Two effects may occur among children who develop hydrocarbon pneumonitis: residual fibrosis in the airways may cause airway obstruction; and changes in alveolar mechanics may result from damage during a period of rapid parenchymal development.

The implications of these manifestations with respect to exposure to other risk factors for chronic obstructive lung disease during adolescence, such as tobacco smoking and air pollution, need to be explored.

Skin exposure to hydrocarbons also occurs in children. Hydrocarbons can cause contact erythema as a result of a defatting action. If the skin is irrigated immediately, serious cutaneous injury or systemic effects are unlikely. However, prolonged skin contact with large volumes of concentrated hydrocarbon solutions can cause severe contact injuries as well as systemic toxicity (Harnsbrough et al., 1985).

Intentional inhalation of hydrocarbons is a growing type of substance abuse among preadolescents and adolescents in the United States and other countries (Adgey et al., 1995; Henretig, 1996; Kurtzman et al., 2001) (see also Chapter 7 for further discussion). Although hydrocarbons are inhaled by adolescents of all socioeconomic groups, the "typical" hydrocarbon user is an adolescent male of lower socioeconomic status with poor school performance and family dysfunction. Volatile hydrocarbons are popular because they are readily available, inexpensive, and legal. They vaporize at room temperature and are deliberately inhaled by sniffing (inhaling directly from the product container), huffing (soaking a cloth with the volatile hydrocarbon and holding it over the nose and/or mouth), or bagging (placing the volatile hydrocarbon in a bag which is held over the mouth and nose). The "high" occurs rapidly and the duration of effect is short. Examples of hydrocarbons that are abused include aliphatic hydrocarbons such as butane, naphtha, gasoline, kerosene, and mineral spirits; halogenated hydrocarbons such as methylene chloride, trichloroethane, trichloroethylene, and fluorinated hydrocarbons (Freon®); and aromatic hydrocarbons such as xylene and toluene.

CNS effects associated with hydrocarbon abuse include ataxia, coma, euphoria, hallucinations, hyperactivity, and seizures. Sudden death with volatile substance abuse is usually the result of cardiovascular toxicity. Although anoxia, respiratory depression, and vagal stimulation play a role, cardiac dysrhythmias due to sensitization of the heart to endogenous catecholamines are the most common cause of death (Shepherd, 1989). Pulmonary irritation may cause coughing, sneezing, and a chemical pneumonitis. Other toxic manifestations that occur with chronic abuse include centrilobular necrosis of the liver (trichloroethylene and toluene), renal tubular acidosis (toluene), bone marrow depression (benzene), and organic lead encephalopathy (gasoline). Treatment includes respiratory support and oxygen administration, cardiovascular monitoring, correction of acidosis and hypokalemia, and administration of antidysrhythmics. Administration of sympathomimetic drugs should be avoided because they increase the risk for cardiac dysrhythmias.

Toxic Alcohol and Glycol Poisonings

Isopropyl alcohol, ethylene glycol, and methanol are the three most toxic alcohols and glycols commonly ingested by both children and adolescents. Isopropyl alcohol is used as a solvent, an antiseptic, and a disinfectant. Methanol is used as a solvent and is found in windshield washing solutions, dry gases, duplicating fluids, and paint removers. Ethylene glycol is the major component of engine antifreeze. In 2000, poison control centers reported 7001 isopropyl alcohol, 393 methanol, and 1622 ethylene glycol exposures among children and adolescents. These exposures included a methanol death involving a 3-month-old infant and an ethylene glycol with boric acid death involving a 13-year-old adolescent (Litovitz et al., 2001).

Isopropyl alcohol. Isopropyl alcohol (isopropanol) is a CNS depressant that produces effects similar to ethanol when acutely ingested. It is rapidly absorbed orally and can also be absorbed through the skin and by inhalation. Significant clinical toxicity has been seen among children when topically applied to the skin to treat fever or when accidentally placed in a humidifier (Arditi & Killner, 1987; Vicas & Beck, 1993). Isopropyl alcohol is metabolized to acetone, which appears in the urine within 30 minutes of ingestion (Lacouture et al., 1989).

Isopropyl alcohol is approximately twice as toxic as ethanol on a milliliter-per-kilogram (ml/kg) basis. An isopropyl alcohol blood concentration of a specific value produces approximately twice the effect of the same blood concentration of ethanol. Isopropyl alcohol blood concentrations are generally available and helpful for evaluating patients who have isopropyl alcohol poisoning. Acetone serum and urine concentrations help to determine whether an isopropyl alcohol ingestion has occurred.

The predominant clinical effects of isopropyl alcohol on the CNS range from sedation to coma. Respiratory depression also can occur. Isopropyl alcohol is more irritating to the GI tract than ethanol. Thus, vomiting and gastritis, including hemorrhagic gastritis, may occur. Although mild hyperglycemia also may occur, children are more likely to be normoglycemic or hypoglycemic. Other effects that may be seen include tachycardia, hypotension, and seizures.

GI decontamination is generally not recommended more than 1 hour following the ingestion of isopropyl alcohol because its absorption from the GI tract is rapid. Although gastric lavage can be performed, the use of ipecac syrup and activated charcoal is not recommended because the onset of CNS depression may be rapid and activated charcoal does not adsorb alcohols. Thus, the mainstay of treatment is symptomatic and supportive medical care, which should include monitoring for and treating hypotension, respiratory depression, and hypoglycemia. Although rarely needed, hemodialysis will remove isopropyl alcohol and should be considered for patients who have high isopropyl alcohol blood concentrations that are unresponsive to traditional therapy.

Methanol. Methanol is an extremely toxic alcohol that produces a severe metabolic acidosis and blindness. Methanol is metabolized to formaldehyde by alcohol dehydrogenase and then by aldehyde dehydrogenase to formic acid. The severe toxicity is produced by the metabolites, formaldehyde and formic acid. The metabolic acidosis is primarily related to formic and lactic acids and the blindness from formaldehyde. The major toxic effects are often delayed by 12–24 hours because they are produced by the metabolites. Both methanol and ethanol are metabolized by alcohol dehydrogenase, although the enzyme has a much higher affinity for ethanol than methanol. This affinity is the basis for using ethanol as an antidote for methanol poisoning. The ethanol provides a substrate other than methanol for alcohol dehydrogenase and, consequently, reduces the production of the toxic metabolites.

Initial clinical effects caused by methanol poisoning include ataxia, confusion, and sedation, which may progress to coma, and a severe anion gap metabolic acidosis. Methanol is irritating to the GI tract, resulting in abdominal pain, nausea, and vomiting. Patients who have severe poisoning develop ADRs that affect vision, including blurred or double vision, decreased visual acuity, whiteness in the visual field, and blindness. Although improvement in vision occurs among some patients, often there are permanent visual sequelae. Tachypnea may occur as a result of the metabolic acidosis. In severe cases, patients also may develop bradycardia, hypotension, respiratory failure, or cardiac failure.

Methanol blood concentrations are important for evaluating patients and determining treatment. Significant toxicity can be seen with methanol blood concentrations in excess of 20 mg/dl. Methanol has a significant osmolal effect. A methanol concentration of 50 mg/dl will raise the serum osmolality by 17 mOsm/liter. In the absence of a methanol blood concentration, an increase in the serum osmolality of 5–10 mOsm/liter or more and the presence of acidosis suggests methanol poisoning. A normal or near normal serum osmolality should not rule out the possibility of methanol poisoning because relatively low methanol blood concentrations are toxic.

Important components of methanol treatment include symptomatic and supportive medical care, GI decontamination in some cases, administration of an antidote to block the production of the toxic metabolites, and hemodialysis to remove methanol. Supportive medical care should include cardiovascular and respiratory support along with the correction of the metabolic acidosis. Metabolic acidosis should be treated with intravenous sodium bicarbonate.

Syrup of ipecac is not recommended for methanol exposures because methanol can produce a rapid loss of consciousness and aspiration may occur. Gastric lavage should be considered within 1 hour of the ingestion. It is important to protect the airway from aspiration by positioning or endotracheal intubation. Methanol is not well adsorbed by activated charcoal.

Both ethanol and fomepizole prevent the metabolism of methanol. One of these antidotes should be administered to patients who have a methanol blood concentration of 20 mg/dl or higher. In the absence of a methanol blood concentration, either ethanol or fomepizole should be considered for patients who have a history of methanol ingestion and metabolic acidosis.

Fomepizole (4-methylpyrazole, 4-MP), an alcohol dehydrogenase inhibitor, prevents methanol and ethylene glycol toxicity by inhibiting the formation of toxic metabolites (Brent et al., 1999; Brent et al., 2001). In the United States, fomepizole is approved for ethylene glycol and methanol poisonings and is sold under the trade name *Antizol®*. A loading dose of 15 mg/kg (up to 1 gram) should be administered, followed by doses of 10 mg/kg every 12 hours for four doses, then 15 mg/kg every 12 hours thereafter until ethylene glycol blood concentrations are below 20 mg/dl. All doses of fomepizole should be administered as a slow intravenous infusion, in at least 100 ml of normal saline or 5% dextrose, over 30 minutes. During hemodialysis, the dosing interval is shortened to every 4 hours. Fomepizole has not been approved for children, but it has been successfully used to manage methanol poisoning among pediatric patients (Fisher & Diaz, 1998).

Alternatively, ethanol can be administered to block methanol metabolism. A loading dose of 7.5–10 ml/kg of 10% ethanol in a 5% dextrose solution is intravenously infused over 30 minutes. The loading dose is followed by a maintenance dose of 1–2 ml/kg/hr of 10% ethanol in D_5W by continuous intravenous infusion. The maintenance dose is increased to 2–3.5 ml/kg/hr if the patient is being dialyzed. Ethanol serum concentrations need to be monitored and the maintenance dose needs to be adjusted to maintain the ethanol blood concentration between 100 and 130 mg/dl. Glucose blood concentrations should be monitored because ethanol can cause hypoglycemia, especially in children.

The advantages of ethanol therapy are its ready availability and low cost. The disadvantages of ethanol therapy include difficulty maintaining desired ethanol blood concentrations and its associated ADRs, including CNS depression and hypoglycemia. The advantages of fomepizole therapy include its easy dosing schedule. The disadvantages include the lack of its availability at some hospitals and its high cost.

Adjunctive therapy includes the administration of leucovorin calcium and folic acid. Folic acid catalyzes the oxidation of formic acid to nontoxic products. Adjunctive management of methanol poisoning begins with leucovorin because it does not require conversion and is metabolically active. The leucovorin therapy is then replaced with the less expensive folic acid therapy. One dose of leucovorin is intravenously infused at 1 mg/kg (up to 50 mg). The leucovorin is followed by folic acid, which is intravenously infused at 1 mg/kg (up to 50 mg/dose) every 4 hours for a total of six doses.

Hemodialysis is an important component of treatment for a seriously ill methanol poisoned patient. It should be considered in any patient with a methanol blood concentration of 50 mg/dl or higher. It should also be considered in patients with lower methanol concentrations, or if a methanol concentration is not available, when severe metabolic acidosis is present. Hemodialysis is frequently used in combination with ethanol or fomepizole treatment. Hemodialysis effectively removes methanol before it is converted to toxic metabolites.

Ethylene Glycol. Ethylene glycol is a sweet tasting liquid most commonly found in automobile antifreeze. It is well-absorbed orally, but is not absorbed through the skin or by the lungs. Ethylene glycol produces a degree of CNS depression that is similar to ethanol. Like methanol, the major toxicity associated with ethylene glycol is the result of its metabolism to more toxic metabolites. Ethylene glycol is primarily first metabolized to glycoaldehyde by alcohol dehydrogenase, then to glycolate, and then to glyoxylate. Glyoxylate is considered to be the most toxic metabolite. Further metabolism to oxalate occurs dependent on the co-factors thiamine and pyridoxine and requires the conversion of NAD to NADH. Diethylene glycol and ethylene glycol ether poisonings may produce similar toxicity.

Three phases have been described for ethylene glycol poisoning. **Phase one** early signs and symptoms occur during the first 12 hours of ethylene glycol poisoning and include ataxia, CNS depression, nausea, the onset of an anion gap metabolic acidosis, slurred speech, and vomiting. Further CNS depression and coma may occur. **Phase two** occurs 12–24 hours after the poisoning and includes cardiopulmonary effects (i.e., cardiogenic pulmonary edema, circulatory collapse, congestive heart failure, tachycardia, tachypnea). Renal toxicity is seen during **phase three** and is characterized by flank pain, acute tubular necrosis, and renal failure. The renal effects are thought to be related to oxalate formation with contributions from glycoaldehyde, glycolic acid, and glyoxylic acid.

The management of ethylene glycol poisoning requires general laboratory monitoring, which should include obtaining serum electrolytes, BUN, serum creatinine, a urinalysis, arterial blood gases, and an ethylene glycol blood concentration. Urine should be evaluated microscopically for oxalate crystals. However, some patients can ingest significant amounts of ethylene glycol without displaying visible oxalate crystals in the urine.

Ipecac syrup is not recommended because CNS depression and aspiration can occur. Gastric lavage may be considered if the ingestion occurred within 1 hour. Activated charcoal does not adsorb ethylene glycol. As with methanol, ethanol or fomepizole will prevent metabolism of ethylene glycol and the production of toxic metabolites. Therapy with either ethanol or fomepizole is indicated for patients who have ethylene glycol blood concentrations of 20 mg/dl or greater. If ethylene glycol blood concentrations are not available, therapy should be initiated upon a history of ethylene glycol exposure and either the presence of oxalate crystals in the urine or an anion gap metabolic acidosis. Fomepizole is approved by the FDA for the treatment of ethylene glycol poisoning for adults; it has been used successfully for pediatric patients who have ethylene glycol poisoning (Harry et al., 1998; Baum et al., 2000; Benitz et al., 2000; Boyer et al., 2001).

Dosing for ethanol and fomepizole is the same as previously discussed for methanol poisoning. Hemodialysis should be considered for patients who have an ethylene glycol blood concentration of 50 mg/dl or greater, a severe metabolic acidosis, or renal failure. Table 4-5 summarizes clinical data concerning the pharmacokinetics, clinical toxicity, and therapy for poisoning involving isopropyl alcohol, methanol, and ethylene glycol.

TABLE 4-5
Isopropyl Alcohol, Ethylene Glycol, and Methanol

	ISOPROPYL ALCOHOL	ETHYLENE GLYCOL	METHANOL
Pharmacokinetics			
Absorption	80%–90% absorbed within 30 min		
Distribution	Distributed in body water: V_d 0.5–0.6 liter/kg		
Renal elimination	20%–50%	20%	2%–5%
Plasma half-life	2–3 hr	3–5 hr	14–20 hr
Plasma half-life with ethanol therapy		17 hr	24–30 hr
Clinical Changes			
Anion gap	Normal	Increased	Increased
Hypocalcemia	No	Yes	No
Oxalate crystals in the urine	No	Yes	No
Renal failure	No	Yes	No
Blindness	No	No	Yes
Therapy			
Ethanol	No	Yes	Yes
Folate	No	No	Yes
Fomepizole	No	Yes	Yes
Leucovorin calcium	No	No	Yes
Thiamine	No	Yes	No
Pyridoxine	No	Yes	No
Hemodialysis	Yes[a]	Yes	Yes

[a] Dialyzable, but most isopropyl alcohol poisonings can be managed without hemodialysis.

Summary

Poisoning is a common pediatric problem. Evaluation of the infant, child, or adolescent who has been exposed to a potentially toxic substance necessitates a thorough history and assessment of symptoms. Treatment may include supportive care, prevention of absorption, enhancement of elimination, and administration of antidotes. Since salicylates, acetaminophen, nonsteroidal anti-inflammatory drugs, iron, antihistamines, caustics, hydrocarbons, and alcohols are frequently involved in childhood poisonings, pediatric healthcare providers should be familiar with the clinical manifestations, inherent toxicity, and treatment of poisonings with these substances. The regional poison control center is a resource that should be consulted to help manage pediatric poisoning.

References

Adgey, A. A. J., Johnston, P. W., & McMechan, S. (1995). Sudden cardiac death and substance abuse. *Resuscitation, 29,* 219–221.

Adler, A. G., Walinsky, P., Krall, R. A., et al. (1980). Death resulting from ipecac syrup. *Journal of the American Medical Association, 243,* 1927–1928.

Albertson, T. E., Derlet, R. W., Foulke, G. E., et al. (1989). Superiority of activated charcoal alone compared with ipecac and activated charcoal in the treatment of acute ingestions. *Annals of Emergency Medicine, 18,* 56–59.

Algren, J. T., & Rodgers, G. C., Jr. (1992). Intravascular hemolysis associated with hydrocarbon poisoning. *Pediatric Emergency Care, 8,* 34–35.

American Academy of Clinical Toxicology; European Association of Poisons Centres and Clinical Toxicologists. (1997). Position statement: Cathartics. *Journal of Toxicology. Clinical Toxicology, 35,* 743–752.

American Academy of Clinical Toxicology; European Association of Poisons Centres and Clinical Toxicologists. (1997). Position statement: Gastric lavage. *Journal of Toxicology. Clinical Toxicology, 35,* 711–719.

American Academy of Clinical Toxicology; European Association of Poisons Centres and Clinical Toxicologists. (1997). Position statement: Ipecac syrup. *Journal of Toxicology. Clinical Toxicology, 35,* 699–709.

American Academy of Clinical Toxicology; European Association of Poisons Centres and Clinical Toxicologists. (1997). Position statement: Single dose activated charcoal. *Journal of Toxicology. Clinical Toxicology, 35,* 721–741.

Anas, N., Namasonthi, V., & Ginsburg, C. M. (1981). Criteria for hospitalizing children who have ingested products containing hydrocarbons. *Journal of the American Medical Association, 346,* 840–843.

Anderson, B. J., Holford, N. H. G., Armishaw, J. C., et al. (1999). Predicting concentrations in children presenting with acetaminophen overdose. *The Journal of Pediatrics, 135,* 290–295.

Anderson, K. D., Rouse, T. M., & Randolph, J. G. (1990). A controlled trial of corticosteroids in children with corrosive injury of the esophagus. *New England Journal of Medicine, 323,* 637–640.

Anene, O., & Castello, F. V. (1994). Myocardial dysfunction after hydrocarbon ingestion. *Critical Care Medicine, 22,* 528–530.

Applequist, P., & Salno, M. (1980). Lye corrosion carcinoma of the esophagus: A review of 63 cases. *Cancer, 45,* 26–55.

Arditi, M., & Killner, M. S. (1987). Coma following use of rubbing alcohol for fever control. *American Journal of Diseases of Children, 141,* 237–238.

Arena, J. M. (1987). Hydrocarbon poisoning—Current management. *Pediatric Annals, 16,* 879–883.

Auerbach, P. S., Osterloh, J., Braun, O., et al. (1986). Efficacy of gastric emptying: Gastric lavage versus emesis induced with ipecac. *Annals of Emergency Medicine, 15,* 692–698.

Bachrach, L., Correa, A., Levin, R., et al. (1979). Iron poisoning: Complications of hypertonic phosphate lavage therapy. *The Journal of Pediatrics, 94,* 147–149.

Banner, W., & Walson, P. D. (1983). Systemic toxicity following gasoline aspiration. *American Journal of Emergency Medicine, 3,* 292–294.

Barer, J., Hill, L. L., Hill, R. M., et al. (1973). Fatal poisoning from salt used as an emetic. *American Journal of Diseases of Children, 125,* 889–890.

Baum, C. R., Langman, C. B., Oker, E. E., et al. (2000). Fomepizole treatment of ethylene glycol poisoning in an infant. *Pediatrics, 106,* 1489–1491.

Beamon, R. F., Siegel, C. J., Landers, G., et al. (1976). Hydrocarbon ingestion in children. A six year retrospective study. *Journal of the American College of Emergency Physicians, 5,* 771–775.

Benitz, J. G., Swanson-Biearman, B., & Krenzelok, E. P. (2000). Nystagmus secondary to fomepizole administration in a pediatric patient. *Journal of Toxicology. Clinical Toxicology, 38,* 795–798.

Black, M. (1984). Acetaminophen hepatotoxicity. *Annual Review of Medicine, 35,* 577–593.

Bond, G. R., Krenzelok, E. P., Normann, S. A., et al. (1994). Acetaminophen ingestion in childhood—Cost and relative risk of alternative referral strategies. *Journal of Toxicology. Clinical Toxicology, 32,* 513–525.

Bond, G. R., Requa, R. K., Krenzelok, E. P., et al. (1993). Influence of time until emesis on the efficacy of decontamination using acetaminophen as a marker in a pediatric population. *Annals of Emergency Medicine, 22,* 1403–1407.

Bosse, G. M., Barefoot, J. A., Pfeifer, M. P., et al. (1995). Comparison of three methods of gut decontamination in tricyclic antidepressant overdose. *Journal of Emergency Medicine, 13,* 203–209.

Boxer, L., Anderson, F. P., & Rowe, D. S. (1969). Comparison of ipecac-induced emesis with gastric lavage in the treatment of acute salicylate ingestion. *The Journal of Pediatrics, 74,* 800–803.

Boyer, E. W., Mejia, M., Woolf, A., et al. (2001). Severe ethylene glycol ingestion treated without hemodialysis. *Pediatrics, 107,* 172–173.

Brent, J., McMartin, K., Phillips, S., et al. (1999). Fomepizole for the treatment of ethylene glycol poisoning. *New England Journal of Medicine, 340,* 879–881.

Brent, J., McMartin, K., Phillips, S., et al. (2001). Fomepizole for the treatment of methanol poisoning. *New England Journal of Medicine, 344,* 424–429.

Brown, J., Burke, B., & Dajani, A. S. (1974). Experimental kerosene pneumonia. Evaluation of some therapeutic regimens. *The Journal of Pediatrics, 84,* 396–401.

Brubacher, J. F., & Hoffman, R. S. (1996). Salicylism from topical salicylates: Review of the literature. *Journal of Toxicology. Clinical Toxicology, 34*(4), 431–436.

Bysani, G. K., Rucoba, R. J., & Noah, Z. L. (1994). Treatment of hydrocarbon pneumonitis. High frequency jet ventilation as an alternative to extracorporeal membrane oxygenation. *Chest, 106,* 300–303.

Campbell, G. S., Burnett, H. F., Ransom, J. M., et al. (1977). Treatment of corrosive burns of the esophagus. *Archives of Surgery, 112,* 495–500.

Campbell, J. W., & Chyka, P. (1992). Physicochemical characteristics of drugs and response to repeat-dose activated charcoal. *American Journal of Emergency Medicine, 10,* 208–210.

Cello, J. P., Fogel, R. P., & Boland, C. R. (1980). Liquid caustic ingestion: Spectrum of injury. *Archives of Internal Medicine, 140,* 501–504.

Ciftci, A. O., Senocak, M. E., Buyukpamukcu, N., et al. (1999). Gastric outlet obstruction due to corrosive ingestion: Incidence and outcome. *Pediatric Surgery International, 15,* 88–91.

Clark, A., & Love, H. (1991). Astemizole-induced ventricular arrhythmias: An unexpected cause of convulsions. *International Journal of Cardiology, 33,* 165–167.

Crain, E. F., Gershel, J. C., & Mezey, A. P. (1984). Caustic ingestions. Symptoms as predictors of esophageal injury. *American Journal of Diseases of Children, 138,* 863–865.

Curry, R. W., Robinson, J. D., & Sughrue, M. J. (1982). Acute renal failure after acetaminophen ingestion. *Journal of the American Medical Association, 247,* 1012–1014.

Curtis, R. A., Barone, J., & Giacono, N. (1984). Efficacy of ipecac and activated charcoal/cathartic. Prevention of salicylate absorption in a simulated overdose. *Archives of Internal Medicine, 144,* 48–52.

Czajka, P. A., Konrad, J. D., & Duffy, J. P. (1981). Iron poisoning: An in vitro comparison of bicarbonate and phosphate lavage solutions. *The Journal of Pediatrics, 98,* 491–494.

Done, A. K. (1978). Aspirin overdosage: Incidence, diagnosis and management. *Pediatrics, 62* (Suppl), 890–897.

Done, A. K. (1968). Treatment of salicylate poisoning. Review of personal and published experiences. *Clinical Toxicology, 1,* 451–467.

Dove, D. J., & Jones, T. (1982). Delayed coma associated with salicylate intoxication. *The Journal of Pediatrics, 100,* 493–496.

Dugandzic, R. M., Tierney, M. G., Dickinson, G. E., et al. (1989). Evaluation of the validity of the Done nomogram in the management of acute salicylate intoxication. *Annals of Emergency Medicine, 18,* 1186–1190.

Eade, N. R., Taussig, L. M., & Marks, M. I. (1974). Hydrocarbon pneumonitis. *Pediatrics, 54,* 351–356.

Eick, T., Blumer, J. L., & Reed, M. D. (2001). Safety of antihistamines in children. *Drug Safety, 24,* 119–147.

Ekins, B. R., Ford, D. C., Thompson, M. I. B., et al. (1987). The effect of activated charcoal on N-acetylcysteine absorption in normal subjects. *American Journal of Emergency Medicine, 5,* 483–487.

Ellenhorn, M. J. (1997). Gut decontamination. In *Ellenhorn's medical toxicology, diagnosis and treatment of human poisoning,* 2nd ed., pp. 66–78. Baltimore, MD: Williams & Wilkins.

Everson, G. W., Bertaccini, E. J., & O'Leary, J. (1991). Use of whole bowel irrigation in an infant following iron overdose. *American Journal of Emergency Medicine, 9,* 366–369.

Farley, T. A. (1986). Severe hypernatremic dehydration after use of an activated charcoal–sorbitol suspension. *The Journal of Pediatrics, 109,* 719–721.

Ferguson, M. K., Migliore, M., Staszak, V. M., et al. (1989). Early evaluation and therapy for caustic esophageal injury. *American Journal of Surgery, 157,* 116–120.

Fernandez, E., & Fernandez-Brito, A. C. (1977). Acetaminophen toxicity. *New England Journal of Medicine, 296,* 577.

Fisher, C. J., Jr., Albertson, T. E., & Foulke, G. E. (1985). Salicylate-induced pulmonary edema: Clinical characteristics in children. *American Journal of Emergency Medicine, 3,* 33–37.

Fisher, D. M., & Diaz, J. E. (1998). Pediatric methanol poisoning treated with fomepizole (Antizol®). [Abstract]. *Journal of Toxicology. Clinical Toxicology, 36,* 512.

Gaudreault, P., Parent, M., McGuigan, M. A., et al. (1983). Predictability of esophageal injury from signs and symptoms. A study of caustic ingestion in 378 children. *Pediatrics, 71,* 767–770.

Gaudreault, P., Temple, A. R., & Lovejoy, F. H. (1982). The relative severity of acute vs. chronic salicylate poisoning in children: A clinical comparison. *Pediatrics, 70*(4), 566–569.

Geffner, M., & Opas, L. (1980). Phosphate poisoning complicating treatment for iron ingestion. *American Journal of Diseases of Children, 134,* 509–510.

Gorman, R. L., Khing-Maung-Gyi, T., Klein-Schwartz, W., et al. (1992). Initial symptoms as predictors of esophageal injury in alkaline corrosive ingestions. *American Journal of Emergency Medicine, 10,* 189–194.

Grbcich, P. A., & Lacouture, P. G. (1987). Administration of charcoal in the home. [Abstract]. AACT/AAPCC Annual Scientific Meeting, Vancouver, Sept. 27, 1987.

Greenblatt, D. J., Allen, M. D., & Koch-Weser, J. (1976). Accidental iron poisoning in childhood: Six cases including one fatality. *Clinical Pediatrics, 15,* 835–838.

Gurwitz, D., Kattan, M., Levison, H., et al. (1978). Pulmonary function abnormalities in asymptomatic children after hydrocarbon pneumonitis. *Pediatrics, 62,* 789–794.

Hall, A. H., Smolinske, S. C., Stover, B., et al. (1992). Ibuprofen overdose in adults. *Journal of Toxicology. Clinical Toxicology, 30,* 23–37.

Haller, J. A., Andrews, H. G., White, J. J., et al. (1971). Pathophysiology and management of corrosive burns of the esophagus: Results of treatment in 285 children. *Journal of Pediatric Surgery, 6,* 578–584.

Halpern, S. M., Fitzpatrick, R., & Volans, G. N. (1993). Ibuprofen toxicity. A review of adverse reactions and overdose. *Adverse Drug Reactions Toxicology Review, 12,* 107–128.

Harnsbrough, J. F., Zapata-Sirvent, R., Dominic, W., et al. (1985). Hydrocarbon contact injuries. *Journal of Trauma, 25,* 250–252.

Harrison, P. M., Keays, R., Bray, G. P., et al. (1990). Improved outcome of paracetamol-induced fulminant hepatic failure by late administration of acetylcysteine. *The Lancet, 335,* 1572–1573.

Harry, P., Jobard, E., Briand, M., et al. (1998). Ethylene glycol poisoning in a child treated with 4-methylpyrazole. *Pediatrics, 102,* E31.

Hawkins, D. B., Demeter, M. J., & Barnett, T. W. (1980). Caustic ingestions: Controversies in management. A review of 214 cases. *Laryngoscope, 90,* 98–109.

Hayllar, J., & Bjarnason, I. (1995). NSAIDs, COX-2 inhibitors, and the gut. *The Lancet, 346,* 1629.

Henretig, F. (1996). Inhalant abuse in children and adolescents. *Pediatric Annals, 25,* 47–52.

Henretig, F. M., Selbst, S. M., Forrest, C., et al. (1989). Repeated acetaminophen overdosing causing hepatotoxicity in children. Clinical reports and literature review. *Clinical Pediatrics, 28,* 525–528.

Heubi, J. E., & Bien, J. P. (1997). Acetaminophen use in children: More is not better. *The Journal of Pediatrics, 130,* 175–177.

Heubi, J. E., Barbacci, M. B., & Zimmerman, H. J. (1998). Therapeutic misadventures with acetaminophen: Hepatotoxicity after multiple doses in children. *The Journal of Pediatrics, 132,* 22–27.

Hoffman, R. S., Howland, M. A., Kamerow, H. N., et al. (1989). Comparison of titratable acid/alkaline reserve and pH in potentially caustic household products. *Clinical Toxicology, 27,* 241–261.

Howell, J. M., Dalsey, W. C., Hartsell, F. W., et al. (1992). Steroids for the treatment of corrosive esophageal injury: A statistical analysis of past studies. *American Journal of Emergency Medicine, 10,* 421–425.

Ilkhanipour, K., Yealy, D. M., & Krenzelok, E. P. (1992). The comparative efficacy of various multiple-dose activated charcoal regimens. *American Journal of Emergency Medicine, 10,* 298–300.

James, J. A. (1970). Acute iron poisoning: Assessment of severity and prognosis. *The Journal of Pediatrics, 77,* 117–119.

Janssen, S., van der Geest, S., Meijer, S., et al. (1988). Impairment of organ function after oral ingestion of refined petrol. *Intensive Care Medicine, 14,* 238–240.

Jones, R. D. M., Lawson, A. D., Andrew, L. J., et al. (1991). Antagonism of the hypnotic effect of midazolam in children: A randomized, double-blind study of placebo and flumazenil administered after midazolam-induced anaesthesia. *British Journal of Anaesthesia, 66,* 660–666.

Kaczorowski, J. M., & Wax, P. (1996). Five days of whole-bowel irrigation in a case of pediatric iron ingestion. *Annals of Emergency Medicine, 27,* 258–263.

Kahn, A., & Blum, D. (1979). Fatal respiratory-distress syndrome and salicylate intoxication in a two-year-old. *The Lancet, 1,* 1131–1132.

Keays, R., Harrison, P. M., Wendon, J. A., et al. (1991). Intravenous acetylcysteine in paracetamol-induced fulminant hepatic failure: A prospective controlled trial. *British Medical Journal, 303,* 1026–1029.

Kelly, C., Egner, J., & **Rubin**, J. (1988). Successful treatment of triazolam overdose with Ro 15-1788 (Anexate). *Southern African Medical Journal, 73,* 442.

Kim, J., Gazarian, M., Verjee, Z., et al. (1995). Acute renal insufficiency in ibuprofen overdose. *Pediatric Emergency Care, 11,* 107–108.

Kirsh, M. M., & Ritter, F. (1976). Caustic ingestion and subsequent damage to the oropharyngeal and digestive passages. *Annals of Thoracic Surgery, 21,* 74–82.

Kirshenbaum, L. A., Mathews, S. C., Sitar, D. S., et al. (1990). Does multiple-dose charcoal therapy enhance salicylate excretion? *Archives of Internal Medicine, 150,* 1281–1283.

Kleinman, J. G., Breitenfield, R. V., & Roth, D. A. (1980). Acute renal failure associated with acetaminophen ingestion: Report of a case and review of the literature. *Clinical Nephrology, 14,* 201–205.

Klein-Schwartz, W., & Oderda, G. M. (1981). Adsorption of oral antidotes for acetaminophen poisoning (methionine and N-acetylcysteine) by activated charcoal. *Clinical Toxicology, 18,* 283–290.

Klein-Schwartz, W., Oderda, G. M., Gorman, R. L., et al. (1990). Assessment of management guidelines. Acute iron ingestion. *Clinical Pediatrics, 29,* 316–321.

Knasel, A. L., & Collins-Barrow, M. D. (1986). Predictability of early indicators of iron toxicity. *Journal of the National Medical Association, 78,* 1037–1040.

Knopp, R. (1979). Caustic ingestions. *Journal of the American College of Emergency Physicians, 8,* 329–336.

Koffler, A., Bernstein, M., LaSette, A., et al. (1978). Fixed-bed charcoal hemoperfusion: Treatment of drug overdose. *Archives of Internal Medicine, 138,* 1691–1694.

Koren, G. (1993). Medications which can kill a toddler with one tablet or teaspoonful. *Journal of Toxicology. Clinical Toxicology, 31,* 407–413.

Kornberg, A. E., & Dolgin, J. (1991). Pediatric ingestions: Charcoal alone versus ipecac and charcoal. *Annals of Emergency Medicine, 20,* 648–651.

Krenzelok, E. P., Keller, R., & Stewart, R. D. (1985). Gastrointestinal transit times of cathartics combined with charcoal. *Annals of Emergency Medicine, 14,* 1152–1155.

Kulig, K., Bar-Or, D., Cantrill, S. V., et al. (1985). Management of acutely poisoned patients without gastric emptying. *Annals of Emergency Medicine, 14,* 562–567.

Kurtzman, T. L., Otsuka, K. N., & Wahl, R. A. (2001). Inhalant abuse by adolescents. *Journal of Adolescent Health, 28,* 170–180.

Lacouture, P. G., Wason, S., Temple, A. R., et al. (1981). Emergency assessment of severity in iron overdose by clinical and laboratory methods. *The Journal of Pediatrics, 99,* 89–91.

Lacouture, P. G., Wason, S., Temple, A. R., et al. (1989). The generation of acetonemia/acetonuria following ingestion of a subtoxic dose of isopropyl alcohol. *American Journal of Emergency Medicine, 7,* 38–40.

Lauterburg, B. H., Vaisnav, Y., Stillwell, W. G., et al. (1980). The effects of age and glutathione depletion on hepatic glutathione turnover in vivo determined by acetaminophen probe analysis. *Journal of Pharmacology and Experimental Therapeutics, 213,* 54–58.

Leape, L. L., Ashcraft, K. W., Scarpelli, D. G., et al. (1971). Hazard to health—Liquid lye. *New England Journal of Medicine, 284,* 578–581.

Liebelt, E. L., & Shannon, M. W. (1993). Small doses, big problems: A selected review of highly toxic common medications. *Pediatric Emergency Care, 9,* 292–297.

Lieh-Lai, M. W., Sarnaik, A. P., Newton, J. F., et al. (1984). Metabolism and pharmacokinetics of acetaminophen in a severely poisoned young child. *The Journal of Pediatrics, 105,* 125–128.

Litovitz, T. L., & Manoguerra, A. (1992). Comparison of pediatric poisoning hazards: An analysis of 3.8 million exposure incidents. *Pediatrics, 89,* 999–1006.

Litovitz, T. L., Klein-Schwartz, W., Oderda, G. M., et al. (1985). Safety and efficacy of ipecac administration in children younger than one year of age. *Pediatrics, 76,* 761–764.

Litovitz, T. L., Klein-Schwartz, W., White, S., et al. (2001). 2000 Annual report of the American Association of Poison Control Centers Toxic Exposure Surveillance System. *American Journal of Emergency Medicine, 19,* 337–395.

Machado, B., Cross, K., & Snodgrass, W. R. (1988). Accidental hydrocarbon ingestion cases telephoned to a regional poison center. *Annals of Emergency Medicine, 17,* 804–807.

Manno, B. R., & Manno, J. E. (1972). Toxicology of ipecac: A review. *Clinical Toxicology, 10,* 221–242.

Mansson, I. (1978). Diagnosis of acute corrosive lesions of the oesophagus. *Journal of Laryngology and Otology, 92,* 499–504.

Marks, M. I., Chicoine, L., Legere, G., et al. (1972). Adrenocorticosteroid treatment of hydrocarbon pneumonia in children: A cooperative study. *The Journal of Pediatrics, 81,* 366–369.

Mayer, A. L., Sitar, D. S., & Tenenbein, M. (1992). Multiple-dose charcoal and whole-bowel irrigation do not increase clearance of absorbed salicylate. *Archives of Internal Medicine, 152,* 393–396.

McCord, M. M. (1987). Toxicity of sorbitol–charcoal suspension. *The Journal of Pediatrics, 110,* 307–308.

McCray, E. A., Bonfiglio, J. F., & Sigell, L. T. (1984). Home administration of syrup of ipecac to infants. *Drug Intelligence and Clinical Pharmacy, 18,* 792–793.

Miller, A. A. (2000). Diphenhydramine toxicity in a newborn: A case report. *Journal of Perinatology, 20,* 390–391.

Miller, R. P., Roberts, R. J., & Fischer, L. J. (1976). Acetaminophen elimination kinetics in neonates, children and adults. *Clinical Pharmacology and Therapeutics, 19,* 284–294.

Miller, T., & Lestina, D. C. (1997). Costs of poisoning in the United States and savings from poison control centers: A benefit cost analysis. *Annals of Emergency Medicine, 29,* 239–245.

Mills, K. C., & Curry, S. C. (1994). Acute iron poisoning. *Emergency Medicine Clinics of North America, 12,* 397–413.

Mitchell, J. R. (1988). Acetaminophen toxicity. *New England Journal of Medicine, 319,* 1601–1602.

Mitchell, J. R., Thorgeirsson, S. S., Potter, W. Z., et al. (1974). Acetaminophen-induced hepatic injury: Protective role of glutathione in man and rationale for therapy. *Clinical Pharmacology and Therapeutics, 16,* 676–684.

Moazam, F., Talbert, J. L., Miller, D., et al. (1987). Caustic ingestion and its sequelae in children. *Southern Medical Journal, 80,* 187–190.

Muhlendahl, K. E., Oberdisse, U., & Krienke, E. G. (1978). Local injuries by accidental ingestion of corrosive substances by children. *Archives of Toxicology, 39,* 299–314.

Mukerji, V., Alpert, M. A., Flaker, G. C., et al. (1986). Cardiac conduction abnormalities and atrial arrhythmias associated with salicylate toxicity. *Pharmacotherapy, 6,* 41–43.

Neuvonen, P. J., Vartianinen, M., & Tokola, O. (1983). Comparison of activated charcoal and ipecac syrup in prevention of drug absorption. *European Journal of Clinical Pharmacology, 24,* 557–562.

Ng, R. W. W., Perry, K., & Martin, D. J. (1979). Iron poisoning. Assessment of radiography in diagnosis and management. *Clinical Pediatrics, 18,* 614–616.

Paloucek, F. P., & Rodvold, D. A. (1988). Evaluation of theophylline overdoses and toxicities. *Annals of Emergency Medicine, 17,* 135–144.

Pei, Y. P. C., & Thompson, D. A. (1987). Severe salicylate intoxication mimicking septic shock. *American Journal of Medicine, 82,* 381–382.

Penna, A., & Buchanan, N. (1991). Paracetamol poisoning in children and hepatotoxicity. *British Journal of Clinical Pharmacology, 32,* 143–149.

Penner, G. E. (1980). Acid ingestion: Toxicology and treatment. *Annals of Emergency Medicine, 9,* 374–379.

Perry, H. E., & Shannon, M. W. (1998). Efficacy of oral versus intravenous N-acetylcysteine in acetaminophen overdose: Results of an open-label, clinical trial. *The Journal of Pediatrics, 132,* 149–152.

Pershad, J., Nichols, M., & King, W. (1999). "The silent killer": Chronic acetaminophen toxicity in a toddler. *Pediatric Emergency Care, 15,* 43–46.

Peterson, C. O., & Fifield, G. C. (1980). Emergency gastrotomy for acute iron poisoning. *Annals of Emergency Medicine, 9,* 262–264.

Peterson, R. G., & Rumack, B. H. (1981). Age as a variable in acetaminophen overdose. *Archives of Internal Medicine, 141,* 390–393.

Piperno, E., Mosher, A. H., Berssenbruegge, D. A., et al. (1978). Pathophysiology of acetaminophen overdosage toxicity: Implications for management. *Pediatrics, 62*(Suppl), 880–889.

Pond, S. M. (1986). Role of repeated oral doses of activated charcoal in clinical toxicology. *Medical Toxicology, 1,* 3–11.

Pond, S. M., Lewis-Driver, D. J., Williams, G. M., et al. (1995). Gastric emptying in acute overdosage: A prospective randomized controlled trial. *Medical Journal of Australia, 163,* 345–349.

Pond, S. M., Olson, K. R., Osterloh, J. D., et al. (1984). Randomized study of the treatment of phenobarbital overdose with repeated doses of activated charcoal. *Journal of the American Medical Association, 251,* 3104–3108.

Pond, S., Rosenberg, J., Benowitz, N. L., et al. (1979). Pharmacokinetics of hemoperfusion for drug overdose. *Clinical Pharmacokinetics, 4,* 329–354.

Prescott, L. F. (1983). Paracetamol overdosage: Pharmacological considerations and clinical management. *Drugs, 25,* 290–314.

Rivera-Penera, T., Gugig, R., Davis, J., et al. (1997). Outcome of acetaminophen overdose in pediatric patients and factors contributing to hepatotoxicity. *The Journal of Pediatrics, 130,* 300–304.

Robertson, W. O. (1979). Syrup of ipecac associated fatality: A case report. *Veterinary and Human Toxicology, 21,* 87–89.

Robotham, J. L., & Lietman, P. S. (1980). Acute iron poisoning. A review. *American Journal of Diseases of Children, 134,* 875.

Roth, S. H. (1988). NSAID and gastropathy: A rheumatologist's review. *Journal of Rheumatology, 15,* 912–919.

Rothstein, F. C. (1986). Caustic injuries to the esophagus in children. *Pediatric Clinics of North America, 33,* 665–674.

Rumack, B. H. (1983). Acetaminophen overdose. *American Journal of Medicine, 75,* 104–112.

Rumack, B. H. (1999). Acetaminophen overdose? A quick answer. *The Journal of Pediatrics, 135,* 269–270.

Rumack, B. H., & Matthew, H. (1975). Acetaminophen poisoning and toxicity. *Pediatrics, 55,* 871–876.

Rumack, B. H., Peterson, R. C., Koch, G. G., et al. (1981). Acetaminophen overdose: 662 cases with evaluation of oral acetylcysteine treatment. *Archives of Internal Medicine, 141,* 380–385.

Scalzo, A. J., Weber, T. R., Jaeger, R. W., et al. (1990). Extracorporeal membrane oxygenation for hydrocarbon aspiration. *American Journal of Diseases of Children, 144,* 867–871.

Schreiner, G. E. (1977). Dialysis of poisons and drugs annual review. *Transactions—American Society for Artificial Internal Organs, 16,* 544–568.

Shepherd, R. T. (1989). Mechanism of sudden death associated with volatile substance abuse. *Human Toxicology, 8,* 287–292.

Smilkstein, M. J., Bronstein, A. C., Linden, C., et al. (1991). Acetaminophen overdose: A 48 hour intravenous N-acetylcysteine treatment protocol. *Annals of Emergency Medicine, 20,* 1058–1063.

Smilkstein, M. J., Knapp, G. L., Kulig, K. W., et al. (1988). Efficacy of oral N-acetylcysteine in the treatment of acetaminophen overdose: Analysis of the national multicenter study (1976 to 1985). *New England Journal of Medicine, 319,* 1557–1562.

Smolinske, S. C., Hall, A. H., Vandenberg, S. A., et al. (1990). Toxic effects of nonsteroidal anti-inflammatory drugs in overdose. Analysis of the national multicenter study (1976 to 1985). *New England Journal of Medicine, 319,* 1557–1562.

Spiller, H. A., & Rodgers, G. C. (1997). Prospective evaluation of administration of activated charcoal (AC) in the home. [Abstract]. *Journal of Toxicology. Clinical Toxicology, 35,* 483.

Stannard, M. W. (1978). Corrosive esophagitis in children. *American Journal of Diseases of Children, 132,* 596–599.

Steele, R. W., Conklin, R. H., & Mark, H. M. (1972). Corticosteroids and antibiotics for the treatment of fulminant hydrocarbon aspiration. *Journal of the American Medical Association, 219,* 1434–1437.

Stein, M., Blayney, D., Feit, T., et al. (1976). Acute iron poisoning in children. *Western Journal of Medicine, 125,* 289–297.

Stiff, G., Alwafi, A., Rees, B. I., et al. (1996). Corrosive injuries of the oesophagus and stomach: Experience in management at a regional paediatric centre. *Annals of the Royal College of Surgeons of England, 78,* 119–123.

Sugawa, C., Mullins, R. J., Lucas, G. E., et al. (1981). The value of early endoscopy following caustic ingestion. *Surgery, Gynecology and Obstetrics, 153,* 553–556.

Tandberg, D., Diven, B. G., & McLeod, J. W. (1986). Ipecac-induced emesis versus gastric lavage: A controlled study in normal adults. *American Journal of Emergency Medicine, 4,* 205–209.

Tenenbein, M. (1991). Multiple doses of activated charcoal: Time for reappraisal? *Annals of Emergency Medicine, 20,* 529–531.

Tenenbein, M. (1987). Whole bowel irrigation in iron poisoning. *The Journal of Pediatrics, 111,* 142–144.

Tenenbein, M., Cohen, S., & Sitar, D. S. (1987a). Efficacy of ipecac-induced emesis, orogastric lavage and activated charcoal for drug overdose. *Annals of Emergency Medicine, 16,* 838–841.

Tenenbein, M., Cohen, S., & Sitar, D. S. (1987b). Whole bowel irrigation as a decontamination procedure after acute drug overdose. *Archives of Internal Medicine, 147,* 905–907.

Tenenbein, M., Kowalsi, S., Sienko, A., et al. (1992). Pulmonary toxic effects of continuous deforoxamine administration in acute iron poisoning. *The Lancet, 339,* 699–701.

Tewfik, T. L., & Schloss, M. D. (1980). Ingestion of lye and other corrosive agents—A study of 86 infant and child cases. *Journal of Otolaryngology, 9,* 72–77.

Tucker, J. A., Turtz, M. L., Silberman, H. D., et al. (1974). Tucker retrograde esophageal dilatation 1924–1974: A historical review. *Annals of Otology, Rhinology, and Laryngology, 83*(Suppl 16), 1–35.

Update: Childhood Poisonings—United States (1985). *Journal of the American Medical Association, 255,* 1857.

Vale, J. A., Rees, A. J., Widdop, B., et al. (1975). Use of charcoal haemoperfusion in the management of severely poisoned patients. *British Medical Journal, 1,* 5–9.

Vicas, I. M., & Beck, R. (1993). Fatal inhalational isopropyl alcohol poisoning in a neonate. *Journal of Toxicology. Clinical Toxicology, 31,* 473–481.

Vital Statistics of the United States, Mortality, CDC Wonder, [*http://wonder.cdc.gov*] 2001.

Wald, P., Wortzman, D., & Notterman, D. (1985). Salicylate-induced pulmonary edema. [Letter]. *American Journal of Emergency Medicine, 3,* 481–482.

Wallace, K. L., Curry, S. C., LoVecchio, F., et al. (1998). Effect of magnesium hydroxide on iron absorption following simulated mild iron overdose in human subjects. *Academy of Emergency Medicine, 5,* 961–965.

Weber, J. L., & Cutz, E. (1980). Liver failure in an infant. *Canadian Medical Association Journal, 123,* 112–117.

Westlin, W. F. (1966). Deferoxamine in the treatment of acute iron poisoning. Clinical experience with 172 children. *Clinical Pediatrics, 5,* 531–535.

Whitten, C. F., Chen, Y. C., & Gibson, G. W. (1966). Studies in acute iron poisoning: II. Further observations on desferrioxamine in the treatment of acute experimental iron poisoning. *Pediatrics, 38,* 102–110.

Wiley, J. F., Gelber, M. L., Henretig, F. M., et al. (1992). Cardiotoxic effects of astemizole overdose in children. *The Journal of Pediatrics, 120,* 799–802.

Wilkinson, S. P., Moodie, H., & Arroyo, V. A. (1977). Frequency of renal impairment in paracetamol overdose compared with other causes of acute liver damage. *Journal of Clinical Pathology, 30,* 141–143.

Winchester, J. F., Gelfand, M. C., Knepshield, J. H., et al. (1977). Dialysis and hemoperfusion of poisons and drugs. *Transactions—American Society for Artificial Internal Organs, 23,* 762–842.

Woolf, A., & Shaw, J. (1998). Childhood injuries from artificial nail primer cosmetic products. *Archives of Pediatrics and Adolescent Medicine, 152,* 41–46.

Woolf, A., Wieler, J., & Greenes, D. (1997). Costs of poison-related hospitalizations at an urban teaching hospital for children. *Archives of Pediatrics and Adolescent Medicine, 151,* 719–723.

Yip, L., Dart, R. C., & Gabow, P. A. (1994). Concepts and controversies in salicylate toxicity. *Emergency Medicine Clinics of North America, 12,* 351–364.

Yip, L., Dart, R. C., & Hurlbut, K. M. (1998). Intravenous administration of oral N-acetylcysteine. *Critical Care Medicine, 26,* 40–43.

Zucker, A. R., Berger, S., & Wood, L. D. H. (1986). Management of kerosene-induced pulmonary injury. *Critical Care Medicine, 14,* 303–304.

5

Adverse Drug Reactions in Neonates, Infants, Children, and Adolescents

Michael J. Rieder

Pediatric clinicians are faced with a number of concerns when a need for drug therapy arises. These concerns include the selection of appropriate drug therapy, its cost, patient compliance, and adverse drug reactions (ADRs). ADRs are the undesirable consequences of drug therapy, which may range from self-limiting effects related to the drug's pharmacologic action to severe and life-threatening effects. The WHO definition of ADRs does not include toxicity related to drug overdosage, although other classifications of ADRs do (e.g., Patterson et al., 1986).

Classification of ADRs

The Patterson et al. (1986) classification system is useful in that it provides a diagnostic framework that can help clinicians understand how the ADR occurred and assist them in planning drug therapy and avoiding future ADRs. This system classifies ADRs as **predictable** (based on current knowledge of the drug's pharmacology) or **unpredictable**.

Predictable ADRs

Predictable ADRs include side effects, secondary effects, drug interactions, and toxic effects. Each type is briefly discussed.

Side effects. Predictable ADRs are undesirable effects, or "side effects," that occur as a consequence of a drug's pharmacology at usual drug dosages and with usual drug serum concentrations. They are often minor and diminish over time. An example of this type of ADR is fine hand tremor associated with the use of beta-adrenergic agonists for the management of asthma.

Secondary effects. These predictable, but not inevitable, effects occur as a consequence of the expected pharmacologic actions of a particular drug. An example is pseudomembranous colitis associated with lincosamide antibiotics, such as clindamycin. This secondary effect can be predicted due to overgrowth of enterotoxin-producing strains of *Clostridium difficile* subsequent to suppression of normal bowel flora as a primary action of the lincosamide antibiotics. However, this effect only occurs in a small minority of patients who are treated with clindamycin.

Drug interactions (see Chapter 6). Desired or undesired effects may occur as a consequence of a drug–drug, drug–food, or drug–disease interaction. One example is bleeding associated with concurrent cimetidine and warfarin pharmacotherapy, which results in the inhibition of warfarin metabolism by cimetidine. Another example is the prolongation of the QT interval during therapy with cisapride and fluconazole. Fluconazole and a number of other drugs inhibit cisapride metabolism and thus increase cisapride serum concentrations, which may prolong the QT interval.

Toxicity. This undesired effect occurs as a consequence of excessive drug accumulation (overdosage) or poisoning. An example is metabolic acidosis and coma produced by salicylate poisoning.

Unpredictable ADRs

Unpredictable ADRs include intolerance, idiosyncratic reactions, and allergic reactions.

Intolerance. Drug intolerance, or exaggerated effects, occur at usual drug dosages and with usual drug serum concentrations in special subsets of patients. The reason for these exaggerated effects is not usually understood. An example of drug intolerance is the severe nausea and vomiting observed among some patients treated with erythromycin.

Idiosyncratic effects. Undesired effects, often very severe, may occur that do not appear to be related to the pharmacology of the drug. Among this diverse group of ADRs are some drug reactions related to the pharmacogenetic or pharmacoanthropologic variations in special subsets of the human population. An example of an idiosyncratic effect is the Stevens-Johnson syndrome, which is associated with the sulfonamide antibiotics.

Allergic effects. Allergic effects occur as a consequence of the drug eliciting an undesirable immune response or possessing characteristics that suggest mediation by the immune system. An example of this type of ADR is the urticaria associated with penicillin therapy.

Risk Factors

In attempting to avoid ADRs, the clinician should appreciate that the risk is not uniform for all patients. Under some circumstances,

TABLE 5-1
Drugs for which Neonates Are at Special Risk for ADRs

Antibiotics (e.g., aminoglycosides, chloramphenicol)
Cardiovascular drugs (e.g., digoxin, dopamine)
Diuretics (e.g., furosemide)
Methylxanthines (e.g., caffeine)
Nutritional components (e.g., amino acid or lipid infusions)

neonates (*see* Tables 5-1 and 5-2), infants, and children are at higher risk for ADRs than are other age groups (Rieder & Matsui, 1998). These risks apply in large part to the developmental biology of the body organs of drug elimination, particularly the liver and kidneys, and in part to risks that apply to other patient groups, such as racial or ethnic groups (*see* Chapter 11).

Other important risk factors for ADRs involving pediatric patients include:

History of previous ADRs: Patients who have had an ADR to one drug appear to be at a higher risk for ADRs involving other drugs. In part, this risk may be due to some other factors, notably those related to alterations in drug elimination.

Polydrug therapy: Polydrug therapy (therapy simultaneously involving more than one drug) carries synergistic, rather than additive, risk for the occurrence of ADRs that may be related to the issue of drug interactions (*see* Chapter 6).

Hepatic or renal dysfunction: Patients with reduced drug elimination, either due to disease or immature body organ function (e.g., neonates, infants, young children) have an increased risk for ADRs, particularly for drugs primarily metabolized or eliminated by the liver or kidneys.

TABLE 5-2
Drugs Implicated in Neonatal Jaundice[a]

Caffeine and sodium benzoate	Novobiocin
Chlorpromazine	Primaquine
Menadione	Salicylates
Nalidixic acid	Sodium benzoate
Nitrofurantoin	Sulfonamides

[a] Avoid the use of these drugs, if possible, in neonates, pregnant adolescent girls who are near term, and in adolescent girls who are breast feeding (*see also* Chapters 2 and 3).

Extremes of age: Neonates, infants, and young children are at substantially increased risk for ADRs (*see* Tables 5-1 and 5-2), primarily because of their immature drug elimination organ function, but also due to differences in other pharmacokinetic factors (e.g., volume of distribution) (*see* Chapter 10). Similarly, at the other end of the age spectrum, elderly patients also are at a substantially increased risk.

Female gender: For reasons that remain unclear, females of almost all ages have an increased risk for ADRs when compared to males. It is unclear as to whether this increased risk occurs prior to, or following, puberty (Tran et al., 1998).

Special populations: Certain groups of patients, for reasons of specific diseases or because they belong to specific ethnic or racial groups, have an increased risk for ADRs. As an example, children with acquired immunodeficiency syndrome (AIDS) have a substantially increased rate of ADRs involving the sulfonamides when compared to the general population. Children of Mediterranean descent have a substantially increased risk for hemolytic anemia from certain drugs such as nalidixic acid or the salicylates related to genetically mediated deficiencies in glucose-6-phosphate dehydrogenase (G-6-PD deficiency).

Special drugs: Certain drugs, notably those with a low therapeutic index (Table 5-3), are associated with a higher risk for ADRs than are drugs in general.

Special care settings: The nature of pediatric drug formulations is such that there is a considerable potential for errors in calculation of drug dose, in preparing doses for individual patients, and in administering prepared doses (*see* Chapter 1). This risk reportedly appears to be significantly higher in certain clinical settings, such as the Neonatal Intensive Care Unit. Risk also is high in clinical situations where infant and child care is provided by personnel who are unfamiliar with pediatric dosages and do not routinely administer drugs to infants and children. There also are healthcare personnel who appear to have particular problems with mathematics and make more calculation errors than do others (Rowe et al., 1998).

Abrupt alterations in drug therapy: The abrupt discontinuation of certain drugs (Table 5-4), notably those that have been used continuously for a long period of time, can be associated with signs and symptoms of withdrawal (e.g., opiates) or with markedly increased disease activity (e.g., corticosteroids).

Establishing ADRs

The approach for determining if an undesirable clinical event is an ADR includes careful assessment of the event and the following important steps.

1. Evaluation of the undesirable event. This evaluation should include a careful history and physical examination, which is supplemented by appropriate laboratory testing. It is key that the suspected ADR is described in as much detail as possible, including its effect on usual patient activities. The history should focus on such details as timing of the undesirable event in relation to the patient's drug therapy, other drug exposures, and other relevant health issues, including the medical disorder for which the drug therapy was prescribed and other concurrent disorders or clinical conditions. The timing of doses and the duration of

TABLE 5-4
Drugs That Require Dose Tapering and for which Abrupt Discontinuation may Produce Significant ADRs

Anticonvulsants (e.g., carbamazepine, phenytoin, valproic acid)
Antihypertensives (e.g., beta-adrenergic blockers, clonidine, methyldopa)
Corticosteroids (e.g., prednisone)
Opiates (e.g., fentanyl, morphine)
Sedative-hypnotics (e.g., barbiturates, benzodiazepines)

TABLE 5-3
Drugs That Have a Low Therapeutic Index

Aminoglycosides (e.g., gentamicin)
Anesthetics (e.g., halothane)
Anticoagulants (e.g., heparin, warfarin)
Anticonvulsants (e.g., phenobarbital, phenytoin)
Antimanics (e.g., lithium)
Antineoplastics (e.g., doxorubicin) (*See* Chapter 12.)
Cardiovascular drugs (e.g., digoxin, lidocaine)
Methylxanthines (e.g., theophylline)

therapy prior to the event are critical, as are the timing and evolution of the adverse event. Other related questions include whether the adverse event improved when the drug therapy was discontinued, and what the time course of improvement was. Additionally, it is impossible to overestimate the importance of a clear understanding of the clinical characteristics of the undesired event; thus, descriptions should be as complete and detailed as possible. Vague descriptions, such as "rash," are of such low specificity as to be nearly useless.

2. Formulation of a differential diagnosis. This step includes the possibility of drug-induced versus nondrug-induced (e.g., disease- or food-induced) events. Part of this consideration is whether the pharmacology of a particular drug would be consistent with the event observed. It may be necessary to obtain additional information in the process of developing a complete differential diagnosis, which may include consultation with a drug information resource, particularly for very unusual events or when recently developed drugs are implicated.

3. Selection of the most probable etiology of the untoward event. In the case of ADRs, this selection is usually done primarily on clinical grounds and the laboratory is often of little help. Part of this deliberation is the consideration whether a careful history supports the onset and time course of the adverse event relative to the timing of drug therapy. The frequently quoted but still very valid doctrine of Occam's Razor ("when all other reasons are ruled out, what is left is probably the cause") is frequently used, with the caveat that unusual adverse events can occur with newly developed drugs in a manner that sometimes cannot be predicted from a knowledge of the preclinical information regarding the pharmacology of the drug. In some cases, it may be useful to obtain a sample of blood, urine, or other suitable biological fluids to determine if the drug might be present in toxic concentrations.

4. Drug therapy and assessment of the goals of drug therapy. The first step is to treat the signs and symptoms of the adverse event, which is largely limited to symptomatic relief and supportive medical care. Given that the untoward event is related to the drug therapy, it is important to review the therapeutic goals for which the drug therapy was prescribed initially, starting with the determination of whether the therapeutic goal was achieved. If the therapeutic goal was achieved (e.g., eradication of a bacterial infection), then further drug therapy may not be needed. If the therapeutic goal was not achieved and the adverse event was not serious and/or was self-limited (e.g., hand tremor associated with the use of beta-adrenergic agonists for the management of asthma), then it may be possible to continue with the drug therapy, ensuring that the patient and his or her parents have a clear understanding as to the presumptive diagnosis of the adverse event and the rationale for continuing the drug therapy. In the event that the ADR was severe and the therapeutic goal was not achieved, then alternative drug therapy should be considered (e.g., anticonvulsant hypersensitivity syndrome in a patient with poorly controlled epilepsy).

5. Confirmation of the adverse event. Confirmatory tests are generally not available except for a few drugs (e.g., penicillin, local anesthetics). In most cases, the diagnosis of an ADR is based on clinical criteria: the patient's signs and symptoms and their relationship to his or her drug therapy.

6. Communication as a key and often neglected aspect of the analysis of ADRs. It is crucial that the patient and his or her parents understand what has occurred, what the offending drug(s) are believed to be, what risk might be involved in regard to future drug therapy, and what the current, revised therapeutic plan is. This process is especially important in pediatrics, because the patient is often dependent on others to convey information to current and future healthcare providers. Additionally, the fact of having had an ADR may affect the patient-clinician relationship, especially for the clinician in primary care practice (e.g., GP, PNP). Clear communication may help to minimize the potentially harmful effects on this relationship. Communication of a suspected ADR with other healthcare providers, especially when patients are infants, children, and adolescents with complex or chronic medical disorders is important in order to optimize their current health status and to prevent a reoccurrence.

7. Reporting the ADR. This step is important, especially for newly developed drugs and when associated ADRs are serious. A report should be made to the responsible drug regulatory agency (Food and Drug Administration, Therapeutic Products Program, Committee for the Safety of Medicines) as well as to the drug manufacturer. Most serious drug hypersensitivities have been reported after the drug has been marketed rather than during Phase I–III testing, and, thus, it is incumbent, particularly on the prescriber and pharmacist, to report unusual or severe ADRs.

As with any clinical problem, prevention is the most desirable approach to ADRs. However, the prevalence and characteristics of ADRs among infants and children is understudied and many common and important problems are not well understood. For example, it has been said that ADRs are less common among pediatric patients than adult patients, but the data are limited and this assertion may not be true. In addition, it is clear that certain groups of pediatric patients—such as those in neonatal intensive care units—have very high rates of ADRs. When specific groups of pediatric patients have been studied in detail, ADR rates have frequently paralleled those of adults (Rieder & Matsui, 1998).

Certain groups of drugs are more likely to be associated with ADRs, and the prescriber of these drugs should be especially vigilant (Tables 5-1 and 5-5). Vigilance is especially critical for drugs with a low therapeutic index, in which calculation or dosing errors are more likely to produce serious ADRs in infants and children, especially neonates (Tables 5-1 and 5-2). As well, certain drugs are likely to produce ADRs when they are abruptly discontinued (Table 5-4). It is also now appreciated that the isozymes of cytochrome P-450 are important determinants of drug metabolism and that drugs that inhibit isozyme-specific P-450 metabolism are associated with a significant risk for ADRs when co-administered with drugs that rely on these pathways for metabolism (see Chapters 6 and 11).

In order to help clinicians prevent or minimize ADRs, two additional tables are provided. Table 5-6 identifies pediatric diseases and conditions that may be mimicked by ADRs, resulting in misdiagnosis. Table 5-7 describes the nature and incidence of ADRs associated with drugs commonly used in promoting childhood and adolescent health.

TABLE 5-5
Drug Classes with a Significant Risk for Producing Serious ADRs in Infants, Children, and Adolescents

Analgesics (e.g., aspirin)
Antibiotics (e.g., aminoglycosides, penicillins)
Anticoagulants (e.g., heparin, warfarin)
Anticonvulsants (e.g., phenytoin, valproic acid)
Antineoplastics (e.g., doxorubicin, methotrexate) (See Chapter 12.)
Cardiovascular drugs (e.g., digoxin)
Methylxanthines (e.g., theophylline)
Vaccines and toxoids (e.g., diphtheria and tetanus toxoids, pertussis vaccine) (See Chapter 9.)

Summary

This chapter has presented an overview of the ADRs associated with the drugs commonly required by pediatric patients with attention to the drug classes that are associated with serious ADRs among neonates, infants, children, and adolescents. These data have been presented in a number of tables for clarity and usefulness. A classification of predictable and unpredictable ADRs also is presented in an effort to help pediatric clinicians understand the mechanism by which the ADR occurred and assist them in planning drug therapy that will avoid, whenever possible, future ADRs. The data presented in this chapter should help pediatric clinicians to recognize the ADRs among their patients when they occur and to prevent and minimize these ADRs whenever possible. Pediatric clinicians are encouraged to be alert for ADRs and to report their occurrences so that their nature and incidence can be better understood in regard to pediatric patients.

TABLE 5-6
Diseases and Clinical Conditions That Can Be Caused by Drugs Used Commonly in the Pediatric Age Group[a]

DISEASE OR CLINICAL CONDITION	POSSIBLE CAUSATIVE DRUGS
Acne	Barbiturates (long term, high dosage), corticosteroids, lithium
Adrenal Insufficiency	Corticosteroids (abrupt withdrawal after prolonged use)
Aggressive Behavior	Alcohol, amphetamines, anabolic steroids, androgens, anticonvulsants (high dosage), cocaine, ethosuximide, triazolam
Akathisia (see also Extrapyramidal reactions)	Antipsychotics (e.g., chlorpromazine, haloperidol)
Akinesia (see also Extrapyramidal reactions)	Antipsychotics (e.g., chlorpromazine, haloperidol)
Anaphylaxis (see also Hypersensitivity reactions)	Amine-class local anesthetics (e.g., lidocaine), cephalosporins, gold sodium thiomalate, nonsteroidal anti-inflammatory drugs (NSAIDs), penicillins, probenecid, salicylates, serums, sulfonamides, tetracyclines, vaccines
Anorexia	Acyclovir, amantadine, amphetamines, amphotericin B, cocaine, digoxin (overdosage), ethosuximide, pemoline. Also, most orally ingested drugs and those that adversely affect the GI system (e.g., erythromycin)
Arthritis	Cefaclor, vaccines (e.g., influenza vaccine)
Asthma (see also Respiratory dysfunction)	Aspirin and other NSAIDs, nonselective beta-adrenergic blockers (e.g., propranolol)
Ataxia	Benzodiazepines, carbamazepine, clonazepam, ethosuximide, phenobarbital, phenytoin, primidone
Behavioral Disturbances	Alcohol and most other psychotropics (e.g., cocaine, tetrahydrocannabinol and other psychedelics) especially in high dosages or with abrupt discontinuation after prolonged use, beta-adrenergic blockers (paradoxical agitation)
Bleeding or Hemorrhage	Anticonvulsants (vitamin K deficiency), aspirin and other NSAIDs, heparin, vitamin E (high dosage), warfarin
Blood Dyscrasias	
Agranulocytosis (white blood cell count <200)	Amphotericin B (injectable), antihistamines, carbamazepine, cimetidine, clindamycin (oral or injectable), clozapine, co-trimoxazole, ethosuximide, gold sodium thiomalate, indomethacin, isoniazid, mebendazole (high dosage), phenothiazines, phenytoin, procainamide, propafenone, quinidine, sulfonamides, tricyclic antidepressants
Anemia	Amphotericin B (injectable), chloramphenicol, flucytosine, furosemide, isoniazid, methotrexate, ribavirin, zidovudine
Aplastic anemia	Chloramphenicol, co-trimoxazole, ethosuximide, indomethacin, phenytoin, quinidine, thiazide diuretics
Eosinophilia	Aztreonam, carbamazepine, co-trimoxazole, erythromycin, hydralazine, isoniazid, phenothiazines
Granulocytopenia	Chloramphenicol, phenytoin, zidovudine
Hemolytic anemia	Cephalosporins, co-trimoxazole, isoniazid, methyldopa, penicillins, quinidine, sulfonamides, vitamin C (high dosages)
Leukocytosis	Haloperidol, lithium, phenothiazines, tetracycline
Leukopenia (white blood cell count ≤3000)	Amphotericin B (injectable), antihistamines, carbamazepine, chloramphenicol, co-trimoxazole, didanosine, ethosuximide, flucytosine, furosemide, ganciclovir, gold sodium thiomalate, haloperidol, indomethacin, methotrexate, phenytoin, primidone, quinidine, trimethoprim
Megaloblastic anemia	Co-trimoxazole, nitrofurantoin, phenobarbital, phenytoin, primidone, triamterene
Methemoglobinemia	Benzocaine, co-trimoxazole, dapsone, lidocaine, nitroglycerin, trimethoprim
Neutropenia (neutrophil count ≤1000)	Clozapine, co-trimoxazole, flucytosine, ganciclovir, griseofulvin, mebendazole (high dosage), nafcillin, phenytoin, trimethoprim, zidovudine
Thrombocytopenia (platelet count ≤150,000)	Amphotericin B (injectable), carbamazepine, chloramphenicol, co-trimoxazole, didanosine, flucytosine, ganciclovir, heparin, indomethacin, isoniazid, mebendazole (high dosage), methotrexate, phenytoin, primidone, quinidine, sulfonamides, tetracycline, trimethoprim, valproic acid
Bronchospasm (see also Respiratory dysfunction)	Iron, injectable (hypersensitivity); noncardioselective beta-adrenergic blockers; drugs commonly associated with hypersensitivity reactions (e.g., aspirin, penicillins)
Candida Infection	Aminoglycosides, beclomethasone (inhalation), chloramphenicol, corticosteroids (topical), penicillins, tetracyclines
Cardiac Dysrhythmias	Anticholinergics, antidysrhythmics, beta-adrenergic agonists, clonidine, cocaine, digoxin, doxyrubicin (long-term therapy), lithium, procainamide, quinidine, ribavirin, theophylline, thyroid hormones, tricyclic antidepressants
Cardiac Failure/Congestive Heart Failure	Amantadine, anthracycline therapy (chronic) (e.g., doxorubicin), beta-adrenergic blockers, chloramphenicol (high dosage, primarily in neonates), disopyramide, lidocaine, propafenone, sodium bicarbonate (high dosage)

[a] Other drugs can cause the listed diseases and clinical conditions, but only the more common examples that have been observed and reported are included.

TABLE 5-6 *continued*

DISEASE OR CLINICAL CONDITION	POSSIBLE CAUSATIVE DRUGS
Cataracts (*see also* Visual dysfunction)	Corticosteroids (ophthalmic), isotretinoin
Constipation	Aluminum hydroxide, anticholinergics (e.g., atropine), antidiarrheals, calcium carbonate, calcium channel blockers, cimetidine, clonidine, disopyramide, diuretics, iron (oral), opiate analgesics, propafenone, verapamil
Convulsions/Seizures	Amantadine, anticonvulsants (abrupt discontinuation after chronic, long-term use), antidepressants, antipsychotics, benzodiazepines, CNS stimulants (e.g., amphetamines, cocaine), haloperidol, iron (injectable), lidocaine, lithium, penicillins (high dosage), propafenone, theophylline, vaccines
Cough (dry, nonproductive)	ACE inhibitors, leukotriene antagonists
Cushing's Syndrome	Corticosteroids
Deafness/Hearing Loss (*see also* Tinnitus)	Aminoglycosides, aspirin, ethacrynic acid, furosemide, griseofulvin, isotretinoin, quinidine
Depression	Amantadine, cimetidine, isotretinoin, sedative-hypnotics
Diarrhea	Amoxicillin–clavulanate, amphotericin B, ampicillin, clindamycin (oral, injectable), digoxin, iron (oral), laxatives, lithium, magnesium carbonate, magnesium hydroxide, methotrexate, potassium chloride, quinidine, tetracyclines, thiazide diuretics, thyroid hormones, vaccines, valproic acid, vitamin C (high dosage)
Encephalopathy	Hexachlorophene (neonates, topical), intrathecal penicillin G, vaccines (e.g., measles, mumps, rubella), toxoids (diphtheria, tetanus)
Epigastric Distress (*see also* Anorexia, Nausea, Peptic ulcers, and Vomiting)	Clindamycin, erythromycin, griseofulvin, iron (oral), isoniazid, methenamine, nalidixic acid, NSAIDs, potassium chloride (oral), protease inhibitors, sulfonamides, tetracyclines, theophylline, valproic acid, vitamin C, zidovudine
Exfoliative Dermatitis (*see also* Stevens-Johnson syndrome and Toxic epidermal necrolysis)	Carbamazepine, co-trimoxazole, phenobarbital, phenytoin, sulfonamides
Extrapyramidal Reactions (*see also* Akathisia and Akinesia)	Haloperidol, methyldopa, metoclopramide, phenothiazines, risperidone
Fever	Anticholinergics, cephalosporins, isoniazid, leukotriene antagonists, penicillins, phenytoin, procainamide, quinidine, sulfonamides, vaccines, vancomycin
Gingival Hyperplasia	Cyclosporine, nifedipine, phenytoin, verapamil
Gingivitis	Gold salts, vitamin A (high dosage)
Glaucoma	Corticosteroids (ophthalmic)
Goiter/Hypothyroidism	Lithium, potassium iodide (saturated solution), thioamides (high dosage)
Gray Baby Syndrome	Chloramphenicol (in neonates and with overdosages in older children)
Growth Suppression	Amphetamines, anabolic steroids, androgens, corticosteroids, methylphenidate, pemoline, quinolone antibiotics, tetracyclines, vitamin D (high dosage)
Hallucinations	Acyclovir, albuterol (salbutamol), alcohol, amantadine, amphetamines, anticholinergics, antihistamine overdosages, beta-adrenergic agonists, cimetidine, cocaine, cyclosporine, digitalis glycosides, phenytoin, procainamide, promethazine, propranolol, psychedelics (LSD, peyote, tetrahydrocannabinol [*see* Chapter 7]), salicylate therapy (chronic, long term), sulfonamides, tricyclic antidepressants, vincristine (high dosage)
Headache	Acyclovir, amphotericin B, anticholinergics, CNS stimulants (hypertensive headache), didanosine, ethosuximide, flecainide, fluconazole, ganciclovir, H_2-receptor antagonists, hydralazine, metronidazole, nitrofurantoin, propafenone, rifampin, theophylline
Hemochromatosis	Iron (high dosage)
Hepatic Dysfunction/Hepatitis	Acetaminophen overdosage, alcohol, aspirin (high dosage), chlorpromazine, cyclophosphamide, docusates, erythromycin, haloperidol, isoniazid, isotretinoin, ketoconazole (oral), methotrexate, methyldopa, pemoline, phenothiazines, phenytoin, propylthiouracil, quinidine, rifampin, sulfonamides, tetracyclines, thiazide diuretics, valproic acid, vitamin A (high dosage)
Hirsutism	Androgens, corticosteroids, cyclosporine, ethosuximide, minoxidil, phenytoin, spironolactone
Hypercalcemia	Calcium salts (high dosage), vitamin A (high dosage), vitamin D (high dosage)
Hyperglycemia	Corticosteroids, diazoxide, ethacrynic acid, furosemide, glucagon (high dosage), sympathomimetic amines, thiazide diuretics
Hypersensitivity Reactions (*see also* Anaphylaxis)	Many drugs, notably penicillin and beta-lactam antibiotics and drug formulations with certain additives (e.g., sulfites)
Hypertension	CNS stimulants (e.g., amphetamines, cocaine, methylphenidate, nicotine), sodium bicarbonate (high dosage), sympathomimetic amines

Footnote on page 288.

TABLE 5-6 continued

DISEASE OR CLINICAL CONDITION	POSSIBLE CAUSATIVE DRUGS
Hypoglycemia	Hypoglycemics, insulin
Hypokalemia	Amphotericin B, corticosteroids, diuretics (excluding potassium-sparing diuretics)
Hypotension	Alcohol, amantadine, antihypertensives, diuretics, flecainide, iron (injectable), lidocaine (injected), lithium, nitroglycerin, phenothiazines, phytonadione (allergic-type reaction), procainamide, quinidine (rapid IV infusion), ribavirin, theophylline (high dosage), vasodilators
Hypothermia	Alcohol, general anesthetics, barbiturates (high dosage or overdosage), beta-adrenergic blockers, clonidine (overdosage), insulin, lithium, opiate analgesics, prazocin, vasodilators
Hypothyroidism	Lithium
Increased Intracranial Pressure/Pseudotumor Cerebri	Isotretinoin, nalidixic acid, tetracycline, vitamin A (high dosage)
Insomnia	Acyclovir (high dosage), beta-adrenergic agonists, CNS stimulants (e.g., amphetamines, caffeine, cocaine, nicotine), SSRIs, theophylline
Jaundice	Erythromycin, methyldopa; in neonates, caffeine/sodium benzoate, chlorpromazine, nalidixic acid, nitrofurantoin, novobiocin, primaquine, salicylates, sodium benzoate, sulfonamides
Learning Impairment (cognitive dysfunction)	Anticonvulsants, beta-adrenergic blockers, CNS depressants (alcohol [acute intoxication, fetal alcohol syndrome], benzodiazepines, and other sedative-hypnotics), cocaine (acute intoxication, fetal cocaine effects), opiate analgesics, tetrahydrocannabinol and other psychedelics
Lymphadenopathy	Iron (injectable), primidone
Nausea	Antineoplastics (see Chapter 12), ethosuximide, ketoconazole, macrolides; some degree of nausea occurs with almost any orally ingested drug
Neuroleptic Malignant Syndrome	Antipsychotics
Nightmares/Night Terrors	Alcohol, benzodiazepines, chloral hydrate, ethosuximide
Nystagmus	Carbamazepine, phenobarbital, phenytoin, primidone
Pancreatitis	Didanosine
Paralysis	Oral polio vaccine
Paranoia (see also Psychosis)	Acyclovir (high dosage), amphetamines, anticholinergics (high dosage), cocaine, corticosteroids, isoniazid, phenylephrine, tetrahydrocannabinol
Peptic Ulcers	Alcohol, caffeine, chloral hydrate, corticosteroids, NSAIDs, tobacco smoking
Peripheral Neuropathy	Didanosine, hydralazine, isoniazid, phenytoin (chronic, long term)
Photosensitivity (see also Visual dysfunction)	Anticholinergics, carbamazepine, coal tar, dacarbazine, haloperidol, nalidixic acid, phenothiazines, sulfonamides, tetracyclines, thiazide diuretics
Pneumonitis (see also Respiratory dysfunction)	Amiodarone, gold salts, nitrofurantoin
Porphyria	Barbiturates
Pseudomembranous Colitis	Chloramphenicol, clindamycin, imipenem–cilastatin, lincosamides (oral or injectable), metronidazole (rare), penicillins (infrequently), tetracyclines
Psychosis	Alcohol, amantadine, amphetamines, anabolic steroids, anticholinergics, ciprofloxacin, cocaine, corticosteroids, ephedrine, isotretinoin, lysergic acid diethylamide (LSD), methylphenidate, oxybutynin
Red Man Syndrome	Vancomycin
Renal Dysfunction	Aminoglycosides, amphotericin B, cisplatin, cyclosporine, furosemide, ifosfamide, isotretinoin, methotrexate (high dosage), NSAIDs, sulfonamides, tetracyclines (outdated), vancomycin, vitamin C (high dosage)
Respiratory Dysfunction (see also Asthma, Bronchospasm, and Pneumonitis)	Cannabis (smoking), clonazepam, diazepam, isoniazid, loperamide, nitrofurantoin, opiate analgesics, pentobarbital, phenobarbital, primidone, propafenone, ribavirin, sedative-hypnotics, tobacco smoking
Reyes' Syndrome	Aspirin (when used for symptomatic management of flulike conditions in children and adolescents)
Rickets	Phenobarbital, phenytoin, primidone
Skin Rash (see also Red man syndrome, Stevens-Johnson syndrome, and Urticaria)	Many drugs, as part of a hypersensitivity syndrome
Staphylococcal Enterocolitis	Chloramphenicol, tetracycline

TABLE 5-6 *continued*

DISEASE OR CLINICAL CONDITION	POSSIBLE CAUSATIVE DRUGS
Stevens-Johnson Syndrome (*see also* Exfoliative dermatitis and Toxic epidermal necrolysis)	Barbiturates, carbamazepine (oral or injectable), clindamycin, ethosuximide, fluoxetine, iodides, penicillins, phenytoin, salicylates, sulfonamides, tetracyclines
Stomatitis, Ulcerative	Methotrexate
Systemic Lupus Erythematosus	Carbamazepine, hydralazine, isoniazid, methyldopa, penicillamine, phenytoin, primidone, procainamide, sulfonamides
Tardive Dyskinesia	Antipsychotics
Thrombophlebitis	Virtually all intravenously administered drugs, especially amphotericin B, cephalosporins, clindamycin, erythromycin, phenytoin, tetracyclines
Tinnitus (*see also* Deafness/Hearing loss)	Aminoglycosides, antimalarials, aspirin, indomethacin, quinidine, tricyclic antidepressants
Tooth Discoloration	Iron (oral liquid formulations), tetracyclines
Tourette's Syndrome	Amphetamines, cocaine, methylphenidate, pemoline
Toxic Epidermal Necrolysis (*see also* Stevens-Johnson syndrome)	Allopurinol, carbamazepine, co-trimoxazole, sulfonamides
Tremor	Amantadine, amphetamines, anticholinergics, antihistamines, hydralazine, lithium, mexiletine, methylphenidate, pemoline, tricyclic antidepressants, SSRIs, theophylline
Urticaria	Aspirin, cephalosporins, penicillins, sulfonamides
Vertigo/Vestibular Dysfunction	Aminoglycosides, haloperidol, indomethacin, minocycline, phenytoin, primidone
Visual Dysfunction (*see also* Cataracts and Photosensitivity)	Alcohol, anticholinergics (and other drugs possessing atropinelike activity), carbamazepine, corticosteroids, digoxin (overdosage), flecainide, NSAIDs, primidone, propafenone, tetrahydrocannabinol and other psychedelics
Vomiting	Virtually all orally administered drugs, especially antineoplastics, erythromycin, ketoconazole, quinidine, vaccines
Xerostomia	Anticholinergics, antihistamines, antipsychotics (e.g., chlorpromazine, haloperidol), tricyclic antidepressants

Footnote on page 288.

TABLE 5-7
Drugs Commonly Required by Infants, Children, and Adolescents: Associated ADRs and Clinical Comments

The ADRs associated with specific drugs commonly required by infants, children, and adolescents are listed. These drugs were included because of their clinical significance in relation to ADRs. The table is not all-inclusive; only the most common drugs and the frequently reported ADRs are listed. For additional information regarding the ADRs associated with a particular drug, readers are encouraged to also consult other tables and chapters of this text as well as other authoritative references.

Some ADRs are ubiquitous with drug therapy. As an illustration, virtually every drug has the potential to cause a hypersensitivity reaction in susceptible patients. In addition, virtually all intravenously administered drugs have the potential to cause phlebitis or thrombophlebitis. Likewise, virtually all orally administered drugs have the potential to cause some degree of GI distress. Generally, these essentially "universal" ADRs are not specifically mentioned unless some special consideration warrants it (e.g., the incidence is particularly high, suggesting that some unique characteristic of the drug is responsible).

To facilitate the use of the table, the drugs have been listed by generic name and arranged according to pharmacologic or therapeutic classification. Drugs that fall into two or more pharmacologic or therapeutic categories have been arbitrarily assigned to only one category (e.g., Hydrochlorothiazide is classified under Diuretics not Antihypertensives). Readers also can use the Index to locate a particular drug and its associated ADRs.

TABLE 5-7 continued

ANALGESICS (*see also* Antiarthritics)

Nonopiates

Acetaminophen (Paracetamol) *(Tempra®, Tylenol®)*

Acetaminophen in recommended dosages is relatively nontoxic. Dermatologic reactions, including pruritic maculopapular rash and urticaria as well as other hypersensitivity reactions, including anaphylaxis, angioedema, and laryngeal edema, have been reported but are uncommon. The most common severe ADR is potentially fatal hepatic necrosis after an overdosage. Hepatic injury also has been reported with the regular long-term use of larger dosages over a prolonged period of time. In addition, excessive alcohol consumption significantly increases the risk for acetaminophen-induced hepatic injury, even at therapeutic dosages. Thus, it is important to evaluate acetaminophen intake from all sources because it is commonly included in many prescription and nonprescription products. Overdosages are treated with acetylcysteine (*see* Chapter 4).

Aspirin (Acetylsalicylic Acid) *(ASA®, Entrophen®)* (*see also* Antiarthritics, Nonsteroidal Anti-Inflammatory Drugs)

GI effects (epigastric distress, dyspepsia, heartburn, nausea, vomiting) occur in 2%–10% of patients receiving analgesic or antipyretic dosages of aspirin. The incidence is higher with anti-inflammatory dosages (*see* Chapter 14); the GI effects can be reduced by giving aspirin with antacids, food, or milk or water (240 ml or more). If GI bleeding occurs, it is usually mild, although chronic, long-term use of aspirin can lead to anemia. Higher dosages may cause gastric ulceration. Tinnitus can occur among susceptible patients at therapeutic dosages but is more usually a sign of high salicylate serum concentrations. However, salicylate poisoning (with metabolic disturbances and toxicity) can occur in the absence of tinnitus. Hypersensitivity reactions (bronchospasm, hypotension, urticaria, rhinitis, rarely angioedema) appear to occur in higher frequency among children with a history of nasal polyps, asthma, or chronic urticaria. A single dose of aspirin can precipitate aspirin-sensitive asthma. The antiplatelet effects of aspirin can predispose patients to bleeding, especially if they are receiving concomitant anticoagulant therapy. Aspirin use in patients with varicella or influenzalike illness should be avoided because it is associated with Reyes' syndrome, a severe and often fatal hepatic encephalopathy. In these patients, acetaminophen usually can be safely substituted.

Chronic high-dose salicylate therapy for juvenile rheumatoid arthritis can result in salicylism. Early signs and symptoms of salicylism include CNS stimulation, hyperthermia, and vomiting, followed by CNS depression, lethargy, and metabolic acidosis (*see* Chapter 4). Salicylism can be confused with Reyes' syndrome among pediatric patients.

Opiates

Note: The long-term use (several weeks) of opiate analgesics can result in habituation (psychological dependence) and addiction (physical dependence), which is characterized by tolerance and the opiate analgesic-withdrawal syndrome.

Codeine

Fentanyl

Meperidine (Pethidine) *(Demerol®)*

Morphine *(M.O.S.®, Morphitec®)*

Opiate analgesics can cause constipation, dizziness, drowsiness, euphoria, mental clouding, miosis, nausea, respiratory depression, sedation, and vomiting. Toxicity is usually dose related, although some patients appear to develop hypersensitivity reactions (e.g., urticaria) with usual therapeutic dosages. Nonfatal overdosages can be treated effectively with the opiate antagonist, naloxone (*see* Chapter 4).

ANTIARTHRITICS

Nonsteroidal Anti-Inflammatory Drugs (NSAIDs)

Aspirin *(ASA®, Entrophen®)* (*see also* Analgesics, Nonopiates)

Ibuprofen *(Advil®, Motrin®)*

Indomethacin *(Indocid®, Indocin®)*

Naproxen *(Anaprox®, Naprosyn®)*

Tolmetin *(Tolectin®)*

Adverse effects of NSAIDs on the GI system range from gastritis to severe perforation and bleeding and are not always symptomatic. The incidence of these ADRs is reportedly higher with indomethacin than with the other NSAIDs; for this reason, indomethacin is generally not recommended for the treatment of juvenile rheumatoid arthritis among children. The mechanism by which the NSAIDs cause ADRs affecting the GI system is believed to be due to inhibition of prostaglandin-mediated GI protection.

ADRs affecting the CNS range from headache (usually worse in the morning) and dizziness to delirium and hallucinations. NSAIDs also can cause ADRs affecting the renal system, including reduced glomerular filtration and sodium retention. In addition, when NSAIDs are used for closure of the ductus arteriosus among neonates, especially preterm neonates, renal dysfunction may occur. Some NSAIDs (particularly indomethacin) are associated with

TABLE 5-7 continued

hematologic ADRs, including serious blood dyscrasias. Cross-hypersensitivity among the various NSAIDs can occur in pediatric patients.

Remittive Agents

Gold Sodium Thiomalate (Sodium Aurothiomalate) *(Myochrysine®)*

Approximately 30% of patients treated with gold sodium thiomalate develop ADRs that require discontinuation of therapy. Gingivitis, glossitis, and stomatitis can occur. Adverse mucocutaneous reactions, including pruritus followed by skin rash, are more common with intramuscular drug delivery. Sunlight can exacerbate dermatitis. Renal effects (e.g., proteinuria and membranous glomerulonephritis) are seen. These ADRs are usually mild and reversible after therapy is discontinued but may be severe and persist with continued use of the drug. Gold also causes blood dyscrasias (e.g., agranulocytosis and leukopenia, which can be fatal), conjunctivitis (rarely), GI distress, and hypersensitivity reactions. Patients must be monitored closely for these ADRs.

Methotrexate (Amethopterin)

The incidence and severity of ADRs from methotrexate are dose related. Common ADRs include abdominal distress, chills, dizziness, fatigue, fever, leukopenia, nausea, and ulcerative stomatitis. Methotrexate also can cause bone marrow suppression and hepatic, renal, and pulmonary toxicities. Sudden death and death caused by interstitial pneumonitis have been reported. Toxic hematopoetic effects can be minimized by treatment ("rescue") with leucovorin (citrovorum factor) *(see* Chapter 12).

Penicillamine *(Cuprimine®, Depen®)*

Penicillamine frequently produces ADRs, including fever, GI distress, joint pain, lymphadenopathy, pruritus, skin rash, and urticaria. A systemic lupuslike reaction or nephrotic syndrome with slight proteinuria may develop; these effects may improve spontaneously or with a reduction in dosage. Hematologic effects (e.g., agranulocytosis, anemia, bone marrow depression, thrombocytopenia) have been reported. Penicillamine also may decrease taste perception.

ANTIBIOTICS

Note: The use of most antibiotics can result in the overgrowth of nonsusceptible organisms and superinfection. Antibiotic selection for severe infections should always be based on culture and sensitivity testing with the exception of initial prescribing for the first several days while awaiting test results. Patients who develop chronic or bloody diarrhea while receiving antibiotic therapy should be assessed for pseudomembranous colitis. The management of pseudomembranous colitis depends on the clinical condition of the patient. However, in most cases, the management includes discontinuation of the causative antibiotic; sigmoidoscopy to confirm the diagnosis of pseudomembranous colitis; appropriate bacteriological studies to positively identify the pathogen; fluid, electrolyte, and protein replacement; and antibiotic therapy, generally oral vancomycin therapy. *(See also* Antifungals, Antivirals.)

Aminoglycosides

Amikacin *(Amikin®)*
Gentamicin *(Garamycin®)*
Neomycin
Netilmicin *(Netromycin®)*
Streptomycin
Tobramycin *(Nebcin®)*

The most serious ADRs associated with aminoglycosides are ototoxicity and nephrotoxicity. Ototoxicity is caused by damage to the eighth cranial nerve and may be manifested by ataxia, dizziness, nystagmus, tinnitus, vertigo, or varying degrees of permanent hearing impairment, including deafness. Nephrotoxicity is usually reversible following discontinuation of aminoglycoside therapy, although deaths from aminoglycoside-induced renal failure have been reported. Both ototoxicity and nephrotoxicity occur when drug serum concentrations are elevated due to reduction in renal drug excretion. Aminoglycoside dosages should be reduced for neonates, infants, and children with renal dysfunction *(see* Chapters 13 and 14) because aminoglycosides are primarily excreted by the kidneys in unchanged form. Prescribing appropriate dosages, limiting therapy to 10 consecutive days or less, and careful therapeutic drug monitoring *(see* Chapters 10 and 14) should reduce the incidence of these serious ADRs.

Cephalosporins

Cefaclor *(Ceclor®)*
Cefadroxil *(Duricef®)*
Cefamandole *(Mandol®)*
Cefazolin *(Ancef®)*
Cefixime *(Suprax®)*
Cefoperazone *(Cefobid®)*
Cefotaxime *(Claforan®)*
Cefoxitin
Cefpodoxime *(Vantin®)*
Ceftazidime *(Fortaz®)*
Ceftizoxime *(Cefizox®)*
Ceftriaxone *(Rocephin®)*
Cefuroxime *(Zinacef®)*
Cefuroxime Axetil *(Ceftin®)*
Cephalexin *(Keflex®)*
Cephalothin *(Ceporacin®)*
Cephapirin *(Cefadyl®)*
Cefprozil *(Cefzil®)*

Hypersensitivity reactions to cephalosporins occur, including angioedema, joint pain, serum sickness, urticaria, and, rarely, fatal anaphylaxis. Fatalities are more common with penicillin allergy, where cross-sensitivity to cephalo-

TABLE 5-7 *continued*

sporins may be present in 10%–30% of patients. However, many patients have been incorrectly identified as penicillin allergic. Delayed-onset serum sickness is more common among children than adults treated with cefaclor, occurring in approximately 0.5% of patients. Hypernatremia may occur when large dosages of cephalosporin sodium salts are administered to patients with renal dysfunction. Intravenous administration frequently causes thrombophlebitis.

Fluoroquinolones

Ciprofloxacin *(Cipro®)*

ADRs associated with ciprofloxacin usually involve the GI system (abdominal pain, diarrhea, nausea, vomiting) or CNS (confusion, dizziness, headache, insomia, lightheadedness, restlessness, seizures, tremor) and may require discontinuation of therapy. Ciprofloxacin is contraindicated for patients with a history of hypersensitivity to any quinolone because of the potential for a fatal hypersensitivity reaction. Ciprofloxacin rarely causes arthralgia and tendonitis (usually involving the fingers), delirium, hallucinations, torsades de pointes, and toxic epidermal necrolysis. The safety of ciprofloxacin in prepubertal children has been questioned because of reports of arthropathy in several species of immature animals; however, this effect has not been observed in several large studies of children treated with ciprofloxacin.

Macrolides

Azithromycin *(Zithromax®)*

Serious ADRs are uncommon. Nausea, vomiting, diarrhea, and abdominal pain can occur, but much less frequently than with erythromycin. Rash can occur; however, true hypersensitivity appears to be quite rare.

Clarithromycin *(Biaxin®)*

Serious ADRs are uncommon. Nausea, vomiting, diarrhea, and abdominal pain can occur, but much less frequently than with erythromycin. May also occasionally cause abnormal taste, dizziness, and headache. Rash can occur, and hypersensitivity can occur rarely.

Erythromycin *(Ery-Tab®, Erythrocin®)*

Epigastric distress (abdominal pain, cramping) is frequently observed during erythromycin therapy, especially after the ingestion of high oral dosages. Nausea, vomiting, and diarrhea also can occur. Hypersensitivity reactions such as skin rash, fever, and eosinophilia rarely occur and are usually mild. Cholestatic jaundice can occur (particularly with erythromycin estolate) and, thus, erythromycin therapy should be generally avoided for patients with hepatic disease.

Penicillins

Amoxicillin *(Amoxil®)*	Nafcillin *(Nafcil®)*
Ampicillin *(Polycillin®)*	Oxacillin *(Prostaphlin®)*
Carbenicillin Indanyl *(Geocillin®)*	Penicillin G
Cloxacillin	Penicillin V
Dicloxacillin *(Dycill®)*	Piperacillin *(Pipracil®)*
Mezlocillin *(Mezlin®)*	Ticarcillin *(Ticar®)*

Hypersensitivity reactions occur in approximately 5%–10% of patients and include angioedema, joint pain, serum sickness, urticaria, and rarely fatal anaphylaxis. There also is an 80% cross-sensitivity with other penicillins. Skin testing with the major and minor determinant mixture is predictive for a serious or life-threatening ADR. Epinephrine (adrenaline) is the drug of choice for a serious hypersensitivity reaction.

ADRs affecting the GI system (diarrhea, epigastric distress, nausea, vomiting) are common during oral penicillin therapy. Amoxicillin has the same spectrum of activity as ampicillin but causes less diarrhea and generally is preferred for pediatric patients. Rash occurs frequently with both amoxicillin and ampicillin. In the presence of renal dysfunction, high dosages of penicillin G can cause excessive serum concentrations and confusion, lethargy, and seizures. High intravenous dosages of the sodium and potassium salts of penicillin should be avoided in patients who have renal dysfunction because of the potential for hypernatremia and hyperkalemia, respectively.

Quinolones

Nalidixic Acid *(NegGram®)*

Nalidixic acid is usually well tolerated, with the usual ADRs being abdominal pain, diarrhea, nausea, and vomiting. These ADRs can be reduced by ingesting each dose of nalidixic acid with food, although each dose is often ingested on an empty stomach to increase absorption. Allergic reactions occur occasionally and usually consist of eosinophilia, fever, photosensitivity, skin rash, or urticaria. Convulsions have been reported in children who had epilepsy when usual therapeutic dosages were used and in children who did not have epilepsy when higher than usual dosages were used.

Increased intracranial pressure with bulging anterior fontanelle, papilledema, and headache have been described in some infants. Hemolytic anemia has been reported among patients who have glucose-6-phosphate dehydrogenase

TABLE 5-7 continued

deficiency. Thus, nalidixic acid should be used with caution, if at all, for patients who have this enzyme deficiency. Contraindications include known hypersensitivity to nalidixic acid or other quinolones and a history of seizures. Patients with severe renal dysfunction may accumulate the drug and experience convulsions, toxic psychosis, and metabolic acidosis. Direct exposure of the skin to sunlight should be avoided during nalidixic acid therapy to reduce photosensitivity reactions. Complete blood counts and renal function tests should be performed periodically when nalidixic acid therapy is required for more than 2 weeks.

Sulfonamides
Sulfamethoxazole *(Gantanol®)*
Sulfisoxazole *(Gantrisin®)*

Common ADRs associated with systemically administered sulfonamides include allergic reactions, anorexia, nausea, and vomiting. Allergic reactions include urticarial reactions that may occur after several days of sulfonamide therapy, maculopapular rashes, and delayed-onset hypersensitivity reactions characterized by fever, photosensitivity, and rash, often toxic epidermal necrolysis or erythema multiforme, and occasionally involvement of lungs, heart, liver, kidneys, and bone marrow. These ADRs can progress to the Stevens-Johnson syndrome and, thus, the sulfonamide should be discontinued immediately if any signs and symptoms of these ADRs develop. It is possible, however, that progression to the Stevens-Johnson syndrome may occur despite the discontinuation of sulfonamide therapy. ADRs involving the hematopoetic system include agranulocytosis, aplastic anemia, eosinophilia, granulocytopenia, hemolytic anemia, hypoprothrombinemia, leukopenia, methemoglobinemia, and thrombocytopenia. Fortunately, these ADRs usually subside with the discontinuation of the offending sulfonamide. Crystalluria may occur if high sulfonamide dosages are administered or if the patient is dehydrated. Crystalluria can be prevented by ensuring adequate hydration. Periodic hematologic monitoring should be conducted during chronic long-term sulfonamide therapy. Sulfonamide therapy generally should be avoided among neonates because of its association with kernicterus.

Tetracyclines
Doxycycline *(Vibramycin®)*
Minocycline *(Minocin®)*
Tetracycline *(Apo-Tetra®, Novo-Tetra®, Nu-Tetra®)*

Common ADRs associated with the tetracyclines include diarrhea, epigastric distress, nausea, photosensitivity, and vomiting. Vomiting occurs most often with minocycline, which also is commonly associated with ADRs involving the CNS such as ataxia, dizziness, drowsiness, fatigue, and lightheadedness. Fatigue occurs generally less commonly with doxycycline. Hypersensitivity reactions are rare. Photosensitivity reactions also have been described, as have bulging fontanels among infants. Tetracycline therapy prior to the formation of the permanent teeth produces dental staining and enamel hypoplasia. Tetracyclines also interfere with the growth of the fibula, but this effect is usually reversible. Due to these effects on dental and bony tissues, tetracycline therapy should be avoided during the last half of pregnancy and in all infants and children younger than 8 years. High-dose tetracycline therapy can cause hepatic damage, especially if administered intravenously. Tetracyclines are catabolic and can cause weight loss in debilitated patients. Superinfection involving *Candida*, staphylococci, or *Clostridium difficile* can occur. Diarrhea occurring during tetracycline therapy should be investigated to rule out potentially fatal staphylococcal enterocolitis or pseudomembranous colitis. Degraded tetracycline products are highly nephrotoxic (capable of causing an acute Fanconilike syndrome) and, thus, outdated tetracycline should not be used. Some tetracycline formulations contain sulfites that may cause hypersensitivity reactions among susceptible pediatric patients (those who have a history of asthma).

Miscellaneous Antibiotics
Aztreonam *(Azactam®)*

Aztreonam is generally well tolerated. However, it has been associated with hypersensitivity reactions (e.g., anaphylaxis), diarrhea, nausea, skin rash, and vomiting. Transient eosinophilia occurs in up to 10% of patients whereas other blood dyscrasias (e.g., anemia, leukopenia, thrombocytopenia) occur in less than 1% of patients. Injectable aztreonam therapy has been associated with phlebitis (intravenous route) or pain at the injection site (intramuscular route) in approximately 3% of patients.

Chloramphenicol *(Pentamycetin®)*

Bone marrow suppression with aplastic anemia, granulocytopenia, leukopenia, and thrombocytopenia is the most feared complication of chloramphenicol therapy. This ADR occurs in two forms: a dose-related form that is reversible when dosages are reduced or when chloramphenicol therapy is discontinued, and an idiosyncratic and irreversible form that does not improve despite the discontinuation of therapy. This latter form is quite uncommon and is not related to the chloramphenicol dosage or duration of therapy. Regular monitoring of blood counts during chloramphenicol therapy is recommended, especially if chronic long-term therapy is required. ADRs also can involve the GI system (diarrhea, nausea, vomiting) and various hypersensitivity reactions, including anaphylactic reactions,

TABLE 5-7 continued

may occur. Chloramphenicol in high dosages can cause the gray baby syndrome among infants, older children, and adolescents. The syndrome starts with abdominal distention and muscle flaccidity and progresses to ashen-gray cyanosis, cardiovascular collapse, and death. Previous serious toxicity or hypersensitivity to chloramphenicol is a contraindication for further therapy. Dosages should be reduced or dosing intervals increased for patients with hepatic failure to avoid drug accumulation. Chloramphenicol serum concentrations should be monitored during therapy and, at the first sign of toxicity, the chloramphenicol should be discontinued because the gray baby syndrome can be reversed if therapy is discontinued early enough. Due to its toxicity, chloramphenicol should be reserved for serious infections unresponsive to less toxic drugs.

Clindamycin *(Cleocin®, Dalacin C®)*

Common ADRs involve the GI system (abdominal pain, diarrhea, nausea, vomiting) and allergic reactions. Skin reactions (maculopapular rash, pruritus, urticaria), fever, hypotension, and, rarely, polyarthritis have been reported. An uncommon, but potentially fatal, ADR is pseudomembranous colitis, which is caused by toxin-producing and antibiotic-resistant clostridia. This ADR is characterized by severe diarrhea and abdominal cramps. Thus, clindamycin should be reserved for serious infections that are not treatable by other, less toxic, drugs. Any serious diarrhea that occurs during clindamycin therapy should be promptly investigated (note that diarrhea, colitis, and pseudomembranous colitis reportedly may begin up to 1-month following the discontinuation of clindamycin therapy).

Co-trimoxazole (trimethoprim and sulfamethoxazole combination product) *(Bactrim®, Septra®)*

Common ADRs include anorexia, nausea, vomiting, and allergic skin reactions (erythema multiforme, maculopapular eruptions, pruritus, urticaria). More serious reactions, such as Stevens-Johnson syndrome or blood dyscrasias (e.g., acute megaloblastic anemia, granulocytopenia, thrombocytopenia), also are possible. Hemolysis may occur in pediatric patients who have glucose-6-phosphate dehydrogenase deficiency (*see also* Sulfonamides).

Imipenem–Cilastatin *(Primaxin®)*

Erythema, pain, phlebitis, and thrombophlebitis may occur at the injection site during imipenem–cilastatin therapy. Nausea, vomiting, and transient hypotension may occur during intravenous infusion. ADRs involving the CNS (e.g., confusion, seizures) are rare, but appear to occur more commonly in patients with underlying CNS disorders. Drug-induced cases of pseudomembranous colitis have been reported.

Isoniazid (Isonicotinic Acid Hydrazide) *(Nydrazid®)*

Approximately 15% of patients treated with isoniazid experience an ADR, particularly those patients who are either slow acetylators of isoniazid (*see* Chapter 11) or pyridoxine (vitamin B_6) deficient. Pyridoxine should be administered to both malnourished infants and children treated with isoniazid and to patients who will be treated with high dosages of isoniazid in order to prevent, or reverse, isoniazid-induced peripheral neuropathy. Blood dyscrasias, epigastric distress, glossitis, hepatitis (potentially fatal), hypersensitivity reactions (fever and skin rash), nausea, vomiting, and peripheral neuropathy have been described. Isoniazid overdosages can produce metabolic acidosis, respiratory distress, and seizures. High dosages of pyridoxine should be used for isoniazid overdosages in addition to standard poisoning management for the treatment of associated seizures (*see* Chapter 4). Severe untreated isoniazid overdosages can result in coma and death.

Methenamine *(Hiprex®, Mandelamine®)*

Approximately 5% of patients treated with methenamine develop ADRs involving the GI system (e.g., anorexia, cramps, diarrhea, stomatitis, vomiting). Large dosages may irritate the urinary bladder, resulting in crystalluria, dysuria, hematuria, proteinuria, urinary frequency, and urinary urgency.

Metronidazole *(Flagyl®)*

Oral metronidazole commonly causes anorexia, headache, a metallic taste, and nausea. It also may cause peripheral neuropathy and seizures, particularly with high cumulative doses. Peripheral neuropathy may be irreversible in some cases. Rarely causes a profound neurological deterioration and pseudomembranous colitis.

Nitrofurantoin *(MacroBID®, Macrodantin®)*

The most common ADRs associated with nitrofurantoin therapy are anorexia, discoloration of the urine (rust yellow to brown), nausea, and vomiting. Abdominal pain, allergic skin reactions, diarrhea, dizziness, drowsiness, headache, nystagmus, peripheral neuropathy (including optic neuritis), and vertigo are reported less frequently. Hemolytic anemia may occur during nitrofurantoin therapy in neonates related to their immature glutathione enzyme systems. The hemolytic anemia predisposes these neonates to kernicterus. Older infants and children with glucose-6-phosphate dehydrogenase deficiency experience hemolysis (rare), and, thus, nitrofurantoin therapy should be used with caution in patients with this enzyme deficiency. Acute, subacute, and chronic pulmonary reactions (potentially fatal) have been reported. These reactions (diffuse interstitial pneumonitis, pulmonary fibrosis), which develop insidiously, occur rarely, particularly among patients who are receiving chronic long-term nitrofurantoin therapy (therapy lasting 6 months or longer).

TABLE 5-7 continued

Rifampin *(Rifadin®, Rimactane®)*

    Rifampin therapy is associated with anorexia, intestinal cramps, epigastric distress, elevation of hepatic enzymes (*see* Chapter 6), fatigue, headache, mental confusion, nausea, and skin rash. Rarely causes jaundice. High-dosage therapy produces a flulike syndrome in up to 50% of patients. May discolor cerebrospinal fluid, contact lenses, feces, saliva, sweat, tears, and urine red–orange.

Trimethoprim *(Proloprim®)*

    Trimethoprim therapy has been associated with epigastric distress, glossitis, nausea, skin rash, and vomiting in up to 5% of patients. It may also cause blood dyscrasias including megaloblastic anemia, neutropenia, and thrombocytopenia.

Vancomycin *(Vancocin®)*

    Vancomycin therapy is frequently associated with chills and fever. It also can cause nephrotoxicity and ototoxicity when therapy is prolonged or when large dosages are required, particularly among patients who have renal dysfunction. Serial monitoring of renal and auditory function should be performed if long-term, chronic therapy is planned. Rapid intravenous infusion is associated with the red man (red neck) syndrome, which may include sudden hypotension; an erythematous rash and flushing of the face, neck, chest, and upper extremities; pruritus; dyspnea; urticaria; and wheezing. Infusion rates slower than 10 mg/min are associated with fewer infusion-related ADRs. Pain and phlebitis may occur at the infusion site.

ANTICHOLINERGICS

Atropine
Glycopyrrolate
Ipratropium Bromide *(Atrovent®)*
Scopolamine (Hyoscine)

    Common ADRs associated with the systemic use of anticholinergics include blurred vision, constipation, drowsiness, dry mouth, photophobia, tachycardia, and urinary retention. Other ADRs include confusion, dizziness, headache, hypersensitivity reactions, and tremor. Inhibited perspiration (anhidrosis) also can occur and can produce hyperthermia in patients in a hot environment. Infants and small children (especially those with Downs' syndrome, acquired brain injury, or spasticity) may be more susceptible to anticholinergic-induced ADRs. Physostigmine salicylate is an effective antidote for poisonings involving the anticholinergics (*see* Chapters 4 and 14).

ANTICOAGULANTS

Note: Blood clotting times (prothrombin time [PT] or international normalized ratio [INR] for warfarin therapy, or activated partial thromboplastin time [aPTT] for heparin therapy) should be monitored during anticoagulant therapy, as appropriate, to optimize therapeutic effect and minimize the incidence of ADRs.

Injectable

Heparin

    Hemorrhage (bleeding) is the most common ADR associated with heparin therapy and is estimated to occur in up to 10% of treated patients. Heparin is administered intravenously. Intramuscular administration should be avoided in order to prevent associated hematoma formation in the muscle and bleeding at the injection site (*see* Chapter 1). Heparin should be dosed conservatively and the concurrent use of aspirin and other drugs that have anticoagulant or antiplatelet effects should be avoided whenever possible (*see* Chapter 6). Reversible thrombocytopenia may develop, usually during the first 3 weeks of heparin therapy. Heparin-induced thrombocytopenia (HIT) is believed to be an allergic-type reaction. Two forms of HIT may occur, a mild form associated with less severe ADRs and a much more severe form in which patients may "paradoxically" develop potentially fatal thrombotic complications, including arterial thrombosis, disseminated intravascular coagulation, gangrene, myocardial infarction, and stroke. The thrombosis is due to "white clots" comprised of fibrin and platelets. Thus, pediatric patients who are receiving acute heparin therapy should have their platelet counts monitored at least every 2 or 3 days and should be otherwise closely clinically monitored. Hypersensitivity reactions, probably caused by preservatives in certain heparin formulations, have been reported and include chills, fever, urticaria, and, rarely, anaphylactic shock. It is important to individualize the heparin dosage by monitoring activated partial thromboplastin time (aPTT). Protamine sulfate is used intravenously as an antidote for excessive bleeding caused by heparin overdosage (*see* Chapter 14).

    The low-molecular-weight heparin formulations are increasingly replacing conventional heparin formulations. Although clinical experience involving pediatric patients is limited, the rate of ADRs with the low-molecular-weight heparin formulations is reportedly low.

Oral

Warfarin *(Coumadin®)*

    Serious bleeding can occur with excessive warfarin dosages. Warfarin should be avoided in pediatric patients with active peptic ulcer disease, cerebral thrombosis, or severe hypertension. Anticoagulation response should be

TABLE 5-7 continued

monitored closely using PT or INR, particularly when warfarin therapy is initiated or adjusted. Phytonadione (vitamin K_1) is a specific antidote for warfarin overdosages (*see* Chapter 14). Avoid, or carefully monitor, the concurrent use of drugs that interact with warfarin (*see* Chapter 6).

ANTICONVULSANTS

Note: Therapeutic drug monitoring should be performed during anticonvulsant therapy to optimize therapeutic effect and to minimize the incidence of ADRs (*see* Chapters 10 and 14). Abrupt discontinuation of anticonvulsant therapy, particularly in pediatric patients who have been receiving chronic long-term, high-dosage therapy, may result in status epilepticus.

Benzodiazepines (*see also* Sedative-Hypnotics)

Clobazam *(Frisium®)*

Clonazepam *(Klonopin®, Rivotril®)*

Diazepam *(Valium®)*

Lorazepam *(Ativan®)*

Nitrazepam *(Mogadon®)*

Ataxia, dizziness, drowsiness, lightheadedness, and sedation are common dose-related ADRs associated with the benzodiazepines. These ADRs occur in approximately 50% of patients. However, they usually subside with the continuation of the benzodiazepine therapy. Behavioral effects (e.g., aggression, hyperactivity, irritability, difficulty concentrating, learning impairment) occur in approximately 25% of patients and can be troublesome. Psychological or physical dependence (habituation and addiction) may develop with chronic long-term benzodiazepine therapy, even at recommended dosages.

Miscellaneous Anticonvulsants

Carbamazepine *(Tegretol®)*

The most common ADRs associated with carbamazepine therapy include ataxia, blurred vision, diplopia, dizziness, drowsiness, nausea, and nystagmus. Tolerance to these ADRs tends to develop with continued carbamazepine therapy. Hypersensitivity-related skin rash occurs in up to 3% of patients and includes altered pigmentation, photosensitivity, exfoliative dermatitis, Stevens-Johnson syndrome, and aggravation of existing systemic lupus erythematosus. Blood dyscrasias (e.g., aplastic anemia, agranulocytosis, eosinophilia, leukopenia, thrombocytopenia) also have been associated with carbamazepine use. Carbamazepine and the tricyclic antidepressants are chemically related and, thus, share some of the same ADRs (anticholinergic effects) and precautions. Contraindications to carbamazepine therapy include a history of hypersensitivity to carbamazepine or a tricyclic antidepressant. Carbamazepine therapy should be initiated with low dosages and serum concentrations should be monitored to achieve and maintain a therapeutic range between 4 and 10 µg/ml (17–43 µmol/liter) (*see* Chapter 14). Moderate carbamazepine overdosages may paradoxically increase seizure activity. Complete blood counts, renal and hepatic function, and vision should be monitored frequently during therapy to detect carbamazepine toxicity. Whenever possible, carbamazepine therapy should be discontinued gradually to minimize the risk for status epilepticus.

Ethosuximide *(Zarontin®)*

ADRs commonly associated with ethosuximide therapy include dizziness, drowsiness, GI distress (e.g., abdominal pain, anorexia, cramps, nausea, vomiting), headache, hiccups, and lethargy. Tolerance to these ADRs typically develops with continued therapy. Photophobia and blurred vision also may occur. Periodic complete blood counts are recommended because ethosuximide has been associated with blood dyscrasias (e.g., agranulocytosis, aplastic anemia, leukopenia). Ethosuximide therapy also has been associated with the occurrence of behavioral/mental disorders (aggressiveness, inability to concentrate, night terrors) and should be discontinued if ataxia or behavioral/mental disorders occur. In addition, skin rash, Stevens-Johnson syndrome, systemic lupus erythematosus, and urticaria have been reported. Ethosuximide therapy is contraindicated for patients who have had a hypersensitivity reaction to ethosuximide or other succinimides. ADRs involving the GI system can be minimized by ingesting each dose of ethosuximide with food or milk. Ethosuximide is used primarily for management of absence seizures and may increase the frequency of grand mal seizures if it is used alone for the management of mixed seizures. Whenever possible, ethosuximide therapy should be gradually discontinued in order to avoid precipitation of absence seizures. Ethosuximide serum concentrations should be monitored to minimize dose-related ADRs; the optimal serum concentration for seizure control is 40–100 mg/liter (280–710 µmol/liter) (*see* Chapter 14).

Paraldehyde

Psychological and physical dependence (habituation and addiction) may develop with chronic long-term paraldehyde therapy. Paraldehyde has a strong, characteristic, and unpleasant odor, which can be detected on the breath for up to 24 hours after use. Overdosage is associated with fatal metabolic acidosis. Paraldehyde therapy is usually reserved for the management of seizure disorders refractory to other anticonvulsant therapy.

TABLE 5-7 *continued*

Phenobarbital (*see also* Sedative-Hypnotics)

Drowsiness and sedation are the principle ADRs associated with phenobarbital therapy. However, paradoxical excitement resembling attention-deficit/hyperactivity disorder occurs in approximately 10% of young children treated with phenobarbital. Phenobarbital suppresses rapid eye movement sleep. Mild skin reactions develop in 1%–3% of patients and serious skin reactions, such as exfoliative dermatitis and Stevens Johnson syndrome, occur rarely. Ataxia, nystagmus, and respiratory depression occur with higher dosages. Osteomalacia and rickets occur rarely as a result of chronic, long-term phenobarbital therapy and its effect on the metabolism of vitamin D. Phenobarbital is contraindicated for patients who have a history of hypersensitivity to barbiturates, hepatic dysfunction, severe respiratory disease, or porphyria. Dosing should be individualized based on phenobarbital serum concentrations to reduce the incidence and severity of ADRs, with optimal serum concentrations for seizure control being 10–40 µg/ml (43–172 µmol/liter) (*see* Chapter 14). Whenever possible, phenobarbital should be discontinued gradually to avoid precipitation of status epilepticus. Physical and psychological dependence (addiction and habituation) can develop with chronic, long-term barbiturate therapy, even at recommended dosages. Barbiturate therapy is not generally recommended for pediatric patients because of the potential for ADRs, including addiction and habituation, and the availability of safer alternative drug therapy (e.g., benzodiazepine therapy).

Phenytoin (Diphenylhydantoin) *(Dilantin®)*

The most common ADRs associated with oral phenytoin therapy include GI disturbances (e.g., constipation, nausea, vomiting), gingival hyperplasia, hirsutism, and skin rash. Meticulous oral hygiene, including brushing of the teeth with a soft toothbrush after every meal, may lessen the severity of gingival hyperplasia. Potentially fatal hematological disorders, including agranulocytosis, aplastic anemia, granulocytopenia, leukopenia, neutropenia, and thrombocytopenia occur occasionally. Chronic long-term use of high phenytoin dosages may cause peripheral neuropathy and may also cause folate deficiency and megaloblastic anemia. Rare complications of phenytoin therapy include Stevens-Johnson syndrome, systemic lupus erythematosus, and fatal hepatic necrosis. Neonates do not absorb phenytoin well and may require substantial oral dosages to maintain therapeutic phenytoin serum concentrations. The most notable ADRs associated with intravenous phenytoin therapy are cardiovascular collapse and CNS depression. Rapid IV administration can cause hypotension. Dosing should be individualized by monitoring phenytoin serum concentrations to reduce the risk for ADRs and to optimize therapeutic efficacy. The generally recommended serum concentration for optimal seizure control is 10–20 µg/ml (40–80 µmol/liter) (*see* Chapter 14). Special caution is merited when increasing phenytoin dosages because phenytoin follows zero-order kinetics throughout the dosing range. Thus, modest increases in dosage can produce significant increases in serum concentration. Moderate overdosages produce various CNS effects (e.g., ataxia, blurred vision, confusion, hallucinations, hyperactive tendon reflexes, hyperactivity, mydriasis, sedation, vertigo). During initial phenytoin therapy, many patients experience occasional ataxia and a mild maculopapular rash which, if therapy is increased in very small increments, will decrease in severity over time. Whenever possible, phenytoin should be discontinued gradually to avoid precipitation of status epilepticus. (*See also* Phenytoin under Cardiovascular Drugs, Antidysrhythmics.)

Primidone *(Mysoline®)*

Common ADRs associated with primidone therapy include ataxia, diplopia, dizziness, nausea, nystagmus, sedation, vertigo, and vomiting. Acute psychotic reactions have been reported in patients with temporal lobe epilepsy. Dosing should be individualized by monitoring primidone serum concentrations. The recommended serum concentration for optimal seizure control is 4–12 µg/ml (18–55 µmol/liter) (*see* Chapter 14). Primidone is converted to two active metabolites, phenobarbital and phenylethylmalonamide. Thus, phenobarbital serum concentrations also may be monitored to reduce the risk for ADRs and optimize therapeutic effect. (*See also* Phenobarbital.)

Valproic Acid (Valproate Sodium) *(Depakene®)*

ADRs associated with valproic acid therapy involve the GI system (e.g., anorexia, diarrhea, nausea, vomiting). These ADRs occur frequently when therapy is initiated, but they can be minimized by ingesting each oral dose of valproic acid with food. Temporary hair loss, fine tremor, and insomnia also occur. The incidence of sedation, lethargy, and ataxia from valproic acid is lower than with other anticonvulsants. Contraindications to valproic acid therapy include a history of hypersensitivity to valproic acid and hepatic disease. It is advisable to monitor patients periodically for increased bleeding time, increased ammonia blood concentrations, decreased hepatic function, and decreased platelet counts because they are early signs of valproic acid toxicity. Hepatic injury and fatal hepatic necrosis have been described, usually among infants and children younger than 5 years treated with multiple drugs for a neurological disorder. Dosing should be individualized by monitoring valproic acid serum concentrations. The recommended serum concentration for optimal seizure control is 40–100 µg/ml (280–700 µmol/liter) (*see* Chapter 14).

ANTIDEPRESSANTS

Note: All patients who are diagnosed with depression should be thoroughly evaluated for suicide risk prior to the initiation of antidepressant therapy and should be monitored regularly during therapy. Appropriate management of suicide risk before the initiation of antidepressant therapy, during therapy, and after the discontinuation of therapy is prudent. The abrupt discontinuation of antidepressant therapy may result in the return of the signs and symptoms of

TABLE 5-7 continued

depression and/or an acute withdrawal syndrome. Signs and symptoms of the acute withdrawal syndrome include anxiety, dizziness, GI distress, headache, hypomania, and nausea. In order to avoid the occurrence of this syndrome, whenever possible, gradually taper the dosage of the antidepressant, particularly for patients who have received long-term chronic antidepressant therapy or therapy with antidepressants that have a short half-life of elimination. Therapeutic dosages may cause seizures in up to 1% of patients. Seizure risk is greatest for those patients who have a pre-existing seizure disorder.

Selective Serotonin Reuptake Inhibitors (SSRIs)

Fluoxetine *(Prozac®)*

Paroxetine *(Paxil®)*

Sertraline *(Zoloft®)*

ADRs associated with the SSRIs are common and can be serious. These ADRs include diarrhea, fatigue, headache, insomnia, malaise, nausea, nervousness, tremor, sexual dysfunction, somnolence, and weight loss. The SSRIs may also cause abnormal dreams, abdominal pain, anorexia, dizziness, dysmenorrhea, dyspnea, joint pain, palpitation, rashes, sweating, and yawning. The serotonin syndrome, an uncommon but severe ADR characterized by an altered level of consciousness, autonomic instability, GI dysfunction, and myoclonus, has been described in association with SSRI therapy, notably when two or more serotonergic drugs (e.g., MAOIs, SSRIs) are used concurrently (*see* Chapter 6). There is no specific antidote for the management of the serotonin syndrome and the best available therapy is supportive medical care.

Tricyclic Antidepressants (TCAs)

Amitriptyline *(Elavil®)*

The TCAs generally have a more significant ADR profile than do the other available classes of antidepressants. Commonly occurring ADRs include anticholinergic effects (e.g., blurred vision, confusion, constipation, drowsiness, dry mouth, urinary retention) and those that affect the cardiovascular system (e.g., hypotension, palpitation, quinidinelike effects), CNS (e.g., ataxia, dizziness, drowsiness, insomnia, tremor), and GI system (e.g., diarrhea, nausea, vomiting). The TCAs may also cause bone marrow depression, gynecomastia, hypersensitivity reactions, and photosensitivity reactions.

ANTIDIABETICS

Insulins

Hypoglycemia is the most common ADR associated with insulin therapy for the management of insulin-dependent diabetes mellitus and is related to dosage, duration of action of the insulin product, and dietary intake and exercise. Localized allergic reactions with itching, redness, swelling, stinging, and warmth at the injection site may develop, but these ADRs usually disappear within a few weeks. Lipodystrophy with atrophy or hypertrophy of subcutaneous fat tissue was a problem with earlier insulin formulations, but the newer human insulins have a low potential for allergic reactions and lipodystrophy. Insulin dosage should be individualized by monitoring glucose blood or urine concentrations. Children and adolescents should wear a medical alert bracelet indicating that they have diabetes and should carry a ready source of carbohydrates (candy or sugar cubes) in the event that a hypoglycemic reaction occurs. Glucagon is the antidote for the hypoglycemia associated with insulin overdosage.

ANTIFUNGALS (*see also* Antibiotics, Antivirals)

Amphotericin B (injection) *(Fungizone®)*

ADRs associated with the intravenous infusion of amphotericin B are common and can be severe. A test dose is frequently administered to determine patient response prior to commencing therapy. Common ADRs associated with amphotericin B intravenous therapy include abdominal cramping, anorexia, azotemia, diarrhea, generalized pain, headache, hypokalemia, nausea, phlebitis, renal tubular acidosis, shaking chills, thrombophlebitis, and vomiting. Alternate-day therapy may decrease the severity of some ADRs, such as anorexia and phlebitis. Uncommon ADRs associated with amphotericin B include blood dyscrasias, cardiac dysrhythmias, hearing loss, pruritus, and skin rash.

Fluconazole *(Diflucan®)*

ADRs associated with fluconazole therapy occur in up to 20% of patients and include abdominal pain, diarrhea, headache, nausea, skin rash, and vomiting. Exfoliative skin disorders and hepatocellular damage are uncommon, but serious ADRs associated with fluconazole.

Flucytosine *(Ancobon®)*

Flucytosine therapy has been associated with blood dyscrasias, diarrhea, nausea, skin rash, and vomiting. Elevation of blood urea nitrogen, serum hepatic enzyme concentrations, and serum creatinine also may be observed.

Griseofulvin *(Fulvicin®)*

Griseofulvin therapy has been associated with epigastric distress, headache, skin rash, urticaria, and vomiting. Monitoring of hematological, hepatic, and renal function should be performed periodically during long-term, high-dosage griseofulvin therapy because ADRs involving these systems, while uncommon, can be serious.

TABLE 5-7 continued

Ketoconazole (oral) *(Nizoral®)*

Oral ketoconazole is associated with nausea and vomiting in up to 10% of patients. Most ADRs are mild and transient. However, hepatotoxicity, although uncommon, can be severe and even fatal. Hepatic function should be monitored prior to and periodically during long-term ketoconazole oral therapy.

Nystatin (oral) *(Mycostatin®)*

Large oral dosages of nystatin occasionally are associated with ADRs affecting the GI system (e.g., diarrhea, nausea, vomiting). There are very few other significant ADRs (e.g., rash) associated with oral nystatin.

ANTIHISTAMINES

Chlorpheniramine *(Chlor-Tripolon®)*

Dimenhydrinate

Diphenhydramine *(Benadryl®)*

Hydroxyzine *(Atarax®)*

Promethazine *(Phenergan®)*

Sedative-hypnotic effects, ranging from drowsiness to deep sleep, are common ADRs associated with antihistamines. These ADRs are more likely to occur when antihistamines are used concurrently with other drugs that have CNS depressant effects. Anticholinergic effects (e.g., blurred vision, constipation, dizziness, dry mouth, urinary retention) also may occur. Other ADRs that involve the GI system include anorexia, diarrhea, epigastric distress, nausea, and vomiting. Allergic dermatitis occurs more often with topical rather than oral antihistamine use. Paradoxical agitation or excitement may rarely occur among children, primarily toddlers.

Significant toxicity, which may be fatal, has been reported with the topical application of antihistamines (e.g., diphenhydramine) and their subsequent systemic absorption among young infants. Topical application of dermatologic products that contain significant amounts of antihistamines to large areas of abraided or denuded skin should be avoided (do not apply to chickenpox or measles lesions, or large areas of skin), particularly when treating infants. Occlusive dressing and disposable diapers and plastic pants likewise should be avoided over treated areas.

ANTIHYPERTENSIVES *(see also* Diuretics)

Note: ADRs associated with antihypertensive therapy can result from a direct pharmacologic effect or as a secondary consequence of a reduction in blood pressure. ADRs associated with a reduction in blood pressure are shared by all drugs in this class and include dizziness, lightheadedness, and syncope. ADRs also can occur with the sudden discontinuation of antihypertensive therapy.

Angiotensin-Converting Enzyme (ACE) Inhibitors

Captopril *(Capoten®)*

Enalapril *(Vasotec®)*

ADRs are reported in up to 2% of patients receiving ACE inhibitors and include abdominal pain, chest pain, cough, diarrhea, dizziness, dysgeusia, headache, hyperkalemia, hypotension, insomnia, palpitation, pruritus, and vomiting. Maculopapular skin rash also has been reported in up to 10% of patients. A dry, persistent cough also may occur with ACE inhibitors. This ADR is unrelated to dosage and resolves when the ACE inhibitor is discontinued. Ace inhibitors may also cause angioedema, blood dyscrasias (e.g., agranulocytosis, neutropenia), photosensitivity reactions, renal dysfunction, and taste disturbances (e.g., metallic or salty taste).

Beta-Adrenergic Blockers

Atenolol *(Tenormin®)*

Labetalol *(Normodyne®, Trandate®)*

Nadolol *(Corgard®)*

Propranolol *(Inderal®)*

The majority of ADRs associated with beta-adrenergic blockers are related to their pharmacological activity. As an example, reduction in heart rate and cardiac output lowers blood pressure and may cause hypotension and exacerbate congestive heart failure. In addition, $beta_1$-receptor blockade may induce severe bronchospasm and peripheral vasoconstriction and mask signs and symptoms of hypoglycemia. Beta-adrenergic blockers can cause or exacerbate confusion and depression. Contraindications to the use of beta-adrenergic blockers include allergic rhinitis during the pollen season, severe asthma, bronchospasm, cardiogenic shock, heart failure, sinus bradycardia with greater than first-degree heart block, and a history of a hypersensitivity reaction to any one of the beta-adrenergic blockers. The pharmacologic activity of beta-adrenergic blockers varies according to their lipid solubility and cardioselectivity. These properties should be considered when selecting a beta-adrenergic blocker to minimize the likelihood of associated ADRs. When discontinuing beta-adrenergic blocker therapy, gradually taper the dosage, whenever possible, in order to avoid rebound hypertension and/or an associated withdrawal syndrome that includes the following signs and symptoms: headache, malaise, palpitation, sweating, and tremulousness.

TABLE 5-7 continued

Miscellaneous Antihypertensives

Clonidine *(Catapres®)*

Constipation, drowsiness, dry mouth, and sedation are common and sometimes severe ADRs associated with clonidine. Dizziness, headache, fatigue, and weakness also have been reported. These ADRs tend to diminish in severity with continued therapy or improve with a reduction in dosage. Dermatologic reactions are relatively common with transdermal formulations of clonidine. Erythema and pruritus occur more frequently among patients who use an adhesive overlay over the clonidine transdermal drug delivery system, a practice sometimes recommended when the system becomes loose. Dermatologic reactions are generally reversible upon removal of the transdermal system. Rebound hypertension with agitation, anxiety, headache, insomnia, nervousness, palpitation, restlessness, sweating, tachycardia, and tremor may occur after abrupt discontinuation of clonidine, especially after long-term, high-dosage therapy. Pediatric patients and their parents should be instructed to avoid missing doses or discontinuing therapy without medical advisement. When clonidine therapy is discontinued, the dosage should be gradually decreased over 2–4 days to avoid associated rebound hypertension. Clonidine transdermal drug delivery systems should be removed prior to attempting cardioversion or defibrillation to avoid the potential hazard of electrical arcing and resultant burns.

Diazoxide *(Hyperstat®)*

Diazoxide therapy is associated with dizziness, hypotension, nausea, vomiting, and weakness in up to 7% of patients. Sodium retention and hyperglycemia may occur, particularly among diabetic patients, after repeated intravenous injections of diazoxide.

Hydralazine *(Apresoline®)*

Common ADRs associated with hydralazine therapy include anorexia, dizziness, headache, nausea, orthostatic hypotension, reflex tachycardia, and sweating. Hypersensitivity reactions, including eosinophilia, fever, pruritus, skin rash, and urticaria, may occur. A syndrome resembling systemic lupus erythematosus or arthritis has been described. Peripheral neuropathy also has been described, but this ADR can be prevented or treated with dietary supplements of pyridoxine (vitamin B_6). Concurrent therapy with a beta-adrenergic blocker prevents associated tachycardia and reduces the hydralazine dosage required to control blood pressure. The incidence of ADRs from hydralazine generally is related to dosage, and, thus, the lowest possible dosage at which a therapeutic effect is achieved should be used.

Methyldopa *(Aldomet®)*

Sedation is the most common ADR associated with methyldopa. Other ADRs include edema, decreased mental acuity, nasal stuffiness, nightmares, orthostatic hypotension, mental depression, and vertigo. Of patients receiving chronic long-term methyldopa therapy, 10%–20% develop a positive Coomb's test, but autoimmune hemolytic anemia and pancytopenia only occur infrequently. Drug-induced fever, which may be accompanied by a flulike syndrome and hepatic abnormalities, typically occurs within 3 weeks of the initiation of therapy. Common ADRs involving the GI system include abdominal distention, constipation, dry mouth, flatulence, nausea, sore or black tongue, and vomiting.

Minoxidil (oral) *(Loniten®, Minox®)*

Hypertrichosis occurs in up to 80% of hypertensive patients treated with minoxidil. Manifestations (new hair growth) generally appear within 3–6 weeks after initiating minoxidil oral therapy and may require up to 6 months to revert to pretreatment appearance after discontinuation of therapy. Reversible changes in the direction and magnitude of the T-wave on the ECG occur in a majority of patients. Pericardial effusion and tamponade have been reported in up to 3% of patients treated with minoxidil, particularly patients with renal dysfunction. Careful monitoring, with particular attention to such signs and symptoms as difficulty breathing, increased heart rate, and rapid weight gain, is required.

Nitroprusside *(Nitropress®)*

Nitroprusside is a rapidly acting and potent antihypertensive, and, therefore, hypotension commonly occurs. Other ADRs, such as apprehension, dizziness, headache, nausea, and palpitation, generally are related to the rate of the intravenous infusion of nitroprusside and can be prevented or minimized by slowing the infusion rate. Excessive dosages of nitroprusside may cause cyanide toxicity with blurred vision, delirium, and tinnitus.

Prazosin *(Minipress®)*

Prazosin therapy should be initiated using a low dosage that should be increased gradually to avoid postural hypotension and syncope. Dizziness, drowsiness, edema, headache, lack of energy, lightheadedness, nausea, nervousness, palpitation, and weakness are common ADRs and may diminish with continued prazosin therapy or a reduction in dosage.

ANTIMANICS

Lithium Salts

Lithium has a low therapeutic index, and dosing must be individualized in relation to lithium serum concentrations and patient response (*see* Chapters 10 and 14). The use of lithium has declined somewhat as alternative treatments have been developed that have a higher therapeutic index than does lithium. Patients who require lithium therapy must maintain a relatively constant fluid and sodium intake. Any drug that affects sodium serum concentra-

TABLE 5-7 *continued*

tions will have an opposite effect on lithium serum concentrations because they are inversely related (as the sodium concentration increases, the lithium concentration decreases and as the sodium concentration decreases, the lithium concentration increases—without any change in the lithium dosage). As many as 50% of patients treated with lithium salts will experience one or more of the following ADRs: dry mouth, edema, fatigue, hand tremor (generally benign), lethargy, leukocytosis (reversible), mental confusion, muscle weakness, nephrogenic diabetes insipidus (with polyuria and polydypsia), and T-wave depression on the ECG (benign and reversible). ADRs affecting the GI system (e.g., abdominal pain, anorexia, bloating, diarrhea, nausea, vomiting) occur initially among approximately 25% of patients but generally resolve during continued lithium therapy. Lithium-induced acneform eruptions and symptomatic hypothyroidism occur in approximately 1% of patients.

ANTINEOPLASTICS (*see* Chapter 12)

ANTIPSYCHOTICS

Note: All antipsychotics have the potential to cause both minor and major ADRs. Anticholinergic effects and extrapyramidal reactions, including movement disorders, parkinsonian signs and symptoms, and tardive dyskinesia, occur with varying severity, depending on the antipsychotic drug, dosage, and duration of therapy. The neuroleptic malignant syndrome may also occur (rarely).

Butyrophenones

Haloperidol *(Haldol®)*

Anticholinergic effects, including dry mouth, hypotension, sedation, and urinary retention, are less frequently observed with haloperidol than with the phenothiazines. However, haloperidol has a greater tendency to cause extrapyramidal reactions, including acute dystonic reactions, akathisia, aphasia, parkinsonian tremor, and tardive dyskinesia. Agitation, anorexia, confusion, hallucinations, headache, insomnia, nausea, vertigo, and vomiting may occur.

Phenothiazines

Chlorpromazine *(Largactil®, Thorazine®)*

Common ADRs associated with the phenothiazines include dizziness, drowsiness, extrapyramidal reactions, orthostatic hypotension, sedation, skin rash, and tachycardia. Anticholinergic effects (e.g., blurred vision, constipation, dry mouth, urinary retention) also may occur. Extrapyramidal reactions include acute dystonic reactions, akathisia, parkinsonian signs and symptoms, perioral tremor, neuroleptic malignant syndrome, and tardive dyskinesia. The incidence of extrapyramidal reactions is significantly higher among children with acute viral infections (e.g., varicella-zoster, measles) than among children who do not have viral infections. Severe extrapyramidal reactions can be managed with antiparkinsonian drugs or amantadine. Levodopa therapy should be avoided because it tends to aggravate the psychotic disorder. Phenothiazines may cause seizures in patients with epilepsy and is not generally recommended for pediatric patients who are younger than 2 years because of the reported association with sleep apnea and the sudden infant death syndrome. If a phenothiazine is required for a patient in this age group, apnea monitoring should be performed. Phenothiazines may also cause agranulocytosis, cholestatic jaundice, gynecomastia, photosensitivity reactions, and retinopathy.

ANTIULCER DRUGS

Antacids

Aluminum Hydroxide *(Alu-Cap®, Amphojel®)*

Constipation is the most common ADR associated with aluminum hydroxide. This ADR can be managed by alternating aluminum hydroxide with magnesium hydroxide, which has a laxative effect, or by using combination products (e.g., *Maalox®, Mylanta®*) containing both aluminum hydroxide and magnesium hydroxide.

Calcium Carbonate *(Alka-Mints®, Tums®)*

Constipation may occur in patients receiving calcium carbonate. Milk–alkali syndrome with hypercalcemia, metabolic alkalosis, and, rarely, renal insufficiency may occur with chronic long-term calcium carbonate use or in patients with pre-existing renal dysfunction. Eructation occurs as a result of the formation of carbon dioxide when calcium carbonate reacts with hydrochloric acid in the stomach and may be bothersome.

Magnesium Hydroxide (Milk of Magnesia)

Diarrhea is a common ADR associated with magnesium hydroxide. Thus, magnesium hydroxide is generally used in combination with aluminum hydroxide (*see* Aluminum Hydroxide). The chronic long-term use of magnesium-containing antacids in patients with renal dysfunction can result in hypermagnesemia characterized by coma, ECG changes, hypotension, nausea, respiratory and mental depression, and vomiting.

H_2-Receptor Antagonists

Cimetidine *(Tagamet®)*

Reversible confusional states manifested by agitation, anxiety, confusion, depression, disorientation, hallucinations, and psychosis have occurred after administration of high dosages of cimetidine to children, particularly chil-

TABLE 5-7 continued

dren with severe illness or renal or hepatic dysfunction. These confusional states usually resolve within 3–4 days after discontinuation of cimetidine therapy. Headache (sometimes severe), transient skin rash, and diarrhea also may occur. Rapid intravenous administration of cimetidine has been associated with sinus bradycardia and hypotension. Cimetidine inhibits hepatic cytochrome P-450 2D6 and 1A2 isoenzymes and, thus, interacts with many drugs that are metabolized in the liver and may cause significant adverse drug interactions (*see* Chapter 6).

Famotidine *(Pepcid®)*

Ranitidine *(Zantac®)*

Famotidine and ranitidine are generally well tolerated, although headaches, which can be severe, have been reported in up to 5% of patients. Constipation, diarrhea, dizziness, insomnia, malaise, somnolence, and vertigo are reported less frequently than headache. Ranitidine does not inhibit cytochrome P-450 isoenzymes to the same extent as does cimetidine and, thus, is less likely than cimetidine to cause significant adverse drug interactions.

ANTIVIRALS (*see also* Antibiotics, Antifungals)

Acyclovir *(Zovirax®)*

Oral acyclovir has been associated with arthralgia, diarrhea, dizziness, leg pain, nausea, skin rash, and vomiting in up to 5% of patients. Intravenous acyclovir has been associated with inflammation and phlebitis at the injection site in up to 15% of patients. Elevated serum creatinine concentrations are seen in up to 5% of patients. Diaphoresis, encephalopathic changes, headache, and nervousness occur in up to 1% of patients.

Amantadine *(Symmetrel®)*

Common ADRs associated with amantadine therapy include anorexia, anxiety, ataxia, congestive heart failure, depression, irritability, orthostatic hypotension, psychosis, and urinary retention. Seizures are rare but are seen more commonly among patients with a history of seizure disorders. Renal dysfunction may predispose pediatric patients to amantadine-induced neurotoxicity.

Didanosine (Dideoxyinosine) *(Videx®)*

Didanosine may cause potentially fatal pancreatitis in up to 10% of patients. Peripheral neuropathy develops in approximately 33% of patients and may be severe enough to require a modification in didanosine dosage or discontinuation of therapy. Other common ADRs associated with didanosine include abdominal pain, diarrhea, headache, leukopenia, nausea, pruritus, and skin rash. Other ADRs reported in up to 10% of patients include alopecia, anemia, arthritis, dizziness, dry mouth, hepatic function test abnormalities, hyperuricemia, myalgia, and thrombocytopenia.

Ganciclovir *(Cytovene®)*

Ganciclovir therapy is commonly associated with leukopenia, neutropenia, and thrombocytopenia, which may require discontinuation of therapy. It also is associated with anemia, chills, edema, fever, hepatic function test abnormalities, headache, malaise, nausea, nervousness, paresthesia, skin rash, somnolence, and tremor in up to 2% of patients. Rapid intravenous injection is associated with a high incidence of ADRs.

Ribavirin *(Virazole®)*

Ribavirin therapy has been associated with anemia, cardiac arrest, hypotension, worsening of respiratory status (e.g., dyspnea), and skin rash. Many of these ADRs occurred among severely ill infants receiving assisted ventilation, and, thus, the precise role of ribavirin is not clear.

Zidovudine (Azidothymidine, AZT) *(Retrovir®)*

Zidovudine therapy is commonly associated with abdominal pain, anemia, asthenia, fever, GI pain, granulocytopenia, headache, nausea, and skin rash. The anemia and granulocytopenia usually develop after 4 weeks of zidovudine therapy and have been severe enough to necessitate a reduction in dosage or discontinuation of therapy in more than 40% of patients. Anorexia, diaphoresis, diarrhea, dizziness, dyspepsia, dyspnea, insomnia, malaise, myalgia, paresthesia, somnolence, taste disturbances, and vomiting occur in 5%–10% of patients.

Protease Inhibitors

Indinavir *(Crixivan®)*

Nelfinavir *(Viracept®)*

Ritonavir *(Norvir®)*

ADRs associated with the protease inhibitors are common, and their evaluation is complex because they are typically used in combination with a number of other drugs. Common ADRs that occur during the first weeks of protease inhibitor therapy include abdominal pain, diarrhea, dyspepsia, nausea, taste disturbances, and vomiting. Hypersensitivity reactions can occur within the first 6 weeks of therapy. Chronic long-term protease inhibitor therapy is associated with insulin resistance, lipodystrophy, and peripheral fat wasting. Hypercholesterolemia and hyperlipidemia also are seen with long-term therapy, most markedly with ritonavir.

TABLE 5-7 *continued*

BRONCHODILATORS
Beta-Adrenergic Agonists
- Albuterol (Salbutamol) *(Ventolin®)*
- Epinephrine (Adrenaline) *(Adrenalin®)*
- Isoproterenol (Isoprenaline) *(Isuprel®)*
- Metaproterenol (Orciprenaline) *(Alupent®)*
- Terbutaline *(Brethine®, Bricanyl®)*

The beta-adrenergic agonists are associated with several ADRs affecting the CNS. These ADRs include anxiety, confusion, hallucinations, insomnia, muscle tremor, and nervousness. Tremor, although initially distressing, tends to diminish over time. ADRs affecting the cardiovascular system include dysrhythmias, palpitation, and tachycardia. Epinephrine may increase blood pressure. Selective beta$_2$-receptor agonists, such as albuterol, metaproterenol, and terbutaline, are less likely to cause ADRs affecting the cardiovascular system. Paradoxical increases in airway resistance may develop with excessive use of beta-adrenergic agonists. Hypokalemia has been described in association with albuterol.

Miscellaneous Bronchodilators
- Aminophylline (Theophylline Ethylenediamine) *(Phyllocontin®)*
- Theophylline *(Aerolate®, Theo-Dur®, Theolair®)*

Theophylline has a low therapeutic index and commonly causes abdominal discomfort, anxiety, epigastric pain, headache, insomnia, nausea, nervousness, tremor, and vomiting when the serum concentrations exceed 20 µg/ml (110 µmol/liter). Among infants and young children, cardiac dysrhythmias, hyperglycemia, hypotension, and tachycardia can be seen as serum concentrations reach 30 µg/ml (165 µmol/liter) and CNS excitement and seizures may occur as serum concentrations near 40 µg/ml (220 µmol/liter). Cardiorespiratory arrest and fatal seizures most often occur at serum concentrations exceeding 40 µg/ml (220 µmol/liter), but may occur at serum concentrations as low as 25 µg/ml (140 µmol/liter). Dizziness is common when theophylline therapy is initiated, but it tends to disappear with continued therapy. Up to 15% of patients reportedly cannot tolerate oral theophylline, even with relatively low serum concentrations (<85 µmol/liter). The theophylline dosage should be individualized by monitoring serum concentrations (*see* Chapters 10 and 14). The use of theophylline has been largely replaced by the use of other bronchodilators that have a better ADR profile and a higher therapeutic index.

- Cromolyn Sodium (Sodium Cromoglycate) *(Intal®)*

Note: Cromolyn sodium, an inhaled powder, is indicated for the prophylactic management of bronchoconstriction associated with chronic asthma only. It has no direct bronchodilating action or place in the therapy of acute asthma attacks or status asthmaticus.

Cromolyn sodium generally is well tolerated. The most common ADRs relate to direct irritation from the inhaled powder and include bronchospasm, cough, nasal congestion, pharyngeal irritation, and wheezing. These ADRs are more commonly encountered in pediatric patients who have concurrent upper respiratory infections. Mild drowsiness, nausea, and skin rash occur in some patients.

Leukotriene Antagonists
- Montelukast *(Singulair®)*
- Zafirlukast *(Accolate®)*

Leukotriene antagonists act to modulate inflammation associated with asthma and have some additive bronchodilatory effects. These drugs are well tolerated. The most common ADRs include cough, fever, gastritis, headache, pharyngitis, and rhinitis.

CARDIOVASCULAR DRUGS (*see also* Anticoagulants, Antihypertensives, and Diuretics)
Antidysrhythmics

Note: Antidysrhythmics have a narrow therapeutic window, so ECG and therapeutic drug monitoring should be performed to minimize the incidence of serious ADRs (*see* Chapters 10 and 14). All antidysrhythmics have the potential to worsen existing dysrhythmias or to cause new dysrhythmias.

- Amiodarone *(Cordarone®)*

ADRs associated with amiodarone therapy are common and can be fatal. Thus, amiodarone therapy should be reserved for life-threatening ventricular dysrhythmias unresponsive to other, less toxic antidysrhythmics. In up to 5% of patients treated with amiodarone, significant bradycardia, exacerbation of dysrhythmias, and hepatic dysfunction have been reported. Up to 15% of patients may experience a potentially fatal syndrome of progressive pulmonary toxicity (alveolitis, interstitial pneumonitis) and dyspnea. Other less severe, but more common ADRs associated with amiodarone therapy include abnormal hepatic function tests, asymptomatic corneal microdeposits, dizziness, movement disorders (e.g., abnormal gait, tremor), nausea, and vomiting. Overall, ADRs necessitate the discontinuation of amiodarone therapy in up to 20% of patients.

TABLE 5-7 continued

Disopyramide *(Rythmodan®, Norpace®)*

Abdominal pain, anticholinergic effects (e.g., constipation, dry mouth, urinary hesitancy) and nausea are fairly common ADRs associated with disopyramide therapy. Depression of ventricular function may be noted in patients with latent or overt congestive heart failure.

Flecainide *(Tambocor®)*

Flecainide therapy is commonly associated with blurred vision, dizziness, faintness, and syncope. Additional ADRs observed among up to 10% of patients include abdominal pain, anorexia, asthenia, atrioventricular block, cardiac dysrhythmias, chest pain, constipation, dyspnea, edema, fatigue, headache, insomnia, malaise, nausea, palpitation, tremor, and vomiting.

Lidocaine *(Xylocaine®)*

Serious ADRs are not commonly associated with lidocaine therapy. Lidocaine can cause blurred vision, bradycardia, cardiovascular collapse, confusion, convulsions, dizziness, drowsiness, hypotension, lightheadedness, and respiratory depression when administered intravenously. These ADRs are usually related to dosage. ADRs affecting the cardiovascular system occur predominantly with higher dosages or among patients who have myocardial conduction defects.

Mexiletine *(Mexitil®)*

Mexiletine therapy is commonly associated with dizziness, heartburn, nausea, and vomiting. Blurred vision, chest pain, diarrhea, dry mouth, dyspnea, incoordination, lightheadedness, nervousness, sleep disturbances, and tremor occur in up to 10% of patients. Convulsions are rare and generally occur with a higher frequency among patients who have a history of a seizure disorder.

Phenytoin (Diphenylhydantoin) *(Dilantin®)*

Phenytoin therapy is associated with ataxia, drowsiness, nausea, nystagmus, and vertigo. Rapid intravenous injection (bolus injection) can cause hypotension and cardiac collapse. Intravenous injections of phenytoin should be administered at a rate not exceeding 50 mg/min or 3 mg/kg/min, whichever rate is slower. Phenytoin therapy also may cause various dermatologic reactions, including morbilliform and scarlatiniform rashes, and potentially fatal Stevens-Johnson syndrome and toxic epidermal necrolysis. (*See also* Anticonvulsants.)

Procainamide *(Pronestyl®)*

Hypersensitivity reactions (e.g., agranulocytosis, angioedema, fever, myalgias, skin rash, systemic lupus erythematosuslike syndromes, thrombocytopenia) occur rarely. Procainamide and its N-acetylprocainamide metabolite also cause hypotension and pruritus. ADRs involving the CNS occur occasionally and include giddiness, mental depression, and psychosis. ADRs involving the GI system include anorexia, diarrhea, nausea, and vomiting. ADRs are more likely to occur and can be severe among patients who have slow acetylator phenotypes (*see* Chapter 11). Procainamide dosage should be individualized by monitoring the ECG and drug serum concentrations (*see* Chapters 10 and 14). Initiation of procainamide therapy by the intravenous route should be done cautiously to avoid excessive hypotension.

Propafenone *(Rythmol®)*

Propafenone can cause angina, blurred vision, congestive heart failure, constipation, dizziness, dypsnea, fatigue, headache, nausea, taste disturbances, ventricular tachycardia, and vomiting in up to 10% of patients. These ADRs are usually related to dosage. In addition, agranulocytosis, apnea, cholestasis, elevation of liver enzymes, increased bleeding time, hyponatremia, lupus erythematosis, and seizures reportedly occur in up to 0.5% of patients.

Quinidine *(Biquin®, Cardioquin®)*

The ADRs associated with quinidine therapy commonly affect the GI system and include abdominal pain, anorexia, cramping, diarrhea, nausea, and vomiting. These ADRs occur in approximately 30% of patients and are the most common reasons for discontinuing quinidine therapy. Hypersensitivity reactions, manifested as angioedema, anaphylactic shock, bronchospasm, exfoliative rash, and fever occur rarely but can be serious. Patients should be monitored during the first few weeks of quinidine therapy for hypersensitivity reactions. Excessive quinidine dosages may cause cinchonism (disturbed vision, fever, headache, nausea, tinnitus, vertigo). The quinidine dosage should be decreased if these signs and symptoms appear. Blood dyscrasias (e.g., agranulocytosis, aplastic anemia, hemolytic anemia, leukopenia, thrombocytopenia) and cardiac dysrhythmias, including torsades de pointes, ventricular tachycardia or fibrillation with syncope, may also occur. If syncope is observed, quinidine therapy should be discontinued. The quinidine dosage should be individualized by monitoring the ECG (e.g., discontinue quinidine if the duration of the QRS complex increases more than 25%) and drug serum concentrations. Intravenous quinidine should be infused slowly to avoid hypotension and should be accompanied by continuous blood pressure and ECG monitoring.

Calcium-Channel Blockers

Nifedipine *(Adalat®)*

Verapamil *(Calan®, Isoptin®)*

TABLE 5-7 *continued*

The calcium channel blockers are generally well tolerated. ADRs tend to be related to dosage and occur most often during periods of dose titration. Blood pressure must be closely monitored for hypotension during these periods of dose titration. Constipation, dizziness, edema, flushing, headache, lethargy, lightheadedness, and nausea occur fairly frequently during calcium-channel blocker therapy. ADRs affecting the cardiovascular system include angina, bradycardia, congestive heart failure, hypotension, palpitation, pedal edema, syncope, and tachycardia. ADRs affecting the cutaneous system may occur, including skin rash, petechiae, pruritus, and urticaria. Gingival hyperplasia also may occur (most often with nifedipine). These ADRs may be transient and generally resolve with continued calcium-channel blocker therapy. However, skin reactions may progress to more serious ADRs, such as erythema muliforme and exfoliative dermatitis. If adverse skin reactions persist, calcium-channel blocker therapy should be discontinued.

Positive Inotropic Drugs

Digoxin *(Lanoxin®)*

Digoxin has a low therapeutic index and, thus, toxic effects are common unless therapy is carefully individualized. Early signs and symptoms of toxicity in neonates, infants, and young children differ from those seen in adults and include atrial dysrhythmias, atrial ectopic rhythms, and paroxysmal atrial tachycardia with varying degrees of atrioventricular block. In contrast to adults, nausea, vomiting, neurologic and visual disturbances, and ventricular dysrhythmias are unusual consequences of digoxin overdosage in pediatric patients. Prolongation of the PR interval on the ECG is a useful sign of impending toxicity in premature infants, although it is relatively benign in older infants and children.

Cardiac toxicity includes potentially serious rhythm disturbances. Hypokalemia and hypercalcemia potentiate digoxin-induced cardiac toxicity. Common causes of hypokalemia include chronic long-term use of potassium-wasting diuretics, prolonged diarrhea, excessive laxative use, and inadequate dietary potassium intake. Severe cardiac dysrhythmias can be treated by administering potassium, phenytoin, or lidocaine. However, potassium should be administered with caution because hyperkalemia can occur and lead to complete atrioventricular block and cardiac arrest. Atropine can be used to control excessive sinus bradycardia and second- and third-degree atrioventricular block (*see* Chapter 14).

Anorexia or nausea may indicate digitalis toxicity. Vision problems are rare and include decreased visual acuity and hazy vision. Older children occasionally report seeing halos around lights or yellowing of vision. Toxicity involving the CNS is often vague and atypical, ranging from lethargy, confusion, and depression to hallucinations, incoherent speech, and paranoia. Digoxin overdosage or poisoning can be treated with digoxin immune Fab (*see* Chapters 4 and 14). Dosing must be individualized by monitoring the ECG and digoxin serum concentrations (*see* Chapters 10 and 14).

Vasodilators

Nitroglycerin

ADRs associated with nitroglycerin therapy are caused primarily by the vasodilating effect of the drug. Headaches, which may be severe, occur among approximately 50% of patients when nitroglycerin therapy is initiated. The headaches generally resolve within a few days of continued therapy. However, generally they may be treated, if necessary, with acetaminophen. Flushing, postural hypotension, and syncope also may occur. Abrupt discontinuation of nitroglycerin therapy may result in nitroglycerin-withdrawal reactions, including angina, acute myocardial infarction, and sudden death.

CNS STIMULANTS

Methylphenidate *(Ritalin®)*
Mixed Amphetamines *(Adderall®)*
Pemoline *(Cylert®)*

CNS stimulant therapy can be associated with anorexia, dizziness, euphoria, growth suppression, hypertension, insomnia, tachycardia, tremor, and weight loss. Tachycardia and hypertension are more commonly associated with methylphenidate than pemoline. All CNS stimulants can aggravate seizure disorders and precipitate Tourette's syndrome or tics in susceptible patients. Pemoline therapy is associated with potentially fatal hepatic dysfunction and, for this reason, is unavailable in some countries. Physical and psychological dependence (addiction and habituation) may develop after long-term chronic use of these drugs. The incidence and severity of ADRs can be minimized by ensuring that a correct diagnosis of attention-deficit/hyperactivity disorder has been made and that the lowest effective dosage is used. Although growth suppression has been noted with the use of CNS stimulant therapy for the management of attention-deficit/hyperactivity disorder, there is no apparent effect on the ultimate adult height achieved.

CORTICOSTEROIDS

Beclomethasone *(Vancenase®, Vanceril®)*
Dexamethasone *(Decadron®)*
Hydrocortisone

TABLE 5-7 continued

Methylprednisolone *(Medrol®)*

Prednisolone

Prednisone

Triamcinolone *(Aristocort®)*

Systemic corticosteroid therapy has been used to treat severe juvenile rheumatoid arthritis and other inflammatory conditions. The major ADRs associated with corticosteroid therapy relate to suppression of the hypothalamic–pituitary–adrenal (HPA) axis. After prolonged daily use of corticosteroids, the body becomes dependent on exogenous corticosteroid supply; serious and possibly life-threatening reactions can occur if corticosteroid therapy is discontinued abruptly or if the patient experiences a stressful event (e.g., major trauma, surgery). HPA-axis suppression can develop within as little as 6 weeks of daily corticosteroid use. Most of the ADRs associated with the corticosteroids are a consequence of prolonged HPA-axis suppression.

Chronic long-term corticosteroid therapy is associated with a myriad of potentially severe ADRs, including abnormalities in glucose metabolism (hyperglycemia), cataract formation, Cushing's syndrome, electrolyte disturbances (hypernatremia, hypocalcemia, and hypokalemia), impaired wound healing, increased susceptibility to infection, myopathy, osteoporosis, and peptic ulcer activation. Corticosteroid therapy also can precipitate diabetes mellitus. Toxic CNS effects include behavioral disturbances, changes in mood, insomnia, and nervousness. Corticosteroid-induced psychosis reportedly occurs in approximately 20% of patients receiving a daily dosage equivalent to 40 mg of prednisone and in up to 90% of patients receiving a daily dosage equivalent to 80 mg of prednisone.

Administration of live virus vaccines (*see* Chapter 9) to pediatric patients receiving chronic long-term corticosteroid therapy can result in disseminated infection and death related to the immunosuppressive actions of the corticosteroids. Whenever possible, the use of systemic corticosteroids should be limited to periods not exceeding 1 week. When chronic, long-term therapy is required, corticosteroids with the shortest half-life of elimination (e.g., prednisone, prednisolone) should be selected and the longest possible dosing interval (e.g., 24 or 48 hours or alternate-day dosing) should be used.

DIURETICS

Note: ADRs associated with diuretic therapy include dehydration, electrolyte imbalances, hypovolemia, and related sequelae.

Loop Diuretics

Ethacrynic Acid (Ethacrynate Sodium) *(Edecrin®)*

Furosemide (Frusemide) *(Lasix®)*

The ADRs associated with loop diuretic therapy include hyperglycemia in diabetic patients and hyperuricemia. Transient deafness may occur after intravenous administration. Furosemide is a potent diuretic that can readily produce alkalosis, dehydration, hypokalemia, and hyponatremia. Dosages should be individualized and electrolyte serum concentrations monitored regularly to ensure that electrolyte imbalances can be readily corrected if they occur. Dietary potassium and potassium supplements may be required to prevent hypokalemia.

Potassium-Sparing Diuretics

Note: Hyperkalemia is the most serious ADR associated with potassium-sparing diuretics, particularly in pediatric patients with renal failure or those who excessively consume potassium-rich foods (e.g., bananas, orange juice).

Spironolactone *(Aldactone®)*

Abdominal cramping, diarrhea, nausea, and vomiting may occur during spironolactone therapy. However, these ADRs are usually mild.

Triamterene *(Dyrenium®)*

The most serious ADR observed during triamterene therapy is hypokalemia. Other common ADRs include azotemia (mild), dizziness, headache, leg cramps, nausea, and vomiting.

Thiazide Diuretics

Hydrochlorothiazide *(HydroDIURIL®)*

Hydrochlorothiazide therapy is associated with hypokalemia in some patients. Thus, potassium serum concentrations should be monitored regularly during therapy. Inclusion of foods high in potassium (e.g., bananas; broccoli; brussel sprouts; dried apricots and peaches; orange, pineapple, and tomato juice; potatoes; winter squash; yams) in the diet or the use of potassium supplements may be necessary. Hyperuricemia may occur but is usually asymptomatic. Diabetic patients may experience glycosuria and hyperglycemia. Rare hypersensitivity reactions, including cholestatic jaundice, photosensitivity reactions, bone marrow depression, necrotizing vasculitis, and interstitial nephritis have been associated with hydrochlorothiazide therapy. Thiazide diuretic therapy also may precipitate or exacerbate azotemia, hepatic coma, and systemic lupus erythematosus.

TABLE 5-7 continued

HORMONES
Thyroid Hormones
> Levothyroxine *(Synthroid®)*
>> The major levothyroxine ADR, hyperthyroidism, is associated with excessive dosage and is characterized by anxiety, diarrhea, heat intolerance, hyperactivity, insomnia, and tachycardia. Dosage adjustments should be determined by individual clinical response and laboratory tests of thyroid function.

LAXATIVES
Note: Excessive use of laxatives can result in dehydration, diarrhea, electrolyte loss, and laxative dependence (cathartic colon).

Emollient
> Docusate Calcium (Dioctyl Calcium Sulfosuccinate) *(Surfak®)*
> Docusate Sodium (Dioctyl Sodium Sulfosuccinate) *(Colace®)*
>> Docusate calcium and docusate sodium are associated with few ADRs other than abdominal cramps, which are occasionally reported. Prolonged use has been associated with hepatic injury. Calcium and sodium can be absorbed from the calcium and sodium docusate salts. Adequate hydration is required to promote drug action.

Lubricant
> Mineral Oil
>> The use of mineral oil as a laxative for long-term chronic therapy for the management of constipation is not recommended because such use may lead to deficiencies of vitamins A, D, E, and K. Lipoid pneumonitis may result from aspiration of mineral oil droplets during ingestion. Leakage of mineral oil past the anal sphincter can be annoying to children and adolescents and is occasionally the cause of pruritus ani.

Saline
> Magnesium Citrate (Citrate of Magnesia)
> Magnesium Hydroxide (Milk of Magnesia)
>> Magnesium citrate and magnesium hydroxide therapy for the management of constipation may cause diarrhea and hypermagnesemia, particularly among patients with renal dysfunction. Adequate hydration is required to promote bowel function.

Stimulant
> Bisacodyl *(Dulcolax®)*
> Cascara Sagrada
> Glycerin (rectal suppositories)
> Senna (Sennosides) *(Ex-Lax®, Senokot®)*
>> Excessive dosages of stimulant laxatives may produce dehydration, diarrhea, flatulence, griping, hypokalemia, hyponatremia, nausea, palpitation, and weakness. Rectal irritation (usually mild) may occur with bisacodyl and glycerin rectal suppositories. Pink-to-red–brown discoloration of the urine (depending on the pH of the urine) may occur with cascara sagrada or senna. Children and adolescents should be informed of this harmless ADR to avoid unnecessary anxiety. Chronic long-term use of stimulant laxatives can result in laxative dependence (cathartic colon) and should be discouraged. Adequate hydration is required to promote bowel function.

NONDEPOLARIZING NEUROMUSCULAR BLOCKERS
> Atracurium
>> The ADRs associated with atracurium are uncommon, occurring in less than 1% of patients. Allergic reactions, bronchospasm, hypotension, and skin rash appear to be related to atracurium-induced histamine release. Reversal of neuromuscular blockade in cases of overdosage can be achieved by administering an anticholinesterase (e.g., edrophonium) or an anticholinergic (e.g., atropine).

SEDATIVE-HYPNOTICS
Note: Sedative-hypnotic drugs can cause respiratory depression and CNS depression with cognitive and psychomotor impairment. Chronic long-term sedative-hypnotic therapy can lead to psychological dependence (habituation) and physical dependence (addiction) (*see* Chapter 7).

Barbiturates
> Pentobarbital *(Nembutal®)*
> Phenobarbital (*see also* Anticonvulsants)
>> Once popular as sedative-hypnotics, the barbiturates have been largely replaced by the benzodiazepines due to their significantly higher therapeutic index. Barbiturates continue to be used, however, for the management of seizure disorders among infants, children, and adolescents and for preoperative sedation. Oversedation and respiratory depression are the most common ADRs associated with the barbiturates. Physical dependence (addiction) and psy-

TABLE 5-7 continued

chological dependence (habituation) can develop with chronic long-term use (generally in excess of 2 months) and can be severe. In addition, the barbiturates, particularly phenobarbital, are hepatic microsomal enzyme inducers and are, thus, capable of increasing the clearance of many drugs that are metabolized by the liver (see Chapter 6).

Benzodiazepines (see also Anticonvulsants)

Chlordiazepoxide *(Librium®)*
Diazepam *(Valium®)*
Lorazepam *(Ativan®)*
Midazolam *(Versed®)*

Benzodiazepines have a high therapeutic index and are, thus, the generally preferred sedative-hypnotic. The most common ADRs affect the CNS (e.g., ataxia, dizziness, drowsiness, fatigue, lightheadedness, weakness) and are related to dosage. Other ADRs involving the CNS include confusion and impaired memory and psychomotor performance. Physical dependence (addiction) may occur, particularly with chronic long-term therapy with high dosages. Psychological dependence (habituation) also may develop with chronic long-term therapy, even at recommended dosages. Anxiety, hostility, and paradoxical excitement have been reported. Tolerance develops rapidly with continuous use over 4–8 weeks. If possible, benzodiazepines should be used on an "as needed" basis (e.g., occasionally for help falling asleep) rather than daily. Abrupt discontinuation of benzodiazepines should be avoided in patients who have been taking them routinely for more than a month, and the dosage should be gradually reduced over a few weeks to avoid the benzodiazepine-withdrawal syndrome. Severe overdosages involving the benzodiazepines can be treated with flumazenil (see Chapter 4).

Miscellaneous Sedative-Hypnotics

Chloral Hydrate

The most common ADRs associated with the use of chloral hydrate affect the GI system and include diarrhea, nausea, stomach pain, and vomiting. Other ADRs include aggravation of peptic ulcers, ataxia, confusion, headache, lightheadedness, malaise, nightmares, and an unpleasant taste in the mouth. Physical and psychological dependence (addiction and habituation) can develop with chronic long-term use. Epigastric distress associated with the oral ingestion of chloral hydrate can be reduced by diluting each dose in water or milk before ingestion. Additive CNS depressant effects can be expected with concurrent use of chloral hydrate and alcohol or other CNS depressants. High dosages of chloral hydrate can cause potentially fatal respiratory depression, particularly among infants and young children.

VACCINES (see Chapter 9)

VITAMINS AND MINERALS

Ascorbic Acid (Vitamin C)

Vitamin C is a relatively nontoxic substance, but ADRs have been reported with chronic long-term use of high dosages (1–10 grams/day). The most common ADRs associated with vitamin C involve the GI system and include abdominal cramps, diarrhea, nausea, and vomiting. Hyperuricemia can occur, and oxalate renal stones have been reported. Rebound scurvy occurs occasionally with chronic long-term use of high dosages (1–10 grams/day) of vitamin C are abruptly discontinued. The recommended daily allowance of vitamin C is 30 mg for infants at birth. This amount gradually increases to 50 mg by 14 years of age. However, premature infants may require larger amounts. As the amount of vitamin C ingested increases, absorption efficiency decreases (e.g., 100% of a 50-mg dose is absorbed compared to only 20% of a 10-gram dose). The excess vitamin C that is not absorbed acts as an osmotic agent and can induce diarrhea. Large dosages of vitamin C can cause hemolysis in patients with glucose-6-phosphate dehydrogenase deficiency.

Iron Dextran (injectable) *(Dexiron®, INFeD®)*

Injectable iron can cause bronchospasm, headache, hypertension, muscle and joint pain, malaise, nausea, tachycardia, and vomiting. These ADRs are more common after intravenous than after intramuscular administration. Allergiclike reactions occur occasionally and include bronchospasm, fever, skin rash, urticaria, and rarely anaphylactic shock. Generalized or local lymphadenopathy and seizures also have been reported. Due to their greater toxicity, injectable iron formulations should only be used in patients who cannot tolerate or do not respond to oral iron formulations. It is advisable to administer a small test dose to check for idiosyncratic or allergiclike reactions before administering larger amounts. Intravenous doses should be administered slowly (20–50 mg/min) to reduce the incidence and severity of ADRs. Intramuscular injection of iron can cause persistent pain and skin discoloration at the injection site; these effects can be avoided by using the "z-track" technique (see Chapter 1).

Iron (oral)

The most common ADRs associated with oral iron therapy involve the GI system and include constipation, cramping, diarrhea, epigastric distress, heartburn, and nausea. Ingesting each dose of oral iron with meals or after

TABLE 5-7 continued

meals minimizes these ADRs but also decreases iron absorption. Vitamin C increases oral iron absorption. Oral iron blackens the stools; pediatric patients and their families should be informed about this harmless effect to avoid unnecessary anxiety. Chronic, excessive oral iron use may lead to hemochromatosis. Overdosages are treated with deferoxamine (*see* Chapter 4).

Phytonadione (Vitamin K_1)

Severe allergic-type ADRs, including severe hypotension, anaphylaxis, and death, have been described during and immediately following intravenous administration of phytonadione. Therefore, intravenous administration should be avoided if possible. Allergic reactions consisting of skin rash and urticaria also may occur occasionally with the oral, intramuscular, and subcutaneous routes of administration and anaphylactic reactions also are possible. Less severe ADRs include occasional gastric upset with headache, nausea, and vomiting following oral administration.

Vitamin A

Generally well tolerated and nontoxic at recommended dosages. Chronic, long-term use of high dosages of vitamin A supplements and excessive vitamin A ingestion from food sources can cause vitamin A toxicity, with anorexia, drowsiness, gingivitis, headache, hemorrhagic papilledema, hepatic damage, increased cerebrospinal fluid pressure, irritability, loss of body hair, mouth fissures, pseudotumor cerebri, skin dryness and desquamation, spleen enlargement, and vomiting. The recommended daily allowance is 2100 IU (375 µg RE in the United States) beginning at birth and gradually increases to 3500 IU (700 µg RE in the United States) by the age of 10 years. One IU is equivalent to 0.3 µg of retinol, and 1 retinol equivalent (RE) has the same activity as 1 µg of retinol. Vitamin A is fat soluble and accumulates in the body when excessive amounts are ingested. Vitamin A supplements are not generally required unless a pediatric patient is malnourished or suffers from a condition that impairs the GI absorption of the vitamin.

Vitamin D

Vitamin D is fat soluble and, thus, chronic long-term vitamin D ingestion from vitamin supplements or excessive ingestion from food sources may cause toxic reactions. Generally, pediatric patients with normal sensitivity to the vitamin do not require supplementation. Initial signs and symptoms of vitamin D toxicity are related to hypercalcemia and include fatigue, headache, nausea, vomiting, and weakness. Hypercalcemia associated with vitamin D results from excessive GI absorption of calcium, increased resorption of bone, and decreased renal excretion of calcium. Prolonged hypercalcemia causes deposition of calcium in soft tissues and in the blood vessels, heart, kidneys, lungs, and skin. It also is associated with anemia, impaired growth among children, nephrocalcinosis, pancreatitis, and renal dysfunction. Death can occur as a result of cardiac or renal damage.

References[1]

Adverse reactions associated with immunizing agents. (1991). *Canada Diseases Weekly Report, 17,* 147–158.

Alexopoulos, E. (1998). Drug-induced acute interstitial nephritis. *Renal Failure, 20,* 809–819.

Aranda, J. V. (1983). Factors associated with adverse drug reactions in the newborn. *Pediatric Pharmacology, 3,* 245–249.

Aranda, J. V., Portugeuz-Malavasi, A., Collinge, J. M., et al. (1982). Epidemiology of adverse drug reactions in the newborn. *Developmental Pharmacology and Therapeutics, 5,* 173–184.

Banner, W. (1986). Clinical toxicology in the neonatal intensive care unit. *Medical Toxicology, 1,* 225–235.

Bonn, D. (1998). Adverse drug reactions remain a major cause of death. *The Lancet, 351,* 1183.

Carbone, J. R. (2000). The neuroleptic malignant and serotonin syndromes. *Emergency Medical Clinics of North America, 18,* 317–325.

Chan, T. C., Evans, S. D., & Clark, R. F. (1997). Drug-induced hyperthermia. *Critical Care Clinics, 13,* 785–808.

Corso, D. M., Pucino, F., DeLeo, J. M., et al. (1992). Development of a questionnaire for detecting potential adverse drug reactions. *DICP: The Annals of Pharmacotherapy, 26,* 890–892.

---

1. The references listed are meant to provide the reader with some benchmarks only and are not intended to be exhaustive. The ADRs reported in this chapter involving infants, children, and adolescents have been compiled from several sources. These sources include current articles and case studies, references cited in the previous editions of this text, current product monographs, and the clinical experience of the author. Because published work in the area of ADRs among infants, children, and adolescents is generally lacking, pediatric clinicians are encouraged to observe for, formally report, and publish ADRs that they note among their pediatric patients.

Doig, J. C. (1997). Drug-induced cardiac arrhythmias: Incidence, prevention and management. *Drug Safety: An International Journal of Medical Toxicology and Drug Experience, 17,* 265–275.

Drugs that cause psychiatric symptoms. (1993). *The Medical Letter on Drugs and Therapeutics, 35,* 65–70.

Epstein, J. H., & Wintroub, B. U. (1985). Photosensitivity due to drugs. *Drugs, 30,* 42–57.

Fasano, M. B., Wood, R. A., Cooke, S. K., et al. (1992). Egg hypersensitivity and adverse reactions to measles, mumps and rubella vaccine. *The Journal of Pediatrics, 120,* 878–881.

Gillman, P. K. (1999). The serotonin syndrome and its treatment. *Journal of Psychopharmacology, 13,* 100–109.

Gonzalez-Martin, G., Caroca, C. M., & Paris, E. (1998). Adverse drug reactions in hospitalized pediatric patients: A prospective study. *International Journal of Clinical Pharmacology and Therapeutics, 36,* 530–533.

Gupta, A. K., & Waldhauser, L. K. (1997). Adverse drug reactions from birth to early childhood. *Pediatric Clinics of North America, 44,* 79–92.

Gupta, A. K., Katz, H. I., & Shear, N. H. (1999). Drug interactions with itraconazole, fluconazole and terbinafine and their management. *Journal of the American Academy of Dermatology, 41,* 237–249.

Hannan, T. J. (1999). Detecting adverse drug reactions to improve patient outcomes. *International Journal of Medical Informatics, 55,* 61–64.

Harris, J. M. (1990). Clonidine patch toxicity. *DICP: The Annals of Pharmacotherapy, 24,* 1191–1194.

Jonville, A. P., Autret, E., Bavoux, F., et al. (1991). Characteristics of medication errors in pediatrics. *DICP: The Annals of Pharmacotherapy, 25,* 1113–1118.

Kassner, E. G. (1991). Drug-related complications in infants and children: Imaging features. *American Journal of Roentgenology, 157,* 1039–1049.

Kaul, D. R., Cinti, S. K., Carver, P. L., et al. (1999). HIV protease inhibitors: Advances in therapy and adverse reactions, including metabolic complications. *Pharmacotherapy, 19,* 281–298.

Kearns, G. L., Wheeler, J. G., Rieder, M. J., et al. (1998). Serum sickness-like reactions to cefaclor: Lack of in vitro cross-reactivity with loracarbef. *Clinical Pharmacology and Therapeutics, 63,* 686–693.

Kimayi-Asadi, A., Harris, J. C., & Nousari, H. C. (1999). Critical overview: Adverse cutaneous reactions to psychotropic medications. *Journal of Clinical Psychiatry, 60,* 714–725.

Knowles, S., Shapiro, L., & Shear, N. H. (1997). Serious dermatologic reactions in children. *Current Opinion in Pediatrics, 9,* 388–395.

Koch, K. E. (1990). Use of standardized screening procedures to identify adverse drug reactions. *American Journal of Hospital Pharmacy, 47,* 1314–1320.

Leeder, J. S., & Kearns, G. L. (1997). Pharmacogenetics in pediatrics. Implications for practice. *Pediatric Clinics of North America, 44,* 55–77.

Manasse, H. R. Jr. (1989). Medication use in a imperfect world: Drug misadventure as an issue of public policy, part 1. *American Journal of Hospital Pharmacy, 46,* 929–944.

Manasse, H. R. Jr. (1989). Medication use in an imperfect world: Drug misadventure as an issue of public policy, part 2. *American Journal of Hospital Pharmacy, 46,* 1141–1142.

Martinez-Mir, I., Garcia-Lopez, M., Palop, V., et al. (1999). A prospective study of adverse drug reactions in hospitalized children. *British Journal of Clinical Pharmacology, 47,* 681–689.

Pagliaro, L. A. (1992). The straight dope: Focusing on learning—Interpreting the interpretations. *Psynopsis, 14,* 7.

Patterson, R., DeSwarte, R. D., Greenberger, P. A., et al. (1986). Drug allergy and protocols for management of drug allergies. *New England Review of Allergy Proceedings, 7,* 325–342.

Pederson-Bjergaard, U., Anderson, M., & Hansen, P. B. (1998). Drug-specific characteristics of thrombocytopenia caused by non-cytotoxic drugs. *European Journal of Clinical Pharmacology, 54,* 701–706.

Pena, B. M., & Krauss, B. (1999). Adverse events of procedural sedation and analgesia in a pediatric emergency department. *Annals of Emergency Medicine, 34,* 483–491.

Pirmohamed, M., & Park, B. K. (1999). The adverse effects of drugs. *Hospital Medicine, 60,* 348–352.

Price, D. L. (2000). Tolerability of montelukast. *Drugs, 59*(Suppl 1), 35–42.

Ravnskov, U. (1999). Glomerular, tubular and interstitial nephritis associated with nonsteroidal anti-inflammatory drugs: Evidence of a common mechanism. *British Journal of Clinical Pharmacology, 47,* 203–210.

Revuz, J. E., & Roujeau, J. C. (1996). Advances in toxic epidermal necrolysis. *Seminars in Cutaneous Medicine and Surgery, 15,* 258–266.

Rieder, M. J. (1997). In vivo and in vitro testing for adverse drug reactions. *Pediatric Clinics of North America, 44,* 93–111.

Rieder, M. J., & Matsui, D. M. (1998). Adverse drug reactions in paediatrics: A rational approach. *Ballière's Clinical Paediatrics, 6*(3), 505–519.

Rieder, M. J., King, S. M., & Read, S. (1997). Adverse reactions to trimethoprim-sulfamethoxazole among children with human immunodeficiency virus infection. *Pediatric Infectious Disease Journal, 16,* 1028–1031.

Rogers, A. S. (1994). The role of cytochrome P450 in developmental pharmacology. *Journal of Adolescent Health, 15,* 635–640.

Roujeau, J. C. (1997). Severe drug-induced blistering disorders. *Reviews in Rheumatology (English Edition), 64,* 5–9.

Rowe, C., Koren, T., & Koren, G. (1998). Errors by paediatric residents in calculating drug doses. *Archives of Disease in Childhood, 79,* 56–58.

Rzany, B., Correia, O., Kelly, J. P., et al. (1999). Risk of Stevens-Johnson syndrome and toxic epidermal necrolysis during first weeks of antiepileptic therapy: A case-control study. Study group of the international case control study on severe cutaneous adverse reactions. *The Lancet, 353,* 2190–2194.

Schumock, G. T., & Thornton, J. P. (1992). Focusing on the preventability of adverse drug reactions. *Hospital Pharmacy, 27,* 538.

Shah, K. (1999). Drug-induced hepatoxicity: Pharmacokinetic perspectives and strategy for risk reduction. *Adverse Drug Reactions and Toxicology Research, 18,* 181–233.

Spector, S. L. (1996). Management of asthma with zafirlukast. Clinical experience and tolerability profile. *Drugs, 52*(Suppl 6), 36–46.

Spigset, O. (1999). Adverse reactions of selective serotonin reuptake inhibitors: Reports from a spontaneous reporting system. *Drug Safety, 20,* 227–287.

Tanaka, E. (1998). In vivo age-related changes in hepatic drug-oxidizing capacity in humans. *Journal of Clinical Pharmacology and Therapeutics, 23,* 247–255.

Theis, J. G., Koren, G., Daneman, R., et al. (1997). Interactions of clobazam with conventional antiepileptics in children. *Journal of Childhood Neurology, 12,* 208–213.

Tran, C., Knowles, S. R., Liu, B. A., et al. (1998). Gender differences in adverse drug reactions. *Journal of Clinical Pharmacology, 38,* 1003–1009.

Turner, S., Nunn, A. J., Felding, K., et al. (1999). Adverse drug reactions to unlicensed and off-label drugs on paediatric wards: A prospective study. *Acta Paediatrica, 88,* 965–968.

van der Anker, J. N. (1996). Pharmacokinetics and renal function in preterm infants. *Acta Paediatrica, 85,* 1393–1399.

Venkatakrishnan, K., von Moltke, L. I., & Greenblatt, D. J. (2000). Effects of the antifungal agents on oxidative drug metabolism: Clinical relevance. *Clinical Pharmacokinetics, 38,* 111–180.

White, T. J., Arkelian, A., & Rho, J. P. (1999). Counting the costs of drug-related adverse events. *Pharmacoeconomics, 15,* 445–458.

Whyte, J., & Greenan, E. (1977). Drug usage and adverse drug reactions in paediatric patients. *Acta Paediatrica Scandinavica, 66,* 767–775.

Williams, D., Kelly, A., & Feely, J. (2000). Drug interactions avoided—A useful indicator of good prescribing practice. *British Journal of Clinical Pharmacology, 49,* 369–372.

Wutschert, R., Piletta, P., & Bounameaux, H. (1999). Adverse skin reactions to low molecular weight heparins: Frequency, management and prevention. *Drug Safety, 20,* 515–525.

Young, C. R., Bowers, M. B. Jr., & Mazure, C. M. (1998). Management of the adverse effects of clozapine. *Schizophrenia Bulletin, 24,* 381–390.

6

Pediatric Drug Interactions

Philip D. Hansten

Although adult patients, particularly geriatric patients, are generally considered at high risk for developing adverse drug interactions, pediatric patients also can be at significant risk. Chronic diseases (e.g., asthma, cancer, juvenile rheumatoid arthritis, seizure disorders) require drugs (e.g., anticonvulsants, corticosteroids, salicylates, theophylline) known to interact with other drugs. Unfortunately, the published literature on drug interactions in pediatric patients is scant when compared with that involving adults. Thus, extrapolation of adult data is often required. However, such extrapolation requires careful consideration because some drugs may display significant age effects in regard to drug interactions. For example, amiodarone *(Cordarone®)* produces a much greater increase in digoxin *(Lanoxin®)* serum concentrations in children than it does in adults (Koren et al., 1984). It also seems likely that other differences exist between children and adults with regard to the incidence and severity of drug interactions.

Several major lawsuits have involved adverse drug interactions among pediatric patients. For example, a 5-year-old boy from Tennessee who was receiving theophylline (200 mg three times daily) was given erythromycin (400 mg four times daily). Six days after initiating the erythromycin, the child suffered severe theophylline toxicity, resulting in seizures and permanent brain damage (LeBlang, 1991). Erythromycin is known to inhibit the hepatic metabolism of theophylline, and the boy's parents sued both the physicians and the pharmacy. In another example, a 7-year-old Baltimore boy who was maintained on both theophylline and carbamazepine developed severe theophylline toxicity with seizures and permanent brain damage after the carbamazepine was discontinued. Carbamazepine can stimulate the hepatic metabolism of theophylline, and the plaintiff claimed that discontinuing the carbamazepine resulted in a dangerous increase in the theophylline serum concentration (Bor, 1990). These two cases demonstrate the potential seriousness of drug interactions in pediatric patients and the importance of anticipating adverse drug interactions and taking appropriate measures to prevent them.

Sites of Drug Interactions

Drugs can interact at a variety of sites in the human body (Figure 6-1). An understanding of the principal sites of drug interactions can assist pediatric clinicians to predict and prevent the occurrence of drug interactions and effectively manage those drug interactions that do occur among their pediatric patients.

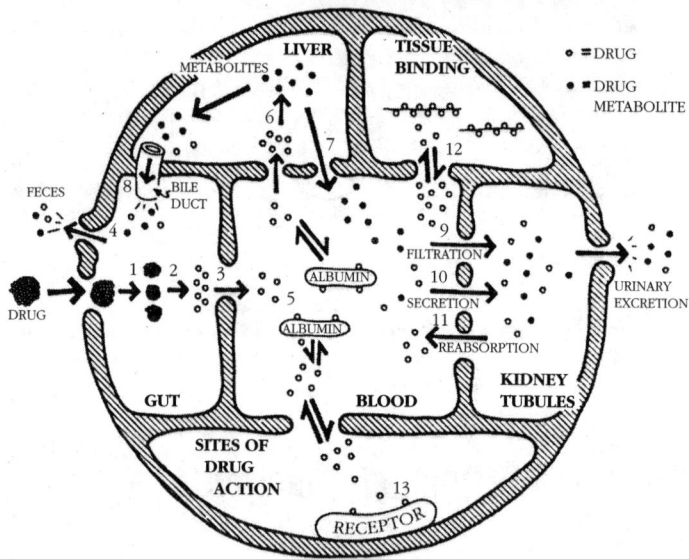

FIGURE 6-1
Principal Sites of Drug Interactions

As illustrated in Figure 6-1, the GI absorption of orally ingested drugs is influenced by the processes of disintegration (1), dissolution (2), and absorption across the gut wall (3). Elimination of the drug and its metabolites in the feces (4) may be affected by concomitant drug therapy. Some drugs bind to serum proteins (principally albumin) (5) and may be displaced from protein binding sites by other drugs. Hepatic metabolism (6) of certain drugs may be enhanced or inhibited by concurrent drug therapy (*see* Table 6-1). Metabolites formed in the liver may return to the circulatory system (7) or undergo biliary excretion (8); these processes may be affected by other drugs. Renal drug elimination processes that are affected by concomitant drug therapy include glomerular filtration (9), active tubular secretion (10), and passive tubular reabsorption (11). Tissue binding (12) of one drug may be affected by another. Drug interactions that involve these 12 sites are often referred to as **pharmacokinetic interactions** because they affect absorption, distribution, metabolism, and excretion. Drugs may have synergistic or antagonistic pharmacologic effects at the receptor site (13). Drug interactions involving the receptor site are often referred to as **pharmacodynamic interactions**.

Drug Interactions and QT Prolongation

Over the past decade, a number of cases of cardiac toxicity have been reported in association with drugs that prolong the QT interval of the ECG (Hoppu et al., 1991; Smith, 1994; Tobin et al., 1991). The QT interval indicates how long it takes the heart to repolarize after each heartbeat. Prolongation of the QT interval (due to slowed cardiac repolarization) is desired when using antidysrhythmic drugs such as amiodarone (*Cordarone*) or sotalol (*Sotacor®*). However, a number of noncardiac drugs have also demonstrated this pharmacologic action. When the QT prolongation is small, the risk is usually negligible. However, extensive prolongation of the QT can be associated with serious ventricular dysrhythmias (e.g., torsades de pointes) in both adults and children (Smith, 1994; Tobin et al., 1991; Viskin, 1999). Sudden death has occurred.

A European agency (EMEA) has developed guidelines for assessing the clinical importance of QT prolongation due to drugs (De Ponti et al., 2000):

Below 30 msec: Unlikely to result in dysrhythmias

(Continued on page 318)

TABLE 6-1
Drug Interactions Involving Hepatic Cytochrome P-450 Isoenzymes[a]

SUBSTRATES		INHIBITORS	INDUCERS
CYP1A2			
Caffeine	Ondansetron *(Zofran®)*	Cimetidine *(Tagamet®)*	Charcoal-broiled meat
Clomipramine *(Anafranil®)*	Ropinirole *(Requip®)*	Ciprofloxacin *(Cipro®)*	Tobacco smoking
Clozapine *(Clozaril®)*	Tacrine *(Cognex®)*	Enoxacin *(Penetrex®)*	
Flutamide *(Eulexin®)*	Theophylline	Ethinyl Estradiol	
Imipramine *(Tofranil®)*	R-Warfarin *(Coumadin®)*	Fluvoxamine *(Luvox®)*	
Olanzapine *(Zyprexa®)*	Zileuton *(Zyflo®)*	Isoniazid *(INH®)*	
		Mexiletine *(Mexitil®)*	
		Norethindrone	
		Tacrine *(Cognex®)*	
		Zileuton *(Zyflo®)*	
CYP2C9			
Celecoxib *(Celebrex®)*	Montelukast *(Singulair®)*	Amiodarone *(Cordarone®)*	Aminoglutethimide
Diclofenac *(Voltaren®)*	Naproxen *(Naprosyn®)*	Clopidogrel *(Plavix®)*	*(Cytadren®)*
Dronabinol *(Marinol®)*	Phenytoin *(Dilantin®)*	Disulfiram *(Antabuse®)*	Barbiturates
Flurbiprofen *(Ansaid®)*	Piroxicam *(Feldene®)*	Efavirenz *(Sustiva®)*	Carbamazepine *(Tegretol®)*
Fluvastatin *(Lescol®)*	Rosiglitazone *(Avandia®)*	Fluconazole *(Diflucan®)*	Griseofulvin *(Fulvicin®)*
Glimepiride *(Amaryl®)*	Tolbutamide *(Orinase®)*	Fluvastatin *(Lescol®)*	Nafcillin *(Unipen®)*
Ibuprofen *(Motrin®)*	Torsemide *(Demadex®)*	Fluvoxamine *(Luvox®)*	Phenytoin *(Dilantin®)*
Indomethacin *(Indocin®)*	S-Warfarin *(Coumadin®)*	Isoniazid *(INH®)*	Primidone *(Mysoline®)*
Losartan *(Cozaar®)*	Zafirlukast *(Accolate®)*	Itraconazole *(Sporanox®)*	Rifampin *(Rimactane®)*
		Ketoconazole *(Nizoral®)*	
		Metronidazole *(Flagyl®)*	
		Sulfinpyrazone *(Anturane®)*	
		Ticlopidine *(Ticlid®)*	
		Trimethoprim–Sulfamethoxazole *(Bactrim®)*	
		Zafirlukast *(Accolate®)*	
CYP2C19			
Amitriptyline *(Elavil®)*	Pantoprazole *(Protonix®)*	Efavirenz *(Sustiva®)*	
Carisoprodol *(Soma®)*	Pentamidine *(Pentam®)*	Felbamate *(Felbatol®)*	
Chloroguanide *(Paludrine®)*	Olanzapine *(Zyprexa®)*	Fluconazole *(Diflucan®)*	
Citalopram *(Celexa®)*	Omeprazole *(Prilosec®)*	Fluoxetine *(Prozac®)*	
Clomipramine *(Anafranil®)*	Phenytoin *(Dilantin®)*	Fluvoxamine *(Luvox®)*	
Diazepam *(Valium®)*	(minor pathway)	Omeprazole *(Prilosec®)*	
Imipramine *(Tofranil®)*	Rabeprazole *(AcipHex®)*	Ticlopidine *(Ticlid®)*	
Lansoprazole *(Prevacid®)*	R-Warfarin *(Coumadin®)*		
Mephenytoin			
CYP2D6			
Amitriptyline *(Elavil®)*	Maprotiline *(Ludiomil®)*	Amiodarone *(Cordarone®)*	NOTE: CYP2D6 appears
Carvedilol *(Coreg®)*	Methamphetamine *(Desoxyn®)*	Chloroquine *(Aralen®)*	relatively resistant to
Clomipramine *(Anafranil®)*	Metoprolol *(Lopressor®)*	Cimetidine *(Tagamet®)*	enzyme induction.
Codeine → Morphine	Mexiletine *(Mexitil®)*	Diphenhydramine *(Benadryl®)*	
Desipramine *(Norpramin®)*	Nortriptyline *(Pamelor®)*	Fluoxetine *(Prozac®)*	
Dexfenfluramine *(Redux®)*	Oxycodone *(Percocet®)*	Haloperidol *(Haldol®)*	
Dextromethorphan *(Bonylin DM®)*	Paroxetine *(Paxil®)*	Mibefradil *(Posicor®)*	
Dihydrocodeine	Perphenazine *(Trilafon®)*	Paroxetine *(Paxil®)*	
Efavirenz *(Sustiva®)*	Propafenone *(Rhythmol®)*	Perphenazine *(Trilafon®)*	
Encainide	Propranolol *(Inderal®)*	Propafenone *(Rhythmol®)*	
Flecainide *(Tambocor®)*	Risperidone *(Risperdal®)*	Propoxyphene *(Darvon®)*	
Fluoxetine *(Prozac®)*	Thioridazine *(Mellaril®)*	Quinacrine	
Fluvoxamine *(Luvox®)*	Timolol *(Blocadren®)*	Quinidine *(Quinidex®)*	
Haloperidol *(Haldol®)*	Tolterodine *(Detrol®)*	Quinine	
Hydrocodone *(Hycodan®)*	Tramadol *(Ultram®)*	Ritonavir *(Norvir®)*	
Imipramine *(Tofranil®)*	Trazodone *(Desyrel®)*	Terbinafine *(Lamasil®)*	
	Venlafaxine *(Effexor®)*	Thioridazine *(Mellaril®)*	
CYP3A4			
Alfentanil *(Alfenta®)*	Atorvastatin *(Lipitor®)*	Amprenavir *(Agenerase®)*	Aminoglutethimide
Alprazolam *(Xanax®)*	Bepridil *(Vascor®)*	Clarithromycin *(Biaxin®)*	*(Cytadren®)*
Amiodarone *(Cordarone®)*	Bromocriptine *(Parlodel®)*	Cyclosporine *(Neoral®)*	Barbiturates
Amlodipine *(Norvasc®)*	Buspirone *(Buspar®)*	Danazol *(Danocrine®)*	Carbamazepine *(Tegretol®)*
Astemizole	Carbamazepine *(Tegretol®)*	Delavirdine *(Rescriptor®)*	Dexamethasone

TABLE 6-1 continued

SUBSTRATES		INHIBITORS	INDUCERS
CYP3A4 continued			
Cisapride (Propulsid®)	Midazolam (Versed®)	Diltiazem (Cardizem®)	Efavirenz (Sustiva®)
Citalopram (Celexa®)	Montelukast (Singulair®)	Erythromycin (E-Mycin®)	Glutethimide
Clarithromycin (Blaxin®)	Nefazodone (Serzone®)	Ethinyl Estradiol	Griseofulvin (Fulvicin®)
Cyclophosphamide (Cytoxan®)	Nicardipine (Cardene®)	Fluvoxamine (Luvox®)	Nevirapine (Viramune®)
Cyclosporine (Neoral®)	Nifedipine (Adalat®)	Grapefruit juice	Phenytoin (Dilantin®)
Dapsone (Avlosulfon®)	Nimodipine (Nimotop®)	Indinavir (Crixivan®)	Primidone (Mysoline®)
Delavirdine (Rescriptor®)	Nisoldipine (Sular®)	Isoniazid (INH®)	Rifabutin (Mycobutin®)
Dexamethasone (Decadron®)	Nitrendipine	Itraconazole (Sporanox®)	Rifampin (Rimactane®)
Diazepam (Valium®)	Paclitaxel (Taxol®)	Ketoconazole (Nizoral®)	St. John's Wort
Diltiazem (Cardizem®)	Pimozide (Orap®)	Methylprednisolone (Medrol®)	(Hypericum®)
Disopyramide (Norpace®)	Pioglitazone (Actos®)	Metronidazole (Flagyl®)	Troglitazone (Rezulin®)
Dofetilide (Tikosyn®)	Prednisolone	Miconazole (Monistat®)	
Doxorubicin (Adriamycin®)	Quetiapine (Seroquel®)	Nefazodone (Serzone®)	
Efavirenz (Sustiva®)	Quinidine (Quinidex®)	Nelfinavir (Viracept®)	
Ergotamine (Ergomar®)	Quinine	Norethindrone	
Erythromycin (E-Mycin®)	Rifabutin (Mycobutin®)	Oxiconazole (Oxistat®)	
Ethinyl Estradiol	Ritonavir (Norvir®)	Prednisone	
Etoposide (VePesid®)	Saquinavir (Invirase®)	Quinupristin/dalforpristin	
Felodipine (Plendil®)	Sertraline (Zoloft®)	(Synercid®)	
Fentanyl (Sublimaze®)	Sibutramine (Meridia®)	Ritonavir (Norvir®)	
Finasteride (Propecia®)	Sildenafil (Viagra®)	Saquinavir (Invirase®)	
Flutamide (Eulexin®)	Simvastatin (Zocor®)	Troleandomycin (TAO®)	
Ifosfamide (Ifex®)	Sirolimus (Rapamune®)	Verapamil (Calan®)	
Indinavir (Crixivan®)	Tacrolimus (Prograf®)	Zafirlukast (Accolate®)	
Isradipine (DynaCirc®)	Tamoxifen (Nolvadex®)	Zileuton	
Itraconazole (Sporanox®)	Terfenadine		
Ketoconazole (Nizoral®)	Testosterone		
Lidocaine (Xylocaine®)	Theophylline (minor pathway)		
Loratadine (Claritin®)	Triazolam (Halcion®)		
Losartan (Cozaar®)	Verapamil (Calan®)		
Lovastatin (Mevacor®)	Vinblastine (Velban®)		
Methadone (Dolophine®)	Vincristine (Oncovin®)		
Methylprednisolone (Medrol®)	R-Warfarin (Coumadin®)		
Miconazole (Monistat®)	Zolpidem (Ambien®)		

[a] **Substrates** represent the drugs that are metabolized by the specified hepatic cytochrome P-450 isoenzymes (CYP1A2, CYP2C9, etc.). **Inhibitors** are drugs (e.g., cimetidine [Tagamet®], fluoxetine [Prozac®], and foods (e.g., grapefruit juice) that can significantly decrease (inhibit) the production of specific hepatic cytochrome P-450 isoenzymes. **Inducers**, conversely, are drugs (e.g., barbiturates, carbamazepine [Tegretol®]) or foods (e.g., charcoal-broiled meat) that can significantly increase (induce) the production of specific hepatic cytochrome P-450 isoenzymes.

30–60 msec: Raises some concern about potential risk of dysrhythmias

Above 60 msec: Clear concern about risk of dysrhythmias

Only a few drugs are capable of producing QT prolongations longer than 30 msec in the absence of excessive doses or drug interactions, but some patients are predisposed through disease or other factors:

- Anorexia nervosa
- Bradycardia (< 50 beats per minute)
- Cardiac hypertrophy
- Congenital QT_c syndrome
- Female gender (QT_c interval generally is longer in women than in men)
- Heart failure
- Hypokalemia
- Hypomagnesemia
- Hypothyroidism
- Impaired hepatic function
- Impaired renal function

Most drugs that increase the QT interval do so in a dose-dependent manner. Therefore, drug interactions that result in large increases in the serum concentrations of a QT prolonging drug can have serious consequences (Table 6-2). For example, the withdrawal of the antihistamines terfenadine (Seldane®) and astemizole (Hismanal®) from the market was largely due to failure to avoid concurrent use of these drugs with CYP3A4 inhibitors (see Table 6-1).

TABLE 6-2
Drug Interactions Resulting in QT Prolongation

QT PROLONGING DRUGS	INTERACTING DRUGS	COMMENTS
Astemizole[a] *(Hismanal®)*	CYP3A4 inhibitors Other drugs that prolong the QT interval[c]	Fatal cardiac dysrhythmias reported when combined with CYP3A4 inhibitors.
Cisapride[b] *(Prepulsid®; Propulsid®)*	CYP3A4 inhibitors Other drugs that prolong the QT interval[c]	Fatal cardiac dysrhythmias reported when combined with CYP3A4 inhibitors.
Moxifloxacin *(Avelox®)*	Other drugs that prolong the QT interval[c]	Sparfloxacin also prolongs the QT interval, but other fluoroquinolones appear to have minimal effects.
Pimozide *(Orap®)*	CYP3A4 inhibitors Other drugs that prolong the QT interval[c]	Fatal cardiac dysrhythmias reported when combined with CYP3A4 inhibitors such as clarithromycin.
Sparfloxacin *(Zagam®)*	Other drugs that prolong the QT interval[c]	Moxifloxacin also prolongs the QT interval, but other fluoroquinolones appear to have minimal effects.
Terfenadine[a] *(Seldane®)*	CYP3A4 inhibitors Other drugs that prolong the QT interval[c]	Fatal cardiac dysrhythmias reported when combined with CYP3A4 inhibitors; terfenadine metabolite (fexofenadine) has minimal effects on the QT interval.
Thioridazine *(Mellaril®)*	CYP2D6 inhibitors Other drugs that prolong the QT interval[c]	May be responsible for some sudden deaths.
Ziprasidone *(Geodon®)*	CYP3A4 inhibitors Other drugs that prolong the QT interval[c]	Based on theoretical considerations; ziprasidone effect on QT interval less than with thioridazine.

[a] Withdrawn from the market in the United States and Canada.
[b] Use restricted in the United States; withdrawn from the market in Canada.
[c] Drugs that can increase the QT_c interval when given alone in therapeutic doses include amiodarone, disopyramide, dofetilide, haloperidol, ibutilide, pimozide, procainamide, quinidine, sotalol, sparfloxacin, and ziprasidone.

Drug Interactions in Pediatric Patients

In developing the following list of drug interactions, an effort was made to emphasize the interactions that are most likely to occur in the pediatric patient rather than to present a comprehensive list of all known drug interactions. Interactions that are clinically insignificant, poorly documented, or obviously based on the pharmacologic actions of the drugs (e.g., synergism or antagonism) generally have not been included. However, because of the increasing importance of drug interactions involving the hepatic cytochrome P-450 isoenzymes (*see also* Chapter 11) and a number of drugs commonly required by pediatric patients, a separate table summarizing these interactions has been included (Table 6-1).

Drugs are listed in alphabetical order by nonproprietary (generic) names with cross-referencing to facilitate data retrieval. Common brand/trade names are provided in parenthesis to assist the reader.[1] Each major drug entry is followed by a series of brief, referenced descriptions of empirically validated drug interactions in alphabetical order by generic name. The reader should consult a comprehensive drug interactions reference (e.g., Hansten & Horn, 2001) if a suspected interaction is not addressed in this chapter.

Acetaminophen *(Tylenol®)*

Cholestyramine resin (Questran®). Cholestyramine resin reduces the GI absorption of acetaminophen. Each oral dose of acetaminophen should be ingested at least 1 hour before cholestyramine resin (Dordoni et al., 1973).

Phenytoin. See Phenytoin + Acetaminophen.

Acetazolamide *(Diamox®)*

Phenytoin. See Phenytoin + Acetazolamide.

Primidone. See Primidone + Acetazolamide.

---

1. Note that omission of a brand/trade name usually indicates that the drug generally is available by generic name. Other brand/trade names for the drugs discussed are included in the Index at the end of this text.

Allopurinol *(Zyloprim®)*

Anticoagulants, oral. See Anticoagulants, Oral + Enzyme Inhibitors.

Azathioprine (Imuran®). Allopurinol impedes the inactivation of azathioprine by inhibiting the metabolism of mercaptopurine, the active metabolite of azathioprine. Azathioprine toxicity (e.g., bone marrow suppression) may result. The azathioprine dosage may need to be reduced to about 25% of the recommended dosage (Aach & Kissane, 1970; Nies & Oates, 1971).

Mercaptopurine (Purinethol®). Allopurinol inhibits the inactivation of mercaptopurine and may result in mercaptopurine toxicity (e.g., bone marrow suppression). The mercaptopurine dosage may need to be reduced to about 25% of the recommended dosage (Coffey et al., 1972).

Theophylline. Allopurinol, particularly in large dosages, may increase theophylline serum concentrations, probably by inhibiting theophylline metabolism. Monitor theophylline serum concentrations and patient clinical status for evidence of excessive theophylline serum concentrations when allopurinol is initiated and for evidence of subtherapeutic theophylline serum concentrations when allopurinol is discontinued (Grygiel et al., 1979; Jacobs & Senior, 1974).

Aminoglycosides

Methotrexate. Oral aminoglycosides may decrease the absorption of oral methotrexate, resulting in low methotrexate serum concentrations. Be alert for decreased therapeutic response to oral methotrexate in pediatric patients receiving oral aminoglycosides (Cohen et al., 1976).

Neuromuscular blockers. Aminoglycosides have neuromuscular blocking activity, which may enhance the effects of neuromuscular blockers (e.g., gallamine, tubocurarine); respiratory arrest has been reported with this combination. Intravenous calcium or anticholinesterases may help reverse the effects of this interaction (Pittinger et al., 1970; Warner & Sanders, 1971).

Penicillins. Penicillins, particularly extended-spectrum penicillins, can inactivate aminoglycoside antibiotics both in vivo and in vitro. Penicillins and aminoglycosides should not be mixed together before intravenous infusion. Aminoglycoside serum concentrations may be **falsely** decreased in the presence of penicillins because of inactivation after the blood sample is drawn. The in vivo effect of this interaction is of clinical significance only in pediatric patients who have severely reduced renal function (Ervin et al., 1976; Riff & Jackson, 1972).

Penicillin V. Oral neomycin can decrease the bioavailability of oral penicillin V by causing a malabsorption syndrome. Alternative antibiotics to penicillin V should be considered for pediatric patients receiving oral neomycin. Intramuscular and intravenous penicillin avoids this interaction (Cheng & White, 1962).

Amiodarone *(Cordarone)*

Anticoagulants, oral. See Anticoagulants, Oral + Enzyme Inhibitors.

Digitalis glycosides. Amiodarone increases digoxin serum concentrations, possibly by reducing renal elimination of digoxin. Children given amiodarone manifest greater increases in digoxin serum concentrations than adults (Koren et al., 1984; Moysey et al., 1981).

Anabolic Steroids

Cyclosporine. See Cyclosporine + Anabolic Steroids.

Insulin. Anabolic steroids (e.g., methandrostenolone) may enhance the hypoglycemic effect of insulin. Monitor for altered insulin requirements if anabolic steroids are initiated or discontinued (Sachs & Wolfman, 1968).

Antacids

Fluoroquinolones. Antacids may reduce the absorption of the oral fluoroquinolones (e.g., ciprofloxacin, enoxacin, gatifloxacin, levofloxacin, lomefloxacin, norfloxacin, ofloxacin, sparfloxacin). Each oral dose of fluoroquinolones should be ingested at least 2 hours before or 6 hours after antacids (Gugler & Allgayer, 1990; Nix et al., 1989).

Iron. Antacids may reduce the absorption of oral iron. Doses of antacids and iron should be ingested at times as far apart as possible (Coste et al., 1977; Hall & Davis, 1969; O'Neil-Cutting & Crosby, 1986).

Itraconazole (Sporanox®). Oral itraconazole requires an acidic environment for absorption. Thus, antacids and any other drugs that increase gastric pH, can reduce itraconazole absorption (Katz & Gupta, 1997; May et al., 1994).

Ketoconazole (Nizoral®). Oral ketoconazole requires an acidic environment for absorption. Thus, antacids, and any other drugs that increase gastric pH, can reduce ketoconazole absorption (Carlson et al., 1983; Lelawongs et al., 1988).

Phenytoin. See Phenytoin + Antacids.

Salicylates. Certain antacids (e.g., magnesium and aluminum hydroxides) may alkalinize the urine, thus enhancing renal excretion of salicylates. Monitor for reduced salicylate serum concentration and adjust the salicylate dosage as necessary (Hansten & Hayton, 1980; Levy et al., 1975).

Tetracyclines. See Tetracyclines + Antacids.

Anticoagulants, Oral

Enzyme inducers. Inducers of hepatic microsomal enzymes (e.g., barbiturates, carbamazepine, nafcillin, phenytoin, primidone, rifabutin, rifampin, troglitazone) reduce the serum concentration and effects of oral anticoagulants (e.g., warfarin). Monitor the prothrombin time (PT) or international normalized ratio (INR), and increase or decrease the oral anticoagulant dosage as necessary when initiating or discontinuing, respectively, an enzyme inducer (O'Reilly et al., 1980). (*See also* Table 6-1.)

Enzyme inhibitors. Inhibitors of hepatic microsomal enzymes (e.g., allopurinol, amiodarone, cimetidine, ciprofloxacin, disulfiram, erythromycin, fluconazole, fluoxetine, metronidazole, propafenone, trimethoprim–sulfamethoxazole) increase the serum concentration and effects of oral anticoagulants. Monitor the PT or INR, and decrease or increase the oral anticoagulant dosage as necessary when initiating or discontinuing, respectively, an enzyme inhibitor (Hansten & Horn, 1985a; Kerley & Ali, 1982; O'Reilly, 1983; Puurunen et al., 1980; Seaton et al., 1990; Smith, 1984). (*See also* Table 6-1.)

Salicylates. Large dosages (≥ 2 grams/day) of salicylates (e.g., aspirin) increase the hypoprothrombinemic response to oral anticoagulants. All dosages of aspirin inhibit platelet function and contribute to GI erosion and bleeding. Use these drugs concurrently only when the benefit is judged to exceed the risk for bleeding. For fever or mild-to-moderate pain, acetaminophen generally can be safely substituted for aspirin (Chesebro et al., 1983; Donaldson et al., 1982; Trunet et al., 1980).

Thyroid hormones. Thyroid hormones increase the catabolism of vitamin K-dependent clotting factors and, thus, the hypoprothrombinemic response to oral anticoagulants. Monitor the PT or INR, and increase or decrease the oral anticoagulant dosage as necessary when thyroid hormones are initiated or discontinued, respectively (Hansten, 1980b).

Anticonvulsants

(*See also* Barbiturates, Carbamazepine, Phenytoin, Primidone, and Valproic Acid.)

Antidepressants, tricyclic. Tricyclic antidepressants can lower the seizure threshold. Large dosages can produce seizures among children and adolescents who have seizure disorders. Pediatric patients who have seizure disorders should be monitored for increased seizure activity when a tricyclic antidepressant is initiated (Dallas & Heathfield, 1967; Petti & Campbell, 1975). Moreover, the hepatic metabolism of tricyclic antidepressants may be increased by enzyme-inducing anticonvulsants such as carbamazepine and phenobarbital (Brown et al., 1990). Monitor the patient for reduced antidepressant effect.

Contraceptives, oral. Several anticonvulsants (e.g., carbamazepine, phenobarbital, phenytoin) have enzyme-inducing properties that may increase the metabolism of oral contraceptives and, thereby, decrease their effectiveness. Spotting or breakthrough bleeding is a useful (but not fail-safe) indicator for this interaction. Alternative contraceptive methods may be required (Coulam & Annegers, 1979; McArthur, 1969).

Antidepressants, Tricyclic

Anticonvulsants. See Anticonvulsants + Antidepressants, Tricyclic.

Cimetidine (Tagamet®). Cimetidine may inhibit the metabolism of tricyclic antidepressants, resulting in excessive antidepressant serum concentrations. Monitor for antidepressant toxicity and reduce the dosage as needed (Abernethy et al., 1984; Shapiro, 1984). Other H_2-antagonists (e.g., ranitidine) are less likely to interact with tricyclic antidepressants.

Clonidine (Catapres®). Tricyclic antidepressants may inhibit the antihypertensive effect of clonidine. Monitor blood pressure closely if tricyclic antidepressants are initiated or discontinued among pediatric patients receiving clonidine (Briant et al., 1973; Hui, 1983).

Selective serotonin reuptake inhibitors (SSRIs). Fluoxetine and paroxetine inhibit cytochrome P-450 2D6 (CYP2D6), which is responsible for the metabolism of several tricyclic antidepressants. Increases in tricyclic antidepressant serum concentrations can be marked. Monitor for antidepressant toxicity, and adjust the dosage as needed. Citalopram, fluvoxamine, sertraline, and venlafaxine have much less effect on CYP2D6 (Bergstrom et al., 1992; van Harten, 1993).

Sympathomimetics. Tricyclic antidepressants enhance the pressor response to direct-acting sympathomimetics such as epinephrine, norepinephrine, and phenylephrine. Use these drugs cautiously in pediatric patients receiving tricyclic antidepressants (Boakes et al., 1973; Ghose, 1980).

Azathioprine *(Imuran®)*

Allopurinol. See Allopurinol + Azathioprine.

Astemizole. (*See* Tables 6-1 and 6-2.)

Barbiturates

(*See also* Anticonvulsants.)

Anticoagulants, oral. See Anticoagulants, Oral + Enzyme Inducers.

Carbamazepine. See Carbamazepine + Barbiturates.

Chloramphenicol. See Chloramphenicol + Barbiturates.

Corticosteroids. Barbiturates increase the metabolism of systemic corticosteroids, thus reducing their therapeutic effect. Monitor for inadequate corticosteroid response, and increase the corticosteroid dosage as necessary (Brooks et al., 1972; Gambertoglio et al., 1982).

Cyclosporine. See Cyclosporine + Barbiturates.

Phenytoin. See Phenytoin + Barbiturates.

Primidone. See Primidone + Barbiturates.

Theophylline. See Theophylline + Barbiturates.

Valproic acid. See Valproic Acid + Barbiturates.

BCG Vaccine

Isoniazid. Isoniazid and other antitubercular drugs antagonize *Mycobacterium tuberculosis* reproduction and therefore impair the development of active immunity following the administration of BCG vaccination. If indicated, treatment with antitubercular drugs should take precedence over the use of BCG vaccine (Grabenstein, 1990).

Benzodiazepines

(*See also* Anticonvulsants.)

Valproic acid. See Valproic Acid + Benzodiazepines.

Beta-Adrenergic Blockers

Cimetidine (Tagamet®). Cimetidine inhibits the hepatic metabolism of labetolol, metoprolol, and propranolol (and probably also other beta-adrenergic blockers metabolized by the liver, such as pindolol and timolol). Monitor for excessive beta-adrenergic blocker effect (e.g., bradycardia and severe hypotension), and adjust the dosage as needed. The disposition of beta-adrenergic blockers eliminated by the kidneys, such as atenolol and nadolol, is unlikely to be affected by cimetidine (Feely et al., 1981; Houtzagers et al., 1982).

Insulin. Many insulin-dependent diabetic patients, including children and adolescents, have developed hypoglycemia during concurrent beta-adrenergic blocker therapy. Beta-adrenergic blockers may prolong hypoglycemic episodes, cause hypertension during hypoglycemic episodes, and inhibit tachycardia and CNS stimulation, which are warning signs of hypoglycemia. Cardioselective beta-adrenergic blockers such as acebutolol, atenolol, and metoprolol are less likely to prolong hypoglycemia and cause hypertension and, thus, are preferred for insulin-dependent diabetic patients (Hansten, 1980a; Hesse & Pedersen, 1973; Newman, 1976).

Nonsteroidal anti-inflammatory drugs (NSAIDs). Indomethacin (and probably other NSAIDs) may inhibit the antihypertensive response to beta-adrenergic blockers, particularly in renin-dependent hypertensive states. Monitor blood pressure carefully, and adjust the beta-adrenergic blocker dosage, as necessary (Salvetti et al., 1982; Watkins et al., 1980).

Prazosin (Minipress®). Beta-adrenergic blockers may enhance the "first-dose" hypotensive reaction following prazosin administration. Prazosin should be given with caution to children receiving beta-adrenergic blockers; it may be prudent to give the first dose of prazosin at bedtime (Elliott et al., 1981; Seideman et al., 1982).

Sympathomimetics. Nonselective beta-adrenergic blockers (e.g., nadolol, pindolol, propranolol) enhance the pressor effect of epinephrine on the systemic circulation by blocking the beta (vasodilator) effects, leaving unopposed alpha (vasoconstrictor) effects. Cardioselective beta-adrenergic blockers (e.g., acebutolol, atenolol, metoprolol) do not enhance the pressor response to epinephrine. The effect of beta-adrenergic blockers on the response to other sympathomimetics is not well established, but be alert for evidence of enhanced response (Houben et al., 1979; Van Herwaarden et al., 1977).

Bumetanide

Nonsteroidal anti-inflammatory drugs (NSAIDs). See Furosemide + Nonsteroidal Anti-Inflammatory Drugs.

Carbamazepine *(Tegretol®)*

(*See also* Anticonvulsants.)

Anticoagulants, oral. See Anticoagulants, Oral + Enzyme Inducers.

Barbiturates. Phenobarbital (and probably also other barbiturates) lowers carbamazepine serum concentrations, probably through hepatic microsomal enzyme induction. The clinical significance of this interaction is unclear because phenobarbital also has anticonvulsant activity and may provide protection despite lowered carbamazepine serum concentrations (Christiansen & Dam, 1973).

Clarithromycin (Biaxin®). Clarithromycin inhibits carbamazepine CYP3A4 metabolism and can produce signs and symptoms of carbamazepine toxicity (e.g., ataxia, dizziness, drowsiness, headache, nausea, nystagmus, vomiting). Azithromycin and dirithromycin do not appear to inhibit CYP3A4 (Albani et al., 1993; Yasui et al., 1997).

Corticosteroids. Carbamazepine can reduce the serum concentrations of dexamethasone, prednisolone, and probably other corticosteroids. Corticosteroid dosage requirements may be increased (Olivesi, 1986; Privitera et al., 1982).

Cyclosporine (Sandimmune®). Carbamazepine (and other hepatic microsomal enzyme inducers) appear to enhance the metabolism of cyclosporine, thus reducing cyclosporine serum concentrations. Monitor for altered cyclosporine serum concentrations when initiating or discontinuing carbamazepine therapy (Alvarez et al., 1991; Schofield et al., 1990).

Diltiazem (Cardizem®). *See* Carbamazepine + Verapamil.

Erythromycin. Erythromycin inhibits the CYP3A4 metabolism of carbamazepine, thereby reducing its clearance. Large increases in carbamazepine serum concentrations have been reported. Monitor for signs and symptoms of toxicity (e.g., ataxia, dizziness, drowsiness, headache, nausea, nystagmus, vomiting) when erythromycin is initiated and for increased seizure activity when erythromycin is discontinued. Monitor the carbamazepine serum concentration if possible (Wong et al., 1983).

Fluoxetine (Prozac®). Fluoxetine increases carbamazepine serum concentrations, probably by inhibiting carbamazepine metabolism in the liver. Monitor for signs and symptoms of carbamazepine toxicity (e.g., ataxia, dizziness, drowsiness, headache, nausea, nystagmus, vomiting), and monitor carbamazepine serum concentrations when initiating fluoxetine in pediatric patients receiving carbamazepine (Grimsley et al., 1991; Pearson, 1990).

Isoniazid. Isoniazid increases carbamazepine serum concentrations, probably by inhibition of hepatic metabolism of carbamazepine. Carbamazepine dosage reduction may be needed when isoniazid is initiated. Monitor for signs and symptoms of carbamazepine toxicity (e.g., ataxia, dizziness, drowsiness, headache, nausea, nystagmus, vomiting), and monitor carbamazepine serum concentrations when initiating isoniazid in pediatric patients receiving carbamazepine (Block, 1982; Valsalan & Cooper, 1982).

Lithium salts. The pharmacologic effect of lithium appears to be enhanced by carbamazepine by an unknown mechanism. This effect can be used to therapeutic advantage. However, if lithium and carbamazepine are given together, be alert for signs and symptoms of lithium toxicity (e.g., apathy, coarse hand tremor, confusion, drowsiness, dysarthria, giddiness) even when lithium serum concentrations are below the usual toxic range (Ghose, 1978; Lipinski & Pope, 1982).

Propoxyphene (Darvon®). Propoxyphene can markedly increase carbamazepine serum concentrations. Carbamazepine toxicity is common in patients receiving this combination. Avoid concurrent propoxyphene therapy, if possible, in pediatric patients receiving carbamazepine. When concomitant use is required, monitor carbamazepine serum concentrations and observe patients for signs and symptoms of carbamazepine toxicity (e.g., ataxia, dizziness, drowsiness, headache, nausea, nystagmus, vomiting) when propoxyphene is initiated. Monitor patients for increased seizure activity when propoxyphene is discontinued (Kubacka & Ferrante, 1983; Yu et al., 1986).

Theophylline. *See* Theophylline + Carbamazepine.

Troleandomycin. Troleandomycin increases carbamazepine serum concentrations, probably by inhibiting carbamazepine metabolism in the liver. Carbamazepine toxicity can occur when troleandomycin is initiated in pediatric patients receiving carbamazepine. Alternative antibiotics should be considered for these patients (Mesdjian et al., 1980).

Verapamil (Isoptin®). Verapamil increases carbamazepine serum concentrations, probably by inhibiting carbamazepine metabolism. Carbamazepine toxicity can occur. Diltiazem also can increase carbamazepine serum concentrations, but nifedipine does not appear to do so (Beattie et al., 1988; Macphee et al., 1986).

Carmustine *(BiCNU®)*

Cimetidine. *See* Cimetidine + Carmustine.

Cephalosporins

Probenecid. Probenecid inhibits the renal excretion of cephalosporins, increasing cephalosporin serum concentrations. No special precautions are necessary because cephalosporins have a high therapeutic index (Griffith et al., 1977).

Chloramphenicol *(Chloromycetin®)*

Barbiturates. Barbiturates may enhance chloramphenicol metabolism, resulting in decreased chloramphenicol serum concentrations. Chloramphenicol may inhibit barbiturate metabolism, resulting in increased barbiturate serum concentrations. If barbiturates and chloramphenicol are used concurrently, be alert for reduced chloramphenicol efficacy and increased barbiturate toxicity. Monitor the serum concentrations of both drugs, and adjust the dosages as needed (Bloxham et al., 1979; Koup et al., 1978).

Phenytoin. See Phenytoin + Chloramphenicol.

Chloroquine *(Aralen®)*

Human diploid-cell rabies (HDCR) vaccine. Chloroquine suppresses the antibody response to intradermal HDCR vaccine. If concurrent use cannot be avoided, monitor antibody titers to confirm sufficient production (Bernard et al., 1985; Pappaioanou et al., 1986; Taylor et al., 1984).

Cholestyramine Resin *(Questran®)*

Acetaminophen. See Acetaminophen + Cholestyramine Resin.

Digitalis glycosides. Cholestyramine resin may impair the GI absorption of digitoxin and, to a lesser extent, digoxin. Doses of cholestyramine resin and digitalis glycosides should be given at times as far apart as possible. However, this practice does not completely avoid the interaction with digitoxin because it undergoes enterohepatic recirculation. Be alert for evidence of reduced digitalis effect in pediatric patients receiving cholestyramine resin (Caldwell et al., 1971; Carruthers & Dujovne, 1980). Colestipol may interact with digitalis glycosides in a similar manner, so it is not a suitable alternative.

Furosemide (Lasix®). Cholestyramine can dramatically reduce furosemide absorption. Furosemide should be ingested 2 hours before or 6 hours after cholestyramine. Colestipol interacts with furosemide in a similar manner, so it is not a suitable alternative (Neuvonen et al., 1988).

Thyroid hormones. Cholestyramine resin inhibits the GI absorption of levothyroxine sodium and liothyronine sodium (Northcutt et al., 1969). Oral doses of these thyroid hormones and cholestyramine resin should be ingested at least 4 hours apart. Colestipol *(Colestid®)* may interact with thyroid hormones in a similar manner, so it is not a suitable alternative.

Cimetidine *(Tagamet®)*

(*See also* Tables 6-1 and 6-2.)

Anticoagulants, oral. See Anticoagulants, Oral + Enzyme Inhibitors.

Antidepressants, tricyclic. See Antidepressants, Tricyclic + Cimetidine.

Beta-adrenergic blockers. See Beta-Adrenergic Blockers + Cimetidine.

Carmustine (BiCNU®). Cimetidine may increase the bone marrow suppressive effect of carmustine. Monitor for evidence of excessive bone marrow suppression in pediatric patients receiving this combination (Selker et al., 1978; Volkin et al., 1982).

Itraconazole (Sporanox®). Oral itraconazole requires an acidic environment for absorption. Thus, any drug that increases gastric pH (e.g., antacids, H_2-receptor antagonists, proton pump inhibitors) can reduce itraconazole absorption (Lange et al., 1997; Zimmermann et al., 1994).

Ketoconazole (Nizoral®). Oral ketoconazole requires an acidic environment for absorption. Thus, cimetidine and any other drugs that increase gastric pH (e.g., antacids and omeprazole) can reduce ketoconazole absorption (Carlson et al., 1983; Lelawongs et al., 1988).

Phenytoin (Dilantin®). Cimetidine inhibits the hepatic metabolism of phenytoin, thus increasing phenytoin serum concentrations. Phenytoin toxicity has been reported. Monitor for evidence of phenytoin toxicity when initiating cimetidine in pediatric patients receiving phenytoin. If possible, measure phenytoin serum concentrations. Reduce the phenytoin dose as necessary. The use of famotidine, nizatidine, or ranitidine instead of cimetidine circumvents the interaction (Bartle et al., 1983; Hansten & Horn, 1985b; Salem et al., 1983).

Procainamide (Pronestyl®). Cimetidine appears to reduce the renal clearance of procainamide and N-acetylprocainamide (NAPA), an active metabolite. Monitor for evidence of excessive procainamide and NAPA serum concentrations. Adjust the procainamide dosage as needed. Ranitidine reduces the renal clearance of procainamide to a lesser extent than cimetidine, and famotidine does not appear to affect procainamide clearance (Klotz et al., 1985; Paloucek et al., 1986; Somogyi & Heinzow, 1982).

Quinidine. Cimetidine inhibits the hepatic metabolism of quinidine, thus increasing quinidine serum concentrations. Monitor for excessive quinidine effect, and adjust the quinidine dosage as necessary (Hardy et al., 1983; Polish et al., 1981).

Theophylline. See Theophylline + Cimetidine.

Tricyclic antidepressants. See Antidepressants, Tricyclic + Cimetidine.

Ciprofloxacin *(Cipro®)*

(See Fluoroquinolones.)

Anticoagulants, oral. See Anticoagulants, Oral + Enzyme Inhibitors.

Clarithromycin *(Biaxin®)*

Carbamazepine. See Carbamazepine + Clarithromycin.

Cyclosporine. See Cyclosporine + Clarithromycin.

Clonidine *(Catapres®)*

Antidepressants, tricyclic. See Antidepressants, Tricyclic + Clonidine.

Colestipol *(Colestid®)*

Thyroid hormones. See Cholestyramine Resin + Thyroid Hormones.

Contraceptives, Oral

Anticonvulsants. See Anticonvulsants + Contraceptives, Oral.

Rifampin (Rifadin®). Rifampin enhances the metabolism of oral contraceptives, which may result in menstrual irregularities and rarely in unintended pregnancy. Use another form of birth control in addition to the oral contraceptive during and for 3 weeks following the discontinuation of rifampin. If rifampin therapy is long term, it may be necessary to use an oral contraceptive with a high estrogen content or substitute another method of birth control for the oral contraceptive (Robertson & Johnson, 1976; Skolnick et al., 1976).

Corticosteroids

Barbiturates. See Barbiturates + Corticosteroids.

Insulin. Corticosteroids tend to impair glucose tolerance and may increase insulin requirements (Hunder et al., 1975).

Phenytoin. See Phenytoin + Corticosteroids.

Rifampin. See Rifampin + Corticosteroids.

Salicylates. Corticosteroids have been shown to reduce salicylate serum concentrations in children receiving large salicylate doses. Discontinuation or tapering of corticosteroid therapy during high-dose salicylate therapy may result in salicylate intoxication (Graham et al., 1977; Klinenberg & Miller, 1965).

Cyclosporine *(Sandimmune®)*

Anabolic steroids. Case reports suggest that anabolic steroids can gradually increase cyclosporine serum concentrations, possibly by inhibiting cyclosporine metabolism. Cyclosporine toxicity has occurred. Monitor for altered cyclosporine response if anabolic steroids are initiated or discontinued (Moller & Ekelund, 1985; Ross et al., 1986).

Barbiturates. Barbiturates (and other hepatic microsomal enzyme inducers) probably enhance the metabolism of cyclosporine, thus reducing cyclosporine serum concentrations. Although clinical evidence is limited, it is prudent to monitor for reduced cyclosporine serum concentrations and adjust the dosage, if needed (Carstensen et al., 1986).

Carbamazepine. See Carbamazepine + Cyclosporine.

Clarithromycin (Biaxin®). Clarithromycin inhibits CYP3A4 cyclosporine metabolism and can substantially increase cyclosporine serum concentrations. Azithromycin and dirithromycin do not appear to inhibit CYP3A4 metabolism (Spicer et al., 1997; Watkins et al., 1997).

Erythromycin. Erythromycin inhibits cyclosporine metabolism and can substantially increase cyclosporine serum concentrations. Several cases of nephrotoxicity have been reported. Avoid erythromycin, if possible, in pediatric patients receiving cyclosporine. If this combination cannot be avoided, monitor cyclosporine serum concentrations and renal function closely (Freeman et al., 1986; Kohan, 1986; Ptachcinski et al., 1985).

Ketoconazole (Nizoral®). Ketoconazole may markedly increase cyclosporine serum concentrations, thus increasing the likelihood of cyclosporine-induced nephrotoxicity. If the combination cannot be avoided, closely monitor for elevated cyclosporine serum concentrations and nephrotoxicity (Hansten, 1984).

Nefazodone (Serzone®). Nefazodone inhibits CYP3A4 cyclosporine metabolism and can increase cyclosporine serum concentrations and toxicity. If the combination cannot be avoided, closely monitor for evidence of excessive cyclosporine effect (Helms-Smith et al., 1996).

Nonsteroidal anti-inflammatory drugs (NSAIDs). Several cases of cyclosporine-induced nephrotoxicity have been reported in patients receiving concurrent NSAID therapy. Although the incidence and severity of this interaction is not well established, it is prudent to monitor for cyclosporine toxicity if a NSAID is initiated in a pediatric patient receiving cyclosporine (Lake, 1991; Yee & McGuire, 1990).

Phenytoin (Dilantin®). Phenytoin (and other hepatic microsomal enzyme inducers) appears to enhance the metabolism of cyclosporine, thus reducing cyclosporine serum concentrations. Monitor for reduced cyclosporine serum concentrations and adjust the cyclosporine dosage if needed (Hansten, 1984).

Potassium-sparing diuretics. Cyclosporine has been associated with hyperkalemia, and concurrent cyclosporine pharmacotherapy with potassium-sparing diuretics (e.g., amiloride, spironolactone, triamterene) or potassium supplements may increase this risk. Monitor potassium serum concentrations closely (Hansten, 1984).

Rifampin (Rifadin®). Rifampin enhances cyclosporine metabolism and reduces cyclosporine serum concentrations. Loss of cyclosporine efficacy has been reported. Monitor for altered cyclosporine response if rifampin is initiated or discontinued in a pediatric patient receiving cyclosporine (Hansten & Horn, 1985c; Howard et al., 1985; Offermann et al., 1985).

Trimethoprim–sulfamethoxazole (Co-trimoxazole) (Septra®). The nephrotoxicity of cyclosporine may be increased by concurrent use of trimethoprim–sulfamethoxazole. Monitor renal function closely (Hansten, 1984; Ringden et al., 1984).

Digitalis Glycosides

Amiodarone. See Amiodarone + Digitalis Glycosides.

Cholestyramine resin. See Cholestyramine Resin + Digitalis Glycosides.

Kaolin-pectin. Kaolin–pectin reduces the GI absorption of oral digoxin, thus reducing digoxin serum concentrations. Each oral dose of kaolin–pectin should be ingested 2 hours after oral digoxin to minimize the interaction. Digoxin capsules may be less likely to be affected by kaolin–pectin than digoxin tablets (Allen et al., 1981; Brown & Juhl, 1976).

Quinidine. Quinidine reduces the elimination of digoxin and displaces digoxin from tissue binding sites, thus increasing digoxin serum concentrations about two- to threefold. Monitor for digoxin toxicity, and reduce the digoxin dosage as necessary (Bussey, 1982; Hansten, 1981b; Small & Marshall, 1979).

Verapamil (Isoptin®). Verapamil reduces the elimination of digoxin, thus increasing digoxin serum concentrations. Monitor for digoxin toxicity, and reduce the digoxin dosage as necessary (Belz et al., 1983; Klein et al., 1982).

Disulfiram *(Antabuse®)*

Anticoagulants, oral. See Anticoagulants, Oral + Enzyme Inhibitors.

Diuretics

(*See* Furosemide, Potassium-Sparing Diuretics, and Thiazide Diuretics.)

Dopamine *(Intropin®)*

Phenytoin. See Phenytoin + Dopamine.

Doxycycline *(Doxycin®)*

Phenytoin. See Phenytoin + Doxycycline.

Enzyme Inducers

Anticoagulants, oral. See Anticoagulants, Oral + Enzyme Inducers.
  (*See also* Tables 6-1 and 6-2.)

Enzyme Inhibitors

Anticoagulants, oral. See Anticoagulants, Oral + Enzyme Inhibitors.
  (*See also* Tables 6-1 and 6-2.)

Erythromycin

Anticoagulants, oral. See Anticoagulants, Oral + Enzyme Inhibitors.

Carbamazepine. See Carbamazepine + Erythromycin.

Theophylline. See Theophylline + Erythromycin.

Fluconazole *(Diflucan®)*

Anticoagulants, oral. See Anticoagulants, Oral + Enzyme Inhibitors.

Phenytoin. Fluconazole can substantially increase phenytoin serum concentrations by inhibiting phenytoin metabolism in the liver. Phenytoin toxicity has been reported. Monitor for increased phenytoin serum concentrations and phenytoin toxicity if fluconazole is initiated in a pediatric patient receiving phenytoin. Monitor for increased seizure activity if fluconazole is discontinued (Howitt & Oziemski, 1989; Mitchell & Holland, 1989).

Fluoroquinolones

Antacids. See Antacids + Fluoroquinolones.

Theophylline. See Theophylline + Fluoroquinolones.

Fluoxetine *(Prozac®)*

Anticoagulants, oral. See Anticoagulants, Oral + Enzyme Inhibitors.

Antidepressants, tricyclic. See Antidepressants, Tricyclic + Selective Serotonin Reuptake Inhibitors.

Carbamazepine. See Carbamazepine + Fluoxetine.

Folic Acid

Phenytoin. See Phenytoin + Folic Acid.

Furosemide (Lasix®)

Cholestyramine resin. See Cholestyramine Resin + Furosemide.

Nonsteroidal anti-inflammatory drugs (NSAIDs). The diuretic and antihypertensive effects of furosemide may be reduced by concomitant NSAID therapy because of inhibition of prostaglandin synthesis, which causes sodium retention. If increasing the dosage of furosemide does not produce the desired response, try a different NSAID. The efficacy of bumetanide is probably also impaired by NSAIDs (Allan et al., 1981; Hansten & Horn, 1986; Roberts et al., 1984).

Phenytoin. See Phenytoin + Furosemide.

Ganciclovir (Cytovene®)

Zidovudine (AZT®). Concurrent use of ganciclovir and zidovudine appears to result in a high incidence of hematologic toxicity, probably because of combined pharmacodynamic effects. Foscarnet has been proposed as an alternative to ganciclovir for the treatment of cytomegalovirus infections in pediatric patients receiving zidovudine (Hochster et al., 1990; Jacobson et al., 1991).

Hepatic Microsomal Enzyme Inducers

(*See* Enzyme Inducers.)

Hepatic Microsomal Enzyme Inhibitors

(*See* Enzyme Inhibitors.)

Insulin

Anabolic steroids. See Anabolic Steroids + Insulin.

Beta-adrenergic blockers. See Beta-Adrenergic Blockers + Insulin.

Corticosteroids. See Corticosteroids + Insulin.

Iron

Antacids. See Antacids + Iron.

Tetracyclines. See Tetracyclines + Iron.

Vitamin E. Vitamin E has been reported to impair the hematologic response to iron in pediatric patients with iron-deficiency anemia. If possible, avoid the use of vitamin E in such patients until after the anemia is corrected (Melhorn & Gross, 1969).

Isoniazid (INH®)

BCG vaccine. See BCG Vaccine + Isoniazid.

Carbamazepine. See Carbamazepine + Isoniazid.

Phenytoin. See Phenytoin + Isoniazid.

Primidone. See Primidone + Isoniazid.

Rifampin (Rifadin®). Rifampin may induce the metabolism of isoniazid to toxic metabolites, resulting in hepatotoxicity, although the incidence is probably very low. Both rifampin and isoniazid can be hepatotoxic alone, so be alert to drug-induced hepatotoxicity when they are used concurrently (Bistritzer et al., 1980; Pessayre et al., 1977).

Itraconazole (Sporanox®)

Antacids. See Antacids + Itraconazole.

Cimetidine. See Cimetidine + Itraconazole.

Digitalis glycosides. See Digitalis Glycosides + Kaolin–Pectin.

Ketoconazole (Nizoral®)

Antacids. See Antacids + Ketoconazole.

Cimetidine. See Cimetidine + Ketoconazole.

Cyclosporine. See Cyclosporine + Ketoconazole.

Lithium Salts *(Lithane®)*

Angiotensin-converting enzyme (ACE) inhibitors. Several case reports have described serious lithium toxicity several weeks after an ACE inhibitor was added to lithium therapy. When concomitant use is required, monitor for evidence of excessive lithium serum concentrations and adjust the lithium dosage as necessary (Baldwin & Safferman, 1990; Douste-Blazy et al., 1986).

Carbamazepine. See Carbamazepine + Lithium Salts.

Nonsteroidal anti-inflammatory drugs (NSAIDs). Several NSAIDs increase lithium serum concentrations by reducing renal clearance of lithium. Lithium toxicity has been reported, although the magnitude of the increase in lithium serum concentration varied considerably. Sulindac may slightly decrease lithium serum concentrations. Monitor for evidence of altered lithium serum concentrations, and adjust the lithium dosage accordingly (Frolich et al., 1978; Furnell & Davies, 1985; Ragheb & Powell, 1986a; Ragheb & Powell, 1986b).

Phenytoin. See Phenytoin + Lithium Salts.

Thiazide diuretics. Thiazide diuretics reduce the renal excretion of lithium, resulting in increased lithium serum concentrations. Lithium toxicity has been reported. Monitor for evidence of excessive lithium serum concentrations and reduce the lithium dosage as necessary (Himmelhoch et al., 1977; Jefferson & Kalin, 1979).

Macrolide Antibiotics

(*See* Clarithromycin and Erythromycin.)

Mercaptopurine

Allopurinol. See Allopurinol + Mercaptopurine.

Methotrexate

Aminoglycosides. See Aminoglycosides + Methotrexate.

Nonsteroidal anti-inflammatory drugs (NSAIDs). Several cases of severe methotrexate toxicity (including fatalities) have occurred following NSAID administration. Although the exact role of NSAIDs in these interactions is controversial, the potential severity of the outcome dictates caution. The risk of toxicity is probably higher in pediatric patients receiving antineoplastic dosages of methotrexate than in patients receiving low-dose methotrexate (Singh et al., 1986; Thyss et al., 1986).

Penicillins. See Penicillins + Methotrexate.

Probenecid. Probenecid inhibits the renal excretion of methotrexate, thus substantially increasing methotrexate serum concentrations. Avoid probenecid use in pediatric patients receiving methotrexate. If the combination must be used, monitor for methotrexate toxicity and reduce the methotrexate dosage as needed. Leucovorin calcium rescue may be required for longer periods than what is normally required in the absence of probenecid (Aherne et al., 1978; Howell et al., 1979).

Salicylates. Salicylates may reduce the renal excretion of methotrexate, thus increasing methotrexate serum concentrations and causing toxicity. Closely monitor pediatric patients for methotrexate toxicity, and reduce the methotrexate dosage as necessary (Liegler et al., 1969; Mandel, 1976).

Sulfonamides. See Sulfonamides + Methotrexate.

Metronidazole *(Flagyl®)*

Anticoagulants, oral. See Anticoagulants, Oral + Enzyme Inhibitors.

Moxifloxacin

(*See* Fluoroquinolones.)
(*See also* Table 6-2.)

Nefazodone *(Serzone®)*

Cyclosporine. See Cyclosporine + Nefazodone.

Neuromuscular Blockers

Aminoglycosides. See Aminoglycosides + Neuromuscular Blockers.

Nonsteroidal Anti-Inflammatory Drugs (NSAIDs)

Beta-adrenergic blockers. See Beta-Adrenergic Blockers + NSAIDs.

Cyclosporine. See Cyclosporine + NSAIDs.

Furosemide. See Furosemide + NSAIDs.

Lithium salts. See Lithium Salts + NSAIDs.

Oral Anticoagulants

(*See* Anticoagulants, Oral.)

Oral Contraceptives

(*See* Contraceptives, Oral.)

Paroxetine *(Paxil®)*

(*See* Selective Serotonin Reuptake Inhibitors.)

Penicillins

(*See also* Penicillin V.)

Aminoglycosides. See Aminoglycosides + Penicillins.

Methotrexate. Large dosages of penicillins appear to interfere with the renal tubular secretion of methotrexate, reducing methotrexate clearance. It is prudent to monitor for methotrexate toxicity when large dosages of penicillins are used. Leucovorin calcium rescue may be required for longer periods than what is normally required in the absence of penicillins (Bleyer, 1978; Gibson et al., 1981).

Penicillin V

(*See also* Penicillins.)

Aminoglycosides. See Aminoglycosides + Penicillin V.

Phenobarbital

(*See* Anticonvulsants and Barbiturates.)

Phenytoin *(Dilantin®)*

(*See also* Anticonvulsants.)

Acetaminophen (Tylenol®). Phenytoin appears to induce acetaminophen metabolism, decreasing its half-life of elimination and potentially increasing the rate of production of hepatotoxic metabolites. Large dosages or prolonged use of acetaminophen should be avoided in pediatric patients receiving phenytoin (Neuvonen et al., 1979; Perucca & Richens, 1971).

Acetazolamide (Diamox®). Acetazolamide may accelerate the development of phenytoin-induced osteomalacia by increasing urinary excretion of calcium and phosphate. If osteomalacia develops while a patient is receiving phenytoin and acetazolamide, discontinuation of acetazolamide or supplementation with vitamin D and phosphate may be of benefit (Mallette, 1977; Matsuda et al., 1975).

Antacids. Aluminum- and magnesium-containing antacids may decrease phenytoin bioavailability, thereby lowering phenytoin serum concentrations. The interaction can be avoided by ingesting each dose of the antacid and phenytoin at least 1 hour apart (Yuen, 1984).

Anticoagulants, oral. See Anticoagulants, Oral + Enzyme Inducers.

Barbiturates. Phenobarbital (and probably other barbiturates) can cause both enzyme induction (the predominant effect) and competitive inhibition (a rare effect) of phenytoin metabolism. Depending on the relative degrees of induction and inhibition, an increase, decrease (the most likely effect), or no change in phenytoin serum concentration may be seen. Pediatric patients should be monitored carefully for evidence of changes in phenytoin serum concentrations when barbiturates are initiated or discontinued or when the barbiturate dosage is altered (Buchanan et al., 1962; Hansen, 1974).

Chloramphenicol (Chloromycetin®). Chloramphenicol inhibits the metabolism of phenytoin causing substantial increases in phenytoin serum concentrations and toxicity. If possible, chloramphenicol should be avoided in pediatric patients receiving phenytoin. Phenytoin serum concentrations should be monitored and the phenytoin dosage adjusted as necessary in patients for whom the combination is unavoidable (Christensen & Skovsted, 1969; Greenlaw, 1979).

Cimetidine. See Cimetidine + Phenytoin.

Contraceptives, oral. See Anticonvulsants + Contraceptives, Oral.

Corticosteroids. Phenytoin increases the metabolism of corticosteroids and reduces their therapeutic efficacy. Monitor for inadequate corticosteroid response when corticosteroids and phenytoin (or other hepatic microsomal enzyme inducers) are used concurrently. Increasing the corticosteroid dosage may circumvent this interaction (Petereit & Meikle, 1977; Wassner et al., 1976).

Co-trimoxazole. See Phenytoin + Trimethoprim.

Cyclosporine. See Cyclosporine + Phenytoin.

Dopamine (Intropin®). Pediatric patients receiving dopamine may develop severe hypotension when intravenous phenytoin is administered. When concurrent therapy cannot be avoided, monitor patients closely for cardiovascular collapse when intravenous phenytoin is administered (Bivins et al., 1978).

Doxycycline (Doxycin®). Phenytoin can stimulate the metabolism of doxycycline, shortening its half-life of elimination. If the two drugs are used concurrently, be alert for doxycycline therapeutic failure (Neuvonen et al., 1975; Penttila et al., 1974).

Fluconazole. See Fluconazole + Phenytoin.

Folic acid. Folic acid can reduce phenytoin serum concentrations, probably by inducing phenytoin metabolism or possibly by decreasing the bioavailability of oral phenytoin. Folic acid also may lower the seizure threshold in pediatric patients treated with phenytoin. Most pediatric patients receiving phenytoin are unaffected by the initiation of folic acid supplements, but they should be monitored for a loss of seizure control (Furlanut et al., 1978; Yuen, 1984).

Furosemide (Lasix®). Oral phenytoin reduces the bioavailability of oral furosemide by inhibiting its absorption. An inhibitory effect of phenytoin on the diuretic response to furosemide has been postulated. Pediatric patients receiving both oral phenytoin and oral furosemide should be monitored for decreased diuretic response. Increasing the furosemide dosage may overcome this interaction (Ahmad, 1974; Fine et al., 1977).

Isoniazid (INH®). Isoniazid raises phenytoin serum concentrations by impairing phenytoin metabolism. Pediatric patients receiving phenytoin should be monitored closely for evidence of excessive phenytoin serum concentrations when isoniazid pharmacotherapy is initiated and for increased seizure activity when isoniazid is discontinued. Phenytoin dosage should be adjusted as required (Kutt et al., 1970; Miller et al., 1979).

Lithium salts (Lithane®). Phenytoin may enhance lithium toxicity. Although the mechanism and clinical significance of this interaction have not been determined, it is prudent to monitor for lithium toxicity when phenytoin is initiated (MacCallum, 1980; Speirs & Hirsch, 1978).

Primidone (Mysoline®). Phenytoin increases the metabolism of primidone to its active metabolite, phenobarbital. Excessive phenobarbital serum concentrations may result. No special precautions appear warranted other than remaining alert to the possibility that toxic phenobarbital serum concentrations may occur (*see also* Phenytoin + Barbiturates) (Fincham et al., 1974; Wilson & Wilkinson, 1973).

Pyridoxine. Large doses of pyridoxine stimulate phenytoin metabolism, resulting in decreased serum concentrations. No precautions are needed with the low pyridoxine doses used in multivitamin products. If large pyridoxine dosages are required, then monitor the patient for loss of seizure control (Hansson & Sillanpaa, 1976).

Salicylates. Large salicylate dosages can displace phenytoin from protein binding sites. This displacement results in lower total phenytoin concentrations, but the free concentration is unchanged. Use caution in interpreting total phenytoin concentrations when large dosages of salicylates are required (e.g., treatment of juvenile rheumatoid arthritis). Free phenytoin serum concentrations may be preferred for monitoring phenytoin therapy in pediatric patients receiving high dosages of salicylates. Salicylate dosages less than 2 grams/day probably have minimal effects on phenytoin disposition (Fraser et al., 1980; Paxton, 1980).

Sulfonamides. Sulfamethizole and sulfaphenazole may inhibit the metabolism of phenytoin, resulting in high phenytoin serum concentrations. Sulfisoxazole has been shown to displace phenytoin from protein binding sites in vitro; the clinical importance of this interaction remains unknown. Monitor for evidence of excessive phenytoin serum concentrations when concurrent therapy with sulfamethizole or sulfaphenazole is initiated and for seizures when it is discontinued (Lumholtz et al., 1975; Lunde et al., 1970).

Theophylline. Phenytoin can enhance theophylline metabolism, resulting in inadequate theophylline serum concentrations. Pediatric patients receiving concurrent theophylline and phenytoin therapy may require higher dosages of theophylline. Particular care should be taken to avoid therapeutic failure with theophylline when phenytoin is initiated and to avoid theophylline toxicity when phenytoin is discontinued (Marquis et al., 1982).

Trimethoprim (Proloprim®). Trimethoprim inhibits phenytoin metabolism, resulting in increased phenytoin serum concentrations. Be alert for evidence of excessive phenytoin serum concentrations when trimethoprim (alone or in combination with sulfamethoxazole [co-trimoxazole]) is initiated (Hansen et al., 1979).

Valproic acid (Depakene®). Valproic acid displaces phenytoin from plasma protein binding sites and inhibits phenytoin metabolism. These effects decrease the total phenytoin concentration, but the free phenytoin concentration initially is unchanged. Total phenytoin concentrations tend to return to normal 3–4 weeks after the initiation of valproic acid. Use caution in interpreting total phenytoin concentrations when initiating valproic acid. Do not increase the phenytoin dosage during the first 3–4 weeks unless seizure control is inadequate. Monitoring free phenytoin serum concentrations may be useful during that initial period (Bruni et al., 1979; Dahlqvist et al., 1979; Monks & Richens, 1980).

Pimozide

(*See* Tables 6-1 and 6-2.)

Potassium Salts

Potassium-sparing diuretics. The concurrent use of potassium salts and potassium-sparing diuretics (e.g., amiloride, spironolactone, triamterene) may result in hyperkalemia, especially in pediatric patients with impaired renal function. Use the combination only when clearly indicated, and monitor the potassium serum concentration closely (Greenblatt & Koch-Weser, 1973; Shapiro et al., 1971).

Potassium-Sparing Diuretics

Angiotensin-converting enzyme (ACE) inhibitors. ACE inhibitors, such as benazepril, captopril, enalapril, fosinopril, lisinopril, and ramipril, tend to cause potassium retention. This effect may be additive with the potassium-conserving effect of potassium-sparing diuretics (e.g., amiloride, spironolactone, triamterene). Although hyperkalemia probably occurs rarely and only in predisposed patients, it is prudent to monitor potassium serum concentrations (Burnakis & Mioduch, 1984; Speirs et al., 1988).

Cyclosporine. See Cyclosporine + Potassium-Sparing Diuretics.

Potassium salts. See Potassium Salts + Potassium-Sparing Diuretics.

Prazosin *(Minipress®)*

Beta-adrenergic blockers. See Beta-Adrenergic Blockers + Prazosin.

Primidone *(Mysoline®)*

(*See also* Anticonvulsants.)

Acetazolamide (Diamox®). Acetazolamide appears to reduce the GI absorption of primidone in certain patients, resulting in inadequate serum concentrations of primidone and its active metabolite phenobarbital. Although the combination need not be avoided, be alert for inadequate seizure control. Adjust the primidone dosage as necessary (Syversen et al., 1977).

Anticoagulants, oral. See Anticoagulants, Oral + Enzyme Inducers.

Barbiturates. The concurrent use of phenobarbital and primidone can result in excessive phenobarbital serum concentrations, particularly in patients with renal dysfunction, because primidone is converted to phenobarbital. The combination of primidone and phenobarbital is irrational (Griffin et al., 1976; Wilson & Wilkinson, 1973).

Isoniazid (INH®). Isoniazid inhibits the metabolism of primidone to its active metabolites, phenobarbital and phenylethylmalonamide. The combination of isoniazid and primidone need not be avoided, but be alert for loss of seizure control when initiating isoniazid in pediatric patients receiving primidone (Sutton & Kupferberg, 1975).

Phenytoin. See Phenytoin + Primidone.

Valproic acid (Depakene®). Valproic acid initially increases primidone (and phenobarbital) serum concentrations; however, later they return to previous values. Monitor for evidence of excessive primidone (and phenobarbital) serum concentrations when valproic acid is initiated and for loss of seizure control when it is discontinued (*see also* Valproic Acid + Barbiturates) (Windorfer et al., 1975).

Probenecid *(Benemid®)*

Cephalosporins. See Cephalosporins + Probenecid.

Methotrexate. See Methotrexate + Probenecid.

Procainamide *(Pronestyl®)*

Cimetidine. See Cimetidine + Procainamide.

Propafenone *(Rythmol®)*

Anticoagulants, oral. See Anticoagulants, Oral + Enzyme Inhibitors.

Pyridoxine

Phenytoin. See Phenytoin + Pyridoxine.

Quinidine

Cimetidine. See Cimetidine + Quinidine.

Rifabutin *(Mycobutin®)*

Anticoagulants, oral. See Anticoagulants, Oral + Enzyme Inducers.

Rifampin *(Rifadin®)*

Anticoagulants, oral. See Anticoagulants, Oral + Enzyme Inducers.

Contraceptives, oral. See Contraceptives, Oral + Rifampin.

Corticosteroids. Rifampin enhances the hepatic metabolism of corticosteroids. Monitor for decreased corticosteroid efficacy, and increase the corticosteroid dosage as necessary (Edwards et al., 1974; Yamada & Iwai, 1976).

Cyclosporine. See Cyclosporine + Rifampin.

Isoniazid. See Isoniazid + Rifampin.

Theophylline. See Theophylline + Rifampin.

Salicylates

Antacids. See Antacids + Salicylates.

Anticoagulants, oral. See Anticoagulants, Oral + Salicylates.

Corticosteroids. See Corticosteroids + Salicylates.

Phenytoin. See Phenytoin + Salicylates.

Selective Serotonin Reuptake Inhibitors

(*See* also Fluoxetine.)

Antidepressants, tricyclic. See Antidepressants, Tricyclic + Selective Serotonin Reuptake Inhibitors.

Sparfloxacin

(*See* Fluoroquinolones.)
(*See also* Table 6-2.)

Sulfonamides

Methotrexate. Sulfisoxazole can displace methotrexate from protein binding sites and also may inhibit renal tubular secretion of methotrexate. Methotrexate toxicity can result. Initiate sulfonamides cautiously in pediatric patients receiving methotrexate. Monitor for methotrexate toxicity (Dixon et al., 1965; Liegler et al., 1969).

Phenytoin. See Phenytoin + Sulfonamides.

Sympathomimetics

Beta-adrenergic blockers. See Beta-Adrenergic Blockers + Sympathomimetics.

Tricyclic antidepressants. See Antidepressants, Tricyclic + Sympathomimetics.

Terfenadine

(*See* Tables 6-1 and 6-2.)

Tetracyclines

(*See also* Doxycycline.)

Antacids. Antacids containing divalent cations (e.g., calcium, magnesium) or trivalent cations (e.g., aluminum) chelate tetracyclines and may markedly impair the GI absorption of oral tetracyclines. Oral tetracyclines should be ingested at least 2 hours before or 4–6 hours after antacids (Chin & Lach, 1975; Neuvonen, 1976).

Iron. Oral iron (and other divalent and trivalent cations such as calcium and magnesium) chelate oral tetracyclines, decreasing their bioavailability and efficacy. Oral tetracyclines should be ingested at least 2 hours before or 4–6 hours after oral iron (or other divalent and trivalent cations) (Neuvonen, 1976; Welling et al., 1977).

Phenytoin. See Phenytoin + Doxycycline.

Theophylline

Allopurinol. See Allopurinol + Theophylline.

Barbiturates. Phenobarbital stimulates the metabolism of theophylline, resulting in a gradual reduction in theophylline serum concentration. Monitor for evidence of subtherapeutic theophylline serum concentrations when barbiturates are initiated and for evidence of excessive theophylline serum concentrations when barbiturates are discontinued (Landay et al., 1978).

Carbamazepine (Tegretol®).
Carbamazepine induces the metabolism of theophylline, resulting in decreased theophylline serum concentrations. Monitor for evidence of subtherapeutic theophylline serum concentrations when carbamazepine is initiated and for evidence of excessive theophylline serum concentrations when carbamazepine is discontinued (Rosenberry et al., 1983).

Cimetidine (Tagamet®). Cimetidine inhibits the metabolism of theophylline, increasing theophylline serum concentrations and the likelihood of theophylline toxicity. Monitor for evidence of excessive theophylline serum concentrations when cimetidine is initiated and for evidence of subtherapeutic theophylline serum concentrations when cimetidine is discontinued. Adjust the theophylline dosage as necessary. Alternative therapy with antacids or ranitidine is preferred to cimetidine therapy (Fenje et al., 1982; Jackson et al., 1981).

Erythromycin (Eryc®, EryPed®). Erythromycin appears to inhibit the metabolism of theophylline, increasing theophylline serum concentrations. The increase in theophylline serum concentration usually does not occur for several days after erythromycin is initiated. Monitor for evidence of excessive theophylline serum concentrations when erythromycin is initiated and for evidence of subtherapeutic theophylline serum concentrations when erythromycin is discontinued. Adjust the theophylline dosage as necessary. Alternative antibiotics may be preferred (Hansten, 1981a; Iliopoulou et al., 1982; Renton et al., 1981).

Fluoroquinolones. Ciprofloxacin and enoxacin reduce theophylline clearance and, therefore, increase theophylline serum concentrations. Monitor theophylline serum concentrations and patient response for evidence of theophylline toxicity. Reduce the theophylline dosage as necessary. Other fluoroquinolones such as lamefloxacin, levofloxacin, ofloxacin, and sparfloxacin do not appear to inhibit theophylline metabolism (Karki et al., 1990; Parent & LeBel, 1991).

Phenytoin. See Phenytoin + Theophylline.

Rifampin. Rifampin stimulates the metabolism of theophylline, resulting in reduced theophylline serum concentrations. Monitor for evidence of subtherapeutic theophylline serum concentrations when rifampin is initiated and for evidence of excessive theophylline serum concentrations when rifampin is discontinued (Boyce et al., 1985; Straughn et al., 1984).

Troleandomycin (TAO®). Troleandomycin inhibits theophylline metabolism, resulting in increased theophylline serum concentrations and the likelihood of toxicity. Consider using alternatives to troleandomycin if pediatric patients require theophylline. If the combination of troleandomycin and theophylline cannot be avoided, monitor for evidence of excessive theophylline serum concentrations when troleandomycin is initiated and for evidence of subtherapeutic theophylline serum concentrations when troleandomycin is discontinued. Adjust the theophylline dosage as necessary (Weinberger et al., 1977).

Verapamil (Isoptin®). Verapamil increases theophylline serum concentrations in a dose-dependent manner, probably by inhibiting theophylline metabolism. Monitor for evidence of excessive theophylline serum concentrations when verapamil is initiated and for evidence of subtherapeutic theophylline serum concentrations when verapamil is discontinued. Adjust the theophylline dosage as necessary. Diltiazem and nifedipine appear less likely to increase theophylline serum concentrations (Abernethy et al., 1988; Christopher et al., 1989).

Thiazide Diuretics

Lithium. See Lithium Salts + Thiazide Diuretics.

Thioridazine *(Mellaril®)*

(*See* Tables 6-1 and 6-2.)

Troglitazone *(Rezulin®)*

Anticoagulants, oral. See Anticoagulants, Oral + Enzyme Inducers.

Thyroid Hormones

Anticoagulants, oral. See Anticoagulants, Oral + Thyroid Hormones.

Cholestyramine resin. See Cholestyramine Resin + Thyroid Hormones.

Tricyclic Antidepressants

(*See* Antidepressants, Tricyclic.)

Trimethoprim *(Proloprim®)*

(*See also* Trimethoprim–Sulfamethoxazole.)

Phenytoin. See Phenytoin + Trimethoprim.

Trimethoprim–Sulfamethoxazole (Co-trimoxazole) *(Septra®)*

Anticoagulants, oral. See Anticoagulants, Oral + Enzyme Inhibitors.

Cyclosporine. See Cyclosporine + Trimethoprim–sulfamethoxazole.

Phenytoin. See Phenytoin + Trimethoprim.

Troleandomycin *(TAO®)*

Carbamazepine. See Carbamazepine + Troleandomycin.

Theophylline. See Theophylline + Troleandomycin.

Valproic Acid *(Depakene®)*

(*See also* Anticonvulsants.)

Barbiturates. Valproic acid inhibits the metabolism of phenobarbital (and presumably other barbiturates), resulting in potentially toxic phenobarbital serum concentrations. Monitor for evidence of excessive phenobarbital serum concentrations when valproic acid is initiated and for evidence of subtherapeutic phenobarbital serum concentrations when valproic acid is discontinued. Adjust the phenobarbital dosage as necessary (Kapetanovic et al., 1981; Patel et al., 1980).

Benzodiazepines. Valproic acid can inhibit the metabolism of diazepam (and presumably other benzodiazepines), resulting in high diazepam serum concentrations and increased adverse drug reactions (e.g., sedation). Monitor for evidence of excessive benzodiazepine serum concentrations when valproic acid is initiated and for evidence of subtherapeutic benzodiazepine serum concentrations when valproic acid is discontinued. The combination of valproic acid and clonazepam has been associated with absence seizures. If concurrent use of clonazepam and valproic acid is required, monitor patients for an increase in absence seizures, and use alternative anticonvulsants, if necessary (Browne, 1979; Dhillon & Richens, 1982).

Phenytoin. See Phenytoin + Valproic Acid.

Primidone. See Primidone + Valproic Acid.

Verapamil *(Calan®)*

Carbamazepine. See Carbamazepine + Verapamil.

Digitalis glycosides. See Digitalis Glycosides + Verapamil.

Theophylline. See Theophylline + Verapamil.

Vitamin E

Iron. See Iron + Vitamin E.

Warfarin *(Coumadin®)*

(*See* Anticoagulants, Oral.)

Zidovudine *(AZT®)*

Ganciclovir. See Ganciclovir + Zidovudine.

Ziprasidone

(*See* Tables 6-1 and 6-2.)

Summary

Adverse drug interactions involving both pharmacokinetic and pharmacodynamic interactions are important considerations when planning and managing drug therapy for pediatric patients. This chapter has presented a brief review of the principal sites of drug interactions and a comprehensive overview of the clinically significant drug interactions that are most likely to occur in pediatric patients. Particular attention was given to drug interactions involving prolongation of the QT interval and to drug interactions involving the hepatic cytochrome P-450 isoenzymes.

While published data regarding the incidence and severity of adverse drug interactions among neonates, infants, children, and adolescents remain scant, pediatric clinicians are encouraged to be cognizant of the potential occurrence of adverse drug interactions in their pediatric patients and to prevent or minimize these interactions whenever possible.

References

Aach, R., & Kissane, J. (Eds.). (1970). Clinicopathologic conference: Hypertension and the lupus syndrome. *American Journal of Medicine, 49*, 519–528.

Abernethy, D. R., Egan, J. M., Dickinson, T. H., et al. (1988). Substrate-selective inhibition by verapamil and diltiazem: Differential disposition of antipyrine and theophylline in humans. *Journal of Pharmacology and Experimental Therapeutics, 244*, 994–999.

Abernethy, D. R., Greenblatt, D. J., Shader, R. I., et al. (1984). Imipramine–cimetidine interaction: Impairment of clearance and enhanced bioavailability. *Journal of Pharmacology and Experimental Therapeutics, 229*, 702–705.

Aherne, G. W., Piall, E., Marks, V., et al. (1978). Prolongation and enhancement of serum methotrexate concentrations by probenecid. *British Medical Journal, 1*, 1097–1099.

Ahmad, S. (1974). Renal insensitivity to frusemide caused by chronic anticonvulsant therapy. *British Medical Journal, 3*, 657–659.

Albani, F., Riva, R., & Baruzzi, A. (1993). Clarithromycin–carbamazepine interaction: A case report. *Epilepsia, 34*, 161–162.

Allan, S. G., Knox, J., & Kerr, F. (1981). Interaction between diuretics and indomethacin. [Letter]. *British Medical Journal, 283*, 1611.

Allen, M. D., Greenblatt, D. J., Harmatz, J. S., et al. (1981). Effect of magnesium–aluminum hydroxide and kaolin–pectin on absorption of digoxin from tablets and capsules. *Journal of Clinical Pharmacology, 21*, 26–30.

Alvarez, J. S., Sarcristan Del Castillo, J. A., Alsar Oritz, M. J., et al. (1991). Effect of carbamazepine on cyclosporin blood level. *Nephron, 58*, 235–236.

Baldwin, C. M., & Safferman, A. Z. (1990). A case of lisinopril-induced lithium toxicity. *DICP, The Annals of Pharmacotherapy, 24*, 946–947.

Bartle, W. R., Walker, S. E., & Shapero, T. (1983). Dose-dependent effect of cimetidine on phenytoin kinetics. *Clinical Pharmacology and Therapeutics, 33*, 649–655.

Beattie, B., Biller, J., Mehlhaus, B., & Murray, M. (1988). Verapamil-induced carbamazepine neurotoxicity. A report of two cases. *European Neurology, 28*, 104–105.

Belz, G. G., Doering, W., Munkes, R., et al. (1983). Interaction between digoxin and calcium antagonists and antiarrhythmic drugs. *Clinical Pharmacology and Therapeutics, 33*, 410–417.

Bergstrom, R. F., Peyton, A. L., & Lemberger, L. (1992). Quantification and mechanism of the fluoxetine and tricyclic antidepressants interaction. *Clinical Pharmacology and Therapeutics, 51*, 239–248.

Bernard, K. W., Fishbein, D. B., Miller, K. D., et al. (1985). Pre-exposure rabies immunization with human diploid-cell vaccine: Decreased antibody responses in persons immunized in developing countries. *American Journal of Tropical Medicine and Hygiene, 34*, 633–647.

Bistritzer, T., Barzilay, T., & Jonas, A. (1980). Isoniazid–rifampin-induced fulminant liver disease in an infant. *The Journal of Pediatrics, 97*, 480–482.

Bivins, B. A., Rapp, R. P., Griffen, W. O., et al. (1978). Dopamine–phenytoin interaction. *Archives of Surgery, 113*, 245–249.

Bleyer, W. A. (1978). The clinical pharmacology of methotrexate: New applications of an old drug. *Cancer, 41*, 36–51.

Block, S. H. (1982). Carbamazepine–isoniazid interaction. *Pediatrics, 69*, 494–495.

Bloxham, R. A., Durbin, G. M., Johnson, T., et al. (1979). Chloramphenicol and phenobarbitone—A drug interaction. *Archives of Disease in Childhood, 54*, 76–77.

Boakes, A. J., Laurence, D. R., Teoh, P. C., et al. (1973). Interactions between sympathomimetic amines and antidepressant agents in man. *British Medical Journal, 1*, 311–315.

Bor, J. (1990, November 29). Improper asthma medications led to boy's brain damage, suit claims. *The Baltimore Sun*, pp. 1B, 4B.

Boyce, E. G., Dukes, G. E., Rollins, D. E., et al. (1985). The effect of rifampin on theophylline kinetics. *Clinical Pharmacology and Therapeutics, 37*, 183.

Briant, R. H., Reid, J. L., & Dollery, C. T. (1973). Interaction between clonidine and desipramine in man. *British Medical Journal, 1*, 522–523.

Brooks, S. M., Werk, E. E., Ackerman, S. J., et al. (1972). Adverse effects of phenobarbital on corticosteroid metabolism in patients with bronchial asthma. *New England Journal of Medicine, 286*, 1125–1128.

Brown, C. S., Wells, B. G., Cold, J. A., et al. (1990). Possible influence of carbamazepine on plasma imipramine concentrations in children with attention deficit hyperactivity disorder. *Journal of Clinical Psychopharmacology, 10*, 359–362.

Brown, D. D., & Juhl, R. P. (1976). Decreased bioavailability of digoxin due to antacids and kaolin–pectin. *New England Journal of Medicine, 295*, 1034.

Browne, T. R. (1979). Interaction between clonazepam and sodium valproate. *New England Journal of Medicine, 300*, 679.

Bruni, J., Wilder, B. J., Willmore, L. J., et al. (1979).

Valproic acid and plasma levels of phenytoin. *Neurology, 29,* 904–905.

Buchanan, R. A., Heffelfinger, J. C., & Weiss, C. F. (1962). The effect of phenobarbital on diphenylhydantoin metabolism in children. *Pediatrics, 43,* 114–116.

Burnakis, T. G., & Mioduch, H. J. (1984). Combined therapy with captopril and potassium supplementation: A potential for hyperkalemia. *Archives of Internal Medicine, 144,* 2371–2372.

Bussey, H. I. (1982). The influence of quinidine and other agents on digitalis glycosides. *American Heart Journal, 104,* 289–302.

Caldwell, J. H., Bush, C. A., & Greenberger, N. J. (1971). Interruption of the enterohepatic circulation of digitoxin by cholestyramine. *Journal of Clinical Investigation, 50,* 2638–2644.

Carlson, J. A., Mann, H. J., & Canafax, D. M. (1983). Effect of pH on disintegration and dissolution of ketoconazole tablets. *American Journal of Hospital Pharmacy, 40,* 1334–1336.

Carruthers, S. G., & Dujovne, C. A. (1980). Cholestyramine and spironolactone and their combination in digitoxin elimination. *Clinical Pharmacology and Therapeutics, 27,* 184–187.

Carstensen, H., Jacobsen, N., & Dieperink, H. (1986). Interaction between cyclosporin A and phenobarbitone. [Letter]. *British Journal of Clinical Pharmacology, 21,* 550.

Cheng, S. H., & White, A. (1962). Effect of orally administered neomycin on the absorption of penicillin V. *New England Journal of Medicine, 267,* 1296–1297.

Chesebro, J. H., Fuster, V., Elveback, L. R., et al. (1983). Trial of combined warfarin plus dipyridamole or ASA therapy in prosthetic heart valve replacement: Danger of ASA compared with dipyridamole. *American Journal of Cardiology, 51,* 1537.

Chin, T. F., & Lach, J. L. (1975). Drug diffusion and bioavailability: Tetracycline metallic chelation. *American Journal of Hospital Pharmacy, 32,* 625–629.

Christensen, L. K., & Skovsted, L. (1969). Inhibition of drug metabolism by chloramphenicol. *The Lancet, 2,* 1397–1399.

Christiansen, J., & Dam, M. (1973). Influence of phenobarbital and diphenylhydantoin on plasma carbamazepine levels in patients with epilepsy. *Acta Neurologica Scandinavica, 49,* 543–546.

Christopher, M. A., Harman, E., & Hendeles, L. (1989). Clinical relevance of the interaction of theophylline with diltiazem or nifedipine. *Chest, 95,* 309–313.

Coffey, J. J., White, C. A., Lesk, A. B., et al. (1972). Effect of allopurinol on the pharmacokinetics of 6-mercaptopurine (NSC 755) in cancer patients. *Cancer Research, 32,* 1283–1289.

Cohen, M. H., Creaven, P. J., Fossieck, B. E., et al. (1976). Effect of oral prophylactic broad spectrum nonabsorbable antibiotics on the gastrointestinal absorption of nutrients and methotrexate in small cell bronchogenic carcinoma patients. *Cancer, 38,* 1556–1559.

Coste, J. F., DeBari, V. A., Keil, L. B., et al. (1977). In-vitro interactions of oral hematinics and antacid suspensions. *Therapy and Research, 22,* 205–216.

Coulam, C. B., & Annegers, J. F. (1979). Do anticonvulsants reduce the efficacy of oral contraceptives? *Epilepsia, 20,* 519–526.

Dahlqvist, R., Borga, O., Rane, A., et al. (1979). Decreased plasma protein binding of phenytoin in patients on valproic acid. *British Journal of Clinical Pharmacology, 8,* 547–552.

Dallas, V., & Heathfield, K. (1967). Iatrogenic epilepsy due to antidepressant drugs. *British Medical Journal, 3,* 162.

De Ponte, F., Poluzzi, E., & Montanaro, N. (2000). QT-interval prolongation by non-cardiac drugs. Lessons to be learned from recent experience. *European Journal of Clinical Pharmacology, 56,* 1–18.

Dhillon, S., & Richens, A. (1982). Valproic acid and diazepam interaction in vivo. *British Journal of Clinical Pharmacology, 13,* 553–560.

Dixon, R. L., Henderson, E. S., & Rall, D. P. (1965). Plasma protein binding of methotrexate and its displacement by various drugs. *Federation Proceedings, 24,* 454.

Donaldson, D. R., Srecharan, N., Crow, M. J., et al. (1982). Assessment of the interaction of warfarin with aspirin and dipyridamole. *Thrombosis and Haemostasis, 47,* 77.

Dordoni, B., Wilson, R. A., Thompson, R. P. H., et al. (1973). Reduction of absorption of paracetamol by activated charcoal and cholestyramine: A possible therapeutic measure. *British Medical Journal, 3,* 86–87.

Douste-Blazy, P. H., Rostin, M., Livarek, B., et al. (1986). Angiotensin converting enzyme inhibitors and lithium treatment. [Letter]. *The Lancet, 1,* 1448.

Edwards, O. M., Courtenay-Evans, R. J., Galley, J. M., et al. (1974). Changes in cortisol metabolism following rifampicin therapy. *The Lancet, 2,* 549–551.

Elliott, H. L., McLean, K., Sumner, D. J., et al. (1981). Immediate cardiovascular responses to oral prazosin—Effects of concurrent beta-blockers. *Clinical Pharmacology and Therapeutics, 29,* 303–309.

Ervin, F. R., Bullock, W. E., & Nuttall, C. E. (1976). Inactivation of gentamicin by penicillins in patients with renal failure. *Antimicrobial Agents and Chemotherapy, 9,* 1004–1011.

Feely, J., Wilkinson, G. R., & Wood, A. J. (1981). Reduction of liver blood flow and propranolol metabolism by cimetidine. *New England Journal of Medicine, 304,* 692–695.

Fenje, P. C., Isles, A. F., Baltodano, A., et al. (1982). Interaction of cimetidine and theophylline in two infants. *Canadian Medical Association Journal, 126,* 1178.

Fincham, R. W., Schotelius, D., & Sahs, A. L. (1974). The influence of diphenylhydantoin on primidone metabolism. *Archives of Neurology, 30,* 259–262.

Fine, A., Henderson, I. S., Morgan, D. R., et al. (1977). Malabsorption of frusemide caused by phenytoin. *British Medical Journal, 2,* 1061–1062.

Fraser, D. G., Ludden, T. M., Evans, R. P., et al. (1980). Displacement of phenytoin from plasma binding sites by salicylate. *Clinical Pharmacology and Therapeutics, 27,* 165–169.

Freeman, D. J., Martell, R., Carruthers, S. G., et al. (1986). The effect of erythromycin on the pharmacokinetics of cyclosporine. [Abstract]. *Clinical Pharmacology and Therapeutics, 39,* 193.

Frolich, J. C., Leftwich, R., Ragheb, M., et al. (1978). Indomethacin increases plasma lithium. *British Medical Journal, 1,* 1115–1116.

Furlanut, M., Benettello, P., Avogaro, A., et al. (1978). Effects of folic acid on phenytoin kinetics in healthy subjects. *Clinical Pharmacology and Therapeutics, 24,* 294–297.

Furnell, M. M., & Davies, J. (1985). The effect of sulindac on lithium therapy. *Drug Intelligence and Clinical Pharmacy, 19,* 374–376.

Gambertoglio, J., Kapusnik, J., Holford, N., et al. (1982). Enhancement of prednisone elimination by anticonvulsants in renal transplant recipients. [Abstract]. *Clinical Pharmacology and Therapeutics, 31,* 228.

Ghose, K. (1978). Effect of carbamazepine in polyuria associated with lithium therapy. *Pharmacopsychiatria, 11,* 241–245.

Ghose, K. (1980). Sympathomimetic amines and tricyclic antidepressant drugs. *Neuropharmacology, 19,* 1251–1254.

Gibson, D. L., Blyer, A. W., & Savitch, J. L. (1981, December). Interaction between penicillins and methotrexate. *American Society of Hospital Pharmacists Midyear Clinical Meeting Abstracts* (p. 111, Abstract No. 305). New Orleans.

Grabenstein, J. D. (1990). Drug interactions involving immunologic agents: Part I. Vaccine–vaccine, vaccine–immunoglobulin, and vaccine–drug interactions. *DICP, The Annals of Pharmacotherapy, 24,* 67–81.

Graham, G. G., Champion, G. D., Day, R. O., et al. (1977). Patterns of plasma concentrations and urinary excretion of salicylate in rheumatoid arthritis. *Clinical Pharmacology and Therapeutics, 22,* 410–420.

Greenblatt, D. J., & Koch-Weser, J. (1973). Adverse reactions to spironolactone: A report from The Boston Collaborative Drug Surveillance Program. [Abstract]. *Clinical Pharmacology and Therapeutics, 14,* 136–137.

Greenlaw, C. W. (1979). Chloramphenicol–phenytoin drug interaction. *Drug Intelligence and Clinical Pharmacy, 13,* 609–610.

Griffin, G. D., Heffron, W. A., Ferguson, B., et al. (1976). Primidone–phenobarbital intoxication. *Drug Therapy, 60,* 76–78.

Griffith, R. S., Black, H. R., Brier, G. L., et al. (1977). Effect of probenecid on the blood levels and urinary excretion of cefamandole. *Antimicrobial Agents and Chemotherapy, 11,* 809–812.

Grimsley, S. R., Jann, M. W., Carter, G., et al. (1991). Increased carbamazepine plasma concentrations after fluoxetine coadministration. *Clinical Pharmacology and Therapeutics, 50,* 10–15.

Grygiel, J. J., Wing, L. M. H., Farkas, J., et al. (1979). Effects of allopurinol on theophylline metabolism and clearance. *Clinical Pharmacology and Therapeutics, 26,* 660–667.

Gugler, R., & Allgayer, H. (1990). Effect of antacids on the clinical pharmacokinetics of drugs: An update. *Clinical Pharmacokinetics, 18,* 210–219.

Hall, G. J. L., & Davis, A. E. (1969). Inhibition of iron absorption by magnesium trisilicate. *Medical Journal of Australia, 2,* 95–96.

Hansen, J. M., Kampman, J. P., Siersbaek-Nielsen, K., et al. (1979). The effect of different sulfonamides on phenytoin metabolism in man. *Acta Medica Scandinavica Supplementum, 624,* 106–110.

Hansson, O., & Sillanpaa, M. (1976). Pyridoxine and serum concentrations of phenytoin and phenobarbitone. [Letter]. *The Lancet, 1,* 256.

Hansten, P. D. (1974, October). Interaction between anticonvulsant drugs: Primidone, diphenylhydantoin and phenobarbital. *Northwest Medical Journal, 1,* 17.

Hansten, P. D. (1980a). Beta-blocking agents and antidiabetic drugs. *Drug Intelligence and Clinical Pharmacy, 14,* 46–50.

Hansten, P. D. (1980b). Oral anticoagulants and drugs which alter thyroid function. *Drug Intelligence and Clinical Pharmacy, 14,* 331.

Hansten, P. D. (1981a). Erythromycin and theophylline. *Drug Interactions Newsletter, 1,* 5–6.

Hansten, P. D. (1981b). Quinidine and digoxin. *Drug Interactions Newsletter, 1,* 13–15.

Hansten, P. D. (1984). Cyclosporine interactions. *Drug Interactions Newsletter, 4,* 29.

Hansten, P. D., & Hayton, W. L. (1980). Effect of antacids and ascorbic acid on serum salicylate concentration. *Journal of Clinical Pharmacology, 24,* 326–331.

Hansten, P. D., & Horn, J. R. (1985a). Erythromycin and warfarin. *Drug Interactions Newsletter, 5,* 37–40.

Hansten, P. D., & Horn, J. R. (1985b). Phenytoin interaction. *Drug Interactions Newsletter, 5,* 1–3.

Hansten, P. D., & Horn, J. R. (1985c). Rifampin interactions. *Drug Interactions Newsletter, 5,* 8.

Hansten, P. D., & Horn, J. R. (1986). Diuretics and nonsteroidal anti-inflammatory drugs. *Drug Interactions Newsletter, 6,* 27–29.

Hansten, P. D., & Horn, J. R. (2001). *Drug interactions analysis and management*. St. Louis, MO: Facts & Comparisons.

Hardy, B. G., Zador, I. T., Golden, L., et al. (1983). Effect of cimetidine on the pharmacokinetics and pharmacodynamics of quinidine. *American Journal of Cardiology, 52,* 172–175.

Haverkamp, W., Breithardt, G., Camm, A. J., et al. (2000). The potential for QT prolongation and proarrhythmia by non-antiarrhythmic drugs. Clinical and regulatory implications. *European Heart Journal, 21,* 1216–1231.

Helms-Smith, K. M., Curtis, S. L., & Hatton, R. C. (1996). Apparent interaction between nefazodone and cyclosporine. [Letter]. *Annals of Internal Medicine, 125,* 424.

Hesse, B., & Pedersen, J. T. (1973). Hypoglycemia after propranolol in children. *Acta Medica Scandinavica, 193,* 551–552.

Himmelhoch, J. M., Forrest, J., Neil, J. F., et al. (1977). Thiazide–lithium synergy in refractory mood swings. *American Journal of Psychiatry, 134,* 149–152.

Hochster, H., Dieterich, D., Bozzette, S., et al. (1990). Toxicity of combined ganciclovir and zidovudine for cytomegalovirus disease associated with AIDS. An AIDS clinical trials group study. *Annals of Internal Medicine, 113,* 111–117.

Hoppu, K., Tikanoja, T., Tapanainen, P., et al. (1991). Accidental astemizole overdose in young children. *The Lancet, 338,* 538–540.

Houben, H., Thien, T., DeBoo, T., et al. (1979). Influence of selective and non-selective beta-adrenoreceptor blockade on the haemodynamic effect of adrenaline during combined antihypertensive drug therapy. *Clinical Science, 57*(Suppl 5), 397S–399S.

Houtzagers, J. J., Struerman, O., & Regardh, C. G. (1982). The effect of pretreatment with cimetidine on the bioavailability and disposition of atenolol and metoprolol. *British Journal of Clinical Pharmacology, 14,* 67–72.

Howard, P., Bixler, T. J., & Gill, B. (1985). Cyclosporine–rifampin drug interaction. *Drug Intelligence and Clinical Pharmacy, 19,* 763–764.

Howell, S. B., Olshen, R. A., & Rice, J. A. (1979). Effect of probenecid on cerebrospinal fluid methotrexate kinetics. *Clinical Pharmacology and Therapeutics, 26,* 641–646.

Howitt, K. M., & Oziemski, M. A. (1989). Phenytoin toxicity induced by fluconazole. [Letter]. *Medical Journal of Australia, 151,* 603–604.

Hui, K. K. (1983). Hypertensive crisis induced by interaction of clonidine with imipramine. *Journal of the American Geriatrics Society, 31,* 164–165.

Hoppu, K., Tikanoja, T., Tapanainen, P., et al. (1991). Accidental astemizole overdose in young children. *The Lancet, 338,* 538–540.

Hunder, G. G., Shepps, S. G., & Allen, G. L. (1975). Daily and alternate-day corticosteroid regimens in treatment of giant cell arteritis. Comparison in a prospective study. *Annals of Internal Medicine, 82,* 613–618.

Iliopoulou, A., Aldhous, M. E., Johnston, A., et al. (1982). Pharmacokinetic interaction between theophylline and erythromycin. *British Journal of Clinical Pharmacology, 14,* 495–496.

Jackson, J. E., Powell, J. R., Wandell, M., et al. (1981). Cimetidine decreases theophylline clearance. *American Review of Respiratory Disease, 123,* 615–617.

Jacobs, M. H., & Senior, R. M. (1974). Theophylline toxicity due to impaired theophylline degradation. *American Review of Respiratory Disease, 110,* 342–345.

Jacobson, M. A., Drew, W. L., Feinberg, J., et al. (1991). Foscarnet therapy for ganciclovir-resistant cytomegalovirus retinitis in patients with AIDS. *Journal of Infectious Diseases, 163,* 1348–1351.

Jefferson, J. W., & Kalin, N. H. (1979). Serum lithium levels and long-term diuretic use. *Journal of the American Medical Association, 241,* 1134–1136.

Kapetanovic, I. M., Kupferberg, H. J., Porter, R. J., et al. (1981). Mechanism of valproate–phenobarbital interaction in epileptic patients. *Clinical Pharmacology and Therapeutics, 29,* 480–486.

Karki, S. D., Bentley, D. W., & Raghavan, M. (1990). Seizure with ciprofloxacin and theophylline combined therapy. *Drug Intelligence and Clinical Pharmacy, 24,* 595–596.

Katz, H. I., & Gupta, A. K. (1997). Oral antifungal drug interactions. *Dermatologic Clinics, 15,* 535–544.

Kerley, B., & Ali, M. (1982). Cimetidine potentiation of warfarin action. *Canadian Medical Association Journal, 126,* 116.

Klein, H. O., Lang, R., Weiss, E., et al. (1982). The influence of verapamil on serum digoxin concentration. *Circulation, 65,* 998–1003.

Klinenberg, J. R., & Miller, F. (1965). Effect of corticosteroids on blood salicylate concentration. *Journal of the American Medical Association, 194,* 601–604.

Klotz, U., Arvela, P., & Rosenkranz, B. (1985). Famotidine, a new H_2-receptor antagonist, does not affect hepatic elimination of diazepam or tubular secretion of procainamide. *European Journal of Clinical Pharmacology, 28,* 671–675.

Kohan, D. E. (1986). Possible interaction between cyclosporine and erythromycin. [Letter]. *New England Journal of Medicine, 314,* 448.

Koren, G., Hesslein, P. S., & MacLeod, S. M. (1984). Digoxin toxicity associated with amiodarone therapy in children. *The Journal of Pediatrics, 104,* 467–470.

Koup, J. R., Gibaldi, M., McNamara, P., et al. (1978). Interaction of chloramphenicol with phenytoin and phenobarbital. Case report. *Clin-*

ical *Pharmacology and Therapeutics, 24,* 571–575.

Kubacka, R. T., & Ferrante, J. A. (1983). Carbamazepine–propoxyphene interaction. *Clinical Pharmacy, 2,* 104.

Kutt, H., Brennan, R., Dehejia, H., et al. (1970). Diphenylhydantoin intoxication. A complication of isoniazid therapy. *American Review of Respiratory Disease, 101,* 377–384.

Kutt, H., Winter, W., & McDowell, F. H. (1966). Depression of parahydroxylation of diphenylhydantoin by antituberculosis chemotherapy. *Neurology, 16,* 594–602.

Lake, K. D. (1991). Management of drug interactions with cyclosporine. *Pharmacotherapy, 11*(Suppl), 110S–118S.

Landay, R. A., Gonzalez, M. A., & Taylor, J. C. (1978). Effect of phenobarbital on theophylline disposition. *Journal of Allergy and Clinical Immunology, 62,* 27–29.

Lange, D., Pavao, J. H., Wu, J., & Klausner, M. (1997). Effect of a cola beverage on the bioavailability of itraconazole in the presence of H_2 blockers. *Journal of Clinical Pharmacology, 37,* 535–540.

LeBlang, T. R. (1991, May). Drug interactions and the pharmacist's duty to warn. *American Druggist, 203,* 46–48.

Lelawongs, P., Barone, J. A., Colaizzi, J. L., et al. (1988). Effect of food and gastric acidity on absorption of orally administered ketoconazole. *Clinical Pharmacology, 7,* 228–235.

Levy, G., Lampman, T., Kamath, B. L., et al. (1975). Decreased serum salicylate concentrations in children with rheumatic fever treated with antacid. *New England Journal of Medicine, 293,* 323–325.

Liegler, D. G., Henderson, E. S., Hahn, M. A., et al. (1969). The effect of organic acids on renal clearance of methotrexate in man. *Clinical Pharmacology and Therapeutics, 10,* 849–857.

Lipinski, J. F., & Pope, H. G., Jr. (1982). Possible synergistic action between carbamazepine and lithium carbonate in the treatment of three acutely manic patients. *American Journal of Psychiatry, 139,* 948–949.

Lumholtz, B., Siersbaek–Nielsen, K., & Skovsted, L. (1975). Sulfamethizole-induced inhibition of diphenylhydantoin, tolbutamide, and warfarin metabolism. *Clinical Pharmacology and Therapeutics, 17,* 731–734.

Lunde, P. K. M., Rane, A., Yaffe, S. J., et al. (1970). Plasma protein binding of diphenylhydantoin in man. Interaction with other drugs and the effect of temperature and plasma dilution. *Clinical Pharmacology and Therapeutics, 11,* 846–854.

MacCallum, W. A. G. (1980). Interaction of lithium and phenytoin. *British Medical Journal, 280,* 610–611.

Macphee, G. J., McInnes, G. T., Thompson, G. G., et al. (1986). Verapamil potentiates carbamazepine neurotoxicity: A clinically important inhibitory interaction. *The Lancet, 1,* 700–703.

Mallette, L. E. (1977). Acetazolamide-accelerated anticonvulsant induced osteomalacia. *Archives of Internal Medicine, 137,* 1013–1017.

Mandel, M. A. (1976). The synergistic effect of salicylates on methotrexate toxicity. *Journal of Plastic and Reconstructive Surgery, 57,* 733–737.

Marquis, J. F., Carruthers, S. G., Spence, J. D., et al. (1982). Phenytoin–theophylline interaction. *New England Journal of Medicine, 307,* 1189–1190.

Matsuda, I., Takekoshi, Y., & Shida, N. (1975). Renal tubular acidosis and skeletal demineralization in patients on long-term anticonvulsant therapy. *The Journal of Pediatrics, 87,* 202–205.

May, D. B., Drew, R. H., Yedinak, K. C., et al. (1994). Effect of simultaneous didanosine administration on itraconazole absorption in healthy volunteers. *Pharmacotherapy, 14,* 509–513.

McArthur, J. (1969). Oral contraceptives and epilepsy. *British Medical Journal, 4,* 80.

Melhorn, D. K., & Gross, S. (1969). Relationships between iron–dextran and vitamin E in an iron deficiency anemia in children. *Journal of Laboratory and Clinical Medicine, 74,* 789–801.

Mesdjian, E., Dravet, C., Centraud, B., et al. (1980). Carbamazepine intoxication due to triacetyloleandomycin administration in epileptic patients. *Epilepsia, 21,* 489–496.

Miller, R. R., Porter, J., & Greenblatt, D. J. (1979). Clinical importance of the interaction of phenytoin and isoniazid. *Chest, 75,* 356–358.

Mitchell, A. S., & Holland, J. T. (1989). Fluconazole and phenytoin: A predictable interaction. *British Medical Journal, 298,* 1315.

Moller, B. B., & Ekelund, B. (1985). Toxicity of cyclosporine during treatment with androgens. [Letter]. *New England Journal of Medicine, 313,* 1416.

Monks, A., & Richens, A. (1980). Effect of single doses of sodium valproate on serum phenytoin levels and protein binding in epileptic patients. *Clinical Pharmacology and Therapeutics, 27,* 89–95.

Moysey, J. O., Jaggarao, N. S. V., Grundy, E. N., et al. (1981). Amiodarone increases plasma digoxin concentrations. *British Medical Journal, 282,* 272.

Neuvonen, P. J. (1976). Interactions with the absorption of tetracyclines. *Drugs, 11,* 45–54.

Neuvonen, P. J., Kivisto, K., & Hirvisalo, E. L. (1988). Effects of resins and activated charcoal on the absorption of digoxin, carbamazepine and frusemide. *British Journal of Clinical Pharmacology, 25,* 229–233.

Neuvonen, P. J., Lehtovaara, R., Bardy, A., et al. (1979). Antipyretic analgesics in patients on antiepileptic drug therapy. *European Journal of Clinical Pharmacology, 15,* 263–268.

Neuvonen, P. J., Penttila, O., Lehtovarra, R., et al.

(1975). Effect of antiepileptic drugs on the elimination of various tetracycline derivatives. *European Journal of Clinical Pharmacology, 9,* 147–154.

Newman, R. J. (1976). Comparison of propranolol, metoprolol, and acebutolol on insulin-induced hypoglycaemia. *British Medical Journal, 2,* 447–449.

Nies, A. S., & Oates, J. A. (1971). Clinicopathologic conference: Hypertension and the lupus syndrome revisited. *American Journal of Medicine, 51,* 812–814.

Nix, D. E., Watson, W. A., Lener, M., et al. (1989). Effects of aluminum and magnesium antacids and ranitidine on the absorption of ciprofloxacin. *Clinical Pharmacology and Therapeutics, 46,* 700–705.

Northcutt, R. C., Stiel, J. N., Hollifield, J. W., et al. (1969). The influence of cholestyramine on thyroxine absorption. *Journal of the American Medical Association, 208,* 1857–1861.

Offermann, G., Keller, F., & Molzahn, M. (1985). Low cyclosporin A blood levels and acute graft rejection in a renal transplant recipient during rifampin treatment. *American Journal of Nephrology, 5,* 385–387.

Olivesi, A. (1986). Modified elimination of prednisolone in epileptic patients on carbamazepine monotherapy, and in women using low-dose oral contraceptives. *Biomedicine and Pharmacotherapy, 40,* 301–308.

O'Neil-Cutting, M. A., & Crosby, W. H. (1986). The effect of antacids on the absorption of simultaneously ingested iron. *Journal of the American Medical Association, 255,* 1468–1470.

O'Reilly, R. A. (1983). Comparative interaction of cimetidine and ranitidine with racemic warfarin in man. *Federal Proceedings, 42,* 1175.

O'Reilly, R. A., Trager, W. F., Motley, C. H., et al. (1980). Interaction of secobarbital with warfarin pseudoracemates. *Clinical Pharmacology and Therapeutics, 28,* 187.

Owens, R. C. (2001). Risk assessment for antimicrobial agent-induced Qtc interval prolongation and torsades de pointes. *Pharmacotherapy, 21,* 301–319.

Paloucek, F., Rodrold, K., Jung, D., et al. (1986). The effects of cimetidine and ranitidine on steady-state pharmacokinetics of procainamide. *Journal of Clinical Pharmacology, 26,* 541–560.

Pappaioanou, M., Fishbein, D. B., Dreesen, D. W., et al. (1986). Antibody response to preexposure human diploid-cell rabies vaccine given concurrently with chloroquine. *New England Journal of Medicine, 314,* 280–284.

Parent, M., & LeBel, M. (1991). Meta-analysis of quinolone–theophylline interactions. *Drug Intelligence and Clinical Pharmacy, 25,* 191–194.

Patel, I. H., Levy, R. H., & Culter, R. E. (1980). Phenobarbital–valproic acid interaction. *Clinical Pharmacology and Therapeutics, 27,* 515–521.

Paxton, J. W. (1980). Effects of aspirin on salivary and serum phenytoin kinetics in healthy subjects. *Clinical Pharmacology and Therapeutics, 27,* 170–178.

Pearson, H. J. (1990). Interaction of fluoxetine with carbamazepine. [Letter]. *Journal of Clinical Psychiatry, 51,* 126.

Penttila, O., Neuvonen, P. J., Aho, K., et al. (1974). Interaction between doxycycline and some antiepileptic drugs. *British Medical Journal, 2,* 470–472.

Perucca, E., & Richens, A. (1971). Paracetamol disposition in normal subjects and in patients treated with antiepileptic drugs. *British Journal of Clinical Pharmacology, 7,* 201–206.

Pessayre, D., Bentata, M., & Degott, C. (1977). Isoniazid–rifampin fulminant hepatitis. A possible consequence of the enhancement of isoniazid hepatotoxicity by enzyme induction. *Gastroenterology, 72,* 284–289.

Petereit, L. B., & Meikle, A. W. (1977). Effectiveness of prednisolone during phenytoin therapy. *Clinical Pharmacology and Therapeutics, 22,* 912–916.

Petti, T. A., & Campbell, M. (1975). Imipramine and seizures. *American Journal of Psychiatry, 132,* 538–540.

Pittinger, C. B., Eryasa, Y., & Adamson, R. (1970). Antibiotic-induced paralysis. *Anesthesia and Analgesia, 49,* 487–492.

Polish, L. B., Branch, R. A., & Fitzgerald, G. A. (1981). Digitoxin–quinidine interaction: Potentiation during administration of cimetidine. *Southern Medical Journal, 74,* 633–634.

Pond, S. M. & Kretschmar, K. M. (1981). Effect of phenytoin on meperidine clearance and normeperidine formation. *Clinical Pharmacology and Therapeutics, 30,* 680–686.

Privitera, M. R., Greden, J. F., Gardner, R. W., et al. (1982). Interference by carbamazepine with the dexamethasone suppression test. *Biological Psychiatry, 17,* 611–620.

Ptachcinski, R. J., Carpenter, B. J., Burckart, G. J., et al. (1985). Effect of erythromycin on cyclosporine levels. *New England Journal of Medicine, 313,* 1416–1417.

Puurunen, J., Sotanienni, E., & Pelkonen, O. (1980). Effect of cimetidine on microsomal drug metabolism in man. *European Journal of Clinical Pharmacology, 18,* 185.

Ragheb, M., & Powell, A. L. (1986a). Failure of sulindac to increase serum lithium levels. *Journal of Clinical Psychiatry, 47,* 33–34.

Ragheb, M., & Powell, A. L. (1986b). Lithium interaction with sulindac and naproxen. *Journal of Clinical Psychopharmacology, 6,* 150–154.

Renton, K. W., Gray, D. J., & Hung, O. R. (1981). Depression of theophylline elimination by erythromycin. *Clinical Pharmacology and Therapeutics, 30,* 422–426.

Riff, L. J., & Jackson, G. G. (1972). Laboratory and

clinical conditions for gentamicin inactivation by carbenicillin. *Archives of Internal Medicine, 130,* 887–891.

Ringden, O., Myrenfors, P., Klintmalm, G., et al. (1984). Nephrotoxicity by co-trimoxazole and cyclosporine in transplanted patients. *The Lancet, 1,* 1016–1017.

Roberts, D. G., Gerber, J. G., & Nies, A. S. (1984). Comparative effects of sulindac and indomethacin in humans. [Abstract]. *Clinical Pharmacology and Therapeutics, 35,* 269.

Robertson, Y. R., & Johnson, E. S. (1976). Interactions between oral contraceptives and other drugs: A review. *Current Medical Research and Opinion, 3,* 647–661.

Rosenberry, K. R., Defusco, C. J., Mansmann, H. C., et al. (1983). Reduced theophylline half-life induced by carbamazepine therapy. *The Journal of Pediatrics, 102,* 472–474.

Ross, W. B., Roberts, D., Griffin, P. J. A., et al. (1986). Cyclosporine interaction with danazol and noresthisterone. [Letter]. *The Lancet, 1,* 330.

Sachs, B. A., & Wolfman, L. (1968). Effect of oxandrolone on plasma lipids and lipoproteins of patients with disorders of lipid metabolism. *Metabolism, 17,* 400–410.

Salem, R. B., Breland, B. D., Mishra, S., et al. (1983). Effect of cimetidine on phenytoin serum levels. *Epilepsia, 24,* 284–288.

Salvetti, A., Arzill, F., Pedrinelli, R., et al. (1982). Interaction between oxprenolol and indomethacin on blood pressure in essential hypertensive patients. *European Journal of Clinical Pharmacology, 22,* 197–201.

Schofield, O. M. V., Camp, R. D. R., & Levene, G. M. (1990). Cyclosporin A in psoriasis: Interaction with carbamazepine. [Letter]. *British Journal of Dermatology, 122,* 425–426.

Seaton, T. L., Celum, C. L., & Black, D. J. (1990). Possible potentiation of warfarin by fluconazole. *Drug Intelligence and Clinical Pharmacy, 24,* 1177–1178.

Seideman, P., Grahnen, A., Haglund, K., et al. (1982). Prazosin first dose phenomenon during combined treatment with a beta-adrenoceptor in hypertensive patients. *British Journal of Clinical Pharmacology, 13,* 865–870.

Selker, R. G., Moore, P., & Lodolce, D. (1978). Bone-marrow depression with cimetidine plus carmustine. [Letter]. *New England Journal of Medicine, 299,* 834.

Shapiro, P. A. (1984). Cimetidine–imipramine interaction: Case report and comments. [Letter]. *American Journal of Psychiatry, 141,* 152.

Shapiro, S., Slone, D., Lewis, G. P., et al. (1971). Fatal reactions among medical inpatients. *Journal of the American Medical Association, 216,* 467–472.

Singh, R. R., Malaviya, A. N., Pandey, J. N., et al. (1986). Fatal interaction between methotrexate and naproxen. *The Lancet, 1,* 1390.

Skolnick, J. L., Stoler, B. S., & Katz, D. B. (1976). Rifampin, oral contraceptives, and pregnancy. *Journal of the American Medical Association, 236,* 1382.

Small, R. E., & Marshall, J. H. (1979). Quinidine-digoxin interaction. *Drug Intelligence and Clinical Pharmacy, 13,* 286–289.

Smith, A. G. (1984). Potentiation of oral anticoagulants by ketoconazole. *British Medical Journal, 288,* 188–189.

Smith, S. J. (1994). Cardiovascular toxicity of antihistamines. *Otolaryngology and Head and Neck Surgery, 111,* 348–354.

Somogyi, A., & Heinzow, B. (1982). Cimetidine reduces procainamide elimination. [Letter]. *New England Journal of Medicine, 307,* 1080.

Speirs, C. J., Dollery, C. T., Inman, W. H. W., et al. (1988). Postmarketing surveillance of enalapril: II. Investigation of the potential role of enalapril in deaths with renal failure. *British Medical Journal, 297,* 830–832.

Speirs, J., & Hirsch, S. R. (1978). Severe lithium toxicity within "normal" serum concentrations. *British Medical Journal, 1,* 815–816.

Spicer, S. T., Liddle, C., Chapman, J. R., et al., (1997). The mechanism of cyclosporine toxicity induced by clarithromycin. *British Journal of Clinical Pharmacology, 43,* 194–196.

Straughn, A. B., Henderson, R. P., Lieberman, P. L., et al. (1984). Effect of rifampin on theophylline disposition. *Therapeutic Drug Monitoring, 6,* 153–156.

Sutton, G., & Kupferberg, H. J. (1975). Isoniazid as an inhibitor of primidone metabolism. *Neurology, 25,* 1179–1181.

Syversen, G. B., Morgan, J. P., Weintraubet, M., et al. (1977). Acetazolamide-induced interference with primidone absorption. *Archives of Neurology, 34,* 80–84.

Taylor, D. N., Wasi, C., & Bernard, K. (1984). Chloroquine prophylaxis associated with a poor antibody response to human diploid cell rabies vaccine. [Letter]. *The Lancet, 1,* 1405.

Thyss, A., Milano, G., Kubar, J., et al. (1986). Clinical and pharmacokinetic evidence of a life-threatening interaction between methotrexate and ketoprofen. *The Lancet, 1,* 256.

Tobin, J. R., Doyle, T. P., Ackerman, A. D., et al. (1991). Astemizole-induced cardiac conduction disturbances in a child. *Journal of the American Medical Association, 266,* 2737–2740.

Trunet, P., LeGall, J. R., Lhoste, F., et al. (1980). The role of iatrogenic disease in admissions to intensive care. *Journal of the American Medical Association, 244,* 2617.

Valsalan, V. C., & Cooper, G. L. (1982). Carbamazepine intoxication caused by interaction with isoniazid. *British Medical Journal, 285,* 261–262.

van Harten, J. (1993). Clinical pharmacokinetics of selective serotonin reuptake inhibitors. *Clinical Pharmacokinetics, 24,* 203–220.

Van Herwaarden, C. L. A., Fennis, J. F. M., Binkhorst, R. A., et al. (1977). Haemodynamic effects of adrenaline during treatment of hypertensive patients with propranolol and metoprolol. *European Journal of Clinical Pharmacology, 12,* 397–402.

Viskin, S. (1999). Long QT syndromes and torsade de pointes. *The Lancet, 354,* 1625–1633.

Volkin, R. L., Shadduck, R. K., Winklestein, A., et al. (1982). Potentiation of carmustine-cranial irradiation-induced myelosuppression by cimetidine. *Archives of Internal Medicine, 142,* 243–245.

Warner, W. A., & Sanders, E. (1971). Neuromuscular blockade associated with gentamicin therapy. *Journal of the American Medical Association, 215,* 1153–1154.

Wassner, S. J., Pennis, A. J., & Malekzadeh, M. H. (1976). The adverse effect of anticonvulsant therapy on renal allograft survival. *The Journal of Pediatrics, 88,* 134–137.

Watkins, J., Abbott, E. C., Hensby, C. N., et al. (1980). Attenuation of hypotensive effect of propranolol and thiazide diuretics by indomethacin. *British Medical Journal, 281,* 702–705.

Watkins, V. S., Polk, R. E., & Stotka, J. L. (1997). Drug interactions of macrolides: Emphasis on dirithromycin. *Annals of Pharmacotherapy, 31,* 349–356.

Weinberger, M., Hudgel, D., Spector, S., et al. (1977). Inhibition of theophylline clearance by troleandomycin. *Journal of Allergy and Clinical Immunology, 59,* 228–231.

Welling, P. G., Koch, P. A., Lau, C. C., et al. (1977). Bioavailability of tetracycline and doxycycline in fasted and nonfasted subjects. *Antimicrobial Agents and Chemotherapy, 11,* 462–469.

Wilson, J. T., & Wilkinson, G. R. (1973). Chronic and severe phenobarbital intoxication in a child treated with primidone and diphenylhydantoin. *The Journal of Pediatrics, 83,* 484–489.

Windorfer, A., Sauer, W., & Gadeke, R. (1975). Elevation of diphenylhydantoin and primidone serum concentration by addition of dipropylacetate, a new anticonvulsant drug. *Acta Paediatrica Scandinavica, 64,* 771–772.

Wong, Y. Y., Ludden, T. M., & Bell, R. D. (1983). Effect of erythromycin on carbamazepine kinetics. *Clinical Pharmacology and Therapeutics, 33,* 484–487.

Yamada, S., & Iwai, K. (1976). Induction of hepatic cortisol-6-hydroxylase by rifampicin. *The Lancet, 2,* 366–367.

Yasui, N., Otani, K., Kaneko, S., et al. (1997). Carbamazepine toxicity induced by clarithromycin coadministration in psychiatric patients. *International Clinical Psychopharmacology, 12,* 225–229.

Yee, G. C., & McGuire, T. R. (1990). Pharmacokinetic interactions with cyclosporin. Part I. *Clinical Pharmacokinetics, 19,* 319–332.

Yu, Y. L., Huang, C. Y., Chin, D., et al. (1986). Interaction between carbamazepine and dextropropoxyphene. *Postgraduate Medical Journal, 62,* 321–323.

Yuen, G. J. (1984). Agents affecting phenytoin bioavailability. *Drug Interactions Newsletter, 4,* 37–42.

Zimmermann, T., Yeates, R. A., Laufen, H., et al. (1994). Influence of concomitant food intake on the oral absorption of two triazole antifungal agents, itraconazole and fluconazole. *European Journal of Clinical Pharmacology, 46,* 147–150.

7

Abusable Psychotropic Use among Children and Adolescents

Ann Marie Pagliaro

The use of the various abusable psychotropics (Figure 7-1) during childhood and adolescence is expected to increase over the next decade as a myriad of contributing factors interact in a variety of ways. As the use of these drugs and substances increases among pediatric patients, pediatric clinicians find that they must be increasingly concerned about the growing acceptance of abusable psychotropic use among children and adolescents, both users and nonusers; the morbidity and mortality associated with increasingly problematic patterns of use; and the associated significant costs to society of childhood and adolescent abusable psychotropic use (e.g., healthcare and law enforcement costs; lost or decreased economic productivity; and pain and suffering of parents and other family members) (Pagliaro & Pagliaro, 1996, 2000; Tweed, 1998). This chapter presents an overview of the abusable psychotropics and their general patterns of use among children and adolescents in the United States and Canada. Attention also is given to their adverse drug reactions and toxic effects. The Mega Interactive Model of Abusable Psychotropic Use among Youth is provided as a means to help pediatric clinicians better understand and effectively deal with this serious concern.

The most commonly used abusable psychotropics (Table 7-1) continue to be alcohol, tobacco, and cannabis, although amphetamines, cocaine, heroin, MDMA, and volatile solvents and inhalants also are being used increasingly. Currently, as many as 4 million adolescents in the United States and Canada are personally experiencing serious problems associated with their abusable psychotropic use. These problems include developmental delays; educational failure; and violent behavior, such as family and school violence (Lowry et al., 1999), gang activity (Tweed, 1998), and other violent acts (e.g., physical assaults, rape, suicide) (Pagliaro & Pagliaro, 1996).

The mortality associated with abusable psychotropic use is significant (Onwuachi-Saunders et al., 1999). For example, Neumark et al. (2000) found that people who had a history of abusable psychotropic use were more likely to have died and to have a younger median age at death than those who did not. In fact, the use of alcohol and other abusable psychotropics has been estimated to be related to approximately 40% of accidental or

PROBLEMS IN PEDIATRIC DRUG THERAPY

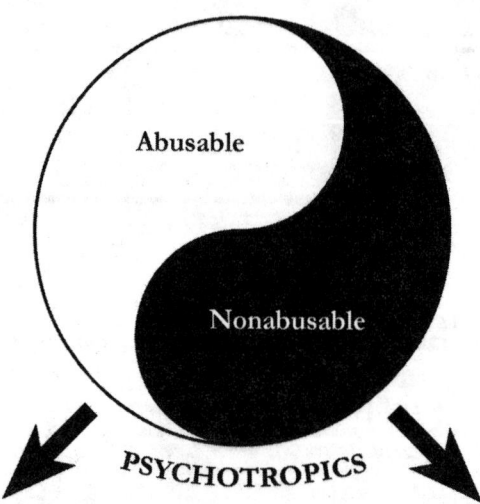

FIGURE 7-1
Abusable and Nonabusable Psychotropics
The term "psychotropics" refers to all exogenous substances (chemicals, drugs, substances, and xenobiotics) that elicit a direct effect on the CNS, resulting in changes in cognition, learning, memory, behavior, perception, or effect. The psychotropics can be further classified, conveniently and parsimoniously, as either abusable or nonabusable. The abusable psychotropics are associated with addiction (the development of tolerance and a withdrawal syndrome upon the discontinuation of use) and habituation. The nonabusable psychotropics have not been consistently associated with addiction and habituation phenomena and, thus, are not considered in this chapter.

TABLE 7-1
Major Abusable Psychotropics[a]

CNS Depressants
- Opiates (e.g., codeine, heroin, meperidine, methadone, morphine)
- Sedative-hypnotics (e.g., alcohol, barbiturates, benzodiazepines, miscellaneous sedative-hypnotics [e.g., chloral hydrate])
- Volatile solvents and inhalants (e.g., gasoline, glue, nitrous oxide, propane)

CNS Stimulants
- Amphetamines (amphetamine, dextroamphetamine, methamphetamine) and other related CNS stimulants (e.g., methylphenidate *[Ritalin®]*)
- Caffeine
- Cocaine
- Nicotine (as a constituent of tobacco)

Psychedelics
- Anesthetics, dissociative (ketamine *[Ketajet®, Ketalar®, Ketavet®]*; phencyclidine [PCP])
- Lysergic acid diethylamide (LSD)
- 3,4-methylenedioxymethamphetamine (MDMA)
- Mescaline (peyote cactus)
- Psilocybin (conocybe and psilocybe mushrooms)
- Tetrahydrocannabinol (cannabis: marijuana, hashish, hashish oil)

[a] Based on that proposed by A. M. Pagliaro, 1990, 1991; anabolic steroids have not been included in this table or this chapter because they are not classified as abusable psychotropics. In addition, other drugs (e.g., dextromethorphan) abused by specific age groups of children and adolescents in specific geographic regions but not widely or consistently abused are not discussed in this chapter.

unintentional deaths, 30% of homicides,[1] and 20% of suicides[2] among adolescents. Alcohol-related accidents alone are the leading cause of death for adolescents 15–20 years of age. In the United States, motor vehicle crashes, other unintentional injuries (e.g., boating accidents, snowmobile crashes), homicide, and suicide account for 73.6% of all deaths among adolescents and young adults 10–24 years of age (Grunbaum et al., 1999). The use of alcohol and other abusable psychotropics also is associated with unprotected sexual intercourse with multiple partners sharing contaminated needles and syringes; and other behaviors that may place children and adolescents at increased risk for unintentional pregnancy and becoming infected with human immunodeficiency virus (HIV), and, subsequently, dying of acquired immune deficiency syndrome (AIDS) or related sequelae (Melzer-Lange, 1998; Pagliaro & Pagliaro, 2000).

---

1. Homicides account for a significant percentage of the annual deaths of inner city boys and men (Grunbaum et al., 1999; Onwuachi-Saunders et al., 1999; Pagliaro & Pagliaro, 1996; Shahpar & Li, 1999). One study (Mclaughlin et al., 2000) found that 52% of murders were committed by juveniles involved in drug selling, and 28% of the murders were otherwise drug related. Adolescent boys who were involved with the sale and distribution of illegal drugs comprised a significant percentage of those who were incarcerated for murder, supporting the link between abusable psychotropic use, drug selling, and homicide.

2. Abusable psychotropic use has long been directly linked to suicide, which is now the second leading cause of death among 15–19-year-olds in the United States (Jones, 1997; Lester, 1999; Mino et al., 1999; Pagliaro & Pagliaro, 1995). In one study (Windle & Windle, 1997), persistently high levels of problem drinking and de-

Interactive Model of Abusable Psychotropic Use

To help pediatric clinicians understand and effectively deal with the complex phenomenon of childhood and adolescent abusable psychotropic use, the Mega Interactive Model of Abusable Psychotropic Use among Youth (MIMAPUY) (Pagliaro & Pagliaro, 1993, 1996) has been developed (Figure 7-2). It can be used for assessing children and adolescents and for devising, delivering, and evaluating individualized prevention and treatment programs for children and adolescents who have problems related to their potential or actual abusable psychotropic use.

The model consists of four interacting dimensions: (1) young person dimension, (2) societal dimension, (3) abusable psychotropic dimension, and (4) time dimension. The abusable psychotropic use milieu for an individual youth at a particular time is represented in Figure 7-2 as the interaction of the young person, societal, and abusable psychotropic dimensions. The phenomenon of abusable psychotropic use displayed by an individual young person is represented as a unit coterie. A collection of unit coteries represents the larger social group or community to which the individual child or adolescent belongs (e.g., a particular peer group or gang, junior high school class, a high school basketball team, a group of runaway street youth).[3] Thus, the model is useful for both individual and group assessment and intervention.

MIMAPUY accounts for the multidimensional etiology of abusable psychotropic use without the imposition of a singular, restrictive theoretical focus or classification system (e.g., *Diagnostic and statistical manual of mental disorders–text revision* [American Psychiatric Association, 2000]). This approach is important in interdisciplinary pediatric healthcare settings. MIMAPUY can be used as a generic theoretical framework by clinicians from a variety of disciplines and theoretical perspectives when diagnosing actual or potential abusable psychotropic use and when planning, implementing, and evaluating the interdisciplinary and multimodal therapy that is often required.

The complexity of MIMAPUY reflects the nature of abusable psychotropic use. Abusable psychotropic use always has been and always will be a complex phenomenon. Thus, a single simple solution cannot be found. The multifactorial etiology of abusable psychotropic use and the myriad of possible interacting and confounding variables that clinicians and researchers must consider have been incorporated into the MIMAPUY.[4] Clinicians should abandon stereotypical thinking in relation to the etiology and treatment of abusable psychotropic use and be encour-

---

pressive symptoms were associated with more thoughts of suicide and more attempts. Adolescents who attempted suicide reported lower levels of family social support, a greater use of the abusable psychotropics to cope with stress, and more abusable psychotropic-using peers.

The use of alcohol and other abusable psychotropics (e.g., heroin, volatile solvents and inhalants) may also predict subsequent suicide attempts (Borges et al., 2000). However, the number of abusable psychotropics used, rather than the type used, seems to be the more important variable. Pediatric clinicians need to be aware that the use of abusable psychotropics may place adolescent suicide ideators at risk for unplanned suicide attempts, and this possibility should be considered during every clinical examination of an adolescent who uses, or is suspected of using, abusable psychotropics (Mino et al., 1999). In addition, several other studies (e.g., Fergusson et al., 1999; Garofalo et al., 1999; Lock & Steiner, 1999) have noted a high risk for suicide among gay, lesbian, and bisexual youth who use abusable psychotropics.

3. Children and adolescents give names to the peer groups they identify with. Peer group self-identification may delineate children and adolescents who are at risk for, or who already display, problematic patterns of abusable psychotropic use (e.g., gang members, runaway street youth). Group self-identification also is one of several variables related to abusable psychotropic use and violence (Sussman et al., 2000).

4. For a comprehensive review of the number of theories that have been produced in an attempt to explain childhood and adolescent abusable psychotropic use, *see* Bhattacharya, 1998; Carvajal et al., 1997; Dembo et al., 1998; Howard et al., 1997; Kim et al., 1998; Oetting & Donnermeyer, 1998; Oetting et al., 1998; Pagliaro & Pagliaro, 1996; and Wahlgren et al., 1997.

Young Person Dimension

Physical Variables
age
gender
general health status (e.g.,
  robust versus frail)
genetic predisposition (e.g.,
  family history of alcoholism)
physical impairment or
  handicap
race

Psychological Variables
aggressiveness
anxiety
attitudes
boredom
cognitive function
depression
developmental level
fears and phobias
general mental health
impulse control
intelligence
loneliness
personality disorders (e.g.,
  antisocial personality)
psychological adjustment
religiosity
risk-taking behavior
self-esteem
sexual orientation/preference
stress

Social Variables
culture
death of parent
delinquency
divorce of parents
dysfunctional family
economic status (e.g., poverty)
education
employment status
ethnic background
gang membership
homelessness
major life events or
  lifestyle changes (e.g.,
  receiving failing grades at school)
moral values
parental attitudes toward
  abusable psychotropic use
peer pressure
physical abuse
religion
sexual abuse
social competence
social stability
social support (e.g., family, school,
  and other social networks)
treatment experiences

Time Dimension

Time Variables
historic period (e.g., 1960s versus 1990s)
length of time of abusable psychotropic use
period of user's life (e.g., childhood
  versus adolescence)

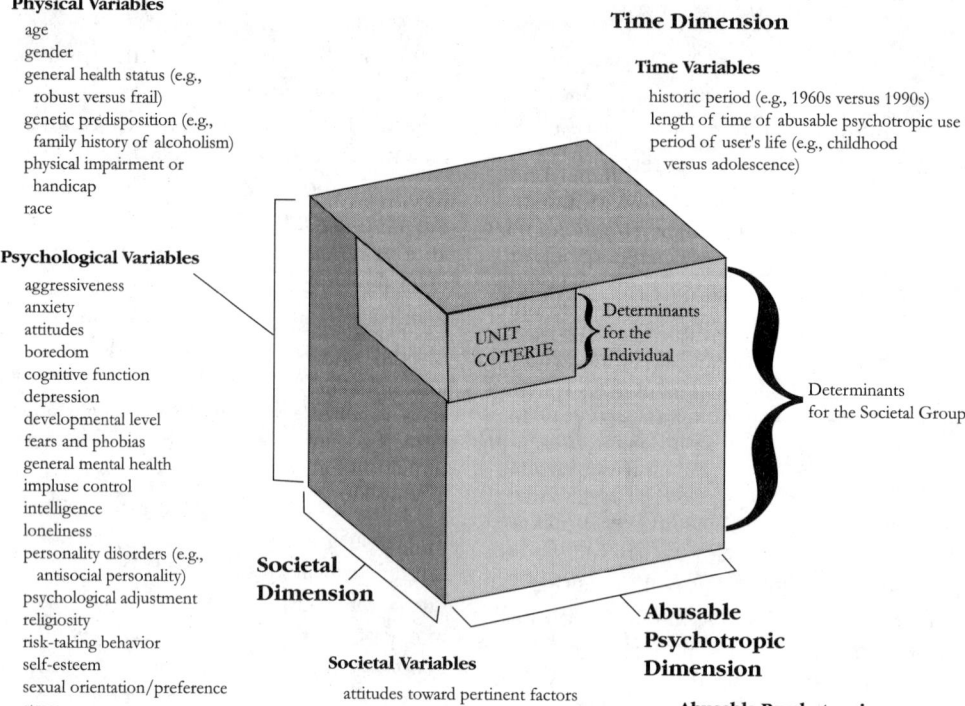

Societal Dimension

Societal Variables
attitudes toward pertinent factors
  (e.g., ageism, sexism, and abusable
  psychotropic use)
community structure
cultures
economy (e.g., availability of jobs)
educational systems
professional ethics
healthcare system
"Law of the Land" (e.g.,
  legal age for purchase
  of alcohol and tobacco)
media influence (e.g., movies,
  rock videos, and rap songs)
professional ethics
realms of professional practice
religions
school system
social controls
social mores
social programs
treatment availability (e.g., access and cost)
youth correctional/detention facilities

Abusable Psychotropic Dimension

Abusable Psychotropic Variables
abuse liability
addiction potential
availability
amount used
  (e.g., individual dose
  and frequency)
cost
interactions
legal status
method of use
pharmacokinetics
pharmacology
toxicology

Pattern-of-Use Variables
nonuse
initial use
social use
habitual use
abuse
compulsive use
resumed nonuse
controlled use
relapsed use

FIGURE 7-2
Mega Interactive Model of Abusable Psychotropic Use among Youth (MIMAPUY)

aged to use MIMAPUY to develop a more individually tailored approach for dealing with this complex problem. The following example illustrates the use of MIMAPUY and an individually tailored approach.

J. B., a 17-year-old boy, consumes alcoholic beverages excessively on a regular basis. In a traditional clinical setting, he would be diagnosed as having alcoholism and would be referred to a generic treatment program for alcoholics. Alternatively, J. B.'s alcohol-consuming behavior could be characterized in the context of the four dimensions of MIMAPUY. The pediatric clinician would identify relevant variables to address when developing and implementing an individualized treatment plan. Consider, for example, that J. B. developed an alcohol problem as a preadolescent after the death of his father from alcohol-related cardiomyopathy. J. B. received bereavement counseling and had abstained from alcohol use until 6 months ago when he and his girlfriend broke up. Given this context, the use of the previously successful treatment, which involved resolution of grief, the development and strengthening of coping abilities, and the provision of alternative support systems, might do much toward the alleviation of the current problem.

MIMAPUY serves as a heuristic device to help pediatric clinicians identify the variables associated with abusable psychotropic use among youth and to better understand the complexity of the phenomenon. MIMAPUY offers the clinician insight into important considerations involving the four interactive dimensions: youth, societal, time, and abusable psychotropic. Although the primary focus of this chapter will be on the abusable psychotropic dimension, a brief overview of the other three dimensions is included.

Young Person Dimension

Almost two decades ago, Andrew Weil (1983) noted that "It's a real problem when you classify drugs as good and bad . . . Drugs are drugs (i.e., inanimate objects without any inherent goodness or badness). The only point that good and bad comes in is in the individual use of drugs." Thus, the use of morphine to relieve severe cancer pain for a terminally ill adolescent is considered good. However, the use of morphine as a dare from a peer that results in a fatal overdose is considered bad. MIMAPUY encourages a scientific (rational and logical) approach to abusable psychotropic use by youth that goes well beyond the abusable psychotropic dimension to include further consideration of the physical, psychological, and social characteristics of the youth.

The influence of the physical, psychological, and social variables on the youth dimension is significant. These variables must be fully addressed when assessing children and adolescents and when planning and implementing abusable psychotropic use prevention and treatment programs. For example, the effective approach and treatment plan for a young "alcoholic" differ greatly for (1) a 12-year-old, middle class, Native American boy who previously performed well academically in school and is living in a stable, supportive family unit, but who has a family history of alcoholism in both maternal and paternal grandfathers and a paternal uncle; (2) a 9-year-old Nicaraguan girl who is clinically depressed and living in a foster home in which she is being sexually abused; (3) a 16-year-old Haitian girl who is a sex trade worker and is currently pregnant and living on her own in a youth emergency shelter; (4) a 17-year-old Hispanic boy who is a gang member living in the inner city and who is the principal source of financial support for his girlfriend and her baby as well as for his mother, grandmother, and four siblings; (5) a 14-year-old boy of above-average intelligence who recently immigrated to the United States from China, does not speak English well, and is not happy in his new country; and (6) a 17-year-old Cuban boy who is an illegal immigrant without any family or social support, works as a male prostitute, and is HIV positive.

Clearly, all children and adolescents who have alcoholism are not alike. Consideration of the variables associated with the young person dimension can assist clinicians in differentiating the unique aspects of each pediatric patient. Such variables as living in a single-parent family, lacking constructive hobbies, having a mental disorder, and having an aggressive delinquent lifestyle are associated with truancy, deficits in school performance, and alcohol and other abusable psychotropic use (Miller & Plant, 1999). This differentiation and appropriate multidisciplinary intervention encourages individualization of assessment and treatment and facilitates optimal therapeutic outcomes for children and adolescents who have problematic patterns of abusable psychotropic use.

Physical variables. Age (Friedman & Glassman, 2000), race (Friedman & Glassman, 2000; Wallace et al., 1999), and gender (Zickler, 2001b) are important physical variables in regard to childhood and adolescent abusable psychotropic use. Gender differences were noted in a study of stages of drug involvement among children and adolescents 12 years of age and older (Van Etten et al., 1999). Boys were more likely than girls to have the initial opportunity to use various abusable psychotropics. However, when presented with an opportunity to use an abusable psychotropic, few male–female differences were observed (Moon et al., 1999). Previously documented male excess in rates of abusable psychotropic use may be due to greater male exposure to opportunities to try drugs, rather than to greater chance of progressing from initial opportunity to actual use (Van Etten & Anthony, 1999). Gender differences also are likely in regard to accepting an abusable psychotropic when it is offered. For example, girls who provide explanations for not accepting an abusable psychotropic may succumb to counterexplanations and ultimately use an abusable psychotropic whereas boys generally do not (Zickler, 2001b). Thus, these findings suggest that sex differences involving abusable psychotropic use emerge early and require attention in regard to gender-sensitive primary prevention programs.

Oftentimes, the physical variables interact with the abusable psychotropic variables in ways that increase the risk for serious outcome. For example, in relation to teratogenic or fetotoxic effects, the risk only becomes apparent when a young girl reaches menarche. The right gender, the right age, and the right drug are required before risk is increased for abusable psychotropic-induced teratogenic or fetotoxic effects (*see* Chapter 2). However, the escalating rates of both chronic alcohol use by adolescent girls and teenage pregnancy require special mention because of the increased risk for fetal alcohol syndrome (FAS). FAS has been, for past quarter century, the most common preventable cause of mental retardation in North America (Abel, 1995; Pagliaro & Pagliaro, 1996, 2000; Pietrantoni & Knuppel, 1991; Streissguth et al., 1991). Cocaine use also has increased among adolescent girls over the past two decades, and attention is only now focusing on the learning deficits and other developmental problems observed among children exposed to cocaine in utero (the sequelae of a possible fetal cocaine syndrome among crack babies) (Pagliaro, 1992a; Pagliaro & Pagliaro, 1996, 2000; Swanson et al., 1999; Walker et al., 1999).

As use patterns change among adolescent girls, the teratogenic and fetotoxic effects of other abusable psychotropics must also be investigated. For example, prospective follow-up of 136 babies exposed in utero to MDMA (ecstasy, chemically similar to methamphetamine and mescaline) indicated that this abusable psychotropic may be associated with a significant risk for congenital anomalies, particularly cardiovascular and musculoskeletal anomalies (McElhatton et al., 1999). More data are needed because most MDMA users also use other abusable psychotropics (Pedersen & Skrondal, 1999) and definitive identification of the actual drugs and substances they may be using while clubbing or at raves generally is not possible.

Psychological variables. Several psychological variables are associated with abusable psychotropic use among children and adolescents. For example, stressful life events, including past physical or sexual assault or being a witness to violence, appear to be important risk factors for abusable psychotropic use among 12–17-year-olds (Clarke et al.,

1999; Kilpatrick et al., 2000; Palacios et al., 1999). Stress-related variables (e.g., family conflict, loss of a parent, coming from a lower socioeconomic status, past history of victimization), perceived stress, and beliefs about the ability of abusable psychotropics to manage stress were significantly related to child and adolescent abusable psychotropic use (Sussman & Dent, 2000). Similarly, when examining abusable psychotropic use during early and midadolescence, Hoffman et al. (2000) found that a cumulative effect of stressful life experiences over time led to a steep escalation of abusable psychotropic use during adolescence. Crimmins et al. (2000) found that the traumatic experiences of children may have a significant influence on their later abusable psychotropic use and participation in violent crimes. These relationships were moderated, however, by family attachment. Personality traits and IQ also play a major moderating role (Martin et al., 1999; Pagliaro & Pagliaro, 1996).

Social variables. When alcohol use was examined with attention to the sociocultural diversity of youth in Hawaii, adolescent boys who were Caucasian, Hawaiian, or Filipino and who had lower educational attainment were at higher risk than other adolescents (Hishinuma et al., 2000). Factors associated with different rates of alcohol use included accessibility, ability to resist offers, parental use of alcohol, parental sanctions, peer influence and use, attitudes and beliefs (e.g., dangerousness, perceived normal drinking), religious affiliation, social occasions, and school interventions.

The relationship of peer and parental attitudes and peer use of alcohol and marijuana was studied in regard to decision-making and self-reinforcement skills of adolescents (Botvin et al., 1999). Social risk factors were strongly associated with increased alcohol and marijuana use among adolescents who had poor interpersonal skills. However, good decision-making and self-reinforcement skills diminished the influence of social risk factors on abusable psychotropic use. These data may be useful in guiding school-based prevention programs. Children and adolescents who had post-traumatic stress disorder also were found to be at increased risk for marijuana and other "hard" abusable psychotropic use (Kilpatrick et al., 2000).

Data from 4111 boys and 4085 girls participating in 10 HIV/AIDS service demonstration projects were presented (Huba et al., 2000). The sample was diverse in age, ethnicity, gender, HIV status, and risk for HIV transmission. Those participants who were most likely to have a history of abusable psychotropic use were boys who were younger and had a sexually transmitted disease; engaged in survival sex; and participated in risky sex with men, women, and drug injectors. For girls, these predictors, with the exception of having a sexually transmitted disease, also were significant. Information about sexual and other risk factors was highly predictive of abusable psychotropic use issues among youth.[5]

Societal Dimension

The societal dimension is often given less attention than the other dimensions by clinicians. This dimension reflects the law of the land (legal restrictions); professional ethics; realms of professional practice; customs, mores, and attitudes toward abusable psychotropic use; and a myriad of other variables. The societal dimension has a significant impact on the prevention and treatment programs that are available for and provided to children and adolescents. Westermeyer (1999) observed that young people were protected from addictive disorders for many centuries and only recently has widespread addiction occurred, reflecting a failure of social institutions and a need for institutional changes.

---

5. Conversely, it should be kept in mind that abusable psychotropic use is itself a major risk factor for engaging in high-risk sexual behaviors (e.g., having multiple sexual partners, needle sharing, engaging in unprotected sexual intercourse) (Inciardi et al., 1999; McNall & Remafedi, 1999; Pagliaro et al., 1993; Tortu et al., 2000).

The availability of treatment programs in terms of access and cost (some programs are available only to children and adolescents whose parents are affluent or who have the necessary insurance coverage) needs to be considered when planning or recommending intervention at the local, state or provincial, and national levels. Other societal variables, such as the dominant culture of a community or city, also can have a significant effect on treatment outcomes. Children and adolescents are more likely to seek, enter, and complete treatment if the treatment program is consonant with their cultural and other social needs (Pagliaro & Pagliaro, 1996). Although the variables in the societal dimension of MIMAPUY are generally not amenable to immediate change, they significantly affect the availability of treatment. Therefore, they must be realistically and appropriately addressed at both the local and national levels.

Religiosity has been generally identified as a "protective" factor in relation to abusable psychotropic use (D'Onofrio et al., 1999). Miller et al. (2000) found an inverse relationship between religiosity (devotion or a personal relationship with the Divine) and affiliation and abusable psychotropic use. Pullen et al. (1999) found that as attendance at religious services by 12–19-year-olds increased, alcohol and other abusable psychotropic use decreased. However, most available data suggest a significant decrease in measures of religiosity for adolescents over the past decade.

Time Dimension

The time dimension usually receives insufficient attention. The time dimension includes such variables as the historic period during which a particular abusable psychotropic is used, the length of time during which it is used in relation to its pattern of use, and the specific period of the user's life. The time dimension plays a significant role in terms of the historic context of abusable psychotropic use in relation to each of the other dimensions. It also affects the consequences associated with the use of a particular abusable psychotropic. For example, the consequences of cannabis use in North America during the 1800s were significantly different from today because cannabis use was then legal. Although cocaine was available in various forms for oral ingestion as a beverage (e.g., Vin Mariani® and, later, Coca Cola®) during the late 19th and early 20th centuries, the crack form of cocaine, now widely abused by youth in North America, was not abused at that time because it had not yet been formulated. New abusable psychotropics (e.g., designer drugs) and new methods for using currently available abusable psychotropics can be expected in the future.

Abusable Psychotropic Dimension

The abusable psychotropic dimension comprises two major types of variables: (1) the abusable psychotropic variables and (2) the pattern-of-use variables. This dimension has obvious relevance for pediatric clinicians. Such factors as the pharmacology, pharmacokinetics, toxicology, abuse liability, and addiction potential of a particular abusable psychotropic are critical factors that continue to receive a great deal of attention in relation to the antecedents and consequences of abusable psychotropic use.

Abusable Psychotropic Variables

North American children and adolescents currently use a variety of abusable psychotropics, including alcohol, amphetamines, cannabis, cocaine, LSD (lysergic acid diethylamide), MDMA (ecstasy), nicotine (tobacco), opiates (e.g., heroin), and volatile solvents and inhalants (e.g., gasoline, glue). This discussion addresses the common patterns of use observed among American and Canadian youth; however, there are regional differences and annual fluctuations in patterns of use (DeWitt, 1991). In addition, the use of various abusable psychotropics by certain groups of children and adolescents (e.g., incarcerated, inner city, reservation Native American, street) is significantly higher than what is reported for the general population (Howard et al., 1999).

For example, a Toronto study reported that more than 90% of street youth use both alcohol and illicit drugs (Smart et al., 1990).

Reports have suggested, sometimes for seemingly political reasons, that abusable psychotropic use by particular groups of youth or in particular geographic regions in North America has decreased (Hauschildt, 1992). However, reports of serious abusable psychotropic use patterns, including abuse and compulsive use (use associated with a high frequency and severity of harm to self and others) and adolescent admissions to alcohol and drug treatment centers are currently at an all-time high (Mathias, 2001; Pagliaro & Pagliaro, 1996).

CNS Depressants

The most commonly used abusable psychotropic among children and adolescents is alcohol. However, other CNS depressants also are used, including volatile solvents and inhalants. Of increasing concern is the more recent trend among adolescents of opiate (heroin) use.

Alcohol. The use of alcohol is a common part of adult socializing and is often viewed by American and Canadian youth as a sign of maturity. Boys and girls who develop patterns of alcohol use generally begin drinking alcoholic beverages in the form of beer, wine, or distilled spirits during their early- or mid-teen years.[6] By their senior year of high school, more than 75% of adolescents report having used alcohol (Pagliaro & Pagliaro, 1996). The major factors contributing to the inappropriate use of alcohol by youth are thought to include: (1) a desire to be more "adultlike" (alcohol is legal only for adults to use); (2) peer pressure; (3) risk-taking behavior; (4) desire for sexual activity (alcohol decreases social inhibitions as a direct psychopharmacologic effect); (5) availability; and (6) societal attitudes that encourage its use (advertisements) (Pagliaro, 1993). Alcohol is the abusable psychotropic used most widely by black adolescents 13–19 years old, followed by tobacco and marijuana (Wallace et al., 1999). The use of alcohol by children and adolescents is often underestimated by pediatric clinicians (Morrison et al., 1995). For example, Gentilello et al. (1999), in a study of hospitalized trauma patients, found that 23% of acutely intoxicated patients were not identified by physicians, thus necessitating the recommendation that formal alcohol screening be done routinely.

The inappropriate use of alcohol by children and adolescents is responsible for more physiologic, psychologic, and sociologic harm than all other abusable psychotropics combined. In addition to the adverse effects noted earlier (e.g., fetal alcohol syndrome and fatal motor vehicle crashes), inappropriate use of alcohol has been associated with up to 70% of criminal assaults, armed robberies, drownings, and murders and up to 50% of child abuse cases, rapes, and suicides (Pagliaro & Pagliaro, 1996). The net effects of the inappropriate use of alcohol are staggering in terms of emotional and economic costs (e.g., lost productivity and direct healthcare costs). In the New Mexico county with the second highest rate of alcohol-related problems in the United States, "at least one person was killed every day in an alcohol-related traffic accident" and no one "was untouched by drunk driving deaths" (United States General Accounting Office . . . , 1992).

Abusable psychotropic use has been related to unintentional injury, which is the leading cause of death for infants, children, and adolescents. A third of these injuries are associated with alcohol use (Hingson et al., 2000). The majority of fatal motor vehicle crashes involving adolescents are the result of alcohol and cannabis intoxication (Pagliaro & Pagliaro, 1996, 2002; Smith et al., 1999). More than 60% of patients injured in alcohol-related motor vehicle crashes attributed their injury partly or totally to the use of alcohol (Sommers et al., 2000). A 0.2% increase in the alcohol blood concentration more than doubled the relative risk of fatal single-vehicle crash injury in 16–20-year-old male drivers (Zador et al., 2000). The drunk driver is not always the fatal victim and chil-

---

6. The reported mean age for alcohol intoxication (being drunk) for a sample of incarcerated children was 12 years of age (Young et al., 1999).

dren who are passengers often bear the consequences of their parents' drunken behavior. The majority of drinking driver-related child passenger deaths in the United States involves a child riding unrestrained in the same vehicle with a drinking driver (Quinlan et al., 2000).

The use of alcohol also has been implicated in a growing number of bicycling accidents involving children and adolescents 10 years of age and older (Li et al., 1996) and fatal snowmobile accidents and crashes (Landen et al., 1999). Chronic abusable psychotropic users visit emergency departments about 30% more often compared with nonusers (McGeary & French, 2000). Accidental deaths also can occur in conjunction with the use of other abusable psychotropics, including opiates (Unintentional. . . , 2000), volatile solvents and inhalants (Bowen et al., 1999; Shepherd & Klein-Schwartz, 1998), and overdosages involving polyabusable psychotropic use (Gill & Stajic, 2000).

Alcoholism is rooted in the classic disease theory and may be defined as sporadic or continuous inappropriate use of alcohol that harms or interferes with a person's physical or mental health, work, family, and/or social life. Alcoholism can be characterized as: (1) progressive (the condition slowly becomes more serious over time); (2) chronic (whether alcohol use is sporadic or continuous, the pattern of inappropriate use occurs over long periods and, in some cases, over a lifetime); and (3) insidious (even though most friends, relatives, and teachers are aware of a drinking problem, alcoholics themselves are usually unable to recognize that they are alcoholics without external assistance). The classic signs and symptoms of alcoholism include: (1) starting the day with a drink; (2) drinking alone; (3) gulping down drinks (as is commonly done with "shooters"); (4) increased tolerance to alcohol; (5) blackouts; and (6) personality changes. These signs and symptoms are observed among adolescents in increasing numbers (Pagliaro & Pagliaro, 1996). Although problems with alcohol use generally become clearly recognizable by 20 years of age (Swartz, 1991), problems are being

TABLE 7-2
Common Adverse Effects Generally Associated with Acute Alcohol Intoxication among Children and Adolescents

- Accidents, general (e.g., drowning)
- Abusive and aggressive behavior, physical and psychological
- Cognitive dysfunction
- Criminal behavior
- Delinquency
- Depression
- Learning impairment
- Memory dysfunction
- Motorized land and water vehicle crashes (e.g., automobile, motorcycle, power boat, truck, SeaDoo®, and snowmobile crashes)
- Psychomotor impairment
- Psychosis
- Self-neglect
- Social problems (e.g., arguments with family members, truancy)
- Suicide
- Violent behavior, including assault, homicide, and rape
- Violent injuries and death

documented more frequently for preadolescents (Pagliaro & Pagliaro, 1996).

There are two major types of young alcoholics: (1) "bender" or "binge" drinkers who heavily drink for short periods, such as on weekends ("TGIF") or after a major school sporting event (e.g., a basketball, football, or hockey game), and (2) daily or chronic drinkers who heavily drink every day or whenever alcohol is available. Problems can be associated with both drinking patterns. Arrests for impaired driving; aggressive or violent behavior (e.g., date rape), often involving peers or family members (Macdonald et al., 1999; Pelletier & Coutu, 1992); expulsion from school; and job firings occur. Acute alcohol intoxication may also result in cognitive, learning, and memory impairment (Pagliaro & Pagliaro, 1996; Tate et al., 1999). The major adverse effects related to acute alcohol intoxication among children and adolescents are listed in Table 7-2.

Opiates. The opiates comprise a group of natural (e.g., morphine) and synthetic (e.g., heroin [diacetylmorphine]) derivatives of opium (the resin obtained from the unripe seed pod of the plant *Papaver somniferum—*

"poppy that causes sleep"). When "hardcore" intravenous drug users are asked to name the first drug that they injected and their age at the time they first injected, they generally report that they first injected heroin (or cocaine) when they were about 16 or 17 years of age (Pagliaro et al., 1993). During the 1970s, 1980s, and the first half of the 1990s, the reported use of heroin within the previous year by high school seniors remained fairly stable (0.5%; U.S. Department of Justice, 1994). However, this figure rose significantly[7] during the latter half of the 1990s as more adolescents began to "chase the dragon." Chasing the dragon refers to heating high-purity heroin (alone or in combination with crack cocaine) and inhaling the trail of smoke through a tube. The increased percent purity of the heroin that has become generally available and its low cost have contributed to this rise in heroin use and its noninjectable methods of use. In the Southwestern United States, the increased purity, increased availability, and decreased cost of heroin have contributed to making intranasal insufflation the major initial route for heroin use among adolescents. As a result, the use of heroin (and other opiates) has become a more recent and serious trend in adolescent abusable psychotropic use (Schwartz, 1998). The short-term physiological effects of opiates are listed in Table 7-3, and the sequence of events related to acute opiate overdosage are presented in Table 7-4.[8] Acute overdosages are treated with the opiate antagonist naloxone (*Narcan®*) along with appropriate emergency medical support of body systems (Pagliaro & Pagliaro, 1999).

Volatile solvents and inhalants. Many different volatile solvents and inhalants (Table 7-5) can be deliberately inhaled to produce a state of intoxication. As with other abusable psychotropics, physiological and psychological effects of volatile solvents and inhalants vary depending on many factors, such as the solvent or inhalant used, amount inhaled, method of inhalation, user, and circumstances of use. Typically, the user experiences an initial sensation of excitation followed by varying degrees of CNS depression and then recovery. The effects of most volatile solvents and inhalants appear and disappear within minutes of use. Use may be accompanied by headache, dizziness, and nausea.

Although volatile solvent and inhalant use has been noted among adults, it is predominantly a youthful practice, with the majority

TABLE 7-3
Short-Term Physiological Effects of Opiates

CNS Depression[a]
- Constriction of the pupils of the eyes (miosis)
- Decreased GI activity and constipation[a]

Depression of the Cough Reflex[a]
- Dilation of the superficial blood vessels and a warming of the skin ("rush")
- Increased perspiration
- Nausea
- Reduced respiratory rate (hypoventilation)
- Reduced cardiovascular activity

[a] These potential adverse effects are often used therapeutically for the medical management of such conditions as cough, diarrhea, or pain.

TABLE 7-4
Signs and Symptoms of Acute Opiate Overdosage

- Pupils: generally constricted (pinpoint pupils); however, with meperidine use, or in cases of extreme hypoxia, may be dilated
- Blood pressure: decreased (shock)
- Body temperature: subnormal
- Respirations: decreased, or absent with accompanying cyanosis
- Reflexes: diminished or absent
- CNS status: stupor or coma; however, convulsions may occur with anoxia or with meperidine and propoxyphene use
- Miscellaneous: constipation, pulmonary edema

---

7. For example, data reported by the National Institute on Drug Abuse indicated that in 1997 more than 2% of American high school seniors (12th graders) had used heroin (Schwartz, 1998).

8. The incidence of unintentional opiate overdosages, primarily due to the increased availability of high-purity heroin at street levels, during the last decade increased from 100% to 300% in various North American cities, including Seattle and Vancouver (Unintentional..., 2000).

TABLE 7-5
Commonly Abused Volatile Solvents and Inhalants

VOLATILE SOLVENT OR INHALANT	MAJOR CHEMICAL INGREDIENTS
Aerosols	Difluorodichloromethane
	Freon
	Isobutane
	Methylene chloride
	Trichlorofluoromethane
Butane lighter fluid	Butane
Dry cleaning fluid	Trichloroethane
Fire extinguishant	Bromochlorodifluoromethane
	Dibromotetrafluoroethane
	Trifluorobromomethane
Gasoline	Benzene
	Heptane
	Hexane
	Hydrocarbons
	Naphthalene
	Tetraethyl lead
	Toluene
	Xylene
Glue	Acetone
	Benzene
	Ethyl acetate
	Heptane
	Hexane
	Isopropyl acetate
	Methyl ethyl ketone
	Naphtha
	Toluene
	Trichloroethane
	Xylene
Kerosene	Hydrocarbons
Nail polish remover	Acetone
	Amyl acetate
Nitrous oxide	Nitrous oxide
Paint thinner	Ethyl acetate
	Isopropanol
	Methanol
	Methylene chloride
	Toluene
	Trichloroethylene
Propane	Propane
Shoe polish	Chlorinated hydrocarbons
	Toluene
Typewriter correction fluid	Amyl acetate
	Trichloroethane

of users being 12–15 years of age. The mean reported age of initial experimentation among a sample of incarcerated children was 9.7 years of age (Young et al., 1999) and in another study it was 13 years (McGarvey et al., 1999). Thus, there appears to be considerable variability in reported age of initial use. However, the use of volatile solvents and inhalants by children as young as 6 years has been documented (Pagliaro & Pagliaro, 1996).

The prevalence of volatile solvent and inhalant use among children and adolescents varies with the historical period, geographic region, culture, ethnicity, and socioeconomic status. Thus, although approximately 15% of all North American youth report having used volatile solvents and inhalants, use may be reported by up to 50% of youth in low socioeconomic groups. Antecedents to the use of volatile solvents and inhalants appear to be highly correlated with social, educational, and economic deprivation (Meadows & Verghese, 1996). A gender effect also has been reported, with a consistent two- to threefold higher incidence of volatile solvent and inhalant use by boys than girls. Adolescents who use volatile solvents and inhalants tend to have higher measures of delinquent behavior (e.g., minor criminal activity, such as breaking windows or stealing) (Mackesy-Amiti & Fendrich, 1999).

Volatile solvents and inhalants are popular among children and adolescents because of their low cost, peer influences, universal availability, rapid effects, and small concealable packaging (e.g., tube of glue). In addition, they generally can be directly purchased by children because they are legal (Espeland, 1995; Pagliaro & Pagliaro, 1996).

More recently, McGarvey et al. (1999) surveyed 285 boys and girls in Virginia juvenile correctional facilities. When compared with other minority and nonminority adolescents in their study, these researchers found that black adolescent boys and girls are significantly less likely to use inhalants. Among boys and girls who used inhalants, use generally begins around 13 years of age and usually occurs at a friend's home, at the user's home, or on the street. "Huffing" is the preferred method of use. Gasoline is most often used, followed in descending order by Freon®, butane lighter fluid, glue, and nitrous oxide. No gender effects were found in regard to age of onset, preferred method of inhalant use, lifetime frequency of inhalant use, frequency of inhalant use in the past year, or preferred inhalant.

For the most part, volatile solvent and inhalant use results in no permanent brain or other body organ damage. However, acute toxicity (e.g., cardiac dysrhythmias associated with fluorinated hydrocarbon propellants) can be fatal (Bowen et al., 1999). In addition, chronic abuse of toluene-containing products and of chlorinated solvents can produce severe body organ damage, particularly affecting the brain, liver, and kidneys (Flanagan & Ives, 1994). Asphyxiation is associated with loss of consciousness while sniffing glue from a plastic bag held over the nose and mouth (Espeland, 1997). In addition, several other adverse effects have been associated with volatile solvent and inhalant abuse (Table 7-6).

The most commonly abused volatile solvents and inhalants are gasoline and glue. However, other solvents and inhalants commonly found in the home also may be used (Table 7-7).

TABLE 7-7
Common Household Products Abused by Children and Adolescents

Bathroom
- Air fresheners
- Hair spray
- Nail polish remover
- Spray deodorants

Garage
- Automobile polish
- Glues and adhesives
- Paint thinner
- Refrigerants (Freon)
- Rust removers
- Spray paint and other pressurized aerosolized sprays

Home Office
- Correction fluid
- Felt-tip markers

Kitchen
- Cooking spray
- Floor wax
- Furniture polish
- Oven cleaners

Laundry Room
- Fabric protectors

TABLE 7-6
Common Adverse Effects Generally Associated with Volatile Solvent and Inhalant Use

- Accidents
- Dizziness
- Headache
- Injury (e.g., burns associated with the inadvertent ignition of gasoline or other flammable volatile solvents and inhalants)
- Loss of balance
- Mood changes
- Slurred and slowed speech
- Sudden sniffing death (fatal cardiac arrest may occur as a result of increased sensitivity to adrenaline and sudden fear, excitement, or surprise [e.g., being found huffing by a teacher or parent]; a sudden adrenaline response combined with inhalant use may make the heart stop pumping suddenly, a situation responsible for one-half of all the deaths associated with inhalant use, particularly the use of fluorocarbon propellants)

Gasoline. Gasoline, a virtually universally available volatile solvent, is composed of a mixture of aliphatic and aromatic hydrocarbons. It also generally contains several additives, including benzene and, in the past, lead, as a result of the petrochemical refining process or to improve engine performance. Children and adolescents usually inhale gasoline fumes directly from a gasoline container (e.g., gasoline can) or from a plastic bag filled with gasoline. Fumes also can be inhaled from a gasoline-soaked rag held over the nose and mouth, and this method has been used by some parents to quiet crying infants (Pagliaro & Pagliaro, 2000).

The inhalation of gasoline fumes causes CNS depression similar to that associated with alcohol ingestion (e.g., dizziness). Inhalation can result in high levels of exposure to gasoline fumes, and consequently in coma and death (Andrews & Snyder, 1991). Additives commonly found in gasoline, particularly lead (where leaded gasolines are still available), are a major source of toxicity for youth who chronically inhale gasoline fumes.

Glue. Glue is the volatile solvent most widely used by children and adolescents. It is composed of several volatile organic constituents (Table 7-7). Glue is generally self-administered by holding the glue container adjacent to the nostrils and inhaling or by placing some glue in a small plastic bag (e.g., plastic sandwich bag), placing the opening of the bag tightly over the nose and mouth, and inhaling. The glue container or plastic bag is often heated (e.g., by holding it in the hands or close to a radiator) to increase the volatility of the glue. When so used, glue produces euphoriant effects and toxicities that generally resemble those associated with the inhalation of gasoline fumes. Glue sniffing has been linked to sudden sniffing death and to chronic damage to the heart, kidneys, liver, lungs, and peripheral nerves (Meadows & Verghese, 1996).

CNS Stimulants

The CNS stimulants most commonly used by children and adolescents are caffeine and nicotine in the form of generally available caffeinated beverages and tobacco products, respectively. Children and adolescents may also use amphetamine, dextroamphetamine, methamphetamine, and other closely related CNS stimulants (e.g., methylphenidate *[Ritalin®]*). These abusable psychotropics may have been prescribed for the symptomatic management of eating disorders and attention-deficit hyperactivity disorder (A-D/HD), or they may have been secured by other means for illicit use. Children and adolescents also may use cocaine in its various forms. These CNS stimulants—amphetamines, cocaine, and nicotine—are discussed in the following sections.

Amphetamines and other related CNS stimulants. The amphetamines, including amphetamine (crank, speed), dextroamphetamine (bennies, truck-drivers), and methamphetamine (crystal, meth, ice) are generally used by adolescents illicitly, particularly for their CNS stimulant effects (e.g., promoting the ability to stay awake). However, they also may be prescribed for the clinical management of selected mental disorders. Approximately 10% of children and adolescents have used amphetamines within the previous year.

Amphetamine. Although methylphenidate has been the drug of choice for the symptomatic management of A-D/HD for several decades, children are increasingly being prescribed amphetamine (e.g., mixed amphetamines *[Adderall®]*)[9] for the symptomatic management of this mental disorder.[10] The general availability of both methylphenidate and the amphetamines among school-age children and adolescents has resulted in a related trend: the illicit use of these drugs by children and adolescents not diagnosed with A-D/HD. These children and adolescents seek, obtain (often from children diagnosed with A-D/HD), and use these abusable psychotropics illicitly for their stimulant effects. In one study, Musser et al. (1998) noted that 16% of children had been

---

9. The mixed amphetamines contain amphetamine aspartate, amphetamine sulfate, dextroamphetamine saccharate, and dextroamphetamine sulfate.

10. As we have noted for some years now (Pagliaro & Pagliaro, 1996), A-D/HD remains one of the most frequently misdiagnosed mental disorders among children and adolescents. In order to increase the validity of diagnosis, we strongly encourage pediatric clinicians to observe the child's or adolescent's reported troublesome behavior in the actual classroom setting and not rely solely on parent or teacher reports of behaviors reflective of DSM-IV-TR criteria or other stipulated criteria. Expert clinical assessment and diagnosis are essential in this regard. In addition, when CNS stimulants are required, we strongly recommend that the selected drug be prescribed at only 80% efficacy in terms of behavioral effects (we do not attempt to totally control all of the problematic behavior pharmacologically, but rather use the drug to render these behaviors manageable by other means [e.g., cognitive behavioral therapy; family therapy]). The use of this reduced dosage, whenever possible, enables us to minimize the associated reduction in the child's or adolescent's functional capacity for learning and memory that is associated with the use of higher CNS stimulant dosages.

asked to sell, give, or trade their methylphenidate to others. Pediatric clinicians must educate parents, and their children and adolescents, about the appropriate use and potential abuse of methylphenidate and other CNS stimulants prescribed for the symptomatic management of A-D/HD. Monitoring the use of these drugs by children and adolescents who require them for the management of this mental disorder, and continuing to educate parents, teachers, and other children and adolescents, who may be interested in trying these drugs, should be essential components of a multimodal treatment plan for the management of this mental disorder.

While concern has been raised about the addiction potential of long-term amphetamine pharmacotherapy, children and adolescents who are appropriately receiving amphetamines or methylphenidate for the symptomatic management of A-D/HD do not appear to become addicted to them. Most published findings (e.g., Biederman et al., 1999) support the hypothesis that these patients do not become addicted, reportedly because of the slow rate of absorption associated with the oral ingestion of the drug (peak blood concentrations are achieved in the brain 60 minutes after oral ingestion, compared with 5 minutes after the injection of cocaine or 9 minutes after the injection of methylphenidate). These findings also seem to explain why non-A-D/HD youth become addicted to CNS stimulants when injected intravenously or when the tablet formulations are crushed and the powder insufflated (insufflation also is associated with the rapid achievement of peak blood concentrations in the brain).[11]

However, some concerns regarding the development of problematic patterns of abusable psychotropic use later during adulthood have been raised. As noted (Levin & Kleber, 1995), hyperactive adults with histories of A-D/HD are more likely than controls to have substance-use disorders. Recent studies suggest that adults who have substance-use disorders, particularly cocaine-use disorders, may be more likely than the general population to have a childhood history of A-D/HD. Schubiner et al. (2000) also found that women with A-D/HD had a higher number of treatments for alcohol abuse than did women who were not diagnosed with A-D/HD.

Dextroamphetamine. Dextroamphetamine (*Dexedrine®*) may be prescribed for the symptomatic management of eating disorders (obesity) among adolescent girls. Aggressive conduct was reported among adolescent girls receiving dextroamphetamine for eating disorders (Thompson et al., 1999); the constellation of eating disorders and aggressive behavior was associated, in turn, with a greater risk for other abusable psychotropic use and attempted suicide. The adverse effects associated with the use of dextroamphetamine and the other amphetamines are listed in Table 7-8.

Methamphetamine. Methamphetamine use is epidemic in North America. It is readily available to youth (and adults) who seek it for its long-acting CNS stimulant effects, which may last up to 12 hours (Bonné, 2001). As with other amphetamines, its use is associated with psychosis (Buffenstein et al., 1999), severe depression, and other noted adverse effects (Table 7-8). Of particular concern is the possibility of long-term neurotoxicities, which may be irreversible because of neuron damage or loss (Ernst et al., 2000; Zickler, 2000, 2001a). Traditionally, methamphetamine was known on the street as "speed" and was injected intravenously. This method of use became associated with sharing contaminated needles and syringes (Molitor et al., 1999) and, thus, an increased risk for infection with the HIV and other blood-borne pathogens.

In the early 1990s, a new form of methamphetamine became widely available. The "West Coast" form was produced as a "rock" similar to the rock form of cocaine (crack cocaine) and also could be smoked. Now known as crystal or ice, it produces pharma-

---

11. Also of interest are the findings of Disney et al. (1999), who studied 626 pairs of 17-year-old twin adolescent girls and boys. A diagnosis of conduct disorder (CD) increased the risk for illicit abusable psychotropic use regardless of gender, whereas a diagnosis of A-D/HD did not.

TABLE 7-8
Common Adverse Effects Generally Associated with Amphetamine Use

- Anorexia
- Blurred vision
- Bruxism
- Cardiomyopathy
- Chilliness
- Dizziness
- Emotional lability
- Hallucinations
- Headaches
- Hypertension
- Insomnia
- Irritability
- Nausea
- Nervousness
- Paranoid ideation
- Physical dependence (addiction)
- Psychological dependence (habituation)
- Psychosis
- Rhabdomyolysis
- Seizures
- Tachycardia
- Talkativeness
- Vomiting

cologic effects similar to crack cocaine except that the effects last for up to 12 hours instead of for just 30 minutes. Thus, adolescents who wanted an instant and lasting CNS stimulant effect and disliked needles or injecting themselves now had a ready means to achieve these desired effects.[12]

Cocaine. Cocaine has been used by approximately 20% of North American children and adolescents. However, this percentage is expected to increase significantly during this decade, primarily because of the ready availability of crack cocaine and its low cost (Pagliaro & Pagliaro, 1996).[13] Other data indicate that the use of cocaine by children and adolescents is significantly related to the incidence of attempted suicides and completed suicides in these age groups (Marzuk et al., 1992). In an effort to "innoculate" children against cocaine and other abusable psychotropic use, early intervention programs are increasingly targeting children younger than 5 years in order to deter later abusable psychotropic use. Unfortunately, these prevention efforts have been characterized by a lack of appropriate experimental research design (Hall & Zigler, 1997), and demonstrated efficacy is often lacking.

Cocaine use during pregnancy is often underestimated (Offidani et al., 1995) and has increased dramatically during the past decade (Rizk et al., 1996). Although confounding variables (e.g., inadequate prenatal care, the concurrent use of several abusable psychotropics during pregnancy) make it difficult to determine the direct effects of perinatal cocaine use on maternal and fetal outcome, the use of cocaine during pregnancy has been associated with maternal hypertension, placental abruptions, spontaneous abortion, and poor weight gain associated with malnutrition secondary to cocaine-induced appetite suppression. The effects on the offspring of maternal cocaine use during pregnancy may include in utero growth retardation, cephalic hemorrhage, fetal edema, altered body composition, congenital malformations (e.g., cardiac malformations), preterm delivery, low birth weight, minor anomalies of the nervous system, and pre- and postnatal death (Rizk et al., 1996). The offspring of adolescent girls who use cocaine during pregnancy also can exhibit a variety of behavioral, visual, hearing, and language disorders during infancy and childhood (Church et al., 1998; Gerber et al., 1995). (*See also* Chapter 2.)

Across different developmental ages and tasks, behavioral and neurophysiological findings suggest that children prenatally exposed to cocaine are more likely to exhibit disrupted arousal regulation; this effect has important implications (Mayes et al., 1998). Impaired arousal orientation may adversely affect ongoing information processing, learning, and memory because arousal regulation serves as a gating mechanism to optimize ori-

---

12. Subsequently, as both availability and use of the rock form increased, adolescents also began to crush the "rocks" and use nasal insufflation ("snorting") as a preferred method of methamphetamine administration.

13. This forecasted increase in cocaine use may be assuaged, at least partially, by an increase in methamphetamine use (*see* Methamphetamine).

entation and attention. In addition, impaired arousal regulation predisposes children to a lower threshold for the activation of stress circuits. This lower threshold may increase their vulnerability to the developmentally detrimental effects of stressful conditions, particularly if these children are exposed to the environmental conditions often found in families who display problematic patterns of abusable psychotropic use.

The adverse effects of cocaine use are listed in Table 7-9. The intravenous injection of cocaine and the sharing of needles (with the associated risk of transmission of HIV and subsequent development of AIDS) has been a major concern over the past decade (Pagliaro et al., 1993). The transmission of HIV continues to increase among intravenous drug users in North America and poses one of the greatest risks of transmission of the virus among heterosexuals, women, and children. In addition, the relationship between cocaine (and other abusable psychotropic) use and an increase in sexual experimentation has important public health implications with respect to the current AIDS pandemic and the spread of other sexually transmitted diseases (e.g., genital ulcers, syphilis) (Pagliaro et al., 1993; Pagliaro & Pagliaro, 2000).

Sexual favors are frequently exchanged for cocaine (Rolfs et al., 1990; Schwarcz et al., 1992). Prostitution usually involves girls, but also may involve boys, and is used as a means to support the cost of cocaine use (L. A. Pagliaro et al., 1992). The phenomenon of "popcorn pimping," in which older adolescents (often girls) pimp for younger adolescents and children to support their own cocaine use, also is becoming increasingly common (author clinical research files).

Nicotine. Nicotine, an autonomic ganglionic stimulant, is one of more than 4000 chemicals inhaled with tobacco smoke. It is primarily absorbed through the pulmonary system (lungs), but also is absorbed buccally in association with the use of chewing tobacco, cigars, and pipe tobacco (cigar and pipe tobacco generally are air cured and, thus, have an alkaline pH that is conducive to buccal absorption).[14]

Nicotine is regularly used in the form of tobacco cigarettes by approximately 4 million North American children and adolescents (Smith & Fiore, 1999). Current tobacco use ranges from 15.1% among middle school students to 34.5% among high school students. Tobacco cigarette smoking is the most prevalent form of tobacco use, followed by cigar smoking and smokeless tobacco use.

Tobacco use among children and adolescents has been increasing throughout each of the past three decades (An et al., 1999; Cigarette smoking. . . , 1999; Kumra & Markoff, 2000). For example, the *Morbidity and Mortality Weekly Report* (Tobacco use among. . . , 1998) reported that cigarette smoking among U.S. high school students increased from 27.5% in 1991 to 36.4% in 1997.[15]

TABLE 7-9
Common Adverse Effects Generally Associated with Cocaine Use, According to Method of Use

General (independent of method of use)
- Cardiac dysrhythmias
- Compulsive use
- Convulsions
- Hyperpyrexia
- Pseudohallucinations (e.g., cocaine bugs, snow lights)
- Psychosis, including hypervigilance and paranoia

Cocaine HCl Intravenous Injection
- Abscess formation
- Embolism
- Infection (e.g., hepatitis, HIV, septicemia)
- Phlebitis

Cocaine HCl Nasal Insufflation
- Erosion of nasal septum
- Nasal congestion

---

14. Nicotine is widely used therapeutically as part of smoking reduction/cessation programs. In this context, it is absorbed buccally with the use of nicotine chewing gum (e.g., *Nicorette®*), nasally from nasal spray formulations (e.g., *Nicotrol NS®*), and transdermally from specialized transdermal nicotine delivery systems (e.g., *Habitrol®, Nicoderm®*) (Pagliaro & Pagliaro, 1999).

15. The prevalence of tobacco smoking nationwide among high school students increased during the 1990s, peaked during 1996–1997, and then began a gradual decline (Youth Tobacco Surveillance, 2001).

Despite age restrictions in regard to the purchase of tobacco products, most children and adolescents do not consider it difficult to purchase these products (Hersch, 1998). Approximately 69% of middle school and 58% of high school students who currently smoke tobacco cigarettes were not asked to show proof of age when they bought or tried to buy cigarettes (Youth Tobacco Surveillance, 2001). Each day more than 3000 American children begin to use tobacco, generally in response to peer pressure and social role models (Cigarette smoking. . . , 1999; Hunter et al., 1991; Iannotti & Bush, 1992; Lamkin & Houston, 1998). In fact, 60% of current cigarette smokers began smoking tobacco before they were 14 years of age;[16] and this percentage increases to 80% by 18 years of age (Youth Tobacco Surveillance. . . , 2001).

The prevalence of regular cigarette smoking among 12th grade girls is about 28%, with the highest rates reported for girls of European descent and the lowest for girls of African and Asian descent.[17] Adolescent girls who do not have plans to go to college are more likely to smoke tobacco cigarettes than those who have college plans (French & Perry, 1996). These adolescent girls usually initiate tobacco smoking to attain a desired self-image that includes feelings of maturity, independence, sexuality, and sociability. They also may smoke tobacco cigarettes because of tobacco advertisements (Hawkins & Hane, 2000; Redmond, 1999) designed to extol the weight-controlling benefits of smoking and exploit the concerns of European American, middle-class adolescents (and women) about attaining and maintaining their desired body weight, which is below the usual parameters for age and height (Seguire & Chalmers, 2000; Tomeo et al., 1999). Parents, peers, and friends also may influence the norms that support (or discourage) tobacco smoking.

Among male and female high school seniors, heavy cigarette use (smoking one or more packages of cigarettes daily) has been associated with starting to smoke at an earlier age, having many peers who smoke cigarettes, having a mother who smokes cigarettes, and poor academic performance (Griffin et al., 1999). The heaviest tobacco use has been generally reported among youth and young adults of European descent, particularly those from a lower socioeconomic status. One study (Winkleby et al., 1999) found that 77% of young men and 61% of young women (18–24 years) from low socioeconomic status were smokers.

Tobacco smoking is the largest single preventable cause of illness and death in North America and is, in fact, responsible for ap-

---

16. A study of incarcerated children by Young et al. (1999) found a mean age of 11.2 years for initial experimentation with tobacco cigarettes. A study of U.S. high school students who smoked found that more than 11% of these students began to smoke at 10 years of age or younger; the younger the age of onset, the more cigarettes smoked per day (Everett et al., 1999).

17. It should be noted, however, that common tobacco cigarettes are not the only types of tobacco cigarettes used by children and adolescents, particularly children and adolescents from ethnic minorities. According to a report in the *Morbidity and Mortality Weekly Report* (Bidi use among. . . , 1999), several variations in tobacco smoking are being observed among many ethnic minority adolescents. For example, the use of "bidis," first observed in Canada during the mid-1980s (Pagliaro & Pagliaro, patient files) and, subsequently, in the United States during the mid-1990s, seems to have become widespread among North American ethnic minority adolescents. Bidis are small, brown, hand-rolled cigarettes that are primarily made in India and other Southeast Asian countries. They consist of tobacco wrapped in a tendu or temburni leaf and are available in cherry, chocolate, mango, and other flavors. One package of twenty bidis generally can be purchased for $1.50 to $4.00.

Another trend has been the use of **kreteks**, tobacco cigarettes that contain a commonly used spice, clove. These cigarettes (60% tobacco and 40% shredded clove buds) are generally imported into North America from Indonesia. Kretek use became a fad in North America in the early 1980s and their use has been associated with severe pulmonary toxicity among adolescents and young adults. The toxicity has been associated with eugenol, a natural compound found in high concentrations in clove buds (Guidotti, 1989). Currently, kreteks are the sixth most prevalent form of tobacco used by North American youth, and they are used more often by boys than girls (Youth Tobacco Surveillance, 2001).

proximately 15% of all deaths in North America (Smith & Fiore, 1999). A large number of deaths from coronary heart disease (25%) and cancer (30% of all cancer deaths and 87% of lung cancer deaths) are attributed to tobacco smoking (Collishaw & Leahy, 1991; Selected tobacco-use . . . , 1992; Smoking-attributable mortality . . . , 1991).

Children and adolescents smoke 1.1 billion packages of cigarettes annually and will account for more than $200 billion in future healthcare costs (Woolf, 1997). Although coronary heart disease and lung cancer may not be noted until middle or late adulthood, a range of adverse effects (e.g., atherosclerosis) may be detected among adolescent tobacco smokers, which extend into adulthood. Exposure to secondhand smoke, or environmental tobacco smoke, is substantially higher among both middle school and high school students (Youth Tobacco Surveillance, 2001). Children and adolescents who are exposed to passive smoke are at risk for the adverse effects of smoking, including alterations in lipid profiles, atherosclerosis, and lung cancer (Feldman et al., 1991; Lesmes & Donofrio, 1992). Through the effects of environmental (sidestream or secondhand) smoke or smoking during pregnancy,[18] adolescent smokers also affect the health of their friends, family members, unborn babies, infants, and children (Woolf, 1997).

Infants of mothers who smoke may receive greater exposure to the products of tobacco smoke through breast milk than through environmental exposure (Mascola et al., 1998). Urine levels of continine, a substance produced by the metabolism of nicotine, were 10 times higher among breast-fed infants of smoking mothers than among bottle-fed infants of smoking mothers. In addition, significantly higher continine levels were found among infants of nonsmoking mothers exposed to secondhand smoke by another household member.

Bronchitis, impaired respiratory function, nasal irritation, respiratory infections, sinus disease, and sudden infant death syndrome (SIDS) occur significantly more often among children whose parents smoke in comparison with children whose parents never smoked (Benninger, 1999; Pagliaro & Pagliaro, 2000; Stone, 1992; Ugnat et al., 1990; Weitzman et al., 1990). The majority of the adverse effects associated with tobacco smoking (e.g., respiratory tract irritation, lung cancer) are related to the constituents in tobacco smoke other than the principal psychotropic, nicotine (Altarac et al., 2000; Marcus et al., 2000; Washington, 1999; Winkleby et al., 1999) (Table 7-10). The adverse effects specifically associated with nicotine are listed in Table 7-11. The use of chewing tobacco also is associated with adverse effects, including oral cancers and dental root surface caries (Tomar & Winn, 1999).

Psychedelics

The psychedelic most commonly used by children and adolescents is cannabis, fol-

TABLE 7-10
Common Adverse Effects Generally Associated with Tobacco Smoking

- Accidental injury
- Atherosclerosis
- Breast cancer
- Chronic obstructive pulmonary disease
- Coronary heart disease
- Increased incidence of respiratory infections
- Lung cancer

TABLE 7-11
Common Adverse Effects Generally Associated with Nicotine Use

- Addiction (physical dependence)
- Blood pressure increase
- Heart rate increase
- Nausea
- Coronary heart disease
- Tremor
- Vomiting

---

18. The adverse neonatal effects of maternal smoking during pregnancy are primarily confined to the third trimester of pregnancy and include low birth weight and preterm delivery (Cigarette smoking. . . , 1999; Moore & Zaccaro, 2000). (*See* Chapter 2.)

lowed by LSD. However, increasing numbers of older adolescents are becoming attracted to the club scene and the use of MDMA. Raving with MDMA also is becoming increasingly common. These psychedelics and their use by children and adolescents are discussed in this section.

Cannabis. Cannabis in its plant form (marijuana), resin form (hashish), or extracted oil form (hashish oil) has been used by approximately 25% of North Americans (Pagliaro, 1993). In fact, marijuana is the illicit drug that is most frequently used by adolescents (Heyman et al., 1999), and more than half of high school seniors report that they have used marijuana at least once (American Academy, 1991; Pagliaro & Pagliaro, 1996). The use of cannabis by children and adolescents is significantly higher than is its use by adults. Although use statistics vary significantly by state, province, and city, it is estimated that approximately 40% of American and Canadian teenagers used marijuana within the previous year and 20% used it within the previous month (Pagliaro & Pagliaro, 1996).

Significant factors associated with an increased probability of cannabis use by adolescents include being a white male, associating with peers who use cannabis, and having access to this psychedelic (Yarnold & Patterson, 1998). Significant variables inhibiting cannabis use are religion, a father in residence, and high academic success (obtaining A's and B's on their report cards).

Another study (Brook et al., 1998) examined factors linked to cannabis use, such as personality, family traits, peer factors, and cultural/economic factors. Some gender effects were reported, and a family interactional model was supported. The domains of family, personality, and peers reportedly had a direct effect on adolescent cannabis use.

Early adolescent marijuana use, at least for North American adolescents of African or Puerto Rican descent, increased the risk during late adolescence for not graduating from high school; being delinquent; having multiple sexual partners; not always using condoms; perceiving drugs as not harmful; having problems with alcohol, cigarettes, and marijuana; and having more friends who exhibit deviant behavior (Brook et al., 1999).

These findings led the researchers to conclude that marijuana use during early adolescence is related to problems during later adolescence that may limit the acquisition of the skills necessary for employment and heighten the risks for contracting HIV infection and abusing legal and illegal abusable psychotropics. They recommend that assessments of marijuana use during early adolescence and its treatment be incorporated into clinical practice.

Ellickson & Morton (1999) examined early risk factors for the initiation of serious patterns of abusable psychotropic ("hard drug") use among adolescents of diverse racial and ethnic backgrounds and found that specific risk factors had a stronger influence for some groups than for others. These differences in major predictors of hard drug use included the following: early marijuana use was the strongest predictor for adolescents of Asian, European, and Hispanic descent, whereas the strongest predictors for adolescents of African descent were social influences to use drugs and intentions to use them. Other factors reflecting racial/ethnic influences were poor parent communication (adolescents of Asian and Hispanic descent [family disruption and limited parental education were associated with an increase in risk for adolescents of European descent, factors that had the opposite effect for adolescents of African or Hispanic descent]), being offered drugs (adolescents of African, Asian, and European descent), and doing poorly in school (Asian descent).

These findings led the researchers to conclude that preventing the early initiation of marijuana (and cigarette) use and reducing social influences and attitudes associated with adolescent abusable psychotropic use may help to decrease the risk for the development of more serious patterns of abusable psychotropic use. They also recommended that prevention programs be sensitive to racial and ethnic differences among adolescents.

Kandel & Chen (2000) followed a sample of marijuana users from adolescence to 35 years of age. Four marijuana-use clusters were identified: early onset–heavy use, early onset–light use, mid-onset–heavy use, and late onset–light use. The groups differed from each other in degree of involvement in marijuana and other abusable psychotropic use and sociodemographic and lifestyle characteristics. The majority of early onset users did not become heavily involved in marijuana use. However, unique factors were associated with membership in each group. Factors differentiating early onset–heavy use from mid-onset–heavy use included association with marijuana-using peers and having had a mental disorder. Peer delinquency was an additional factor differentiating early initiators who became heavy users from those who did not.

Novins & Mitchell (1998) examined the characteristics of marijuana users among a large sample of Native American Indian high school students (n = 1464). Forty percent of the students in their study had used marijuana at least once during the last month. The factors associated with marijuana use varied by gender and with the frequency of use. Low frequency use among girls was associated with peers who encouraged alcohol use and the use of alcohol with cocaine. For boys, low-frequency use was associated with alcohol use, greater positive alcohol expectancies, and lower grades in school. For girls and boys, high frequency marijuana use was associated with alcohol and cocaine (and other stimulant) use. High frequency use among girls also was associated with higher scores on an antisocial behavior scale.

The adverse effects associated with cannabis use are listed in Table 7-12. Contrary to popular beliefs about cannabis, its use does not cause permanent brain injury or damage as portrayed in the cult classic movie *Reefer Madness* (Meade et al., 1937). Nor does its use appear to be directly related to suicide attempts (Beautrais et al., 1999).

However, the use of cannabis has been associated with four well-defined toxicities that are particularly significant for children and adolescents: (1) respiratory disease; (2) impaired ability to operate a motor vehicle or other hazardous machinery; (3) amotivational

---

**TABLE 7-12
Common Adverse Effects Generally Associated with Acute and Chronic Cannabis Use**

Acute
- Paranoia
- Panic reaction
- Psychomotor impairment, often associated with motor vehicle crashes
- Psychosis
- Tachycardia
- Toxic delirium

Chronic
- Amotivational syndrome
- Habituation (psychological dependence)
- Learning disabilities (e.g., disruption of short-term memory)
- Respiratory irritation and lung disease (e.g., asthma, bronchitis)

---

syndrome; and (4) learning impairment. In addition, psychological effects (e.g., panic attacks, paranoia, psychosis, psychological dependence) (Dalmau et al., 1999; Pagliaro & Pagliaro, 1996) may occur among users. The occurrence of these toxicities appears to depend on a genetic and/or psychological predisposition.

Respiratory disease. A number of studies have documented the direct irritant effects (coughing, dry mouth, sore throat) of cannabis smoke on the respiratory tract and its negative effects on pulmonary function, including chronic obstructive pulmonary diseases such as asthma and bronchitis. The severity of the associated respiratory disease appears to be clearly related to the smoking techniques employed by cannabis smokers (inhaling deeply and holding the smoke in the deepest areas of the respiratory tract for several seconds to obtain maximal psychotropic effects). Several researchers have noted a high risk of lung cancer among cannabis users and that, in terms of respiratory toxicity, smoking one marijuana joint is roughly equivalent to smoking 20 tobacco cigarettes.

Impaired ability to operate a motor vehicle or other hazardous machinery. The use of even moderate amounts of cannabis produces an acute state of intoxication and a dose-related impairment in the ability to drive a motor vehicle or to operate other complex and hazardous machinery. This impairment is related primarily to the following effects of tetrahydrocannabinol (the principal active psychotropic ingredient in cannabis): (1) time–space distortion, (2) impaired visual accommodation, (3) decreased muscular coordination, and (4) impaired short-term memory. These effects impair perceptual-motor skills and performance on decision-making tasks and, hence, the ability to operate a motor vehicle or other hazardous equipment. These adverse effects are significantly exacerbated by the concurrent ingestion of alcohol, a commonly observed practice among cannabis users (Pagliaro & Pagliaro, 1996).

Amotivational syndrome. The amotivational syndrome was originally associated with the chronic abuse of the barbiturates during the 1950s. However, since the 1970s the amotivational syndrome has been predominantly associated with chronic cannabis use among preadolescents (10–12 years of age) (Pagliaro & Pagliaro, 1996). Cannabis users with amotivational syndrome typically lack the motivation and drive observed among other youth of the same age and background who do not use cannabis. They generally spend an inordinate amount of time alone stoned, listening to music or watching television, and are often referred to by their peers as being burned or burned out. A major psychological problem faced by these young cannabis users is that they increasingly use cannabis as a means for coping with the various problems that they encounter in their daily lives. This pattern of use does not encourage the development of the normal coping skills necessary to progress psychologically from childhood to adulthood and leaves them ill-prepared to function adequately in the adult world.

Learning impairment. Cannabis use adversely affects learning in several ways. For example, it impairs short-term memory and, hence, the retention of what is presented by teachers in the classroom (Pagliaro, 1992a, 1993). In addition, the amotivational syndrome associated with chronic, high-dose use of cannabis is a significant impediment to learning because children and adolescents who display this pattern of use are frequently absent from school and do not appear to be able to adequately address the tasks associated with learning (e.g., attention, perception, motivation, cognitive processing, memory) when they are in attendance (Pagliaro, 1992a).

Despite growing concerns by pediatric clinicians about the physical and psychological effects of cannabis, survey data show that increasing numbers of children and adolescents are using it as they (and in many cases, their parents or legal guardians) become less concerned about its harmful effects (Heyman et al., 1999; Mathias, 2001). Current efforts to legalize cannabis also appear to have increased the acceptability associated with the use of this abusable psychotropic.

LSD. Ten percent of North American children and adolescents reportedly have used LSD, a psychedelic drug originally popularized during the 1960s and 1970s by the writings of Harvard professors Timothy Leary and Richard Alpert and by the music of the Beatles, Jimi Hendrix, Jefferson Airplane, and others during the height of the acid rock years. The use of LSD waned during the 1980s, but LSD has now been rediscovered by the grandchildren and great grandchildren of the Hippie generation who use it on Bart Simpson window panes, often as they gather worldwide in groups of thousands to rave. Another psychedelic drug, MDMA (3,4-methylenedioxymethamphetamine or ecstasy), also is used in this social context (author files; Randall, 1992a, 1992b).

Various types of toxicity have been linked to LSD use, but virtually all of the major physical toxicities postulated since its formulation and "discovery" by Albert Hoffman in the 1940s have been refuted. It is now recognized that LSD is not a human teratogen (*see* Chapter 2).

Although it is not addictive, the use of LSD can result in bad trips (panic reactions) and other psychological sequelae, including psychosis (Table 7-13), particularly among children and adolescents who are predisposed to, or have a history of, mental illness (Hurlbut, 1991).

TABLE 7-13
Common Adverse Effects Generally Associated with LSD Use

- Bad trips (panic reactions)
- Flashbacks
- Psychosis

MDMA. MDMA (3,4-methylenedioxymethamphetamine) is another psychedelic drug used in the social context of clubbing and raves (author clinical files; Randall, 1992a, 1992b). Also known as Adam, clarity, E, ecstasy, essence, XTC, it has a chemical structure similar to methamphetamine and mescaline with similar but milder CNS stimulant and psychedelic effects. Inadvertently produced during the early 1900s by German scientists who were developing a vasoconstrictor, hydrastinine, MDMA did not gain much attention until the late 1970s, when it was touted by many psychotherapists as being more effective for their patients than years of intensive psychotherapy because of its reported ability to induce empathy and encourage deep emotional feelings.[19] During this time, MDMA also began to be used within the rave scene in the United Kingdom. (A similar, more potent abusable psychotropic, methylenedioxyamphetamine [MDA] may also be used by ravers.) By 1985, it was designated a schedule I drug by the U.S. Drug Enforcement Agency and, thus, became illegal in North America. However, it had already become popular and inculcated on university and college campuses and in dance clubs. MDMA continues to be so used and is now competing with cocaine as the second most popular illicit abusable psychotropic after marijuana.

MDMA is used by young adults during all-night parties at night clubs and raves (Weir, 2000).[20] Most often used in the tablet form, MDMA is usually ingested orally. It also is available as a powder and may be insufflated or smoked; it is rarely injected. As noted (NIDA Notes, 1999), 3.6% of 12th graders, 3.3% of 10th graders, and 1.8% of 8th graders reported that they had used MDMA during the past year. In a follow-up study of a group of graduates from each surveyed high school class, the number of college students who had used ecstasy during the past year rose from 0.9% in 1991 to 2.4% in 1997. The annual use for young adults increased from 0.8% to 2.1% during the same period. By 1998, the use of MDMA by adolescents and young adults in nightclubs and raves had increased in 21 major U.S. cities.

The main psychotropic action of MDMA is believed to be related to the release of serotonin, which may have effects on the regulation of appetite, mood, sex drive, and sleep. Serotonin also is thought to produce elation, feelings of love, increased sensitivity to environmental stimuli, and feelings of increased energy. These pharmacologic actions have led to its identification in the lay media as the hug drug, love drug, or feel good chemical. Although considered by many people to be nonaddictive and relatively safe, the use of MDMA has been associated with several adverse effects, including many adverse effects that can be fatal (Andreu et al., 1998; Gouzoulis-Mayfrank et al., 2000; Parrott et al., 1998) (Table 7-14).

In addition, several studies have suggested that chronic MDMA use may result in significant depletion of serotonin, damage to related neurotransmitters, and resultant neurotoxicity (Gerra et al., 1998; Parrott et al., 1998, 2000; Williams et al., 1998). The neurotoxic effects may be prolonged even after the use of the MDMA has been discon-

---

19. In November 2001, the FDA approved the clinical testing of MDMA for the symptomatic management of post-traumatic stress disorder (PTSD).

20. Raves may be attended by large numbers of ravers, sometimes in excess of 20,000. They are international in scope and are characterized by clandestine venues, hypnotic electronic music, and the use of several other drugs (e.g., GHB [gamma-hydroxybutyrate], ketamine) in addition to MDMA (Weir, 2000). Ketamine, also known as K or Special K, is a dissociative anesthetic available generally for clinical use in Canada and for veterinary use only in the United States. It produces CNS depressant effects similar to those produced by alcohol and hallucinations (Cloud, 2001).

TABLE 7-14
Common Adverse Effects Generally Associated with MDMA Use

- Anxiety
- Bruxism (grinding of the teeth)
- Blurred vision
- Chills or profuse sweating
- Confusion
- Death, although rare, may occur as a result of associated CNS stimulation that enables users to dance for extended periods in hot, crowded rave conditions, which may result in severe dehydration and hyperthermia (see Heat stroke). Death usually occurs as a result of associated cardiac, hepatic, or renal failure.
- Depression
- Faintness
- Heat stroke, associated with inadequate hydration and not taking rest breaks from dancing; the heat stroke may be fatal as a result of associated hepatic and renal failure.[a]
- Hypertension
- Insomnia
- Memory impairment; may be persistent with heavy use
- Muscle tension
- Nausea
- Neurotoxicity (risk appears to be significant for high-dose and long-term users)
- Psychosis, including paranoia during, and sometimes weeks after, use
- Seizures (risk for seizures is particularly significant for children and adolescents who have a prior history of seizure disorders)
- Tachycardia
- Teeth-clenching, involuntary

[a] Fatalities also have been associated with consuming too much water and failing to urinate, resulting in either cerebral edema from hyponatremia or a ruptured bladder from excessive urine volume.

tinued (Gerra et al., 2000; Tuchtenhagen et al., 2000). However, more data are needed (Leshner, 2000; News Update, 2000a).

Seizures also are being increasingly associated with MDMA use, although these reported associations are inconclusive as to the exact role played by MDMA and that played by environmental and other factors (e.g., neurological status of MDMA users) (Burgess et al., 2000; Man treated for ecstasy seizure, 2001; Zickler, 2000, 2001a). In addition, MDMA use in dance clubs has been associated with high-risk sexual behavior (e.g., unprotected anal intercourse with multiple partners) among older, gay adolescent boys (Klitzman et al., 2000). This high-risk behavior is consistent with the relationship that is generally noted between abusable psychotropic use and high-risk sexual activity (Huba et al., 2000).

Pattern-of-Use Variables

The importance of the abusable psychotropic dimension and its associated variables cannot be denied. However, quantitative as well as qualitative descriptions of abusable psychotropic use behavior are required, since varying degrees of use are observed. The pattern-of-use variables are particularly useful and pragmatic for quantifying and qualifying abusable psychotropic use among children and adolescents.

Over the past several decades, children and adolescents have increasingly experimented with and have widely used abusable psychotropics such as alcohol, nicotine, cannabis, and cocaine. Children and adolescents today are perhaps not unlike previous generations who used these and other abusable psychotropics, such as peace pills (phencyclidine [PCP]) and LSD. However, current use patterns have been associated with increasing harm to the individual user and to other people. This situation is expected to worsen significantly during the current decade as the use of abusable psychotropics by children and adolescents continues to increase despite the well-documented risks and costs to society (Pagliaro & Pagliaro, 1996). They also are using more than one type of abusable psychotropic and these abusable psychotropics may be used concurrently or concomitantly. This section first discusses polyabusable psychotropic use and then describes the specific patterns of abusable psychotropic use observed among children and adolescents.

Polyabusable Psychotropic Use

During the 1980s, the trend of polyabusable psychotropic use among children and adolescents—using several different abusable psychotropics concurrently—became firmly established, and the trend continued during the 1990s (Fiegelman et al., 1990; Pagliaro & Pagliaro, 1996) and into the new millenium.

Polyabusable psychotropic use is characterized by: (1) the concurrent use of more than one abusable psychotropic; and (2) the use of different abusable psychotropics at different times predicated primarily upon availability and cost. Polyabusable psychotropic use by children and adolescents appears to be significantly influenced by peer pressure and behavioral group norms (Pagliaro & Pagliaro, 1996).

Alcohol, cannabis, and nicotine are often used together and with other abusable psychotropics. High school seniors who drink alcohol and smoke tobacco cigarettes are at increased risk for using cannabis, and those who do also have an increased risk for using still other abusable psychotropics (Lewinsohn et al., 1999; Merrill et al., 1999). Many specific patterns of combined use have been identified. For example, alcohol is commonly used with cocaine, not only in social contexts, but also to come down and get straight from a cocaine high. Alcohol also is commonly used at the same time as LSD as part of a popular ritual of use, as a vehicle to facilitate the oral ingestion of the LSD blotter dosage forms (doses adsorbed to paper), and to mellow out the LSD "head stone." Another common example of polyabusable psychotropic use involves the use of tobacco as a vehicle for cannabis use (e.g., putting hashish oil on a tobacco cigarette; mixing marijuana or hashish and tobacco together and rolling it into a cigarette or smoking the mixture in a pipe) (Pagliaro & Pagliaro, 1993, 1996).

Patterns of Abusable Psychotropic Use

There are several well-defined patterns of abusable psychotropic use: nonuse, initial use, social use, habitual use, abuse, and compulsive use. These patterns of use represent a continuum of increasingly more harmful and compulsive abusable psychotropic use behavior. There are also patterns of controlled use, resumed nonuse, and relapsed use. The latter two may occur in somewhat predictable cycles ultimately resulting in a long-term return to either patterns of compulsive use or nonuse (abstinence) (Figure 7-3).

Obviously, initial and social use do not always progress to abuse and compulsive use patterns and some youth may resume a pattern of nonuse without relapsing to a previous pattern of use. They also may display different patterns of use for different abusable psychotropics (e.g., social use for LSD, resumed nonuse for alcohol, compulsive use for tobacco cigarettes). This model offers a means for identifying the nature and severity of actual or potential problems that require different treatment approaches. The focus of this approach is on the overall pattern of

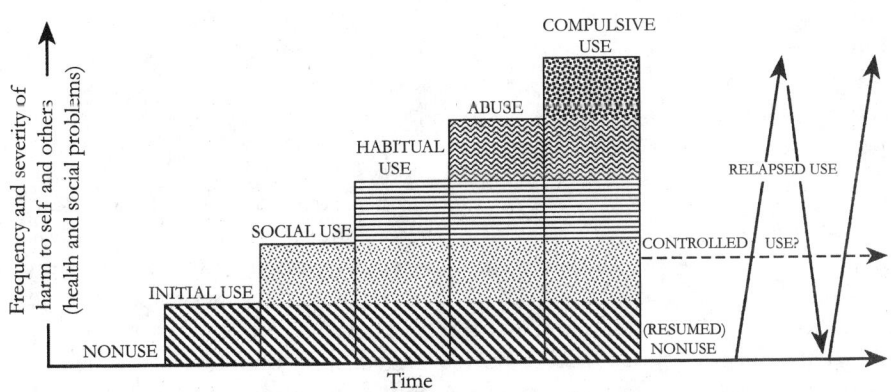

FIGURE 7-3
Patterns of Abusable Psychotropic Use

abusable psychotropic use instead of simply the characteristics of the specific abusable psychotropic.

Initial use. The first-time use of a particular abusable psychotropic generally involves some degree of curiosity and experimentation. For most children and adolescents, this pattern of use usually does not develop into a pattern of abuse. As many emergency department personnel and pediatric clinicians know, admission to a hospital or morgue can result from the initial use of a particular abusable psychotropic by a particular child or adolescent; fortunately, these consequences are uncommon.

Most children and adolescents are curious about the effects of an abusable psychotropic and use it only once (or a couple of times), when the opportunity presents itself, without any long-term adverse effects. A school-age child might try a cigarette or take a puff of crack cocaine with the encouragement of an older sibling. Younger children, including toddlers and preschoolers, may be given a sip of beer or a toke from a marijuana joint by older siblings and their friends just to see the child's reaction. Initial use may also be prompted by a parent, an adult relative, or a family friend (Numbers, 2000).

Social use. The second pattern of use is social use. Although the abusable psychotropic is actively sought, there are no major adverse effects associated with its use. An example of this pattern of use is drinking an alcoholic beverage for fun at a friend's house when the parents are away, or drinking spiked punch at a school dance. In these situations, the child or adolescent did not go to the friend's house or school dance primarily for the alcohol, but sought and used it after his or her arrival.

Habitual use. Habitual use involves the establishment of a definite pattern of abusable psychotropic use (e.g., smoking marijuana every day after school or drinking with the guys every Friday and Saturday night). The characteristics of this pattern of use include the absence of major adverse effects and the absence of physical dependence (addiction). However, psychological dependence (habituation) is an integral feature of this pattern of abusable psychotropic use.

Abuse. In the abuse pattern, the abusable psychotropic is actively sought. For example, alcohol may be brought to school in a Thermos® so that it will be available throughout the day between classes. Abusable psychotropic use continues despite harmful effects. Examples of this pattern of use include an adolescent who has had seizures associated with the use of MDMA but continues to use it; an adolescent with asthma controlled by bronchodilators who continues to smoke cigarettes; and a pregnant adolescent who continues to drink alcohol, even though she has been warned about the dangers to the fetus. In this pattern of use, the negative consequences of abusable psychotropic use generally are well recognized, but the abusable psychotropic still continues to be actively sought.

Compulsive use. The most serious pattern of abusable psychotropic use is compulsive use. This pattern of use is characterized by a complete lack of control over the use of an abusable psychotropic. Children and adolescents who display this pattern of use say that they just cannot help themselves. The abusable psychotropic, regardless of whether it is alcohol, cocaine, nicotine, or some other abusable psychotropic, becomes the major focus of these children and adolescents. Compulsive users spend most of their time thinking about, obtaining, and using the abusable psychotropic.

Resumed nonuse, controlled use, and relapsed use. Once the pattern of compulsive use is reached, return to previous and less severe patterns of use traditionally has been thought to be virtually impossible. Complete abstinence is the accepted therapeutic goal for compulsive use. This goal has been challenged and continues to be debated by experts (Levy, 1992; Littrell, 1991). Until further research produces clear evidence to the contrary, complete abstinence is recommended as the only way to effectively control compulsive use (Pagliaro & Pagliaro, 2000). This therapeutic goal appears to apply to all abusable psychotropics and to all children and adolescents (Pagliaro & Pagliaro, 1996).

These patterns of abusable psychotropic use are steps in the progressive development of physical and psychological dependence. A better understanding of these patterns of abusable psychotropic use will enable pediatric clinicians to appropriately assess children and adolescents for potential and actual problems related to abusable psychotropic use. Pediatric clinicians also will be able to devise prevention and treatment strategies that meet the needs of individual children and adolescents who either have or are developing problematic patterns of abuse or compulsive use. Attention should be given to abstinence and relapse prevention programs specifically designed for children and adolescents to reduce the extremely high recidivism rates (in excess of 70%) that are routinely encountered 12 months after the completion of most treatment programs (Pagliaro & Pagliaro, 1996).

Treatment

Pharmacologic advances in the prevention and treatment of abusable psychotropic use have been significant and include methadone maintenance programs and the use of naltrexone for the treatment of opiate addiction; clonidine-assisted opiate detoxification; naloxone for the treatment of opiate overdosage; flumazenil for the treatment of benzodiazepine overdosage; and disulfiram for the treatment of alcoholism (Pagliaro & Pagliaro, 1996, 2000).

Pharmaceutical advances also include the development of dosage forms that prevent or help reduce the illicit use of abusable psychotropics. For example, the illicit intravenous use of pentazocine has been all but eliminated in the United States by the development of the combination pentazocine and naloxone tablets *(Talwin-Nx®)* (Pagliaro, 1992b; Pagliaro & Pagliaro, 1996, 1999, 2000).

Advances also have been made in the pharmacologic management of the withdrawal phenomenon associated with several abusable psychotropics (e.g., bromocriptine or fluoxetine for the symptomatic management of cocaine withdrawal [L. A. Pagliaro et al., 1992] and buspirone for the symptomatic management of nicotine withdrawal [Hilleman et al., 1992]). Transdermal nicotine delivery systems have become important adjuncts to smoking cessation programs (Pagliaro & Pagliaro, 1999; Tonnesen et al., 1991).

Although healthcare providers have become knowledgeable about the pharmacology, toxicology, abuse potential, and addiction liability of abusable psychotropics among adults, increased attention must be directed toward the prevention and treatment of abusable psychotropic use among children and adolescents. In addition, new alternative approaches to drug education, particularly in regard to risk and protective factors known to be predictive of the onset of abusable psychotropic use, will be needed (Hansen & McNeal, 1999). Clinicians must recognize that:

- certain abusable psychotropics are particularly attractive to children and adolescents and are used preferentially for a variety of reasons (e.g., major psychotropic effect, availability, social norms);
- children and adolescents are at particular risk for social problems associated with abusable psychotropic use (e.g., overdose death; morbidity and mortality associated with automobile crashes; learning disorders; incarceration for drug-related offenses, such as possession of illicit substances, breaking and entering, and prostitution; family violence and incest; teenage pregnancy; suicide; and transmission of sexually transmitted diseases, including gonorrhea, syphilis, and HIV); and
- because of its heterogeneity, this age group requires individualized and diverse prevention and treatment approaches (what works for a 14-year-old

pregnant Laotian girl from a poor, single-parent family living in a large inner city, who is a gang member and is addicted to crack cocaine, probably will not work for a 16-year-old boy of Japanese ancestry from an upper-middle class, two-parent family living in the suburbs, who is addicted to alcohol).

It is generally agreed that multimodal prevention and treatment approaches have the greatest potential for success and that increased participation by pediatric clinicians in both prevention and treatment can deter or curtail the use of abusable psychotropics by children and adolescents. Obviously the best treatment for abusable psychotropic use is prevention, and considerable effort has been made in this regard. Primary prevention efforts should begin in various ways with children and adolescents of all ages and with their parents.[21]

Pediatric clinicians must be knowledgeable about abusable psychotropic use and be comfortable talking with children and adolescents and their parents about it. Early prevention should be incorporated into regular pediatric health maintenance programs. On a regular basis, clinicians should ask children and adolescents what they are learning in school about abusable psychotropics and if they have used any of these drugs. Parents and other family members can be asked about their own use of alcohol, tobacco, or other abusable psychotropics and educated about the relationships between smoking and common illnesses (e.g., asthma, respiratory infections).

Parenting abilities also can be assessed: for example, accidents, child abuse or neglect, and child behavioral problems may be related to parental abusable psychotropic use (Pagliaro & Pagliaro, 2000). Clinicians must be extremely conscious of the family dynamics and parenting styles that their patient is subject to.

To achieve maximal success in the treatment of the young abusable psychotropic user, the approach must be tailored to meet his or her individual needs (Kaminer, 1999). The use of MIMAPUY can help clinicians plan treatment by identifying the variables in each dimension that are in need of change. For example, if the abusable psychotropic is identified as particularly harmful in the abusable psychotropic dimension, a less harmful substance from the same pharmacologic classification might be substituted (e.g., methadone for heroin). If the method of administration is identified as particularly dangerous, a less dangerous method might be used (e.g., substituting heroin cigarettes for heroin injections, as has been done in the United Kingdom).

Similarly, if specific stresses and maladaptive coping mechanisms are identified among the psychological variables in the young person dimension, techniques for stress reduction and the development of better coping abilities would be an integral component of the treatment plan. If lack of family support is identified as a major contributing factor to abusable psychotropic use among the social variables in the young person dimension, intervention might include attempts to increase family or other support (family counseling might be considered).[22] If a lack of adequate healthcare resources (e.g., youth programs with appropriately trained staff) is identified

---

21. For culturally sensitive and curricular treatment approaches, see Baldwin et al. (1996) and Ramirez et al. (1997). For a more detailed review of treatment strategies, see Pagliaro & Pagliaro (1996, 2000).

22. The social factor of the young person dimension is receiving more attention, with the family being considered both a major contributing factor for abusable psychotropic use among youth and the potential cure. The U.S. Department of Justice developed a family skills training program for parents and children in 1983, The Strengthening Families Program (SFP). Since its development, it has been modified for use for diverse families across the United States (Kumpfer & Tait, 2000) and emphasizes improving family relations and parenting skills. Other approaches include public media announcements. For example, some success has been achieved with televised public service announcements (PSAs) targeted specifically to youth. A 26.7% drop in marijuana use among the targeted adolescent population was documented (Palmgreen et al., 2001).

as a major factor in the societal dimension that contributes to abusable psychotropic use, intervention might include attempts to increase social assistance (develop specific social programs for children and adolescents) and training of pediatric psychologists, social workers, and other professionals to specifically deal with abusable psychotropic use among children and adolescents.

Evaluation of treatment is one of the most crucial and yet perhaps the most frequently overlooked step in the treatment process. It is useless for pediatric clinicians to plan treatment or for children and adolescents to follow a plan of treatment if the treatment is ineffective. Evaluation can be readily performed using MIMAPUY by comparing the variables before treatment (baseline evaluation), during treatment (formative evaluation), and at predetermined intervals after treatment is completed (summative evaluation).

For example, if unemployment is a social variable in the young person dimension that is identified as a major contributing factor in an adolescent's history of abusable psychotropic use and if job training and employment strategies are not adequately addressed, the prognosis will not be favorable despite other treatment interventions. Although program evaluators and researchers are often particularly interested in the summative evaluation in terms of program success and recidivism rates, the pediatric clinician should be most interested in the formative evaluation because the treatment plan can be modified midstream to optimize therapeutic outcome.

The MIMAPUY also is useful because it can reveal factors that may, for a particular young person, contribute to relapse if not addressed. Such factors include abusable psychotropic use related to inadequate coping when the youth is faced with significant stressors such as the death of a loved one, a diagnosis of cancer, or an arrest. In addition, MIMAPUY can be used as a framework for helping young people understand the factors affecting their abusable psychotropic use and for enabling them to participate in their healthcare planning and treatment. General guidelines (with demonstrated effectiveness) for the treatment of young abusable psychotropic users are listed in Table 7-15.

TABLE 7-15
Abusable Psychotropic Use: Guidelines for Treating Children and Adolescents

- Individualize treatment.
- Recognize that different types of treatment may be required.
- Be nonjudgmental in approaching treatment.
- Remember that success or failure is ultimately the youth's responsibility.
- Assess for (and treat, or refer for treatment, as appropriate) any accompanying mental disorders (other DSM-IV-TR axis diagnoses and dual diagnoses).
- Break the denial regarding abusable psychotropic use problems.
- Respect children and adolescents; do not treat them in a condescending manner.
- Provide treatment in a straightforward, unbiased manner that is appropriately tailored to developmental, learning, and social needs and abilities.
- Work toward mutually agreed upon, realistic, and achievable goals.
- Remember that reasons for abusable psychotropic use may differ from one child or adolescent to another and even for the same individual over time.
- Address underlying problems (e.g., depression, lack of self-esteem, sexual abuse).
- Involve family, friends, and other people as appropriate in confrontation, treatment planning, and program implementation.
- Use peer groups (place youth in treatment groups according to age and gender).
- Use community social agencies designed for youth.
- Make referrals to other appropriate health and social care agencies.
- Provide appropriate follow-up services.

Summary

The use of abusable psychotropics is a significant problem among North American children and adolescents that shows no indication of abatement. The major abusable psychotropics used by children and adolescents are alcohol, amphetamines, cannabis, cocaine, LSD, MDMA, nicotine, opiates (heroin), and volatile solvents and inhalants. MIMAPUY is a heuristic device that helps pediatric clinicians analyze the myriad of variables associated with abusable psychotropic use. Pediatric clinicians can use MIMAPUY both to increase their understanding of the complex phenomenon of abusable psychotropic use among youth and to provide more effective prevention and treatment interventions for their pediatric patients.

References[23]

Abel, E. L. (1995). An update on incidence of FAS: FAS is not an equal opportunity birth defect. *Neurotoxicology and Teratology, 17*(4), 437–443.

Adler, M. W. (1998). Nathan B. Eddy Award Lecture. *NIDA Research Monographs, 178,* 11–22.

Agurell, S., Halldin, M., Lingren, J., et al. (1986). Pharmacokinetics and metabolism of delta-1-tetrahydrocannabinol and other cannabinoids with emphasis on man. *Pharmacological Review, 38,* 21–43.

Alexander, C. S., Allen, P., Crawford, M. A., et al. (1999). Taking a first puff: Cigarette smoking experiences among ethnically diverse adolescents. *Ethnic Health, 4*(4), 245–257.

Altarac, M., Gardner, J. W., Popovich, R. M., et al. (2000). Cigarette smoking and exercise-related injuries among young men and women. *American Journal of Preventive Medicine, 18*(3, Suppl), 96–102.

American Academy of Pediatrics Committee on Adolescence, Committee on Substance Abuse. (1991). Marijuana: A continuing concern for pediatricians. *Pediatrics, 88,* 1070–1072.

An, L. C., O'Malley, P. M., Schulenberg, J. E., et al. (1999). Changes at the high end of risk in cigarette smoking among US high school seniors, 1976–1995. *American Journal of Public Health, 89*(5), 699–705.

Andreu, V., Mas, A., Bruguera, M., et al. (1998). Ecstasy: A common cause of severe acute hepatotoxicity. *Journal of Hepatology, 29*(3), 394–397.

Andrews, L. S., & Snyder, R. (1991). Toxic effects of solvents and vapors. In *Casarett and Doull's toxicology: The basic science of poisons,* 4th ed., M. O. Amdur, J. Doull, & C. D. Klaassen, Eds., New York: Pergamon.

Arellano, C. M. (1996). Child maltreatment and substance use: A review of the literature. *Substance Use & Misuse, 31*(7), 927–935.

Baldwin, J. A., Rolf, J. E., Johnson, J., et al. (1996). Developing culturally sensitive HIV/AIDS and substance abuse prevention curricula for Native American Youth. *Journal of School Health, 66*(9), 322–327.

Bauman, K. E., & Ennett, S. T. (1996). On the importance of peer influence for adolescent drug use: Commonly neglected considerations. *Addiction, 91*(2), 185–198.

Beautrais, A. L., Joyce, P. R., & Mulder, R. T. (1999). Cannabis abuse and serious suicide attempts. *Addiction, 94*(8), 1155–1164.

Beauvais, F. (1992). Trends in Indian adolescent drug and alcohol use. *American Indian Alaskan Native Mental Health Research, 5,* 1–12.

Beilman, G. J., Brasel, K. J., Dittrich, K., et al. (1999). Risk factors and patterns of injury in snowmobile crashes. *Wilderness and Environmental Medicine, 10*(4), 226–232.

Beman, D. S. (1995). Risk factors leading to adolescent substance abuse. *Adolescence, 30*(117), 201–208.

Benninger, M. S. (1999). The impact of cigarette smoking and environmental tobacco smoke on nasal and sinus disease: A review of the literature. *American Journal of Rhinology, 13*(6), 435–438.

Bhattacharya, G. (1998). Drug use among Asian-Indian adolescents: Identifying protective/risk factors. *Adolescence, 33*(129), 169–184.

Bidi use among urban youth—Massachusetts. (1999). *MMWR Morbidity and Mortality Weekly Report, 48*(36), 796–799.

Biederman, J., Wilens, T., Mick, E., et al. (1999). Pharmacotherapy of attention-deficit/hyperactivity disorder reduces risk for substance use disorder. *Pediatrics, 104*(2), e20.

Bonné, J. (2001). Meth's deadly buzz. [on line]. Available: Http://www.msnbc.com/news/

Borges, G., Walters, E. E., & Kessler, R. C. (2000). Associations of substance use, abuse, and dependence with subsequent suicidal behavior. *American Journal of Epidemiology, 151*(18), 781–789.

Botvin, G. J., Griffin, K. W., Diaz, T., et al. (1999). Smoking initiation and escalation in early adolescent girls: One-year follow-up of a school-based prevention intervention for minority youth. *Journal of the American Medical Women's Association, 54*(3), 139–143, 152.

Botvin, G. J., Malgady, R. G., Griffin, K. W., et al. (1998). Alcohol and marijuana use among rural youth: Interaction of social and intrapersonal influences. *Addictive Behaviors, 23*(3), 379–387.

Bowen, S. E., Daniel, J., & Balster, R. L. (1999). Deaths associated with inhalant abuse in Virginia from 1987 to 1996. *Drug and Alcohol Dependence, 53*(3), 239–245.

Boyle, M. H., & Offord, D. R. (1991). Psychiatric disorder and substance use in adolescence. *Canadian Journal of Psychiatry, 36,* 699–705.

Brook, J. S., Balka, E. B., & Whiteman, M. (1999). The risks for late adolescence of early adolescent marijuana use. *American Journal of Public Health, 89*(10), 1549–1554.

Brook, J. S., Brook, D. W., De La Rosa, M., et al. (1998). Pathways to marijuana use among adolescents: Cultural/ecological, family, peer, and personality influences. *Journal of the American Academy of Child and Adolescent Psychiatry, 37*(7), 759–766.

Buffenstein, A., Heaster, J., & Ko, P. (1999).

---

23. In addition to current reference citations, some earlier original and classic works also have been cited. For a more comprehensive listing of earlier related references, readers are referred to Pagliaro & Pagliaro, 1996, 2000.

Chronic psychotic illness from methamphetamine. *American Journal of Psychiatry, 156*(4), 662.

Burgess, C., O'Donohoe, A., & Gill, M. (2000). Agony and ecstasy: A review of MDMA effects and toxicity. *European Psychiatry, 15*(5), 287–294.

Carroll, J. F., Malloy, T. E., Hannigan, P., et al. (1977). Meaning and evolution of the term "multiple substance use." *Contemporary Drug Problems, 6,* 101–134.

Carvajal, S. C., Photiades, J. R., Evans, R. I., et al. (1997). Relating a social influence model to the role of acculturation in substance use among Latino adolescents. *Journal of Applied Social Psychology, 27*(18), 1617–1628.

Chick, J., Gough, K., Falkowski, W., et al. (1992). Disulfiram treatment of alcoholism. *British Journal of Psychiatry, 161,* 84–89.

Child abuse and neglect a national emergency, U.S. advisory board declares in first report. (1991). *Hospital and Community Psychiatry, 42,* 101–102.

Church, M. W., Crossland, W. J., Holmes, P. A., et al. (1998). Effects of prenatal cocaine on hearing, vision, growth, and behavior. *Annals of the New York Academy of Science, 846,* 12–28.

Cigarette smoking among high school students—11 states, 1991–1997. (1999). *MMWR Morbidity and Mortality Weekly Reports, 48*(31), 686–692.

Cigarette smoking during the last 3 months of pregnancy among women who gave birth to live infants—Maine, 1988–1997. *MMWR Morbidity and Mortality Weekly Report, 48*(20), 421–425.

Clarke, J., Stein, M. D., Sobota, M., et al. (1999). Victims as victimizers: Physical aggression by persons with a history of childhood abuse. *Archives of Internal Medicine, 159*(16), 1920–1924.

Cloud, J. (2001). Recreational pharmaceuticals. *Time, 157*(2), 68.

Coke emergencies up, DAWN report. (1992). *The Journal, 21,* 3.

Collins, R. L., Ellickson, P. L., & Bell, R. M. (1998). Simultaneous polydrug use among teens: Prevalence and predictors. *Journal of Substance Abuse, 10*(3), 233–253.

Collishaw, N., & Leahy, K. (1991). Mortality attributable to tobacco use in Canada. *Chronic Diseases in Canada, 12,* 46.

Crimmins, S. M., Cleary, S. D., Brownstein, H. H., et al. (2000). Trauma, drugs and violence among juvenile offenders. *Journal of Psychoactive Drugs, 32*(1), 43–54.

Dalmau, A., Bergman, B., & Brismar, B. (1999). Psychotic disorders among inpatients with abuse of cannabis, amphetamine and opiates. Do dopaminergic stimulants facilitate psychiatric illness? *European Psychiatry, 14*(7), 366–371.

Dembo, R., Schmeidler, J., Sue, C. C., et al. (1998). Psychosocial, substance use, and delinquency differences among Anglo, Hispanic White, and African-American male youths entering a juvenile assessment center. *Substance Use & Misuse, 33*(7), 1481–1510.

Dembo, R., Williams, L., Schmeidler, J., et al. (1991). Juvenile crime and drug abuse: A prospective study of high risk youth. *Journal of Addictive Disorders, 11*(2), 5–31.

DeWitt, C. B. (1991, June). Drug use forecasting. *Research in Action* (U.S. Department of Justice), pp. 1–8.

DeWitt, C. B., O'Neil, J. A., & Baldau, V. (1991, August). Drug use forecasting: Drugs & crime 1990 annual report. *Research in Action* (U.S. Department of Justice), pp. 1–24.

Disney, E. R., Elkins, I. J., McGue, M., et al. (1999). Effects of ADHD, conduct disorder, and gender on substance use and abuse in adolescence. *American Journal of Psychiatry, 156*(10), 1515–1521.

D'Onofrio, B. M., Murrelle, L., Eaves, L. J., et al. (1999). Adolescent religiousness and its influence on substance use: Preliminary findings from the mid-Atlantic school age twin study. *Twin Research, 2*(2), 156–168.

Ellickson, P. L., & Morton, S. C. (1999). Identifying adolescents at risk for hard drug use: Racial/ethnic variations. *Journal of Adolescent Health, 25*(6), 382–395.

Epps, R. P., & Manley, M. W. (1991). A physician's guide to preventing tobacco use during childhood and adolescence. *Pediatrics, 88,* 140–144.

Ernst, T., Chang, L., Leonido-Lee, M., et al. (2000). Evidence for long-term neurotoxicity associated with methamphetamine abuse: A 1H MRS study. *Neurology, 54*(6), 1344–1349.

Espeland, K. (1995). Identifying the manifestations of inhalant abuse. *Nurse Practitioner, 20*(5), 49–50, 53.

Espeland, K. E. (1997). Inhalants: The instant, but deadly high. *Pediatric Nursing, 23*(1), 82–86.

Everett, S. A., Warren, C. W., Sharp, D., et al. (1999). Initiation of cigarette smoking and subsequent smoking behavior among U.S. high school students. *Preventive Medicine, 29*(5), 327–333.

Feldman, J., Shenker, I. R., Etzel, R. A., et al. (1991). Passive smoking alters lipid profiles in adolescents. *Pediatrics, 88,* 259–264.

Felts, W. M., Chenier, T., & Barnes, R. (1991). Drug use and suicide ideation and behavior among North Carolina public school students. *American Journal of Public Health, 82,* 870–872.

Fergusson, D. M., Horwood, L. J., & Beautrais, A. L. (1999). Is sexual orientation related to mental health problems and suicidality in young people? *Archives of General Psychiatry, 56*(10), 876–880.

Fiegelman, W., Hyman, M. M., Amann, K., et al (1990). Correlates of persisting drug use among former youth multiple drug abuse patients. *Journal of Psychoactive Drugs, 22,* 63–75.

Finke, L. M., & Bowman, C. A. (1997). Factors in childhood drug and alcohol use: A review of the literature. *Journal of Child and Adolescent Psychiatric Nursing, 10*(3), 29–34.

Finke, L., & Williams, J. (1999). Alcohol and drug use of inter-city versus rural school age children. *Journal of Drug Education, 29*(3), 279–291.

Fisher, L. (2000). Bidis—The latest trend in U. S. teen tobacco use. *Cancer Causes Control, 11*(6), 577–578.

Flanagan, R. J., & Ives, R. J. (1994). Volatile substance abuse. *Bulletin on Narcotics, 46*(2), 49–78.

Flumazenil. (1992). *The Medical Letter on Drugs and Therapeutics, 34,* 66–68.

Forster, J. L., Hourigan, M., & McGovern, P. (1992). Availability of cigarettes to underage youth in three communities. *Preventive Medicine, 21*(3), 320–328.

French, S. A., & Perry, C. L. (1996). Smoking among adolescent girls: Prevalence and etiology. *Journal of the American Medical Women's Association, 51*(1-2), 25–28.

Friedman, A. S., & Glassman, K. (2000). Family risk factors versus peer risk factors for drug abuse. A longitudinal study of an African American urban community sample. *Journal of Substance Abuse Treatment, 18*(3), 267–275.

Fromme, K., & D'Amico, E. J. (2000). Measuring adolescents' alcohol outcome expectancies. *Psychology of Addictive Behavior, 14*(2), 206–212.

Garofalo, R., Wolf, R. C., Wissow, L. S., et al. (1999). Sexual orientation and risk of suicide attempts among a representative sample of youth. *Archives of Pediatric and Adolescent Medicine, 153*(5), 487–493.

Generali, J. A. (1992). Nicotine transdermal patches. *Facts and Comparisons Drug Newsletter, 11,* 33–34.

Gentilello, L. M., Villaveces, A., Ries, R. R., et al. (1999). Detection of acute alcohol intoxication and chronic alcohol dependence by trauma center staff. *Journal of Trauma, 47*(6), 1131–1135.

Gerber, S. E., Epstein, L., & Mencher, L. S. (1995). Recent changes in the etiology of hearing disorders: Perinatal drug exposure. *Journal of the American Academy of Audiology, 6*(5), 371–377.

Gerra, G., Zaimovic, A., Ferri, M., et al. (2000). Long-lasting effects of (+/−)3,4-methylenedioxymethamphetamine (ecstasy) on serotonin system function in humans. *Biological Psychiatry, 47*(2), 127–136.

Gerra, G., Zaimovic, A., Giucastro, G., et al. (1998). Serotonergic function after (+/−)3,4-methylenedioxymethamphetamine ("Ecstasy") in humans. *International Clinical Psychopharmacology, 13*(1), 1–9.

Gill, J. R., & Stajic, M. (2000). Ketamine in non-hospital and hospital deaths in New York City. *Journal of Forensic Sciences, 45*(3), 655–658.

Giovino, G. A. (1999). Epidemiology of tobacco use among US adolescents. *Nicotine and Tobacco Research, 1*(Suppl 1), S31–S40.

Gouzoulis-Mayfrank, E., Daumann, J., Tuchtenhagen, F., et al. (2000). Impaired cognitive performance in drug free users of recreational ecstasy. *Journal of Neurology, Neurosurgery, and Psychiatry, 68*(6), 719–725.

Gravey, M. (1990). Information and alternatives: The role of a youth non-government organization in drug abuse control. *Bulletin of Narcotics, 43,* 29–33.

Greenbaum, P. E., Foster-Johnson, L., & Petrila, A. (1996). Co-occurring addictive and mental disorders among adolescents: Prevalence research and future directions. *American Journal of Orthopsychiatry, 66*(1), 52–60.

Griffin, K. W., Botvin, G. J., Doyle, M. M., et al. (1999). A six-year follow-up study of determinants of heavy cigarette smoking among high-school seniors. *Journal of Behavioral Medicine, 22*(3), 271–284.

Griffin, K. W., Botvin, G. J., Scheier, L. M., et al. (2000). Parenting practices as predictors of substance use, delinquency, and aggression among urban minority youth: Moderating effects of family structure and gender. *Psychology of Addictive Behaviors, 14*(2), 174–184.

Grisso, J. A., Schwarz, D. F., Hirschinger, N., et al. (1999). Violent injuries among women in an urban area. *New England Journal of Medicine, 341*(25), 1899–1905.

Gritz, E. R., Prokhorov, A. V., Hudmon, K. S., et al. (1998). Cigarette smoking in a multiethnic population of youth: Methods and baseline findings. *Preventive Medicine, 27*(3), 365–384.

Grunbaum, J. A., Kann, L., Kinchen, S. A., et al. (1999). Youth risk behavior surveillance—National alternative high school youth risk behavior survey, United States, 1998. *MMWR Morbidity and Mortality Weekly Report CDC Surveillance Summary, 48*(7), 1–44.

Guidotti, T. L. (1989). Critique of available studies on the toxicology of kretek smoke and its constituents by routes of entry involving the respiratory tract. *Archives of Toxicology, 63*(1), 7–12.

Hall, N. W., & Zigler, E. (1997). Drug-abuse prevention efforts for young children: A review and critique of existing programs. *American Journal of Orthopsychiatry, 67*(1), 134–143.

Hansen, W. B., & McNeal, R. B., Jr. (1999). Drug education practice: Results of an observational study. *Health Education Research, 14*(1), 85–97.

Harper, G. W., & Robinson, W. L. (1999). Pathways to risk among inner-city African-American adolescent females: The influence of gang membership. *American Journal of Community Psychology, 27*(3), 383–404.

Hauschildt, E. (1992, October/November). Massive U.S. drug 'war' a failure: Policy group. *The Journal, 21,* 5.

Hawke, J. M., Jainchill, N., & De Leon, G. (2000).

Adolescent amphetamine users in treatment: Client profiles and treatment outcomes. *Journal of Psychoactive Drugs, 32*(1), 95–105.

Hawkins, K., & Hane, A. C. (2000). Adolescents' perceptions of print cigarette advertising: A case for counteradvertising. *Journal of Health Communication, 5*(1), 83–96.

Hersch, J. (1998). Teen smoking behavior and the regulatory environment. *Duke Law Journal, 47*(6), 1143–1170.

Heyman, R. B., Anglin, T. M., Copperman, S. M., et al. (1999). American Academy of Pediatrics. Committee on Substance Abuse. Marijuana: A continuing concern for pediatricians. *Pediatrics, 104*(4, Part 1), 982–985.

Hilleman, D. E., Mohiuddin, S. M., Del Core, M. G., et al. (1992). Effect of buspirone on withdrawal symptoms associated with smoking cessation. *Archives of Internal Medicine, 152,* 350–352.

Hingson, R. W., Heeren, T., Jamanka, A., et al. (2000). Age of drinking onset and unintentional injury involvement after drinking. *Journal of the American Medical Association, 284*(12), 1527–1533.

Hishinuma, E. S., Nishimura, S. T., Miyamoto, R. H., et al. (2000). Alcohol use in Hawaii. *Hawaii Medical Journal, 59*(8), 329–335.

Hoffman, J. P., Cerbone, F. G., & Su, S. S. (2000). A growth curve analysis of stress and adolescent drug use. *Substance Use & Misuse, 35*(5), 687–716.

Howard, M. O., Kivlahan, D., & Walker, R. D. (1997). Cloninger's tridimensional theory of personality and psychopathology: Applications to substance use disorders. *Journal of Studies on Alcohol, 58*(1), 48–66.

Howard, M. O., Walker, R. D., Walker, P. S., et al. (1999). Inhalant use among urban American Indian youth. *Addiction, 94*(1), 83–95.

Huba, G. J., Melchoir, L. A., Greenberg, B., et al. (2000). Predicting substance abuse among youth with, or at high risk for, HIV. *Psychology of Addictive Behavior, 14*(2), 197–205.

Hug, T. E., Fitzgerald, K. M., & Cibis, G. W. (2000). Clinical and electroretinographic findings in fetal alcohol syndrome. *Journal of the American Academy of Pediatric Ophthalmologists and Surgeons, 4*(4), 200–204.

Hunter, S. M., Vizelberg, I. A., & Berenson, G. S. (1991). Identifying mechanisms of adoption of tobacco and alcohol use among youth: The Bogalusa heart study. *Social Networks, 13,* 91–104.

Hurlbut, K. M. (1991). Drug-induced psychoses. *Emergency Medicine Clinics of North America, 9,* 31–52.

Iannotti, R. J., & Bush, P. J. (1992). Perceived vs. actual friends' use of alcohol, cigarettes, marijuana, and cocaine: Which has the most influence. *Journal of Youth and Adolescence, 21,* 375–389.

Inciardi, J. A., Surratt, H. L., Colon, H. M., et al. (1999). Drug use and HIV risks among migrant workers on the DelMarVa Peninsula. *Substance Use & Misuse, 34*(4-5), 653–666.

It's an important form of entertainment for kids: Winnipeg solvent sniffers receiving little aid. (1986). *The Addiction Research Foundation Journal, 15*(8), 3.

Johnson, B. D., Dunlap, E., & Maher, L. (1998). Nurturing for careers in drug use and crime: Conduct norms for children and juveniles in crack-using households. *Substance Use & Misuse, 33*(7), 1511–1546.

Johnson, E. M. (1990). Chemical dependency and black America: The government responds. *Journal of the National Black Nurses Association, 4,* 47–56.

Johnson, E. M., Davis, D. J., & Denniston, R. W. (1991). *Prevention plus II: Assessing alcohol and other drug prevention programs at the school and community level (ADM91-1817).* Rockville, MD: Office for Substance Abuse Prevention.

Jones, G. D. (1997). The role of drugs and alcohol in urban minority adolescent suicide attempts. *Death Studies, 21*(2), 189–202.

Kaminer, Y. (1999). Addictive disorders in adolescents. *Psychiatric Clinics of North America, 22*(2), 275–288.

Kandel, D. B., & Chen, K. (2000). Types of marijuana users by longitudinal course. *Journal of Studies on Alcohol, 61*(3), 367–378.

Karavokiros, K. A., & Tsipis, G. B. (1990). Flumazenil: A benzodiazepine antagonist. *DICP Annals of Pharmacotherapy, 24,* 976–981.

Kelleher, K. J., Rickert, V. I., Hardin, B. H., et al. (1992). Rurality and gender: Effects on early adolescent alcohol use. *American Journal of Diseases of Children, 146,* 317–322.

Kilpatrick, D. G., Acierno, R., Saunders, B., et al. (2000). Risk factors for adolescent substance abuse and dependence: Data from a national sample. *Journal of Consulting and Clinical Psychology, 68*(1), 19–30.

Kim, S., Crutchfield, C., Williams, C., et al. (1998). Toward a new paradigm in substance abuse and other problem behavior prevention for youth: Youth development and empowerment approach. *Journal of Drug Education, 28*(1), 1–17.

Klitzman, R. L., Pope, H. G., & Hudson, J. I. (2000). MDMA ("Ecstasy") abuse and high-risk sexual behaviors among 169 gay and bisexual men. *American Journal of Psychiatry, 157*(7), 1162–1164.

Kumpfer, K. L., & Tait, C. M. (2000, April). Family skills training for parents and children. *Juvenile Justice Bulletin,* pp. 1–11.

Kumra, V., & Markoff, B. A. (2000). Who's smoking now? The epidemiology of tobacco use in the United States and abroad. *Clinics in Chest Medicine, 21*(1), 1–9, vii.

Lamkin, L. P., & Houston, T. P. (1998). Nicotine dependency and adolescents: Preventing and treating. *Primary Care; Clinics in Office Practice, 25*(1), 123–135.

Landen, M. G., Middaugh, J., & Dannenberg, A. L. (1999). Injuries associated with snow-mobiles, Alaska, 1993–1994. *Public Health Report, 114*(1), 48–52.

Latimer, W. W., Winters, K. C., Stinchfield, R., et al. (2000). Demographic, individual, and interpersonal predictors of adolescent alcohol and marijuana use following treatment. *Psychology of Addictive Behaviors, 14*(2), 162–173.

Leshner, A. I. (2000). A club drug alert. *NIDA Notes, 14*(6), 3–4.

Lesmes, G. R., & Donofrio, D. K. (1992). Passive smoking: The medical and economic issues. *American Journal of Medicine, 93*(Suppl 1A), 38S–42S.

Lester, D. (1999). Suicidality and risk-taking behaviors: An ecological study of youth behaviors in 29 states. *Perceptual and Motor Skills, 88*(3, Part 2), 1299–1300.

Levin, F. R., & Kleber, H. D. (1995). Attention-deficit hyperactivity disorder and substance abuse: Relationships and implications for treatment. *Harvard Review of Psychiatry, 2*(5), 246–258.

Levy, M. (1992). Alcohol and addictions. [Letter]. *American Journal of Psychiatry, 149*(8), 1117–1118.

Lewinsohn, P. M., Rohde, P., & Brown, R. A. (1999). Level of current and past adolescent cigarette smoking as predictors of future substance use disorders in young adulthood. *Addiction, 94*(6), 913–921.

Li, G., Baker, S. P., Sterling, S., et al. (1996). A comparative analysis of alcohol in fatal and nonfatal bicycling injuries. *Alcoholism, Clinical and Experimental Research, 20*(9), 1553–1559.

Lindenbaum, G. A., Carroll, S. F., Daskal, I., et al. (1989). Patterns of alcohol and drug abuse in an urban trauma center: The increasing role of cocaine abuse. *Journal of Trauma, 29*, 1654–1658.

Littrell, J. (1991). *Understanding and treating alcoholism.* Hillsdale, NH: Lawrence Erlbaum.

Lock, J., & Steiner, H. (1999). Gay, lesbian, and bisexual youth risks for emotional, physical and social problems: Results from a community-based survey. *Journal of the American Academy of Child and Adolescent Psychiatry, 38*(3), 297–304.

Lowry, R., Cohen, L. R., Modzeleski, W., et al. (1999). School violence, substance use, and availability of illegal drugs on school property among US high school students. *Journal of School Health, 69*(9), 347–355.

Macdonald, S., Wells, S., Giesbrecht, N., et al. (1999). Demographic and substance use factors related to violent and accidental injuries: Results from an emergency room study. *Drug and Alcohol Dependence, 55*(1-2), 53–61.

Mackesy-Amiti, M. E., & Fendrich, M. (1999). Inhalant use and delinquent behavior among adolescents: A comparison of inhalant users and other drug users. *Addiction, 94*(4), 555–564.

MacKinnon, D. P., Nohre, L., Pentz, M. A., et al. (2000). The alcohol warning and adolescents: 5-year effects. *American Journal of Public Health, 90*(10), 1589–1594.

Man treated for ecstasy seizure. (2001, January 22) Available: http://www2.alberta.com/news/

Marcus, P. M., Newman, B., Millikan, R. C., et al. (2000). The association of adolescent cigarette smoking, alcoholic beverage consumption, environmental tobacco smoke, and ionizing radiation with subsequent breast cancer risk (United States). *Cancer Causes Control, 11*(3), 271–278.

Martin, C. S., Lynch, K. G., Pollock, N. K., et al. (2000). Gender differences and similarities in the personality correlates of adolescent alcohol problems. *Psychology of Addictive Behaviors, 14*(2), 121–133.

Martin, S. L., Clark, K. A., Lynch, S. R., et al. (1999). Violence in the lives of pregnant teenage women: Associations with multiple substance use. *American Journal of Drug and Alcohol Abuse, 25*(3), 425–440.

Marzuk, P. M., Tardiff, K., Leon, A. C., et al. (1992). Prevalence of cocaine use among residents of New York City who committed suicide during a one-year period. *American Journal of Psychiatry, 149*, 371–375.

Mascola, M. A., Van Vunakis, H., Tager, I. B., et al. (1998). Exposure of young infants to environmental tobacco smoke: Breast-feeding among smoking mothers. *American Journal of Public Health, 88*(6), 893–896.

Mathias, R. (2001). Cocaine, marijuana, and heroin abuse up, methamphetamine abuse down. *NIDA Notes, 15*(3), 4–5.

Mayes, L. C., Grillon, C., Granger, R., et al. (1998). Regulation of arousal and attention in preschool children exposed to cocaine prenatally. *Annals of the New York Academy of Science, 846*, 126–143.

McBride, N., Midford, R., Farringdon, F., et al. (2000). Early results from a school alcohol harm minimization study: The School Health and Alcohol Harm Reduction Project. *Addiction, 95*(7), 1021–1042.

McElhatton, P. R., Bateman, D. N., Evans, C., et al. (1999). Congenital anomalies after prenatal ecstasy exposure. *The Lancet, 354*(9188), 1441–1442.

McGarvey, E. L., Clavet, G. J., Mason, W., et al. (1999). Adolescent inhalant abuse: Environments of use. *American Journal of Drug and Alcohol Abuse, 25*(4), 731–741.

McGeary, K. A., & French, M. T. (2000). Illicit drug use and emergency room utilization. *Health Services Research, 35*(1, Part 1), 153–169.

Mclaughlin, C. R., Daniel, J., & Joost, T. F. (2000). The relationship between substance use, drug selling, and lethal violence in 25 juvenile murderers. *Journal of Forensic Sciences, 45*(2), 349–353.

McNall, M., & Remafedi, G. (1999). Relationship of amphetamine and other substance use to unprotected intercourse among young men who have sex with men. *Archives of Pediatric and Adolescent Medicine, 153*(11), 1130–1135.

Meade, L. (Author), Hirliman, G. (Producer), & Gasnier, L. (Director). (1937). *Reefer madness* (film). Mt. Morris, IL: High Times Video.

Meadows, R., & Verghese, A. (1996). Medical complications of glue sniffing. *Southern Medical Journal, 89*(5), 455–462.

Melzer-Lange, M. D. (1998). Violence and associated high-risk health behavior in adolescents. Substance abuse, sexually transmitted diseases, and pregnancy of adolescents. *Pediatric Clinics of North America, 45*(2), 307–317.

Merrill, J. C., Kleber, H. D., Shwartz, M., et al. (1999). Cigarettes, alcohol, marijuana, other risk behaviors, and American youth. *Drug and Alcohol Dependence, 56*(3), 205–212.

Miller, L., Davies, M., & Greenwald, S. (2000). Religiosity and substance use and abuse among adolescents in the National Comorbidity Survey. *Journal of the American Academy of Child and Adolescent Psychiatry, 39*(9), 1190–1197.

Miller, P., & Plant, M. (1999). Truancy and perceived school performance: An alcohol and drug study of UK teenagers. *British Journal on Alcohol and Alcoholism, 34*(6), 886–893.

Miller-Tutzauer, C., Leonard, K. E., & Windle, M. (1991). Marriage and alcohol use: A longitudinal study of "maturing out." *Journal of Studies on Alcohol, 52,* 434–440.

Mino, A., Bousquet, A., & Broers, B. (1999). Substance abuse and drug-related death, suicidal ideation, and suicide: A review. *Crisis, 20*(1), 28–35.

Molitor, F., Ruiz, J. D., Flynn, N., et al. (1999). Methamphetamine use and sexual and injection risk behaviors among out-of-treatment injection drug users. *American Journal of Drug and Alcohol Abuse, 25*(3), 475–493.

Moon, D. G., Hecht, M. L., Jackson, K. M., et al. (1999). Ethnic and gender differences and similarities in adolescent drug use and refusals of drug offers. *Substance Use & Misuse, 34*(8), 1059–1083.

Moore, M. L., & Zaccaro, D. J. (2000). Cigarette smoking, low birth weight, and preterm births in low-income African American women. *Journal of Perinatology, 20*(3), 176–180.

Morrison, S. F., Rogers, P. D., & Thomas, M. H. (1995). Alcohol and adolescents. *Pediatric Clinics of North America, 42*(2), 371–387.

Musser, C. J., Ahmann, P. A., Theye, F. W., et al. (1998). Stimulant use and the potential for abuse in Wisconsin as reported by school administrators and longitudinally followed children. *Journal of Developmental and Behavioral Pediatrics, 19*(3), 187–192.

Naum, G. P., Yarian, D. O., & McKenna, J. P. (1995). Cigarette availability to minors. *Journal of the American Osteopathic Association, 95*(11), 663–665.

Neumark, Y. D., Van Etten, M. L., & Anthony, J. C. (2000). "Drug dependence" and death: Survival analysis of the Baltimore ECA sample from 1981 to 1995. *Substance Use & Misuse, 35*(3), 313–327.

News Update (2000a). *Child and Adolescent Psychopharmacology, 2*(9), 2.

News Update (2000b). *Child and Adolescent Psychopharmacology, 2*(12), 3.

Nicotine patches. (1992). *The Medical Letter on Drugs and Therapeutics, 34,* 37–38.

Novins, D. K., & Mitchell, C. M. (1998). Factors associated with marijuana use among American Indian adolescents. *Addiction, 93*(11), 1693–1702.

Numbers. (2000). *Time Magazine,* September 4, p. 9.

Oetting, E. R., & Beauvais, F. C. (1991). Critical incidents: Failure in prevention. *International Journal of the Addictions, 26,* 797–820.

Oetting, E. R., & Donnermeyer, J. F. (1998). Primary socialization theory. The etiology of drug use and deviance. I. *Substance Use & Misuse, 33*(4), 995–1026.

Oetting, E. R., Donnermeyer, J. F., & Deffenbacher, J. L. (1998). Primary socialization theory. The influence of the community on drug use and deviance. III. *Substance Use & Misuse, 33*(8), 1629–1665.

Offidani, C., Pomini, F., Caruso, A., et al. (1995). Cocaine during pregnancy: A critical review of the literature. *Minerva Ginecologica, 47*(9), 381–390.

Onwuachi-Saunders, C., Forjuoh, S. N., West, P., et al. (1999). Child death reviews: A gold mine for injury prevention and control. *Injury Prevention: Journal of the International Society for Child and Adolescent Injury Prevention, 5*(4), 276–279.

Ornstein, T. J., Iddon, J. L., Baldacchino, A. M., et al. (2000). Profiles of cognitive dysfunction in chronic amphetamine and heroin abusers *Neuropsychopharmacology, 23*(2), 113–126.

Pagliaro, A. M. (1990). Addiction as disease: The life and death of a theory of drug and substance abuse. [Abstract]. *Proceedings of the Western Pharmacology Society, 33,* 286.

Pagliaro, A. M. (1991). The contributions of psychologic theories to the understanding of substance abuse phenomenon. [Abstract]. *Canadian Journal of Psychology, 32,* 334.

Pagliaro, A. M., & Pagliaro, L. A. (1996). *Substance use among children and adolescents: Its nature, extent, and effects from conception to adulthood.* New York: John Wiley.

Pagliaro, A. M., & Pagliaro, L. A. (2000). *Substance*

use among women. Philadelphia, PA: Brunner/Mazel.

Pagliaro, A. M., & Pagliaro, L. A. (2002). Addictionologists' perspective on catastrophic injury. In K. Anchor, Ed., *The handbook of catastrophic injury*. Nashville, TN: American Board of Disability Analysts.

Pagliaro, A. M., Pagliaro, L. A., Thauberger, P. C., et al. (1992, May 28). *Knowledge, behaviours, and risk perceptions of intravenous drug users in relation to HIV infection and AIDS*. Poster presented at the Second Annual Conference of the Canadian Association for HIV Research, Vancouver, British Columbia, Canada.

Pagliaro, A. M., Pagliaro, L. A., Thauberger, P. C., et al. (1993). Knowledge, behaviors, and risk perceptions of intravenous drug users in relation to HIV infection and AIDS: The PIARG projects. *Advances in Medical Psychotherapy, 6*, 1–28.

Pagliaro, L. A. (1990). Overview of the problem of drug abuse in Canada. [Abstract]. *Alberta Psychology, 19*(3), 11.

Pagliaro, L. A. (1991a). The straight dope: Cannibalism, birth defects, homosexuality, and other myths associated with drug and substance abuse. *Psynopsis, 13*(4), 8.

Pagliaro, L. A. (1991b). The straight dope. *Psynopsis, 13*(2), 7.

Pagliaro, L. A. (1992a). Focus on learning—Interpreting the interpretations. *Psynopsis, 14*(2), 7.

Pagliaro, L. A. (1992b). The straight dope: Predictions for 1992. *Psynopsis, 14*(1), 8.

Pagliaro, L. A. (1993). Issues in substance abuse for Canadian teachers. In *Contemporary educational issues: The Canadian mosaic*, 2nd ed., L. Stewin & S. McCann, Eds., pp. 207–222, Toronto: Stewart.

Pagliaro, L. A., & Pagliaro, A. M. (1993). The phenomenon of abusable psychotropic use among North American youth. *Journal of Clinical Pharmacology, 33*, 676–690.

Pagliaro, L. A., & Pagliaro, A. M. (1999). *Psychologists' psychotropic drug reference*. Philadelphia, PA: Brunner/Mazel.

Pagliaro, L. A., Jaglalsingh, L. H., & Pagliaro, A. M. (1992). Cocaine use and depression. *Canadian Medical Association Journal, 147*, 1636–1637.

Palacios, W. R., Urmann, C. F., Newel, R., et al. (1999). Developing a sociological framework for dually diagnosed women. *Journal of Substance Abuse Treatment, 17*(1-2), 91–102.

Palmgreen, P., Donohew, L., Lorch, E. P., et al. (2001). Television campaigns and adolescent marijuana use: Tests of sensation seeking targeting. *American Journal of Public Health, 91*(2), 292–296.

Parrott, A. C., Lees, A., Garnham, N. J., et al. (1998). Cognitive performance in recreational users of MDMA or "ecstasy." Evidence for memory deficits. *Journal of Psychopharmacology, 12*(1), 79–83.

Parrott, A. C., Sisk, E., & Turner, J. J. (2000). Psychobiological problems in heavy "ecstasy" (MDMA) polydrug users. *Drug and Alcohol Dependence, 60*(1), 105–110.

Pedersen, W., & Skrondal, A. (1999). Ecstasy and new patterns of drug use: A normal population study. *Addiction, 94*(11), 1695–1706.

Pelletier, D., & Coutu, D. (1992). Substance abuse and family violence in adolescents. *Canadian Mental Health, 40*(2), 6–12.

Pietrantoni, M., & Knuppel, R. A. (1991). Alcohol use in pregnancy. *Clinics in Perinatology, 18*, 93–111.

Pribor, E. F., & Dinwiddie, S. H. (1992). Psychiatric correlates of incest in childhood. *American Journal of Psychiatry, 149*, 52–56.

Pullen, L., Modrcin-Talbott, M. A., West, W. R., et al. (1999). Spiritual high vs high on spirits: Is religiosity related to adolescent alcohol and drug abuse? *Journal of Psychiatric and Mental Health Nursing, 6*(1), 3–8.

Quinlan, K. P., Brewer, R. D., Sleet, D. A., et al. (2000). Characteristics of child passenger deaths and injuries involving drinking drivers. *Journal of the American Medical Association, 283*(17), 2249–2252.

Ramirez, A. G., Gallion, K. J., Espinoza, R., et al. (1997). Developing a media- and school-based program for substance abuse prevention among Hispanic youth: A case study of Mirame!/Look at me! *Nicotine & Tobacco Research: Official Journal of the Society for Research on Nicotine and Tobacco, 1*(Suppl 1), S99–104.

Randall, T. (1992a). "Rave" scene, ecstasy use, leap Atlantic. *Journal of the American Medical Association, 268*, 1506.

Randall, T. (1992b). Ecstasy-fueled "rave" parties become dances of death for English youths. *Journal of the American Medical Association, 268*, 1505–1506.

Redmond, W. H. (1999). Effects of sales promotion on smoking among U.S. ninth graders. *Preventive Medicine, 28*(3), 243–250.

Rizk, B., Atterbury, J. L., & Groome, L. J. (1996). Reproductive risks of cocaine. *Human Reproduction Update, 2*(1), 43–55.

Rolfs, R. T., Goldberg, M., & Sharrar, R. G. (1990). Risk factors for syphilis: Cocaine use and prostitution. *American Journal of Public Health, 80*, 853–857.

Rose, S. M., Peabody, C. G., & Stratigeas, B. (1991). Undetected abuse among intensive case management clients. *Hospital and Community Psychiatry, 42*, 499–503.

Ruegg, R. (1991). The International Catholic Child Bureau and drug abuse: Contributions to drug abuse prevention by a non-government organization concerned with children. *Bulletin on Narcotics, 43*, 9–15.

Safer, D. J., Zito, J. M., & Gardner, J. F. (2000). Trends in pemoline treatment and adverse drug reactions in youths. Presented at the 47th annual Meeting of the American Academy of Child and Adolescent Psychiatry, New York, October 2000.

Sarvela, P. D., Pape, D. J., Odulana, J., et al. (1990). Drinking, drug use, and driving among rural midwestern youth. *Journal of School Health, 60,* 215–219.

Schor, E. L. (1996). Adolescent alcohol use: Social determinants and the case for early family-centered prevention. Family-focused prevention of adolescent drinking. *Bulletin of the New York Academy of Medicine, 73*(2), 335–356.

Schubiner, H., Tzelepis, A., Milberger, S., et al. (2000). Prevalence of attention-deficit/hyperactivity disorder and conduct disorder among substance abusers. *Journal of Clinical Psychiatry, 61*(4), 244–251.

Schwarcz, S. K., Bolan, G. A., Fullilove, M., et al. (1992). Crack cocaine and the exchange of sex for money or drugs: Risk factors for gonorrhea among black adolescents in San Francisco. *Sexually Transmitted Diseases, 19,* 7–13.

Schwartz, R. H. (1998). Adolescent heroin use: A review. *Pediatrics, 102*(6), 1461–1466.

Segal, B. (1990). Comparisons: Alaska and the lower-48 states. In *Drug-taking behavior among school-aged youth: The Alaska experience and comparisons with lower-48 states,* pp. 101–111. Binghamton, NY: Haworth.

Segal, B. M., & Stewart, J. C. (1996). Substance use and abuse in adolescence: An overview. *Child Psychiatry and Human Development, 26*(4), 193.

Seguire, M., & Chalmers, K. I. (2000). Late adolescent female smoking. *Journal of Advanced Nursing, 31*(6), 1422–1429.

Selected tobacco-use behaviors and dietary patterns among high school students—United States, 1991. (1992). *MMWR Morbidity and Mortality Weekly Report, 41,* 417–421.

Shahpar, C., & Li, G. (1999). Homicide mortality in the United States, 1935–1994, age, period, and cohort effects. *American Journal of Epidemiology, 150*(11), 1213–1222.

Shepherd, G., & Klein-Schwartz, W. (1998). Accidental and suicidal adolescent poisoning deaths in the United States, 1979–1994. *Archives of Pediatric and Adolescent Medicine, 152*(12), 1181–1185.

Sherman, D. J. (1992). The neglected health care needs of street youth. *Public Health Reports, 107,* 433–440.

Smart, R. G., Adlaf, E. M., Porterfield, K. M., et al. (1990). *Drugs, youth and the street.* Toronto: Addiction Research Foundation.

Smith, G. S., Branas, C. C., & Miller, T. R. (1999). Fatal nontraffic injuries involving alcohol: A metaanalysis. *Annals of Emergency Medicine, 33*(6), 659–668.

Smith, S. S., & Fiore, M. C. (1999). The epidemiology of tobacco use, dependence, and cessation in the United States. *Primary Care; Clinics in Office Practice, 26*(3), 433–461.

Smoking-attributable mortality and years of potential life lost—United States, 1988. (1991). *MMWR Morbidity and Mortality Weekly Report, 40,* 62–63, 69–71.

Sommers, M. S., Dyehouse, J. M., Howe, S. R., et al. (2000). Attribution of injury to alcohol involvement in young adults seriously injured in alcohol-related motor vehicle crashes. *American Journal of Critical Care, 9*(1), 28–35.

Soueifm, M. I., Darweesh, Z. A., & Taha, H. S. (1985). The non-medical use of prescription psychotropic drugs by school boys in greater Cairo. *Drugs and Alcohol Dependence, 15,* 193–201.

Stone, R. (1992). Bad news on second-hand smoke. *Science, 257,* 607.

Streissguth, A. P., Aase, J. M., Clarren, S. K., et al. (1991). Fetal alcohol syndrome in adolescents and adults. *Journal of the American Medical Association, 265,* 1961–1967.

Sussman, S., & Dent, C. W. (2000). One-year prospective prediction of drug use from stress-related variables. *Substance Use & Misuse, 35*(5), 717–735.

Sussman, S., Dent, C. W., & McCullar, W. J. (2000). Group self-identification as a prospective predictor of drug use and violence in high-risk youth. *Psychology of Addictive Behaviors, 14*(2), 192–196.

Swanson, M. W., Streissguth, A. P., Sampson, P. D., et al. (1999). *Journal of Developmental and Behavioral Pediatrics, 20*(5), 325–334.

Swartz, J. (1991). *Report III: Implications of the drug use forecasting data for TASC programs.* Washington, DC: Bureau of Justice Assistance.

Tapert, S. F., Brown, S. A., Myers, M. G., et al. (1999). The role of neurocognitive abilities in coping with adolescent relapse to alcohol and drug use. *Journal of Studies on Alcohol, 60*(4), 500–508.

Tate, P. S., Freed, D. M., Bombardier, C. H., et al. (1999). Traumatic brain injury: Influence of blood alcohol level on post-acute cognitive function. *Brain Injury, 13*(10), 767–784.

Thompson, K. M., Wonderlich, S. A., Crosby, R. D., et al. (1999). The neglected link between eating disturbances and aggressive behavior in girls. *Journal of the American Academy of Child and Adolescent Psychiatry, 38*(10), 1277–1284.

Tobacco, alcohol, and other drug use among high school students—United States, 1991. (1992). *MMWR Morbidity and Mortality Weekly Report, 41,* 698–703.

Tobacco use among high school students—United States, 1997. (1998). *MMWR Morbidity and Mortality Weekly Report, 47*(12), 229–233.

Tomar, S. L., & Winn, D. M. (1999). Chewing tobacco use and dental caries among U.S. men.

Journal of the American Dental Association, 130(11), 1601–1610.

Tomeo, C. A., Field, A. E., Berkey, C. S., et al. (1999). Weight concerns, weight control behaviors, and smoking initiation. Pediatrics, 104(4, Part 1), 918–924.

Tonnesen, P., Norregaard, J., Simonsen, K., et al. (1991). A double-blind trial of a 16-hour transdermal nicotine patch in smoking cessation. New England Journal of Medicine, 325, 311–315.

Tortu, S., Beardsley, M., Deren, S., et al. (2000). HIV infection and patterns of risk among women drug injectors and crack users in low and high sero-prevalence sites. AIDS Care, 12(1), 65–76.

Tuchtenhagen, F., Daumann, J., Norra, C., et al. (2000). High intensity dependence of auditory evoked dipole source activity indicates decreased serotonergic activity in abstinent ecstasy (MDMA) users. Neuropsychopharmacology, 22(6), 608–617.

Tweed, S. H. (1998). Intervening in adolescent substance abuse. Nursing Clinics of North America, 33(1), 29–45.

Ugnat, A., Mao, Y., Miller, A. B., et al. (1990). Effects of residential exposure to environmental tobacco smoke on Canadian children. Canadian Journal of Public Health, 81, 345–349.

Unintentional opiate overdose deaths—King County, Washington, 1990–1999. (2000). MMWR Morbidity and Mortality Weekly Report, 49(28), 636–640.

United States General Accounting Office: Report to the Chairman, Subcommittee on Labor, Health and Human Services, Education, and Related Agencies, Committee on Appropriations, House of Representatives. (1992, January). Adolescent Drug Use Prevention (pp. 10–20). Common features of promising community programs (GAO/PEMD-92-2).

Van Etten, M. L., & Anthony, J. C. (1999). Comparative epidemiology of initial drug opportunities and transitions to first use: Marijuana, cocaine, hallucinogens and heroin. Drug and Alcohol Dependence, 54, 117–125.

Van Etten, M. L., Neumark, Y. D., & Anthony, J. C. (1999). Male–female differences in the earliest stages of drug involvement. Addiction, 94(9), 1413–1419.

Wahlgren, D. R., Hovell, M. F., Slymen, D. J., et al. (1997). Predictors of tobacco use initiation in adolescents: A two-year prospective study and theoretical discussion. Tobacco Control, 6(2), 95–103.

Walker, A., Rosenberg, M., & Balaban-Gil, K. (1999). Child and Adolescent Psychiatric Clinics of North America, 8(4), 845–867.

Wallace, J. M., Forman, T. A., Guthrie, B. J., et al. (1999). The epidemiology of alcohol, tobacco and other drug use among black youth. Journal of Studies on Alcohol, 60(6), 800–809.

Washington, R. L. (1999). Interventions to reduce cardiovascular risk factors in children and adolescents. American Family Physician, 59(8), 2211–2218.

Wegman, D. H., & Davis, L. K. (1999). Protecting youth at work. American Journal of Industrial Medicine, 36(5), 579–583.

Weil, A. (1983). No bad drugs. Newservice, 1, 22–35.

Weinberg, N. Z., Rahdert, E., Colliver, J. D., et al. (1998). Adolescent substance abuse: A review of the past 10 years. Journal of the American Academy of Child and Adolescent Psychiatry, 37(3), 252–261.

Weir, E. (2000). Raves: A review of the culture, the drugs and the prevention of harm. CMAJ, Canadian Medical Association Journal, 162(13), 1843–1848.

Weitzman, M., Gortmaker, S., Walker, D. K., et al. (1990). Maternal smoking and childhood asthma. Pediatrics, 85, 505–511.

Westermeyer, J. (1999). The role of cultural and social factors in the cause of addictive disorders. Psychiatric Clinics of North America, 22(2), 253–273.

White, H. R. (1997). Longitudinal perspective on alcohol use and aggression during adolescence. Recent Developments in Alcoholism, 13, 81–103.

Wilens, T. E., & Biederman, J. (1993). Psychopathology in preadolescent children at high risk for substance abuse: A review of the literature. Harvard Review of Psychiatry, 1(4), 207–218.

Williams, H., Dratcu, L., Taylor, R., et al. (1998). "Saturday night fever": Ecstasy related problems in a London accident and emergency department. Journal of Accidents and Emergency Medicine, 15(5), 322–326.

Windle, R. C., & Windle, M. (1997). An investigation of adolescents' substance use behaviors, depressed affect, and suicidal behaviors. Journal of Child Psychology and Psychiatry and Allied Disciplines, 38(8), 921–929.

Winkleby, M. A., Robinson, T. N., Sundquist, J., et al. (1999). Ethnic variation in cardiovascular disease risk factors among children and young adults: Findings from the Third National Health and Nutrition Examination Survey, 1988–1994. Journal of the American Medical Association, 281(11), 1006–1013.

Woolf, A. D. (1997). Smoking and nicotine addiction: A pediatric epidemic with sequelae in adulthood. Current Opinion in Pediatrics, 9(5), 470–477.

Yarnold, B. M., & Patterson, V. (1998). Marijuana use among Miami's adolescents, 1992. Journal of Health and Social Policy, 10(1), 65–79.

Yee, B. W., Castro, F. G., Hammond, W. R., et al. (1995). Risk-taking and abusive behaviors among ethnic minorities. Health Psychology, 14(7), 622–631.

Young, S. J., Longstaffe, S., & Tenenbein, M. (1999). Inhalant abuse and the abuse of other drugs. *American Journal of Drug and Alcohol Abuse, 25*(2), 371–375.

Youth and alcohol: Dangerous and deadly consequences. (1992). Washington, DC: Department of Health and Human Services (pp. 1–9).

Youth Tobacco Surveillance—United States, 2000. (2000). Office on Smoking and Health, National Center for Chronic Disease Prevention and Health Promotion (pp. 1–88). American Legacy Foundation, Washington D.C., and CDC Foundation, Atlanta, Georgia. Available: http://www.cdc.gov/mmwr/preview/mmwrhtml/ss5004a1.htm

Zador, P. L., Krawchuk, S. A., & Voas, R. B. (2000). Alcohol-related relative risk of driver fatalities and driver involvement in fatal crashes in relation to driver age and gender: An update using 1996 data. *Journal of Studies on Alcohol, 61*(3), 387–395.

Zickler, P. (2000). NIDA launches initiative to combat club drugs. *NIDA Notes, 14*(6), 1, 5.

Zickler, P. (2001a). Brain imaging studies show long-term damage from methamphetamine abuse. *NIDA Notes, 5*(3), 11, 13.

Zickler, P. (2001b). Gender differences in prevalence of drug abuse traced to opportunities to use. *NIDA Notes, 15*(4), 6–7.

Zickler, P. (2001c). New clinical guidelines describe proven treatments for nicotine addiction. *NIDA Notes, 15*(4), 13.

Intravenous Drugs for Neonates, Infants, Children, and Adolescents: Preparation, Storage, and Administration

Dawn R. Butler, Carla Wallace, Tamara K. Hutson, and John J. Piecoro, Jr.

Preparing, storing, and administering intravenous (IV) drugs to neonates, infants, and children involves several related considerations. These can be divided into intrinsic factors that relate to the effect of the apparatus on drug delivery and extrinsic factors that relate to drug administration procedures (Leff & Roberts, 1992).

General Considerations

Intrinsic factors include equipment and cost considerations. Extrinsic factors affecting drug delivery are the optimal rate and method of drug delivery, drug dilution and fluid volume restrictions required by pediatric patients, and physicochemical properties of IV drugs and fluids that influence administration and storage (e.g., pH, specific gravity, solubility).

Equipment and Cost

Specific equipment (e.g., electronic infusion devices [EID]) may be required for administration of IV drugs. The cost of this equipment can be a limiting factor that affects availability. In choosing the most cost-effective equipment for the administration of IV drugs to infants and children, pediatric clinicians should evaluate both infusion device specifications and reports of problems associated with their use.

The most effective, practical, and safe methods for administering IV drugs are the manual system (antegrade or retrograde addition of a drug into the tubing of an established IV infusion) and the EID. Clinical investigations have shown that the manual system may be used when the drug volume is small, the IV flow rate is slow (<20 ml/hr), or the drug can be administered by IV push. EIDs are preferred when the primary IV flow rate is incompatible with optimal drug delivery (too fast or too slow), the drug volume exceeds the volume of the IV tubing, or the drug, while possible to administer intravenously, cannot be given IV push. Whenever possible, the use of low-volume IV tubing (an intraluminal diameter of 0.06–0.14 cm) and the use of the terminal injection site (the site closest to the patient) should be encouraged to improve the dependability of drug delivery to pediatric patients. To lessen the risk of concentration-dependent phlebitis, the osmolality of the drug should be less than 500 mOsm/kg water.

By using the IV flow rate, drug administration rate, and the osmolalities of both the IV solution and the IV drug, the concentration and osmolality of the final infusate can be calculated. Thus, a maximum drug infusion rate can be determined that will consider these factors and avoid an excessively high osmolality and resultant phlebitis.

Rate and Method of Drug Delivery

Intravenous drugs are administered by rapid or slow IV push or by infusion. Drugs can be administered by **rapid** (less than 30 sec) and **slow** (over 3–5 min) IV push directly into a vein to achieve the desired therapeutic effect. When IV drugs are administered by infusion, they may be administered either intermittently or continuously. **Intermittent infusion** refers to the periodic administration of a drug, often diluted in a small volume of compatible IV solution in a syringe, bag, or bottle, over a period of 10 min to several hours. **Continuous infusion** refers to the IV administration of a drug usually in a large volume of compatible IV solution over 24 hours or longer. (For detailed, specific information on IV drug administration techniques, the reader is referred to Chapter 1.)

Drug Dilution and Fluid Volume Restriction

IV drugs are supplied either in a commercially diluted form ready for use or in a form (e.g., dry, lyophilized powder) that requires reconstitution with a compatible diluent prior to use. Some drugs may require further dilution prior to their IV injection or infusion. The type and volume of IV solution required and the ability of a neonate, infant, or child to tolerate the required solution are important considerations. Some drugs (e.g., acetylcysteine, amphotericin B lipid complex) may be diluted only in dextrose 5% in water (D_5W) for infusion. However, patients who are severely hyperglycemic may not be able to tolerate the dextrose load. Other drugs, such as vidarabine, must be diluted in a particular volume of solution to ensure dissolution. However, pediatric patients with the syndrome of inappropriate antidiuretic hormone (SIADH) may not tolerate the additional volume needed to properly dilute and administer the drug. In addition, neonates with compromised respiratory function may require fluid restriction. Fluid balance regulating mechanisms may be immature, particularly in children younger than 2 years.

Physicochemical Properties: pH Adjustment and Specific Gravity

The pH of IV drugs has been implicated as a contributing factor in phlebitis. Adjustment of the pH to a near physiologic level (7.4) may decrease the incidence of phlebitis. The specific gravity of the reconstituted drug may affect the rate of drug delivery. If the specific gravity of an IV solution and a drug solution differ significantly, the drug solution may "layer out" within the IV tubing, thereby altering the drug infusion time. The specific gravity can be predicted in a manner similar to that used for osmolality.

Skills and Training of Pediatric Clinicians

Most IV drugs can be safely administered by nurses. However, there are certain drugs that can cause acute life-threatening adverse drug reactions (ADRs) upon administration and, thus, warrant administration by a pediatric clinician with specialized education and training. For a small number of drugs that have a much greater than normal chance to induce life-threatening effects, administration by physicians only is required by policy in some institutions. Physicians are often guided by specific protocols and procedures for medication administration that may vary regionally and from institution to institution. Pediatric clinicians must maintain their current skills and training in the administration of IV drugs and know their limits of practice while striving to promote optimal drug therapy for their patients.

Summary

IV drug therapy is often required during childhood for the treatment of disease and the promotion of health. This chapter identifies important considerations for pediatric clinicians and presents in Table 8-1 the major factors that require consideration when drugs are administered intravenously to neonates, infants, or children. These factors include information regarding dosage form availability (commercial dilution versus lyophilized powder), requirements for further dilution before administration, storage and stability information, recommendations for IV injection and infusion rate, and compatible infusion solutions. The information in this chapter will enable pediatric clinicians to optimize therapy and minimize adverse effects to neonates, infants, and children by safely preparing, storing, and administering drugs.

(Table begins on page 390.)

TABLE 8-1
Intravenous Drug Administration Guidelines for Infants and Children

DRUG[a,b] (TRADE NAME)	COMMERCIAL DILUTION OR RECONSTITUTION AND pH[c]	METHOD OF ADMINISTRATION, FURTHER DILUTION, AND RECOMMENDED RATE OF INFUSION[d]	COMPATIBLE INFUSION SOLUTIONS[e]	CAUTIONS, COMMENTS, AND INCOMPATIBILITIES[f,g,h]	REFERENCES[i]
Acetazolamide Sodium (*Diamox®*)	Reconstitute with sterile water for injection to yield 100 mg/ml. Stable for 3 days under refrigeration, but recommend using within 24 hr of reconstitution due to lack of preservatives. pH: 9.2	**IV push (preferred):** Inject without further dilution over 60 sec. *Maximum rate:* 500 mg/min. **Intermittent infusion:** Infuse without further dilution, or further dilute as desired, and infuse over 15–60 min. **Continuous infusion:** Dilute as desired and infuse over 24 hr. *Maximum concentration:* 100 mg/ml.	D_5W $D_{10}W$ D_5W/LR Dextran 6%/ D_5W or NS Dextrose/ saline combinations LR NS R	Observe for anorexia, crystalluria, dysuria, electrolyte disturbances, GI irritation, headache, paresthesias, and weakness. Incompatible with total parenteral (TPN) solution. Avoid IM route because of pain associated with alkaline pH.	Gura 1999 Hebel 1999 McEvoy 2001 Trissel 2001
Acetylcysteine (*Mucomyst®*)	Available as 200 mg/ml pH: 6–7.5	**Continuous infusion:** Dilute to 50 mg/ml with D_5W and infuse loading dose over 15 min, then dilute to >1.3 mg/ml with D_5W, and infuse dose over 20 hr.	D_5W	May cause nausea, vomiting, and other GI symptoms. Hypersensitivity reactions (bronchospasm, facial edema, hypotension, rashes, urticaria) may occur. Injectable form is not commercially available in the U.S.	Bailey 1998 Reynolds 1993
Acyclovir Sodium (*Zovirax®*)	Reconstitute powder for injection with sterile water for injection to yield 50 mg/ml. pH: 10.5–11.6	**Intermittent infusion:** Dilute to <7 mg/ml and infuse over 60 min. Dilutions should be used within 24 hr. Solutions up to 10 mg/ml have been administered to fluid-restricted patients through a central line.	D_5W D_5W Dextrose/ saline combinations LR NS	Rapid IV injection is associated with crystalluria, elevation in serum creatinine, and renal tubular damage. Extravasation may cause inflammation and phlebitis. Incompatible with amifostine and ondansetron. Incompatible with blood products and solutions containing protein. Do not admix with other drugs. A yellowish discoloration may occur if diluted with >10% dextrose, but this does not affect potency.	Gura 1999 McEvoy 2001 Taketomo 2000 Trissel 2001
Adenosine (*Adenocard®*)	Available as 3 mg/ml (2-ml vials) Do not refrigerate because crystallization may occur. pH: 5.5–7.5	**IV push:** Inject without further dilution over 1–2 sec at closest injection site to patient, preferably a peripheral line. Follow immediately with a saline flush. Doses <600 μg, dilute with NS to 300 μg/ml.	NS	Observe for asystole, dysrhythmias, or flushing (may last a few seconds). May also cause heart block and bradycardia, may exacerbate asthma. Administer to patient with ECG monitoring. Do not admix with any other drugs.	Gura 1999 Hebel 1999 Phelps 1996 Taketomo 2000
Albumin [Normal Human Serum Albumin]	Available as 50 mg/ml (5%) and 250 mg/ml (25%). Use within 4 hr of opening vial. pH: 6.4–7.4	**IV push (slow):** Dilute as desired, inject at 0.05–0.1 gram/min. If blood volume is greater than normal, inject slowly (1 ml/min of 25% solution or 2–4 ml/min of 5% solution).	D_5W $D_{10}W$ Dextrose/ saline combinations	Observe for chills, fever, hypotension, nausea, rash, and vomiting. Rapid infusion may cause vascular overload. Do not infuse if solution is turbid. Avoid 25% in preterm neonates due to risk of intraventricular hemorrhage. If	Gura 1999 Hebel 1999 McEvoy 2001 Trissel 2001

---

[a] Approved clinical protocols are generally the most recent and best guidelines for administering antineoplastic drugs to infants and children. *See* Chapter 12.

[b] Solutions containing benzyl alcohol are contraindicated in neonates because of association with convulsions, hypotension, intracranial hemorrhage, metabolic acidosis, respiratory distress, and possibly death (Gershanik et al., 1982).

[c] The pH values provided correspond to those of commercially diluted solutions or to the dry products after reconstitution with the recommended diluents.

[d] The method of administration, dilution, and rate of infusion are predicated on the condition of the infant or child and should always be guided by individual response.

[e] More detailed compatibility information is provided in the *Handbook on Injectable Drugs*, published by the American Society of Health-System Pharmacists (Trissel, 2001).

[f] For additional detailed information on cautions and adverse drug reactions, the reader is referred to the dosing chapters (Chapters 12, 13, and 14) and to the adverse drug reaction chapter (Chapter 5).

[g] Generally, drugs with a low (acidic) pH are **not** physically compatible with drugs with a high (alkaline) pH; sodium or potassium salts are **not** compatible with hydrochloride or sulfate salts.

[h] Solutions containing propylene glycol and other glycols may cause vasodilation and with rapid administration lower blood pressure.

[i] Only the first author and year of publication are provided in the table. For complete reference citations, *see* References.

TABLE 8-1 continued

DRUG[a,b] (TRADE NAME)	COMMERCIAL DILUTION OR RECONSTITUTION AND pH[c]	METHOD OF ADMINISTRATION, FURTHER DILUTION, AND RECOMMENDED RATE OF INFUSION[d]	COMPATIBLE INFUSION SOLUTIONS[e]	CAUTIONS, COMMENTS, AND INCOMPATIBILITIES[f,g,h]	REFERENCES[i]
Albumin *continued*			NR 1/2 NS NS R TPN	diluting 25% to 5%, use NS or D_5W as diluent. Do not use sterile water. 5% albumin = 300 mOsm/liter, 25% albumin = 1500 mOsm/liter; sodium content 130–160 mEq/liter.	
Albuterol [Salbutamol] *(Ventolin®)*	Available as 0.5 mg/ml pH: 3.5	**IV push:** Inject without further dilution over 5–10 min. **Continuous infusion:** Infuse at 5 µg/min.	D_5W NS	Monitor blood pressure, ECG, glucose, heart rate, and potassium serum concentrations during IV infusion. Monitor hepatic and renal function. Injectable form is not commercially available in the U.S.	Repchinsky 2002
Alprostadil [Prostaglandin E_1] *(Prostin VR Pediatric®)*	Available as 500 µg/ml in anhydrous ethanol Keep refrigerated. pH: Information not available	**Continuous infusion:** Dilute to 2–20 µg/ml. **Usual rate of infusion:** 0.05–0.1 µg/kg/min (range 0.01–0.4 µg/kg/min). Dilution stable for 24 hr.	D_5W NS	Dilute prior to administration. Monitor respiratory and cardiac status because apnea and hypotension are common. Extravasation may cause tissue sloughing and necrosis because of the drug's high osmolality (330–920 mOsm/kg).	Gura 1999 Phelps 1996 Taketomo 2000
Alteplase *(Ativase®)*	Reconstitute powder for injection with sterile water for injection to yield 1 mg/ml. Do not use bacteriostatic water for injection. Use within 8 hr. pH: 7.3	**Intermittent infusion:** Dilute to ≥0.5 mg/ml in D_5W or NS. Concentrations <0.5 mg/ml may precipitate.	D_5W NS (preferred)	Avoid extravasation. Monitor bleeding from venipuncture sites, blood pressure, and bruising. Do not shake. Use controlled infusion device. Incompatible with dobutamine, dopamine, heparin, and nitroglycerin. 50 mg = 29 million IU.	Gura 1999 McEvoy 2001 Trissel 2001
Amifostine *(Ethyol®)*	Reconstitute powder for injection with NS for injection to yield 50 mg/ml. pH: 7	**Intermittent infusion:** Dilute to 5–40 mg/ml with NS and infuse over 15 min, 30 min prior to chemotherapy. Reconstituted solutions and solutions diluted in NS are stable for 5 hr at room temperature and 24 hr refrigerated.	NS	Keep patients supine during infusion. Monitor blood pressure every 3–5 min during infusion. If hypotension develops, stop infusion. Do not prolong infusion as this worsens side effects. Patients should be well hydrated prior to infusion. Incompatible with acyclovir, amphotericin B, chlorpromazine, cisplatin, ganciclovir, hydroxyzine, and prochlorperazine.	McEvoy 2001 Taketomo 2000 Trissel 2001
Amikacin Sulfate *(Amikin®)*	Available as 50 and 250 mg/ml pH: 3.5–5.5	**IV push:** Inject without further dilution over 2–5 min (not preferred because associated with high peak serum concentrations). **Intermittent infusion (preferred):** Dilute to at least 5–10 mg/ml; infuse over 30–60 min. 5 mg/ml stable 24 hr at room temperature.	D_5W $D_{10}W$ D_5W/1/2 NS D_5W/NS LR Mannitol 20% 1/2 NS NS	Observe for hypersensitivity reactions, possible ototoxicity, and renal toxicity. Inactivated by penicillins, so should not be administered within 1 hr of IV penicillin.	Gura 1999 McEvoy 2001 Sifton 2002 Taketomo 2000 Trissel 2001
Aminocaproic Acid *(Amicar®)*	Available as 250 mg/ml pH: 6–7.6	**Continuous infusion:** Dilute as desired (maximum concentration 20 mg/ml), infuse at initial rate of 100 mg/kg (3 grams/m²) during first hour, then 33.3 mg/kg/hr (1 gram/m²/hr) (total dose not to exceed 18 grams/m²/24 hr).	D_5W D_5W/NS NS R	Observe for bradycardia, cardiac dysrhythmias, and hypotension. Incompatible with fructose infusion solutions.	McEvoy 2001 Taketomo 2000 Trissel 2001
Aminophylline [Theophylline Ethylene Diamine]	Available as 25 mg/ml pH: 8.6–9.0	**Intermittent infusion:** Dilute with at least an equal volume of IV solution, and infuse over 20–30 min. **Continuous infusion:** Dilute with at least an equal volume of IV solution and adjust infusion rate according to drug serum concentrations. Do not administer by continuous infusion to neonates.	D_5W D_5W/1/2 NS D_5W/NS LR NS R	Observe for cardiac dysrhythmias, hypertension, and sinus tachycardia. Incompatible with alkali-labile drugs (erythromycin, penicillin G).	Gura 1999 Hebel 1999 McEvoy 2001 Phelps 1996 Reynolds 1993 Taketomo 2000 Trissel 2001

Footnotes are on page 390.

TABLE 8-1 continued

DRUG[a,b] (TRADE NAME)	COMMERCIAL DILUTION OR RECONSTITUTION AND pH[c]	METHOD OF ADMINISTRATION, FURTHER DILUTION, AND RECOMMENDED RATE OF INFUSION[d]	COMPATIBLE INFUSION SOLUTIONS[e]	CAUTIONS, COMMENTS, AND INCOMPATIBILITIES[f,g,h]	REFER- ENCES[i]
Amiodarone (*Cordarone®*)	Available as 50 mg/ml pH: 4	Divide loading dose into approximately five doses and inject each over 5–10 min at 1–6 mg/ml. May repeat doses every 30 min as needed.	D_5W	Infusions of greater than 2 hr should be dispensed in glass bottles. Use an in-line filter. Concentrations greater than 2 mg/ml must be administered via a central venous line. Inhibitor of cytochrome P-450, therefore use with caution with other drugs metabolized by it.	Gura 1999 Taketomo 2000 Trissel 2001
Ammonium Chloride (Abbott)	Available as 265 mg/ml (5 mEq/ml) pH: 4–6	**Intermittent infusion:** Dilute to 1 mEq/5 ml and infuse at <1 mEq/kg/hr (52 mg/kg/hr) over a minimum of 3 hr. *Maximum concentration:* 0.4 mEq/ml.	$D_{2.5}W$ D_5W $D_{10}W$ D_5W/LR Dextran 6% Dextrose/ saline combinations LR 1/2 NS NS	Observe for apnea, bradycardia, confusion, dysrhythmias, hyperventilation, irregular breathing, metabolic acidosis (from increased chloride), pain, phlebitis, and rash. Incompatible with most drugs. Avoid rapid IV administration, which may cause ammonia toxicity. Solutions may precipitate at cold temperatures.	Gura 1999 McEvoy 2001 Taketomo 2000 Trissel 2001
Amphotericin B (*Fungizone®*)	Reconstitute lyophilized powder for injection with sterile water for injection (without preservatives) to yield 5 mg/ml. Reconstituted solutions are stable 24 hr at room temperature and 1 week refrigerated. pH: 5.7	**Intermittent infusion:** Dilute to <0.1 mg/ml in D_5W only and infuse over 2–6 hr (1–2-hr infusion is also well tolerated). An in-line filter (>1 μm mean pore diameter) may be used. 0.5 mg/ml has been administered to fluid-restricted patients through a central line.	D_5W preferred Solutions of $D_{10}W$ up to $D_{20}W$ have been used.	Observe for chills, fever, phlebitis, renal toxicity (can decrease renal toxicity by salt loading with 10 ml/kg NS), and phlebitis. Monitor electrolyte serum concentrations and blood pressure. Benzyl alcohol, sodium chloride, and other electrolyte solutions may cause precipitation. Compatible with heparin sodium and hydrocortisone. Incompatible with total parenteral nutrition (TPN) and lipids, amifostine, amikacin, cefepime, chlorpromazine, diphenhydramine, dopamine, meropenem, penicillin, and ranitidine. Exposure to light <24 hr does not appreciably affect potency. Pretreat with acetaminophen and/or diphenhydramine 30–60 min prior to administration.	Gura 1999 McEvoy 2001 Taketomo 2000 Trissel 2001
Amphotericin B Lipid Complex (*Abelcet®*)	Available as 5 mg/ml refrigerated suspension. Diluted solutions stable up to 48 hr refrigerated. pH: 5–7	**Intermittent infusion:** Dilute to 1 mg/ml with D_5W and infuse at a maximum rate of 2.5 mg/kg/hr. Do not use <5-μm filter. In fluid-restricted patients, 2 mg/ml has been used.	D_5W	Management of side effects similar to amphotericin B. If infusion time exceeds 2 hr, mix contents by rotating infusion bag. Do not mix with saline or electrolyte solutions. Incompatible with TPN.	Gura 1999 McEvoy 2001 Taketomo 2000
Amphotericin B Liposome (*AmBisome®*)	Reconstitute powder for injection with sterile water to yield 4 mg/ml. Stable for 72 hr at room temperature when diluted with $D_{10}W$ or $D_{20}W$. Stable in D_5W for 14 days when refrigerated. pH: 5–6	**Intermittent infusion:** Dilute to 0.5–2.2 mg/ml and infuse over 2 hr. Do not use in-line filters of <1-μm mean pore diameter.	D_5W $D_{10}W$ $D_{20}W$	Management of side effects similar to amphotericin B. Do not mix with saline or electrolyte solutions. Incompatible with TPN.	McEvoy 2001 Taketomo 2000
Ampicillin Sodium	Reconstitute powder for injection with sterile or bacteriostatic water for injection to yield 100 mg/ml. pH: 8–10	**IV push (slow):** Dilute to 100 mg/ml and infuse no faster than 100 mg/min (may dilute in sterile water for injection up to 200 mg/ml). **Intermittent infusion (preferred):** Dilute to <30 mg/ml with compatible diluent and	$D_5W/1/4$ NS $D_5W/1/2$ NS LR NS	Observe for hypersensitivity reactions. Stability is greatly decreased in highly concentrated dextrose solutions. Generally avoid admixing with other drugs; administer at least 1 hr before or after IV aminoglycosides because ampicillin can inactivate the aminoglycoside.	Gura 1999 Hebel 1999 McEvoy 2001 Phelps 1996 Sifton 2002

TABLE 8-1 *continued*

DRUG[a,b] (TRADE NAME)	COMMERCIAL DILUTION OR RECONSTITUTION AND pH[c]	METHOD OF ADMINISTRATION, FURTHER DILUTION, AND RECOMMENDED RATE OF INFUSION[d]	COMPATIBLE INFUSION SOLUTIONS[e]	CAUTIONS, COMMENTS, AND INCOMPATIBILITIES[f,g,h]	REFERENCES[i]
Ampicillin Sodium *continued*		infuse diluted solution over 10–15 min. Solutions >30 mg/ml must be used within 1 hr after reconstitution.			Taketomo 2000 Trissel 2001
Ampicillin–Sulbactam (*Unasyn®*)	Reconstitute powder for injection with sterile water for injection to yield 100 mg/ml (ampicillin). pH: 8–10	**IV push:** Dilute to <30 mg/ml (ampicillin) and inject over 10–15 min. **Intermittent infusion:** Dilute as for IV push and infuse over 15–30 min.	D_5W D_5W/1/2 NS LR NS	Observe for diarrhea, phlebitis, pseudomembranous colitis, and rash. 3-gram vial contains 2 grams ampicillin and 1 gram sulbactam; 1.5-gram vial contains 1 gram ampicillin and 500 mg sulbactam. Administer at least 1 hr before or after IV aminoglycosides because ampicillin can inactivate the aminoglycoside. Concentrated dextrose solutions can decrease ampicillin stability. Compatible with famotidine.	McEvoy 2001 Taketomo 2000 Trissel 2001
Amsacrine (*AMSA P-D®*)	Mix 1.5-ml ampule with provided diluent (lactic acid) to yield 5 mg/ml. This mixture is stable for 24 hr at room temperature or 72 hr refrigerated when protected from direct exposure to sunlight. pH: Information not available	**Intermittent infusion:** Further dilute in 500 ml and infuse over 1–2 hr. Stable up to 7 days in glass or Abbott plastic.	D_5W	Chemotherapy precautions are required when handling. Myelosuppression is dose limiting, and phlebitis is common. Incompatible with NS and other chloride-containing solutions. Incompatible with acyclovir, amphotericin B, aztreonam, ceftazidime, ceftriaxone, cimetidine, furosemide, ganciclovir, heparin, methylprednisolone, and metoclopramide.	Repchinsky 2002 Reynolds 1993
Asparaginase (*Elspar®, Kidrolase®*)	Reconstitute powder for injection with sterile water or NS for injection to yield 2000 units/ml. Refrigerate reconstituted solutions and discard after 8 hr. pH: 7.4	**Intermittent infusion:** Dilute further and infuse over a minimum of 30 min into free-flowing solutions.	D_5W NS	Skin test prior to initial dose and when a week or more has elapsed between doses. Observe for hypersensitivity reactions. Appropriate agents to treat an anaphylactoid reaction should be readily available. May use a 5-μm filter during administration.	McEvoy 2001 Taketomo 2000 Trissel 2001
Atracurium Besylate	Available as 10 mg/ml Keep refrigerated. Stable at room temperature for 14 days. pH: 3.25–3.65	**IV push:** Inject rapidly without further dilution. (Too slow injection may result in bradycardia.) **Continuous infusion:** Usual dilution for infusion is 0.2–0.5 mg/ml.	D_5W D_5W/NS NS	Rarely, mild histamine response seen. This drug is a paralyzing agent and should be administered by clinicians trained in airway management. Avoid IM injection due to tissue irritation. Do not mix with alkaline solutions. Does not alter level of consciousness; therefore, addition of sedation and/or analgesia is recommended.	Gura 1999 McEvoy 2001 Phelps 1996 Taketomo 2000 Trissel 2001
Atropine Sulfate	Available as 0.1, 0.4, and 1 mg/ml pH: 3–6.5	**IV push:** Inject without further dilution over 1 min.	D_5W $D_{10}W$ D_5W/1/2 NS D_5W/NS LR NS	Slow infusion can cause paradoxical bradycardia; not recommended for neonates because of risk of paradoxical bradycardia. Monitor for confusion, fever, sinus tachycardia, and urinary retention. Incompatible with norepinephrine and sodium bicarbonate.	Gura 1999 McEvoy 2001 Phelps 1996 Taketomo 2000 Trissel 2001
Azathioprine Sodium (*Imuran®*)	Reconstitute with sterile water for injection to yield 10 mg/ml. Stable 2 weeks at room temperature, but	**IV push:** Inject without further dilution over 5 min. **Intermittent infusion:** Dilute to <10 mg/ml and infuse over 15–60 min.	D_5W NS	Observe for fever, nausea, rash, and vomiting. Rare hypersensitivity reaction can occur. Dose-limiting ADR is bone marrow suppression.	Gura 1999 McEvoy 2001 Taketomo 2000 Trissel 2001

(Continued)

Footnotes are on page 390.

TABLE 8-1 continued

DRUG[a,b] (TRADE NAME)	COMMERCIAL DILUTION OR RECONSTITUTION AND pH[c]	METHOD OF ADMINISTRATION, FURTHER DILUTION, AND RECOMMENDED RATE OF INFUSION[d]	COMPATIBLE INFUSION SOLUTIONS[e]	CAUTIONS, COMMENTS, AND INCOMPATIBILITIES[f,g,h]	REFERENCES[i]
Azathioprine Sodium *continued*	since product does not contain preservatives, recommend using within 24 hr of reconstitution. pH: 9.6				
Azithromycin *(Zithromax®)*	Reconstitute powder for injection with sterile water for injection to yield 100 mg/ml. pH: 6.4–6.6	Further dilute to 2 mg/ml with a compatible IV solution. Infuse over 1 hr. Do not administer IV push. 2-mg/ml solutions are stable for 24 hr at room temperature and 7 days at 5°C.	D_5W D_5W/LR D_5W/1/3 NS D_5W/1/2 NS D_5W/1/2 NS + 20 mEq KCl LR Normosol® solutions 1/2 NS NS	Patients who experience allergic reactions to azithromycin may require prolonged periods of observation and symptomatic treatment due to the drug's long tissue half-life. Do not administer to patients receiving cisapride.	Gura 1999 McEvoy 2001 Taketomo 2000
Aztreonam *(Azactam®)*	Available as 20 and 40 mg/ml (frozen) **or** reconstitute powder for injection with sterile water for injection to yield 200 mg/ml; reconstituted solution stable 48 hr at room temperature and 7 days refrigerated. pH: 4.5–7.5	**IV push:** Inject over 3–5 min directly into vein or tubing of a patent IV infusion. *Maximum concentration:* 66 mg/ml. **Intermittent infusion:** Dilute to 5–20 mg/ml and infuse over 20–60 min.	D_5W $D_{10}W$ D_5W/LR Dextrose/ saline combinations NS R Sodium lactate 1/6 M	Observe for allergic reactions, discomfort at injection site, phlebitis, and thrombophlebitis. Frozen solutions are iso-osmotic.	McEvoy 2001 Taketomo 2000
Bleomycin Sulfate[a] *(Blenoxane®)*	Reconstitute powder for injection with NS for injection to yield 3 units/ml. Reconstituted solutions stable for 24 hr at room temperature. pH: 4.5–6	**IV push:** Dilute if desired to <3 units/ml and inject slowly over 10 min. *Maximum:* 1 unit/min **Intermittent infusion:** Dilute with 50–100 ml D_5W or NS (preferred) and infuse over 10–30 min.	D_5W NS	A 1-unit test dose is recommended for lymphoma patients for the first two doses to assess for possible hypersensitivity. Pulmonary toxicity has occurred at a total dose of 100 units/m² in young patients. Observe for anaphylactic reactions, cough, leukopenia, phlebitis, rash, shortness of breath, stomatitis, thrombocytopenia, and wheezing. Monitor vital signs every 15 min. Compatible with most chemotherapeutic agents.	McEvoy 2001 Taketomo 2000 Trissel 2001
Bumetanide	Available as 0.25 mg/ml pH: 6.8–7.8	**IV push:** Inject without further dilution over 1–2 min. **Intermittent infusion:** Dilute as desired and infuse over 10 min.	D_5W LR NS	Observe for dizziness, hyperglycemia, hypotension, nausea, vomiting, and weakness. Monitor creatinine, chloride, potassium, and uric acid serum concentrations. May alter hepatic function tests. Use with caution in patients with sulfa allergies as cross-hypersensitivity may occur. Contains benzyl alcohol. Protect from light.	Gura 1999 Phelps 1996 Taketomo 2000 Trissel 2001
Caffeine Citrate *(Cafcit®)*	Available as 10 mg/ml pH: 3–4	**Intermittent infusion:** Dilute with at least an equal volume of IV solution and infuse over 20–30 min.	D_5W $D_{10}W$	Observe for cardiac dysrhythmias, including sinus tachycardia and hypertension during administration. Do not use commercially available caffeine/sodium benzoate for pediatric patients and neonates.	Gershanik 1982 Nahata 1987 Wojtynek 1999

TABLE 8-1 continued

DRUG[a,b] (TRADE NAME)	COMMERCIAL DILUTION OR RECONSTITUTION AND pH[c]	METHOD OF ADMINISTRATION, FURTHER DILUTION, AND RECOMMENDED RATE OF INFUSION[d]	COMPATIBLE INFUSION SOLUTIONS[e]	CAUTIONS, COMMENTS, AND INCOMPATIBILITIES[f,g,h]	REFER- ENCES[i]
Calcium Chloride	Available as 100 mg/ml (1.36 mEq/ml elemental calcium) pH: 6.5–8	**IV push:** Inject no faster than 1 ml/min (100 mg/min). **Intermittent infusion:** Dilute to ≤20 mg/ml and infuse over at least 30 min. **Continuous infusion:** Dilute to ≤20 mg/ml and infuse over 24 hr (adjust infusion rate according to calcium serum concentration).	D_5W $D_{10}W$ $D_5W/1/3$ NS $D_5W/1/2$ NS D_5W/NS LR	Administer through a small-bore needle into a large vein. Rapid IV administration may cause bradycardia, hypotension, and vasodilation. Extravasation may cause local tissue necrosis. Monitor ionized calcium in neonates, critically ill infants, and children. Do not admix with bicarbonates, catecholamines, or phosphates. Do not use small scalp veins or small hand and foot veins due to risk of extravasation.	Gura 1999 McEvoy 2001 Phelps 1996 Taketomo 2000 Trissel 2001
Calcium Gluconate	Available as 100 mg/ml (0.46 mEq/ml elemental calcium) pH: 6–8.2	**IV push:** Inject without further dilution no faster than 100 mg/min. **Intermittent infusion:** Dilute to <50 mg/ml and infuse over at least 30 min. **Continuous infusion (preferred):** Dilute to <50 mg/ml and infuse over 24 hr if possible (adjust infusion rate according to calcium serum concentration).	D_5W $D_{10}W$ Dextrose/ saline combina- tions LR	Observe for bradycardia, cardiac dysrhythmias, and hypotension. Extravasation may cause necrosis and sloughing. Do not infuse through scalp vein in infants. Use caution when infusing with TPN due to the possibility of precipitation with phosphate in TPN.	Hebel 1999 McEvoy 2001 Phelps 1996 Taketomo 2000 Trissel 2001
Carboplatin[a] *(Paraplatin®, Paraplatin-AQ®)*	Reconstitute powder for injection with sterile water for injection, D_5W, or NS to yield 10 mg/ml. Reconstituted solution stable for 8 hr at room temperature. pH: 5–7	**Intermittent infusion:** Dilute to 0.5–2 mg/ml with D_5W or NS and infuse over 15–60 min. Diluted solutions of 2 mg/ml stable for 24 hr under refrigeration.	D_5W $D_5W/1/4$ NS $D_5W/1/2$ NS D_5W/NS NS	Observe for alopecia, anemia, leukopenia, nausea, nephrotoxicity, neutropenia, ototoxicity, peripheral neuropathy, rash, thrombocytopenia, and vomiting. Monitor calcium and magnesium serum concentrations. Avoid contact with aluminum. Incompatible with fluorouracil and mesna.	McEvoy 2001 Taketomo 2000 Trissel 2001
Carmustine[a] *(BiCNU®)*	Reconstitute powder for injection with absolute ethyl alcohol and sterile water for injection to yield 3.3 mg/ml in 10% ethyl alcohol. When in glass and protected from light, reconstituted solutions are stable for 8 hr at room temperature and 24 hr refrigerated. pH: 5.6–6	**Intermittent infusion:** Dilute to 0.2–1 mg/ml with D_5W or NS and infuse over 1–2 hr. Dilutions to 0.2 mg/ml in D_5W or NS are stable for 48 hr refrigerated in glass and protected from light and for 8 hr at room temperature in regular light.	D_5W NS	Observe for dermatitis, flushing, hepatotoxicity, myelosuppression, nausea, pulmonary fibrosis, renal failure, thrombophlebitis, and vomiting. Avoid contact with skin. Administration over <1 hr may cause phlebitis and flushing. Use glass bottles (avoid plastic). Protect from light. Incompatible with allopurinol and sodium bicarbonate.	McEvoy 2001 Taketomo 2000 Trissel 2001
Cefamandole Nafate *(Mandol®)*	Reconstitute powder for injection with sterile water for injection, NS, or D_5W to yield 100 mg/ml. pH: 6–8.5	**IV push:** Inject without further dilution over 3–5 min. **Intermittent infusion (preferred):** Dilute to 20 mg/ml and infuse over 30–60 min. 20- and 100-mg/ml solutions stable 24 hr at room temperature and 96 hr at 4–8°C.	D_5W $D_{10}W$ Dextrose/ saline combina- tions NS Sodium lactate 1/6 M	Observe for vein irritation. Do not use in neonates. Use cautiously in penicillin-sensitive patients. Do not admix with other drugs. Contains N-methyltetrazolethiol side chain that may be responsible for certain hematologic adverse effects.	McEvoy 2001 Phelps 1996 Sifton 2002 Trissel 2001

Footnotes are on page 390.

TABLE 8-1 continued

DRUG[a,b] (TRADE NAME)	COMMERCIAL DILUTION OR RECONSTITUTION AND pH[c]	METHOD OF ADMINISTRATION, FURTHER DILUTION, AND RECOMMENDED RATE OF INFUSION[d]	COMPATIBLE INFUSION SOLUTIONS[e]	CAUTIONS, COMMENTS, AND INCOMPATIBILITIES[f,g,h]	REFERENCES[i]
Cefazolin Sodium (Ancef®, Kefzol®)	Reconstitute powder for injection with sterile water for injection, bacteriostatic water for injection, or NS to yield 100 mg/ml. Reconstituted solutions stable 24 hr at room temperature and 96 hr at 4–8°C. pH: 4.8–6	**IV push:** Dilute to 50–100 mg/ml and inject over 3–5 min. **Intermittent infusion (preferred):** Dilute to 20 mg/ml and infuse over 10–60 min.	D_5W $D_{10}W$ Dextrose/saline combinations LR NS TPN	Observe for phlebitis. Do not admix with other drugs.	Gura 1999 McEvoy 2001 Phelps 1996 Sifton 2002 Taketomo 2000 Trissel 2001
Cefepime Hydrochloride (Maxipime®)	Reconstitute powder for injection with sterile water for injection, NS, or D_5W to yield 100 mg/ml. pH: 4–6	**Intermittent infusion:** Dilute to 1–40 mg/ml and infuse over 30 min. 1–40-mg/ml solutions stable 24 hr at room temperature and 7 days refrigerated at 2–8°C in compatible IV solution.	D_5LR D_5W $D_{10}W$ Dextrose/saline combinations Normosol solutions Sodium lactate 1/6 M	Administer separately from aminoglycosides, ampicillin (>40 mg/ml), metronidazole, and vancomycin. May cause pain/phlebitis, rash.	Gura 1999 McEvoy 2001 Taketomo 2000 Trissel 2001
Cefoperazone Sodium (Cefobid®)	Reconstitute powder for injection with D_5W, dextrose/saline combinations, or NS to yield 100 mg/ml. pH: 4.5–6.5	**Intermittent infusion:** Dilute to 50 mg/ml with suitable IV solution and infuse over 15–60 min. **Continuous infusion:** Dilute to 2–25 mg/ml and infuse over 24 hr. 2–300-mg/ml solutions stable 24 hr at room temperature or 5 days at 2–8°C.	D_5W $D_{10}W$ D_5W/LR Dextrose/saline combinations LR Normosol solutions NS	Observe for vein irritation. Use cautiously in penicillin-sensitive patients. Do not admix with other drugs. Contains N-methyltetrazolethiol side chain that may be responsible for certain hematologic adverse effects	McEvoy 2001 Phelps 1996 Sifton 2002 Trissel 2001
Cefotaxime Sodium (Claforan®)	Reconstitute powder for injection with sterile water for injection to yield 100 mg/ml. pH: 4.5–6.5	**IV push:** Dilute to <100 mg/ml and inject over 3–5 min. **Intermittent infusion:** Dilute as for IV push and infuse over 15–30 min. Solutions <100 mg/ml are stable 24 hr at room temperature and 5 days refrigerated at 5°C or lower.	D_5W $D_{10}W$ $D_5W/1/4$ NS $D_5W/1/2$ NS D_5W/NS LR NS	Observe for diarrhea, fever, headache, nausea, phlebitis, rash, thrombocytopenia, and vomiting. Do not admix with alkaline solutions, aminoglycosides, or aminophylline.	Gura 1999 Hebel 1999 McEvoy 2001 Phelps 1996 Sifton 2002 Taketomo 2000 Trissel 2001
Cefoxitin Sodium (Mefoxin®)	Reconstitute powder for injection with sterile water for injection to yield 100 mg/ml. 100-mg/ml solution stable 24 hr at room temperature and 7 days refrigerated at <5°C. pH: 4.2–8	**IV push:** Inject without further dilution over 3–5 min. **Intermittent infusion (preferred):** Dilute to <20 mg/ml and infuse over 10–60 min. *Maximum concentration:* 40 mg/ml.	D_5W $D_{10}W$ Dextrose/saline combinations LR NS	Observe for phlebitis. Not recommended for infants <3 months of age. Do not admix with aminoglycosides. Stability is decreased when admixed with alkaline solutions.	McEvoy 2001 Phelps 1996 Sifton 2002 Trissel 2001
Ceftazidime (Ceptaz®, Fortaz®, Tazicef®, Tazidime®)	Reconstitute powder for injection with sterile water for injection or bacteriostatic water for injection to yield 100 or 200 mg/ml.	**IV push:** Dilute to <100 mg/ml and inject over 3–5 min. **Intermittent infusion:** Dilute to <40 mg/ml and infuse over 15–30 min. 40-mg/ml solution stable 24 hr at room temperature and for 7 days refrigerated in	D_5W $D_{10}W$ D_5W/NS LR NS	Observe for eosinophilia, fever, hemolytic anemia, leukopenia, nausea, phlebitis, pseudomembranous colitis, rash, thrombocytopenia, and vomiting. Use a venting needle while reconstituting ceftazidime because carbon dioxide gas is formed and must be removed prior to	Gura 1999 McEvoy 2001 Taketomo 2000 Trissel 2001

TABLE 8-1 continued

DRUG[a,b] (TRADE NAME)	COMMERCIAL DILUTION OR RECONSTITUTION AND pH[c]	METHOD OF ADMINISTRATION, FURTHER DILUTION, AND RECOMMENDED RATE OF INFUSION[d]	COMPATIBLE INFUSION SOLUTIONS[e]	CAUTIONS, COMMENTS, AND INCOMPATIBILITIES[f,g,h]	REFERENCES[i]
Ceftazidime *continued*	Stable 7 days refrigerated. pH: 5–8	a compatible IV solution.		administration. Do not admix with aminoglycosides. Compatible with acyclovir sodium, ciprofloxacin, clindamycin, esmolol HCl, and famotidine. Stable in dialysis solution.	
Ceftizoxime Sodium *(Cefizox®)*	Available as 20 and 40 mg/ml (frozen) **or** reconstitute powder for injection with sterile water for injection, D_5W, or NS to yield 100 mg/ml. pH: 5.5–8	**IV push:** Inject without further dilution over 3–5 min. **Intermittent infusion (preferred):** Dilute to 20–40 mg/ml and infuse over 30–60 min. **Continuous infusion:** Dilute to 20–40 mg/ml and infuse over 24 hr. Frozen solution stable 48 hr at room temperature and 21 days refrigerated. Reconstituted solutions stable 24 hr at room temperature and 96 hr at 5°C.	D_5W $D_{10}W$ Dextrose/saline combinations Invert sugar 10%/W LR NS R Sodium bicarbonate 5%	Observe for vein irritation. Use cautiously in penicillin-sensitive patients. Do not admix with other drugs.	McEvoy 2001 Sifton 2002 Trissel 2001
Ceftriaxone Sodium *(Rocephin®)*	Reconstitute powder for injection with sterile water for injection, NS, or D_5W to yield 100 mg/ml. pH: 6.7	**IV push:** Dilute to <40 mg/ml and inject over 2–4 min. *Maximum concentration:* 40 mg/ml. **Intermittent infusion (preferred):** Dilute to 40 mg/ml and infuse over 10–30 min *Maximum concentration:* 40 mg/ml. Stability depends on IV solution used for further dilution.	D_5W $D_{10}W$ $D_5W/1/2$ NS D_5W/NS NS	Observe for hypersensitivity reaction. Not recommended for infants with hyperbilirubinemia. Do not admix with aminoglycosides. Stability is decreased when admixed with alkaline solutions. Compatible with TPN.	Gura 1999 Hebel 1999 McEvoy 2001 Phelps 1996 Sifton 2002 Trissel 2001
Cefuroxime Sodium *(Zinacef®)*	Reconstitute powder for injection with sterile water for injection, NS, or D_5W to yield 100 mg/ml. pH: 6–8.5	**IV push:** Dilute to 50–100 mg/ml and inject over 3–5 min. **Intermittent infusion (preferred):** Dilute to 1–30 mg/ml and infuse over 15–60 min. *Maximum concentration:* 30 mg/ml.	D_5W $D_{10}W$ Dextrose/saline combinations LR NS R	Observe for phlebitis and hypersensitivity reaction. Not recommended for infants <3 months of age. Do not admix with aminoglycosides. Compatible with TPN.	Gura 1999 Hebel 1999 McEvoy 2001 Phelps 1996 Sifton 2002 Trissel 2001
Chloramphenicol Sodium Succinate *(Chloromycetin®)*	Reconstitute powder for injection with sterile water for injection or D_5W to yield 100 mg/ml. pH: 6.4–7	**IV push:** Inject without further dilution over 3–5 min. *Maximum concentration:* 100 mg/ml. **Intermittent infusion:** Dilute as desired to a maximum concentration of 20 mg/ml and infuse over 15–30 min.	D_5W $D_{10}W$ $D_5W/1/4$ NS $D_5W/1/2$ NS D_5W/NS Dextran solutions LR NS	Observe for aplastic anemia, diarrhea, nausea, and phlebitis. Incompatible with phenothiazines and vancomycin. Adjust dose based on serum levels.	Gura 1999 Repchinsky 2002 Taketomo 2000
Chlorothiazide *(Diuril®)*	Reconstitute powder for injection with sterile water for injection to yield 25 mg/ml. Stable for 24 hr at room temperature. pH: 9.2–10	**IV push:** Inject without further dilution over 3–5 min. **Intermittent infusion:** Infuse over 30 min.	D_5W $D_{10}W$ Dextrose/saline combinations LR NS R	Do not infuse with blood or blood products. Monitor for electrolyte disturbances and hypotension. Do not administer IM because of pain associated with alkaline pH.	Gura 1999 McEvoy 2001 Taketomo 2000 Trissel 2001

Footnotes are on page 390.

TABLE 8-1 continued

DRUG[a,b] (TRADE NAME)	COMMERCIAL DILUTION OR RECONSTITUTION AND pH[c]	METHOD OF ADMINISTRATION, FURTHER DILUTION, AND RECOMMENDED RATE OF INFUSION[d]	COMPATIBLE INFUSION SOLUTIONS[e]	CAUTIONS, COMMENTS, AND INCOMPATIBILITIES[f,g,h]	REFERENCES[i]
Chlorpromazine Hydrochloride (*Largactil®, Thorazine®*)	Available as 25 mg/ml pH: 3–5	**IV push (slow):** Dilute <1 mg/ml with NS and infuse at 0.5 mg/min in children; <1 mg/min in adults. Diluted solutions of 1 mg/ml stored at room temperature and protected from light are stable for 30 days.	D_5LR D_5R D_5W $D_{10}W$ Dextran 6%/D_5W or NS Dextrose/saline combinations LR 1/2 NS NS R TPN	Observe for hypotension; monitor ECG and blood pressure during infusion. May cause agranulocytosis and leukopenia (with large doses for long periods), blurred vision, constipation, dry mouth, dysrhythmias, extrapyramidal reactions, neuroleptic malignant syndrome, rash, sedation, seizures, tachycardia, and urinary retention. Incompatible with barbiturate salts and other alkaline media. Give IV infusion only when no alternative route is available because the drug is very irritating to veins. Protect from light.	Gura 1999 McEvoy 2001 Taketomo 2000 Trissel 2001
Cimetidine (*Tagamet®*)	Available as 150 mg/ml pH: 3.8–7	**IV push:** Dilute to 15 mg/ml and inject over at least 5 min. **Intermittent infusion (preferred):** Dilute to 6 mg/ml and infuse over 15–30 min.	D_5W $D_{10}W$ D_5W/LR D_5W/NS $D_5W/1/3$ NS $D_5W/1/2$ NS IL LR NS TPN	Do not administer by rapid IV push because hypotension and cardiac arrest have been reported. Observe for dizziness, mental confusion, neutropenia, and rash. Do not refrigerate. Incompatible with barbiturates and some cephalosporins. Inhibits the cytochrome P-450 enzyme system, therefore use cautiously with other medications metabolized by the P-450 enzyme.	Gura 1999 McEvoy 2001 Phelps 1996 Taketomo 2000 Trissel 2001
Ciprofloxacin (*Cipro®*)	Available as 1% and 2% pharmacy bulk packages that must be diluted to 0.5–2 mg/ml prior to administration. Also available as 10-mg/ml vials and 2-mg/ml ready-to-use minibags. pH: 3.3–3.9	**Intermittent infusion:** Slow IV infusion over 60 min. *Maximum concentration:* 2 mg/ml. Injection further diluted to 0.5–2 mg/ml is stable for 14 days at room temperature or refrigerated.	D_5W $D_{10}W$ $D_5W/1/4$ NS $D_5W/1/2$ NS LR NS R	Observe for venous irritation during infusion. Infuse in a large vein to minimize discomfort (burning, irritation, pain, thrombophlebitis) that occurs with rapid infusion. Do not Y-site into other infusion solutions.	Gura 1999 Hebel 1999 McEvoy 2001 Taketomo 2000 Trissel 2001
Cisatracurium (*Nimbex®*)	Available as 2 and 10 mg/ml. Keep refrigerated, protect from light, stable 21 days at room temperature. pH: 3.25–3.65	**IV push:** Inject without further dilution over 5–10 sec. **Continuous infusion:** Dilute to 0.1–0.4 mg/ml and infuse at 1–5 µg/kg/min. 0.1 mg/ml is stable for 24 hr refrigerated.	D_5NS D_5W NS	Should be administered by clinicians trained in airway management. Avoid IM injection due to tissue irritation. Does not alter level of consciousness; therefore, addition of sedation and/or analgesia is recommended. Incompatible with lactated Ringer's solution, ketorolac, and propofol.	Hebel 1999 Repchinsky 2002 Taketomo 2000
Cisplatin[a] (*CISplatin®*)	Reconstitute with sterile water for injection to yield 1 mg/ml. Stable for 20 hr at room temperature after reconstitution. If using bacteriostatic water for injection containing benzyl alcohol or parabens, 1-mg/ml solutions are stable 72 hr at room temperature. pH: 3.5–5.5	**IV push:** Associated with increased nephrotoxicity. **Intermittent infusion:** Dilute as desired (usually add mannitol per protocol) and infuse over 15–20 min, 1 mg/min, or up to 6–24 hr.	D_5W/NS $D_5W/1/2$ NS $D_5W/1/2$ NS/1.875% mannitol $D_5W/1/3$ NS/1.875% mannitol/20 mEq KCl/liter 1/3 NS 1/2 NS NS	Nausea and vomiting invariably occur. Observe for nephrotoxicity, monitor serum electrolyte concentrations. May cause anaphylactic reaction, elevation of hepatic enzymes, myelosuppression, peripheral neuropathy, phlebitis, and seizures. Hydrate patient before and for 24 hr after administration. Maintain good urine output. Avoid contact with aluminum. Protect from light. Do not refrigerate. Incompatible with alkaline solutions and solutions with a low chloride concentration (0.2% NaCl).	McEvoy 2001 Taketomo 2000 Trissel 2001

TABLE 8-1 continued

DRUG[a,b] (TRADE NAME)	COMMERCIAL DILUTION OR RECONSTITUTION AND pH[c]	METHOD OF ADMINISTRATION, FURTHER DILUTION, AND RECOMMENDED RATE OF INFUSION[d]	COMPATIBLE INFUSION SOLUTIONS[e]	CAUTIONS, COMMENTS, AND INCOMPATIBILITIES[f,g,h]	REFER- ENCES[i]
Cladribine (*Leustatin®*)	Reconstitute with diluent provided to yield 1 mg/ml. Solutions should be administered immediately after initial dilution or stored under refrigeration for <8 hr. pH: 5.5–8	**Intermittent or continuous infusion over 24 hr:** Further dilute with NS for injection to 500 ml. **7-Day continuous infusion:** Further dilute with bacteriostatic NS to 100 ml.	NS (Do **not** use D_5W.)	Dose-limiting toxicity is myelosuppression. Do not infuse with other IV medications or additives. Use 0.22-μm filter when preparing 7-day infusion.	McEvoy 2001 Sifton 2002 Taketomo 2000
Clindamycin Phosphate[b] (*Cleocin®*)	Available as 150 mg/ml pH: 5.5–6.7	**Intermittent infusion:** Dilute to 6–12 mg/ml and infuse over 10–60 min (do not exceed 18 mg/ml or 30 mg/min). Concentrations of 6–12 mg/ml stable 16 days at 25°C and 32 days refrigerated at 4°C.	D_5W LR NS	Do not administer IV push. Observe for local erythema, pain, swelling, phlebitis, and thrombophlebitis. Hypotension and cardiac arrest may occur with rapid administration.	Gura 1999 Hebel 1999 McEvoy 2001 Phelps 1996 Sifton 2002 Trissel 2001
Cyclophos- phamide (*Cytoxan®, Procytox®*)	Reconstitute powder for injection with sterile water or bacteriostatic water for injection to yield 20–25 mg/ml. Stable for 24 hr at room temperature and 6 days refrigerated. If reconstituting with sterile water without preservatives, use within 6 hr. pH: 3–9	May be given IV push, intermittent infusion, or continuous infusion per protocol.	D_5W D_5W/NS D_5W/R LR 1/2 NS	Maintain high fluid intake and urine output to minimize hemorrhagic cystitis.	McEvoy 2001 Repchinsky 2002 Taketomo 2000 Trissel 2001
Cyclosporine (*Sandimmune®*)	Available as 50 mg/ml in polyoxyethylated castor oil/ethanol vehicle. Dilutions stable 24 hr in D_5W and 12 hr in NS (glass) or 6 hr in NS (PVC). Store at room temperature protected from light. pH: Information not available	**Intermittent infusion:** Dilute to 0.5–2.5 mg/ml and infuse slowly over 2–6 hr. **Continuous infusion:** Dilute to 2–5 mg/ml with D_5W only (unstable in NS) and infuse over 24 hr.	D_5W NS	Must be diluted prior to administration. Draw levels from different line than where drug infused. May bind to plastic tubing and polyvinyl chloride (PVC) bags. Non-PVC containers and administration sets should be used. Glass containers are preferred. Observe for flushing, gingival hyperplasia, headache, hypersensitivity, hypertension, hypomagnesemia, nephrotoxicity, and seizures.	Gura 1999 McEvoy 2001 Taketomo 2000 Trissel 2001
Cytarabine (*Cytosar®*)	Reconstitute powder for injection with bacteriostatic water for injection to yield 20–100 mg/ml. Store reconstituted solutions at room temperature for up to 48 hr. Discard hazy solutions. pH: 5–7.4	**IV push:** May inject without further dilution. **Intermittent infusion:** Dilute to 0.5–5 mg/ml and infuse over 1–3 hr.	D_5W D_5W/NS LR NS	Observe for cerebellar dysfunction. Use steroid eye drops with high doses and monitor for respiratory distress. Incompatible with allopurinol, fluorouracil, ganciclovir, heparin, insulin, methotrexate, methylprednisolone, nafcillin, and penicillin G.	McEvoy 2001 Repchinsky 2002 Taketomo 2000 Trissel 2001

Footnotes are on page 390.

TABLE 8-1 continued

DRUG[a,b] (TRADE NAME)	COMMERCIAL DILUTION OR RECONSTITUTION AND pH[c]	METHOD OF ADMINISTRATION, FURTHER DILUTION, AND RECOMMENDED RATE OF INFUSION[d]	COMPATIBLE INFUSION SOLUTIONS[e]	CAUTIONS, COMMENTS, AND INCOMPATIBILITIES[f,g,h]	REFERENCES[i]
Dacarbazine[a] (*DTIC-Dome®*)	Reconstitute powder for injection with sterile water for injection to yield 10 mg/ml. Stable for 8 hr at room temperature and 72 hr refrigerated. pH: 3–4	**IV push:** Dilute in 5–10 ml IV solution, if desired, and infuse over 2–3 min. May also give by direct infusion over 1 min. **Intermittent infusion (preferred):** Dilute in 50–250 ml IV solution and infuse over 15–30 min (or per protocol). Dilutions up to 500 ml are stable for 8 hr at room temperature and 72 hr refrigerated.	D_5W NS	Specially trained pediatric clinician should be present for IV push; avoid extravasation. Observe for fever, malaise, nausea, phlebitis, and vomiting (common on the first day of administration). Protect from light; change in color of solution signifies decomposition. Incompatible with allopurinol, cefepime, hydrocortisone, and piperacillin–tazobactam.	McEvoy 2001 Taketomo 2000 Trissel 2001
Dactinomycin[a] [Actinomycin D] (*Cosmegen®*)	Reconstitute powder for injection with sterile or nonbacteriostatic water for injection (without preservatives) to yield 500 µg/ml. Discard unused portions of reconstituted drug immediately. pH: 5.5–7	**IV push:** Dilute in 3–5 ml IV solution and inject over 1–3 min, then follow with a 5–10-ml flush of D_5W or NS. May also inject, by direct infusion, into the side-port of a free-flowing IV solution	D_5W NS	Do not filter final solution. Specially trained pediatric clinician should be present for IV push. Avoid extravasation. Dose-limiting side effect is bone marrow suppression (particularly leukopenia and thrombocytopenia). Observe for alopecia, diarrhea, nausea, stomatitis (particularly with concurrent radiation therapy), and vomiting (which may require interruption in course of therapy). Compatible with dacarbazine. Incompatible with filgrastim.	McEvoy 2001 Taketomo 2000 Trissel 2001
Dantrolene Sodium (*Dantrium®*)	Reconstitute powder for injection with sterile or nonbacteriostatic water for injection to yield 0.33 mg/ml. pH: 9.5	**IV push:** Inject without further dilution over 1–2 min. **Intermittent infusion:** Dilute as desired and infuse over 60 min. Solution stable for 6 hr at 15–30°C.	Nonbacteriostatic water for injection Sterile water for injection	Avoid extravasation. Each 20 mg of dantrolene sodium solution contains 3 grams of mannitol. Monitor hepatic transaminases for hepatotoxicity. Monitor patient for confusion, diarrhea, drowsiness, muscle weakness, nausea, pleural effusion with pericarditis, rash, seizures, and vomiting. Protect from light. Incompatible with bacteriostatic water, D_5W, and NS.	McEvoy 2001 Rapp 1988 Taketomo 2000 Sifton 2002
Daunorubicin Hydrochloride[a] (*Cerubidine®*)	Reconstitute powder for injection with sterile water for injection or NS to yield 5 mg/ml. When protected from light, the reconstituted solution is stable to 24 hr at room temperature and 48 hr refrigerated. pH: 4.5–6.5	**IV push:** Dilute with 10–15 ml NS and inject over 2–3 min into tubing of free-flowing IV solution. **Intermittent infusion:** Dilute with 100 ml IV solution and infuse over 30–45 min. Unstable in solutions with a pH >8. If color changes from red to blue–purple, decomposition has occurred.	D_5W D_5W/NS LR NS	Specially trained pediatric clinician should be present for administration; avoid extravasation. Dose-limiting side effect is bone marrow suppression. Observe for fever, mucositis, nausea, rash, thrombophlebitis, and vomiting. Cardiotoxicity based on cumulative dose (400 mg/m^2 in patients receiving chest radiation; 10 mg/kg in children <2 yr; 300 mg/m^2 in children >2 yr). Incompatible with allopurinol, cefepime, dexamethasone, fludarabine, fluorouracil, heparin, piperacillin–tazobactam, and sodium bicarbonate.	McEvoy 2001 Taketomo 2000 Trissel 2001
Deferoxamine Mesylate (*Desferal®*)	Reconstitute powder for injection with sterile water for injection to yield 250 mg/ml. Reconstituted solutions are stable for 7 days at room temperature, protected from light. Discard turbid solutions. pH: Information not available	**Continuous infusion:** Dilute dose to 10 mg/ml in NS and infuse <15 mg/kg/hr. In treatment of acute iron intoxication, 35 mg/kg/hr has been used. *Maximum concentration:* 250 mg/ml.	D_5W LR NS	Rapid IV administration is associated with edema, flushing, hypotension, shock, and urticaria. Monitor for cataracts, fever, hearing loss, hypersensitivity reaction, leg cramps, rash, and tachycardia.	Gura 1999 McEvoy 2001 Taketomo 2000 Trissel 2001

TABLE 8-1 continued

DRUG[a,b] (TRADE NAME)	COMMERCIAL DILUTION OR RECONSTITUTION AND pH[c]	METHOD OF ADMINISTRATION, FURTHER DILUTION, AND RECOMMENDED RATE OF INFUSION[d]	COMPATIBLE INFUSION SOLUTIONS[e]	CAUTIONS, COMMENTS, AND INCOMPATIBILITIES[f,g,h]	REFERENCES[i]
Desmopressin Acetate (DDAVP®)	Available as 4 and 15 µg/ml. Store at 2–8°C. pH: 4	**IV push.** Inject 4 µg/ml over 1 min. **Intermittent infusion:** Dilute to a maximum of 0.5 µg/ml and infuse over 15–30 min.	NS	Observe for abdominal cramps, flushing, headache, hypertension, hyponatremia, nausea, phlebitis, and water intoxication.	Gura 1999 McEvoy 2001 Taketomo 2000
Dexamethasone Sodium Phosphate (Decadron®)	Available as 4, 10, and 24 mg/ml pH: 7–8.5	**IV push:** Inject <10 mg/ml over 1–5 min. **Intermittent infusion:** Dilute with at least an equal volume of IV solution and infuse over at least 15–30 min.	D_5W Dextrose/saline combinations NS	May cause fluid and electrolyte imbalances. Observe for GI upset or bleeding.	Gura 1999 Hebel 1999 McEvoy 2001 Phelps 1996
Dexrazoxane (Zinecard®)	Reconstitute with diluent provided to 10 mg/ml. Reconstituted solution stable for 6 hr at room temperature or refrigerated. pH: 3.5–5.5	**IV push:** Inject slowly. **Intermittent infusion:** Dilute to 1.3–5 mg/ml in NS or D_5W and infuse over 15–30 min.	D_5W NS	Handle, prepare, and dispense as an antineoplastic agent. Administer doxorubicin within 30 min from the beginning of the dexrazoxane infusion. Degrades rapidly at pH >7.	McEvoy 2001 Sifton 2002 Taketomo 2000
Dextrose	Available as: 2.5%, 5%, 10%, 20%, 25%, 30%, 40%, 50%, 60%, and 70% pH: 3.5–6.5	**IV push:** Solutions up to 25% may be injected at 200 mg/kg over 1 min. **Intermittent and continuous infusions:** Solutions of ≤10% may be infused through a peripheral IV, solutions ≤30% may be infused through a central line.	LR NS R	Infusion >10% can be irritating to the veins. Monitor for hyperglycemia, which causes osmotic fluid shifts, and may result in rapid dehydration. Rebound hypoglycemia may occur following hyperglycemia as a result of the stimulation of insulin secretion.	McEvoy 2001 Phelps 1996
Diazepam (Valium®)	Available as 5 mg/ml pH: 6.2–6.9	**IV push:** Inject without further dilution over at least 3 min. Do not exceed 5 mg/min. **Continuous infusion:** Not recommended, but 0.2 mg/ml in D_5W or NS has been used at 0.8–1.6 mg/kg/hr.	D_5W NS	Specially trained pediatric clinician should be present. Avoid extravasation. Observe closely for hypotension and respiratory depression. Incompatible with most IV solutions. Protect from light. Contains benzyl alcohol. Do not inject intra-arterially.	Gura 1999 Hebel 1999 McEvoy 2001 Phelps 1996 Taketomo 2000 Trissel 2001
Diazoxide (Hyperstat®)	Available as 15 mg/ml pH: 11.6	**IV push:** Inject without further dilution over 10–30 sec.	Do not dilute.	Avoid extravasation. Observe for cardiac arrest, cardiac dysrhythmias, dizziness, flushing, headache, hyperglycemia, hypotension, nausea, seizures, sodium and water retention, tachycardia, vomiting, and weakness. Slow administration may reduce antihypertensive response. Do not admix with other drugs; avoid use for >4–5 days. Administer through peripheral IVs to decrease the risk of dysrhythmias. Do not give IM.	Gura 1999 Hebel 1999 Phelps 1996 Repchinsky 2002 Taketomo 2000
Digoxin (Lanoxin®)	Available as 100 and 250 µg/ml pH: 6.8–7.2	**IV push:** Inject without further dilution over at least 5 min. **Intermittent infusion:** Dilute to ≤25 µg/ml and infuse over 30 min. *Maximum concentration:* 100 µg/ml for pediatric patients.	D_5W $D_{10}W$ Dextran 6%/D_5W or NS Dextrose/saline combinations IL LR NS TPN	Monitor cardiac status closely with periodic ECGs; monitor serum electrolytes since abnormalities can predispose to digoxin toxicity. Do not admix with other drugs. If dilution is desired, the manufacturer recommends at least a fourfold dilution to prevent precipitation; a 10-fold dilution may improve accuracy of dose measurements. Protect from light.	Gura 1999 McEvoy 2001 Phelps 1996 Taketomo 2000 Trissel 2001

Footnotes are on page 390.

TABLE 8-1 continued

DRUG[a,b] (TRADE NAME)	COMMERCIAL DILUTION OR RECONSTITUTION AND pH[c]	METHOD OF ADMINISTRATION, FURTHER DILUTION, AND RECOMMENDED RATE OF INFUSION[d]	COMPATIBLE INFUSION SOLUTIONS[e]	CAUTIONS, COMMENTS, AND INCOMPATIBILITIES[f,g,h]	REFER- ENCES[i]
Digoxin Immune Fab (*Digibind®*)	Reconstitute powder for injection with 4 ml sterile water for injection to yield ~9.5 mg/ml. pH: 6–8	**Intermittent infusion:** Infuse 1 mg/ml over 15–60 min through a 0.22-μm filter; may give more rapidly if cardiac arrest is imminent.	NS	Administer intradermal test dose (0.1 ml of 1:100 dilution), wait 20 min for reaction. Continuous ECG monitoring is required. Observe for worsening of cardiac output and hypokalemia. Each 38-mg vial will bind ~0.5 mg digoxin.	Gura 1999 McEvoy 2001 Phelps 1996 Taketomo 2000
Dimen- hydrinate (*Gravol®*)	Available as 50 mg/ml pH: 6.4–7.2	**IV push:** Dilute dose to <5 mg/ml and inject over at least 2–3 min.	D_5W $D_{10}W$ D_5W/LR Dextran 6%/D_5W Dextrose/ saline combina- tions LR NS	Observe for sedation and somnolence or paradoxical CNS stimulation. Compatible drugs include amikacin sulfate, calcium gluconate, chloramphenicol sodium succinate, heparin sodium, hydroxyzine HCl, methicillin sodium, penicillin G potassium, potassium chloride, prochlorperazine edisylate, and vancomycin HCl. Incompatible with aminophylline, ammonium chloride, barbiturates, hydrocortisone, phenytoin, and tetracycline. Injection contains benzyl alcohol.	Repchinsky 2002 Taketomo 2000
Diphen- hydramine Hydro- chloride (*Benadryl®*)	Available as 10 and 50 mg/ml pH: 5–6	**IV push:** Inject without further dilution over 5 min. **Intermittent infusion:** Dilute as desired and infuse over 15 min. Rate not to exceed 25 mg/min. Store preparations at room temperature.	D_5W $D_{10}W$ D_5W/LR D_5W/R Dextran 6%/D_5W or NS Dextrose/ saline combina- tions IL LR 1/2 NS NS R TPN	Observe for dizziness, hypotension, palpitations, paradoxical excitement, sedation, tremors, and urinary retention. Incompatible with allopurinol, amphotericin B, cefepime, foscarnet, pentobarbital, phenytoin, and thiopental. Protect from light.	Gura 1999 McEvoy 2001 Taketomo 2000 Trissel 2001
Dobutamine Hydrochlo- ride (*Dobutrex®*)	Available as 12.5 mg/ml pH: 2.5–5.5	**Continuous infusion:** Dilute to ≤5 mg/ml and infuse at 2.5–40 μg/kg/min.	D_5W D_5W/LR $D_5W/1/2$ NS D_5W/NS LR 1/2 NS NS TPN	Administer with electronic infusion device. Avoid extravasation as it may cause tissue sloughing and necrosis. Solution may exhibit pink discoloration without loss of potency for up to 24 hr at room temperature. Closely monitor blood pressure, cardiac output, ECG, and heart rate. Observe for dysrhythmias, hypertension, and tachycardia. Incompatible with alkaline solutions and heparin. Compatible with dopamine, epinephrine, isoproterenol, and lidocaine.	Gura 1999 McEvoy 2001 Phelps 1996 Sodorff 1999 Taketomo 2000 Trissel 2001
Docetaxel (*Taxotere®*)	Available as 40-mg/ml concentrate to be diluted to 10 mg/ml with provided diluent (13% ethanol in water for injection). Remove from refrigerator and let stand 5 min before adding diluent. Stable for 8 hr at room temperature or refrigerated. pH: Information not available	**Intermittent infusion:** Dilute to 0.3–0.9 mg/ml with D_5W or NS and infuse over 1 hr.	D_5W NS	Dose-limiting toxicity is myelo- suppression. Protect from bright light. Avoid PVC-containing equipment. Hypersensitivity reactions are common. Premedication with dexamethasone is recommended.	McEvoy 2001 Repchinsky 2002 Sifton 2002

TABLE 8-1 *continued*

DRUG[a,b] (TRADE NAME)	COMMERCIAL DILUTION OR RECONSTITUTION AND pH[c]	METHOD OF ADMINISTRATION, FURTHER DILUTION, AND RECOMMENDED RATE OF INFUSION[d]	COMPATIBLE INFUSION SOLUTIONS[e]	CAUTIONS, COMMENTS, AND INCOMPATIBILITIES[f,g,h]	REFERENCES[i]
Dolasetron (Anzemet®)	Available as 20 mg/ml After dilution, stable 24 hr at room temperature and 48 hr refrigerated. Manufacturer recommends immediate use after dilution. pH: 3.2–3.8	**IV push:** Inject undiluted over 30 sec. **Intermittent infusion:** Dilute in 50 ml and infuse over <15 min.	D_5W $D_5W/1/2$ NS D_5W/LR NS LR Mannitol 10%	Do not mix with other medications. Caution in patients who are prone to prolongation of the QTc interval (patients with hypokalemia or hypomagnesemia, and patients who have received high cumulative doses of anthracyclines). *See also* Chapter 6.	Taketomo 2000
Dopamine Hydrochloride (Intropin®)	Available as 40, 80, and 160 mg/ml pH: 2.5–5 (depending on brand)	**Continuous infusion:** Dilute to ≤3.2 mg/ml in IV solution and infuse at 2–20 µg/kg/min. Concentrations as high as 6 mg/ml have been infused into large veins in cases of extreme fluid restriction.	D_5W D_5W/LR $D_5W/1/2$ NS D_5W/NS IL LR Mannitol 20% NS R TPN	Administer by electronic infusion device. Closely monitor blood pressure, cardiac output, ECG, and heart rate. Observe for cardiac dysrhythmias, dyspnea, headache, hypotension, nausea, tachycardia, vasoconstriction, and vomiting. Do not administer discolored solutions (darker than slightly yellow). Extravasation may cause local tissue necrosis and sloughing. Compatible with dobutamine, epinephrine, lidocaine, and nitroglycerin. Incompatible with sodium bicarbonate and other alkaline IV solutions. Do not administer via umbilical artery catheter.	Gura 1999 Phelps 1996 Repchinsky 2002 Sodorff 1999 Taketomo 2000
Doxapram Hydrochloride[b] (Dopram®)	Available as 20 mg/ml pH: 3.5–5	**Continuous infusion:** Dilute to 1 mg/ml and infuse at 1.5 mg/kg/hr for 24 hr, then titrate to lowest effective dose. *Maximum concentration:* 2 mg/ml.	D_5W $D_{10}W$ NS	Monitor blood pressure, CNS status, heart rate, and reflexes. Incompatible with alkaline solutions. Contains benzyl alcohol. Store at 15–30°C.	Gura 1999 McEvoy 2001 Phelps 1996 Taketomo 2000 Trissel 2001
Doxorubicin Hydrochloride[a] (Adriamycin®)	Available as 2 mg/ml **or** reconstitute with sterile water for injection (without preservatives), D_5W, or NS to yield 2 mg/ml. Reconstituted vials stable for 24 hr at room temperature and 48 hr refrigerated. pH: 2.5–4.5 (solution) pH: 3.8–6.5 (powder for injection)	**IV push:** Inject without further dilution, or dilute further with at least 1/2 of the initial volume, and inject over 3–5 min. **Intermittent infusion:** Dilute as desired (not to exceed 2 mg/ml) and infuse over 1–4 hr (for large doses). Solutions prepared from the multidose vial can be stored for up to 7 days at room temperature under normal light or 15 days refrigerated. Unstable in solutions with pH <3 or >7.	D_5W LR *Normosol R®* NS	Specially trained pediatric clinician should be present for IV push; avoid extravasation. Pediatric patients are at increased risk for developing late cardiac toxicity and CHF during early adulthood. Monitor for cardiotoxicity, extravasation, hyperuricemia, leukopenia, mucositis, and thrombocytopenia. Avoid contact with aluminum. Protect from prolonged exposure to sunlight. Incompatible with allopurinol, aminophylline, cefepime, fluorouracil, furosemide, ganciclovir, heparin, and piperacillin–tazobactam.	McEvoy 2001 Taketomo 2000 Trissel 2001
Doxorubicin Hydrochloride Liposomal (Doxil®)	Available as 2-mg/ml concentrate for IV infusion. Concentrate should be refrigerated at 2–8°C and protected from freezing. pH: 6.5	Appropriate dose (up to a maximum of 90 mg) should be diluted in 250 ml D_5W. Diluted solutions are stable 24 hr when refrigerated at 2–8°C. Infuse slowly over 30 min. In-line filters should not be used.	D_5W	If infusion reactions such as chills, facial edema, flushing, or shortness of breath occur, slow the rate of infusion or stop the infusion. Monitor for extravasation. Diluents containing preservatives should not be used to dilute doxorubicin liposomal.	Hebel 1999 McEvoy 2001

Footnotes are on page 390.

TABLE 8-1 continued

DRUG[a,b] (TRADE NAME)	COMMERCIAL DILUTION OR RECONSTITUTION AND pH[c]	METHOD OF ADMINISTRATION, FURTHER DILUTION, AND RECOMMENDED RATE OF INFUSION[d]	COMPATIBLE INFUSION SOLUTIONS[e]	CAUTIONS, COMMENTS, AND INCOMPATIBILITIES[f,g,h]	REFER- ENCES[i]
Droperidol	Available as 2.5 mg/ml pH: 3–3.8	**IV push (slow):** Inject over 2–5 min.	D_5W LR	Observe for dystonic reaction, hallucinations, hypotension, respiratory depression, sedation, and tachycardia. Incompatible with allopurinol, barbiturates, cefepime, foscarnet, furosemide, and piperacillin–tazobactam.	McEvoy 2001 Taketomo 2000 Trissel 2001
Edrophonium Chloride (Enlon®, Reversol®, Tensilon®)	Available as 10 mg/ml pH: 5.4	**IV push:** Inject rapidly without further dilution.	D_5W D_5W/LR D_5W/R LR NS R	Overdose can result in cholinergic crisis. Antidote is atropine. Monitor blood pressure, heart rate, muscle strength, and respiratory rate. Contains phenol and sodium sulfite as preservatives.	McEvoy 2001 Taketomo 2000 Trissel 2001
Enalaprilat (Vasotec®)	Available as 1.25 mg/ml For neonates, recommended concentration is 25 µg/ml. pH: 6.5–7.5	**IV push:** Inject without further dilution over 5 min (adjust dose according to response).	D_5W D_5W/LR D_5W/NS NS	Monitor blood pressure. Sodium and/or volume depletion may lead to severe hypotension; use small initial doses to prevent hemodynamic side effects. Discontinue if angioedema occurs. Contains benzyl alcohol.	Gura 1999 Phelps 1996 Taketomo 2000 Trissel 2001
Epinephrine Hydrochloride (Adrenalin®)	Available as 1:10,000 (0.1 mg/ml) and 1:1000 (1 mg/ml) pH: 2.5–5	**IV push:** Inject 0.01 mg/kg without further dilution over 1–3 min. **Continuous infusion:** Dilute further to ≤64 µg/ml and infuse at 0.02–1 µg/kg/min.	D_5W $D_{10}W$ D_5W/LR D_5W/NS $D_5W/1/4\ NS$ $D_5W/1/2\ NS$ Dextran solutions LR NS	Specially trained pediatric clinician must be present for IV push. Observe for cardiac dysrhythmias and hypertension. Do not use discolored solutions. Incompatible with alkaline solutions. Do not administer intra-arterially. An infusion pump should be used to administer continuous infusions.	Gura 1999 McEvoy 2001 Phelps 1996 Sodorff 1999 Taketomo 2000 Trissel 2001
Epoetin Alfa (Epogen®)	Available as 2000, 3000, 4000, and 10,000 units/ml pH: 6.6–7.2	**IV push:** Inject without further dilution into venous return line of dialysis tubing over 5 min (at end of dialysis session for dialysis patients). Can be diluted with an equal volume of NS and injected over 1–3 min if not on dialysis.	NS	Monitor blood pressure, Hct, and iron serum concentrations. Supplemental iron is often required. Do not freeze or shake the solution.	McEvoy 2001 Taketomo 2000 Trissel 2001
Erythromycin[b] Lactobionate (Erythrocin®)	Reconstitute powder for injection with sterile water for injection (without preservatives) to yield 50 mg/ml. pH: 6–8	**Intermittent infusion:** Dilute to 1–5 mg/ml and infuse over 20–60 min. Prolonging infusion >60 min may decrease cardiac effects. Use diluted solutions within 8 hr stored at room temperature or within 24 hr stored at 2–8°C.	Buffered dextrose solutions D_5W/NS LR Normosol R NS	Observe for phlebitis and thrombophlebitis. Addition of sodium bicarbonate buffer is necessary if pH <5.5 (unstable in acidic solutions). Incompatible with sodium salts of most antibiotics. Contraindicated in patients receiving cisapride. Contains benzyl alcohol.	Phelps 1996 Repchinsky 2002 Taketomo 2000
Esmolol Hydrochloride (Brevibloc®)	Available as 10 and 250 mg/ml pH: 3.5–5.5	**IV push:** Dilute to 10 mg/ml and inject loading dose over 1–2 min. **Continuous infusion:** After the loading dose, infuse 10 mg/ml at 50–500 µg/kg/min, titrating the dose for appropriate response.	D_5W D_5W/LR D_5W/NS $D_5W/1/2\ NS$ D_5W/R LR 1/2 NS NS	Monitor blood pressure, ECG, heart rate, IV site, and respiratory rate. If hypotension occurs, decrease dose or discontinue. Avoid extravasation. Avoid abrupt discontinuation of therapy. Once stopped, effects last 2–16 min.	Gura 1999 McEvoy 2001 Phelps 1996 Sodorff 1999 Taketomo 2000 Trissel 2001
Ethacrynate Sodium (Edecrin®)	Reconstitute with D_5W or NS to yield 1 mg/ml. pH: 6.3–7.7	**IV push:** Inject without further dilution over 10 min. (Too rapid infusion is associated with tinnitus and deafness.) **Intermittent infusion:** Infuse over 20–30 min. *Maximum concentration:* 2 mg/ml in D_5W only.	D_5W D_5W/NS LR NS	Observe for phlebitis and thrombophlebitis. Discard hazy or opalescent solutions. Incompatible with solutions or drugs with a final pH <5 and with blood products.	Gura 1999 McEvoy 2001 Phelps 1996 Taketomo 2000 Trissel 2001

TABLE 8-1 continued

DRUG[a,b] (TRADE NAME)	COMMERCIAL DILUTION OR RECONSTITUTION AND pH[c]	METHOD OF ADMINISTRATION, FURTHER DILUTION, AND RECOMMENDED RATE OF INFUSION[d]	COMPATIBLE INFUSION SOLUTIONS[e]	CAUTIONS, COMMENTS, AND INCOMPATIBILITIES[f,g,h]	REFER- ENCES[i]
Etoposide[a,b] *(VePesid®)*	Available as 20 mg/ml **or** reconstitute with bacteriostatic water for injection, bacteriostatic sodium chloride for injection, D$_5$W, NS, or sterile water for injection to yield 10–20 mg/ml. pH: 3–4	**Intermittent infusion:** Dilute to 0.2–0.4 mg/ml and infuse slowly over at least 30–60 min to minimize risk of bronchospasm and hypotension. Rate not to exceed 100 mg/m^2/hr or 3.3 mg/kg/hr. Stability is concentration dependent (D$_5$W or NS). *Concentration / Stability* 0.2 mg/ml — 96 hr 0.4 mg/ml — 48 hr 1 mg/ml — 2 hr 2 mg/ml — 1 hr Only stable for 8 hr in LR. Discard solution if cloudy.	D$_5$W LR NS	Hematologic toxicity is the dose-limiting side effect. Monitor for anaphylactoid reactions and hypotension. Follow CBC with differential, renal function tests, and serum bilirubin. May use an in-line 0.22-μm filter. Incompatible with cefepime and idarubicin.	McEvoy 2001 Taketomo 2000 Trissel 2001
Factor IX Complex *(BeneFix®, Hemonyne®, Konyne®–80, Profilnine® SD, Proplex® T)*	Reconstitute powder for injection with diluent provided (sterile water for injection) warmed to room temperature. Store unopened vials refrigerated. Reconstituted solution is stable 12 hr at room temperature, but to decrease the risk of bacterial contamination, it should be administered within 3 hr of reconstitution. Do **not** refrigerate reconstituted product. pH: Information not available	**IV infusion (slow):** Rates vary with product. Most manufacturers recommend adjusting the infusion rate to the comfort of the patient, but in general should not exceed 3 ml/min.		Solutions should be drawn into syringes using a filter needle. Use a separate filter needle for each vial. Prepared from pooled human plasma; risk of viral infections is not totally eliminated. Do not administer with aminocaproic acid as the rate of thrombosis is increased. If headache, flushing, or changes in heart rate or blood pressure occur, the infusion rate should be slowed and/or stopped.	Lacy 1999 McEvoy 2001 Sifton 2002
Factor IX (Human) *(Immunine VH®, Mononine®)*	Reconstitute powder for injection with diluent provided (sterile water for injection). Reconstituted solution should be administered within 3 hr of mixing. pH: Information not available.	**IV infusion:** Rate should be adjusted to the response and comfort of the patient; 2 ml/min is generally well tolerated in adults. Rate should not exceed 2 ml/min.		Solutions should be drawn into syringes using a filter spike. Use a separate filter spike for each vial. Do not inject air into the vial prior to drug removal. Prepared from pooled human plasma; risk of viral infections is not totally eliminated. Do not administer with aminocaproic acid as the rate of thrombosis is increased. Use with caution in patients with liver disease, postoperatively, neonates, patients at risk of thromboembolic phenomena, or disseminated intravascular coagulopathy due to the increased risk of thromboembolic complications.	Lacy 1999 McEvoy 2001 Repchinsky 2002 Sifton 2002
Famotidine *(Pepcid®)*	Available as 10 mg/ml Dilutions with D$_5$W or NS are stable for 48 hr at room temperature. pH: 5–5.6	**IV push:** Dilute to 2 mg/ml and inject over <10 min, not to exceed 10 mg/min. *Maximum concentration:* 4 mg/ml. **Intermittent infusion:** Dilute to 0.5 mg/ml.	D$_5$W D$_{10}$W LR NS TPN	Monitor renal and hepatic function. Incompatible with cefepime and piperacillin–tazobactam.	Gura 1999 McEvoy 2001 Taketomo 2000 Trissel 2001

Footnotes are on page 390.

TABLE 8-1 continued

DRUG[a,b] (TRADE NAME)	COMMERCIAL DILUTION OR RECONSTITUTION AND pH[c]	METHOD OF ADMINISTRATION, FURTHER DILUTION, AND RECOMMENDED RATE OF INFUSION[d]	COMPATIBLE INFUSION SOLUTIONS[e]	CAUTIONS, COMMENTS, AND INCOMPATIBILITIES[f,g,h]	REFERENCES[i]
Fat Emulsion (*Intralipid®*)	Available as 10%, 20%, and 30% emulsion. Stable until the manufacturer's expiration date when stored in the intact container at room temperature. pH: 7.5–8	Daily dose of fat emulsion (0.5–4 grams/kg) should preferably be administered over 24 hr via electronic infusion device. In-line filters should not be used. Remaining contents of a partially used bottle must be discarded and should not be saved for later use.	Manufacturer recommends not mixing fat emulsion in other solutions for infusion.	Very-low-birth-weight infants and small-for-gestational age infants clear IV lipids more slowly and are at greater risk for developing hyperlipidemia. Due to lack of experience, 30% fat emulsion is not recommended for use in infants and children.	Repchinsky 2002 Trissel 2001
Fentanyl Citrate	Available as 50 µg/ml pH: 4–7.5	**IV push:** Inject without further dilution slowly over 3–5 min (titrate to desired level of sedation). **Continuous infusion:** Infuse 1–20 µg/kg/hr.	D_5W LR NS	Monitor blood pressure, heart rate, and respiratory rate. Rapid administration can result in skeletal muscle and chest wall rigidity that may require a non-depolarizing skeletal muscle relaxant. Observe for apnea and seizures. Naloxone should be readily available to reverse significant respiratory and CNS depression associated with overdoses. Peak respiratory depression occurs ~5–15 min after a dose. Adheres to ECMO circuit and may necessitate larger doses.	Gura 1999 Phelps 1996 Taketomo 2000 Trissel 2001
Filgrastim [G-CSF] (*Neupogen®*)	Available as 300 µg/ml Refrigerate; discard vials after 24 hr at room temperature. pH: 4	**Intermittent infusion:** Dilute with 50–100 ml and infuse over 15–60 min (usually 30 min). **Continuous infusion:** Dilute with 50–100 ml and infuse over 24 hr. Most stable at concentrations >15 µg/ml. Dilutions from 2 to 15 µg/ml should have albumin added to yield a final albumin concentration of 2 mg/ml. Dilutions stable for 7 days refrigerated, but sterility may be a concern because preservatives are not added. Do not dilute to <2 µg/ml.	D_5W	Do not administer within 24 hr of cancer chemotherapy. Monitor platelet count and uric acid concentration. Perform CBC with differential, hepatic function tests, and urinalysis. Observe for bone pain. Do not shake. Incompatible with amphotericin B, cefepime, cefotaxime, cefuroxime, clindamycin, etoposide, furosemide, heparin, methylprednisolone, metronidazole, NS, and piperacillin–tazobactam.	Gura 1999 McEvoy 2001 Taketomo 2000 Trissel 2001
Fluconazole (*Diflucan®*)	Available as 2 mg/ml pH: 4–8	**Intermittent infusion:** Infuse over 2 hr.	D_5W NS	Monitor hepatic and renal function. Avoid admixing with other drugs. Contraindicated in patients receiving cisapride. Do not freeze.	McEvoy 2001 Taketomo 2000 Trissel 2001
Fludarabine (*Fludara®*)	Available as sterile powder for injection, 50 mg. Reconstitute in sterile water for injection to 25 mg/ml. Stable for at least 16 days at room temperature and normal light conditions. However, contains no preservative and should be used within 8 hr after preparation. pH: Information not available	**Intermittent infusion:** Dilute appropriate dose of drug to <1 mg/ml in compatible IV solution. Infuse over 30 min. **Continuous infusion:** May be infused over 48 hr.	D_5W NS	Many toxic effects are dose related, with more serious adverse effects occurring at relatively high doses. Not used routinely in children, although studied for pediatric cancers.	Hebel 1999 McEvoy 2001

TABLE 8-1 continued

DRUG[a,b] (TRADE NAME)	COMMERCIAL DILUTION OR RECONSTITUTION AND pH[c]	METHOD OF ADMINISTRATION, FURTHER DILUTION, AND RECOMMENDED RATE OF INFUSION[d]	COMPATIBLE INFUSION SOLUTIONS[e]	CAUTIONS, COMMENTS, AND INCOMPATIBILITIES[f,g,h]	REFERENCES[i]
Flumazenil (Anexate®, Romazicon®)	Available as 0.1 mg/ml pH: 4	**IV push:** Inject without further dilution over 30 sec into a free-flowing IV. *Maximum rate:* 0.2 mg/ml. Doses may be repeated every minute up to a total dose of 2 mg.	D_5W LR NS	Specially trained pediatric clinician should be present. Relatively short half-life of elimination (~1 hr) may necessitate re-administration. Generally well tolerated, but may induce convulsions in benzodiazepine-dependent epileptic infants and children.	Gura 1999 Phelps 1996 McEvoy 2001 Taketomo 2000 Trissel 2001
Fluorouracil[a] (Adrucil®)	Available as 50 mg/ml, discard opened vials after 1 hr. Slight discoloration (very pale yellow) does not affect potency. Marked discoloration indicates that degradation has occurred and that the solution should not be used. May adsorb to glass. Warm (60°C) the solution carefully with vigorous shaking if it is cloudy; allow to cool to body temperature before administration. pH: 9.2	**IV push:** Inject undiluted over 1–5 min. **Intermittent infusion:** Infuse over several hours (up to 24 hr).	D_5W D_5W/LR NS TPN	Specially trained pediatric clinician should be present for IV push. Avoid extravasation. Monitor CBC, hepatic and renal function, and fluid intake and output. Do not admix with acidic drugs or drugs that decompose in alkaline solutions. Incompatible with cytarabine, diazepam, doxorubicin, and methotrexate.	McEvoy 2001 Taketomo 2000 Trissel 2001
Folic Acid	Available as 5 mg/ml pH: 8–11	**Continuous infusion:** Dilute to <0.1 mg/ml and infuse over 1–2 hr.	TPN	Protect from light. Incompatible with oxidizing and reducing agents, heavy metal ions, and riboflavin.	McEvoy 2001 Trissel 2001
Fosphenytoin (Cerebyx®)	Available as 50 mg phenytoin equivalents (PE)/ml. Concentrations of 1.5–25 mg PE/ml in D_5W or NS, stable for 8 hr at room temperature or 24 hr refrigerated. pH: 8.6–9	**IV push:** Dilute with D_5W or NS to 1.5–25 mg PE/ml. *Maximum rate:* 150 mg PE/min.	D_5W $D_{10}W$ D_5W/LR D_5W/1/2 NS LR NS	Monitor blood pressure and ECG with loading doses. Discontinue if rash or acute hepatotoxicity occurs.	Gura 1999 Repchinsky 2002 Sifton 2002 Taketomo 2000
Furosemide (Lasix®)	Available as 10 mg/ml pH: 8–9.3	**IV push:** Inject without further dilution over 1–2 min. *Maximum rate:* 0.5 mg/kg/min or 4 mg/min, whichever is less. **Intermittent infusion:** Dilute in at least an equal volume of compatible IV solution and infuse at 0.5 mg/kg/min. *Maximum rate:* 4 mg/min. *Maximum concentration for administration:* 10 mg/ml. **Continuous infusion:** Dilute to 1–2 mg/ml and infuse at 0.1–0.4 mg/kg/hr. *Maximum concentration:* 10 mg/ml.	D_5W D_5W/LR D_5W/NS IL 3% NaCl NS TPN	Ototoxicity is associated with infusion rate >4 mg/min. Incompatible with acidic solutions (pH <5.5), some brands of dopamine, meperidine, and morphine. Follow urine output and serum electrolytes carefully. Protect from light.	Gura 1999 Hebel 1999 McEvoy 2001 Phelps 1996 Taketomo 2000 Trissel 2001
Ganciclovir (Cytovene®)	Reconstitute 500 mg powder for injection with 10 ml sterile water for injection	**Intermittent infusion:** Dilute to <10 mg/ml and infuse slowly over at least 1 hr. Concentrations of 5–10 mg/ml in D_5W or NS are	D_5W LR NS R	Monitor CBC with differential platelet count, and SCr. Rapid infusions are associated with toxic plasma levels. Avoid contact with skin. May cause	Gura 1999 McEvoy 2001 Taketomo *(Continued)*

Footnotes are on page 390.

TABLE 8-1 continued

DRUG[a,b] (TRADE NAME)	COMMERCIAL DILUTION OR RECONSTITUTION AND pH[c]	METHOD OF ADMINISTRATION, FURTHER DILUTION, AND RECOMMENDED RATE OF INFUSION[d]	COMPATIBLE INFUSION SOLUTIONS[e]	CAUTIONS, COMMENTS, AND INCOMPATIBILITIES[f,g,h]	REFERENCES[i]
Ganciclovir *continued*	(not bacteriostatic water for injection because it is incompatible and a precipitate may form) to yield 50 mg/ml. Reconstituted solutions stable for 12 hr at room temperature. Do not refrigerate. pH: 11	stable for 28 days refrigerated, but manufacturer recommends discarding after 24 hr due to risk of bacterial contamination.		phlebitis. May use in-line 0.22-μm filter. Incompatible with amifostine, aztreonam, cefepime, cytarabine, doxorubicin, fludarabine, foscarnet, ondansetron, piperacillin–tazobactam, and sargramostim.	2000 Trissel 2001
Gentamicin Sulfate *(Garamycin®)*	Available as 10 and 40 mg/ml pH: 3–5.5	**Intermittent infusion:** Dilute to a convenient concentration and infuse over 30–120 min (usually 30 min). Dilute solution stable 24 hr at room temperature.	D_5W LR NS *Normosol* products TPN	Monitor BUN, SCr, urine output, and CBC periodically. Inactivated by IV penicillins. Do not admix with other drugs.	Gura 1999 McEvoy 2001 Phelps 1996 Trissel 2001
Glucagon	Reconstitute with special diluent provided by manufacturer to yield 1 mg/ml. (1 mg = 1 IU = 1 USP unit.) Doses >2 mg should be diluted with sterile water, not the diluent provided by the manufacturer. pH: 2.5–3	**IV push:** Inject without further dilution over 3–5 min.	Dextrose solutions only	Initial administration under direct medical supervision. Do not delay initiation of dextrose infusion while awaiting the effect of glucagon. Incompatible with saline and any solution pH 3–9.5.	Hebel 1999 McEvoy 2001 Taketomo 2000
Glycopyrrolate[b] *(Robinul®)*	Available as 0.2 mg/ml pH: 2–3	**IV push:** Inject without further dilution into tubing of a patent IV infusion. **Intermittent infusion:** Dilute to 2 μg/ml and infuse over 15–20 min.	D_5W $D_{10}W$ $D_5W/1/2$ NS NS R	Observe for anticholinergic side effects, excitation, and nervousness. Compatible with atropine sulfate, benzquinamide HCl, chlorpromazine HCl, codeine phosphate, diphenhydramine HCl, droperidol, fentanyl citrate, hydromorphone HCl, hydroxyzine HCl, levorphanol tartrate, lidocaine HCl, meperidine HCl, midazolam HCl, morphine sulfate, nalbuphine HCl, neostigmine methylsulfate, oxymorphone, procaine HCl, prochlorperazine edisylate, promazine HCl, promethazine HCl, pyridostigmine bromide, scopolamine hydrobromide, triflupromazine HCl, and trimethobenzamide HCl. Incompatible with alkaline drugs (pH >6).	Gura 1999 McEvoy 2001 Trissel 2001
Gonadorelin[b] Hydrochloride *(Factrel®)*	Reconstitute powder for injection with special diluent (2% benzyl alcohol in sterile water) provided by the manufacturer to yield 100 or 250 μg/ml. pH: Information not available	**IV push:** Dilute with 3 ml NS and inject over 30 sec. Prepare immediately before use. Store at room temperature and use within 24 hr.	NS	Monitor FSH and LH.	Taketomo 2000
Granisetron *(Kytril®)*	Available as 1 mg/ml pH: 4.7–7.3	**IV push:** Not recommended, but has been given undiluted over 30 sec, or diluted in small volume D_5W or NS and given slow IV push over 5 min.	D_5W Dextrose/ saline combinations	Infuse 30 min before the start of chemotherapy. Observe for constipation and headache. Incompatible with amphotericin B.	Gura 1999 Taketomo 2000 Trissel 2001

DRUG[a,b] (TRADE NAME)	COMMERCIAL DILUTION OR RECONSTITUTION AND pH[c]	METHOD OF ADMINISTRATION, FURTHER DILUTION, AND RECOMMENDED RATE OF INFUSION[d]	COMPATIBLE INFUSION SOLUTIONS[e]	CAUTIONS, COMMENTS, AND INCOMPATIBILITIES[f,g,h]	REFER-ENCES[i]
Granisetron *continued*		**Intermittent infusion:** Dilute in 20–50 ml D$_5$W or NS and infuse over 30–60 min. Stable in D$_5$W or NS for 24 hr at room temperature.	NS TPN		
Heparin Sodium	Available as 10, 100, 1000, 5000, 10,000, 20,000, and 40,000 units/ml pH: 5–8	**Intermittent or continuous infusion:** Dilute to desired concentration and infuse at 15–25 units/kg/hr (adjust rate to maintain PTT 1.5 times normal).	D$_5$W D$_{10}$W D$_5$W/LR D$_5$W/1/2 NS D$_5$W/NS Dextran 6%/D$_5$W or fat emulsion 10% IL LR 1/2 NS NS TPN	Protamine sulfate should be available to reverse excessive anticoagulation associated with overdose. Incompatible with aminoglycosides, ciprofloxacin, phenytoin, promethazine HCl, and vancomycin HCl. Monitor CBC and platelet count, aPTT, and for signs of bleeding. Do not check aPTT any sooner than 4 hr after a bolus or increase in dose.	Gura 1999 Hebel 1999 McEvoy 2001 Phelps 1996 Taketomo 2000 Trissel 2001
Hydralazine Hydrochloride *(Apresoline®)*	Available as 20 mg/ml pH: 3.4–4	**IV push:** Inject without further dilution over 1–2 min. *Maximum rate:* 5 mg/min or 0.2 mg/kg/min, whichever is less.	D$_5$W D$_5$W/LR D$_5$W/1/2 NS D$_5$W/NS Dextran 6%/D$_5$W or NS NS 1/2 NS TPN	Monitor blood pressure and heart rate for 30–60 min after dose. Do not admix with other drugs.	Gura 1999 McEvoy 2001 Phelps 1996 Taketomo 2000 Trissel 2001
Hydrocortisone Sodium Phosphate *(Hydrocortone®)*	Available as 50 mg/ml pH: 7.5–8.5	**IV push:** Inject without further dilution over 30 sec for doses <100 mg or over 10 min for doses >500 mg. **Intermittent infusion:** Dilute to 1 mg/ml and infuse over at least 30 min. *Maximum concentration:* 5 mg/ml.	D$_5$W Dextrose/saline solutions Fat emulsion 1/2 NS NS TPN	Monitor blood pressure and glucose levels. Incompatible with sargramostim.	Gura 1999 Taketomo 2000 Trissel 2001
Hydrocortisone Sodium Succinate[b] *(Solu-Cortef®)*	Reconstitute powder for injection with bacteriostatic water for injection or bacteriostatic sodium chloride injection (both contain benzyl alcohol) to yield 50 mg/ml. Reconstituted solutions stable at room temperature if protected from light. pH: 7–8	**IV push:** Inject without further dilution over 30 sec for doses <100 mg or over 10 min for doses >500 mg. **Intermittent infusion:** May dilute to <1 mg/ml and infuse over at least 30 min. *Maximum concentration:* 125 mg/ml.	D$_{2.5}$W D$_5$W D$_{10}$W D$_{20}$W D$_5$W/LR D$_5$W/R Dextran solutions Dextrose/saline solutions Fat emulsion 1/2 NS NS 3% NaCl TPN	Monitor blood pressure and serum glucose. Incompatible with barbiturates, bleomycin, ciprofloxacin, hydralazine, idarubicin, midazolam, nafcillin, phenytoin, promethazine, and sargramostim.	Gura 1999 Taketomo 2000 Trissel 2001
Hydromorphone *(Dilaudid®)*	Available as 1, 2, 4, and 10 mg/ml. Store at room temperature. Protect from light. pH: 4–5.5	**IV push:** May be injected over 2–3 min.	D$_5$W D$_5$W/LR D$_5$W/NS LR 1/2 NS NS TPN	Incompatible with sodium bicarbonate and thiopental.	McEvoy 2001 Taketomo 2000

Footnotes are on page 390.

TABLE 8-1 continued

DRUG[a,b] (TRADE NAME)	COMMERCIAL DILUTION OR RECONSTITUTION AND pH[c]	METHOD OF ADMINISTRATION, FURTHER DILUTION, AND RECOMMENDED RATE OF INFUSION[d]	COMPATIBLE INFUSION SOLUTIONS[e]	CAUTIONS, COMMENTS, AND INCOMPATIBILITIES[f,g,h]	REFER-ENCES[i]
Idarubicin (*Idamycin®*)	Reconstitute powder for injection to 1 mg/ml; do not use bacteriostatic diluent. Reconstituted solutions stable for 3 days at room temperature and 7 days refrigerated. pH: 5–7	**Intermittent infusion:** Infuse undiluted over 10–30 min into a free-flowing IV.	D_5W D_5W/NS LR NS	Specially trained pediatric clinician should be present for IV push. Maximum lifetime anthracycline dose ~137.5 mg/m². Monitor for cardiotoxicity (ECG, ECHO), extravasation, and myelosuppression. Unstable in alkaline solutions.	Taketomo 2000 Trissel 2001
Ifosfamide[a] (*Ifex®*)	Reconstitute powder for injection with sterile or bacteriostatic water for injection to yield 50 mg/ml. Reconstituted solution is stable for 7 days at room temperature and 21 days refrigerated. pH: 6	**Intermittent infusion:** Dilute to <40 mg/ml and infuse slowly over at least 30 min. **Continuous infusion:** Dilute to 0.6–20 mg/ml and infuse over 24 hr. Diluted solutions are stable 1 week at room temperature and 6 weeks refrigerated, but the manufacturer recommends using within 24 hr.	$D_{2.5}W$ D_5W D_5W/NS D_5W/R LR 1/2 NS NS Sterile water for injection	Provide adequate hydration and administer with mesna. Monitor CBC with differential, hepatic and renal function, urine output, and urinalysis. Incompatible with cefepime and methotrexate.	McEvoy 2001 Taketomo 2000 Trissel 2001
Imipenem–Cilastatin (*Primaxin®*)	Reconstitute powder for injection with sterile water for injection or NS to yield 2.5 or 5 mg/ml of each drug pH: 6.5	**Intermittent infusion:** Dilute to <5 mg/ml of each drug and infuse over 30–60 min (if nausea or vomiting occurs during administration, decrease rate). When diluted with compatible IV solution, the solution is stable for 4 hr at room temperature or 24 hr refrigerated.	D_5W $D_{10}W$ Dextrose/saline combinations NS	Monitor hematologic, hepatic, and renal functions. Monitor for seizure activity in patients with a history of seizures or with meningitis. Contains 3.2 mEq of sodium per gram imipenem.	McEvoy 2001 Taketomo 2000 Trissel 2001
Immune Globulin (*Gamimune N®**, *Gammagard® S/D***, *Gammar-P® IV***, *Iveegam® IV***, *Polygam® S/D***, *Venoglobulin-S®***, *Sandoglobulin®****)	Available as 50 mg/ml **or** reconstitute with diluent supplied by manufacturer to yield 30 or 60 mg/ml. *Gammagard S/D* and *Polygam S/D* should be used within 2 hr after reconstitution. *Sandoglobulin* is stable for 24 hr if refrigerated after reconstitution. *pH: 4–4.5 **pH: 6.4–7.2 ***pH: 6.4–6.8	**Intermittent infusion:** Infuse *Gamimune N* (maximum concentration 10%) at 0.01–0.02 ml/kg/min for 30 min and, if no adverse effects are observed, increase rate gradually to maximum of 0.08 ml/kg/min (may dilute with D_5W); filter and infuse *Gammagard S/D* (maximum concentration 5%) and *Polygam S/D* (maximum concentration 10%) at 0.5 ml/kg/hr and, if no adverse effects occur, gradually increase rate to maximum of 4 ml/kg/hr; infuse *Gammar-P IV* (maximum concentration 5%) at 0.6 ml/kg/hr for 15–30 min and then increase rate gradually to 1.8–3.6 ml/kg/hr; infuse *Iveegam* (maximum concentration 5%) at 60–120 ml/hr; infuse *Sandoglobulin* at 0.5–1 ml/min for 15–30 min and then increase the rate to 1.5–2.5 ml/min (if tolerated, subsequent doses may be infused at 2–2.5 ml/min); infuse *Venoglobulin-S* (maximum concentration 10%) at 0.6–1.2 ml/kg/hr for 30 min and, if tolerated, increase to 2.4 ml/kg/hr.	D_5W NS	Observe for hypotension and anaphylaxis, have epinephrine available; if hypotension observed, decrease rate or stop infusion until reaction subsides; then resume at slower rate as tolerated by patient. Do not admix with other drugs. Do not shake preparations. Give by separate infusion line.	Sifton 2002

CHAPTER 8: INTRAVENOUS DRUGS FOR NEONATES, INFANTS, CHILDREN, AND ADOLESCENTS

TABLE 8-1 continued

DRUG[a,b] (TRADE NAME)	COMMERCIAL DILUTION OR RECONSTITUTION AND pH[c]	METHOD OF ADMINISTRATION, FURTHER DILUTION, AND RECOMMENDED RATE OF INFUSION[d]	COMPATIBLE INFUSION SOLUTIONS[e]	CAUTIONS, COMMENTS, AND INCOMPATIBILITIES[f,g,h]	REFERENCES[i]
Indomethacin (*Indocin®*)	Reconstitute powder for injection with sterile water for injection to yield 1 mg/ml. pH: 6–7.5	**IV push:** Dilute to 0.5 mg/ml and inject over 5–10 sec. **Intermittent infusion (preferred):** Dilute to 0.5–1 mg/ml and infuse over 20–30 min. Contains no preservatives; reconstitute just prior to use.	NS Sterile water for injection	Administer through a central or large vein; avoid extravasation. Use solution within 1 hr after preparation. Monitor BUN, CBC, hepatic enzymes, platelet count, and SCr. Do not admix with dextrose. Rapid infusion may result in decreased mesenteric artery blood flow.	Gura 1999 McEvoy 2001 Taketomo 2000 Trissel 2001
Insulin, Regular Human (*Humulin R®, Novolin R®*)	Available as 100 units/ml. Stable at room temperature up to 1 month; stable refrigerated for 3 months. pH: 7–7.8	**IV push:** Inject slowly without further dilution not to exceed 30 units/min. **Intermittent or continuous infusion:** Dilute to 0.2–1 unit/ml in NS and infuse at 0.05–0.1 unit/kg/hr.	NS TPN	Do not administer if turbid, discolored, or unusually viscous. Insulin adsorbs to glass and plastic IV containers, IV tubing, and filters. If new tubing is needed for infusion, flush with insulin solution, wait 30 min, then flush again before starting infusion. Incompatible with aminophylline, barbiturates, chlorothiazide, cytarabine, dobutamine, dopamine, norepinephrine, and phenytoin.	Gura 1999 McEvoy 2001 Taketomo 2000 Trissel 2001
Irinotecan Hydrochloride (*Camptosar®*)	Available as 20 mg/ml pH: 3–3.8	**Intermittent infusion:** Dilute in D_5W to 0.12–2.8 mg/ml. NS may also be used. Infuse over 90 min to decrease the likelihood of cholinergic symptoms developing. Solutions diluted in D_5W should be used within 24 hr if refrigerated or within 6 hr if stored at room temperature. Solutions prepared in NS should **not** be refrigerated because of the possible formation of visible particulates; they should be stored at room temperature and used within 6 hr.	D_5W (preferred) NS	Must be diluted prior to administration. Observe for particulate matter in the vial and again in the syringe when transferring drug solution to prepare admixtures. Use under the supervision of physician experienced with antineoplastic agents.	Hebel 1999 McEvoy 2001 Repchinsky 2002 Trissel 2001
Iron Dextran (*INFeD®*)	Available as 50 mg/ml pH: 5.2–6.5	**IV push (not recommended):** Inject without further dilution very slowly (<50 mg/min). **Intermittent infusion:** Dilute with NS to a maximum concentration of 50 mg/ml and infuse 25 mg as a test dose over 5 min; if no reaction occurs, then infuse remainder of dose over 1–6 hr. Flush with NS following infusion. Store at controlled room temperature.	NS TPN	Observe for anaphylaxis. When diluted with D_5W, phlebitis is more common.	Gura 1999 McEvoy 2001
Isoproterenol Hydrochloride	Available as 0.2 mg/ml (1:5000) pH: 2.5–4.5	**Continuous infusion:** Dilute to 4–12 µg/ml (D_5W preferred) and infuse at 0.1–1 µg/kg/min (may use more concentrated solution, up to 64 µg/ml, if patient is severely fluid restricted).	D_5W D_5W/LR D_5W/1/4 NS D_5W/1/2 NS D_5W/NS Dextran 6%/D_5W or NS 1/2 NS NS TPN	Administer with electronic infusion device. Titrate dose to response. Monitor blood pressure, ECG, and heart rate (avoid heart rate >180 beats/min). Can cause myocardial ischemia. If using for bronchodilation, taper over 24 hr to avoid rebound bronchospasm. Incompatible with alkaline solutions.	Gura 1999 Hebel 1999 McEvoy 2001 Phelps 1996 Sodorff 1999 Taketomo 2000 Trissel 2001

Footnotes are on page 390.

TABLE 8-1 continued

DRUG[a,b] (TRADE NAME)	COMMERCIAL DILUTION OR RECONSTITUTION AND pH[c]	METHOD OF ADMINISTRATION, FURTHER DILUTION, AND RECOMMENDED RATE OF INFUSION[d]	COMPATIBLE INFUSION SOLUTIONS[e]	CAUTIONS, COMMENTS, AND INCOMPATIBILITIES[f,g,h]	REFERENCES[i]
Kanamycin Sulfate (*Kantrex®*)	Available as 37.5, 250, and 333 mg/ml pH: 4.5	**Intermittent infusion:** Dilute to 2.5–5 mg/ml and infuse over 30–60 min (30 min preferred).	D_5W D_5W/NS LR NS TPN	Avoid admixing with other antibacterial agents. Inactivated by penicillin.	Hebel 1999 McEvoy 2001 Trissel 2001
Ketamine Hydrochloride (*Ketalar®*)	Available as 10, 50, and 100 mg/ml pH: 3.5–5.5	**IV push:** Dilute to ≤10 mg/ml and inject over ≥60 sec. **Intermittent infusion:** Dilute to ≤2 mg/ml and infuse at 0.5 mg/kg/min. **Continuous infusion:** Dilute to a maximum concentration of 2 mg/ml and infuse at 1–2 mg/kg/hr for anesthesia.	D_5W NS Sterile water for injection	Monitor blood pressure and heart rate. Do not use in patients with glaucoma, hypertension, or increased intracranial pressure. Patients may experience hallucinations; a low dose of a benzodiazepine can help prevent this.	Phelps 1996 Taketomo 2000 Trissel 2001
Labetalol Hydrochloride (*Normodyne®*)	Available as 5 mg/ml pH: 3–4	**IV push:** Inject without further dilution over 2 min. *Maximum rate:* 2 mg/min. **Continuous infusion:** Dilute to 1 mg/ml and infuse at 0.4–1 mg/kg/hr. *Maximum rate for hypertensive emergencies:* 3 mg/kg/hr.	D_5W NS	Monitor blood pressure, heart rate, and respiratory rate. Concentrations of up to 5 mg/ml have been used safely in a small number of adult patients who were fluid restricted.	Gura 1999 Phelps 1996 Taketomo 2000 Trissel 2001
Leucovorin Calcium	Available as 5 mg/ml **or** reconstitute with bacteriostatic water for injection containing benzyl alcohol[b] or sterile water for injection to yield 10 or 20 mg/ml. When doses >10 mg/m² are used, prepare with preservative-free sterile water. Once reconstituted with preservative, stable for 7 days at room temperature. Solutions further diluted with 50 ml D_5W are stable 24 hr at room temperature. pH: 8.1	**IV push:** Maximum rate 160 mg/min. **Intermittent infusion:** Dilute to <20 mg/ml and infuse at <160 mg/min.	D_5W $D_{10}W$ $D_{10}W/NS$ LR NS R TPN	Monitor for erythema, pruritus, and rash. Leucovorin may enhance the toxicity of fluorouracil. Not adversely affected by room light. Incompatible with droperidol, fluorouracil, foscarnet, and sodium bicarbonate.	Gura 1999 McEvoy 2001 Taketomo 2000 Trissel 2001
Levothyroxine Sodium (*Synthroid®*)	Reconstitute *Synthroid* with NS or bacteriostatic sodium chloride injection with benzyl alcohol[b] to yield 40 or 100 μg/ml. pH: Information not available	**IV push:** Inject without further dilution over 2–3 min.	NS	Use reconstituted solution immediately. Adverse reactions result from overdose and are manifested primarily as symptoms of hyperthyroidism. Protect from light. Incompatible with other drugs and solutions. Do not switch brands without physician knowledge. IV dose = 1/2 oral dose	Hebel 1999 McEvoy 2001 Taketomo 2000

TABLE 8-1 continued

DRUG[a,b] (TRADE NAME)	COMMERCIAL DILUTION OR RECONSTITUTION AND pH[c]	METHOD OF ADMINISTRATION, FURTHER DILUTION, AND RECOMMENDED RATE OF INFUSION[d]	COMPATIBLE INFUSION SOLUTIONS[e]	CAUTIONS, COMMENTS, AND INCOMPATIBILITIES[f,g,h]	REFERENCES[i]
Lidocaine Hydrochloride (Xylocaine®)	Available as 2, 4, 5, 10, 15, 20, 40, 100, and 200 mg/ml pH: 5–7 pH: 3.5–6 (premixed in D_5W)	**IV push:** Inject 10 or 20 mg/ml slowly over 2–4 min. *Maximum rate:* 0.7 mg/kg/min or 50 mg/min. **Continuous infusion:** Dilute to 4 µg/ml (D_5W preferred) and infuse at 10–50 µg/kg/min (may use more concentrated solution, up to 8 mg/ml, if patient is fluid restricted).	D_5W D_5W/LR D_5W/NS LR NS TPN	Administer with electronic infusion device. Monitor ECG continuously. Observe for agitation, bradycardia, cardiac dysrhythmias, hypotension, loss of consciousness, and seizures. Avoid admixing. Compatible with bretylium, calcium chloride, dexamethasone, dobutamine, dopamine, heparin, hydrocortisone, insulin (regular), potassium chloride, ranitidine, sodium bicarbonate, and sodium succinate.	McEvoy 2001 Phelps 1996 Sodorff 1999 Taketomo 2000 Trissel 2001
Lincomycin Hydrochloride[b] (Lincocin®)	Available as 300 mg/ml pH: 3–5.5	**Intermittent infusion:** Dilute to <10 mg/ml and infuse over at least 1 hr.	D_5W $D_{10}W$ D_5W/NS $D_{10}W$/NS NS R Sodium lactate 1/6 M	Monitor blood pressure during infusion. Avoid admixing. Incompatible with kanamycin sulfate.	Hebel 1999 McEvoy 2001 Trissel 2001
Lorazepam (Ativan®)	Available as 2 and 4 mg/ml. Stable 8 weeks at room temperature. pH: 6.4	**IV push:** Dilute with an equal volume of IV solution and inject slowly over 2–5 min. *Maximum rate:* 0.05 mg/kg over 2–5 min up to 2 mg/min. *Maximum concentration:* 4 mg/ml.	D_5W NS Sterile water for injection	Monitor respiratory function. Do not use if solution is discolored. Injectable solution contains benzyl alcohol, polyethylene glycol, and propylene glycol. Toxicity has been noted in neonates and patients receiving high doses. Avoid intra-arterial administration.	Gura 1999 Phelps 1996 Taketomo 2000 Trissel 2001
Lymphocyte Immune Globulin (Atgam®)	Available as 50 mg/ml. Dilutions at 4 mg/ml are stable 24 hr refrigerated. pH: 6.8	**Intermittent infusion:** Dilute with NS or 1/2 NS to <1 mg/ml and infuse through an in-line filter (pore size 0.2–1 µm) over 4–8 hr. *Maximum concentration:* 4 mg/ml.	D_5W/1/4 NS D_5W/1/2 NS 1/2 NS NS	Infuse through a central line to minimize phlebitis and thrombosis. Monitor CBC with differential, platelet count, renal function, and vital signs. Pretreatment with antihistamines, antipyretics, and corticosteroids is usually necessary. Observe for allergic reactions. Avoid admixing with acidic solutions. Solutions must contain some saline to avoid precipitation.	Gura 1999 McEvoy 2001 Taketomo 2000 Trissel 2001
Magnesium Sulfate	Available as 100 mg/ml (0.8 mEq/ml), 125 mg/ml (1 mEq/ml), 250 mg/ml (2 mEq/ml), and 500 mg/ml (4 mEq/ml) pH: 5.5–7	**IV push:** Inject without further dilution over 3–5 min, not to exceed 150 mg/min. **Intermittent infusion:** Dilute to a maximum concentration of 200 mg/ml and infuse over at least 15–30 min (preferably over 2–4 hr).	D_5W D_5W/LR LR NS TPN	Monitor blood pressure, deep tendon reflexes, ECG, and magnesium serum levels. Observe for hypotension and respiratory depression. Incompatible with alkali carbonates and bicarbonates and concentrated phosphate solutions.	Gura 1999 Hebel 1999 McEvoy 2001 Phelps 1996 Taketomo 2000 Trissel 2001
Mannitol	Available as 50 mg/ml (5%), 100 mg/ml (10%), 150 mg/ml (15%), 200 mg/ml (20%), and 250 mg/ml (25%) pH: 4.5–7	**IV push (for oliguria or acute increase in ICP):** Inject without further dilution slowly over 3–5 min. **Intermittent infusion (for increased intracranial pressure):** Infuse without further dilution at 0.25–0.5 gram/kg over 30–60 min. May give up to 2 grams/kg as prophylaxis for neurosurgery.	NS	Monitor renal function and serum osmolality. The osmolarity of the 25% solution is 1373 mOsm/liter, 20% solution is 1100 mOsm/liter. Solutions ≥20% should be filtered and not be admixed with KCl or NaCl. Do not use solutions containing crystals (warm the solution to resolubilize the crystals, but cool to body temperature prior to use). Incompatible with blood, strongly acidic solutions, and strongly alkaline solutions.	Gura 1999 McEvoy 2001 Phelps 1996 Taketomo 2000 Trissel 2001

Footnotes are on page 390.

TABLE 8-1 continued

DRUG[a,b] (TRADE NAME)	COMMERCIAL DILUTION OR RECONSTITUTION AND pH[c]	METHOD OF ADMINISTRATION, FURTHER DILUTION, AND RECOMMENDED RATE OF INFUSION[d]	COMPATIBLE INFUSION SOLUTIONS[e]	CAUTIONS, COMMENTS, AND INCOMPATIBILITIES[f,g,h]	REFER- ENCES[i]
Mechlor- ethamine Hydrochlo- ride [Nitrogen Mustard] *(Mustargen®)*	Reconstitute powder for injection with sterile water for injection or NS to yield 1 mg/ml. Use immediately after reconstitution. Discard any unused drug after 60 min. pH: 3–5	**IV push:** Inject without further dilution over 1–3 min and follow with flush.	NS	Hematologic toxicities are dose limiting. Monitor CBC, platelet count, and uric acid serum concentration. Unstable in neutral or alkaline solutions. Avoid extravasation. Incompatible with allopurinol and cefepime.	McEvoy 2001 Taketomo 2000 Trissel 2001
Melphalan *(Alkeran®)*	Reconstitute powder for injection with provided diluent to 5 mg/ml; stable 90 min at room temperature. Further dilute with NS to a concentration ≤2 mg/ml prior to administration; must complete administration within 1 hr. Do not refrigerate because a precipitate may form. pH: Information not available	**Intermittent infusion:** Infuse over 15–30 min (rate not to exceed 10 mg/min). Dilute with NS to >2 mg/ml for central lines or 0.45 mg/ml for peripheral lines. May filter through a 0.45-μm Millex-HV filter	NS	Observe for cystitis, hemorrhagic leukopenia, hypersensitivity reactions, hypotension, rash, and thrombocytopenia. Hematologic toxicities are dose limiting. Incompatible with amphotericin B, chlorpromazine, D_5W, and LR.	McEvoy 2001 Taketomo 2000 Trissel 2001
Meperidine Hydrochlo- ride *(Demerol®)*	Available as 10, 25, 50, 75, and 100 mg/ml pH: 3.5–6	**IV push:** Dilute to 10 mg/ml and inject slowly over >5 min. **Intermittent infusion (usually not recommended):** Dilute to 1 mg/ml and infuse over at least 15–30 min. **Continuous infusion:** Dilute to 1 mg/ml and infuse at 0.3–1.5 mg/kg/hr.	D_5W $D_{10}W$ D_5W/LR D_5W/R Dextran 6%/D_5W or NS Dextrose/ saline combinations *Ionosol®* products LR 1/2 NS NS R	Observe for respiratory depression and have naloxone available to reverse effects. Incompatible with allopurinol, aminophylline, cefepime, furosemide, heparin, idarubicin, piperacillin–tazobactam, phenobarbital, phenytoin, and sodium bicarbonate.	Gura 1999 McEvoy 2001 Taketomo 2000 Trissel 2001
Meropenem *(Merrem® IV)*	Reconstitute powder for injection with NS to 50 mg/ml. pH: 7.3–8.3	**IV push:** Inject without further dilution over 3–5 min. Solution stable 2 hr at room temperature and up to 18 hr refrigerated. **Intermittent infusion:** Dilute to 5–10 mg/ml and infuse over 15–30 min. *Maximum concentration:* 10 mg/ml. Solution stable 4 hr at room temperature and 24 hr refrigerated.	D_5W NS Sterile water for injection	Use with caution in patients with a history of seizures, CNS disease, CNS infection, and/or compromised renal function. Observe for pain/inflammation at the injection site. Sodium content 3.92 mEq/gram.	Gura 1999 McEvoy 2001 Taketomo 2000

TABLE 8-1 continued

DRUG[a,b] (TRADE NAME)	COMMERCIAL DILUTION OR RECONSTITUTION AND pH[c]	METHOD OF ADMINISTRATION, FURTHER DILUTION, AND RECOMMENDED RATE OF INFUSION[d]	COMPATIBLE INFUSION SOLUTIONS[e]	CAUTIONS, COMMENTS, AND INCOMPATIBILITIES[f,g,h]	REFERENCES[i]
Mesna[a] (Mesnex®, Uromitexan®)	Available as 100 mg/ml. Diluted solutions stable for 24 hr at room temperature, but it is generally recommended to store under refrigeration and to use within 6 hr. pH: 6.5–8.5	**IV push:** Dilute to 20 mg/ml and inject over 1 min. **Intermittent infusion:** Dilute to 20 mg/ml and infuse over 15–30 min. May also be given as a continuous infusion.	D_5W $D_5W/1/2$ NS D_5W/NS LR NS TPN	Used for prophylaxis of cyclophosphamide- or ifosfamide-induced hemorrhagic cystitis. Mesna is administered 15 min before ifosfamide or cyclophosphamide and 4 and 8 hr after each dose. May also be given every 3 hr for three to six doses. At recommended dosages, ADRs are uncommon. Compatible for 24 hr when mixed with ifosfamide or cyclophosphamide. Incompatible with cisplatin and carboplatin.	McEvoy 2001 Taketomo 2000 Trissel 2001
Methohexital Sodium (Brevital®)	Reconstitute with sterile water for injection (preferred), D_5W, or NS (do not use a bacteriostatic diluent) to yield 10 mg/ml. pH: 10–11 (10 mg/ml) pH: 9.5–10.5 (2 mg/ml in D_5W)	**IV push:** Inject without further dilution. **Intermittent infusion:** Infuse 10 mg/ml at 2–4 ml/min. **Continuous infusion:** Dilute to 2 mg/ml with D_5W or NS and infuse at 3 ml/min (individualize dose based on patient response). Stable 24 hr at room temperature.	D_5W D_5W/NS NS	Specially trained pediatric clinician should be present for IV push. Observe for hypotension, respiratory depression, seizures, and thrombophlebitis. Avoid contact with rubber stoppers or silicone. Do not admix with acidic solutions or alkali-labile drugs.	McEvoy 2001 Taketomo 2000 Trissel 2001
Methotrexate Sodium[a,b]	Available as 25 mg/ml **or** reconstitute powder for injection with preservative-free D_5W or NS for injection to yield 25 or 50 mg/ml. Stable in D_5W, NS, or D_5W/NS for 1 week at room temperature. Protect from light. pH: 8.5 (preservative free) pH: 7–8.8 (preserved)	**IV push:** Inject without further dilution over 1 min. **Intermittent infusion:** Dilute in 50 ml D_5W and infuse over 15 min (or as per protocol). **Continuous infusion:** Dilute according to protocol and infuse over 24 hr (usually for doses >100–300 mg/m² and followed by leucovorin).	D_5W D_5W/NS NS	Specially trained pediatric clinician should be present for IV push. Monitor CBC, renal and hepatic function, and urinalysis. High doses should be avoided in patients with CrCl <50%–75% of normal. Administer leucovorin rescue, monitor methotrexate concentrations (especially with high doses to guide further leucovorin rescue). Methotrexate serum levels $>1 \times 10^{-7}$ mol/liter for >40 hr are toxic. Use with caution in patients with renal or liver impairment, ascites, or pleural effusion. Incompatible with bleomycin, chlorpromazine, cytarabine, droperidol, fluorouracil, idarubicin, ifosfamide, midazolam, prednisolone, promethazine, propofol, and sodium phosphate.	McEvoy 2001 Taketomo 2000 Trissel 2001
Methyldopate Hydrochloride (Aldomet®)	Available as 50 mg/ml pH: 3–4.2	**IV push:** Not recommended. **Intermittent infusion:** Dilute to ≤10 mg/ml (D_5W preferred), infuse over 30–60 min. Stable 24 hr at room temperature.	D_5W D_5W/NS Dextran 6%/NS LR Normosol M/D_5W NS Sodium bicarbonate 5% TPN	Observe for drug fever, orthostatic hypotension, and sedation. Incompatible with acid-labile drugs.	McEvoy 2001 Phelps 1996 Repchinsky 2002 Taketomo 2000 Trissel 2001
Methylene Blue	Available as 10 mg/ml pH: 3–4.5	**IV push:** Inject without further dilution over 5–10 min.	NS	Large dose may cause cyanosis, dizziness, hypertension, mental confusion, and sweating. May discolor feces and urine blue–green.	McEvoy 2001 Taketomo 2000

Footnotes are on page 390.

TABLE 8-1 continued

DRUG[a,b] (TRADE NAME)	COMMERCIAL DILUTION OR RECONSTITUTION AND pH[c]	METHOD OF ADMINISTRATION, FURTHER DILUTION, AND RECOMMENDED RATE OF INFUSION[d]	COMPATIBLE INFUSION SOLUTIONS[e]	CAUTIONS, COMMENTS, AND INCOMPATIBILITIES[f,g,h]	REFERENCES[i]
Methyl-prednisolone Sodium Succinate[b] (Solu-Medrol® A)	Reconstitute powder for injection with diluent supplied by manufacturer (bacteriostatic water for injection containing 0.9% benzyl alcohol[b]) to yield 40, 62.5, or 125 mg/ml. Discard after 48 hr. pH: 7–8	**Intermittent infusion:** Dilute to <62.5 mg/ml and infuse as follows: if dose <1.8 mg/kg or <125 mg, give over 3–15 min; if dose >2 mg/kg or 250 mg, give over 15–30 min; if 15 mg/kg or >500 mg/dose, give over at least 30 min. Doses >1 gram, give over >1 hr.	D_5W D_5W/NS LR NS TPN	Hypotension, cardiac dysrhythmia, and sudden death have been reported in patients given high doses IV push over <10 min. Incompatible with allopurinol, calcium gluconate, ciprofloxacin, filgrastim, nafcillin, ondansetron, penicillin G, propofol, and sargramostim.	Gura 1999 McEvoy 2001 Taketomo 2000 Trissel 2001
Metoclo-pramide Hydro-chloride (Reglan®)	Available as 5 mg/ml. Dilutions stable for 48 hr protected from light and refrigerated. If exposed to regular light, stable for 24 hr. pH: 3–6.5	**IV push:** Inject without further dilution over 1–2 min slowly. **Intermittent infusion:** Dilute to 0.2 mg/ml and infuse over at least 15 min. *Maximum rate:* 5 mg/min.	D_5W $D_5W/1/2$ NS LR NS (preferred) R TPN	Observe for extrapyramidal side effects (dystonic reactions) that are more prevalent in children than adults; treat dystonic reactions with diphenhydramine. Rapid IV administration is associated with a transient, but intense, feeling of anxiety and restlessness, followed by drowsiness. Incompatible with allopurinol, ampicillin, calcium gluconate, cefepime, erythromycin, fluorouracil, furosemide, penicillin G, and sodium bicarbonate.	Gura 1999 McEvoy 2001 Taketomo 2000 Trissel 2001
Metoprolol (Lopressor®)	Available as 1 mg/ml pH: 7.5	**IV push:** Inject without further dilution and give over 2–3 min. May repeat dose every 15 min as necessary. 0.3 mg/ml stable 24 hr at room temperature.	D_5W NS	Avoid using in patients with COPD or asthma. Monitor blood pressure and heart rate closely. Limited data exist on use in pediatrics.	Hebel 1999 McEvoy 2001 Repchinsky 2002 Trissel 2001
Metro-nidazole (Flagyl IV RTU®)	Available as 5 mg/ml Do not refrigerate. pH: 4.5–7	**Intermittent infusion:** Infuse over 1 hr.	D_5W LR NS	Observe for abdominal cramping, seizures, nausea, thrombophlebitis, unpleasant metallic taste, and vomiting. Do not admix with other drugs or solutions. Solution interaction with aluminum hub needles may cause solution discoloration. Sodium content 28 mEq/gram.	Gura 1999 Hebel 1999 McEvoy 2001 Taketomo 2000 Trissel 2001
Metro-nidazole Hydro-chloride	Available as 5 mg/ml (ready-to-use solution) and as powder for reconstitution. Reconstitute powder for injection with sterile water for injection, bacteriostatic water for injection, NS, or bacteriostatic NS to yield 100 mg/ml. pH: 6–7	**Intermittent infusion:** Dilute reconstituted solution to 8 mg/ml with NS, D_5W, or LR, then neutralize with 5 mEq sodium bicarbonate per 500 mg metronidazole, and infuse over 30–60 min. Store solutions of <8 mg/ml at room temperature and use within 24 hr.	D_5W LR NS	Observe for abdominal cramping, nausea, seizures, thrombophlebitis, unpleasant metallic taste, and vomiting. Do not admix with other drugs or solutions. Sodium content 28 mEq/gram.	Gura 1999 Hebel 1999 McEvoy 2001 Repchinsky 2002 Taketomo 2000 Trissel 2001
Midazolam Hydro-chloride[b] (Versed®)	Available as 1 and 5 mg/ml pH: 3	**IV push:** Inject without further dilution over 20–30 sec for anesthesia induction, wait 2 min, and further titrate dosage in up to three small increments. **Intermittent infusion:** Infuse over at least 2 min, wait 2 min, and evaluate patient; titrate as needed in small increments over at least 2 min.	D_5W LR NS TPN	Specially trained pediatric clinician should be present for IV push. Equipment, drugs, and skilled personnel should be available for assisted or controlled respiration and cardiovascular support. Monitor cardiac and respiratory functions continuously for early signs of apnea or underventilation because hypoxia and cardiac arrest can occur. Have flumazenil available for overdoses	Gura 1999 McEvoy 2001 Phelps 1996 Taketomo 2000 Trissel 2001

CHAPTER 8: INTRAVENOUS DRUGS FOR NEONATES, INFANTS, CHILDREN, AND ADOLESCENTS

TABLE 8-1 *continued*

DRUG[a,b] (TRADE NAME)	COMMERCIAL DILUTION OR RECONSTITUTION AND pH[c]	METHOD OF ADMINISTRATION, FURTHER DILUTION, AND RECOMMENDED RATE OF INFUSION[d]	COMPATIBLE INFUSION SOLUTIONS[e]	CAUTIONS, COMMENTS, AND INCOMPATIBILITIES[f,g,h]	REFER-ENCES[i]
Midazolam Hydro-chloride[b] *continued*		**Continuous infusion:** Infuse loading dose over 2–3 min, then follow with continuous infusion at 0.05–0.1 mg/kg/hr. Titrate to desired effect (0.02–0.4 mg/kg/hr).		or reversal of oversedation. Compatible with atropine, fentanyl, meperidine, and morphine for ≤4 hr. Do not inject intra-arterially. Contains benzyl alcohol.	
Milrinone (*Primacor®*)	Available as 1 mg/ml. Store diluted solutions at room temperature and use within 24 hr. pH: 3.2–4	**IV push:** May inject undiluted, slowly over 15 min. **Continuous infusion:** Dilute to ≤200 µg/ml and infuse at 0.5 µg/kg/min. Titrate to desired effect (0.25–0.75 µg/kg/min).	D_5W 1/2 NS NS	Limited studies in pediatric patients. Use with caution and adjust dose in patients with impaired renal function. Monitor for hypotension and ventricular dysrhythmias.	Hebel 1999 Taketomo 2000
Minocycline (*Minocin®*)	Available as sterile powder for injection, 100 mg. Reconstitute in sterile water for injection to 20 mg/ml. Reconstituted solution stable 24 hr at room temperature. pH: 2–2.8	**Intermittent infusion:** Dilute to 0.1–0.2 mg/ml. Infuse over 6 hr; begin infusion of diluted solutions immediately after preparation.	D_5W Dextrose/saline combinations LR NS R	Incompatible with calcium-containing solutions.	McEvoy 2001 Trissel 2001
Mitomycin[a] (*Mutamycin®*)	Reconstitute powder for injection with sterile water for injection to yield 500 µg/ml. Reconstituted solutions stable 1 week at room temperature and 2 weeks refrigerated. If not used within 24 hr, protect from light. Diluted solutions (20–40 µg/ml) stable at room temperature for 3 hr in D_5W, 12 hr in NS, and 24 hr in LR. pH: 6–8	**IV push:** Inject over 5–10 min. **Intermittent infusion:** Dilute in 50–250 ml of IV solution (to yield 20–40 µg/ml) and infuse through an IV catheter or the tubing of an IV infusion over 30–60 min.	D_5W LR NS	Highly toxic with a low therapeutic index, use only under constant supervision by experienced clinicians and administer only to hospitalized patients who receive frequent determinations of hematopoietic, renal, and pulmonary function. Monitor for life-threatening thrombocytopenia. Avoid extravasation because cellulitis, tissue sloughing, and ulceration may occur.	McEvoy 2001 Taketomo 2000 Trissel 2001
Mitoxantrone Hydro-chloride[a] (*Novantrone®*)	Available as 2 mg/ml. Stable 7 days at room temperature and 14 days refrigerated after opening. pH: 3–4.5	**IV push:** Dilute three or four times with NS or D_5W and inject over at least 3 min into the tubing of a free-running IV infusion. **Intermittent infusion:** Infuse over 15–30 min. **Continuous infusion:** Infuse at 0.02–0.5 mg/ml in NS or D_5W.	D_5W D_5W/NS NS	Highly toxic with a low therapeutic index, use only under constant supervision by experienced clinicians and administer only to hospitalized patients who receive frequent determinations of hematopoietic, cardiac, and pulmonary function. Avoid extravasation because cellulitis, tissue sloughing, and ulceration may occur. Incompatible with aztreonam, cefepime, heparin, piperacillin–tazobactam, and propofol.	McEvoy 2001 Taketomo 2000 Trissel 2001
Morphine Sulfate	Available as 0.5, 1, 2, 4, 5, 8, 10, and 15 mg/ml pH: 2.5–7 (depending on manufacturer)	**IV push:** Dilute, if necessary, to ≤5 mg/ml and inject over 4–5 min. **Intermittent or continuous infusion:** Dilute to a maximum concentration of 1 mg/ml and infuse at a rate of 0.025–2 mg/kg/hr, titrating to desired response	D_5W $D_{10}W$ Dextran 6%/ D_5W or NS Dextrose/saline combinations	Use electronic infusion device for continuous infusion. Observe for hypotension and respiratory depression. Have naloxone available for overdose and respiratory depression. Compatible with atropine, diphenhydramine, glycopyrrolate, hydroxyzine, and metoclopramide. Incompatible	Gura 1999 McEvoy 2001 Phelps 1996 Taketomo 2000 Trissel 2001

(Continued)

Footnotes are on page 390.

TABLE 8-1 continued

DRUG[a,b] (TRADE NAME)	COMMERCIAL DILUTION OR RECONSTITUTION AND pH[c]	METHOD OF ADMINISTRATION, FURTHER DILUTION, AND RECOMMENDED RATE OF INFUSION[d]	COMPATIBLE INFUSION SOLUTIONS[e]	CAUTIONS, COMMENTS, AND INCOMPATIBILITIES[f,g,h]	REFERENCES[i]
Morphine Sulfate *continued*		or until adverse effects occur.	*Inosol* products LR NS TPN	with alkalis, bromides, iodides, and iron salts.	
Muromonab-CD3 *(Orthoclone OKT3®)*	Available as 1 mg/ml. Store under refrigeration. Do not shake. Use immediately after opening. pH: Information not available	**IV push:** Inject without further dilution over <1 min through a low protein-binding 0.22-μm filter.	Do not dilute.	Monitor CBC, chest X-ray, vital signs, and weight. Most patients experience chills and pyrexia, which lessen on successive days of therapy. Anaphylaxis can occur with any dose. Recommend decreasing the dose of azathioprine and cyclosporine by ~50% while patient is receiving muromonab-CD3, and decreasing prednisone dose.	Gura 1999 Hebel 1999 Phelps 1996 Taketomo 2000
Nafcillin Sodium[b]	Reconstitute powder for injection with sterile water for injection, NS, or bacteriostatic water for injection to yield 250 mg/ml. Stable for 3 days at room temperature, 7 days when refrigerated. pH: 6–8.5	**IV push:** Dilute with 15–30 ml IV solution and inject over 5–10 min. **Intermittent infusion (preferred):** Dilute to <40 mg/ml and infuse over 30–60 min *Maximum:* 200 mg/min. Diluted solution stable for 24 hr at room temperature and 96 hr refrigerated.	D_5W Dextran 40/ 10% D_5W Dextrose/ saline combinations LR NS Normosol M Normosol R	Observe for hypersensitivity and thrombophlebitis. Avoid admixing with other drugs. Incompatible with aminoglycosides and additives resulting in final pH <5 or >8, including ascorbic acid, succinylcholine, and tetracyclines. Sodium content: 2.9 mEq/gram.	Hebel 1999 McEvoy 2001 Phelps 1996 Trissel 2001
Naloxone Hydrochloride *(Narcan®)*	Available as 0.02, 0.4, and 1 mg/ml. Stable 24 hr at 4 μg/ml in D_5W and NS. pH: 3–4	**IV push:** Inject 0.1 mg/kg without further dilution over 30 sec. **Continuous infusion:** Dilute to <4 μg/ml and infuse over 24 hr (0.04–0.16 mg/kg/hr), titrating to patient response (preferred for overdose with long-acting opiates such as methadone or propoxyphene).	D_5W NS	Monitor blood pressure, heart rate, and respiratory rate. Do not admix with alkaline solutions. Protect from light. Do not use if solution discolored; 0.02 mg/ml not recommended by the AAP for use secondary to fluid overload when multiple doses are given.	Gura 1999 McEvoy 2001 Taketomo 2000 Trissel 2001
Neostigmine Methylsulfate *(Prostigmin®)*	Available as 0.25, 0.5, and 1 mg/ml pH: 5.9	**IV push:** Inject slowly without further dilution.	D_5W D_5W/LR D_5W/R LR NS	Administer IV atropine to counteract the muscarinic adverse effects (abdominal cramps, bradycardia, bronchospasm, diarrhea, excessive salivation and sweating, increased bronchial secretions, miosis, nausea, vomiting). Provide assisted ventilation if neostigmine is used during surgery. Monitor heart rate, muscle strength, and respiratory rate.	McEvoy 2001 Taketomo 2000 Trissel 2001
Netilmicin Sulfate[b] *(Netromycin®)*	Available as 50 and 100 mg/ml pH: 3.5–6	**Intermittent infusion:** Dilute to 1–6 mg/ml in NS, D_5W, or LR and infuse over 30–60 min. Stable for 24 hr at room temperature or 48 hr refrigerated.	D_5W $D_{10}W$ D_5W/NS LR NS R	Compatible at Y-site with aminophylline and calcium gluconate. Incompatible with furosemide, heparin sodium, and mezlocillin. Adjust doses based on serum peak and trough concentrations.	Hebel 1999 McEvoy 2001 Repchinsky 2002 Trissel 2001
Nicardipine *(Cardene®)*	Available as 2.5 mg/ml pH: 3.5	**Continuous infusion:** Dilute to 0.1 mg/ml and infuse at 0.5–3 μg/kg/min. Stable 24 hr at room temperature when diluted to 0.1 mg/ml. Concentrations of 0.5 and 1 mg/ml have been used in clinical trials; however, it was not specified whether the patients had peripheral or central IV access.	D_5W D_5W/1/2 NS D_5W/NS 1/2 NS NS	Monitor blood pressure and heart rate closely. If administered via a peripheral IV, the maximum recommended concentration is 0.1 mg/ml, and the site should be changed every 12 hr due to venous irritation. Visually compatible for 4 hr at Y-site with dobutamine, dopamine, fentanyl, labetalol, midazolam, milrinone, morphine, nitroglycerin, and vecuronium. Incompatible with furosemide and heparin.	McEvoy 2001 Trissel 2001

TABLE 8-1 continued

DRUG[a,b] (TRADE NAME)	COMMERCIAL DILUTION OR RECONSTITUTION AND pH[c]	METHOD OF ADMINISTRATION, FURTHER DILUTION, AND RECOMMENDED RATE OF INFUSION[d]	COMPATIBLE INFUSION SOLUTIONS[e]	CAUTIONS, COMMENTS, AND INCOMPATIBILITIES[f,g,h]	REFERENCES[i]
Nitroglycerin	Available as 0.5, 0.8, 5, and 10 mg/ml pH: 3–6.5	**Continuous infusion:** Dilute to ≤400 µg/ml in D_5W or NS and infuse at 0.5 µg/kg/min, titrating until blood pressure response is obtained (usual dose 1–3 µg/kg/min). Dilution requirements and infusion rates differ among commercial nitroglycerin products, so follow the manufacturer's specific instructions. Stable up to 48 hr at room temperature in D_5W or NS.	D_5W D_5W/LR D_5W/1/2 NS D_5W/NS LR 1/2 NS NS	Readily migrates into many plastics; use glass IV bottles, and avoid filters, which adsorb the drug. The type of IV administration set used, polyvinyl chloride (PVC) or non-PVC, must be considered (when PVC tubing is used, higher dosages may be required). Monitor blood pressure and heart rate continuously. Do not admix with other drugs.	Gura 1999 McEvoy 2001 Phelps 1996 Repchinsky 2002 Sodorff 1999 Taketomo 2000 Trissel 2001
Norepinephrine Bitartrate [Noradrenaline] (*Levophed*®)	Available as 1 mg/ml pH: 3–4.5	**Continuous infusion:** Dilute to 4–16 µg/ml with D_5W and infuse at 0.05–0.1 µg/kg/min, then titrate to desired effect (maximum 1–2 µg/kg/min). Stable 24 hr at room temperature at ≤8 µg/ml.	D_5W D_5W/NS IL LR TPN	Monitor ECG and hemodynamic status. Provide adequate fluid volume replacement. Avoid extravasation because may cause tissue sloughing and necrosis. Phentolamine may be infiltrated with a fine hypodermic needle around the extravasated area (use within 12 hr of extravasation). Administer with infusion pump. Protect from light. Do not use if solution is pinkish or darker than slightly yellow. Not stable with alkaline solutions. Duration of effect: 1–2 min after discontinuation of drip.	McEvoy 2001 Phelps 1996 Repchinsky 2002 Sodorff 1999 Taketomo 2000 Trissel 2001
Ondansetron (*Zofran*®)	Available as 2 mg/ml. When diluted, stable for 7 days at room temperature or refrigerated. Unstable under intense light, but stable in daylight. pH: 3.3–4	**IV push:** Inject without dilution over 2–5 min. **Intermittent infusion:** Dilute to 0.6 mg/ml with D_5W or NS and infuse over 15 min *Maximum:* 1 mg/ml.	D_5W D_5W/NS LR NS R TPN	Observe for constipation, diarrhea, and headache. Incompatible with acyclovir, allopurinol, aminophylline, amphotericin B, ampicillin, ampicillin–sulbactam, cefepime, furosemide, ganciclovir, lorazepam, methylprednisolone, piperacillin, sargramostim, and sodium bicarbonate.	Gura 1999 McEvoy 2001 Taketomo 2000 Trissel 2001
Oxacillin Sodium	Reconstitute powder for injection with sterile water for injection or NS to yield 100 mg/ml; stable 24 hr at room temperature. pH: 6–8.5	**IV push:** Inject without further dilution over 10 min. **Intermittent infusion:** Dilute to <100 mg/ml and infuse over 15–30 min. Solutions containing 10–100 mg/ml are stable for 7 days at room temperature in saline solutions and 1–2 days in dextrose or LR solutions. All are stable 8 days refrigerated.	D_5W $D_{10}W$ D_5W/LR D_5W/NS LR NS	Monitor BUN, CBC, and SCr periodically. Sodium content 2.8–3.1 mEq/gram oxacillin. Incompatible with aminoglycosides.	Gura 1999 McEvoy 2001 Phelps 1996 Taketomo 2000 Trissel 2001
Paclitaxel (*Taxol*®)	Available as 6 mg/ml in dehydrated ethanol and polyethoxyethylated castor oil. Stable up to 27 hr at room temperature when diluted to 0.3–1.2 mg/ml. pH: Information not available.	**Intermittent infusion:** Dilute to 0.3–1.2 mg/ml and infuse over 3 hr. **Continuous infusion:** Dilute to 0.3–1.2 mg/ml and infuse over 24, 72, and 96 hr and up to 14 days	D_5W D_5W/NS D_5W/R NS	Must be diluted prior to administration. Dose-limiting toxicity is myelosuppression. Do not administer if baseline neutrophil count < 1500/mm³. Hypersensitivity reactions are common. Premedication with dexamethasone, diphenhydramine, and an H_2-receptor antagonist is recommended. Use a 0.22-µm in-line filter. Avoid contact with PVC. Incompatible with amphotericin B, chlorpromazine, hydroxyzine, methylprednisolone, and mitoxantrone.	McEvoy 2001 Sifton 2002 Taketomo 2000

Footnotes are on page 390.

TABLE 8-1 continued

DRUG[a,b] (TRADE NAME)	COMMERCIAL DILUTION OR RECONSTITUTION AND pH[c]	METHOD OF ADMINISTRATION, FURTHER DILUTION, AND RECOMMENDED RATE OF INFUSION[d]	COMPATIBLE INFUSION SOLUTIONS[e]	CAUTIONS, COMMENTS, AND INCOMPATIBILITIES[f,g,h]	REFERENCES[i]
Pancuronium Bromide[b]	Available as 1 and 2 mg/ml. Refrigerate. Stable 6 months at room temperature. pH: 4	**IV push:** Inject slowly without further dilution. **Continuous infusion:** Dilute to a maximum 0.8 mg/ml and infuse at ~0.1 mg/kg/hr.	D_5W D_5W/NS LR NS	Monitor blood pressure, ECG, and heart rate. Concurrent administration with aminoglycosides, clindamycin, corticosteroids, ketamine, and vancomycin may prolong the neuromuscular blocking effect. This drug is a paralyzing agent and should be administered by clinicians trained in airway management. Does not alter level of consciousness; therefore, addition of sedation and/or analgesia is recommended.	Hebel 1999 McEvoy 2001 Phelps 1996 Taketomo 2000 Trissel 2001
Paraldehyde	Available as 1 gram/ml pH: Information not available	**Intermittent infusion:** Dilute in a volume of NS 10–20 times the volume of the paraldehyde and infuse at 0.1–0.15 ml/kg/hr.	NS only	Use IV in emergency only; observe for cardiac depression, coughing, cyanosis, hypotension, pulmonary edema, and respiratory depression. Avoid contact with plastic and rubber. Do not use discolored solution or solutions with a sharp odor of acetic acid. Use only freshly opened vials, and discard any unused contents after 24 hr. Do not admix with other drugs. Injectable form not available in the U.S.	McEvoy 2001 Reynolds 1993
Penicillin G Potassium	Reconstitute powder for injection with sterile water for injection, D_5W, or NS to yield 100,000, 200,000, 250,000, or 500,000 units/ml. pH: 6.6–8.5	**Intermittent infusion:** Dilute to 100,000–500,000 units/ml and infuse over 15–60 min. Stable for 7 days refrigerated.	D_5W Dextran 6%/D_5W LR NS R	Contains 1.7 mEq potassium and 0.3 mEq sodium per million units of penicillin G. Monitor CBC, hepatic and renal function, and serum electrolytes. Incompatible with aminoglycosides. Inactivated in acid and alkaline solutions.	Gura 1999 Hebel 1999 McEvoy 2001 Phelps 1996 Sifton 2002 Taketomo 2000 Trissel 2001
Pentamidine Isethionate (*Pentacarinat®*)	Reconstitute powder for injection with sterile water for injection to yield 100 mg/ml. After reconstitution with sterile water, stable for 48 hr at room temperature. Solutions of 2 mg/ml in D_5W stable for 24 hr at room temperature. pH: 4.1–5.4	**Intermittent infusion:** Dilute to 2 mg/ml, and infuse over at least 60 min (maximum 6 mg/ml in severely fluid-restricted patients).	D_5W NS	Administer with electronic infusion device. Hypotensive reactions have occurred when the drug was administered too rapidly; patients should be in a supine position, and blood pressure should be monitored closely during and after administration until stable. If hypotension occurs, increase infusion time from 1 to 2 hr. Monitor ECG, renal function, and respiratory rate. Incompatible with cefotaxime, cefoxitin, ceftazidime, ceftriaxone, fluconazole, and foscarnet. Do not admix with other drugs or solutions. Protect from light.	Gura 1999 McEvoy 2001 Repchinsky 2002 Taketomo 2000 Trissel 2001
Pentobarbital Sodium[h] (*Nembutal®*)	Available as 50 mg/ml pH: 9.5	**Intermittent infusion:** Infuse without further dilution slowly over 10–30 min (at <50 mg/min). **Continuous infusion:** Infuse loading dose slowly over 1–2 hr; then infuse 1 mg/kg/hr, titrating up to 2–3 mg/kg/hr.	D_5W LR NS R	Monitor blood pressure and respiratory rate. Low pH may cause precipitation; use clear solutions only. Incompatible with clindamycin, diphenhydramine, droperidol, fentanyl, insulin, meperidine, methadone, norepinephrine, pancuronium, phenytoin, promethazine, ranitidine, and vancomycin. Protect from light.	McEvoy 2001 Taketomo 2000 Trissel 2001
Phenobarbital Sodium[h]	Available as 30, 60, 65, and 130 mg/ml (some preparations contain alcohols, including propylene glycol) pH: 9.2–10.2	**IV push:** Inject without further dilution slowly at <1 mg/kg/min (maximum 30 mg/min in infants and children, 60 mg/min in adults).	D_5W LR NS R TPN	Monitor phenobarbital serum concentrations. Observe for hypotension and respiratory depression. Do not administer intra-arterially. Do not admix with acidic solutions because precipitation may occur; use clear solutions only. Incompatible with chlorpromazine, clinda-	Gura 1999 McEvoy 2001 Taketomo 2000 Trissel 2001

CHAPTER 8: INTRAVENOUS DRUGS FOR NEONATES, INFANTS, CHILDREN, AND ADOLESCENTS

TABLE 8-1 continued

DRUG[a,b] (TRADE NAME)	COMMERCIAL DILUTION OR RECONSTITUTION AND pH[c]	METHOD OF ADMINISTRATION, FURTHER DILUTION, AND RECOMMENDED RATE OF INFUSION[d]	COMPATIBLE INFUSION SOLUTIONS[e]	CAUTIONS, COMMENTS, AND INCOMPATIBILITIES[f,g,h]	REFERENCES[i]
Phenobarbital Sodium[h] *continued*				mycin, diphenhydramine, hydralazine, hydrocortisone, insulin, meperidine, methadone, morphine, norepinephrine, pancuronium, promethazine, ranitidine, and vancomycin.	
Phenylephrine Hydrochloride	Available as 10 mg/ml pH: 3–6.5	**IV push:** Dilute to 1 mg/ml and inject slowly over 20–30 sec. **Continuous infusion:** Dilute to 0.02–0.1 mg/ml and infuse at 0.1–0.5 µg/kg/min, titrating to desired response. Stable 48 hr at room temperature when mixed with D_5W at 1 mg/ml.	D_5W/NS LR NS R Sterile water for injection	Use a large vein for infusion. Avoid extravasation. Phentolamine may be infiltrated with a fine hypodermic needle around the extravasated area (use within 12 hr of extravasation). Monitor blood pressure, heart rate, and renal function. May contain sulfites, which cause allergic reactions in some patients. Do not use if solution turns brown or contains a precipitate. Incompatible with alkaline fluids.	McEvoy 2001 Sodorff 1999 Taketomo 2000 Trissel 2001
Phenytoin Sodium[h] [Diphenylhydantoin Sodium] *(Dilantin®)*	Available as 50 mg/ml pH: 10–12.3	**IV push:** Inject without further dilution at 0.5 mg/kg/min for neonates, 1–3 mg/kg/min for infants and children; maximum 50 mg/min in adults and adolescents, then flush IV tubing or catheter with NS. May dilute with NS, but only to a concentration of <6 mg/ml.	NS	Avoid extravasation. Monitor blood pressure. Do not refrigerate. Slightly yellow solutions may be used, but discard if hazy. Contains benzyl alcohol. Use 0.22-µm in-line filter. Incompatible with D_5W, LR, TPN, amikacin, barbiturates, ciprofloxacin, dobutamine, heparin, insulin, meperidine, morphine, norepinephrine, potassium chloride, and propofol.	Gura 1999 McEvoy 2001 Taketomo 2000 Trissel 2001
Physostigmine Salicylate *(Antilirium®)*	Available as 1 mg/ml pH: 2–4	**IV push:** Inject slowly without further dilution at a rate of 0.5 mg/min in children, adolescents, and adults. *Maximum:* 2 mg/dose.	D_5W NS	Avoid rapid administration. Monitor heart rate (bradycardia is common). Do not admix with other drug solutions or IV solutions. Do not use if solution is dark.	Hebel 1999 Phelps 1996 Taketomo 2000
Phytonadione[b] [Vitamin K_1] *(AquaMEPHYTON®)*	Available as 2 and 10 mg/ml pH: 5–7	**IV infusion:** Dilute in preservative-free D_5W or NS and infuse at <1 mg/min (preferred 15–30 min).	D_5W D_5W/NS NS	Monitor PT. Contains benzyl alcohol. IV route indicated only when other routes of administration are not feasible. Protect from light.	Gura 1999 Hebel 1999 McEvoy 2001 Phelps 1996 Sifton 2002 Taketomo 2000
Piperacillin Sodium *(Pipracil®)*	Reconstitute powder for injection with sterile water for injection, NS, bacteriostatic sterile water for injection, or bacteriostatic NS to yield 400 mg/ml. pH: 5.5–7.5	**IV push:** Inject without further dilution over 3–5 min. **Intermittent infusion:** Dilute to <20 mg/ml and infuse over 30 min. Stable for 24 hr at room temperature and 7 days refrigerated.	D_5W D_5W/NS LR NS	Monitor for vein irritation. Monitor bleeding time, CBC, and serum electrolytes. Sodium content: 1.85 mEq/gram piperacillin. Incompatible with aminoglycosides.	Hebel 1999 McEvoy 2001 Phelps 1996 Sifton 2002 Taketomo 2000 Trissel 2001
Piperacillin–Tazobactam *(Zosyn®)*	Reconstitute powder for injection with compatible diluent to 200 mg/ml. pH: 4.5–6.8	**Intermittent infusion:** Dilute to <200 mg/ml and infuse over 30 min. Stable 24 hr at room temperature and 48 hr at 2–8°C.	D_5W NS Sterile water for injection	Observe for vein irritation. Sodium content: 2.35 mEq/gram; dose based on the piperacillin component.	Gura 1999 McEvoy 2001 Taketomo 2000 Trissel 2001
Plicamycin[a] [Mithramycin] *(Mithracin®)*	Reconstitute powder for injection with sterile water for injection to yield 500 µg/ml. Reconstituted solution stable 24 hr at room temperature and 48 hr refrigerated. pH: 7	**Intermittent infusion:** Dilute with 1000 ml D_5W or NS and infuse over 4–6 hr or dilute in 100–150 ml D_5W and infuse over 30–60 min.	D_5W NS	Causes hemorrhagic toxicity, marked facial flushing, persistent epistaxis, prolonged prothrombin time, thrombocytopenia, and a substantial increase in fibrinolytic activity. Watch for extravasation. Avoid rapid IV push. Incompatible with cefepime and unstable at pH <4.	McEvoy 2001 Taketomo 2000 Trissel 2001

Footnotes are on page 390.

TABLE 8-1 continued

DRUG[a,b] (TRADE NAME)	COMMERCIAL DILUTION OR RECONSTITUTION AND pH[c]	METHOD OF ADMINISTRATION, FURTHER DILUTION, AND RECOMMENDED RATE OF INFUSION[d]	COMPATIBLE INFUSION SOLUTIONS[e]	CAUTIONS, COMMENTS, AND INCOMPATIBILITIES[f,g,h]	REFERENCES[i]
Potassium Chloride	Available as 1.5 and 2 mEq/ml. Store at room temperature. Use admixtures within 24 hr after preparation. pH: 4–8	**Intermittent infusion:** Dilute to <200 mEq/liter for central IV, or <80 mEq/liter for peripheral IV, and infuse at <0.25 mEq/kg/hr. In severe hypokalemia rates up to 1 mEq/kg/hr have been used, but a cardiac monitor must be utilized.	Dextrose/saline combinations LR R TPN	Do not administer IV push. Administer only to patients with adequate urine output; dilute injection before IV use (do not administer without further dilution). Incompatible with amphotericin B, diazepam, and phenytoin.	McEvoy 2001 Taketomo 2000 Trissel 2001
Potassium Phosphate	Available as 3 mmol/ml (phosphate) and 4.4 mEq/ml potassium. Store at room temperature. Stable for 24 hr at room temperature. pH: 7–7.8	**Intermittent infusion:** Dilute to <0.05 mmol/ml for peripheral and <0.12 mmol/ml for central line infusion. *Maximum rate of infusion:* 0.06 mmol/kg/hr.	D_5W NS	Administer only to patients with adequate urine output. Use caution if mixing with calcium products. Incompatible with dobutamine.	McEvoy 2001 Taketomo 2000 Trissel 2001
Pralidoxime Chloride (*Protopam®*)	Reconstitute with sterile water (preservative free) to yield 50 mg/ml. pH: 3.5–4.5	**IV push:** Inject without further dilution over 5 min. **Intermittent infusion:** Infuse over 15–30 min. **Continuous infusion:** Dilute to 10–20 mg/ml with NS, and infuse at 10–20 mg/kg/hr.	NS	Observe for blurred vision, headache, hyperventilation, muscle weakness, and tachycardia. Rapid infusion may cause transient neuromuscular blockade or laryngospasm. Used for treatment of organophosphate poisoning. Use with caution in patients with myasthenia gravis.	McEvoy 2001 Phelps 1996 Taketomo 2000
Procainamide Hydrochloride (*Pronestyl®*)	Available as 100 mg/ml pH: 4–6	**IV push:** Dilute to 20–30 mg/ml and inject loading dose of 3–6 mg/kg over 5 min (maximum 100 mg/dose). May repeat every 5–10 min, up to 15 mg/kg maximum total loading dose. **Continuous infusion:** Dilute to ≤4 mg/ml and infuse at 20–80 µg/kg/min (maximum 2 grams/24 hr). Stable for 24 hr at room temperature in D_5W.	D_5W (preferred) NS	Administer with infusion pump. Monitor blood pressure, CBC with differential, ECG, and platelet count. Use only clear or slightly yellow solutions.	McEvoy 2001 Phelps 1996 Repchinsky 2002 Taketomo 2000 Trissel 2001
Promethazine Hydrochloride (*Phenergan®*)	Available as 25 mg/ml pH: 4–5.5	**IV push:** Dilute to <25 mg/ml, and inject at <25 mg/min.	D_5W Dextrose/saline combinations LR NS TPN	Do not administer SC or intra-arterially because necrotic lesions may occur. Avoid extravasation. Observe for dystonic reactions, and monitor blood pressure. Protect from light. Incompatible with allopurinol, aminophylline, cefepime, cefotetan, foscarnet, furosemide, heparin, hydrocortisone, methotrexate, penicillin G, pentobarbital, phenobarbital, and piperacillin–tazobactam.	Gura 1999 McEvoy 2001 Taketomo 2000 Trissel 2001
Propofol (*Diprivan®*)	Available as 1% solution (10 mg/ml) [oil-in-water emulsion] pH: 7–8.5 (Diprivan) pH: 4.5–6.5 (Baxter product)	**IV push:** May dilute to ≥2 mg/ml with D_5W or inject undiluted over 20–30 sec. Titrate to onset of anesthesia. **Continuous infusion:** May dilute to ≥2 mg/ml with D_5W or infuse undiluted at 50–200 µg/kg/min.	D_5W D_5W/LR D_5W/1/4 NS D_5W/1/2 NS LR	Based on recent reviews of new clinical data, the U.S. Food and Drug Administration has determined that there may be safety concerns when propofol is used for sedation in pediatric ICU patients. Propofol is not approved for sedation in pediatric ICU patients in the United States and the manufacturer does not recommend its use in this manner. Rapid IV injection can cause hypotension and bradycardia. Only clinicians trained in general anesthesia should administer this drug. Equipment, drugs, and skilled personnel should be available for assisted or controlled respiration and cardiovascular support. Monitor cardiac and respir-	Gura 1999 Phelps 1996 Taketomo 2000 Trissel 2001

TABLE 8-1 continued

DRUG[a,b] (TRADE NAME)	COMMERCIAL DILUTION OR RECONSTITUTION AND pH[c]	METHOD OF ADMINISTRATION, FURTHER DILUTION, AND RECOMMENDED RATE OF INFUSION[d]	COMPATIBLE INFUSION SOLUTIONS[e]	CAUTIONS, COMMENTS, AND INCOMPATIBILITIES[f,g,h]	REFERENCES[i]
Propofol *continued*				atory functions continuously. Excitatory phenomena manifested as jerking of arms, feet, hands, and legs, and spontaneous musculoskeletal movements and twitching occur in 33%–90% of pediatric patients. Flushing, local pain, and rash may occur at the site of injection. May turn urine green. Lipid content is 10%; therefore, monitor patients for elevated triglycerides. Do not filter or admix with other drugs or coadminister through the same IV catheter with blood or plasma. Do not use if there is evidence of separation of the phases of the emulsion. Careful aseptic technique is necessary when preparing this product because the lipid base is a good medium for promoting bacterial growth. If transferred to a syringe or other container, administration should be completed within 6 hr after the container is opened. Do not refrigerate. Baxter product contains sodium metabisulfite, which can cause allergic reactions in sulfite-sensitive patients.	
Propranolol Hydrochloride (Inderal®)	Available as 1 mg/ml pH: 2.8–3.5	**IV push:** Inject slowly without further dilution over 10 min. Do not exceed 1 mg/min.	D_5W LR NS	Monitor blood pressure and ECG. Not significantly removed by hemodialysis. Decomposes rapidly at alkaline pH.	Gura 1999 McEvoy 2001 Phelps 1996 Taketomo 2000 Trissel 2001
Protamine Sulfate[b]	Available as 10 mg/ml pH: 6–7	**IV push:** Inject without further dilution slowly at <5 mg/min. Store in refrigerator. Stable for 10 days at room temperature.	D_5W NS	Observe for bradycardia, dyspnea, flushing, and hypotension, especially with rapid infusion. Use with caution in patients allergic to fish. Do not admix with other drugs.	Gura 1999 McEvoy 2001 Taketomo 2000
Pyridoxine Hydrochloride [Vitamin B_6]	Available as 100 mg/ml pH: 2–3.8	**IV push:** Inject without further dilution over 3–5 min. **Intermittent infusion:** Infuse slowly over 3 hr. Protect from light; store at 15–30°C.	D_5W D_5W/NS NS	Large doses (>1 gram) may cause changes in blood pressure, heart rate, and respiratory rate. Protect from light.	McEvoy 2001 Taketomo 2000 Trissel 2001
Quinidine Gluconate (Lilly)	Available as 80 mg/ml pH: 5.5–7	**Intermittent infusion:** Dilute to 16 mg/ml and infuse at <10 mg/min. Stable 24 hr at room temperature and 48 hr refrigerated.	D_5W	Use IV route only in emergencies. Administer IM dose to test for idiosyncratic reaction. Monitor blood pressure, digoxin serum concentration in patients receiving digoxin, ECG, and hepatic function. Do not admix with other drugs.	McEvoy 2001 Taketomo 2000 Trissel 2001
Ranitidine Hydrochloride (Zantac®)	Available as 25 and 1 mg/ml premix in 1/2 NS. Stable for 48 hr at room temperature or 30 days when frozen in D_5W or NS. Stable for 24 hr in TPN and TPN with lipids. pH: 6.7–7.3	**IV push (not recommended):** Dilute to <2.5 mg/ml (usual concentration 0.5 mg/ml), and inject over at least 5 min, not to exceed 10 mg/min. **Intermittent infusion (preferred):** Dilute to <2 mg/ml and infuse over 15–30 min. **Continuous infusion:** Dilute with IV solution or TPN, and infuse over 24 hr.	D_5W $D_{10}W$ Dextrose/saline combinations (any) LR 1/2 NS NS TPN	IV push is not recommended because of an increased risk of bradycardia. Monitor hepatic and renal function. Incompatible with amphotericin B, ceftazidime, and phenobarbital. Protect from light.	Gura 1999 McEvoy 2001 Phelps 1996 Taketomo 2000 Trissel 2001

Footnotes are on page 390.

TABLE 8-1 continued

DRUG[a,b] (TRADE NAME)	COMMERCIAL DILUTION OR RECONSTITUTION AND pH[c]	METHOD OF ADMINISTRATION, FURTHER DILUTION, AND RECOMMENDED RATE OF INFUSION[d]	COMPATIBLE INFUSION SOLUTIONS[e]	CAUTIONS, COMMENTS, AND INCOMPATIBILITIES[f,g,h]	REFERENCES[i]
Rifampin (*Rifadin*®)	Reconstitute powder for injection with NS to yield 60 mg/ml. Stable 24 hr at room temperature. pH: Information not available	**Intermittent infusion:** Dilute to <6 mg/ml and infuse over 30–180 min.	D_5W NS	If local irritation or inflammation occurs at the injection site, discontinue the infusion and restart it at another site. Causes discoloration of urine and other body fluids.	McEvoy 2001 Taketomo 2000
Rituximab (*Rituxan*®)	Available as 10 mg/ml. Keep refrigerated. Diluted solution (1–4 mg/ml) is stable 24 hr refrigerated and an additional 12 hr at room temperature. pH: Information not available	**IV infusion:** Dilute to 1–4 mg/ml with D_5W or NS and infuse as follows. Initial infusion rate is 50 mg/hr; if no hypotension or hypersensitivity reactions occur, rate may be increased by 50 mg/hr every 30 min to a maximum of 400 mg/hr. If no adverse reactions occurred during the initial infusion, subsequent infusions may be initiated at 100 mg/hr and increased by 100 mg/hr every 30 min to a maximum of 400 mg/hr.	D_5W NS	Contraindicated in patients with a history of allergic reactions to murine proteins. Do not infuse with any other medications running in the same line/lumen. To minimize hypersensitivity reactions or infusion-related symptoms, administration of acetaminophen and diphenhydramine should be considered before each dose. Medications for the treatment of acute hypersensitivity reactions (epinephrine, antihistamine, and corticosteroids) should be available during administration. Since blood pressure might decrease transiently during the infusion of rituximab, consideration should be given to holding the administration of antihypertensive medications for 12 hr prior to administration of rituximab. Vital signs should be monitored frequently during the infusion. CBC and platelets should be monitored regularly during treatment with rituximab. Protect from light	Lacy 1999 McEvoy 2001
Rocuronium (*Zemuron*®)	Available as 10 mg/ml. Keep refrigerated. Unopened vials are stable 60 days at room temperature, opened vials are stable 30 days at room temperature. pH: Information not available	**IV push:** Inject undiluted by rapid IV injection. May repeat every 20–30 min as needed to maintain neuromuscular blockade. **Continuous infusion:** Dilute to 0.5–1 mg/ml and infuse at 10–12 µg/kg/min.	D_5W LR NS	Monitor blood pressure, ECG, and heart rate. Concurrent administration with aminoglycosides, clindamycin, corticosteroids, ketamine, and vancomycin may prolong the neuromuscular blocking effect. This drug is a paralyzing agent and should be administered by clinicians trained in airway management. Do not mix with alkali solutions. Does not alter level of consciousness; therefore, addition of sedation and/or analgesia is recommended.	Hebel 1999 McEvoy 2001 Taketomo 2000
Sargramostim [GM-CSF] (*Leukine*®)	Available as both 500-µg/ml solution containing benzyl alcohol[b] and as a lyophilized powder (250 µg/vial). Reconstitute powder for injection with 1 ml sterile water for injection with or without preservatives to yield 250 µg/single-dose vial. If reconstituted with sterile water without preservatives, discard after 6 hr. If reconstituted with bacteriostatic water, use within 20 days if refrigerated. Diluted	**Intermittent infusion:** Dilute and infuse over 0.5–4 hr. If dilution expected to result in a concentration <10 µg/ml, then 0.1% albumin human (e.g., 1 ml of 5% albumin human added to 50 ml of NS) must be added to the NS prior to the dilution of sargramostim to prevent adsorption of sargramostim to the components of the drug delivery system.	D_5W NS (preferred)	Do not use an in-line filter or admix with other drugs (unless compatibility is confirmed). Monitor CBC twice weekly for excessive leukocytosis. Observe for dyspnea and fluid retention. May cause flulike syndrome. Do not shake vial. Incompatible with acyclovir, ampicillin, ampicillin–sulbactam, chlorpromazine, haloperidol, hydrocortisone, hydromorphone, imipenem–cilastatin, lorazepam, methylprednisolone, morphine, ondansetron, sodium bicarbonate, and tobramycin.	Gura 1999 McEvoy 2001 Taketomo 2000 Trissel 2001

TABLE 8-1 continued

DRUG[a,b] (TRADE NAME)	COMMERCIAL DILUTION OR RECONSTITUTION AND pH[c]	METHOD OF ADMINISTRATION, FURTHER DILUTION, AND RECOMMENDED RATE OF INFUSION[d]	COMPATIBLE INFUSION SOLUTIONS[e]	CAUTIONS, COMMENTS, AND INCOMPATIBILITIES[f,g,h]	REFERENCES[i]
Sargramostim *continued*	solutions of 2.5, 8, or 12 µg/ml are stable for 48 hr refrigerated or stored at room temperature. pH: 7.1–7.7				
Scopolamine Hydrobromide [Hyoscine Hydrobromide]	Available as 0.3, 0.4, 0.86, and 1 mg/ml pH: 3.5–6.5	**IV push:** Dilute with equal volume of sterile water and inject over 2–3 min.	D_5W NS Sterile water	Observe for blurred vision, CNS confusion, dry mouth, tachycardia, and urinary retention. Protect from light. Incompatible with alkali.	McEvoy 2001 Taketomo 2000 Trissel 2001
Secobarbital Sodium[h]	Available as 50 mg/ml. Stable for 1 month at room temperature, stable 9 months in Tubex. pH: 9.5–10.5	**IV push:** Inject with or without further dilution at <50 mg/15 sec. Do not dilute with solutions containing bacteriostatic agents.	NS R Sterile water for injection	Avoid intra-arterial injection and IV route except in an emergency (e.g., seizures resulting from tetanus). Observe for hypotension and respiratory depression. Incompatible with atracurium, hydrocortisone, insulin, LR, norepinephrine, pancuronium, succinylcholine, sodium bicarbonate, and vancomycin. May precipitate at pH <9.2, so avoid diluting in LR. Store in refrigerator. Protect from light.	McEvoy 2001 Taketomo 2000 Trissel 2001
Sodium Bicarbonate	Available as 0.5 mEq/ml (4.2%), 0.892 mEq/ml (7.5%), and 1 mEq/ml (8.4%). May dilute the 1-mEq/ml solution 1:1 with sterile water for injection (if 0.5 mEq/ml is unavailable). pH: 7–8.5	**IV push for emergencies only:** Infants and children, use 0.5 mEq/ml and inject 1 mEq/kg slowly (<1–2 mEq/kg/min), then 0.5 mEq/kg every 10 min. **Intermittent infusion:** Dilute to 0.5 mEq/ml in dextrose and infuse over 2 hr. **Continuous infusion:** Dilute to 0.5 mEq/ml for ages <2 years and 1 mEq/ml >2 years.	D_5W Dextrose/ saline combinations LR NS R	Avoid extravasation. Do not admix with acidic salts, acids, calcium salts, or catecholamines. Incompatible with amiodarone, atropine, carboplatin, cefotaxime, ciprofloxacin, cisplatin, dobutamine, imipenem–cilastatin, magnesium sulfate, and ticarcillin–clavulanate. Monitor acid–base status. Each gram of sodium bicarbonate provides ~12 mEq of sodium and bicarbonate ions.	Gura 1999 McEvoy 2001 Taketomo 2000 Trissel 2001
Sodium Chloride	Commercially diluted and available as 0.45%, 0.9%, 3%, and 5% pH: 4.5–7	**Intermittent infusion:** Infuse 10–20 ml/kg NS over 15–20 min (maximum 1 mEq/kg/hr) to increase intravascular volume. Adjust dosage according to fluid and electrolyte status. **Continuous infusion:** Infuse 2–4 mEq/kg/day (maximum 100–150 mEq/day).	Dextrose LR R	Avoid administering IV push. Monitor chloride, potassium, and sodium levels. Observe for fluid retention. NS contains 154 mEq of both chloride and sodium per liter. Do not admix with mannitol or streptomycin sulfate.	Hebel 1999 McEvoy 2001 Phelps 1996 Taketomo 2000 Trissel 2001
Sodium Nitroprusside	Available as 25 mg/ml pH: Information not available	**Continuous infusion:** Dilute in D_5W before infusion. Infuse at 0.5–10 µg/kg/min, then titrate to desired effect (usual dose 3 µg/kg/min; maximum 10 µg/kg/min). Do **not** administer at maximum rate for longer than 10 min. Usual maximum concentration is ≤200 µg/ml, although concentrations up to 1 mg/ml have been used in fluid-restricted patients.	D_5W	Avoid extravasation. Monitor blood pressure. Monitor thiocyanate serum concentration if patient is in renal failure or therapy >2 days. Protect IV container from light; it is not necessary to wrap the administration set. Administer with an infusion pump. Discard solution 24 hr after reconstitution. Do not admix with other drugs.	Gura 1999 McEvoy 2001 Sifton 2002 Sodorff 1999 Taketomo 2000 Trissel 2001

Footnotes are on page 390.

TABLE 8-1 continued

DRUG[a,b] (TRADE NAME)	COMMERCIAL DILUTION OR RECONSTITUTION AND pH[c]	METHOD OF ADMINISTRATION, FURTHER DILUTION, AND RECOMMENDED RATE OF INFUSION[d]	COMPATIBLE INFUSION SOLUTIONS[e]	CAUTIONS, COMMENTS, AND INCOMPATIBILITIES[f,g,h]	REFER- ENCES[i]
Streptoki- nase (*Streptase*®)	Reconstitute powder for injection with D_5W or NS (preferred) to yield 50,000, 100,000, or 150,000 IU/ml. Store reconstituted solutions refrigerated, use within 24 hr. pH: 6–8	**Continuous infusion:** Administer loading dose over 30 min, then infuse for 24–72 hr. *Maximum:* 1.5 million units in 50 ml.	D_5W NS	Use an electronic infusion device for administration. Measure thrombin time (TT) and activated partial thromboplastin time (aPTT) before initiating treatment. If heparin is used before or after streptokinase, TT or aPTT should be less than twice the normal control value. To prevent rethrombosis after streptokinase, continuous heparin is recommended. Allergic reactions, including anaphylaxis, may occur. Monitor blood pressure closely. Compatible with dobutamine, dopamine, heparin sodium, lidocaine, and nitroglycerin. Incompatible with dextrans. Do not shake solution.	McEvoy 2001 Taketomo 2000 Trissel 2001
Succinyl- choline Chloride (*Anectine*®)	Available as 20, 50, and 100 mg/ml. Refrigerate. Stable for 14 days at room temperature. pH: 3–4.5	**IV push:** Inject without further dilution over 10–30 sec. May repeat every 5–10 min as needed.	D_5W D_5W/NS LR NS	Continuous infusion not recommended for pediatric patients due to increased risk of malignant hyperthermia. Do not use in patients with severe trauma, extensive burns, or neuromuscular disorders due to increased risk of hyperkalemia. Monitor for bradycardia and hypotension. Pretreatment with atropine may reduce risk of bradycardia. This drug is a paralyzing agent and should be administered by clinicians trained in airway management. Do not admix with alkaline solutions, barbiturates, nafcillin, or sodium bicarbonate. Concurrent administration with aminoglycosides, clindamycin, and vancomycin may prolong the neuromuscular blocking effect. Does not alter level of consciousness; therefore, addition of sedation and/or analgesia is recommended.	McEvoy 2001 Phelps 1996 Taketomo 2000 Trissel 2001
Teniposide (*Vumon*®)	Available as 10 mg/ml in benzyl alcohol[b], ethanol, and polyoxyethylated castor oil. Refrigerate. Stable 24 hr at room temperature. pH: Information not available	**IV infusion:** Dilute to 0.1, 0.2, 0.4, or 1 mg/ml with D_5W or NS and infuse over at least 30–60 min. Prepare in glass or other non-DEHP-containers (e.g., polyolefin containers). PVC containers not recommended.	D_5W NS	Must be diluted prior to administration. Severe hypersensitivity reactions occur in ~5% of patients (this incidence is higher in patients with neuroblastoma or brain tumors), therefore, medications to treat such reactions should be available. If patients have a reaction, pretreatment with a corticosteroid and antihistamine is recommended with subsequent doses. Extravasation may result in local tissue necrosis and/or thrombophlebitis. Severe myelosuppression can occur. Patients with Down's syndrome are particularly sensitive to the myelosuppressive effects, and the initial dose should be reduced. Incompatible with heparin. Do not use in-line filters.	Lacy 1999 McEvoy 2001 Repchinsky 2002
Thiamine Hydrochlo- ride [Vitamin B_1]	Available as 100 and 200 mg/ml pH: 2.5–4.5	**IV push:** Inject without further dilution over several minutes.	D_5W $D_{10}W$ D_5W/LR D_5W/R Dextran 6%/D_5W Dextran 6%/NS	May cause allergic reactions with symptoms ranging from feeling of warmth, rash, or tingling to angioedema, cardiovascular collapse, and death. An intradermal test dose may be administered to patients with suspected sensitivity.	McEvoy 2001 Taketomo 2000 Trissel 2001

TABLE 8-1 *continued*

DRUG[a,b] (TRADE NAME)	COMMERCIAL DILUTION OR RECONSTITUTION AND pH[c]	METHOD OF ADMINISTRATION, FURTHER DILUTION, AND RECOMMENDED RATE OF INFUSION[d]	COMPATIBLE INFUSION SOLUTIONS[e]	CAUTIONS, COMMENTS, AND INCOMPATIBILITIES[f,g,h]	REFER- ENCES[i]
Thiamine Hydrochloride *continued*			Dextrose/saline combinations LR NS R		
Thiopental Sodium *(Pentothal®)*	Reconstitute powder for injection with sterile water for injection, NS, or D$_5$W to yield 20–50 mg/ml. Reconstituted solutions stable 3 days at room temperature and 7 days refrigerated. pH: 10–11	**IV infusion:** Inject without further dilution over 10–60 min (avoid rapid IV injection).	D$_5$W NS	Avoid extravasation and intra-arterial injection. Monitor vital signs for hypotension and respiratory depression. Incompatible with atropine, chlorpromazine, diphenhydramine, fentanyl, methadone, morphine, promethazine, succinylcholine, and tubocurarine.	Repchinsky 2002 Taketomo 2000 Trissel 2001
Thiotepa[a] *(Thioplex®)*	Reconstitute powder for injection with 1.5 ml sterile water for injection to yield 10 mg/ml. Refrigerate reconstituted solutions. Manufacturer recommends use within 8 hr. Dilute with NS prior to use. Concentrations of 1–3 mg/ml in NS stable 24 hr at room temperature or 48 hr refrigerated. Stable 24 hr at 5 mg/ml. Once diluted with NS, the manufacturer recommends immediate use. pH: 5.5–7.5	**IV push:** Inject without further dilution over 5 min. **Intermittent infusion:** Dilute with NS to <10 mg/ml and infuse slowly.	Dextrose solutions Dextrose/saline combinations LR NS R	Store under refrigeration and protect from light. Reconstituted solutions should be clear to slightly opaque. Monitor CBC and serum uric acid. Thiotepa is a highly toxic drug with a low therapeutic index, so it must be used only under constant supervision by experienced clinicians. Use 0.22-μm filter (Millex-GS) prior to administration. Unstable in acidic medium. Incompatible with cisplatin and filgrastim.	McEvoy 2001 Sifton 2002 Taketomo 2000 Trissel 2001
Ticarcillin (T) Disodium and Clavulanate (C) Potassium *(Timentin®)*	Available frozen as 300 mg/ml (T) and 10 mg/ml (C) **or** reconstitute powder for injection with sterile water for injection or NS to yield 200 mg/ml (T) and 6.7–13.4 mg/ml (C). pH: 5.5–7.5	**Intermittent infusion:** Dilute to 10–100 mg/ml (T) and infuse over 30 min. Stable for 24 hr at room temperature and 4 days refrigerated.	D$_5$W LR NS Sterile water for injection	Observe for hypersensitivity reaction and phlebitis. Sodium content 4.75 mEq/gram *Timentin*. Do not admix with other antibiotics or sodium bicarbonate.	Gura 1999 Hebel 1999 McEvoy 2001 Taketomo 2000 Trissel 2001
Tobramycin Sulfate *(Nebcin®)*	Available as 10 and 40 mg/ml pH: 3–6.5	**Intermittent infusion:** Dilute to 2–40 mg/ml and infuse over 30–60 min. Stable for 24 hr at room temperature.	D$_5$W LR NS R	Monitor BUN, CBC, SCr, and urine output periodically. Incompatible with cephalosporins and penicillins; administer at least 1 hr apart or with adequate flushing of IV tubing. Adjust doses based on serum peak and trough concentrations.	Gura 1999 McEvoy 2001 Phelps 1996 Sifton 2002 Taketomo 2000 Trissel 2001

Footnotes are on page 390.

TABLE 8-1 continued

DRUG[a,b] (TRADE NAME)	COMMERCIAL DILUTION OR RECONSTITUTION AND pH[c]	METHOD OF ADMINISTRATION, FURTHER DILUTION, AND RECOMMENDED RATE OF INFUSION[d]	COMPATIBLE INFUSION SOLUTIONS[e]	CAUTIONS, COMMENTS, AND INCOMPATIBILITIES[f,g,h]	REFERENCES[i]
Topotecan (Hycamtin®)	Reconstitute powder for injection with 4 ml of sterile water for injection to 1 mg/ml. This solution is stable for 24 hr at room temperature. Dilute with NS or D_5W prior to administration. Solutions of 10–500 µg/ml are stable for 24 hr at room temperature. pH: 2.5–3.5	**IV infusion:** Dilute to 10–500 µg/ml with NS or D_5W and infuse over 30 min.	D_5W NS	Avoid extravasation that can cause mild erythema and bruising. Monitor CBC frequently during therapy. Before treatment is initiated, patients should have a neutrophil count $\geq 1500/mm^3$, platelet count $\geq 100,000/mm^3$, and hemoglobin ≥ 9 mg/dl. No pediatric data are available for dosage adjustments, but adult data indicate that the dosage should be reduced by $\sim 50\%$ in patients with mild-to-moderate renal impairment. Use with caution in patients with CrCl <40 ml/min.	Lacy 1999 McEvoy 2001
Tranexamic Acid (Cyklokapron®)	Available as 100 mg/ml. Store at room temperature. pH: 6.5–7.5	**IV push:** Inject without further dilution at maximum rate of 100 mg/min (over at least 5 min). **Continuous infusion:** Infuse 10 mg/kg/hr.	D_5W $D_{10}W$ Dextrose/saline combinations NS	Contraindicated in patients with active intravascular clotting process. Ophthalmic examination should be performed on patients treated for several weeks (baseline and periodic exams). Discontinue treatment if disturbances of color vision are noted. Do not admix with blood or infusion solutions containing penicillins.	Micromedex 1999 Repchinsky 2002 Taketomo 2000
Trastuzumab (Herceptin®)	Reconstitute the lyophilized powder for injection with 20 ml bacteriostatic water for injection to yield 21 mg/ml. Reconstituted solution stable for 28 days refrigerated. If unpreserved sterile water for injection is used for reconstitution, the product should be used immediately. pH: 6	**Intermittent infusion:** Infuse initial loading dose of 4 mg/kg as a 90-min infusion. The weekly maintenance dose is 2 mg/kg infused over 30 min if initial loading dose was well tolerated.	Saline solutions (Do **not** administer with dextrose-containing solutions.)	Do not administer as an IV push or bolus. Observe patients for fever, chills, and other infusion-related symptoms. Do not admix with other drugs.	Micromedex 1999 Repchinsky 2002
Trimethoprim (T) + Sulfamethoxazole (S) (Septra®)	Available as 16 mg/ml (T) and 80 mg/ml (S) pH: 10	**Intermittent infusion:** Dilute each milliliter of drug with 25 ml of diluent and infuse over 60–90 min. This concentration is stable for 48 hr in D_5W and NS. For fluid-restricted patients, dilute each milliliter of drug with 15 ml diluent. This concentration is stable for 4 hr in D_5W and only 2 hr in NS. Manufacturer recommends only D_5W for dilution and infusion, but NS has been used.	D_5W (preferred) D_5W/1/2 NS LR 1/2 NS NS	Must be diluted. Rapid infusion must be avoided. Observe for pain and phlebitis. Adequate fluid intake must be maintained to prevent crystalluria. Use with caution in infants <2 months of age. Avoid use in infants with jaundice. Incompatible with fluconazole, foscarnet, and midazolam. Do not admix with other drugs.	Gura 1999 McEvoy 2001 Taketomo 2000 Trissel 2001
Tubocurarine Chloride	Available as 3 mg/ml pH: 2.5–5	**IV push:** Inject without further dilution over 60–90 sec and flush IV cannula with NS or D_5W.	D_5W LR NS R	Monitor blood pressure, ECG, and heart rate. Have atropine and edrophonium available to reverse the effects. This drug is a paralyzing agent and should be administered by clinicians trained in airway management. Concurrent administration with aminoglycosides, clindamycin, and magnesium may prolong the neuromuscular blocking effect. Avoid admixing with alkaline solutions. Discard solution if discolored. Does not alter level of consciousness; therefore, addition of sedation and/or analgesia is recommended.	McEvoy 2001 Phelps 1996 Taketomo 2000 Trissel 2001

CHAPTER 8: INTRAVENOUS DRUGS FOR NEONATES, INFANTS, CHILDREN, AND ADOLESCENTS

TABLE 8-1 continued

DRUG[a,b] (TRADE NAME)	COMMERCIAL DILUTION OR RECONSTITUTION AND pH[c]	METHOD OF ADMINISTRATION, FURTHER DILUTION, AND RECOMMENDED RATE OF INFUSION[d]	COMPATIBLE INFUSION SOLUTIONS[e]	CAUTIONS, COMMENTS, AND INCOMPATIBILITIES[f,g,h]	REFERENCES[i]
Valproate Sodium (Depacon®, Epiject IV®)	Available as 100 mg/ml. Stable 24 hr at room temperature when diluted in D₅W, LR, or NS. pH: 7.6	**Intermittent infusion:** Dilute with 50 ml to 2 mg/ml and infuse over 1 hr. *Maximum rate:* 10 mg/min. Doses >250 mg should be divided in two.	D₅W LR NS	Monitor drug levels, platelet count, and LFTs. Watch closely during infusion for hypotension. Total daily IV dose is equal to the oral dose, but should be divided with a frequency of every 6 hr. Patients should be changed to oral product as soon as possible.	Gura 1999 Repchinsky 2002 Taketomo 2000
Vancomycin Hydrochloride (Vancocin®)	Reconstitute powder for injection with sterile water for injection or NS to yield 50 mg/ml. Refrigerate and use within 2 weeks after reconstitution. pH: 2.5–4.5	**Intermittent infusion:** Dilute to <5 mg/ml and infuse over 60 min (decrease infusion rate and concentration and pretreat with antihistamine before subsequent doses if "red neck/red man" syndrome occurs).	D₅W NS	Avoid extravasation. Monitor BUN, CBC, and SCr periodically. Peak and trough serum concentrations may aid in dosage adjustments. Incompatible with ceftazidime, heparin, and phenobarbital.	Gura 1999 Hebel 1999 McEvoy 2001 Phelps 1996 Taketomo 2000
Vecuronium Bromide[b] (Norcuron®)	Reconstitute with sterile water for injection to yield 1 mg/ml. Stable up to 5 days at room temperature if bacteriostatic water is used; use within 24 hr of preparation if sterile water for injection is used and refrigerate. pH: 4	**IV push:** Inject slowly without further dilution over 1–2 min. **Continuous infusion:** Dilute to a maximum concentration of 1 mg/ml and infuse at 0.05–0.1 mg/kg/hr beginning 20–40 min after IV push. Titrate to desired effect.	D₅W D₅W/NS LR NS	Use electronic infusion device for administration. Monitor vital signs frequently (every 15 min until stable). This drug is a paralyzing agent and should be administered by clinicians trained in airway management. Do not administer IM. Concurrent administration with aminoglycosides, clindamycin, corticosteroids, and vancomycin may prolong the neuromuscular blocking effect. Do not mix with alkali solutions. A cholinesterase inhibitor (edrophonium, neostigmine, pyridostigmine) may reverse the neuromuscular blockade induced by vecuronium. Does not alter level of consciousness; therefore, addition of sedation and/or analgesia is recommended.	Gura 1999 McEvoy 2001 Taketomo 2000 Trissel 2001
Verapamil Hydrochloride (Isoptin®)	Available as 2.5 mg/ml pH: 4.1–6	**IV push:** Inject without further dilution over 2–4 min.	Solutions with pH 3–6 Dextrose solutions R Saline solutions	Monitor blood pressure and ECG. Store at room temperature; protect from heat and freezing. Use only clear solutions; precipitation occurs in solutions with pH >6. Incompatible with albumin, amphotericin B, hydralazine, sulfamethoxazole, and trimethoprim.	Gura 1999 McEvoy 2001 Repchinsky 2002 Taketomo 2000 Trissel 2001
Vinblastine Sulfate[a,b] (Velban®)	Available as 1 mg/ml **or** reconstitute with NS (with preservatives) to yield 1 mg/ml. Reconstituted 1-mg/ml solutions in NS are stable 30 days refrigerated and protected from light. pH: 3–5.5	**IV push:** Inject without further dilution into vein or tubing of a patent IV over 1 min (according to protocol). **Continuous infusion:** Dilute each day's dose in 1 liter D₅W or NS and infuse over 24 hr.	D₅W NS	Avoid extravasation. Monitor CBC with differential, hepatic function, platelet count, and uric acid serum concentration. Incompatible with cefepime and furosemide.	McEvoy 2001 Taketomo 2000 Trissel 2001
Vincristine Sulfate[a] (Oncovin®)	Available as 1 mg/ml. Store in refrigerator; stable for 1 month at room temperature. Protect from light. pH: 3.5–5.5	**IV push:** Use without dilution (1 mg/ml) or dilute in a small volume of D₅W or NS only and inject into large vein or tubing of a patent IV over 1 min (or according to protocol).	D₅W LR NS	Avoid extravasation. Monitor CBC and uric acid serum concentration. Observe for ataxia, constipation, foot or wrist drop, neurotoxicity, numbness, and tingling sensation. Incompatible with cefepime, furosemide, idarubicin, and sodium bicarbonate.	McEvoy 2001 Taketomo 2000 Trissel 2001

Footnotes are on page 390

TABLE 8-1 continued

DRUG[a,b] (TRADE NAME)	COMMERCIAL DILUTION OR RECONSTITUTION AND pH[c]	METHOD OF ADMINISTRATION, FURTHER DILUTION, AND RECOMMENDED RATE OF INFUSION[d]	COMPATIBLE INFUSION SOLUTIONS[e]	CAUTIONS, COMMENTS, AND INCOMPATIBILITIES[f,g,h]	REFERENCES[i]
Vitamins, multiple (MVI Pediatric®)	Reconstitute contents of MVI Pediatric vial with 5 ml of sterile water for injection, NS, or D_5W. Use immediately after preparation. pH: Information not available	**Continuous infusion:** Dilute in at least 100 ml of IV solution and infuse over 24 hr.	D_5W NS TPN	Must be diluted prior to administration. Observe for anaphylaxis. Incompatible with acetazolamide, chlorothiazide, and tetracycline. Note that shortages have occurred periodically in the U.S.	McEvoy 2001 Phelps 1996
Zidovudine [AZT] (Retrovir®)	Available as 10 mg/ml pH: 5.5	**Intermittent infusion:** Dilute to ≤4 mg/ml and infuse over 60 min. **Continuous infusion:** Dilute total daily dose in IV solution (≤4 mg/ml) and infuse over 24 hr. Solutions containing ≤4 mg/ml are stable for 24 hr at room temperature and 48 hr refrigerated at 2–8°C.	D_5W NS	Obtain blood cell counts and indices of anemia (hemoglobin and mean corpuscular volume) before and during therapy. Avoid IM, IV push, and rapid IV infusion. May cause pain/irritation at the injection site.	Gura 1999 McEvoy 2001 Phelps 1996 Taketomo 2000

References[1]

Bailey, B., & McGuigan, M. A. (1998). Management of anaphylactoid reactions to intravenous N-acetylcysteine. *Annals of Emergency Medicine, 31,* 710–715.

Gershanik, J. J., Beecher, B., George, W., et al. (1982). Neonatal deaths associated with use of benzyl alcohol–United States. *Morbidity and Mortality Weekly Report, 31*(22), 290–291.

Gura, K. M. (1999). Intravenous medication administration guidelines for pediatric patients. *Journal of Pediatric Pharmacy Practice, 4*(2), 80–106.

Hebel, S. K. (Ed.). (1999). *Facts and comparisons.* St. Louis, MO: Lippincott.

Lacy, C., Armstrong, L. L., Ingrim, N. B., et al. (Eds.) (1999). *Drug information handbook,* Cleveland, OH: Lexi-Comp.

Leff, R., & Roberts, R. J. (1992). *Practical aspects of intravenous drug administration: Principles and techniques for nurses, pharmacists, and physicians.* Bethesda, MD: American Society of Hospital Pharmacists.

McEvoy, G. K. (Ed.). (2001). *American Hospital Formulary Service—Drug Information '00.* Bethesda, MD: American Society of Health-System Pharmacists.

Micromedex Drugdex. (1999). Tranexamic Acid, Micromedex, Inc.

Nahata, M. C., Roberts, D. L., & Hipple, T. F. (1987). Formulation of caffeine injection for IV administration. *American Journal of Hospital Pharmacy, 44,* 1308–1312.

Phelps, S. J., & Hak, E. B. (1996). *Guidelines for administration of intravenous medications to pediatric patients.* Bethesda, MD: American Society of Health-System Pharmacists.

Rapp, R. P., Butts, J. D., & Piecoro, J. J., Jr. (1988). Guidelines for the administration of commonly used intravenous drugs: 1988 update. *Journal of Pharmacological Technology, 7,* 14–32.

Repchinsky, C. (Ed.). (2002). *Compendium of pharmaceuticals and specialties.* Ottawa, ON: Canadian Pharmacists Association.

Reynolds, J. E. F. (Ed.). (1993). *Martindale: The extra pharmacopoeia,* 30th ed., London, England: The Pharmaceutical Press.

Sifton, D. W. (Ed). (2002). *Physicians' desk reference,* 56th ed., Montvale, NJ: Medical Economics Data.

Sodorff, M. M., Galt, K. A., Galt, M., et al. (1999). Recommended maximum concentrations of common acute care parenteral admixtures. *Hospital Pharmacy, 34,* 937–942.

---

1. Current product package inserts and prescribing information have been utilized in addition to the references cited here.

Taketomo, C. K., Hodding, J. H., & Kraus, D. M. (2000). *Pediatric dosage handbook,* 7th ed. Cleveland, OH: Lexi-Comp.

Trissel, L. A. (2001). *Handbook on injectable drugs,* 10th ed., Bethesda, MD: American Society of Health-System Pharmacists.

Wojtynek, J. (1999). Caffeine citrate injection. *Pharmacy Phax Phacts,* 6, 1–2.

9

Pediatric Immunizations

David W. Scheifele

Childhood immunization programs are the single most effective preventive healthcare measure available (Centers for Disease Control and Prevention, 1999). The vaccines that are now used routinely for infants and children generally are safe and effective, although none is completely safe or effective. Appropriate use of vaccines substantially influences their margin of safety and effectiveness.

General Cautions

Several factors should be considered when planning immunizations for infants and children (Centers for Disease Control and Prevention Advisory Committee on Immunization Practices, 1994). These factors include the presence of minor infections; eczema and atopic dermatitis; allergies to vaccine components; use of live viral vaccines; pregnancy; breast feeding; immunization of infants and children with neurological disorders; concurrent immunosuppressive therapy; human immunodeficiency virus infection; hemophilia; immunization of premature neonates; timing of vaccine administration; use of vaccine combinations; interference by immune globulin, blood, and plasma infusions; and proper storage and handling of immunizing products.

Minor infections are prevalent among infants and children. All vaccines can be administered to children with minor illnesses, such as the common cold or diarrhea, with or without low-grade fever. However, an illness with a moderate or severe fever is sufficient reason to defer immunization. Vaccination can proceed as soon as the child has recovered from the febrile condition. Routine physical examinations and temperature measurements are not prerequisites for immunizing infants and children who appear healthy. Current antibiotic therapy is not a contraindication to vaccination and neither is recent exposure to a contagious disease.

Eczema and atopic disease generally are not contraindications to immunization unless the infant or child is allergic to a specific vaccine component.

Allergy to vaccine components is rare among infants and children. Some vaccines contain preservatives, stabilizers, or trace amounts of antibiotics (e.g., neomycin) to which infants and children may be hypersensitive. The presence of such additives or excipients can be determined from the product labeling. No currently recommended vaccine contains penicillin or its derivatives. Vaccines, which are prepared in embryonated chicken eggs (e.g., influenza virus vaccine), should not be administered to infants and children who are hypersensitive to eggs unless special procedures are followed (James et al., 1998). Measles and mumps vaccines are usually prepared in chick embryo cell cultures and contain little egg antigen.

Egg-allergic children can generally be administered measles and mumps vaccines without special procedures provided that adequate facilities are available to manage rare instances of anaphylaxis (James et al., 1995). Some anaphylactic reactions are triggered by gelatin, a commonly used stabilizer in measles, mumps, and rubella (MMR) and varicella vaccines.

Live viral vaccines (e.g., MMR, varicella) must not be administered to infants and children with impaired immunity, except as indicated. Oral poliovirus vaccine (OPV) is contraindicated in children with impaired immunity or who reside in the household of an immunocompromised person. Inactivated poliomyelitis vaccine (IPV) is indicated in such circumstances.

Pregnancy is a contraindication to administration of live viral vaccines (e.g., MMR, varicella) because of the theoretical risk to the developing fetus. Conception should be avoided by the recipient for 1 month after measles or mumps vaccination and for 3 months after rubella vaccination (Centers for Disease Control and Prevention Advisory Committee on Immunization Practices, 1998). Inactivated viral and bacterial vaccines may be administered to pregnant women if indicated (if the woman is at immediate risk), although it is preferable to defer immunization until after delivery. Varicella vaccine and the combined MMR vaccine may be administered safely to infants and children living in the same household with a pregnant woman.

Breast feeding does not interfere with or serve as a substitute for immunization. Therefore, infants who are breast fed should receive all recommended immunizations at the usual times. Mothers who are breast feeding can receive live viral vaccines without interrupting the feeding schedule.

Immunization of infants and children with neurologic disorders (e.g., epilepsy) is usually recommended because the advantages of protection against disease generally outweigh the risks of immunization. Fever resulting from immunization may trigger convulsions in predisposed infants and children, although prophylaxis strategies are available for some situations (e.g., reduction of fever risk with acetaminophen administered prophylactically after killed vaccines). Acellular pertussis-containing vaccines are much less likely to trigger febrile convulsions or hypotonic–hyporesponsive episodes than older, whole cell pertussis-containing vaccines, making the more recently developed vaccines more suitable for use in children with neurologic disorders.

Immunosuppressive therapy may blunt the response to active immunization. Immunization should be deferred until short-term immunosuppressive treatment is completed. Inactivated vaccines may be used for infants and children receiving long-term immunosuppressive therapy but live vaccines should be deferred. A similar caution is required following completion of antineoplastic drug therapy (*see* Chapter 12) and after bone marrow transplantation (Centers for Disease Control and Prevention Advisory Committee on Immunization Practices, 1993).

Infants and children who are infected with **human immunodeficiency virus (HIV)** are particularly likely to benefit from the timely administration of routine immunizations. Inactivated poliomyelitis vaccine (IPV) should be used, in preference to OPV. BCG vaccine should be avoided. Other vaccines routinely recommended for HIV-infected children include diphtheria, tetanus, and pertussis (DTP or DTaP); *Haemophilus influenzae* type b conjugate (HbCV); hepatitis B (HB); and MMR. The MMR has proven safe even in children with symptomatic immunodeficiency but is contraindicated in those who are severely immunocompromised (with low CD4 and T-lymphocyte counts). Pneumococcal conjugate vaccine is recommended for HIV-infected children younger than 59 months and pneumococcal polysaccharide vaccine is recommended for children 5 years of age and older. Influenza virus vaccine is recommended annually for HIV-infected children and their household members. Varicella vaccine can be considered for use in children with mildly symptomatic HIV infection.

Children who have **hemophilia** can be safely immunized if firm pressure is applied to the injection site for at least 5 minutes immediately after injecting the immunizing agent. For additional safety, immunization injections can be scheduled shortly after administration of antihemophilic therapy.

Premature infants respond adequately to routinely used vaccines and should be vaccinated at the same chronological age and according to the same schedule and precautions as full-term infants, provided that they are in stable condition. The full recommended dose of each vaccine should be used, but only inactivated poliovirus vaccine should be used. Responses to hepatitis B vaccination may be suboptimal in infants weighing less than 2000 grams (Lau et al., 1992).

Timing of vaccine administration is important. Administration of live virus vaccines at an earlier age than what is recommended increases the likelihood that the response will be blunted by residual maternal antibodies, whereas delayed administration prolongs the risk of exposure to naturally acquired viruses. Administration of vaccines that require a series of doses for complete immunization at shorter than recommended intervals may result in suboptimal antibody response. In contrast, dosing intervals that are longer than what is recommended do not diminish antibody concentrations. Therefore, interruption of a series of immunizations for whatever reason does not necessitate starting the series over or adding extra booster doses.

Vaccine combinations have obvious practical advantages. Most commonly used vaccines can be administered safely at the same time without impairing the immune response to any component. Commercially prepared vaccine combinations are convenient to use, store, and record. In addition, the use of combined vaccines reduces exposure to preservatives (e.g., thimerosal).

Immune globulin, blood, and plasma infusions can interfere with the response to live virus vaccines for up to 3 months after the infusion (up to 10 months in the case of high-dose intravenous immunoglobulin [IVIG]) (Centers for Disease Control and Prevention Advisory Committee on Immunization Practices, 1993). They generally do not interfere with the response to inactivated vaccines, provided that different anatomic injection sites are used.

Storage and handling of immunizing products should be performed in accordance with the manufacturer's recommendations. Storage temperature is particularly important. Alum-adsorbed vaccines should never be frozen, whereas varicella vaccine requires storage at $-15°C$ or colder. Correct handling of multiple-dose containers is essential if loss of potency and bacterial contamination are to be avoided. Vaccine providers should ensure that their refrigerator/freezer maintains appropriate temperature and that products are used prior to their expiry date (Bell et al., 2001).

Immunization Records

A permanent personal immunization record should be established when a child receives his or her first immunization. The child's parents should bring the record when taking the child for subsequent immunizations or other healthcare. The vaccine provider should maintain a separate, permanent immunization record for the child, including the name of the vaccine, date administered, dose, route of administration, site, manufacturer, lot number, and any immediate reaction. Providers should strive to adhere to the Standards for Pediatric Immunization Practices (Centers for Disease Control and Prevention, 1993) that address the importance of tracking systems and the use of audits to monitor immunization coverage levels among their patients.

Adverse Drug Reactions

Local or systemic adverse drug reactions (ADRs) may occur after immunization. Most reactions are mild, predictable, and self-limited and occur shortly after vaccination. Rarely, serious or unexpected ADRs may occur. Some apparent reactions may be the result of coincidental illness (Peltola & Heinonen, 1986) or previously undetected disease.

Pediatric clinicians should be aware of the incidence and nature of ADRs to vaccines and inform parents about these risks in rela-

VAERS

VACCINE ADVERSE EVENT REPORTING SYSTEM
24 Hour Toll Free Information 1-800-822-7967
P.O. Box 1100, Rockville, MD 20849-1100
PATIENT IDENTITY KEPT CONFIDENTIAL

For CDC/FDA Use Only
VAERS Number ____________
Date Received ____________

Patient Name:	Vaccine administered by (Name):	Form completed by (Name):
Last First M.I.	Responsible Physician ____________	Relation to Patient ☐ Vaccine Provider ☐ Patient/Parent ☐ Manufacturer ☐ Other
Address	Facility Name/Address	Address *(if different from patient or provider)*
City State Zip	City State Zip	City State Zip
Telephone no. (___) ____________	Telephone no. (___) ____________	Telephone no. (___) ____________

1. State
2. County where administered
3. Date of birth __/__/__ (mm dd yy)
4. Patient age
5. Sex ☐ M ☐ F
6. Date form completed __/__/__ (mm dd yy)

7. Describe adverse events(s) (symptoms, signs, time course) and treatment, if any

8. Check all appropriate:
- ☐ Patient died (date __/__/__ mm dd yy)
- ☐ Life threatening illness
- ☐ Required emergency room/doctor visit
- ☐ Required hospitalization (______days)
- ☐ Resulted in prolongation of hospitalization
- ☐ Resulted in permanent disability
- ☐ None of the above

9. Patient recovered ☐ YES ☐ NO ☐ UNKNOWN

10. Date of vaccination __/__/__ (mm dd yy) Time ________ AM PM

11. Adverse event onset __/__/__ (mm dd yy) Time ________ AM PM

12. Relevant diagnostic tests/laboratory data

13. Enter all vaccines given on date listed in no. 10

	Vaccine (type)	Manufacturer	Lot number	Route/Site	No. Previous Doses
a.					
b.					
c.					
d.					

14. Any other vaccinations within 4 weeks prior to the date listed in no. 10

	Vaccine (type)	Manufacturer	Lot number	Route/Site	No. Previous doses	Date given
a.						
b.						

15. Vaccinated at:
☐ Private doctor's office/hospital ☐ Military clinic/hospital
☐ Public health clinic/hospital ☐ Other/unknown

16. Vaccine purchased with:
☐ Private funds ☐ Military funds
☐ Public funds ☐ Other/unknown

17. Other medications

18. Illness at time of vaccination (specify)

19. Pre-existing physician-diagnosed allergies, birth defects, medial conditions(specify)

20. Have you reported this adverse event previously? ☐ No ☐ To health department ☐ To doctor ☐ To manufacturer

Only for children 5 and under

22. Birth weight ________ lb. ________ oz.

23. No. of brother and sisters

21. Adverse event following prior vaccination (check all applicable, specify)

	Adverse Event	Onset Age	Type Vaccine	Dose no. in series
☐ In patient				
☐ In brother or sister				

Only for reports submitted by manufacturer/immunization project

24. Mfr./imm. proj. report no.

25. Date received by mfr./imm.proj.

26. 15 day report? ☐ Yes ☐ No

27. Report type ☐ Initial ☐ Follow-Up

Health care providers and manufacturers are required by law (42 USC 300aa-25) to report reactions to vaccines listed in the Table of Reportable Events Following Immunization
Reports for reactions to other vaccines are voluntary except when required as a condition of immunization grant awards.

FIGURE 9-1

Form for Reporting Adverse Reactions to Vaccines

tion to the benefits of immunization and the risks associated with target diseases. Parents should be encouraged to report any ADRs. Clinicians should report ADRs (particularly severe or unusual ones) to the local health department, the manufacturer, and in the United States, to the Vaccine Adverse Event Reporting System (VAERS) (Figure 9-1).

Local ADRs usually consist of swelling, redness, and tenderness at the injection site. More severe local reactions (e.g., infection, abscess formation) occasionally occur. Booster doses of bacterial vaccines (e.g., DTP or DTaP) more often cause local reactions than do primary doses.

Systemic ADRs include fever, rash, joint or muscle pain, fainting, and fever-associated seizures. Most of these reactions subside within 48 hours. Allergic reactions such as urticaria, bronchospasm, and anaphylaxis are rare, but potentially life threatening. Risk management strategies must include screening for a history of relevant allergies and preparedness to treat immediate reactions when they occur.

Severe ADRs, whether local or systemic, should prompt the clinician to postpone additional doses, report the reaction, and seek expert advice.

References

Bell, K. N., Hogue, C. J. R., Manning, G., et al. (2001). Risk factors for improper vaccine storage and handling in private provider offices. *Pediatrics, 107,* 100.

Centers for Disease Control and Prevention Advisory Committee on Immunization Practices. (1994). General recommendations on immunization. *Morbidity and Mortality Weekly Report, 43,* RR-I, 1–38.

Centers for Disease Control and Prevention Advisory Committee on Immunization Practices. (1998). Measles, mumps and rubella: Vaccine use and strategies for elimination of measles, rubella, and congenital rubella syndrome and control of mumps. *Morbidity and Mortality Weekly Report, 47,* RR-8.

Centers for Disease Control and Prevention Advisory Committee on Immunization Practices. (1993). Use of vaccines and immune globulins in persons with altered immunocompetence. *Morbidity and Mortality Weekly Report, 42,* RR-4.

Centers for Disease Control and Prevention. (1999). Impact of vaccines universally recommended for children–United States, 1900–1998. *Morbidity and Mortality Weekly Report, 48,* 243–248.

Centers for Disease Control and Prevention. (1993). Standards for pediatric immunization practices recommended by the National Vaccine Advisory Committee. *Morbidity and Mortality Weekly Report, 42,* 1–13.

James, J. M., Burks, A. W., Robertson, P. K., et al. (1995). Safe administration of the measles vaccine to children allergic to eggs. *New England Journal of Medicine, 332,* 1262–1266.

James, J. M., Zeiger, R. S., Lester, M. R., et al. (1998). Safe administration of influenza vaccine to patients with egg allergy. *The Journal of Pediatrics, 133,* 624–628.

Lau, Y. L., Tan, A. Y. C., Ng, K. W., et al. (1992). Response of pre-term infants to hepatitis B vaccine. *The Journal of Pediatrics, 121,* 962–965.

Peltola, H., & Heinonen, O. P. (1986). Frequency of true adverse reactions to measles-mumps-rubella vaccine: A double-blind, placebo-controlled trial in twins. *The Lancet, 1,* 939–942.

Active Immunization Schedules and Monographs for Vaccines and Toxoids

The following schedules and monographs provide the pediatric clinician with essential information for providing childhood immunization. Each monograph includes information on the formulations used for immunization, recommended use, ADRs, contraindications, and current references.

Schedules for active immunization of normal infants and children (Tables 9-1 and 9-2a and 2b) were harmonized in 1999 among the U.S. Public Health Service, the American Academy of Pediatrics, and the American Academy of Family Physicians. Schedules contain considerable flexibility for local program variations or provider preferences. Schedules used in Canada are similar to those shown, but product availability may differ. Immunization schedules evolve frequently, so pediatric clinicians should ensure that the current version is followed.

It is essential that the manufacturer's labeling (package insert) be consulted for instructions on storage, handling, and administration. The characteristics of vaccines prepared by different manufacturers vary, and a manufacturer's product may change over time.

Diphtheria Toxoid

Diphtheria is a serious communicable disease caused by toxigenic strains of *Corynebacterium diphtheriae* (Hodes, 1979). Mortality is as high as 10% in untreated, susceptible patients, with high death rates in the very young. Routine immunization against diphtheria in in-

TABLE 9-1
Recommended Childhood Immunization Schedule in the United States, January–December 2002[a]

	BIRTH	1 MONTH	2 MONTHS	4 MONTHS	6 MONTHS	12 MONTHS	15 MONTHS	18 MONTHS	24 MONTHS	4–6 YEARS	11–12 YEARS	14–18 YEARS
Hepatitis B[b]		HBV										
			HBV			HBV					HBV	
Diphtheria, Tetanus, and Pertussis (DTP)			DTaP	DTaP	DTaP		DTaP[c]			DTaP		Td
H. influenzae Type b[d]			Hib	Hib	Hib	Hib						
Polio[e]			IPV	IPV		Polio[e]				Polio		
Pneumococcal Conjugate			PVC	PVC	PVC	PVC						
Measles, Mumps, and Rubella (MMR)						MMR				MMR[f]	MMR	
Varicella[g]						Var					Var	
Hepatitis A[h]										Hep A in selected areas		

[a] Currently licensed vaccines are listed under routinely recommended ages. Bars indicate range of recommended ages of immunization. Any dose not administered at the recommended age should be administered as a "catch-up" immunization at any subsequent visit when indicated and feasible. Shaded cells indicate vaccines to be administered if previously recommended doses were missed or administered earlier than the recommended minimum age. Combination vaccines may be used whenever any components of the combination are indicated and its other components are not contraindicated. Approved by the Advisory Committee on Immunization Practices (ACIP), the American Academy of Pediatrics (AAP), and the American Academy of Family Physicians (AAFP).

[b] All U.S. newborns should be vaccinated against hepatitis B before leaving the hospital. Infants born to HBsAg-negative mothers should receive the second dose of hepatitis B vaccine (HBV) at least 1 month after the first dose. The third dose should be administered at least 4 months after the first dose and at least 2 months after the second dose, but not before 6 months of age for infants.

Infants born to HBsAg-positive mothers should receive HBV vaccine and 0.5 ml of hepatitis B immune globulin (HBIG) within 12 hours of birth at separate sites. The second dose is recommended at 1–2 months of age and the third dose at 6 months of age. Infants born to mothers whose HBsAg status is unknown should receive HBV vaccine within 12 hours of birth. Maternal blood should be drawn at the time of delivery to determine the mother's HBsAg status; if the HBsAg test is positive, the infant should receive HBIG as soon as possible (no later than 1 week of age). All children and adolescents (through 18 years of age) who have not been immunized against hepatitis B may begin the series during any visit. Special efforts should be made to immunize children who were born in or whose parents were born in areas of the world with moderate or high endemicity of hepatitis B virus infection.

[c] DTaP (diphtheria and tetanus toxoids and acellular pertussis vaccine) is the preferred vaccine for all doses in the immunization series. The fourth dose may be administered as early as 12 months of age, provided 6 months have elapsed since the third dose and if the child is unlikely to return at 15–18 months. Td is recommended at 11–12 years of age if at least 5 years have elapsed since the last dose of DTP, DTaP, or DT. Subsequent routine Td boosters are recommended every 10 years.

[d] Three *Haemophilus influenzae* type b (Hib) conjugate vaccines are licensed for infant use. If PRP-OMP (*PedvaxHIB* or *ComVax*, Merck) is administered at 2 and 4 months of age, a dose at 6 months is not required.

[e] Inactivated poliovirus (IPV) vaccine is preferred for all doses. The third dose can be administered at 6 months or at 12–18 months.

[f] The second dose of measles, mumps, and rubella (MMR) vaccine is recommended routinely at 4–6 years of age but may be administered during any visit, provided at least 4 weeks have elapsed since receipt of the first dose and that both doses are administered beginning at or after 12 months of age. Those who have not previously received the second dose should complete the schedule by the 11–12-year visit.

[g] Varicella (Var) vaccine is recommended at any visit on or after the first birthday for susceptible children, i.e., those who lack a reliable history of chickenpox and who have not been immunized. Susceptible persons 13 years of age or older should receive two doses, administered at least 4 weeks apart.

[h] Hepatitis A vaccine (Hep A) is recommended for use in selected states and/or regions and for certain high-risk groups.

fancy and childhood during the past 50 years has virtually eradicated the disease in Canada and the United States. However, toxigenic strains of diphtheria bacilli are still detected each year in asymptomatic carriers, indicating the need to maintain protection against the disease. A lapse in control programs in states of the former Soviet Union resulted in a major epidemic during the 1990s, with more than 100,000 cases (Vitek & Wharton, 1998).

Formulations. Diphtheria toxoid is a cell-free preparation of the toxin produced by diphtheria bacilli; the toxin is neutralized with formaldehyde. The immunity conferred is antitoxic (not antibacterial), protecting against the systemic effects of diphtheria toxin but not directly against local infection. Immunity persists for at least 10 years after immunization.

Most diphtheria toxoids are adsorbed onto aluminum salts because such preparations induce higher antitoxin titers and more durable protection (Centers for Disease Control and Prevention . . . , 2000). Diphtheria toxoid is available alone and in combination with tetanus toxoid and pertussis and poliomyelitis

TABLE 9-2a
Routine Immunization Schedule for Children less than 7 Years of Age Who Were *Not* Immunized during the First 15 Months of Life[a]

TIMING	DTaP	IPV	HIB	MMR	TD	HBV
First visit	X	X	X	X		
2 months later	X	X				
2 months later	X	(X)[b]				
6–12 months later	X	X				
4–6 years	X[c]	X[c]		X[d]		
11–16 years					X	X[e]

[a] Modified from Canadian Immunization Guide, 1998.
[b] This dose is not needed routinely but can be included for convenience.
[c] Omit these doses if the previous doses of DTaP and IPV were administered after the 4th birthday.
[d] The second dose can be administered as soon as 1 month after the first dose.
[e] The three-dose series of HBV vaccinations can be administered in preadolescence (11–12 years) or starting at any earlier age if the child is at increased risk of exposure.

vaccines. Preparations with smaller amounts of diphtheria toxoid (generally designated Td) are intended for use in children 7 years of age or older and adults because of their greater susceptibility to ADRs. Preparations for infants and younger children (designated DTP) contain larger amounts of diphtheria toxoid.

Recommended use. Routine immunization against diphtheria is recommended for all infants and children. Products in which diphtheria toxoid is combined with tetanus toxoid and pertussis vaccine (DTP or DTaP) are preferred for primary immunization of infants and children under 7 years of age. The primary immunizing course of diphtheria toxoid consists of four doses, ideally begun at 2 months of age (Table 9–1). The intervals between the first three doses are preferably 8 weeks; the fourth dose is administered 1 year after the third dose. The fourth dose also can be administered at 15 months of age concurrently with MMR, IPV, and HbCV. A booster dose should be administered at 4–6 years of age (at or before school entry). The "adult" vaccine (Td) should be administered 10 years later.

Active immunization should be carried out during convalescence from diphtheria. The disease does not necessarily confer immunity.

Adsorbed vaccines such as diphtheria toxoid must be injected intramuscularly. Adsorbed vaccines must not be frozen during shipping or storage. The manufacturer's recommendations in the product labeling should be followed.

ADRs. Life-threatening reactions to diphtheria toxoid are extremely rare. Local and febrile

TABLE 9-2b
Routine Immunization Schedule for Children 7 Years of Age or Older Who Were *Not* Immunized in Early Infancy[a]

TIMING	Td[b]	IPV	MMR	HBV
First visit	X	X	X	Preadolescence[c]
2 months later	X	X	X[d]	
6–12 months later	X	X		
4–6 years later	X	X		
10 years later	X			

[a] Modified from Canadian Immunization Guide, 1998.
[b] The availability of Td.aP vaccines may result in a recommendation for immunization against pertussis in this age group.
[c] The three-dose series of HBV vaccinations can be administered in preadolescence (11–12 years) or at any earlier age if the child is at increased risk of exposure.
[d] The minimum interval between first and second MMR doses is 4 weeks.

reactions are uncommon in infants and children younger than 7 years of age (Cody et al., 1981). Td booster doses administered at 14–16 years of age cause local reactions in about 25% of recipients, most of whom consider the reactions tolerable (Scheifele et al., 1998).

Contraindications. Children 7 years of age and older should be administered only the "adult" formulation (Td). Before giving a combination vaccine, it is important to ensure that there are no contraindications (e.g., hypersensitivity) to the administration of any of the components.

Centers for Disease Control and Prevention Advisory Committee on Immunization Practices. (2000). Use of diphtheria toxoid–tetanus toxoid–acellular pertussis vaccine as a five dose series. *Morbidity and Mortality Weekly Report, 49,* RR-13.

Cody, C. L., Baraff, L. J., Cherry, J. D., et al. (1981). Nature and rates of adverse reactions associated with DTP and DT immunizations in infants and children. *Pediatrics, 68,* 650–660.

Hodes, H. L. (1979). Diphtheria. *Pediatric Clinics of North America, 26,* 445–459.

Scheifele, D. W., Dobson, S., Kallos, A., et al. (1998). Comparative safety of tetanus-diphtheria toxoids booster immunization in students in grades 6 and 9. *Pediatric Infectious Diseases Journal, 17,* 1121–1126.

Vitek, C. R., & Wharton, M. (1998). Diphtheria in the former Soviet Union: Re-emergence of a pandemic disease. *Emerging Infectious Diseases, 4,* 539–549.

Haemophilus Influenzae Type b Conjugate Vaccine

Haemophilus influenzae type b (Hib) was, until recently, the most common cause of bacterial meningitis and a leading cause of serious, invasive infections in infants and young children. Approximately 1 in 200 children suffered a systemic Hib infection before 5 years of age (Cochi & Broome, 1986; Force et al., 1992). The risk was greatest among children attending day-care facilities (Istre et al., 1985); pediatric patients with splenic dysfunction, sickle cell anemia, or antibody deficiency; and Innuit (aboriginal Alaskan) children (Ward et al., 1981). About 60% of affected infants and children developed meningitis and the other 40% experienced bacteremia, epiglottitis, cellulitis, pneumonia, or septic arthritis (American Academy of Pediatrics, 1997). The peak incidence occurred among infants between the ages of 6 and 12 months (Cochi & Broome, 1986). The risk of Hib infection has been greatly reduced by the universal immunization of infants according to recommended guidelines (Centers for Disease Control and Prevention . . . , 1991; Bisgard et al., 1998).

Formulations. Several different Hib conjugate vaccines (HbCV) are used. Each vaccine contains purified Hib capsular polysaccharide, a polymer of ribose, ribitol, and phosphate, chemically linked to a protein carrier. These formulations differ in the size and number of polysaccharide molecules per dose and in the nature of the protein carrier. Products recommended for young infants elicit protective responses following a series of two or three primary doses (Table 9-3). Immunization with HbCV reduces nasopharyngeal Hib colonization.

Efficacy of currently used HbCV formulations exceeds 95%. Immunity conferred is specific to type b organisms, but other types of *H. influenzae* rarely cause invasive infection. Immunity appears to be long-lasting following completion of the recommended dose series (Scheifele et al., 1999).

HbCV vaccines are available in combinations with other routinely used vaccines. Examples include DTP-HbCV and HB-HbCV. In Canada, a DTaP-IPV-HbCV combination is widely used (National Advisory Committee . . . , 1998).

Recommended use. HbCV is recommended for all infants and children 2–59 months old (National Advisory Committee . . . , 1998). Priority is given to 2-month-old infants to elicit active protection before maternally derived protection wanes at about 6 months of age. A series of two or three (depending on the product) primary doses is administered (usually with DTP for convenience) at 2, 4, and, for some products, 6 months of age. HbCV can be administered concurrently with MMR vaccine (in separate syringes at separate sites). A booster dose of HbCV is recommended at ages varying from 12 to 18 months, depending on the product used (American Academy of Pediatrics, 1997).

TABLE 9-3
Hib Conjugate Vaccines Suitable for Infants

PRODUCT (MANUFACTURER)	CARRIER PROTEIN	RECOMMENDED AGES FOR PRIMARY DOSES	RECOMMENDED AGES FOR BOOSTER DOSE
HibTITER (Wyeth–Ayerst)	A nontoxic 2, 4, and mutant diphtheria toxin	2, 4, and 6 months	15–18 months
PedvaxHIB (Merck)	Outer membrane complex from *Neisseria meningitidis*	2 and 4 months	12–15 months
ActHIB (Pasteur Merieux Connaught)	Tetanus toxoid	2, 4, and 6 months	15–18 months

Children who are older when Hib immunization is initiated require fewer HbCV doses; after 15 months of age, only one dose is required. The product labeling details the abbreviated dosing schedules for infants and children who are 7–14 months of age. Infants and children who develop Hib infection before 24 months of age do not develop reliable immunity to Hib and should be immunized with HbCV after they recover from their illness. HbCV is also indicated for unimmunized children older than 5 years of age who have an increased risk of Hib infection associated with chronic illness (e.g., asplenia, sickle cell disease).

ADRs. ADRs to HbCV are uncommon and usually mild, consisting primarily of local soreness at the injection site and fever. Systemic reactions other than fever are rare.

Contraindications. HbCV should not be administered to infants and children who are allergic to any constituent of the formulation.

American Academy of Pediatrics. (1997). *Report of the committee on infectious diseases*, 24th ed., pp. 220–231. Elk Grove Village, IL: American Academy of Pediatrics.

Bisgard, K. M., Kao, A., Leake, J., et al. (1998). Haemophilus influenzae invasive disease in the United States, 1994–1995: Near disappearance of a vaccine-preventable childhood disease. *Emerging Infectious Diseases, 4*, 229–237.

Centers for Disease Control and Prevention Advisory Committee on Immunization Practices. (1991). Haemophilus b conjugate vaccines for prevention of Haemophilus influenzae type b disease among infants and children two months of age and older. *Morbidity and Mortality Weekly Report, 40*(Suppl RR-1), 1–7.

Cochi, S. L., & Broome, C. V. (1986). Vaccine prevention of Haemophilus influenzae type b disease—Past, present and future. *Pediatric Infectious Disease, 5*, 12–19.

Force, R. W., Lugo, R. A., & Nahata, M. C. (1992). Haemophilus influenzae type b conjugate vaccines. *DICP Annals of Pharmacotherapy, 26*, 1429–1440.

Istre, G. R., Conner, J. S., Broome, C. V., et al. (1985). Risk factors for primary invasive Haemophilus influenzae disease: Increased risk from day-care attendance and in school age household members. *The Journal of Pediatrics, 106*, 190–195.

National Advisory Committee on Immunization. (1998). *Canadian immunization guide*, 5th ed., pp. 78–82. Ottawa, ON: Health Canada.

Scheifele, D. W., Halperin, S. A., Guasparini, R., et al. (1999). Extended follow-up of antibody levels and antigen responsiveness after 2 Haemophilus influenzae type b conjugate vaccines. *The Journal of Pediatrics, 135*, 240–245.

Ward, J. I., Margolis, H. S., Lum, M. K., et al. (1981). Haemophilus influenzae disease in Alaskan Eskimos: Characteristics of a population with an unusual incidence of invasive disease. *The Lancet, 1*, 1281–1285.

Hepatitis A Vaccine

Hepatitis A virus (HAV) infection (Koff, 1998) is responsible for most cases of acute hepatitis in the United States and Canada. The severity of illness increases with age. Young children are often mildly ill or asymptomatic but readily spread infection to contacts. Recovery may take several months but no chronic infection state occurs. Fulminant hepatitis occasionally occurs, particularly in older adults with pre-existing liver disease.

Vaccination programs target people at increased risk of infection and communities with high rates or recurrent outbreaks of infection.

Formulations. Licensed vaccines contain inactivated HAV, which has been grown in human fibroblast cultures, inactivated with formalin and adsorbed to alum adjuvant

(Lemon & Thomas, 1997; Furesz et al., 1995). Pediatric formulations of HAV vaccines are appropriately used from 1–18 or 2–17 years of age, depending on the product and country. Products may contain trace amounts of neomycin.

A single intramuscular dose elicits protective levels of antibodies within 4 weeks in more than 97% of recipients. A second dose is recommended 6–18 months later for long-term protection (extending 10 years or more) (Wiedermann et al., 1997).

A combined HAV–HBV vaccine is available in a pediatric formulation for children needing protection against both infections (Diaz-Mitoma et al., 1999). Three doses are recommended, at 0, 1, and 6 months.

Recommended use. Universal HAV immunization of children is recommended in states with higher than average rates of HAV infection. Alaska and Oklahoma have established programs requiring children to be immunized prior to entering school or day-care facilities. Immunization is started after the second birthday. Earlier administration is not recommended because maternally derived anti-HAV interferes with the response to vaccination.

Other potential candidates for vaccination (American Academy of Pediatrics . . . , 1996) are travelers to countries where hepatitis A is endemic; residents of communities with high endemic rates or recurrent outbreaks of HAV; youth with lifestyle-determined risks of infection (Villano et al., 1997), including use of oral or intravenous illicit drugs in unsanitary conditions and men who have sex with men; children with hemophilia A or B receiving plasma-derived clotting factors (Mah et al., 1994); children with chronic liver disease or a transplanted liver, who may be at increased risk of fulminant hepatitis A (Vento et al., 1998); and children attending day-care facilities may be at increased risk in some areas.

HAV vaccine can be administered concurrently with other childhood vaccines, at separate anatomic injection sites.

ADRs. ADRs after HAV vaccination are generally infrequent, mild and short-lived, and limited to soreness and redness at the injection site (Furesz et al., 1995). Rare instances of anaphylaxis have been reported.

Contraindications. HAV vaccine should not be administered to children or adolescents who have had an anaphylactic reaction to a previous dose. Caution is required for pediatric patients who are allergic to neomycin.

American Academy of Pediatrics Committee on Infectious Diseases. (1996). Prevention of hepatitis A infections: Guidelines for use of hepatitis A vaccine and immune globulin. *Pediatrics, 98,* 1207–1215.

Diaz-Mitoma, F., Law, B., & Parsons, J. (1999). A combined vaccine against hepatitis A and B in children and adolescents. *Pediatric Infectious Disease Journal, 18,* 109–114.

Furesz, J., Scheifele, D. W., & Palkonyay, L. (1995). Safety and effectiveness of the new inactivated hepatitis A virus vaccine. *Canadian Medical Association Journal, 152,* 343–348.

Koff, R. S. (1998). Hepatitis A. *The Lancet, 341,* 1643–1649.

Lemon, S. M., & Thomas, D. L. (1997). Vaccines to prevent viral hepatitis. *New England Journal of Medicine, 336,* 196–204.

Mah, M. W., Royce, R. A., Rathouz, P. J., et al. (1994). Prevalence of hepatitis A antibodies in hemophiliacs: Preliminary results from the Southeastern Delta Hepatitis Study. *Vox Sanguinous, 67*(Suppl 1), 21–23.

Vento, S., Garofano, T., Renzini, C., et al. (1998). Fulminant hepatitis associated with hepatitis A virus superinfection in patients with chronic hepatitis C. *New England Journal of Medicine, 338,* 286–290.

Villano, S. A., Nelson, K. E., Vlahov, D., et al. (1997). Hepatitis A among homosexual men and injection drug users: More evidence for vaccination. *Clinical Infectious Diseases, 25,* 726–728.

Wiedermann, G., Kundi, M., Ambrosch, F., et al. (1997). Inactivated hepatitis A vaccine: Long-term antibody persistence. *Vaccine, 15,* 612–615.

Hepatitis B Virus Vaccine

Hepatitis B virus (HBV) causes both acute and chronic hepatitis. Children are especially likely to develop chronic infection, known as the chronic carrier state, which is associated with long-term risks of cirrhosis and hepatocellular carcinoma (Mahoney, 1999). Children most often become infected during birth to an infected mother or through close contact with infected household members. Adolescents and youth are at risk of exposure through sexual activity and intravenous use of abusable psychotropics (*see* Chapter 7).

Immunization programs in the United States and Canada are directed at individuals at high risk of exposure to HBV and at groups targeted for universal vaccination (Mast et al., 1998).

Formulations. HBV vaccines consist of highly purified, alum-adsorbed hepatitis B surface antigen (HBsAg) prepared from cultures of yeast containing recombinant hepatitis B viral DNA (Lemon & Thomas, 1997). HBV vaccine is free of other HBV components. In response to concerns about the safety of thimerosal preservative (a mercurial salt), thimerosal-free formulations are now available. Recombinant vaccines from different companies have similar immunogenicity and can be used interchangeably. However, pediatric clinicians must be cognizant of differences in age-related dose volumes (see product labeling for details).

Some combined vaccines are available (e.g., HbCV, HBV vaccine) and more are being developed to facilitate use (e.g., DTaP-IPV-HbCV-HBV vaccine).

Recommended use. Universal HBV vaccination is recommended for certain children in Canada, and all United States newborns must be vaccinated before leaving the hospital. Infants are the primary target of U.S. programs, but children 11–12 years old also are targeted for catch-up vaccination (Mast et al., 1998). In Canada, school-based programs for adolescents have been established in all provinces, with considerable success (Dobson et al., 1995). Some jurisdictions have extended their programs to include infants, but this will become more practical when combination vaccines are available.

Individuals of any age at increased risk of HBV infection are also targeted for vaccination (American Academy of Pediatrics, 1997), including students in healthcare and emergency service settings; residents of institutions for the developmentally disabled; homosexual and bisexual males; heterosexual men or women with multiple sexual partners or with a recent history of a sexually transmitted disease; intravenous drug users; hemophiliacs and others receiving repeated infusions of blood or blood products; hemodialysis patients; household and sexual contacts of acute HBV cases and HBV carriers, including infected adoptees, children whose families have emigrated from areas where there is a high prevalence of HBV infection and children who are likely to be exposed to HBV carriers in their extended families (Mahoney et al., 1995); certain travelers to hepatitis B endemic areas; children in child-care settings; and communities or populations in which HBV is highly endemic. Not all of these situations are necessarily included in local programs or facilitated by free supplies of vaccine.

Postexposure prophylaxis is another important use of HBV vaccine. All infants born to infected mothers should be identified by routine screening programs for pregnant women or by testing at delivery. These infants should receive 0.5 ml hepatitis B immune globulin (HBIG) and start a course of three doses of HBV vaccine within 12 hours after birth (American Academy of Pediatrics, 1997). HBIG and HBV vaccine can be administered concurrently, at separate anatomic injection sites.

HBV-susceptible children who injure themselves with discarded needles will generally require postexposure prophylaxis with HBIG and HBV vaccination, as will victims of sexual assault if the HBsAg status of the assailant cannot be determined (National Advisory Committee . . . , 1998).

HBV vaccines are administered by intramuscular injection. The usual schedule recommends doses at birth and at 1 and 6 months of age, but numerous alternative schedules exist, depending upon the urgency of the situation. HBV vaccines can be administered concurrently with other childhood vaccines, at separate anatomic injection sites. A two-dose schedule has been approved for adolescents (Poland, 2001).

Routine booster doses are not recommended. Protection lasts at least 15 years.

ADRs. HBV vaccines are well tolerated, causing only minor local reactions. Anaphylactic reactions occur rarely. A causative link between hepatitis B vaccination and demyelinating diseases of the CNS has been alleged from case anecdotes but is not substantiated by epidemiologic data (Sadovnick & Scheifele, 2000).

Contraindications. HBV vaccine should not be administered to a child or adolescent who has experienced an anaphylactic reaction to a previous dose. Pregnancy is not considered a contraindication to vaccine use when indicated.

American Academy of Pediatrics. (1997). *Report of the committee on infectious diseases,* 24th ed., pp. 247–260. Elk Grove Village, IL: American Academy of Pediatrics.

Dobson, S., Scheifele, D. W., & Bell, A. (1995). Assessment of a universal, school-based hepatitis B vaccination program. *Journal of the American Medical Association, 274,* 1209–1213.

Lemon, S. M., & Thomas, D. L. (1997). Vaccines to prevent viral hepatitis. *New England Journal of Medicine, 336,* 196–204.

Mahoney, F. J. (1999). Update on diagnosis, management, and prevention of hepatitis B virus infection. *Clinical Microbiology Reviews, 12,* 351–366.

Mahoney, F. J., Lawrence, M., Scott, C., et al. (1995). Continuing risk of hepatitis B virus transmission among Southeast Asian infants in Louisiana. *Pediatrics, 96,* 1113–1116.

Mast, E. E., Mahoney, F. J., Alter, M. J., et al. (1998). Progress towards elimination of hepatitis B virus transmission in the United States. *Vaccine, 16,* S48–S51.

National Advisory Committee on Immunization. (1998). *Canadian immunization guide,* 5th ed., pp. 90–102. Ottawa, ON: Health Canada.

Poland, G. A. (2001). Adolescent hepatitis B immunization: Making it simpler. *Pediatrics, 107,* 771–772.

Sadovnick, A. D., & Scheifele, D. W. (2000). No evidence for an increased frequency of adolescent multiple sclerosis with a school-based hepatitis B vaccination programme for grade 6 students. *The Lancet, 355,* 549–550.

Influenza Virus Vaccine

Influenza is one of the more severe forms of viral respiratory tract infection, causing high fever, aching, and prostration that last for several days (Glezen & Couch, 1997). Complications occur frequently and include otitis media, sinusitis, bronchitis, and bronchopneumonia (MacDonald, 1995). Influenza is highly contagious, spreading readily among school children and household members. The outcome is benign for most children but influenza causes substantial morbidity in children who have chronic lung disease and other chronic illnesses (Serwint et al., 1991). Immunization should be offered to such children on an annual basis.

Formulations. Influenza virus vaccines are reformulated annually to keep abreast of changes in circulating strains (Centers for Disease Control and Prevention . . . , 2001). Classical influenza virus vaccines are suspensions of several strains of virus that have been inactivated (usually with formalin) after cultivation in hen's eggs. Coverage for both A and B strains is provided in all formulations. Chemically disrupted "split virus" (subvirion) vaccine formulations are recommended for children because they are better tolerated than whole virus formulations (now largely obsolete). Inactivated influenza vaccine is about 70%–90% effective in children for preventing infection by influenza virus during the year after its administration. The vaccine is administered by intramuscular injection. Two doses, at least 4 weeks apart, are recommended for first-time recipients of influenza vaccine who are less than 9 years old. In subsequent years, a single annual dose suffices. The minimum age for vaccination is 6 months. The dosage is 0.25 ml for infants and children 6–35 months of age and 0.5 ml for children 3 years of age and older.

A live, attenuated, trivalent influenza vaccine was developed in the United States for use in children (Belshe et al., 1998). It is administered intranasally and causes minimal ADRs. Protection extends for at least two winters, barring major changes in circulating strains. This combination of convenient, painless administration and multiyear effectiveness raises the prospect of universal immunization of children, a development that would substantially reduce the circulation of influenza viruses among people of all ages, given the central role of children in disseminating the infection (Mathias, 1996).

Recommended use. Immunization each autumn is advised for children who are likely to suffer severe illness or death from influenza (Centers for Disease Control and Prevention . . . , 2001). Because influenza virus vaccines are reformulated annually, pediatric clinicians should consult current recommendations. Predisposing conditions for severe influenza include chronic heart disease; chronic lung disease (e.g., cystic fibrosis, bronchopulmonary dysplasia, and asthma) requiring regular medical follow-up; chronic renal disease, especially with azotemia, and the nephrotic syndrome; immunosuppression, including symptomatic HIV infection and immunosuppression caused by drug therapy (responses in such children may be sufficient to favorably modify the course of natural infection [Jackson et al., 1997]); and other chronic conditions such as insulin-dependent diabetes, severe anemia, and conditions treated for long periods with aspirin (acetylsalicylic acid) (because of a risk of Reye's syndrome after influenza).

Utilization of influenza vaccine in children is typically poor unless pediatric clinicians make an effort to acquaint parents with its benefits and promote its use each autumn (Szilagyi & Rodewald, 1992).

Immunization is recommended for close contacts of children at high risk from influenza, including siblings and care providers. Health professionals who are in routine contact with pediatric patients should be immunized (Centers for Disease Control and Prevention . . . , 2001).

Influenza vaccine can be administered concurrently with routine childhood vaccines, at separate anatomic injection sites.

ADRs. Fever, malaise, and myalgia occur within a day or two after administration of inactivated, "split" vaccines in a small percentage of children. Transient injection site soreness, redness, or swelling occur in about one-third of vaccine recipients. Immediate hypersensitivity reactions are rare, even with repeated annual exposure.

Contraindications. Children who are allergic to eggs or thimerosal should not receive influenza virus vaccine, unless special measures are followed (James et al., 1998). Revaccination is contraindicated in children who have experienced an anaphylactic reaction to a previous dose of influenza vaccine.

Belshe, R. B., Mendelman, P. M., Treanor, J., et al. (1998). The efficacy of live, attenuated, cold-adapted, trivalent intranasal influenza virus vaccine in children. *New England Journal of Medicine, 338,* 1405–1412.

Centers for Disease Control and Prevention Advisory Committee on Immunization Practices. (2001). Prevention and control of influenza. *Morbidity and Mortality Weekly Report, 50,* RR–4.

Glezen, W. P., & Couch, R. B. (1997). Influenza viruses. In *Viral infections of humans—epidemiology and control,* 4th ed., pp. 473–505. A. S. Evans & R. A. Kaslow, Eds., New York: Plenum Medical.

Jackson, C. R., Vavro, C. L., Valentine, M. E., et al. (1997). Effect of influenza immunization on immunologic and virologic characteristics of pediatric patients infected with human immunodeficiency virus. *Pediatric Infectious Disease Journal, 16,* 200–204.

James, J. M., Zeiger, R. S., Lester, M. R., et al. (1998). Safe administration of influenza vaccine to patients with egg allergy. *The Journal of Pediatrics, 133,* 624–628.

MacDonald, J. C. (1995). Influenza in children. *The Canadian Journal of Pediatrics, 2,* 266–269.

Mathias, R. G. (1996). Influenza immunization—Should everyone receive it? *Canadian Journal of Public Health, 87,* 295–296.

Serwint, J. R., Miller, R. M., & Korsch, B. M. (1991). Influenza type A and B infections in hospitalized pediatric patients—Who should be immunized? *American Journal of Diseases of Children, 145,* 623–626.

Szilagyi, P. G., & Rodewald, L. E. (1992). Missed opportunities for influenza vaccination among children with asthma. *Pediatric Infectious Disease Journal, 11,* 705–708.

Measles Virus Vaccine

Measles is an uncomfortable, week-long illness with fever, cough, and rash. Complications include otitis media, pneumonia, and encephalitis (acute and chronic). Mass immunization has eliminated indigenous cycles of transmission in the United States and limited the impact of imported infections to small clusters of cases (Centers for Disease Control and Prevention, 1999). Strenuous efforts are being made to eradicate indigenous measles in all countries of the Americas (de Quadros et al., 1996). Continuation of vaccination efforts is necessary to prevent the reappearance of the disease.

Formulations. Measles virus vaccine is generally used in combination with mumps and rubella vaccines (MMR), but it is available alone for outbreak control campaigns. Such products should be administered only by the subcutaneous route. Measles virus vaccines consist of live, attenuated measles virus grown in tissue culture and extensively purified. In the case of MMR products, measles vaccine virus is grown in chick fibroblast cultures and may contain residual traces of ovalbumenlike protein and neomycin. Gelatin is present as a stabilizer. Measles virus vaccines should be refrigerated and protected from light.

Measles virus vaccine induces an antibody response in 90%–95% of recipients after one dose and in about 98% after a second dose administered at least 4 weeks later. Efficacy is reduced by improper storage and by administration to infants younger than 12 months of age or within 3 months after receiving blood products (up to 10 months after high dose IVIG treatment). Protection after successful vaccination is long-lasting.

Recommended use. Two doses of measles vaccine should be administered (National Advisory Committee . . . , 1996a, American Academy of Pediatrics. . . , 1998). The first dose of measles virus vaccine is recommended for all children at 12 months (Canada) or 15 months (U.S.) of age, or as soon thereafter as possible. A second dose of measles vaccine (i.e., revaccination) is recommended to raise population seropositivity rates as near to 100% as possible, a measure necessitated by the extreme contagiousness of measles infection. The target age for second doses varies from the second year of life to school entry (4–6 years old), depending on the jurisdiction.

Administration of measles virus vaccine within 3 days after exposure to natural measles prevents illness in most (68%) household-exposed susceptible children. Intramuscular human immune globulin (0.25 ml/kg) is preferred for protection of exposed infants younger than 12 months of age. A higher dose (0.5 ml/kg) is recommended for immunocompromised infants.

MMR can be administered concurrently with other childhood vaccines, at separate anatomic sites.

ADRs. Immunization induces a low-grade, noncommunicable infection that is generally asymptomatic. However, 5%–15% of recipients of a first dose will develop a fever, generally beginning the sixth to twelfth day after immunization and lasting for up to 5 days. Children who are predisposed to febrile seizures may experience seizures after measles immunization. A transient rash may occur, but other signs and symptoms are uncommon (Duclos & Ward, 1998). Thrombocytopenia and encephalitis are rare complications, occurring much less often after vaccination than after contracting natural measles. ADRs are much less common after a second measles vaccination and tend to occur only in those not protected by the first dose.

Contraindications. Measles vaccine is contraindicated in infants and children whose immune function is impaired (Centers for Disease Control and Prevention . . . , 1998). HIV-infected children are an exception: vaccination should be administered unless they are severely immunocompromised, as judged by an expert in the care of patients with HIV. Measles vaccine is contraindicated in children who have experienced an anaphylactic reaction or thrombocytopenia following a previous dose or who are allergic to a vaccine component such as gelatin. Children with a history of anaphylactic reaction (hives, swelling of the mouth and throat, difficulty breathing, hypotension) to eggs do not usually react to the small quantity of ovalbumenlike protein in the vaccine. Such children can be vaccinated in the usual fashion (James et al., 1995), but in a setting where an anaphylactic reaction can be appropriately managed. Those at risk should be observed for 30 minutes after vaccination for any sign or symptom of an allergic reaction (National Advisory Committee . . . , 1996b).

Measles vaccine should not be administered during pregnancy.

American Academy of Pediatrics Committee on Infectious Diseases. (1998). Age for routine admin-

istration of the second dose of measles-mumps-rubella vaccine. *Pediatrics, 101,* 129–133.
Centers for Disease Control and Prevention Advisory Committee on Immunization Practices. (1998). Measles, mumps and rubella—Vaccine use and strategies for elimination of measles and rubella and congenital rubella syndrome and control of mumps. *Morbidity and Mortality Weekly Report, 47,* RR–8.
Centers for Disease Control. (1999). Epidemiology of measles—United States, 1998. *Morbidity and Mortality Weekly Report, 48,* 749–753.
de Quadros, C. A., Olivé, J. M., Hersh, B. A., et al. (1996). Measles elimination in the Americas: Evolving strategies. *Journal of the American Medical Association, 275,* 224–229.
Duclos, P., & Ward, B. J. (1998). Measles vaccines—A review of adverse events. *Drug Safety, 1998,* 435–454.
James, J. M., Burks, A. W., Roberson, P. K., et al. (1995). Safe administration of the measles vaccine to children allergic to eggs. *New England Journal of Medicine, 332,* 1262–1266.
National Advisory Committee on Immunization. (1996a). Supplementary statement on measles elimination in Canada. *Canada Communicable Disease Report, 22,* 9–15.
National Advisory Committee on Immunization. (1996b). Supplementary statement on MMR vaccine and anaphylactic hypersensitivity to egg or egg-related antigens. *Canada Communicable Disease Report, 22,* 113–115.

Meningococcal Vaccine

Neisseria meningitidis (meningococcus) is a significant cause of sepsis and meningitis among children and adolescents. Infection can progress rapidly, threatening survival. Cases most often involve infants, adolescents, and young adults. Risk factors for infection in adolescents and young adults include tobacco smoke exposure, bar patronage, and crowded living conditions, such as college dormitories (Harrison et al., 1999). Infecting strains are most often of serogroups B, C, and Y in the United States and Canada.

Formulations. Meningococcal vaccines (Peltola, 1998) contain purified capsular polysaccharides from groups A, C, Y, and W-135. No vaccine is licensed for use against group B strains. Among children (≥2 years of age), A and C polysaccharide vaccines are 80%–90% effective in preventing disease caused by the constituent groups in outbreak settings. A single dose is protective for at least 2 years, but responses wane thereafter, declining faster in children than in adolescents or young adults (King et al., 1996).

Newer vaccines have been developed involving conjugates of group A and C polysaccharides with carrier proteins, such as diphtheria and tetanus toxoids (Peltola, 1998). Formulations with one or both groups are able to elicit antibody responses in young infants, including establishment of immunological memory for durable protection. Universal immunization of children with group C conjugate was implemented in the United Kingdom in 1999 (MacLennan, 2001) and could follow in Canada and the United States. Candidate group B vaccines based on outer membrane proteins are being evaluated.

Recommended use. Starting in the autumn of 1999, U.S. health authorities recommended that students attending colleges and universities, particularly those who will live in dormitories or similar settings, should consider receiving quadrivalent meningococcal polysaccharide vaccine (American Academy . . . , 2000).

Use of meningococcal polysaccharide vaccines is otherwise limited to selected individuals at increased risk of acquiring infection and for control of outbreaks caused by serogroups present in the vaccines. Individuals recommended for vaccination (Centers for Disease Control and Prevention . . . , 1997) include children 2 years of age or older with functional or anatomic asplenia (who have increased risk of fulminant meningococcal infection) and children 2 years of age or older traveling to a country in which there is a high incidence of meningococcal disease.

A single dose of polysaccharide vaccine is administered to children 2 years or older. The vaccine is injected subcutaneously or intramuscularly. Repeat doses may be needed for those children who are at continuing risk.

ADRs. Local redness, swelling, and pain occur frequently but these reactions are not severe and usually resolve within a few days

(Scheifele et al., 1994). Systemic ADRs are uncommon, consisting mainly of low-grade fever (Yergeau et al., 1996).

Contraindications. Repeat vaccination is contraindicated following an anaphylactic reaction to a previous dose. Pregnancy is not a contraindication to vaccination.

American Academy of Pediatrics Committee on Infectious Diseases. (2000). Meningococcal disease prevention and control strategies for practice-based physicians (Addendum: Recommendations for college students). *Pediatrics, 106,* 1500–1504.

Centers for Disease Control and Prevention Advisory Committee on Immunization Practices. (1997). Control and prevention of meningococcal disease. *Morbidity and Mortality Weekly Report, 46,* RR–5.

Harrison, L. H., Dwyer, D. M., Maples, C. T., et al. (1999). Risk of meningococcal infection in college students. *Journal of the American Medical Association, 281,* 1906–1910.

King, W. J., MacDonald, N. E., Wells, G., et al. (1996). Total and functional antibody response to a quadrivalent meningococcal polysaccharide vaccine among children. *The Journal of Pediatrics, 128,* 196–202.

MacLennan, J. (2001). Meningococcal group C conjugate vaccines. *Archives of Disease in Childhood, 84,* 383–386.

Peltola, H. (1998). Meningococcal vaccines–Current status and future possibilities. *Drugs, 55,* 347–366.

Scheifele, D. W., Bjornson, G., & Boraston, S. (1994). Local adverse effects of meningococcal vaccine. *Canadian Medical Association Journal, 150,* 14–15.

Yergeau, A., Alain, L., Pless, R., et al. (1996). Adverse events temporally associated with meningococcal vaccines. *Canadian Medical Association Journal, 154,* 503–507.

Mumps Virus Vaccine

Mumps is a highly communicable disease that is generally mild, but that can lead to complications such as meningoencephalitis, deafness, orchitis, and oophritis. Extensive vaccination programs using measles-mumps-rubella (MMR) vaccine have reduced mumps incidence to very low levels in the United States (Van Loon et al., 1995) and Canada.

Formulations. Mumps virus vaccine contains live, attenuated virus grown in chick fibroblast cultures. It is supplied alone or in combination with measles and rubella vaccines. Mumps vaccine is safe and highly effective (Centers for Disease Control and Prevention . . . , 1998). A single dose produces an antibody response in more than 95% of susceptible children. Antibody responses persist for at least 20 years; booster doses are not required. Use of mumps vaccine is most cost-effective when a combined MMR product is used.

Recommended use. Mumps virus vaccine is recommended for all susceptible children 12 months (Canada) or 15 months (U.S.) of age or older. The subcutaneous route of administration is usual. Mumps vaccine should usually be administered in combination with measles and rubella vaccines.

Mumps vaccination administered after exposure to mumps virus may not prevent the disease but is not harmful.

ADRs. ADRs after mumps vaccination are rare. Viral meningitis without sequelae and parotitis have been reported.

Contraindications. Mumps virus vaccine (and other live vaccines) should not be administered to children who have impaired immunity. An exception is children with HIV infection, who should receive MMR vaccine unless they are severely immunocompromised (as judged by an expert in the care of patients with HIV).

Children with a severe hypersensitivity to neomycin or who developed anaphylaxis after a previous dose of MMR vaccine should not be administered mumps or MMR vaccine.

Children with a history of anaphylactic reaction to eggs do not usually react to the small quantity of ovalbumenlike protein in the vaccine. Such children can be vaccinated in the usual fashion (James et al., 1995) but in a setting where an anaphylactic reaction can be managed properly. Those children who are determined to be at risk should be observed for 30 minutes after vaccination for any sign or symptom of an allergic reaction.

Mumps virus vaccine should not be administered during pregnancy.

Centers for Disease Control and Prevention Advisory Committee on Immunization Practices.

(1998). Measles, mumps, rubella—Vaccine use and strategies for elimination of measles, rubella and congenital rubella syndrome and control of mumps. *Morbidity and Mortality Weekly Report, 47,* RR–8.

James, J. M., Burks, A. W., Roberson, P. K., et al. (1995). Safe administration of the measles vaccine to children allergic to eggs. *New England Journal of Medicine, 332,* 1262–1266.

Van Loon, F. P. L., Holmes, S. J., Sirotkin, B. I., et al. (1995). Mumps surveillance–United States, 1988–1993. *Morbidity and Mortality Weekly Report, 44,* SS-3, 1–14.

Passive Immunization

Immune globulin. Immune globulin (IG) is prepared from large pools of plasma of healthy, screened donors and contains immunoglobulin (IgG) antibodies specific for a wide variety of pathogens. Preparations of IG can be used to prevent or modify the course of certain infections when administered prior to exposure or shortly afterward.

While hepatitis A vaccination is preferred for pre-exposure prophylaxis, IG can be used instead for children too young to vaccinate or whose immune response is unreliable. A dose of IG of 0.02 ml/kg will prevent HAV infection for up to 3 months. A similar dose administered within 2 weeks of exposure (preferably within 72 hours) to hepatitis A usually prevents or modifies the course of the illness.

Susceptible children exposed to measles are usually best protected by immediate immunization with measles (MMR) vaccine. However, in situations where vaccine use is not desirable (e.g., infants younger than 1 year of age and immunocompromised children), IG should be administered. The IG dosage is 0.25 ml/kg for normal children and 0.5 ml/kg for immunocompromised children, to a maximum dose of 15 ml.

Hyperimmune globulins. Hyperimmune globulin formulations have much higher antibody titers against specific pathogens than IG because they are prepared from plasma from specifically immunized donors or from selected plasma units with high titers. Such formulations are generally used for postexposure prophylaxis of potentially serious infections.

Varicella-zoster immune globulin human. Varicella-zoster immune globulin human (VZIG) administered within 4 days after exposure can prevent or modify the course of varicella in susceptible children at risk for serious, disseminated illness. Candidates include immunocompromised children and neonates born to mothers who developed varicella within 5 days before or 2 days after delivery. The recommended dosage of VZIG is one vial (125 units) per 10 kg of body weight (rounded up to the nearest 10 kg) administered intramuscularly. The incubation period for varicella can be prolonged to 28 days in children who receive VZIG.

Hepatitis B immune globulin human. Hepatitis B immune globulin human (HBIG) is used for postexposure prophylaxis of susceptible individuals, typically infants born to HBsAg-positive mothers and children injured with discarded hypodermic needles. The dose for neonates is 0.5 ml and for children it is 0.06 ml/kg. HBIG is injected intramuscularly. Children administered HBIG should be started on a course of HBV vaccinations at the same time, using a separate anatomic site.

Rabies immune globulin human. Rabies immune globulin (RIG) is used in combination with rabies vaccine to provide protection between the time of injury (bite) and the onset of active antibody production. The recommended RIG dose is 20 IU/kg. Approximately one-half of the RIG dose is infiltrated around the wound; the other half is administered intramuscularly. There are no known contraindications to RIG use.

Tetanus immune globulin human. Tetanus immune globulin human (TIG) is used for postinjury prophylaxis for tetanus-prone wounds in patients who have not been fully immunized with tetanus toxoid (if two or fewer doses were administered). The recommended TIG dose is 250 units intramuscularly. Tetanus active immunization should be initiated concurrently. TIG and tetanus toxoid should be injected at separate anatomic injection sites.

ADRs. The main problems with the use of IG and hyperimmune globulins are limited supply, high cost, and pain on injection. Thus, they should be used only when clearly indicated. Serious ADRs are uncommon, but anaphylaxis has been reported. Despite the extensive screening currently applied to blood products, the absence of transmissible pathogens (e.g., HIV) cannot be guaranteed.

Pertussis Vaccine

Pertussis (whooping cough) is a highly communicable bacterial disease caused by *Bordetella pertussis*. It is characterized by a prolonged course and severe coughing spells. Major complications include bronchopneumonia, airway obstruction, and encephalopathy. Protective measures should be initiated as early in life as possible because the severity of and fatality from the disease are greatest during infancy. Many infants are highly susceptible to infection because their mothers lack sufficient immunity.

A vaccine containing killed, whole pertussis organisms of common serotypes was widely used in Canada and the United States during the past 50 years, and the incidence of, and mortality from, pertussis have declined remarkably (National Advisory Committee . . . , 1998). However, whole cell vaccines were moderately reactogenic, causing injection site pain and temperature elevation greater than 38°C in about 50% of infants (Cody et al., 1981). Acellular pertussis vaccines were more recently introduced and are preferred over whole cell vaccines (American Academy of Pediatrics . . . , 1997) because of their greatly improved safety profile (Edwards & Decker, 1996) and demonstrated protective efficacy (Cherry, 1997). Whole cell vaccines continue to be used in countries unable to afford the higher cost of acellular pertussis vaccines.

Formulations. Acellular pertussis (aP) vaccines contain one or more purified components derived from *B. pertussis*. All formulations contain detoxified pertussis toxin (PT) and some contain up to four additional components including filamentous hemagglutinin (FHA), pertactin (69 kD outer membrane protein), and fimbrial proteins. When directly compared, formulations with three to five antigens were more efficacious than those with two antigens (Cherry, 1997). Components are adsorbed on aluminum salts. Acellular pertussis vaccine is usually administered in combination with other immunizing drugs, such as diphtheria and tetanus toxoids (DTaP). In Canada, a combined vaccine containing DTaP-IPV and HbCV is widely used. The ideal formulation for infants would also include hepatitis B vaccine.

Recommended use. Primary immunization consists of four doses of the vaccine, usually administered as a combined preparation (e.g., DTaP-Polio). The first three doses are administered at intervals of 8 weeks beginning at 2 months of age, and a fourth dose is administered 1 year after the third dose. The fourth dose can be administered at 15–18 months of age, concurrently with MMR, IPV, and HbCV. A booster dose is administered to children 4–6 years of age (at or before school entry) (Centers for Disease Control and Prevention . . . , 2000). Because protection wanes in late adolescence, products are currently being introduced for booster immunization of adolescents and young adults, using a combination of Td and aP vaccines. This option did not exist with whole cell pertussis vaccines because of excessive reactogenicity in persons older than 7 years, but aP vaccines are well tolerated by this age group (Keitel et al., 1999).

Monovalent aP vaccine is available for "catch-up" immunization of children who require only a pertussis vaccine.

The manufacturer's recommendations for dosage and route of administration should be followed. Adsorbed preparations such as DTP or DTaP are administered intramuscularly. Routine use of acetaminophen (15 mg/kg/dose) at the time of immunization and 4 and 8 hours afterward to reduce the incidence of febrile reactions is no longer necessary when acellular pertussis-based vaccines are used, but this practice may still be of benefit for infants and children at increased risk of febrile seizures or with low pain tolerance.

ADRs. Acellular pertussis-containing vaccines (DTaP) are generally no more reactogenic

TABLE 9-4
Adverse Drug Reactions Associated with Pertussis Vaccines[a]

ADVERSE REACTION	PERCENTAGE REPORTING WITHIN 72 HOURS OF AN INFANT VACCINATION			
	DT	DTaP1	DTaP2	DTP
Tenderness	22.2	21.8	22.2	80.5
Erythema ≥ 2 cm	3.5	3.1	4.8	14.6
Fever ≥ 38°C	34.8	35.2	36.9	90.4
Fever ≥ 40°C	0.09	0.05	0.03	0.5
Persistent crying				
≥ 1 hr	4.9	5.4	4.9	20.1
≥ 3 hr	0.01	0.03	0.05	3.4
Convulsions	0.03	0.03	0.00	0.02
Hypotonic–hyporesponsive episode	0.00	0.00	0.01	0.08

[a] Modified from National Advisory Committee . . . , 1998.

than DT toxoids alone and are considerably less reactogenic than DTP vaccines (Table 9-4). The improvements in DTaP over DTP vaccines include lower rates of both commonly occurring ADRs (e.g., fever and injection site pain) and of less commonly occurring ADRs (e.g., persistent crying and hypotonic–hyporesponsive episodes). Although injection site reactions are infrequent and mild after primary doses, they increase in frequency and severity after booster doses. Among children receiving a fifth consecutive dose of DTaP at 4–6 years of age, over half developed injection site swelling and redness; however, few were reportedly distressed by these ADRs (Halperin et al., 1999). The immunologic basis of such reactions remains undefined. Td.aP or aP vaccine alone has been well tolerated by adolescents and adults (Keitel et al., 1999).

Contraindications. Pertussis vaccine should not be administered to pediatric patients who have had an anaphylactic reaction to a previous dose or to any constituent of the vaccine.

Certain other events temporally associated with whole-cell pertussis vaccination were once considered contraindications to further pertussis immunization, but **with use of acellular pertussis vaccine they are no longer considered contraindications** (National Advisory Committee . . . , 1998). These events include the following:

- High fever within 48 hours after vaccination not attributable to intercurrent illness is not a contraindication. Fever may recur in such infants with subsequent doses, but the risk is reducible with acetaminophen prophylaxis.
- Febrile convulsion is more likely in children who experience postvaccination fever but there are no sequelae, permitting vaccination to continue with the described precautions.
- Afebrile convulsions have not been shown to be caused by pertussis vaccine and are not a contraindication to pertussis vaccination.
- Persistent, inconsolable crying and high-pitched crying after pertussis vaccination are not associated with any sequelae and are likely responses to pain at the injection site. These reactions do not preclude further pertussis vaccination. Acetaminophen prophylaxis may reduce discomfort with subsequent doses.
- Hypotonic–hyporesponsive episodes are not a contraindication to the use of acellular pertussis vaccine. These episodes occur with similar frequency after DTaP and DT vaccines, making it difficult to attribute causation in recipients of DTaP to the pertussis component. Continued immunization with all antigens is recommended.
- Onset of encephalopathy temporally related to pertussis vaccination does not indicate that the vaccine was the cause. Encephalopathy from whatever cause is

not a contraindication to pertussis vaccination.

- Deferral of pertussis immunization for children with evolving neurologic conditions is no longer necessary because the incidence of ADRs is no greater with DTaP than with DT vaccines. Modern methods of diagnosis and treatment of neurologic conditions leave little room for natural disease progressions to be misinterpreted as immunization-related events.

American Academy of Pediatrics Committee on Infectious Diseases. (1997). Acellular pertussis vaccine: Recommendations for use as the initial series in infants and children. *Pediatrics, 99,* 282–288.

Centers for Disease Control and Prevention Advisory Committee on Immunization Practices. (2000). Use of diphtheria toxoid-tetanus toxoid-acellular pertussis vaccine in a five-dose series. *Morbidity and Mortality Weekly Report, 44,* RR–13.

Cherry, J. D. (1997). Comparative efficacy of acellular pertussis vaccines: An analysis of recent trials. *Pediatric Infectious Disease Journal, 16,* S90–S96.

Cody, C. L., Baraff, L. J., Cherry, J. D., et al. (1981). Nature and rates of adverse reactions associated with DTP and DT immunizations in infants and children. *Pediatrics, 68,* 650–660.

Edwards, K. M., & Decker, M. D. (1996). Acellular pertussis vaccines for infants. *New England Journal of Medicine, 334,* 391–392.

Halperin, S. A., Scheifele, D. W., Barreto, L., et al. (1999). Comparison of a fifth dose of a five-component acellular or whole cell pertussis vaccine in children four to six years of age. *Pediatric Infectious Disease Journal, 18,* 772–779.

Keitel, W. A., Muenz, L. R., Decker, M. D., et al. (1999). A randomized clinical trial of acellular pertussis vaccines in healthy adults: Dose-response comparisons of 5 vaccines and implications for booster immunization. *Journal of Infectious Diseases, 180,* 397–403.

National Advisory Committee on Immunization. (1998). *Canadian immunization guide,* 5th ed., pp. 133–139. Ottawa, ON: Health Canada.

Pneumococcal Vaccine

Streptococcus pneumoniae (pneumococcus) is a leading cause of otitis media, pneumonia, bacteremia, and meningitis among children (Kaplan et al., 1998). Serious pneumococcal infections are more common in children with splenic dysfunction, sickle cell anemia (Wong et al., 1992), or immunosuppression (including HIV infection). Resistance to penicillin and other commonly used antibiotics is rapidly increasing in frequency, complicating the selection of drugs for empiric therapy (McCracken, 1995). Of the 90 known pneumococcal serotypes, fewer than a dozen account for the majority of infections in children.

Formulations. Two types of pneumococcal vaccine are currently available. One type contains purified capsilar polysaccharides from the 23 types of *S. pneumoniae* most often associated with infection in children and adults. A 0.5-ml dose of vaccine contains 25 µg of each polysaccharide antigen. Pneumococcal polysaccharide vaccine is **not** recommended for use among children who are younger than 2 years because they tend to respond poorly. Antibody responses to this vaccine among young children also are frequently incomplete or weak. At all ages, antibody responses are short-lived because the polysaccharide antigens do not induce immunologic memory.

A newer type of vaccine contains seven or more capsular polysaccharides that are conjugated to carrier proteins such as diphtheria or tetanus toxoids (Eskola & Anttila, 1999). Conjugate vaccines are able to induce antibody responses in infants by using a series of doses, which are typically administered at 2, 4, and 6 months of age. These vaccines also induce immunologic memory for durable protection. A high rate of protection has been demonstrated against invasive infection caused by pneumococcal serotypes included in the vaccine (Black et al., 2000). In both Canada and the United States, the seven serotypes in the currently available vaccine account for more than 80% of invasive infections (Scheifele et al., 2000). Vaccination can also reduce the risk for the development of pneumonia and otitis media; however, the reported risk reduction is small for otitis media (Eskola et al., 2001).

Recommended use. In the United States, conjugate pneumococcal vaccine is recommended for all infants starting at 2 months of age. Conjugate pneumococcal vaccine can be administered concurrently with other infant vaccinations, using separate anatomic injection sites. The recommended dosing schedule is 2, 4, and 6 months of age, with a booster dose to be administered at 12–15 months of age. Catch-up vaccination is recommended for all children 23 months of age or younger. Fewer doses are required for children immunized at 7 months of age or later (Centers for Disease Control and Prevention . . . , 2000). Conjugate pneumococcal vaccine also is recommended for children 24–59 months of age with certain chronic conditions (Centers for Disease Control and Prevention . . . , 2000) and also should be considered for those with other risk factors for pneumococcal disease such as attendance at group day-care centers. Children 4 months of age and older with chronic conditions should be administered two doses of the conjugate pneumococcal vaccine 2 months apart; those in good health require only one dose. Conjugate pneumococcal vaccine is not recommended for children 5 years of age or older because the proportion of invasive pneumococcal infections covered by the seven-valent vaccine is only 50%–60% among older children and adolescents.

The pneumococcal polysaccharide vaccine is recommended only for children 5 years of age or older and adolescents who are at a high risk for invasive pneumococcal infection because of an underlying medical condition, such as asplenia. If such patients have previously been administered a course of pneumococcal conjugate vaccine *prior* to 2 years of age, then a subsequent dose of the pneumococcal polysaccharide vaccine is recommended to broaden serotype coverage (Centers for Disease Control and Prevention . . . , 2000).

Serious pneumococcal infections can occur in children despite having received pneumococcal vaccination because of incomplete serotype coverage, even with the 23-valent polysaccharide pneumococcal vaccine.

ADRs. ADRs after immunization with pneumococcal vaccine generally are mild and include pain and erythema at the injection site and transient low-grade fever. Allergic reactions are rare.

Contraindications. Anaphylactic reaction to pneumococcal vaccine is a contraindication to revaccination.

Black, S., Shinefield, H., Fireman, B., et al. (2000). Efficacy, safety and immunogenicity of heptavalent pneumococcal conjugate vaccine in children. *Pediatric Infectious Disease Journal, 19,* 187–195.

Centers for Disease Control and Prevention Advisory Committee on Immunization Practices. (2000). Prevention of pneumococcal disease among infants and young children. *Morbidity and Mortality Weekly Report, 49,* RR–9.

Eskola, J., & Anttila, M. (1999). Pneumococcal conjugate vaccines. *Pediatric Infectious Diseases Journal, 18,* 543–551.

Eskola, J., Kilpi, T., Palmu, A., et al. (2001). Efficacy of a pneumococcal conjugate vaccine against acute otitis media. *New England Journal of Medicine, 344,* 403–409.

Kaplan, S. L., Mason, E. O., Barson, W. J., et al. (1998). Three-year multicenter surveillance of systemic pneumococcal infections in children. *Pediatrics, 102,* 538–545.

McCracken, G. H. (1995). Emergence of resistant Streptococcus pneumoniae: A problem in pediatrics. *Pediatric Infectious Diseases Journal, 14,* 424–428.

Scheifele, D., Halperin, S., Pelletier, L., et al. (2000). Invasive pneumococcal infections in Canadian children, 1991–1998: Implications for new vaccination strategies. *Clinical Infectious Diseases, 31,* 58–64.

Wong, W. Y., Overturf, G. D., & Powars, D. R. (1992). Infection caused by Streptococcus pneumoniae in children with sickle cell disease: Epidemiology, immunologic mechanisms, prophylaxis and vaccination. *Clinical Infectious Diseases, 14,* 1124–1136.

Poliomyelitis Vaccines

Paralytic poliomyelitis was eliminated from North and South America in 1991 as a result of childhood immunization programs (Centers for Disease Control and Prevention, 1994). The World Health Organization expects that global disease eradication can be achieved within a few years. Concerted efforts are being made to stamp out infection in the remaining hotspots in Africa and Asia, but, until complete success is achieved and verified, all countries need to maintain their polio immunization programs.

Formulations. Two types of poliovirus vaccine are available: the live, oral poliovirus vaccine (OPV) and the enhanced potency inactivated poliomyelitis vaccine (IPV). Both contain polioviruses of types 1, 2, and 3. OPV is ideally suited for mass campaigns in endemic areas. IPV is preferred for use in polio-free areas (Katz, 1996; National Advisory Committee . . . , 1998) because it avoids the rare occurrence of vaccine-induced paralytic disease.

IPV contains polioviruses grown in tissue culture cells and subsequently inactivated with formalin. Modern culture techniques have resulted in products with enhanced potency compared with earlier formulations. IPV is available alone or in combination with diphtheria and tetanus toxoids and pertussis vaccines (e.g., DTaP-IPV, Td.IPV). When used as recommended by the manufacturer, IPV produces immunity to all three polioviruses in more than 90% of recipients after two doses and in nearly 100% after three doses (Vidor et al., 1997). IPV induces secretion of limited amounts of mucosal antibodies in the throat and GI tract and may not block intestinal replication of wild polioviruses. Formulations may contain trace amounts of streptomycin, polymyxin B, or neomycin. IPV-containing products do not contain a thimerosal preservative.

OPV contains attenuated strains of poliovirus grown in tissue cultures. The immune response after OPV administration resembles that induced by natural infection, including the development of secretory antibodies within the GI tract. These antibodies are believed to prevent intestinal infection with wild polioviruses, preventing subsequent dissemination to susceptible people in the community. Fecal excretion of poliovirus occurs after OPV administration and may lead to infection of close contacts. Such indirect "immunization" generally is beneficial but, in rare instances, paralytic disease can occur (Strebel et al., 1992).

Recommended use. Immunization against poliomyelitis is recommended for all children beginning in early infancy. Both OPV and IPV are highly effective. Exclusive use of IPV is recommended in the United States and Canada to avoid rare instances of OPV-associated paralysis. Children who began immunization with OPV may switch to IPV without alteration of the series.

A primary immunization course of IPV consists of three injections (typically at 2, 4, and 6–18 months of age). When combined vaccines are used (e.g., DTaP-IPV), an extra dose of IPV can be administered for convenience at 6 or 18 months, without increasing ADRs. A booster dose is administered at or before school entry (4–6 years of age). The need for a booster dose in adolescence (at 14–16 years of age) is uncertain with enhanced potency vaccines.

ADRs. ADRs associated with IPV (Vidor et al., 1997) generally are limited to minor local reactions, although anaphylactic reactions occur rarely. IPV does not add measurably to the reactogenicity of combination vaccines that contain it.

OPV has rarely been associated with paralytic disease (at a rate of approximately one case per 8 million doses distributed in the U.S.) (Strebel et al., 1992). Paralysis is more likely in immunodeficient patients and non-immunized adult contacts of vaccine recipients. Paralysis results from mutations of the vaccine virus toward greater neurovirulence as it replicates in the GI tract.

Contraindications. IPV should not be administered to pediatric patients who have experienced an anaphylactic reaction to a previous dose of IPV, streptomycin, polymyxin B, or neomycin.

IPV can be administered without risk to those with impaired immunity or who will have close contact with such persons. Suboptimal protection may be induced in those who are immunocompromised.

Centers for Disease Control and Prevention Advisory Committee on Immunization Practices. (1994). Certification of poliomyelitis eradication—the Americas, 1994. *Morbidity and Mortality Weekly Report, 43,* 720–722.

Katz, S. L. (1996). Poliovaccine policy–time for a change. *Pediatrics, 98,* 116–117.

National Advisory Committee on Immunization. (1998). *Canadian immunization guide,* 5th ed., pp. 144–148. Ottawa, ON: Health Canada.

Strebel, P. M., Sutter, R. W., Cochi, S. L., et al. (1992). Epidemiology of poliomyelitis in the United States one decade after the last reported case of indigenous wild virus-associated disease. *Clinical Infectious Diseases, 14,* 568–579.

Vidor, E., Meschevitz, C., & Plotkin, S. (1997). Fifteen years of experience with vero-produced enhanced potency inactivated poliovirus vaccine. *Pediatric Infectious Disease Journal, 16,* 312–322.

Rotavirus Vaccine

Rotaviruses are the leading cause of viral gastroenteritis in infants. Nearly every child has one or more such infections by 2 years of age. A significant proportion of cases require medical attention and 1%–2% require hospital admission (Glass et al., 1996).

In 1998, a rotavirus vaccine was licensed in the United States for routine use in infants (Centers for Disease Control and Prevention, 1999). The vaccine contained live, attenuated (rhesus reassortant) rotaviruses and was administered orally, at 2, 4, and 6 months of age. In the spring of 1999, the use of this vaccine was halted when surveillance data indicated a significant risk of intussusception following vaccination (Centers for Disease Control and Prevention . . . , 1999).

Centers for Disease Control and Prevention Advisory Committee on Immunization Practices. (1999). Rotavirus vaccine for the prevention of rotavirus gastroenteritis among children. *Morbidity and Mortality Weekly Report, 48,* RR-2.

Centers for Disease Control and Prevention. (1999). Intussusception among recipients of rotavirus vaccine–United States, 1998–1999. *Morbidity and Mortality Weekly Report, 48,* 577–581.

Glass, R. I., Kilgore, P. E., Holman, R. C., et al. (1996). The epidemiology of rotavirus diarrhea in the United States: Surveillance and estimates of disease burden. *Journal of Infectious Diseases, 174*(Suppl), S5–S11.

Rubella Virus Vaccine

The major objective of immunization with the rubella virus vaccine is the prevention of rubella infection during pregnancy and of congenital rubella syndrome (CRS) (Grabenstein, 1991). Infection of a fetus by rubella virus from the mother during early pregnancy can cause severe congenital malformations, including bony changes, cardiovascular defects, cataracts, deafness, encephalomyelitis, microcephaly, and thrombocytopenia. In Canada and the United States, efforts have been directed at immunizing infants, adolescent girls, and susceptible postpartum women. CRS incidence has been markedly reduced (Centers for Disease Control and Prevention . . . , 2001).

Formulations. Rubella virus vaccines contain live, attenuated rubella virus (e.g., strain RA27/3) grown in human diploid cell cultures. The vaccine is administered as a subcutaneous injection. Antibody production is induced in more than 97% of vaccine recipients. Long-term immunity is evident, extending more than 20 years (Bottiger & Forsgren, 1997). Rubella vaccine virus is available alone or in combination with measles and mumps vaccines (i.e., MMR vaccine).

Recommended use. Rubella virus vaccine (as MMR) should be administered to all children at 12 months (Canada) or 15 months (U.S.) of age or as soon thereafter as possible. Second doses of MMR are recommended, at least 4 weeks after the first dose. Rubella vaccine is best tolerated prior to puberty. Rubella vaccine also should be administered to all adolescent girls who were not vaccinated as children. A documented history of vaccination is presumptive evidence of immunity. Rubella or MMR vaccines can be administered concurrently with other routinely used vaccines, at separate anatomic injection sites. As with other live virus vaccines, rubella vaccine should not be administered before 12 months of age or within 3 months after receiving blood products (10 months after high-dose IVIG).

ADRs. Serious ADRs to rubella vaccine are uncommon. Rash, fever, lymphadenopathy, and joint pain are uncommon in children; they are more common in postpubertal girls and occur in a pattern similar to natural rubella infection. Joint involvement usually begins 7–21 days after immunization as arthralgia or, less frequently, arthritis, which is usually transient (Tingle et al., 1997). Such signs and symptoms occur much less frequently after vaccination than after natural rubella infection.

Contraindications. Rubella virus vaccine is contraindicated during pregnancy. It should not be administered to immunocompromised children (with the exception of children with

HIV infection associated with nonsevere immunocompromise) or to those known to be hypersensitive to a component of the vaccine (e.g., gelatin, neomycin). Vaccine-induced rubella infection is not communicable to close contacts, including pregnant women. Postpartum immunization of mothers who are breast feeding can result in transmission of vaccine virus to infants in the breast milk, but this transmission has not been associated with any apparent untoward effects.

Bottiger, M., & Forsgren, M. (1997). Twenty years' experience of rubella vaccination in Sweden: 10 years of selective vaccination (of 12-year-old girls and women postpartum) and 13 years of a general two-dose vaccination. *Vaccine, 15,* 1538–1544.

Centers for Disease Control and Prevention Advisory Committee on Immunization Practices. (2001). Control and prevention of rubella: Evaluation and management of suspected outbreaks, rubella in pregnant women and surveillance for congenital rubella syndrome. *Morbidity and Mortality Weekly Report, 50,* RR–12.

Grabenstein, J. D. (1991). Preventing rubella and congenital rubella syndrome. *Hospital Pharmacy, 26,* 553–558.

Tingle, A. J., Mitchell, L. A., Grace, M., et al. (1997). Randomized double-blind placebo-controlled study on adverse effects of rubella immunization in seronegative women. *The Lancet, 349,* 1277–1281.

Tetanus Toxoid

Tetanus is an often fatal disease (Weinstein, 1973) caused by a neurotoxin produced by *Clostridium tetani,* an organism ubiquitous in soil. Immunization is highly effective, provides long-lasting protection, and is recommended for all infants, children, and adolescents.

Formulations. Tetanus toxoid is a cell-free preparation of the neurotoxin that is neutralized with formaldehyde. Most tetanus toxoids are adsorbed onto aluminum salts because such formulations induce higher antitoxin titers and more durable protection (Centers for Disease Control and Prevention . . . , 2000). Tetanus toxoid is available alone and in combination with diphtheria toxoid and pertussis and inactivated poliomyelitis vaccines. All formulations contain comparable amounts of tetanus toxoid.

Recommended use. Routine immunization against tetanus is recommended for all infants and children (Centers for Disease Control and Prevention . . . , 2000). Products in which tetanus toxoid is combined with diphtheria toxoid and pertussis vaccine (DTP or DTaP) are preferred for primary immunization of infants and children younger than 7 years of age. The primary immunizing course of tetanus toxoid consists of four doses, ideally begun at 2 months of age (Table 9-1). The intervals between the first three doses are preferably 8 weeks; the fourth dose is administered 1 year after the third dose. The fourth dose can be administered at 15 months of age concurrently with MMR, IPV, and HbCV. A booster dose should be administered at 4–6 years of age (at or before school entry). Additional doses of tetanus toxoid are recommended at 10-year intervals, preferably using the "adult" (Td) vaccine.

Active immunization should be carried out during convalescence from tetanus because the disease often does not confer immunity.

Adsorbed vaccines such as tetanus toxoid must be injected intramuscularly. Freezing should be avoided during shipping and storage. Follow the manufacturer's recommendations in the product labeling.

Tetanus prophylaxis in wound management. Table 9-5 summarizes the recommended use of tetanus toxoid and tetanus immune globulin (TIG) in wound management. It is important to determine the number of doses of tetanus toxoid previously administered and the time elapsed since the last dose was administered. When a tetanus toxoid booster is required, the opportunity should be taken to administer other needed boosters using a combination vaccine (Td or DTP as appropriate).

ADRs. Serious ADRs to primary immunization with tetanus toxoid are rare (Cody et al., 1981). Local erythema and swelling are common after booster doses (Scheifele et al., 1998). Severe local reactions are often associated with high concentrations of circulating antitoxin (Levine & Edsall, 1981) and may be the result of frequent dosing of tetanus toxoid. Systemic reactions are uncommon.

TABLE 9-5
Guide to Tetanus Prophylaxis in Wound Management
(Centers for Disease Control and Prevention, 1991)

HISTORY OF TETANUS IMMUNIZATION	CLEAN, MINOR WOUNDS		ALL OTHER WOUNDS	
	Td[a]	TIG[b]	Td[a]	TIG[b]
Uncertain or less than three doses	Yes	No	Yes	Yes
Three or more doses	No[c]	No	No[d]	No

[a] Adult tetanus toxoid (full dose) and diphtheria toxoid (reduced dose) in combination.
[b] Tetanus immune globulin human.
[c] Unless more than 10 years have elapsed since the last tetanus toxoid dose.
[d] Unless more than 5 years have elapsed since the last tetanus toxoid dose.

Contraindications. Routine "adult" booster doses should not be administered more frequently than at 10-year intervals (Levine & Edsall, 1981; White et al., 1969). If a dose is administered more frequently, tetanus toxoid can cause severe local and systemic reactions. Tetanus toxoid should not be administered if a severe systemic reaction occurred after a previous dose. Before administering a combined vaccine, it is important to ensure that there are no contraindications (e.g., hypersensitivity) to the administration of any of the components.

Centers for Disease Control and Prevention Advisory Committee on Immunization Practices. (2000). Use of diphtheria toxoid-tetanus toxoid-acellular pertussis vaccine as a five-dose series. *Morbidity and Mortality Weekly Report, 49,* RR-13.
Cody, C., Baraff, L. J., Cherry, J. D., et al. (1981). Nature and rates of adverse reactions associated with DTP and DT immunizations in infants and children. *Pediatrics, 68,* 650–660.
Levine, L., & Edsall, G. (1981). Tetanus toxoid: What determines reaction proneness? *Journal of Infectious Diseases, 144,* 376–377.
Scheifele, D. W., Dobson, S., Kallos, A., et al. (1998). Comparative safety of tetanus-diphtheria toxoids booster immunization in students in grades 6 and 9. *Pediatric Infectious Diseases Journal, 17,* 1121–1126.
Weinstein, L. (1973). Tetanus. *New England Journal of Medicine, 289,* 1293–1296.
White, E. G., Barnes, G. M., Griffith, A. H., et al. (1969). Duration of immunity after active immunization against tetanus. *The Lancet, 2,* 95–96.

Varicella-Zoster Virus Vaccine

Varicella (chickenpox) affects almost all children in the absence of control measures (Arvin, 1996). Most recover uneventfully from the fever and rash, although recovery may take a week or more. Complications include scarring, skin infection, febrile convulsions, pneumonitis, hepatitis, and encephalitis. Zoster (shingles) is a delayed complication (painful neuritis and localized rash) that occurs in 15%–20% of patients after an extended latent period. Infection during early pregnancy can result in fetal malformations.

Varicella-zoster virus (VZV) vaccines are available to prevent chickenpox.

Formulations. Available vaccines contain live, attenuated VZV (Oka strain), prepared in human fibroblast cultures and stabilized with gelatin. Vaccines may contain trace amounts of neomycin.

Recommended use. Universal childhood vaccination against VZV is advocated in the United States (Centers for Disease Control and Prevention . . . , 1996, 1999) and Canada (National Advisory Committee . . . , 1999), but programs have not been fully implemented. Not all pediatric clinicians are convinced of the need to prevent VZV infections (Newman & Taylor, 1998). Cost is a deterrent to others. A high level of uptake may not be achievable without an MMR-VZV combination vaccine.

VZV vaccine is recommended to be administered just after the first birthday. Earlier administration is not recommended because maternally derived antibodies may interfere with the response. A single dose of vaccine is sufficient and is administered subcutaneously. Susceptible children (defined by a negative history of VZV infection) of any age are also candidates for vaccination. Susceptible adolescents are particularly likely to benefit from vaccination because VZV infection is more severe at this age. However, adolescents require two doses of VZV vaccine, spaced 4 weeks or more apart.

Varicella vaccine is effective in preventing illness or reducing its severity if administered within 3 days (and possibly within 5 days) of exposure (Centers for Disease Control and Prevention . . . , 1999).

Available vaccines are about 95% effective in preventing severe varicella during the first 7–10 years after administration (Centers for Disease Control and Prevention . . . , 1996). Breakthrough infections occur in 1%–2% of vaccinated children annually and are generally mild, limited to a few dozen lesions (Johnson et al., 1997). Booster doses are not recommended. Duration of protection is not known, but it extends for at least 15 years.

ADRs. VZV vaccine is generally well tolerated in healthy children. ADRs occur infrequently and are usually mild and transient. Redness and pain occur at the injection site in about 20% of recipients. Up to 4% of vaccinated children develop a few skin lesions 5–26 days after vaccination, consisting of erythematous maculopapules or vesicles. Vesicles may be limited to the injection site. Vaccine strain virus has been detected in vesicular lesions, indicating the possibility of transmission to susceptible contacts, although this has rarely been documented from vaccinated healthy children. Transmission has not been documented in the absence of rash.

VZV vaccine administered to immunocompromised children can result in extensive skin lesions resembling varicella with an increased likelihood of transmission to susceptible contacts (La Russa et al., 1996). However, contact cases with normal immune systems had mild infection, in keeping with the attenuated nature of the vaccine virus.

Recipients of VZV vaccine may subsequently develop zoster (shingles). The rate at which this occurs is lower than after natural infection and the illness is milder, with fewer lesions or evidence of neuritis than with natural zoster (Centers for Disease Control and Prevention . . . , 1999).

Contraindications. VZV vaccine should not be administered to children with impaired cellular immunity. It should not be administered to pregnant women.

Administration of VZV vaccine should be delayed in children who have been administered blood or blood products (for up to 10 months after high-dose IVIG).

Revaccination should be avoided in children and adolescents who experienced an anaphylactic reaction to a previous dose of VZV vaccine. Vaccination is contraindicated in children and adolescents known to be allergic to constituents of the vaccine, including gelatin and neomycin.

Arvin, A. M. (1996). Varicella-zoster virus. *Clinical Microbiology Reviews, 9,* 361–381.

Centers for Disease Control and Prevention Advisory Committee on Immunization Practices. (1996). Prevention of varicella. *Morbidity and Mortality Weekly Report, 45,* RR–11.

Centers for Disease Control and Prevention Advisory Committee on Immunization Practices. (1999). Prevention of varicella updated. *Morbidity and Mortality Weekly Report, 48,* RR–6.

Johnson, C. E., Stancin, T., Fattlar, D., et al. (1997). A long-term prospective study of varicella vaccine in healthy children. *Pediatrics, 100,* 761–766.

La Russa, P., Steinberg, S., & Gershon, A. A. (1996). Varicella vaccine for immunocompromised children: Results of collaborative studies in the United States and Canada. *Journal of Infectious Diseases, 174*(Suppl 3), S320–S323.

National Advisory Committee on Immunization. (1999). Statement on the recommended use of varicella virus vaccine. *Canada Communicable Disease Report, 25,* ACS-1.

Newman, R. D., & Taylor, J. A. (1998). Reactions of pediatricians to the recommendation for universal varicella vaccination. *Archives of Pediatrics and Adolescent Medicine, 152,* 792–796.

10

Pediatric Pharmacokinetics

Clarence T. Ueda and Eric B. Hoie

Pediatric patients represent a unique patient population with respect to their drug therapy needs. Rapid and variable maturational changes in body composition (Behrman, 1992; Friis-Hansen, 1961, 1971, 1983) and body organ function (Aranda & Stern, 1983; Boreus, 1982; Hook & Bailie, 1979) during infancy lead to wide inter- and intra-patient differences in drug disposition. Moreover, because the gestational age determines the physiologic state of neonates, the absorption and disposition characteristics of drugs vary, depending on whether the neonate was born prematurely or at full-term (Morselli, 1976, 1989). Additionally, the degree of drug response in pediatric patients, especially in neonates, may vary with age, possibly due to age-related differences in drug receptor sensitivity and protein binding characteristics (Milsap & Szefler, 1986).

An obvious factor that influences the selection and use of drugs in pediatric patients is the effect of underlying disease states. Many disease states that are known to affect the disposition of drugs in adults also have been shown to alter the distribution, metabolism, and excretion of drugs in pediatric patients. These disease states include hepatic and renal disease (Kauffman & Habersang, 1978; Kunin & Atuk, 1966; Roberts, 1984; Welling et al., 1974), cystic fibrosis (Kuhn & Nahata, 1985), and cardiovascular disorders (Morselli, 1989).

The numerous factors that can affect drug therapy in pediatric patients underscore the importance of individualized drug selection, dosing, and therapeutic drug monitoring (TDM). This chapter presents the important pharmacokinetic factors and principles, including therapeutic monitoring considerations, that apply when providing drug therapy for pediatric patients.

Pharmacokinetic Factors and Drug Effect

The provision of optimal pediatric drug therapy is a complex process that is affected by many different factors. Most notable among the factors that influence drug effect are the pharmacokinetic factors of drug absorption, distribution, metabolism, and excretion. These factors affect drug concentrations and the fate of the drug in the body after administration. Thus, they have a significant influence on the pharmacologic activity of a drug.

In neonates, infants, and children, drug therapy is further complicated by factors unique to this patient group. These factors include natural maturational changes in organ structure and function, enzymatic activity, and body composition; availability of proper or desired dosage forms and appropriate prescribing information; and disease states. Complicating matters even further, maturational changes occur at different rates, depending on the organ system and the type of tissue (Behrman, 1992; Friis-Hansen, 1961, 1971, 1983; Morselli, 1976, 1989; Yaffe & Danish, 1978).

Absorption

Regardless of the route of administration,[1] the rate and extent of drug absorption depend on the physicochemical properties of the drug and its dosage form, the physical and chemical characteristics of the site of administration, the nature of the drug transport mechanism, and the physiological processes that affect the absorption of the drug from the administration site. The interaction of these variables determines the rate and amount of drug absorbed from the site at which a drug is given.[2]

In general, the method of pediatric drug administration varies with age. Premature neonates and young infants (<2 months of age) generally receive drugs intravenously. As they mature, other routes of administration can be used.

Oral administration. Age-related maturational changes in gastric acidity, gastric emptying, intestinal motility, activity of GI enzymes, and biliary function can affect the rate and extent of drug absorption from the GI tract after oral administration (Besunder et al., 1988; Kearns & Reed, 1989; Loebstein & Koren, 1998; Milsap & Szefler, 1986; Morselli, 1989).

With the exception of a short period immediately after birth (a few hours to a few days) when the pH is considerably more acidic, gastric pH is essentially neutral (pH 6–8) because of the immaturity of the gastric mucosa (Agunod et al., 1969; Avery et al., 1966; Koren, 1997; Miller, 1941). The pH of the gastric secretions reaches adult levels usually by 2 years of age but may take as long as 6–7 years (Boreus, 1982). The timing of these changes affects the oral bioavailability of pH-dependent drugs absorbed from the GI tract (e.g., acid-labile drugs and weak acids and bases).

GI drug absorption is highest in the small intestine because of its greater absorptive capacity (large surface area). Therefore, the gastric emptying rate and intestinal motility markedly affect the absorption of drugs after oral administration. The gastric emptying rate is reduced in neonates and infants compared with adults and may also be erratic (Cavell, 1979; Grand et al., 1976; Koren, 1997; Loebstein & Koren, 1998; Signer & Fridrich, 1975). Gastric emptying rates comparable to those in adults are reached by 6–8 months of age (Heimann, 1980; Koren, 1997; Milla & Fenton, 1983; Signer & Fridrich, 1975). Similarly, intestinal motility in neonates and infants is irregular and may be diminished, prolonging intestinal transit time (Milla & Fenton, 1983; Signer & Fridrich, 1975). As with adults, intestinal motility in neonates and infants is influenced by the presence of food in the GI lumen (Milla & Fenton, 1983).

In the neonate, biliary function is immature and the amounts of bile salts in the GI tract are low during the first few months after birth (de Belle et al., 1979; Lebenthal et al., 1983; Murphy & Signer, 1974; Watkins et al., 1973). In addition, the activity of some GI enzymes is diminished during the first year of life (Cavell, 1979; Grand et al., 1976; Hadorn et al., 1968; Zoppi et al., 1972).

Intramuscular administration. Intramuscular drug absorption in pediatric patients is highly dependent on age and physical development. Drug absorption may be slow and erratic in neonates because of low blood flow in the vicinity of the injection site, hemodynamic and/or vasomotor instability, or poor skeletal muscle tone (Koren, 1997; Morselli et al., 1980). The physicochemical properties of the drug and injection vehicle also significantly influence the absorption of drugs given intramuscularly to pediatric patients.

---

1. The exception to this rule pertains, of course, to the intravenous route of administration, for which, by definition absorption is assumed to be complete (i.e., 100%; F = 1.0).

2. *See* Chapter 1 for additional data and discussion.

Rectal administration. In general, the absorption of drugs after rectal administration to pediatric patients is poor and erratic (Gibaldi, 1991). However, bioavailability of some drugs, such as diazepam (Agurell et al., 1975; Dhillon et al., 1982; Dulac et al., 1978), midazolam (Saint-Maurice et al., 1986), and theophylline (Bolme et al., 1979; de Boer et al., 1982) can be quite good, particularly when administered as a rectal solution or a suspension rather than as a rectal suppository. Plasma concentrations of these drugs approximating those obtained after intravenous administration have been attained. Thus, rectal solutions and suspensions are the preferred dosage forms for rectal drug administration in newborns and young infants.

Transdermal administration. Although topical administration of drugs for systemic effects is uncommon in neonates, transdermal fentanyl and clonidine are used in older children. Transdermal absorption of drugs in neonates and infants is higher than in older children because of the relative thinness of the stratum corneum skin layer and high skin hydration (Koren, 1997; Morselli et al., 1980; Radde & McKercher, 1985). Toxic effects have been reported in newborns following skin cleansing with topical drugs, including hexachlorophene and boric acid (Koren, 1997). As the skin layer thickness increases and the skin becomes more cornified with age, the rate and extent of transdermal drug absorption diminish.

Distribution

Drug distribution in the body depends on the physicochemical properties of the drug and the physiologic characteristics of the body, including body water, body fat, and plasma protein binding. The latter factors are particularly important considerations for drug therapy in pediatric patients because of the dramatic maturational changes that take place in these patients (Figure 10-1).

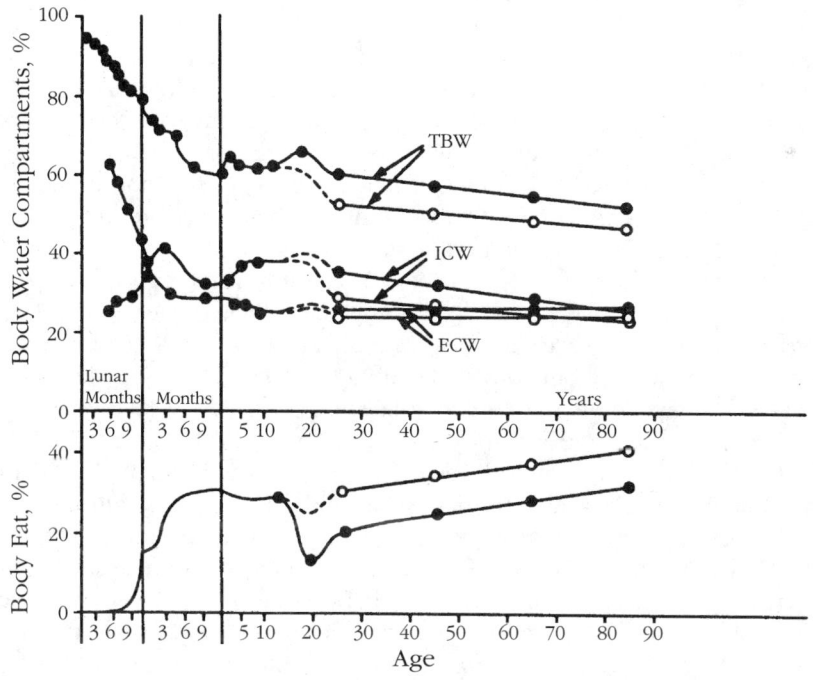

FIGURE 10-1

Maturational Changes in Total Body Water (TBW), Extracellular Water (ECW), Intracellular Water (ICW), and Fat Content of the Body as a Percentage of Total Body Weight by Age and Gender

Key: (●) males and (○) females. (Reprinted with permission from Friis-Hansen, 1971)

Body water. Two important variables affecting drug distribution and, consequently, the outcome of drug therapy are the relative percentages of total body water (TBW) and extracellular water (ECW) in relation to total body weight (Friis-Hansen, 1961, 1971, 1983). Water comprises a much higher percentage of total body weight in neonates than in infants. At birth, TBW may range from 75% to 85% of the total body weight. During the first 12 months after birth, TBW diminishes dramatically and then gradually decreases to adult proportions of approximately 60% of the total weight by 12 years of age (see Figure 10-1).

Pronounced changes in ECW are also observed during the first 12 months after birth (Figure 10-1). ECW decreases from approximately 45%–50% of the total body weight at birth to approximately 25% of the total weight at 1 year of age. For the average adult, ECW represents about 20% of the total body weight. With the exception of the first few months after birth, the percentage of TBW that is intracellular water remains fairly constant.

Body fat. In addition to changes in body water content, the body fat content changes dramatically during the first few months after birth (Figure 10-1). In preterm neonates, fat comprises approximately 1% of the total body weight compared with approximately 15% in term infants (Loebstein & Koren, 1998). Adult body fat levels are generally reached in pediatric patients by 9–12 months of age.

Plasma protein binding. In the vascular system, a drug may be bound to plasma proteins (e.g., albumin, α_1-acid glycoprotein) or it may be unbound (free). Because of the large physical size of the drug–protein complex, the bound form of the drug is unavailable for distribution or elimination. Only free, unbound drug can distribute out of the bloodstream into extravascular tissues and have an effect.

The plasma of neonates contains lower concentrations of total protein (about 80%) and albumin than that of adults (Darrow & Cary, 1933; Ehrnebo et al., 1971; Metcoff & Stare, 1947; Nahata, 1989; Notarianni, 1990; Radde, 1985; Routledge, 1994). Hence, neonatal plasma has a lower capacity to bind drugs. Furthermore, the affinity of the plasma proteins of neonates for some drugs may be reduced (Ehrnebo et al., 1971; Herngren et al., 1983; Koren, 1997; Morselli, 1976; Morselli et al., 1980; Nahata, 1989). These factors cause a decrease in the extent of drug binding and a corresponding increase in the free drug concentration in neonatal plasma.

Endogenous substances such as bilirubin and free fatty acids compete with drugs for binding sites on plasma proteins and may further reduce the protein binding of drugs in neonatal plasma (Koren, 1997; Nahata, 1989; Notarianni, 1990). Conversely, drugs that are highly bound in the plasma (e.g., sulfisoxazole) are capable of displacing bilirubin from albumin (Routledge, 1994; Silverman et al., 1956), thereby potentially predisposing newborns to bilirubin encephalopathy (see "Jaundice" in Table 5-6, Chapter 5). Drug binding by plasma proteins reaches adult levels by approximately 12 months of age (Boreus, 1982; Darrow & Cary, 1933; Metcoff & Stare, 1947).

Metabolism

Drug metabolism takes place in many organs and tissues throughout the body. However, the liver is the principal site of metabolic activity. In the neonate, most of the drug-metabolizing pathways are present at birth, but, because of immaturity, the ability and capacity of these enzymatic processes to metabolize drugs are limited (Aranda & Stern, 1983; Assael, 1982; Boreus, 1982; de Wildt et al., 1999; Gladtke, 1979; Juchau et al., 1980; Leeder & Kearns, 1997; Rane & Tomson, 1980; Tserng et al., 1981). Neonates and young infants metabolize drugs at much slower rates than older infants, children, and adults. The "gray baby" syndrome in infants receiving chloramphenicol is an excellent example of what can happen when a metabolic pathway is deficient and its capacity to remove a potentially toxic drug is exceeded (Friedman et al., 1979; Weiss et al., 1960). In this situation, the decreased ability of infants to form the glucuronide conjugate leads to an accumulation of chloramphenicol to toxic levels (see "Chloramphenicol" in Chapter 5).

Pharmacogenetic studies[3] have shown that genetic variations exist for many drug-metabolizing enzymes (Leeder & Kearns, 1997; Rane, 1999). Several polymorphisms have been identified for important Phase I and Phase II enzymes that determine the metabolizer status of patients (e.g., rapid or slow metabolizers). Complicating matters, drug-metabolizing enzyme development may be enzyme specific and isoform specific (Leeder & Kearns, 1997). Some enzymes reach, and may exceed, adult activity levels when the infant is a few months old while others may take years to reach adult levels. Because metabolic pathways develop at variable rates in infants and children, the ability of a child to metabolize many drugs may not be determinable fully until 12–15 months of age (Rane, 1999).

An example of metabolic differences that exist in enzyme development and metabolic pathway is the conversion of theophylline to caffeine, which is present in neonates and young infants, but not in older infants and children. As hepatic enzymes develop, theophylline clearance increases in infants and children, resulting in a shorter elimination half-life compared to adults (Loebstein & Koren, 1998; Weinberger & Hendeles, 1983). Older infants and children metabolize some drugs more rapidly than adults. Some examples are carbamazepine (Rane et al., 1976); quinidine (Szefler et al., 1982), and phenytoin (Roberts, 1984).

Excretion

The renal excretion of drugs and metabolites in the urine involves two mechanisms: **glomerular filtration** and **tubular secretion.** Renal function at birth is highly dependent on gestational age (Arant, 1978; Koren, 1997; Leake & Trygstad, 1977; Ohning, 1995; Siegel & Oh, 1976). Renal function is much more developed in full-term neonates than in premature infants (Guignard & John, 1986). Nevertheless, glomerular filtration rate and renal tubular secretory activity are both reduced in premature and full-term neonates compared with adults with normal renal function (Aperia & Zetterstrom, 1982; Arant, 1978; Hook & Bailie, 1979; Leake & Trygstad, 1977).

Glomerular filtration is more developed than tubular secretion at birth. This glomerular/tubular imbalance persists for approximately 6–8 months after birth (Barnett, 1950; Braunlich, 1977; Guignard et al., 1975; Houston & Oetliker, 1981; Patrick, 1995; Rubin et al., 1949; Siegel & Oh, 1976). The increase in glomerular filtration rate parallels the increase in renal blood flow in the maturing infant. The glomerular filtration rate reaches adult levels by about 12 months of age in most full-term infants (Hook & Bailie, 1979; Loggie et al., 1975). Premature infants will take longer to reach adult levels.

The renal tubular secretion mechanisms are not fully functional until after the glomerular filtration rate has reached adult levels. There are two different mechanisms that develop at different rates for the secretion of weak acids and bases (Kim et al., 1972). The secretion of organic acids in the proximal tubules is reduced in neonates, compared with adults, accounting for the prolonged half-life of penicillins and cephalosporins in neonates (Assael, 1982; Barnett et al., 1949).

Passive tubular reabsorption also is reduced in neonates compared with adults (Boreus, 1982; Morselli, 1976; Morselli et al., 1980). The renal tubules of neonates have less surface area and the urine-concentrating ability and pH are lower compared to infants, children, and adults (Braunlich, 1977; Yaffe & Stern, 1976). The effect of these differences on renal drug excretion depends on the physicochemical and pharmacokinetic properties of the drug.

Pharmacokinetic Principles

Disposition Parameters

For most drugs, an adequate concentration of drug at the site of action is required for drug therapy to be effective. The plasma (or serum) concentration of the drug is a measurable indicator of this variable.

---

3. *See also* Chapter 11 for additional data and discussion.

Volume of distribution. The amount of drug in the body (X) at any time after a given dose is related to the corresponding concentration of drug in the plasma (C) by the following relationship:

$$X = V \bullet C \qquad \text{(Eq. 10-1)}$$

where the proportionality constant, V, is the **apparent volume of distribution**. The value of V varies with the drug, individual patient physiologic characteristics, which in a given pediatric patient will vary over time due to maturational changes, and disease state. From Equation 10-1, the drug plasma concentration depends on the amount of drug in the body.

The determination of V in pediatric patients is difficult to assess because of the difficulties in obtaining a sufficient number of plasma samples to make the determination. Clinically, V can be estimated in pediatric patients using Equation 10-2:

$$V = \frac{FD}{C_{max}(1 - e^{-K\tau})} \qquad \text{(Eq. 10-2)}$$

where C_{max} is the maximum drug plasma concentration reached at steady state with a fixed dose, D; F is the bioavailability factor, which for an intravenous dose is equal to 1; K is the first-order elimination rate constant and equal to $0.693/T_{1/2}$, where $T_{1/2}$ is the elimination half-life of the drug; and τ is the dosing frequency or interval.

Half-life. The amount of drug in the body after a given dose depends on how much drug has been eliminated by metabolism and/or excretion up to that time. A convenient means to assess this variable is through a knowledge of the **elimination half-life** ($T_{1/2}$) of the drug, which is defined as the time required for the removal of one-half of the amount of the drug in the body at any given time. That is, the amount of drug in the body, and, therefore, the concentration of drug in the plasma, declines 50% every half-life. For most drugs, over a finite period of time, such as a drug treatment period, the value of the elimination half-life remains constant (is unchanged) in a given patient. The relationship between drug plasma concentrations and elimination half-life is shown in Figure 10-2.

Clinically, knowledge of the elimination half-life of a drug in a given patient makes it possible to determine when steady-state conditions (e.g., steady-state drug plasma concentrations) will be reached after continuous (intravenous infusion or multiple dose) drug administration. Steady-state plasma concentrations are attained after approximately 4–5 half-lives. For example, for a drug with a $T_{1/2}$ of 6 hours, steady-state plasma concentrations would be reached with continuous drug administration in approximately 24–30 hours.

The elimination half-life of a drug in a given patient is easily determined by constructing a graph on semilogarithmic graph paper as shown in Figure 10-3. After graphing a minimum of two measured plasma drug concentrations and drawing the best-fitting straight line through the data points, the half-life is determined by simply measuring the time required for a given concentration on the line to fall or decline to one-half that value.

Alternatively, the half-life of the drug in a given patient can be calculated using the following equation:

$$T_{1/2} = \frac{0.693}{\frac{\ln C_1 - \ln C_2}{t_2 - t_1}} \qquad \text{(Eq. 10-3)}$$

where C_1 and C_2 are plasma concentrations obtained at times t_1 and t_2, respectively. In Equation 10-3, the term in the denominator is equivalent to the value of K, the first-order elimination rate constant. Therefore, the expression for $T_{1/2}$ in Equation 10-3 may be rewritten as:

$$T_{1/2} = \frac{0.693}{K} \qquad \text{(Eq. 10-4)}$$

The determination of $T_{1/2}$ by these methods assumes that the pharmacokinetic characteristics of the drug are linear and that $T_{1/2}$ does not change during the treatment period. This is a valid assumption for most drugs. Exceptions include such drugs as phenytoin (Chiba et al., 1980; Richens, 1979), salicylate (Levy, 1975), and theophylline (Weinberger & Ginchansky, 1977). These drugs exhibit nonlinear or dose-dependent pharmacokinetic behavior, and the

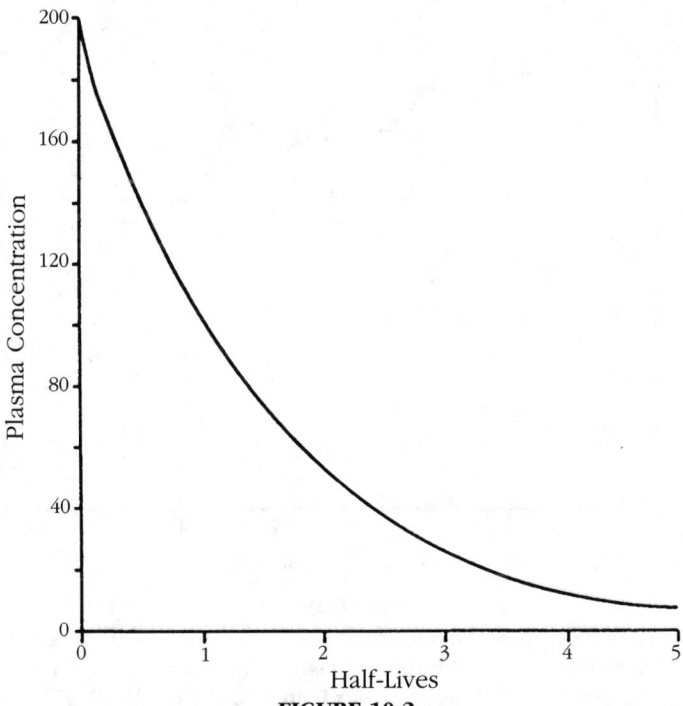

FIGURE 10-2

Relationship between Plasma Drug Concentration and Time Expressed in Terms of Number of Elimination Half-lives

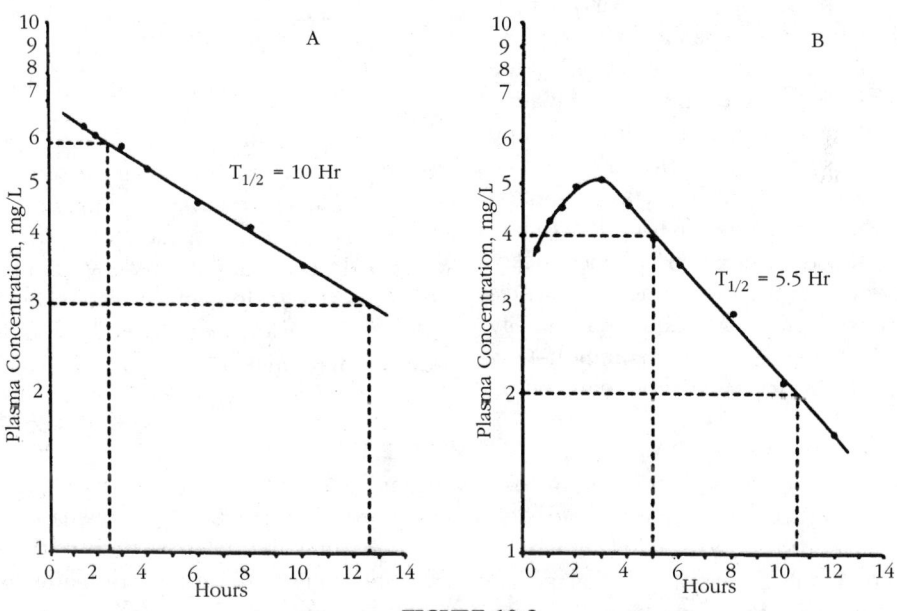

FIGURE 10-3

Determination of the Elimination Half-life, $T_{1/2}$, of Two Hypothetical Drugs using Plasma Drug Concentration *versus* Time Curves Plotted on Semilogarithmic Graph Paper

Key: After (A) rapid intravenous injection and (B) administration by the oral, intramuscular, rectal, or other nonintravenous route with an absorption phase

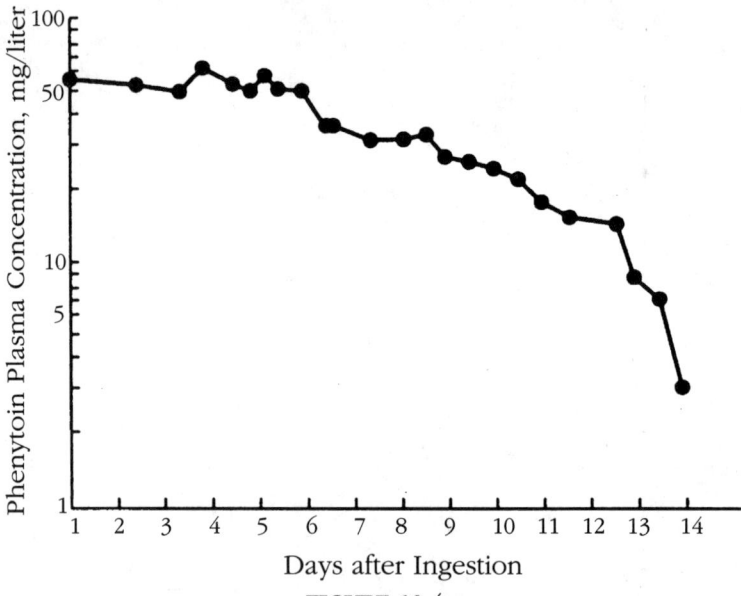

FIGURE 10-4
Plasma Concentration *versus* Time Curve for Phenytoin Illustrating Nonlinear Decline in Phenytoin Plasma Concentration over Time
(Reprinted with permission from Wilson et al., 1979)

"measured" elimination half-life depends on the dose administered and the time when the plasma concentrations are measured.

For drugs that exhibit nonlinear pharmacokinetics, when drug plasma concentrations approach or exceed the capacity (V_{max}) of the enzyme system(s) of the primary eliminating organ (e.g., liver), the concentrations of drug in the plasma will decline nonlinearly or curvilinearly over time when the data are plotted semilogarithmically as shown for phenytoin in Figure 10-4. In contrast, when plasma concentrations are low and the enzyme system(s) is functioning well below its maximum capacity (less than K_m), the plasma concentration–time curve exhibits linear or first-order elimination kinetics (e.g., Figure 10-3).

Clearance. Of the disposition parameters, drug clearance (Cl) is perhaps the most important because it is a measure of the ability of the primary organs responsible for metabolism and excretion (liver and kidneys) to remove the drug from the blood. Clearance is defined as the volume of blood, plasma, or serum from which the drug is totally removed per unit of time. Clearance is related to the apparent volume of distribution, elimination half-life, and elimination rate constant in the following manner.

$$Cl = V \bullet 0.693/T_{1/2} = V \bullet K \quad \text{(Eq. 10-5)}$$

Dosing

Clearance is the proportionality constant that relates the dosage regimen and the drug concentrations in the plasma at steady state. When a drug is administered by continuous intravenous infusion, the relationship between the infusion rate (R) and steady-state drug plasma concentration (C_{ss}) is:

$$R = Cl \bullet C_{ss} \quad \text{(Eq. 10-6)}$$

Thus, a knowledge of the drug clearance and the desired steady-state plasma concentration permits the determination of the infusion rate required to produce or maintain that concentration.

Multiple intermittent dosing of a drug produces fluctuations in plasma concentrations between maximum (peak) and minimum (trough) concentrations. The relationship between the dosing regimen and average steady-state plasma concentration is described by:

$$\frac{FD}{\tau} = Cl \cdot C_{ave} \quad (Eq.\ 10\text{-}7)$$

where FD/τ is the rate of drug administration, τ is the dosing frequency or interval, and C_{ave} is the average drug plasma concentration at steady state. The dose (D) of drug needed to achieve the desired C_{ave} is given by Equation 10-8:

$$D = \frac{ClC_{ave}\tau}{F} \quad (Eq.\ 10\text{-}8)$$

At steady state, the maximum (C_{max}), minimum (C_{min}), and average (C_{ave}) plasma concentrations are related to dose and dosing interval as follows (Gibaldi & Perrier, 1982).

$$C_{max} = \frac{FD}{V(1 - e^{-K\tau})} \quad (Eq.\ 10\text{-}9)$$

$$C_{min} = \frac{FD\ e^{-K\tau}}{V(1 - e^{-K\tau})} \quad (Eq.\ 10\text{-}10)$$

$$C_{ave} = \frac{FD}{VK\tau} = \frac{FD}{Cl\tau} \quad (Eq.\ 10\text{-}11)$$

Increasing or decreasing the dose administered will result in proportionate changes in C_{max}, C_{min}, and C_{ave}. However, increasing the dosing interval, τ, will increase the magnitude of the difference between C_{max} and C_{min} (the peak and trough concentrations). Conversely, decreasing τ will reduce the size of the difference between the peak and trough concentrations.

Dosing drugs with nonlinear or dose-dependent elimination kinetics in pediatric patients can be a significant challenge because the relationship between the dose administered and the steady-state plasma concentration is not linear (not proportionate). A small change in dose can produce a disproportionately greater change in the plasma concentration, depending on the size of the dose administered (Figure 10-5). **Drugs with nonlinear pharmacokinetics require careful dosing and close monitoring.**

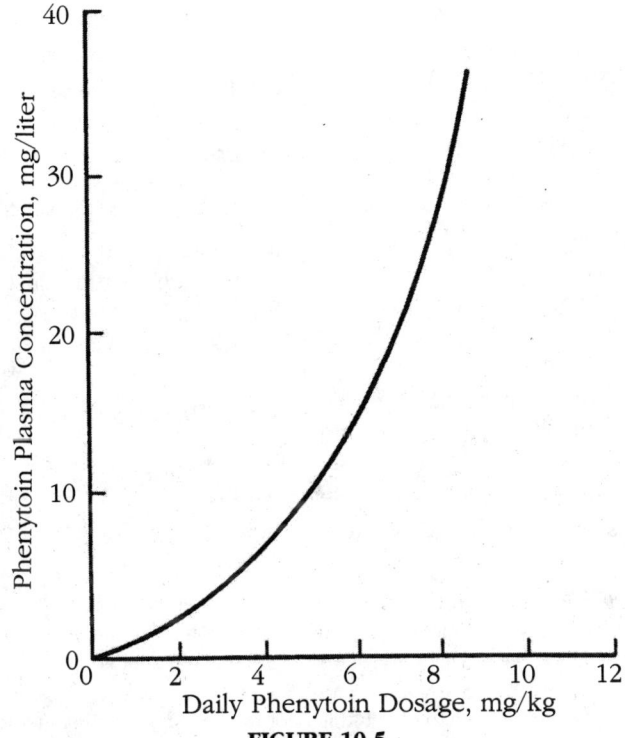

FIGURE 10-5

Nonlinear, Dose-dependent Relationship between Steady-state Plasma Concentration and Daily Dosage for Phenytoin

Therapeutic Monitoring Considerations

Therapeutic drug monitoring is essential for drugs possessing a low therapeutic index to ensure their safe and effective use. For a listing of drugs commonly monitored in pediatric patients, *see* Table 14-3, in Chapter 14.

Although it may not be possible to obtain the desired plasma concentration or therapeutic response initially, measurement of the plasma concentrations, when available, can be used to determine the pharmacokinetic parameters of the drug in the individual pediatric patient. This patient-specific information facilitates the determination of the proper dosing regimen to achieve the desired plasma concentration and, thus, desired therapeutic response.

As an example, assume that, during a 15-mg/hr continuous intravenous infusion of theophylline in a 5-year-old child weighing 25 kg, a steady-state plasma concentration of 8 mg/liter was obtained. By using this information and rearranging Equation 10-6 to solve for Cl, the calculated Cl for theophylline in this patient is 1.88 liter/hr. Therefore, to achieve a C_{ss} of 12 mg/liter in this patient, the theophylline infusion rate would need to be increased to 22–23 mg/hr.

As another example, a 3-day-old infant born at 34 weeks gestation has been receiving gentamicin 2.5 mg/kg intravenous intermittent infusion over 30 minutes every 12 hours. Gentamicin serum concentrations measured 30 minutes before and 30 minutes after the fourth dose[4] are reported from the clinical laboratory as 2.8 and 6.2 mg/liter, respectively. From Equation 10-3, the estimated half-life for gentamicin in this patient is 9.6 hours, and with Equation 10-2, the value for V is 0.70 liter/kg. With this information, several possible dosage adjustments could be considered that would provide safe and effective gentamicin serum concentrations in this patient. Rearranging Equation 10-9 and solving for D, an intravenous gentamicin dose of 3.5 mg/kg administered every 24 hours would produce in this patient peak drug concentrations of 6.1 mg/liter and, using Equation 10-10, trough gentamicin concentrations of 1.1 mg/liter.

When, after applying appropriate pharmacokinetic principles and equations, the desired serum or plasma drug concentration and/or therapeutic response are not achieved, other factors to consider include dose calculation, compounding and/or dispensing errors, underdosing due to loss of drug in the hub of the needle when it is injected by intravenous push or because of inadequate flushing of the intravenous tubing after completion of the intravenous infusion, and blood sampling errors (e.g., collecting the blood sample through the same line used to administer the drug).

Altered Pharmacokinetics in Disease States and with Concurrent Drug Therapy

Various disease states, including cystic fibrosis (Kuhn & Nahata, 1985; Rey et al., 1998) and renal and liver disease (Kauffman & Habersang, 1978; Roberts, 1984) are known to alter drug disposition significantly in pediatric patients. In addition, other concurrently administered drugs may influence the disposition characteristics (*see* Chapter 6). An understanding of these effects is important when selecting and monitoring drug therapy.

Renal Disease/Dysfunction

Renal disease and dysfunction may impair the elimination of drugs and metabolites when their principal means of removal is excretion

---

4. In this example, the time elapsed after the administration of the first dose is 36 hours. Thus, assuming an elimination half-life of 9.6 hours, the time to reach steady-state concentrations would be 5 × 9.6 or 48 hours. Clinically, serum concentration determinations are frequently ordered after administration of a routine or fixed number (e.g., 3 or 4) of doses. While it would be preferable to acquire drug serum concentration data after steady state has been reached, the need to obtain this information in a timely manner to reduce potential risks due to prolonged subtherapeutic or toxic drug concentrations is also an important consideration. In these situations, any dosage adjustments based on drug serum concentrations obtained prior to the achievement of steady state will need to take this factor into consideration.

in the urine. The degree of renal impairment, fraction of the dose that is renally excreted in unchanged form, activity of metabolites that are excreted by the kidneys, and therapeutic index of the drug are factors that should be considered when selecting a drug and designing a drug therapy plan for patients with renal disease and dysfunction (Gibson, 1986).

In general, clearance is reduced and the half-life is prolonged for drugs eliminated primarily by the kidneys in patients with renal dysfunction. These patients generally require lower daily drug dosages, less frequent drug administration, or both. However, the dosage requirements for patients with renal dysfunction may vary greatly depending on the severity of the impairment. This variability is illustrated with the cephalosporins and aminoglycosides, two classes of drugs that are primarily eliminated by the kidneys (Gibson, 1986). In patients with end-stage renal failure, the urinary excretion of drugs in both classes may fall to less than 10% of normal values (Kunin & Atuk, 1966; Lockwood & Bower, 1973; Welling et al., 1974). Drugs with a low therapeutic index (e.g., aminoglycosides) may require significant dosage modifications, even in patients with only moderate renal dysfunction. In contrast, dosage adjustments may not be necessary for drugs with a wide therapeutic index (e.g., cephalosporins) unless renal function is severely impaired.

Renal function may be reduced in premature infants because they are prone to periods of hypoxia and ischemia, and their immature kidneys are especially prone to hypoxia (Dauber et al., 1976; Jones et al., 1979). A reduction in the clearance of renally excreted drugs may also occur in infants with decreased left ventricular output because of decreased renal blood flow and glomerular filtration rate (Castaneda & Mayer, 1990; Huhta, 1990).

Liver Disease/Dysfunction

Liver disease and dysfunction may affect the absorption and disposition of drugs by a number of different mechanisms, depending on the nature and severity of the condition. These mechanisms include alterations in hepatic blood flow, plasma protein concentration, and activity of drug-metabolizing enzymes (Wilkinson, 1986). In general, changes in drug disposition are not observed until the condition becomes moderate to severe. Moreover, acute diseases such as viral hepatitis appear to have little, if any, effect on drug metabolism (Roberts, 1984). However, chronic conditions can have substantial effects. In chronic liver diseases, it is not uncommon to observe reduced drug clearances, altered drug distribution (i.e., volume of distribution), and prolonged elimination half-lives.

Liver disease also can alter the absorption of some oral drugs. The reduced first-pass clearance by the liver of drugs with a high hepatic extraction ratio, such as morphine and propranolol (Rowland & Tozer, 1989), enhances their oral bioavailability (Neal et al., 1979; Wilkinson, 1986; Wood et al., 1978).

Decreases in plasma protein binding may be associated with the reduced plasma albumin concentrations in patients with liver disease (Olsen et al., 1975; Wilkinson, 1986). This effect may alter (increase) drug distribution in the body and may be an important consideration for drugs possessing a narrow therapeutic index.

Cystic Fibrosis

The volume of distribution and renal clearance of many drugs, particularly broad spectrum antibiotics, are increased in pediatric patients with cystic fibrosis (Kearns et al., 1982; Kuhn & Nahata, 1985; Rey et al., 1998). Larger doses or more frequent dosing of aminoglycosides, cephalosporins, and penicillins must be used in these patients. Some reports indicate that nonrenal clearance (e.g., hepatic metabolism) of drugs may also be increased in patients with cystic fibrosis (Rey et al., 1998; Spino et al., 1984; Ziemniak et al., 1984).

Concurrent Drug Therapy

Drug disposition may be influenced by concurrent drug therapy. Such drug interactions are commonly observed when a concurrently administered drug stimulates (e.g., phenobarbital) or inhibits (e.g., cimetidine) a drug-metabolizing enzyme system (Powell & Cate, 1986). The inhibition of renal tubular secretion and reduction in the renal clearance of penicillins and cephalosporins by probenecid (Rowland & Tozer, 1989) is another example of a pharmacokinetically mediated drug interaction. (*See also* Chapter 6, for a comprehensive discussion).

Summary

The wide variability in drug absorption, distribution, metabolism, and excretion observed in pediatric patients, coupled with the increased potential for preparation and administration errors with medications used in these patients, underscore the importance of therapeutic drug monitoring, particularly for drugs with a low therapeutic index. Interpatient and intrapatient variabilities in drug absorption, distribution, metabolism, and excretion further increase the risk(s) of toxic or subtherapeutic drug concentrations in neonates, infants, and young children.

The use of drugs for which there is very limited clinical experience in pediatric patients presents additional therapeutic challenges for clinicians. Drugs that have been demonstrated to be safe and effective in adults may produce unexpected toxicities in pediatric patients. Drugs for which pediatric data are lacking should be prescribed and administered with caution until sufficient experience has been gained with their use and only when the potential therapeutic benefits outweigh anticipated risks. In all cases, the pediatric patient should be monitored closely to ensure that the drug therapy is effective and that toxicity is avoided or minimized. The clinical application of pharmacokinetic principles and data can help ensure optimal drug therapy for pediatric patients.

References

Agunod, M., Yamaguchi, N., Lopez, R., et al. (1969). Correlative study of hydrochloric acid, pepsin, and intrinsic factor secretion in newborns and infants. *American Journal of Digestive Disease, 14,* 400–414.

Agurell, S., Berlin, A., Ferngren, H. G., et al. (1975). Plasma levels of diazepam after parenteral and rectal administration to children. *Epilepsia, 16,* 277–283.

Aperia, A., & Zetterstrom, R. (1982). Renal control of fluid homeostasis in the newborn infant. *Clinics in Perinatology, 9,* 523–533.

Aranda, J. V., & Stern, L. (1983). Clinical aspects of developmental pharmacology and toxicology. *Pharmacology and Therapeutics, 20,* 1–51.

Arant, B. S. Jr. (1978). Developmental patterns of renal functional maturation compared in human neonates. *The Journal of Pediatrics, 92,* 705–712.

Assael, B. M. (1982). Pharmacokinetics and drug distribution during postnatal development. *Pharmacology and Therapeutics, 18,* 159–197.

Avery, G. B., Randolph, J. G., & Weaver, T. (1966). Gastric acidity in the first day of life. *Pediatrics, 37,* 1005–1007.

Barnett, H. L. (1950). Kidney function in young infants. *Pediatrics, 5,* 171–179.

Barnett, H. L., McNamara, H., Schultz, S., et al. (1949). Renal clearances of sodium penicillin G, procaine penicillin G and inulin in infants and children. *Pediatrics, 3,* 418–422.

Behrman, R. E. (Ed). (1992). *Nelson textbook of pediatrics.* Philadelphia: Saunders.

Besunder, J. B., Reed, M. D., & Blumer, J. L. (1988). Principles of drug biodisposition in the neonate: A critical evaluation of the pharmacokinetic–pharmacodynamic interface (part I). *Clinical Pharmacokinetics, 14,* 189–216.

Bolme, P., Edlund, P. O., Eriksson, M., et al. (1979). Pharmacokinetics of theophylline in young children with asthma: Comparison of rectal enema and suppositories. *European Journal of Clinical Pharmacology, 16,* 133–139.

Boreus, L. O. (1982). *Principles of pediatric pharmacology.* New York: Churchill Livingstone.

Braunlich, H. (1977). Kidney development—drug elimination mechanisms. In P. L. Morselli, Ed. *Drug disposition during development,* pp. 89–100. New York: Spectrum.

Castaneda, A. R., & Mayer, J. E. (1990). Neonatal repair of transposition of the great arteries. In W. A. Long, Ed. *Fetal and neonatal cardiology,* pp. 789–795. Philadelphia: Saunders.

Cavell, B. (1979). Gastric emptying in preterm infants. *Acta Paediatrica Scandinavica, 68,* 725–730.

Chiba, K., Ishizaki, T., Miura, H., et al. (1980). Michaelis-Menten pharmacokinetics of diphenylhydantoin and application in the pediatric age patient. *The Journal of Pediatrics, 96,* 479–484.

Darrow, D. C., & Cary, M. K. (1933). The serum albumin and globulin of newborn, premature and normal infants. *The Journal of Pediatrics, 3,* 573–579.

Dauber, I. M., Kraus, A. N., Symchych, P. S., et al. (1976). Renal failure following perinatal anoxia. *The Journal of Pediatrics, 88,* 851–855.

de Belle, R. C., Vaupshas, V., Vitullo, B. B., et al. (1979). Intestinal absorption of bile salts: Immature development in the neonate. *The Journal of Pediatrics, 94*, 472–476.

de Boer, A. G., Moolenaar, F., de Leede, L. G. J., et al. (1982). Rectal drug administration: Clinical pharmacokinetic considerations. *Clinical Pharmacokinetics, 7*, 285–311.

de Wildt, S. N., Kearns, G. L., Leeder, J. S., et al. (1999). Cytochrome P450 3A: Ontogeny and drug disposition. *Clinical Pharmacokinetics, 37*, 485–505.

Dhillon, S., Ngwane, E., & Richens, A. (1982). Rectal absorption of diazepam in epileptic children. *Archives of Disease in Childhood, 57*, 264–267.

Dulac, O., Aicardi, J., Rey, E., et al. (1978). Blood levels of diazepam after single rectal administration in infants and children. *The Journal of Pediatrics, 93*, 1039–1041.

Ehrnebo, M., Agurell, S., Jalling, B., et al. (1971). Age differences in drug binding by plasma proteins: Studies on human foetuses, neonates and adults. *European Journal of Clinical Pharmacology, 3*, 189–193.

Friedman, C. A., Lovejoy, F. C., & Smith, A. L. (1979). Chloramphenicol disposition in infants and children. *The Journal of Pediatrics, 95*, 1071–1077.

Friis-Hansen, B. (1961). Body water compartments in children: Changes during growth and related changes in body composition. *Pediatrics, 28*, 169–181.

Friis-Hansen, B. (1971). Body composition during growth: *In vivo* measurements and biochemical data correlated to differential anatomical growth. *Pediatrics, 47*, 264–274.

Friis-Hansen, B. (1983). Water distribution in the foetus and newborn infant. *Acta Paediatrica Scandinavica, 305*(Suppl), 7–11.

Gibaldi, M. (1991). *Biopharmaceutics and clinical pharmacokinetics*. Philadelphia: Lea & Febiger.

Gibaldi, M., & Perrier, D. (1982). *Pharmacokinetics*. New York: Marcel Dekker.

Gibson, T. P. (1986). Influence of renal disease on pharmacokinetics. In W. E. Evans, J. J. Schentag, and W. J. Jusko, Eds. *Applied pharmacokinetics: Principles of therapeutic monitoring*, pp. 83–115. Spokane: Applied Therapeutics.

Gladtke, E. (1979). The importance of pharmacokinetics for paediatrics. *European Journal of Pediatrics, 131*, 85–91.

Grand, R. J., Watkins, J. B., & Torti, F. M. (1976). Development of the human gastrointestinal tract: A review. *Gastroenterology, 70*, 790–810.

Guignard, J. P., & John, E. G. (1986). Renal function in the tiny premature infant. *Clinics in Perinatology, 13*, 377–401.

Guignard, J. P., Torrado, A., Da Cunha, O., et al. (1975). Glomerular filtration rate in the first three weeks of life. *The Journal of Pediatrics, 87*, 268–272.

Hadorn, B., Zoppi, G., Shmerling, D. H., et al. (1968). Quantitative assessment of exocrine pancreatic function in infants and children. *The Journal of Pediatrics, 73*, 39–50.

Heimann, G. (1980). Enteral absorption and bioavailability in children in relation to age. *European Journal of Clinical Pharmacology, 18*, 43–50.

Herngren, L., Ehrnebo, M., & Boreus, L. O. (1983). Drug binding to plasma proteins during human pregnancy and in the perinatal period. *Developmental Pharmacology and Therapeutics, 6*, 110–124.

Hook, J. B., & Bailie, M. D. (1979). Perinatal renal pharmacology. *Annual Review of Pharmacology and Toxicology, 19*, 491–509.

Houston, I. B., & Oetliker, O. (1981). Growth and development of the kidneys. In J. A. Davis and J. Dobbing, Eds. *Scientific foundations of paediatrics*, pp. 486–496. Baltimore: University Park Press.

Huhta, J. C. (1990). Patent ductus arteriosus in the preterm neonate. In W. A. Long, Ed. *Fetal and neonatal cardiology*, pp. 389–400. Philadelphia: Saunders.

Jones, A. S., James, E., Bland, H., et al. (1979). Renal failure in the newborn. *Clinical Pediatrics, 18*, 286–291.

Juchau, M. R., Chao, S. T., & Omiecinski, C. J. (1980). Drug metabolism by the human fetus. *Clinical Pharmacokinetics, 5*, 320–339.

Kauffman, R. E., & Habersang, R. (1978). Modification of dosage regimens in disease states of childhood. In B. L. Mirkin, Ed. *Clinical pharmacology and therapeutics: A pediatric perspective*, pp. 73–88. Chicago: Year Book Medical Publishers.

Kearns, G. L., Hilman, B. C., & Wilson, J. T. (1982). Dosing implications of altered gentamicin disposition in patients with cystic fibrosis. *The Journal of Pediatrics, 100*, 312–318.

Kearns, G. L., & Reed, M. D. (1989). Clinical pharmacokinetics in infants and children: A reappraisal. *Clinical Pharmacokinetics, 17*(Suppl 1), 29–67.

Kim, J. K., Hirsch, G. H., & Hook, J. B. (1972). In vitro analysis of organic ion transport in renal cortex of newborn rat. *Pediatric Research, 6*, 600–605.

Koren, G. (1997). Therapeutic drug monitoring principles in the neonate. *Clinical Chemistry, 43*, 222–227.

Kuhn, R. J., & Nahata, M. C. (1985). Therapeutic management of cystic fibrosis. *Clinical Pharmacy, 4*, 555–565.

Kunin, C. M., & Atuk, N. (1966). Excretion of cephaloridine and cephalothin in patients with renal impairment. *New England Journal of Medicine, 274*, 654–656.

Leake, R. D., & Trygstad, C. W. (1977). Glomerular filtration rate during the period of adaptation to extrauterine life. *Pediatric Research, 11*, 959–962.

Lebenthal, E., Lee, P. C., & Heitlinger, L. A. (1983). Impact of development of the gastrointestinal tract on infant feeding. *The Journal of Pediatrics, 102,* 1–9.

Leeder, J. S., & Kearns, G. L. (1997). Pharmacogenetics in pediatrics. Implications for practice. *Pediatric Clinics of North America, 44,* 55–77.

Levy, G. (1975). Salicylate pharmacokinetics in the human neonate. In P. L. Morselli, S. Garattini, & F. Sereni, Eds. *Basic and therapeutic aspects of perinatal pharmacology,* pp. 319–330. New York: Raven Press.

Lockwood, W. R., & Bower, J. D. (1973). Tobramycin and gentamicin concentrations in the serum of normal and anephric patients. *Antimicrobial Agents and Chemotherapy, 3,* 125–129.

Loebstein, R., & Koren, G. (1998). Clinical pharmacology and therapeutic drug monitoring in neonates and children. *Pediatrics in Review, 19,* 423–428.

Loggie, J. M. H., Kleinman, L. I., & Van Maanen, E. F. (1975). Renal function and diuretic therapy in infants and children. Part I. *The Journal of Pediatrics, 86,* 485–496.

Metcoff, J., & Stare, F. (1947). The physiologic and clinical significance of plasma proteins and protein metabolites. *New England Journal of Medicine, 236,* 26–35.

Milla, P. J., & Fenton, T. R. (1983). Small intestinal motility patterns in the perinatal period. *Journal of Pediatric Gastroenterology and Nutrition, 2*(Suppl 1), S141–S144.

Miller, R. A. (1941). Observations on the gastric acidity during the first month of life. *Archives of Disease in Childhood, 16,* 22–30.

Milsap, R. L., & Szefler, S. J. (1986). Special pharmacokinetic considerations in children. In W. E. Evans, J. J. Schentag, & W. J. Jusko, Eds. *Applied pharmacokinetics: Principles of therapeutic drug monitoring,* pp. 294–330. Spokane: Applied Therapeutics.

Morselli, P. I. (1976). Clinical pharmacokinetics in neonates. *Clinical Pharmacokinetics, 1,* 81–98.

Morselli, P. I. (1989). Clinical pharmacology of the perinatal period and early infancy. *Clinical Pharmacokinetics, 17*(Suppl 1), 13–28.

Morselli, P. I., Franco-Morselli, R., & Bossi, L. (1980). Clinical pharmacokinetics in newborns and infants: Age-related differences and therapeutic implications. *Clinical Pharmacokinetics, 5,* 485–527.

Murphy, G. M., & Signer, E. (1974). Bile acid metabolism in infants and children. *GUT, 15,* 151–163.

Nahata, M. C. (1989). Pediatrics. In J. T. DiPiro, R. L. Talbert, P. E. Hayes, et al., Eds. *Pharmacotherapy: A pathophysiologic approach,* pp. 35–41. New York: Elsevier.

Neal, E. A., Meffin, P. J., Gregory, P. B., et al. (1979). Enhanced bioavailability and decreased clearance of analgesics in patients with cirrhosis. *Gastroenterology, 77,* 96–102.

Notarianni, L. J. (1990). Plasma protein binding of drugs in pregnancy and in neonates. *Clinical Pharmacokinetics, 18,* 20–36.

Ohning, B. L. (1995). Neonatal pharmacodynamics—basic principles II: Drug action and elimination. *Neonatal Network, 14,* 15–19.

Olsen, G. D., Bennett, W. M., & Porter, G. A. (1975). Morphine and phenytoin binding to plasma proteins in renal and hepatic failure. *Clinical Pharmacology and Therapeutics, 17,* 677–684.

Patrick, C. H. (1995). Therapeutic drug monitoring in neonates. *Neonatal Network, 14,* 21–25.

Powell, J. R., & Cate, E. W. (1986). Induction and inhibition of drug metabolism. In W. E. Evans, J. J. Schentag, & W. J. Jusko, Eds. *Applied pharmacokinetics: Principles of therapeutic drug monitoring,* pp. 139–186. Spokane: Applied Therapeutics.

Radde, I. C. (1985). Drugs and protein binding. In S. M. MacLeod & I. C. Radde, Eds. *Textbook of pediatric clinical pharmacology,* pp. 32–43. Littleton: PSG Publishing.

Radde, I. C., & McKercher, H. G. (1985). Transport through membranes and development of membrane transport. In S. M. MacLeod & I. C. Radde, Eds. *Textbook of pediatric clinical pharmacology,* pp. 1–16. Littleton: PSG Publishing.

Rane, A. (1999). Phenotyping of drug metabolism in infants and children: Potentials and problems. *Pediatrics, 104,* 640–643.

Rane, A., Hojer, B., & Wilson, J. T. (1976). Kinetics of carbamazepine and its 10,11-epoxide metabolite in children. *Clinical Pharmacology and Therapeutics, 19,* 276–283.

Rane, A., & Tomson, G. (1980). Prenatal and neonatal drug metabolism in man. *European Journal of Clinical Pharmacology, 18,* 9–15.

Rey, E., Treluyer, J. M., & Pons, G. (1998). Drug disposition in cystic fibrosis. *Clinical Pharmacokinetics, 35,* 313–329.

Richens, A. (1979). Clinical pharmacokinetics of phenytoin. *Clinical Pharmacokinetics, 4,* 153–169.

Roberts, R. J. (1984). *Drug therapy in infants: Pharmacologic principles and clinical experience.* Philadelphia: Saunders.

Routledge, P. A. (1994). Pharmacokinetics in children. *Journal of Antimicrobial Chemotherapy, 34*(Suppl A), 19–24.

Rowland, M., & Tozer, T. N. (1989). *Clinical pharmacokinetics: Concepts and applications.* Philadelphia: Lea and Febiger.

Rubin, M. I., Bruck, E., & Rapoport, M. (1949). Maturation of renal function in childhood: Clearance studies. *Journal of Clinical Investigation, 28,* 1144–1162.

Saint-Maurice, C., Meistelman, C., Rey, E., et al. (1986). The pharmacokinetics of rectal midazolam for premedication in children. *Anesthesiology, 65,* 536–538.

Siegel, S. R., & Oh, W. (1976). Renal function as a

marker of human fetal maturation. *Acta Paediatrica Scandinavica, 65,* 481–485.

Signer, E., & Fridrich, R. (1975). Gastric emptying in newborns and young infants. *Acta Paediatrica Scandinavica, 64,* 525–530.

Silverman, W. A., Anderson, D. H., Blanc, W. A., et al. (1956). A difference in mortality rate and incidence of kernicterus among premature infants allotted to two prophylactic antibacterial regimens. *Pediatrics, 18,* 614–624.

Spino, M., Chai, R. P., Isles, A. F., et al. (1984). Cloxacillin absorption and disposition in cystic fibrosis. *The Journal of Pediatrics, 105,* 829–835.

Szefler, S. J., Pieroni, D. R., Gingell, R. L., et al. (1982). Rapid elimination of quinidine in pediatric patients. *Pediatrics, 70,* 370–375.

Tserng, K. Y., King, K. C., & Takieddine, F. N. (1981). Theophylline metabolism in premature infants. *Clinical Pharmacology and Therapeutics, 29,* 594–600.

Watkins, J. B., Ingall, D., Szczepanik, P., et al. (1973). Bile salt metabolism in the newborn. *New England Journal of Medicine, 288,* 431–434.

Weinberger, M., & Ginchansky, E. (1977). Dose-dependent kinetics of theophylline disposition in asthmatic children. *The Journal of Pediatrics, 91,* 820–824.

Weinberger, M., & Hendeles, L. (1983). Theophylline for chronic asthma: Rationale for treatment, product selection, dosage schedule. *Pediatric Pharmacology, 3,* 273–285.

Weiss, C. F., Glazko, A. J., & Weston, J. K. (1960). Chloramphenicol in the newborn infant, a physiologic explanation of its toxicity when given in excessive doses. *New England Journal of Medicine, 262,* 787–794.

Welling, P. G., Craig, W. A., Amidon, G. L., et al. (1974). Pharmacokinetics of cefazolin in normal and uremic subjects. *Clinical Pharmacology and Therapeutics, 15,* 344–353.

Wilkinson, G. R. (1986). Influence of hepatic disease on pharmacokinetics. In W. E. Evans, J. J. Schentag, & W. J. Jusko, Eds. *Applied pharmacokinetics: Principles of therapeutic drug monitoring,* pp. 116–138. Spokane: Applied Therapeutics.

Wilson, J. T., Huff, J. G., & Kilroy, A. W. (1979). Prolonged toxicity following acute phenytoin overdose in a child. *The Journal of Pediatrics, 95,* 135–138.

Wood, A. J. J., Kornhauser, D. M., Wilkinson, G. R., et al. (1978). The influence of cirrhosis on steady-state blood concentrations of unbound propranolol after oral administration. *Clinical Pharmacokinetics, 3,* 478–487.

Yaffe, S. J., & Danish, M. (1978). Problems of drug administration in the pediatric patient. *Drug Metabolism Reviews, 8,* 303–318.

Yaffe, S. J., & Stern, L. (1976). Clinical implications of perinatal pharmacology. In B. L. Mirkin, Ed. *Perinatal pharmacology and therapeutics,* pp. 355–428. New York: Academic.

Ziemniak, J. A., Assael, B. M., Padoan, R., et al. (1984). The bioavailability and pharmacokinetics of cimetidine and its metabolites in juvenile cystic fibrosis patients: Age-related differences as compared to adults. *European Journal of Clinical Pharmacology, 26,* 183–189.

Zoppi, G., Andreotti, G., Pajno-Ferrara, F., et al. (1972). Exocrine pancreas function in premature and full term neonates. *Pediatric Research, 6,* 880–886.

11

Pediatric Pharmacogenetics

J. Steven Leeder

The pediatric patient has been perceived simplistically in the past as a "miniature" or "small version" adult. More recently, clinicians, researchers, the pharmaceutical industry, and regulatory agencies have come to realize that this perception is erroneous. Rather, infants, children, and adolescents represent distinct subpopulations each with their own unique characteristics, which is not surprising given the rapid growth and development that occurs during the first year of life and the complex changes that mark the transition through adolescence to adulthood. Clearly, the response to drug therapy is a function of development, affecting drug disposition and the interaction of drugs with their pharmacologic targets. Pharmacokinetic studies conducted in neonates, infants, children, and adolescents demonstrate that development influences the absorption, distribution, metabolism, and excretion of many drugs. Furthermore, developmental differences in drug metabolism often produce definable "patterns" in drug clearance that, in some cases, enable pharmacokinetic description of patient subpopulations within the pediatric age group (Kauffman & Kearns, 1992). Developmental patterns of drug transport and receptor expression/function are less well characterized but are equally important for understanding the response to drug therapy throughout childhood.

With regard to heritable traits, no one can deny the role that genetic factors play in influencing a child's potential characteristics such as height, weight, hair color, and behavior. Likewise, genetic factors are important, although not sole, determinants of inter- and intra-individual variability in both drug disposition and response. Pharmacogenetics is an important component of the growth and development processes of pediatric patients, particularly in regard to the enzymes involved in drug biotransformation.

Pharmacogenetic Principles

Pharmacogenetics probably originated about 150 years ago when physiological chemists discovered that foreign substances excreted by humans were chemically altered relative to the forms that had been administered. Coincident with a "rediscovery" of Gregor Mendel's laws of heredity around the turn of the century, investigators in England and France suggested that genetic material played a role in directing these chemical reactions. Notably, Archibald Garrod, through his studies of urinary pigments and sulfonal-induced porphyria, proposed that enzymes were implicated in the detoxification of foreign substances. A key element of his later work was the concept that disproportionate responses to foreign substances could result from deficiency of the required detoxifying enzyme. However, it was not until the 1950s that certain adverse drug reactions (ADRs), such as unusually prolonged respiratory muscle paralysis due to succinylcholine- and isoniazid-induced neurotoxicity, were recognized to be a consequence of inherited variation in enzyme activities. In 1959, Friedrich Vogel coined the term pharmacogenetics to describe the study of genetically determined variations in drug response. Since then, the importance of genetic polymorphisms in drug-metabolizing enzymes has become increasingly apparent, particularly in recent years, because of enhanced awareness of clinically useful drugs that are metabolized by polymorphically expressed enzymes and the increasing proportion of affected patients who are treated with these drugs.

Genetic variability results from gene mutation and the exchange of genetic information between chromosomes during meiosis. With the exception of sex-linked genes (genes occurring on the X or Y chromosome), individuals carry two copies of each gene they possess. However, a specific gene may be present in the population in different forms that do not have identical nucleic acid sequences. Different nucleotides at a given position within a gene contribute to variability and result in gene **polymorphisms,** with single nucleotide polymorphisms (SNPs) rapidly becoming part of the pharmacogenetics vocabulary as sequencing of the human genome approaches completion. In genes where polymorphisms have been detected, alternative forms of the gene are called **alleles.** When the alleles at a particular gene locus are identical, a **homozygous** state exists; whereas a **heterozygous state** refers to the situation where different alleles are present at the same gene locus. The term **genotype** refers to an individual's genetic constitution while the related observable characteristics or physical manifestations constitute the **phenotype,** which is the net consequence of genetic and environmental effects.

To end confusion between genotypic and phenotypic definitions of polymorphism, and to clarify the relationship between genetic concepts and the clinical relevance of a given phenotype, Meyer (1991) proposed the following definition of **pharmacogenetic polymorphism**:

> A pharmacogenetic polymorphism is a monogenic trait that is caused by the presence in the same population of more than one allele at the same locus and more than one phenotype in regard to drug interaction with the organism. The frequency of the least common allele is > 1%.

According to this definition, the key elements of pharmacogenetic polymorphism are heritability, the involvement of a single gene locus, and the fact that distinct phenotypes are observed within the population **only** after drug challenge. Current understanding rests on enzymes responsible for drug biotransformation. Clinically, individuals typically are classified as being "fast," "rapid," or "extensive" metabolizers and "slow" or "poor" metabolizers. However, depending on the particular enzyme, there also may be an intermediate metabolizer group. As described later, pediatric pharmacogenetics involves an added measure of complexity since fetuses and neonates may be phenotypically slow or poor metabolizers for certain drug-metabolizing pathways, acquiring a phenotype consistent with their genotype later in development.

The most common consequence of genetically defective drug-metabolizing enzyme activity is a "functional" overdose due to accumulation of active drug as a result of inefficient elimination by the affected biotransformation pathway. In some cases, an inability to convert a prodrug to its corresponding pharmacologically active moiety may result in lack of efficacy; predisposition to idiosyncratic toxicity unrelated to the intended drug effect is less common. However, not all pharmacogenetic polymorphisms are clinically relevant. The likelihood of a clinically significant event is enhanced if (1) the drug is widely used, (2) the drug has a narrow therapeutic range, (3) the defective metabolic pathway is quantitatively significant in determining the drug's overall fate in the body (limited alternative clearance pathways), and (4) therapeutic alternatives are limited or absent.

Basic Concepts of Drug Biotransformation

Chemical modification of drugs via biotransformation generally terminates biological activity through decreased affinity for receptors or other cellular targets as well as more rapid elimination. Drug biotransformation is complex; lipophilic compounds may be converted to more hydrophilic products in several ways. In general, several important characteristics distinguish enzymes involved in drug biotransformation from other enzymes. First is the concept of broad substrate specificity: a single isozyme may metabolize various chemically diverse compounds. Second, many different enzymes may be involved in the biotransformation of a single drug (enzyme multiplicity). Third, a given drug may undergo several different reaction types. An example is racemic warfarin, for which at least seven hydroxylated metabolites have been identified and are produced by different cytochrome P-450 isoforms (Rettie et al., 1992).

Drug biotransformation reactions are conveniently classified into phase I and phase II reactions, which generally occur sequentially. Phase I reactions introduce or reveal (by oxidation, reduction, or hydrolysis) a functional group within the substrate drug molecule that serves as a site for phase II conjugation. Conjugation with endogenous substrates (acetate, glucuronic acid, glutathione, glycine, sulfate) further increases the polarity of drugs or their intermediate metabolites and thereby enhances their renal excretion. Interindividual variability is a consequence of the complex interplay among genetic (genotype, gender, race/ethnic background), environmental (diet, disease, concurrent medication, other xenobiotic exposure), and developmental (somatic growth in infants, children, and adolescents; senescence in the elderly) factors. Thus, for any individual, the pathway and rate of a given compound's metabolic clearance are functions of that individual's unique phenotype with respect to the forms and amounts of drug-metabolizing enzymes expressed (Wrighton & Stevens, 1992).

The cytochromes P-450 (CYPs) are quantitatively the most important of the phase I enzymes; these heme-containing proteins catalyze the metabolism of many lipophilic endogenous substances (fat-soluble vitamins, fatty acids, leukotrienes, prostaglandins, steroids, thromboxanes) and exogenous compounds such as drugs. The most recent estimate of the full human complement of CYPs is 56 genes and several pseudogenes (Nelson, 1999). CYPs can be functionally divided into two distinct classes: the steroidogenic enzymes expressed in specialized tissues such as the adrenal glands, gonads, and placenta; and the CYPs involved in the metabolism of drugs, pesticides, and environmental contaminants (see Chapter 6).

CYP **nomenclature** is based on evolutionary considerations and uses the root symbol CYP for cytochrome P-450. CYPs that share at least 40% amino acid sequence homology are grouped into families denoted by an Arabic numeral following the CYP root. Subfamilies, designated by a letter, represent clusters of highly related genes. Members of the human CYP2 family, for example, have greater than 67% amino acid sequence homology. Individual CYPs in a subfamily are numbered sequentially (e.g., CYP3A4, CYP3A5). Cytochromes P-450 important in human drug metabolism are predominantly found in the CYP1, CYP2, and CYP3 gene families (Figure 11-1).

Phase II enzymes include arylamine N-acetyltransferases (NAT1 and NAT2), glucuronosyl transferases (UGTs), epoxide hydrolase, glutathione S-transferases (GSTs), sulfotransferases (STs), and methyltransferases (catechol O-methyltransferase, thiopurine S-methyltransferase, several N-methyltransferases). Like the CYPs, UGTs, STs, and GSTs are gene families with multiple individual isoforms; each isoform has its own preferred substrates, mode of regulation, and tissue-specific patterns of expression (Burchell & Coughtrie, 1997; Rushmore & Pickett, 1993).

Pharmacogenetics of Specific Drug-Metabolizing Enzymes

CYP2D6. The best-studied genetic variation in drug response is the debrisoquin–sparteine polymorphism. The CYP2D6 gene locus is

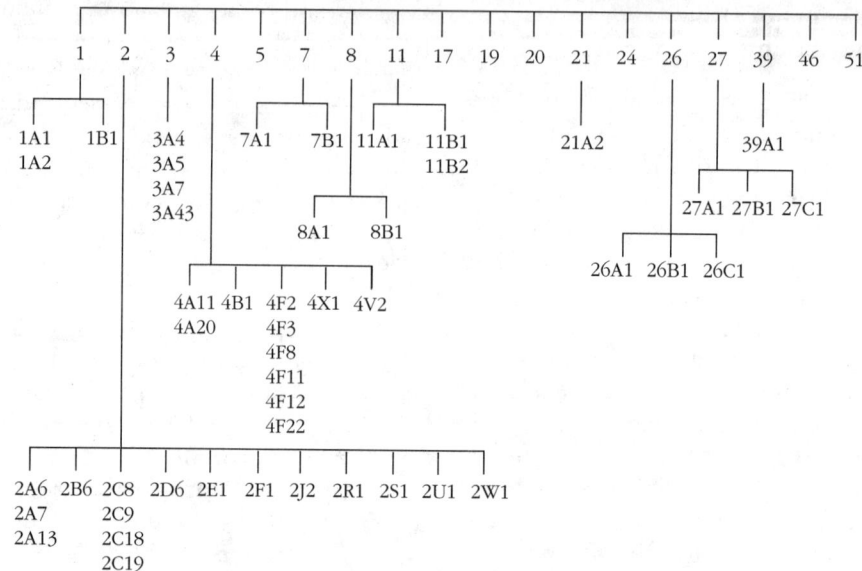

FIGURE 11-1
The Human Cytochrome P-450 (CYP) Superfamily

CYPs that share at least 40% sequence homology are grouped into families (CYP1, CYP2, CYP3 ... CYP51). CYPs with greater than 55% homology are grouped into subfamilies designated by a letter (CYP2A, CYP2B ... CYP2J). Individual CYPs in a subfamily are numbered sequentially (CYP3A4, CYP3A5, CYP3A7). CYPs important in drug biotransformation are found in the CYP1, CYP2, and CYP3 gene families. The other CYP proteins are involved in the synthesis and degradation of endogenous substances such as steroids, fatty acids, fat-soluble vitamins, and eicosanoids. With completion of the draft sequence of the human genome, 56 human CYPs have been identified. A complete listing and human CYP update can be found on the internet at http://drnelson.utmem.edu/human.p450s.html.

highly polymorphic with more than 50 allelic variants (Marez et al., 1997). Individual alleles are designated by the gene name (CYP2D6), followed by an asterisk and an Arabic numeral, i.e., CYP2D6*1 designates, by convention, the fully functional wild-type allele. Allelic variants are a consequence of point mutations, single or multiple base pair deletions or additions, gene rearrangements, or deletion of the entire gene that result in a reduction or complete loss of activity. The CYP2D6 nomenclature presented by Daly et al. (1996) has been widely accepted, and an updated listing of CYP2D6 alleles can be found on the internet (http://www.imm.ki.se/CYPalleles/cyp2d6.htm).

So-called CYP2D6 poor metabolizers possess two recessive loss-of-function alleles: CYP2D6*3, *4, *5, *6, *7, *8, *11, *12, *13, *15, *16, or *18. While poor metabolizers may be homozygous for one particular defective allele (i.e., CYP2D6*4/*4), compound heterozygosity (i.e., CYP2D6*4/*6) is commonly observed. The poor-metabolizer phenotype, found in about 5%–10% of Caucasians and about 1%–2% of Asian subjects, results in inefficient metabolism of more than 40 therapeutic entities, including several ß-receptor antagonists, antidysrhythmics, antidepressants, antipsychotics, and morphine derivatives (Table 11-1). In Caucasians, the *3, *4, *5, and *6 alleles are the most common loss-of-function alleles and account for approximately 98% of poor-metabolizer phenotypes (Gaedigk et al., 1999). Compared to Caucasians, Asian and African-American populations have lower CYP2D6 activities even though the actual incidence of poor metabolizers is less than that observed in the Caucasian population. This apparent paradox is

TABLE 11-1
Some Substrates of Drug-Metabolizing Enzymes in Humans[a]

ENZYME	SUBSTRATE[b]
CYP1A2	Caffeine, clozapine, imipramine, theophylline, R-warfarin
CYP2C9	Fluoxetine,[c] fluvoxamine, ibuprofen (and other nonsteroidal anti-inflammatory drugs), irbesartan, losartan, phenytoin, sertraline, tetrahydrocannabinol, tolbutamide, torsemide, S-warfarin
CYP2C19	Citalopram, diazepam, imipramine, omeprazole[c] (5-hydroxylation)
CYP2D6	Amitriptyline, clomipramine, codeine, desipramine, dextromethorphan, encainide, fenfluramine, flecainide, fluoxetine,[d] fluvoxamine, haloperidol, hydrocodone, imipramine, metoprolol (and other beta adrenergic blockers), nortriptyline, oxycodone, paroxetine, perphenazine, propafenone, risperidone, thioridazine, tramadol
CYP3A4	Alfentanil, alprazolam, amiodarone, astemizole, budesonide, bupropion, carbamazepine, cisapride, cyclosporine, diazepam, diltiazem, erythromycin, ethinyl estradiol, ethosuximide, etoposide, fentanyl, ifosphamide, imipramine, lidocaine, loratidine, lovastatin, meperidine, methadone, midazolam, nefazodone, nifedipine, omeprazole[d] (S-oxidation), quinidine, sertraline, tacrolimus, teniposide, terfenadine, triazolam, verapamil, R-warfarin
UGT1A6	Acetaminophen
UGT1A8	Propofol
UGT2B7	Morphine, S-naproxen (and other nonsteroidal anti-inflammatory drugs), oxazepam
NAT2	Acebutolol, caffeine,[d] clonazepam, dapsone, hydralazine, isoniazid, nitrazepam, procainamide, sulfonamides
TPMT	Azathioprine, mercaptopurine, thioguanine

[a] See also Chapter 6.
[b] Some drugs act as a substrate for more than one CYP isoform.
[c] Quantitatively important CYP pathway.
[d] Secondary pathway.

partially explained by a lower frequency of nonfunctional alleles (*3, *4, *5, *6) and a relatively high frequency of a population-selective allele that is associated with decreased activity relative to the wild-type *1 allele. For example, the CYP2D6*10 occurs in approximately 50% of Asians (Bertilsson, 1995; Johansson et al., 1994) while the *17 allele is present in 30%–35% of black African subjects (Masimirembwa et al., 1996a, 1996b).

Homozygosity for the *10 allele decreased clearance of CYP2D6 substrates such as metoprolol (Huang et al., 1999) and nortriptyline (Yue et al., 1999). Clinical consequences of the *17 allele have been less well studied, but limited in vitro (Oscarson et al., 1997) and in vivo (Droll et al., 1998) data suggest that the intrinsic clearance of CYP2D6 substrates is differentially affected in the presence of the CYP2D6*17 protein. The most common clinically significant consequence of polymorphic CYP2D6 activity is drug accumulation with resultant concentration-dependent toxicities that are observed in those subjects possessing two nonfunctional alleles regardless of ethnic origin. A less common consequence of deficient CYP2D6 activity is the potential for lack of efficacy or therapeutic failure from drugs such as codeine (Sindrup & Brøsen, 1995) and tramadol (Poulsen et al., 1996) that depend on functional CYP2D6 activity for conversion to the pharmacologically active species.

CYP2C19. Originally observed as a marked inability to 4'-hydroxylate the S-enantiomer of mephenytoin, CYP2C19 or mephenytoin hydroxylase deficiency is present in 3%–5% of the Caucasian population and in approximately 20% of Asians. As is the case for CYP2D6, a poor-metabolizer phenotype is conferred by inheritance of two recessive loss-of-function alleles. At least five defective alleles have been identified (Ibeanu et al., 1998). The two most common variant alleles, CYP2C19*2 and *3, result from single base substitutions that introduce premature stop codons and consequently truncated polypeptide chains that possess no functional activity (Goldstein & de Morais, 1994). Several additional alleles that are associated with severely reduced or no functional activity have also been described and an updated listing can be found at http://www.imm.ki.se/CYPalleles/cyp2c19.htm.

Relatively few therapeutic agents depend on CYP2C19 for elimination compared with

CYP2D6 and CYP3A4 (Table 11-1). As a result, its clinical impact is less than that of CYP2D6 deficiency, particularly in Caucasians. However, pronounced pharmacodynamic effects may follow administration of CYP2C19 substrates (omeprazole in Asians) because of the considerably higher frequency of CYP2C19 poor metabolizers in these populations (Furuta et al., 1999). However, as in the case of CYP2D6, drug accumulation and the risk of concentration-dependent toxicity remain the most important consequences of CYP2C19 deficiency.

CYP2C9. Impaired metabolism of several CYP2C9 substrates has also been observed in treated populations, specifically for drugs with low therapeutic indexes (phenytoin [Kutt et al., 1964], tolbutamide [Bhasker et al., 1997; Sullivan-Klose et al., 1996], warfarin [Steward et al., 1997]). Three allelic variants have been observed in population studies. In contrast to the situation for CYP2C19 and CYP2D6, the two mutant allelic variants of CYP2C9 (CYP2C9*2 and *3, *4 and *5) code for proteins with functional, albeit it reduced, activity (Dickman et al., 2001; Stubbins et al., 1996; Sullivan-Klose et al., 1996). Single nucleotide polymorphisms result in amino acid substitutions at position 144 of the CYP2C9 protein for CYP2C9*2, at position 359 for CYP2C9*3 and CYP2C9*4, and at position 360 for CYP2C9*5. Using *S*-warfarin 7-hydroxylation as a measure of CYP2C9 activity, the CYP2C9*2 protein is associated with approximately 5.5-fold decreased intrinsic clearance relative to the wild-type enzyme (Rettie et al., 1994). The conservative isoleucine to leucine change characteristic of the CYP2C9*3 allele occurs within a region of the protein that affects substrate orientation within the active site and, as a result, produces a considerable (27-fold) decrease in intrinsic clearance (Haining et al., 1996). Likewise, clinical and experimental data for tolbutamide (Bhasker et al., 1997), warfarin (Steward et al., 1997), and phenytoin (Mamiya et al., 1998) indicate that the consequences of the CYP2C9*3 allele are likely to be more dramatic than those associated with CYP2C9*2. Given a frequency of approximately 0.07 for the CYP2C9*3 allele in Caucasians (Stubbins et al., 1996; Sullivan-Klose et al., 1996), 0.5% of the population would be homozygous for this allele (CYP2C9*3/*3) and at risk for severe toxicity if exposed to normal doses of substrates with low therapeutic indexes.

CYP2C9*5 appears to be expressed exclusively in Americans of African descent with 3% of individuals carrying this allelic variant. The aspartate to glutamate change at codon 360 results in a protein that has 10%–20% of the activity associated with the fully functional CYP2C9 protein (Dickman et al., 2001).

CYP1A2. CYP1A2 is the sole member of the CYP1A subfamily expressed in human liver. It metabolizes several drugs, procarcinogens (Eaton et al., 1995), and presumably endogenous substrates such as uroporphyrinogen (Lambrecht et al., 1992). Since CYP1A2 activity is responsible for approximately 90% of caffeine systemic clearance (Kalow & Tang, 1993), caffeine has been used extensively to study the pharmacogenetics of CYP1A2 in humans. With caffeine as a phenotyping probe, CYP1A2 activity has been reported to be unimodal (Tang et al., 1994), bimodal (Fuhr & Rost, 1994), and trimodal (Butler et al., 1992). Studies reporting a polymodal distribution analyzed smokers and nonsmokers separately; studies reporting a log normal distribution did not. Smoking increases CYP1A2 activity as do other environmental factors such as consumption of charcoal-broiled beef and cruciferous vegetables. Thus, the analysis of populations with various extrinsic factors capable of altering the activity of a given drug-metabolizing enzyme may mask the presence (or absence) of a specific polymorphism (Eaton et al., 1995). Regardless, CYP1A2 expression shows considerable variability in humans, up to 100-fold or greater for some activities (Butler et al., 1989). To some extent, this variability may be attributed to recently described variation in the regulatory regions of the CYP1A2 gene, resulting in differential inducibility in response to smoking and possibly other inducers (Nakajima et al., 1999).

CYP3A4. The CYP3A subfamily consists of four members in humans (CYP3A4, 3A5, 3A7, and 3A43; Gellner et al., 2001) and is quantitatively the most important group of CYPs in terms of human hepatic drug biotransformation. These isoforms catalyze the oxidation of many different therapeutic entities, several of which are important to pediatric practice (Table 11-1). CYP3A4 is the major isoform expressed in adult liver (Schuetz et al., 1994) and is also abundantly expressed in intestine (Kolars et al., 1994) where it contributes significantly to the first-pass metabolism of substrates such as midazolam (Paine et al., 1996; Thummel et al., 1996). CYP3A5 is polymorphically expressed, being present in approximately 25% of adult liver microsomal samples tested (Wrighton et al., 1989). CYP3A7 is the predominant CYP isoform in fetal liver comprising 30%–50% of total fetal hepatic CYP protein (Wrighton & VandenBranden, 1989).

Several methods have been proposed for CYP3A phenotyping, and the advantages and limitations of each were reviewed (Watkins, 1994). By using these various phenotyping probes, CYP3A4 activity varied widely (up to 50-fold) among individuals but evidence for polymorphic activity has been elusive. The functional consequence of a polymorphism in the CYP3A4 promoter region (Felix et al., 1998; Rebbeck et al., 1998) has not been thoroughly investigated, but it appears to be limited (Ball et al., 1999; Wandel et al., 2000). Several coding region polymorphisms have also been described (http://www.imm.ki.se/CYPalleles/cyp3a4.htm). The CYP3A4*2 allele occurs in 2.7% of Caucasians (Sata et al., 2000) while the frequency of the CYP3A4*3 allele is approximately 1%–4% (Dai et al., 2001; van Schaik et al., 2001). The effects of these polymorphisms on the clinical pharmacokinetics of CYP3A4 substrates have not been evaluated, but in vitro data suggest that clinical significance may be limited (Eiselt et al., 2001). In contrast, newer insights into CYP3A5 expression suggest that its contribution to interindividual variability in CYP3A-dependent drug metabolism may be greater than previously considered (Kuehl et al., 2001).

Other CYP isoforms. Allelic variants of CYP2A6 are associated with amino acid substitutions that lead to deficient or altered catalytic activity (Fernandez-Salguero et al., 1995; Hadidi et al., 1997). However, relatively few drugs used clinically (e.g., nicotine) depend on CYP2A6 as the primary biotransformation pathway. Variability in CYP2E1 expression may be related to variations in the regulatory region of the gene, resulting in differential inducibility in response to ethanol or obesity (McCarver et al., 1998).

Glucuronosyl transferases. Like the CYPs, the glucuronosyl transferases (UGTs) represent a gene superfamily of enzymes that all conjugate their respective substrates with glucuronic acid (Mackenzie et al., 1997). Several mutations in UGT1 genes have been reported. Inheritance of two defective alleles is associated with reduced bilirubin-conjugating activity, giving rise to clinical conditions such as Crigler-Najjar syndrome and Gilbert's syndrome (Mackenzie et al., 1997). Polymorphic activity of UGTs involved in drug biotransformation (UGT2B subfamily) has been suggested (Burchell & Coughtrie, 1997), but the lack of isoform-specific probes analogous to dextromethorphan or debrisoquin for CYP2D6 has hampered investigation.

Arylamine N-acetyltransferases. One of the earliest discovered and most widely recognized genetic polymorphisms is represented by arylamine N-acetyltransferase-2 (NAT2) activity. Approximately 50% of North Americans, of either African or European descent, are phenotypically slow acetylators. This situation places many individuals at increased risk for adverse drug effects such as sulfasalazine-induced hemolysis, hydrazine- or arylamine-induced peripheral neuropathy, drug-induced lupus erythematosus associated with procainamide or isoniazid therapy, and Stevens-Johnson syndrome or toxic epidermal necrolysis associated with sulfonamide administration (May, 1994). NAT2 function is inherited in an autosomal dominant fashion with the inheritance of two slow alleles required for expression of the slow-metabolizer phenotype. The relative proportion of rapid and slow metabolizers varies considerably with ethnic or geographic origin. For example, the percentage of slow acetylators among Canadian Eskimos is 5%, but the level approaches 90% in some Mediterranean populations (Meyer, 1990). According to the standardized NAT2 nomenclature, the wild type and three additional fast alleles give rise to the rapid acetylator phenotype while nine slow alleles have been described. The activity of two additional alleles is unknown (Vatsis et al., 1995).

Thiopurine S-methyltransferase. Thiopurine S-methyltransferase (TPMT) is a cytosolic enzyme that catalyzes the S-methylation of aromatic and heterocyclic sulfur-containing compounds such as azathioprine, mercaptopurine, and thioguanine. While approximately 89% of Caucasians and African-Americans have high TPMT activity and 11% have intermediate activity, 1 in 300 individuals inherits TPMT deficiency as an autosomal recessive trait. TPMT activity is usually measured in blood with activity in erythrocytes reflecting that found in other tissues including liver and leukemic blasts (McLeod et al., 1995b; Szumlanski et al., 1992). In patients with intermediate or low activity, more drug is shunted toward production of cytotoxic thioguanine nucleotides that are required for drug effect. In the small population (0.3%) of treated patients with relative TPMT deficiency, severe and potentially life-threatening myelosuppression can develop with only 10% of the standard thiopurine dose (Lennard et al., 1993, 1997).

Nine different TPMT alleles have been characterized (Otterness et al., 1997). TPMT*1 is defined as the wild-type allele, and the mutant alleles are designated TPMT*2 through TPMT*6. TPMT*3A is the most common mutant allele and is characterized by two nucleotide transition mutations, G460A and A719G, that lead to two amino acid substitutions Ala154Thr and Tyr240Cys (Szumlanski et al., 1996; Tai et al., 1996). Although the *3A allele only has a frequency of 0.03% in the general population, it represents 55% of all mutant alleles. Either mutation alone results in loss of functional activity as a consequence of either loss of protein stability or altered enzymatic activity (Tai et al., 1996). Alleles occurring less frequently include the independent occurrence of the mutations at positions 460 and 719 (designated as TPMT*3B and TPMT*3C, respectively), single nucleotide changes that produce amino acid substitutions in the coding region (TPMT*2, *5, and *6 alleles), and defective intron-exon splicing (TPMT*4 allele) (Krynetski et al., 1995; Otterness et al., 1997). Most recently, a polymorphic locus was identified in the promoter region of the TPMT gene involving four to eight repeats of a specific nucleotide sequence in tandem (Spire-Vayron de la Moureyre et al., 1998). While these repeats appear to modulate TPMT activity when expressed in vitro (Spire-Vayron de la Moureyre et al., 1999), their role in regulating activity in vivo is relatively modest compared to the effect of mutations in the gene coding region (Yan et al., 2000).

The small percentage of patients with low-to-absent TPMT activity is at increased risk for developing severe myelosuppression if treated with routine doses of thiopurines and thus require a 10–15-fold reduction in dose to minimize this risk. Furthermore, these patients may be at increased risk of relapse consequent to inadequate or absent treatment with the thiopurines. Given the expanding use of mercaptopurine and azathioprine in pediatric patients to treat inflammatory bowel disease and juvenile arthritis and to prevent renal allograft rejection, TPMT deficiency is not trivial. In fact, a priori determination of TPMT phenotype or genotype soon may become the standard of care. Anecdotal experience suggests that patients classified as having intermediate TPMT activity frequently require more thiopurine dosage reductions in response to drug-induced myelosuppression. However, the risk of neutropenia or relapse attributable to normal doses of mercaptopurine or azathioprine in such patients has not been extensively evaluated.

Other phase II enzymes. The expression of several additional phase II enzymes is polymorphic in humans, but most are only involved minimally in drug biotransformation or are more important toxicologically. These enzymes include epoxide hydrolase, glutathione S-transferases, sulfotransferases, and methyltransferases (catechol O-methyltransferase, histamine N-methyltransferase, pyridine N-methyltransferase) and will not be discussed further.

Pediatric Considerations

In pediatric patients, genetic and environmental determinants of variability are superimposed on changing development and maturation. These factors further complicate therapy. For example, the weight of a neonate doubles by 5 months of age and triples by 1 year of age, and caloric expenditures increase three- to fourfold over this period. Thus, it is likely that other functions, such as drug biotransformation, undergo profound changes as well. Likewise, the processes occurring during the transition from childhood to adulthood that characterize puberty are exceedingly complex and undoubtedly influence drug biotransformation capacity.

For many years, drug biotransformation capability was considered to be limited at best in the fetus and neonate but to increase over the first year to levels in toddlers and young children that generally exceeded adult capacity. In fact, there are several situations where examination of clinical pharmacokinetic data has revealed discernible patterns of drug clearance related to developmental differences in drug biotransformation. As knowledge of mammalian drug biotransformation processes has increased, it has become apparent that there are developmental differences in expression among drug-metabolizing enzyme families (Table 11-2). Furthermore, individual drug-metabolizing enzymes may have unique developmental profiles (Cresteil, 1998) that influence the response, desired or undesired, to a given drug. Thus, when applied to that proportion of the human population that encompasses the fetus through to adolescence, pediatric pharmacogenetics really seeks to address the changes in phenotype that occur on the background of a fixed genotype as individuals grow and mature.

CYP2D6. While understanding of genetic variation in CYP2D6 activity may exceed that of most other drug-metabolizing enzymes, knowledge regarding its ontogeny is limited. In vitro studies indicate that fetal liver microsomes have limited CYP2D6 activity (approximately 1% of adult values), but CYP2D6 protein is detectable in all samples from neonates up to 7 days of age. Thereafter, both CYP2D6 protein and catalytic activity progressively increase over the first 28 days of life to levels ap-

TABLE 11-2
Developmental Patterns for Drug-Metabolizing Enzymes as Inferred from In Vitro Drug Metabolism Studies and In Vivo Pharmacokinetic Investigations[a]

ENZYME	APPARENT DEVELOPMENTAL PATTERN
CYP1A2	Not present to an appreciable extent in human fetal liver. Adult levels are first reached by 4 months of age and may be exceeded in children by 1–2 years of age. Activity slowly declines to adult levels, which are attained at the conclusion of puberty. Gender differences in activity are possible during puberty.
CYP2C9, CYP2C19	Not apparent in fetal liver. Inferential data using phenytoin disposition as a nonspecific pharmacologic probe suggest low activity in first week of life with adult activity reached by 6 months of age. Peak activity (as reflected by average values for V_{max}) appears to be 1.5–1.8-fold greater than adult values at 3–4 years of age with a gradual decline to adult values by the conclusion of puberty.
CYP2D6	Low to absent in fetal liver but uniformly present at 1 week of postnatal age. Poor activity (~20% of adult) at 1 month of postnatal age. Adult competence attained by approximately 3–5 years of age.
CYP3A4	Low activity in the first month of life; approach of adult levels by 6–12 months of postnatal age. Pharmacokinetic data suggest that adult activity may be exceeded between 1 and 4 years of age. Activity then progressively declines, reaching adult levels at the conclusion of puberty.
UGTs	Ontogeny is isoform specific as reflected by pharmacokinetic data for certain pharmacologic substrates (acetaminophen, chloramphenicol). Generally, adult activity, as reflected from pharmacokinetic data, appears to be achieved by 6–18 months of age.
TPMT	Levels in fetal liver are approximately 30% of adult. In the neonate, activity is approximately 50% higher than in adults with a phenotype distribution that parallels adults. In Korean children, adult activity appears at approximately 7–9 years of age.
NAT2	Some fetal activity present by 16 weeks. Virtually 100% of infants between birth and 2 months of age exhibit the slow-metabolizer phenotype. Adult phenotype distribution reached by 4–6 months of postnatal age with adult activity present by 1–3 years of age.

[a] Data summarized from references presented in the text; CYP = cytochrome P-450; NAT2 = arylamine N-acetyltransferase; TPMT = thiopurine S-methyltransferase; UGTs = glucuronosyl transferases.

proximately 20% of those observed in adults (Treluyer et al., 1991). Preliminary in vivo data using dextromethorphan O-demethylation to dextrorphan as a measure of functional CYP2D6 activity indicate that a phenotype consistent with genotype is achieved by 2 weeks of age (Leeder et al., 1999). However, until these phenotyping data are confirmed by pharmacokinetic studies, neonates should be considered to be poor metabolizers. Dextromethorphan phenotyping data in older children suggest that CYP2D6 catalytic activity comparable to adults is present by 10 years of age and probably much earlier (Relling et al., 1991). In addition, a lower incidence of poor metabolizers was observed in African-Americans (1.9%) as compared to Caucasians (7.7%), similar to the distribution found for American adults of each race.

CYP2C9 and CYP2C19. Phenytoin is used widely for seizure disorders in children and adults. Biotransformation of phenytoin to (*S*)-5-(4-hydroxyphenyl)-5-phenylhydantoin (*S*-HPPH) by CYP2C9 and subsequent conjugation with glucuronic acid represents the principal metabolic pathway by which the drug is eliminated. Phenytoin can also be metabolized by CYP2C19 to yield *R*-HPPH. Under normal conditions, 95% of the HPPH recovered in the urine is the CYP2C9 product *S*-HPPH (Fritz et al., 1987). However, as phenytoin plasma concentrations increase from 5 to 60 µM (from 1.25 to 15 µg/ml), the contribution of CYP2C19 to overall phenytoin biotransformation increases threefold (Bajpai et al., 1996). Nevertheless, changes in phenytoin pharmacokinetics during development provide some insight into the maturation of CYP2C9 function.

In preterm infants, the apparent half-life of phenytoin is prolonged and highly variable (~75 hours) relative to term neonates less than 1 week postnatal age (~20 hours) or term neonates greater than 2 weeks of age (~8 hours) (Loughnan et al., 1977). In vitro, CYP2C9-mediated phenytoin metabolism is saturable (Bajpai et al., 1996). However, saturable phenytoin metabolism does not appear until approximately 10 days postnatal age, suggesting that acquisition of functional CYP2C9 activity is delayed over this period (Bourgeois & Dodson, 1983). Data derived from phenytoin dosage individualization procedures in Japanese children age 6 months to 15 years indicate that the Michaelis-Menten parameter K_m is less than 20 µM (5 µg/ml) in the majority of patients. This finding is consistent with CYP2C9 being primarily responsible for phenytoin elimination in this population (Chiba et al., 1980). Furthermore, while K_m appears to be independent of age in this treated population, V_{max} values declined from 14 mg/kg/day in infancy to 8 mg/kg/day in adolescence. While changes in phenytoin bioavailability may also contribute to this latter finding, cited data indicate that the fractional excretion of HPPH in urine does not vary over the age range studied. This finding implies that the observed reduction in V_{max} is a function of progressively decreasing CYP2C9 activity from infancy to adolescence (Chiba et al., 1980) and would then account for the higher phenytoin dosage requirements (on the basis of body weight) in younger children compared to adults (Leff et al., 1986). Studies with *S*-warfarin (Takahashi et al., 2000) suggest that increased CYP2C9 activity in prepubertal children may be more a function of an increased ratio of liver mass to total body mass in children than to increased expression of functional enzyme (more CYP2C9 molecules per unit area of heptic endoplasmic reticulum, for example).

CYP1A2. The use of prototypic substrates such as caffeine and theophylline has permitted some insight into the changes in CYP1A2 activity during human prenatal development. Functional CYP1A2 does not appear to be present appreciably in either human embryonic or fetal liver (Hakkola et al., 1994; Yang et al., 1995), and activity as measured by caffeine 3-demethylation is very low in neonates. Maturation is delayed compared to other CYP isoforms with in vitro data, suggesting that activity comparable to that observed in adults is achieved by 4 months postnatal age (Cazeneuve et al., 1994).

The developmental profile of caffeine elimination in vivo mirrors that observed in vitro with full 3-demethylation activity observed by

4–6 months of age (Aranda et al., 1979; Le Guennec & Billon, 1987) and possibly delayed in breast-fed infants (Le Guennec & Billon, 1987). Similarly, 3-demethylation of theophylline is also CYP1A2 dependent, but more importantly, 8-hydroxylation to the major metabolite 1,3-dimethyluric acid is also primarily catalyzed by CYP1A2 at physiologic concentrations (Zhang & Kaminsky, 1995). While information concerning the developmental aspects of CYP1A2 activity should be available from theophylline pharmacokinetic data, this is an oversimplification since other P-450s (CYP2E1 and CYP3A4) may also contribute to theophylline 8-hydroxylation. These pathways may, in fact, be quantitatively more important in those individuals with low CYP1A2 activity (premature infants and neonates). Nevertheless, available pharmacokinetic data indicate that theophylline clearance is low at birth and increases linearly over the first year of life (Nassif et al., 1981). A more detailed analysis of theophylline biotransformation suggests that 3-demethylation activity reaches adult levels by approximately 55 weeks postconceptional age (= 4–5 months postnatal age). In older infants and children, theophylline clearance generally exceeds adult capacity (Kraus et al., 1993) as manifested by the higher doses of theophylline required to maintain concentrations in the therapeutic range (Milavetz et al., 1986).

The point at which the relatively higher CYP1A2 activity of children declines to adult levels is not well characterized. Studies using [^{13}C]-caffeine 3-demethylation (caffeine breath test) in adolescents suggests that there are gender-dependent differences in the maturation of CYP1A2 activity. In females, caffeine 3-demethylation decreases to adult levels at Tanner stage II but these levels are not achieved in males until stages IV/V (Lambert et al., 1986). At any pubertal stage, there is considerable intersubject variability, and pubertal stage per se is not necessarily predictive of CYP1A2 activity.

CYP3A4. The term CYP3A is often used to refer to CYPs 3A4, 3A5, and 3A7 collectively since historically, it has been difficult to differentiate one isoform from another based on physical characteristics or catalytic properties. Relatively high levels of a functional CYP3A isoform(s) are present during embryogenesis (days 50–60 of gestation), primarily as catalytically active CYP3A7 (Yang et al., 1994). In vitro studies with fetal liver microsomes indicate that CYP3A activity ranges from 30% to 70% of adult values, depending on the substrate (dextromethorphan or ethylmorphine) used (Jacqz-Aigrain & Cresteil, 1992; Treluyer et al., 1991). Additional in vitro studies using more isoform-specific substrates indicate that CYP3A7-dependent dehydroepiandrosterone (DHEA) 16α-hydroxylase activity is very high in fetal liver and shows maximal activity in the early neonatal period with a progressive decline thereafter. In contrast, CYP3A4 activity as measured by testosterone 6β-hydroxylation is essentially absent in fetal liver, but it increases during the first week of postnatal life (Lacroix et al., 1997).

Interpretation of data obtained in vivo concerning the ontogeny of individual CYP3A isoforms is complicated by issues related to isoform specificity in the biotransformation of putative CYP3A "probes" and tissue-specific localization of CYP3A isoforms (hepatic and intestinal expression of CYP3A4; renal expression of CYP3A5). The relative advantages and disadvantages of several phenotyping measures for CYP3A activity were reviewed (Watkins, 1994). When administered intravenously, midazolam clearance reflects hepatic CYP3A activity (Kinirons et al., 1999). Based on data from a population study of intravenous midazolam pharmacokinetics in critically ill neonates, considerable interindividual variability in midazolam clearance exists in this patient population (Burtin et al., 1994). Clearance (and thus, hepatic CYP3A activity) is markedly lower in neonates (1.2 ml/kg/min in infants <39 weeks of gestation and 1.8 ml/kg/min in infants >39 weeks of gestation) relative to infants greater than 3 months of age (~9 ml/kg/min). Thus, CYP3A activity increases approximately fivefold over the first 3 months of life (Payne et al., 1989). The finding of low concentrations of 1'-hydroxymidazolam in neonates (Burtin et al., 1994) provides further confirmation that functional CYP3A activity is limited in neonates.

Carbamazepine (CBZ) represents an additional therapeutic entity used to follow the maturation of CYP3A function in children since formation of its major metabolite, carbamazepine 10,11-epoxide (CBZ-E), is largely a CYP3A4-mediated process (Kerr et al., 1994). Data from therapeutic drug monitoring databases and pharmacokinetic studies indicate that carbamazepine clearance is higher in children compared with adults (Pynnönen et al., 1977; Riva et al., 1985), thereby necessitating higher doses of the drug on a milligram-per-kilogram basis to achieve and maintain therapeutic concentrations. Korinthenberg et al. (1994) demonstrated that the ratio of CBZ-E to CBZ in plasma decreases over the period spanning the first year of life to 15 years. While factors other than CYP3A4 activity (i.e., microsomal epoxide hydrolase activity) may also influence this ratio, these data are consistent with increased CYP3A4 activity in early childhood with a gradual decline to levels approximating those in the adult around the time of puberty.

Glucuronosyl transferases. The consequences of developmental changes in UGT activity became apparent with the observation that cardiovascular collapse in neonates treated with chloramphenicol (gray baby syndrome) was associated with immaturity of glucuronosyl transferase activity (Weiss et al., 1960; Young & Lietman, 1978). In vitro studies and clinical observations with UGT substrates such as acetaminophen, bilirubin, and morphine are consistent with isoform-specific patterns of development. However, overlapping isoform specificities of available phenotyping probes preclude a clear understanding of UGT ontogeny. Nonetheless, some definable patterns can be inferred from available data (de Wildt et al., 1999).

Conjugation of bilirubin, attributed to UGT1A1, is essentially undetectable in fetal liver but increases immediately after birth and reaches adult levels by 3–6 months of age. Glucuronidation of acetaminophen, a substrate for UGT1A6 and, to a lesser extent, UGT1A9, is impaired in neonates relative to adolescents and adults but is compensated for, to some extent, by increased sulfation. Thus, while the percentage of acetaminophen dose excreted unchanged in urine is similar in neonates and adults, the ratio of glucuronide to sulfate metabolite apparently increases from 0.34 in neonates to 1.8 in adults (Miller et al., 1976). In vitro, fetal liver glucuronidation of morphine, a UGT2B7 substrate, is 10%–20% of that observed in the adult liver (Pacifici et al., 1982). Fetal liver glucuronidation of morphine can be detected in vivo in premature infants as young as 24 weeks of gestation. Morphine clearance is closely correlated with postconceptional age (PCA) and increases approximately fourfold between 27 weeks PCA and term (Scott et al., 1999). Because morphine 6-glucuronide also has analgesic properties, delayed acquisition of morphine glucuronidation activity may have pharmacodynamic ramifications in neonates.

N-Acetyltransferase-2. NAT2 activity can be detected in vitro by 16 weeks of gestation (Peng et al., 1984). When caffeine is used as a phenotyping probe in vivo, all infants between 0 and 55 days of age appear to be phenotypically slow acetylators. In contrast, 50% and 62% of infants between 122 and 224 and 225 and 342 days of age, respectively, can be characterized as fast acetylators (Pariente-Khayat et al., 1991). Maturation of isoniazid acetylation occurs during the first 4 years of life (Pariente-Khayat et al., 1997). Additional studies in normal European children (Hadasova et al., 1990) as well as children of both European and African descent (Evans et al., 1989) confirm that NAT2 phenotypes corresponding to the frequency distributions reported for adults of the same races occur by 3–4 years of age. Thus, NAT2 activity is fully expressed by 3 years of age with competence (as compared to adult values) reached as early as 10–12 months of age.

Thiopurine S-methyltransferase. From a developmental perspective, TPMT appears to be present in human fetal liver at levels approximately one-third those observed in adult liver (Pacifici et al., 1991). In neonates, peripheral blood TPMT activity is 50% greater than in race-matched adults and demonstrates a distribution of activity consistent with the polymorphism characterized in adults (McLeod et al., 1995a). There appears to be a tendency for red blood cell TPMT activity to decrease during childhood. However, no statistically significant correlation with age was observed in a study population of Korean school children (n = 309, 7–9 years of age) in whom TPMT activities were comparable to previously reported adult values (Park-Hah et al., 1996). The higher TPMT activity observed in neonates may well have therapeutic implications, but there are no data to indicate how long this higher activity is maintained or how rapidly adult levels of activity are acquired.

Summary

Cumulative experience with pharmacotherapy in children indicates that it is difficult to prescribe rationally solely on the basis of patient age. Furthermore, the apparent drug biotransformation phenotype may be influenced by disease (infection), exogenous factors (diet, environmental contaminants), and concurrent drug use. However, drug response is a function of the complex interplay among genes involved in drug transport, drug biotransformation, receptors, and signal transduction processes, among others. Completion of the Human Genome Project will result in the enumeration of the sequence of all three billion DNA base pairs of the human genome. There is much anticipation that the established sequence data can be translated into knowledge of how encoded genes and gene products influence the pathogenesis of disease and consequently the development of new therapeutic entities capable of ameliorating these diseases. In this context, optimization of pediatric pharmacotherapy necessarily requires that the developmental regulation of genes involved with drug transport, receptor binding, and signal transduction, as well as drug biotransformation be thoroughly investigated before the promise of pharmacogenetics and pharmacogenomics for rational therapeutics can be realized in children (Evans & Relling, 1999).

References

Aranda, J. V., Collinge, J. M., Zinman, R., et al. (1979). Maturation of caffeine elimination in infancy. *Archives of Disease in Childhood, 54*, 946–949.

Bajpai, M., Roskos, L. K., Shen, D. D., et al. (1996). Roles of cytochrome P4502C9 and cytochrome P4502C19 in the stereoselective metabolism of phenytoin to its major metabolite. *Drug Metabolism and Disposition, 24*, 1401–1403.

Ball, S. E., Scatina, J., Kao, J., et al. (1999). Population distribution and effects on drug metabolism of a genetic variant in the 5′ promoter region of CYP3A4. *Clinical Pharmacology and Therapeutics, 66*, 288–294.

Bertilsson, L. (1995). Geographical/interracial differences in polymorphic drug oxidation. *Clinical Pharmacokinetics, 29*, 192–209.

Bhasker, C. R., Miners, J. O., Coulter, S., et al. (1997). Allelic and functional variability of cytochrome P4502C9. *Pharmacogenetics, 7*, 51–58.

Bourgeois, B. F. D., & Dodson, W. E. (1983). Phenytoin elimination in newborns. *Neurology, 33*, 173–178.

Burchell, B., & Coughtrie, M. W. H. (1997). Genetic and environmental factors associated with variation of human xenobiotic glucuronidation and sulfation. *Environmental Health Perspectives, 105*(Suppl 4), 739–747.

Burtin, P., Jacqz-Aigrain, E., Girard, P., et al. (1994). Population pharmacokinetics of midazolam in neonates. *Clinical Pharmacology and Therapeutics, 56*, 615–625.

Butler, M. A., Iwasaki, M., Guengerich, F. P., et al. (1989). Human cytochrome P450PA (P-450IA2), the phenacetin O-deethylase, is primarily responsible for the hepatic 3-demethylation of caffeine and N-oxidation of carcinogenic arylamines. *Proceedings of the National Academy of Sciences, 86*, 7696–7700.

Butler, M. A., Lang, N. P., Young, J. F., et al. (1992). Determination of CYP1A2 and NAT2 phenotypes in human populations by analysis of caffeine urinary metabolites. *Pharmacogenetics, 2*, 116–127.

Cazeneuve, C., Pons, G., Rey, E., et al. (1994). Biotransformation of caffeine in human liver microsomes from foetuses, neonates, infants and adults. *British Journal of Clinical Pharmacology, 37*, 405–412.

Chiba, K., Ishizaki, T., Miura, H., et al. (1980). Michaelis-Menten pharmacokinetics of diphenylhydantoin and application in the pediatric age patient. *The Journal of Pediatrics, 96*, 479–484.

Cresteil, T. (1998). Onset of xenobiotic metabolism in children: Toxicological implications. *Food Additives and Contaminants, 15*(Suppl), 45–51.

Dai, D., Tang, J., Rose, R., et al. (2001). Identification of variants of CYP3A4 and characterization of their abilities to metabolize testosterone and chlorpyrifos. *Journal of Pharmacology and Experimental Therapeutics, 299*, 825–831.

Daly, A. K., Brockmöller, J., Broly, F., et al. (1996). Nomenclature for human *CYP2D6* alleles. *Pharmacogenetics, 6*, 193–201.

de Wildt, S. N., Kearns, G. L., Leeder, J. S., et al. (1999). Glucuronidation in humans. Pharmacogenetic and developmental aspects. *Clinical Pharmacokinetics, 36*, 439–452.

Dickman, L. J., Rettie, A. E., Kneller, M. B., et al. (2001). Identification and functional characterization of a new CYP2C9 variant (CYP2C9*5) expressed among African Americans. *Molecular Pharmacology, 60*, 382–387.

Droll, K., Bruce-Mensah, K., Otton, S. V., et al. (1998). Comparison of three CYP2D6 probe substrates and genotype in Ghanaians, Chinese and Caucasians. *Pharmacogenetics, 8*, 325–333.

Eaton, D. L., Gallagher, E. P., Bammler, T. K., et al. (1995). Role of cytochrome P4501A2 in chemical carcinogenesis: Implications for human variability in expression and enzyme activity. *Pharmacogenetics, 5*, 259–274.

Eiselt, R., Domanski, T. L., Zibat, A., et al. (2001). Identification and functional characterization of eight CYP3A4 protein variants. *Pharmacogenetics, 11*, 447–458.

Evans, W. E., & Relling, M. V. (1999). Pharmacogenomics: Translating functional genomics into rational therapeutics. *Science, 286*, 487–491.

Evans, W. E., Relling, M. V., Petros, W. P., et al. (1989). Dextromethorphan and caffeine as probes for simultaneous determination of debrisoquin-oxidation and *N*-acetylation phenotypes in children. *Clinical Pharmacology and Therapeutics, 45*, 568–573.

Felix, C. A., Walker, A. H., Lange, B. J., et al. (1998). Association of *CYP3A4* genotype with treatment-related leukemia. *Proceedings of the National Academy of Sciences, 95*, 13176–13181.

Fernandez-Salguero, P., Hoffman, S. M., Cholerton, S., et al. (1995). A genetic polymorphism in coumarin 7-hydroxylation: Sequence of the human CYP2A genes and identification of variant CYP2A6 alleles. *American Journal of Human Genetics, 57*, 651–660.

Fritz, S., Lindner, W., Roots, I., et al. (1987). Stereochemistry of aromatic phenytoin hydroxylation in various drug hydroxylation phenotypes in humans. *Journal of Pharmacology and Experimental Therapeutics, 241*, 615–622.

Fuhr, U., & Rost, K. (1994). Simple and reliable CYP1A2 phenotyping by the paraxanthine/caffeine ratio in plasma and saliva. *Pharmacogenetics, 4*, 109–116.

Furuta, T., Ohashi, K., Kosuge, K., et al. (1999). *CYP2C19* genotype status and effect of omeprazole on intragastric pH in humans. *Clinical Pharmacology and Therapeutics, 65*, 552–561.

Gaedigk, A., Gotschall, R. R., Forbes, N. S., et al. (1999). Optimization of cytochrome P4502D6 (CYP2D6) phenotype assignment using a genotyping algorithm based on allele frequency data. *Pharmacogenetics, 9*, 669–682.

Gellner, K., Eiselt, R., Hustert, E., et al. (2001). Genomic organization of the human *CYP3A* locus: Identification of a new, inducible *CYP3A* gene. *Pharmacogenetics, 11*, 111–121.

Goldstein, J. A., & de Morais, S. M. F. (1994). Biochemistry and molecular biology of the human *CYP2C* subfamily. *Pharmacogenetics, 4*, 285–299.

Hadasova, E., Brysova, V., & Kadlcakova, E. (1990). *N*-Acetylation in healthy and diseased children. *European Journal of Clinical Pharmacology, 39*, 43–47.

Hadidi, H., Zahlsen, K., Idle, J. R., et al. (1997). A single amino acid substitution (Leu160His) in cytochrome P450 CYP2A6 causes switching from 7-hydroxylation to 3-hydroxylation of coumarin. *Food and Chemical Toxicology, 35*, 903–907.

Haining, R. L., Hunter, A. P., Veronese, M. E., et al. (1996). Allelic variants of human cytochrome P450 2C9: Baculovirus-mediated expression, purification, structural characterization, substrate stereospecificity, and prochiral selectivity of the wild-type and I359L mutant forms. *Archives of Biochemistry and Biophysics, 333*, 447–458.

Hakkola, J., Pasanen, M., Purkunen, R., et al. (1994). Expression of xenobiotic-metabolizing cytochrome P450 forms in human adult and fetal liver. *Biochemical Pharmacology, 48*, 59–64.

Huang, J., Chuang, S.-K., Cheng, C. L., et al. (1999). Pharmacokinetics of metoprolol enantiomers in Chinese subjects of major CYP2D6 genotypes. *Clinical Pharmacology and Therapeutics, 65*, 402–407.

Ibeanu, G. C., Goldstein, J. A., Meyer, U., et al. (1998). Identification of new human *CYP2C19* alleles (*CYP2C19*6* and *CYP2C19*2B*) in a Caucasian poor metabolizer of mephenytoin. *Journal of Pharmacology and Experimental Therapeutics, 286*, 1490–1495.

Jacqz-Aigrain, E., & Cresteil, T. (1992). Cytochrome P450-dependent metabolism of dextromethorphan: Fetal and adult studies. *Developmental Pharmacology and Therapeutics, 18*, 161–168.

Johansson, I., Oscarson, M., Yue, Q. Y., et al. (1994). Genetic analysis of the Chinese cytochrome P4502D locus: Characterization of variant CYP2D6 genes present in subjects with diminished capacity for debrisoquine hydroxylation. *Molecular Pharmacology, 46*, 452–459.

Kalow, W., & Tang, B. K. (1993). The use of caffeine for enzyme assays: A critical appraisal. *Clinical Pharmacology and Therapeutics, 53*, 503–514.

Kauffman, R. E., & Kearns, G. L. (1992). Pharmacokinetic studies in pediatric patients: Clinical and ethical considerations. *Clinical Pharmacokinetics, 23,* 10–29.

Kerr, B. M., Thummel, K. E., Wurden, C. J., et al. (1994). Human liver carbamazepine metabolism. Role of CYP3A4 and CYP2C8 in 10,11-epoxide formation. *Biochemical Pharmacology, 47,* 1969–1979.

Kinirons, M. T., O'Shea, D., Kim, R. B., et al. (1999). Failure of erythromycin breath test to correlate with midazolam clearance as a probe of cytochrome P4503A. *Clinical Pharmacology and Therapeutics, 66,* 224–231.

Kolars, J. C., Lown, K. S., Schmiedlin-Ren, P., et al. (1994). CYP3A gene expression in human gut epithelium. *Pharmacogenetics, 4,* 247–259.

Korinthenberg, R., Haug, C., & Hannak, D. (1994). The metabolization of carbamazepine to CBZ-10,11-epoxide in children from the newborn age to adolescence. *Neuropediatrics, 25,* 214–216.

Kraus, D. M., Fischer, J. H., Reitz, S. J., et al. (1993). Alterations in theophylline metabolism during the first year of life. *Clinical Pharmacology and Therapeutics, 54,* 351–359.

Krynetski, E. Y., Schuetz, J. D., Galpin, A. J., et al. (1995). A single point mutation leading to loss of catalytic activity in human thiopurine S-methyltransferase. *Proceedings of the National Academy of Sciences, 92,* 949–953.

Kuehl, P., Zhang, J., Lin, Y., et al. (2001). Sequence diversity in *CYP3A* promoters and characterization of the genetic basis of polymorphic CYP3A5 expression. *Nature Genetics, 27,* 383–391.

Kutt, H., Wolk, M., Scherman, R., et al. (1964). Insufficient parahydroxylation as a cause of diphenylhydantoin toxicity. *Neurology (NY), 14,* 542–548.

Lacroix, D., Sonnier, M., Moncion, A., et al. (1997). Expression of CYP3A in the human liver—Evidence that the shift between CYP3A7 and CYP3A4 occurs immediately after birth. *European Journal of Biochemistry, 247,* 625–634.

Lambert, G. H., Schoeller, D. A., Kotake, A. N., et al. (1986). The effect of age, gender, and sexual maturation on the caffeine breath test. *Developmental Pharmacology and Therapeutics, 9,* 375–388.

Lambrecht, R. W., Sinclair, P. R., Gorman, N., et al. (1992). Uroporphyrinogen oxidation catalyzed by reconstituted cytochrome P4501A2. *Archives of Biochemistry and Biophysics, 294,* 504–510.

Leeder, J. S., Gaedigk, A., Gotschall, R., et al. (1999). Acquisition of functional CYP2D6 activity in the first year of life. *Clinical Pharmacology and Therapeutics, 65,* 176.

Leff, R. D., Fischer, L. J., & Roberts, R. J. (1986). Phenytoin metabolism in infants following intravenous and oral administration. *Developmental Pharmacology and Therapeutics, 9,* 217–223.

Le Guennec, J.-C., & Billon, B. (1987). Delay in caffeine elimination in breast-fed infants. *Pediatrics, 79,* 264–268.

Lennard, L., Gibson, B. E. S., Nicole, T., et al. (1993). Congenital thiopurine methyltransferase deficiency and 6-mercaptopurine toxicity during treatment for acute lymphoblastic leukaemia. *Archives of Disease in Childhood, 69,* 577–579.

Lennard, L., Lewis, I. J., Michelagnoli, M., et al. (1997). Thiopurine methyltransferase deficiency in childhood lymphoblastic leukaemia: 6-Mercaptopurine dosage strategies. *Medical and Pediatric Oncology, 29,* 252–255.

Loughnan, P. M., Greenwald, A., Purton, W. W., et al. (1977). Pharmacokinetic observations of phenytoin disposition in the newborn and young infant. *Archives of Disease in Childhood, 52,* 302–309.

Mackenzie, P. I., Owens, I. S., Burchell, B., et al. (1997). The UDP glucuronosyltransferase gene superfamily: Recommended nomenclature update based on evolutionary divergence. *Pharmacogenetics, 7,* 255–269.

Mamiya, K., Ieiri, I., Shimamoto, J., et al. (1998). The effects of genetic polymorphisms of CYP2C9 and CYP2C19 on phenytoin metabolism in Japanese adult patients with epilepsy: Studies in stereoselective hydroxylation and population pharmacokinetics. *Epilepsia, 39,* 1317–1323.

Marez, D., Legrand, M., Sabbagh, N., et al. (1997). Polymorphism of the cytochrome P450 CYP2D6 gene in a European population: Characterization of 48 mutations and 53 alleles, their frequencies and evolution. *Pharmacogenetics, 7,* 193–202.

Masimirembwa, C., Hasler, J., Bertilsson, L., et al. (1996a). Phenotype and genotype analysis of debrisoquine hydroxylase (CYP2D6) in a black Zimbabwean population. Reduced enzyme activity and evaluation of metabolic correlation of CYP2D6 probe drugs. *European Journal of Clinical Pharmacology, 51,* 117–122.

Masimirembwa, C., Persson, I., Bertilsson, L., et al. (1996b). A novel mutant variant of the CYP2D6 (CYP2D6*17) *gene* common in a black African population: Association with diminished debrisoquine hydroxylase activity. *British Journal of Clinical Pharmacology, 42,* 713–719.

May, G. (1994). Genetic differences in drug disposition. *Journal of Clinical Pharmacology, 34,* 881–897.

McCarver, D. G., Byun, R., Hines, R. N., et al. (1998). A genetic polymorphism in the regulatory sequences of human *CYP2E1*: Association with increased chlorzoxazone hydroxylation in the presence of obesity and ethanol intake. *Toxicology and Applied Pharmacology, 152,* 276–281.

McLeod, H. L., Krynetski, E. Y., Wilimas, J. A., et al. (1995a). Higher activity of polymorphic thiopurine S-methyltransferase in erythrocytes from neonates compared to adults. *Pharmacogenetics, 5,* 281–286.

McLeod, H. L., Relling, M. V., Liu, Q., et al. (1995b). Polymorphic thiopurine methyltransferase activity in erythrocytes is indicative of activity in leukemic blasts from children with acute lymphoblastic leukemia. *Blood, 85,* 1897–1902.

Meyer, U. A. (1990). Genetic polymorphisms of drug metabolism. *Fundamental and Clinical Pharmacology, 4,* 595–615.

Meyer, U. A. (1991). Genotype or phenotype: The definition of a pharmacogenetic polymorphism. *Pharmacogenetics, 1,* 66–67.

Milavetz, G., Vaughan, L. M., Weinberger, M. M., et al. (1986). Evaluation of a scheme for establishing and maintaining dosage of theophylline in ambulatory patients with chronic asthma. *The Journal of Pediatrics, 109,* 351–354.

Miller, R. P., Roberts, R. J., & Fischer, L. J. (1976). Acetaminophen elimination kinetics in neonates, children, and adults. *Clinical Pharmacology and Therapeutics, 19,* 284–294.

Nakajima, M., Yokoi, T., Mizutani, M., et al. (1999). Genetic polymorphism in the 5'-flanking region of human CYP1A2 gene: Effect on the CYP1A2 inducibility in humans. *Journal of Biochemistry, 125,* 803–808.

Nassif, E. G., Weinberger, M. M., Shannon, D., et al. (1981). Theophylline disposition in infancy. *The Journal of Pediatrics, 98,* 158–161.

Nelson, D. R. (1999). Human cytochromes P450. http://drnelson.utmem.edu/human.p450s.html

Oscarson, M., Hildestrand, M., Johansson, I., et al. (1997). A combination of mutations in the CYP2D6*17 (CYP2D6Z) allele causes alterations in enzyme function. *Molecular Pharmacology, 32,* 1034–1040.

Otterness, D., Szumlanski, C., Lennard, L., et al. (1997). Human thiopurine methyltransferase pharmacogenetics: Gene sequence polymorphisms. *Clinical Pharmacology and Therapeutics, 62,* 60–73.

Pacifici, G. M., Romiti, P., Giuliani, L., et al. (1991). Thiopurine methyltransferase in humans: Development and tissue distribution. *Developmental Pharmacology and Therapeutics, 17,* 16–23.

Pacifici, G. M., Säwe, J., Kager, L., et al. (1982). Morphine glucuronidation in human fetal and adult liver. *European Journal of Clinical Pharmacology, 22,* 553–558.

Paine, M. F., Shen, D. D., Kunze, K. L., et al. (1996). First-pass metabolism of midazolam by the human intestine. *Clinical Pharmacology and Therapeutics, 60,* 14–24.

Pariente-Khayat, A., Pons, G., Rey, E., et al. (1991). Caffeine acetylator phenotyping during maturation in infants. *Pediatric Research, 29,* 492–495.

Pariente-Khayat, A., Rey, E., Gendrel, D., et al. (1997). Isoniazid acetylation metabolic ratio during maturation in children. *Clinical Pharmacology and Therapeutics, 62,* 377–383.

Park-Hah, J. O., Klemetsdal, B., Lysaa, R., et al. (1996). Thiopurine methyltransferase activity in a Korean population sample of children. *Clinical Pharmacology and Therapeutics, 60,* 68–74.

Payne, K., Mattheyse, F. J., Liebenberg, D., et al. (1989). The pharmacokinetics of midazolam in paediatric patients. *European Journal of Clinical Pharmacology, 37,* 267–272.

Peng, D. R., Birgersson, C., von Bahr, C., et al. (1984). Polymorphic acetylation of 7-aminoclonazepam in human liver cytosol. *Pediatric Pharmacology, 4,* 155–159.

Poulsen, L., Arendt-Nielsen, L., Brosen, K., et al. (1996). The hypoalgesic effect of tramadol in relation to CYP2D6. *Clinical Pharmacology and Therapeutics, 60,* 636–644.

Pynnönen, S., Sillanpäa, M., Frey, H., et al. (1977). Carbamazepine and its 10,11-epoxide in children and adults with epilepsy. *European Journal of Clinical Pharmacology, 11,* 129–133.

Rebbeck, T. R., Jaffe, J. M., Walker, A. H., et al. (1998). Modification of clinical presentation of prostate tumors by a novel genetic variant in CYP3A4. *Journal of the National Cancer Institute, 90,* 1225–1229.

Relling, M. V., Cherrie, J., Schell, M. J., et al. (1991). Lower prevalence of the debrisoquin oxidative poor metabolizer phenotype in American black versus white subjects. *Clinical Pharmacology and Therapeutics, 50,* 308–313.

Rettie, A. E., Korzekwa, K. R., Kunze, K. L., et al. (1992). Hydroxylation of warfarin by human cDNA-expressed cytochrome P-450: A role for P-4502C9 in the etiology of (S)-warfarin drug interactions. *Chemical Research in Toxicology, 5,* 54–59.

Rettie, A. E., Wienkers, L. C., Gonzalez, F. J., et al. (1994). Impaired (S)-warfarin metabolism catalysed by the R144C allelic variant of CYP2C9. *Pharmacogenetics, 4,* 39–42.

Riva, R., Contin, M., Albani, F., et al. (1985). Free concentration of carbamazepine and carbamazepine-10,11-epoxide in children and adults. Influence of age and phenobarbitone co-medication. *Clinical Pharmacokinetics, 10,* 524–531.

Rushmore, T. H., & Pickett, C. B. (1993). Glutathione S-transferases, structure, regulation, and therapeutic implications. *Journal of Biological Chemistry, 268,* 11475–11478.

Sata, F., Sapone, A., Elizondo, G., et al. (2000). CYP3A4 allelic variants with amino acid substitutions in exons 7 and 12: Evidence for an allelic variant with altered catalytic activity. *Clinical Pharmacology and Therapeutics, 67,* 48–56.

Schuetz, J. D., Beach, D. L., & Guzelian, P. S. (1994). Selective expression of cytochrome P450 CYP3A mRNAs in embryonic and adult human liver. *Pharmacogenetics, 4,* 11–20.

Scott, C. S., Riggs, K. W., Ling, E. W., et al. (1999). Morphine pharmacokinetics and pain assessment in premature newborns. *The Journal of Pediatrics, 135,* 423–429.

Sindrup, S. H., & Brøsen, K. (1995). The pharmacogenetics of codeine hypoalgesia. *Pharmacogenetics, 5*, 335–346.

Spire-Vayron de la Moureyre, C., Debuysère, H., Fazio, F., et al. (1999). Characterization of a variable number tandem repeat region in the thiopurine S-methyltransferase gene promoter. *Pharmacogenetics, 9*, 189–198.

Spire-Vayron de la Moureyre, C., Debuysère, H., Mastain, B., et al. (1998). Genotypic and phenotypic analysis of the polymorphic thiopurine S-methyltransferase gene (TPMT) in a European population. *British Journal of Pharmacology, 125*, 879–887.

Steward, D. J., Haining, R. L., Henne, K. R., et al. (1997). Genetic association between sensitivity to warfarin and expression of CYP2C9*3. *Pharmacogenetics, 7*, 361–367.

Stubbins, M. J., Harries, L. W., Smith, G., et al. (1996). Genetic analysis of the human cytochrome P450 CYP2C9 locus. *Pharmacogenetics, 6*, 429–439.

Sullivan-Klose, T. H., Ghanayem, B. I., Bell, D. A., et al. (1996). The role of the CYP2C9-Leu359 allelic variant in the tolbutamide polymorphism. *Pharmacogenetics, 6*, 341–349.

Szumlanski, C. L., Honchel, R., Scott, M. C., et al. (1992). Human liver thiopurine methyltransferase pharmacogenetics: Biochemical properties, liver erythrocyte correlation and presence of isozymes. *Pharmacogenetics, 2*, 148–159.

Szumlanski, C., Otterness, D., Her, C., et al. (1996). Thiopurine methyltransferase pharmacogenetics: Human gene cloning and characterization of a common polymorphism. *DNA and Cell Biology, 15*, 17–30.

Tai, H.-L., Krynetski, E. Y., Yates, C. R., et al. (1996). Thiopurine S-methyltransferase deficiency: Two nucleotide transitions define the most prevalent mutant allele associated with loss of catalytic activity in Caucasians. *American Journal of Human Genetics, 58*, 694–702.

Takahashi, H., Ishikawa, S., Nomoto, S., et al. (2000). Developmental changes in pharmacokinetics and pharmacodynamics of warfarin enantiomers in Japanese children. *Clinical Pharmacology and Therapeutics, 68*, 541–555.

Tang, B.-K., Zhou, Y., Kadar, D., et al. (1994). Caffeine as a probe for CYP1A2 activity: Potential influence of renal factors on urinary phenotypic trait measurements. *Pharmacogenetics, 4*, 117–124.

Thummel, K. E., O'Shea, D., Paine, M. F., et al. (1996). Oral first-pass elimination of midazolam involves both gastrointestinal and hepatic CYP3A-mediated metabolism. *Clinical Pharmacology and Therapeutics, 59*, 491–502.

Treluyer, J.-M., Jacqz-Aigrain, E., Alvarez, F., et al. (1991). Expression of CYP2D6 in developing human liver. *European Journal of Biochemistry, 202*, 583–588.

Van Schaik, R. H. N., de Wildt, S. N., Brosens, R., et al. (2001). The CYP3A4*3 allele: Is it really rare? *Clinical Chemistry, 47*, 1104–1106.

Vatsis, K. P., Weber, W. W., Bell, D. A., et al. (1995). Nomenclature for N-acetyltransferases. *Pharmacogenetics, 5*, 1–17.

Wandel, C., Witte, J. S., Hall, J. M., et al. (2000). CYP3A activity in African American and European American men. Population differences and functional effect of the CYP3A4*1B 5'-promoter region polymorphism. *Clinical Pharmacology and Therapeutics, 68*, 82–91.

Watkins, P. B. (1994). Noninvasive tests of CYP3A enzymes. *Pharmacogenetics, 4*, 171–184.

Weiss, C. F., Glazko, A. J., Westin, J. K., et al. (1960). Chloramphenicol in the newborn infant. A physiologic explanation of its toxicity when given in excessive doses. *New England Journal of Medicine, 262*, 787–794.

Wrighton, S. A., & Stevens, J. C. (1992). The human hepatic cytochromes P450 involved in drug metabolism. *CRC Critical Reviews in Toxicology, 22*, 1–21.

Wrighton, S. A., & VandenBranden, M. (1989). Isolation and characterization of human fetal liver cytochrome P450HLp2: A third member of the P450III gene family. *Archives of Biochemistry and Biophysics, 268*, 144–151.

Wrighton, S. A., Ring, B. J., Watkins, P. B., et al. (1989). Identification of a polymorphically expressed member of the human cytochrome P-450III family. *Molecular Pharmacology, 36*, 97–105.

Yan, L., Zhang, S., Eiff, B., et al. (2000). Thiopurine methyltransferase polymorphic tandem repeat: Genotype-phenotype correlation analysis. *Clinical Pharmacology and Therapeutics, 68*, 210–219.

Yang, H.-Y. L., Lee, Q. P., Rettie, A. E., et al. (1994). Functional cytochrome P4503A isoforms in human embryonic tissues: Expression during organogenesis. *Molecular Pharmacology, 46*, 922–928.

Yang, H.-Y. L., Namkung, M. J., & Juchau, M. R. (1995). Expression of functional cytochrome P4501A1 in human embryonic hepatic tissues during organogenesis. *Biochemical Pharmacology, 49*, 717–726.

Young III, W. S., & Lietman, P. S. (1978). Chloramphenicol glucuronyl transferase: Assay, ontogeny and inducibility. *Journal of Pharmacology and Experimental Therapeutics, 204*, 203–211.

Yue, Q.-Y., Zhong, Z.-H., Tybring, G., et al. (1999). Pharmacokinetics of nortriptyline and its 10-hydroxy metabolite in Chinese subjects of different CYP2D6 genotypes. *Clinical Pharmacology and Therapeutics, 64*, 384–390.

Zhang, Z.-Y., & Kaminsky, L. S. (1995). Characterization of human cytochromes P450 involved in theophylline 8-hydroxylation. *Biochemical Pharmacology, 50*, 205–211.

12

Pediatric Antineoplastic Drug Therapy

Norman J. Lacayo, Tina Baggott, and Branimir I. Sikic

Until the 1950s most drug dosages used for children were simply "smaller" adult dosages. Unfortunately this approach to pediatric drug dosing resulted in many adverse drug reactions (ADRs). In 1962, the U.S. Food and Drug Administration (FDA) introduced regulations to require safety and efficacy studies among children prior to the approval of drugs for pediatric use. However, by 1992, less than 25% of drugs used in the United States had been tested for safety and efficacy in children (Yaffe & Aranda, 1992).

In contrast, the development and use of antineoplastic drugs for children have been quite different. Sidney Farber and colleagues at the Children's Hospital in Boston (Laszlo, 1995) pioneered the use of antineoplastic drugs for the treatment of childhood leukemia in 1948. The outcome of these clinical studies over the next three decades guided the development of multidrug pediatric antineoplastic drug therapy (for childhood acute lymphoblastic leukemia [ALL], Burkitt's lymphoma), adjuvant therapy (for Wilms' tumor), regional therapy (for intrathecal CNS prophylaxis in childhood leukemia), and neoadjuvant therapy (for osteosarcoma).

In North America (Canada and the U.S.) more than 80% of children with cancer participate in clinical trials sponsored by the Children's Oncology Group (COG, formerly the Children's Cancer Group; the Intergroup Rhabdomyosarcoma Study; the National Wilms' Tumor Study; and the Pediatric Oncology Group). This cooperative group, sponsored by the U.S. National Cancer Institute, includes more than 237 affiliated hospitals in North America and elsewhere.

The participation of children in clinical trials has enabled the rigorous testing of the efficacy of multidrug antineoplastic regimens; the identification of drugs active in specific diseases; and the reduction of long-term toxicity by modifying drug combinations, dosages, and duration of therapy. This research has resulted in a nearly 70% cure rate and a prolonged disease-free survival for most children diagnosed with cancer (SEER Data, NCI, 1999). Furthermore, the outcome of children enrolled in clinical protocols is better than those treated off protocol.

In contrast to the early pioneering work by pediatric oncologists, more recently, the development of new antineoplastic drugs for children has lagged behind that for adults because pediatric patients represent less than 1% of newly diagnosed cases of cancer. Due to high cure rates and prolonged disease-free survival, only a few hundred children are eligible for phase I studies every year. Usually only the most promising antineoplastic drugs identified in adult phase I trials are chosen for

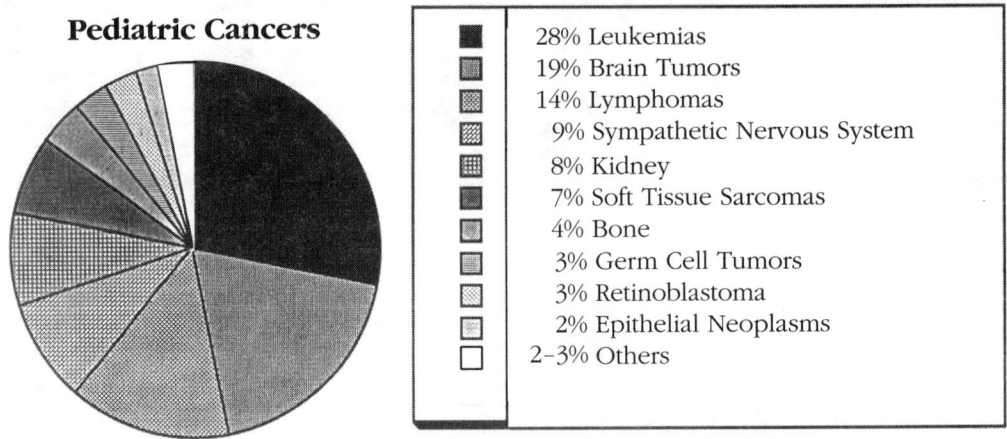

FIGURE 12-1
Relative Incidence of Pediatric Cancers
(adapted from SEER Data, 1974–1993)

pediatric studies. To address this disparity, clinical researchers are incorporating the use of pharmacologically guided dosing and biological surrogate markers to better evaluate the efficacy of new drugs.

There are more than 10,000 new cases of various types of childhood cancer (Figure 12-1) diagnosed every year in North America. The care of children with cancer is provided by a multidisciplinary team involving pediatric medical subspecialists in hematology-oncology, radiation oncology, surgery, and anesthesiology, as well as nurse practitioners, nurses, pharmacists, psychologists, dietitians, and physical and occupational therapists dedicated to the special needs of these children.

Most children are enrolled in open phase III clinical trials or treated according to the superior arm from a completed phase III trial.[1] Antineoplastic drug regimens are outlined in these protocols and should be prescribed and administered as outlined. All prescribed orders for antineoplastic drug therapy should be written by pediatric oncologists and countersigned, usually by another physician. A variety of salvage protocols or "standard of care" therapies[2] have been published in peer-reviewed journals and are available to those who care for children with cancer. These resources are used for the formulation of a therapeutic plan when a patient is ineligible for a clinical trial, refuses participation in a clinical trial, or when no open clinical trial is available at the time of diagnosis. Because most of these protocols are used in multiple institutions, strict adherence is required and they should be modified only as allowed by the instructions in the protocol. In the event of toxicity, dosage modifications are allowed. In addition, other changes are permitted by the principal investigators responsible for these studies to assure optimal patient care. When patients are taken off study, their therapy may follow the current standard of care for their specific disease. Various salvage protocols may be used if the cancer recurs. A limited number of phase I studies are available for patients with refractory cancers.

The information presented in this chapter serves as a guide to the indications, usual

---

1. Phase I trials evaluate the safety and usually identify the maximum tolerated dose (MTD) and dose-limiting toxicity (DLT) of a new drug. Phase II trials test the efficacy of a new drug in a general or specific disease category. Phase III trials test a new drug in a randomized fashion to determine whether or not it increases overall survival (OS).

2. "Salvage protocols" are used to denote combination antineoplastic drug protocols commonly used to treat relapsed patients in order to achieve a second remission. "Standard of care" is used to denote what is considered by experts in the field as the best therapy available and most commonly used.

dosages, dosage forms, and ADRs of specific antineoplastic drugs. These drugs have a narrow therapeutic index and effective doses usually cause severe ADRs, some of them life threatening. Any physician or nurse practitioner participating in the care of children with cancer must be fully familiar with the indications, appropriate dosage, and ADRs of the antineoplastic drugs administered to their patients. In addition, they should be familiar with special considerations regarding age; weight; variations in drug absorption, distribution, metabolism, and excretion secondary to both age and coexisting medical problems (*see also* Chapter 10); and possible pharmacokinetic interactions (*see also* Chapter 6). All members of the team (nurses, pharmacists, physicians) should review antineoplastic drug therapy orders in the patient's chart as well as at the bedside to avoid errors with drug selection, doses, or dosing schedules.

Supportive care guidelines that deal with hydration and urine output requirements, use of drugs to ameliorate toxicity (e.g., antiemetics), therapeutic drug monitoring, and the use of hematopoietic growth factors also should be reviewed carefully. Discussions of drug classification, mechanisms of action, and mechanisms of drug resistance are beyond the scope of this chapter, but the class to which each antineoplastic drug belongs is included.

Pediatric Considerations

The cornerstone of pediatrics is the prevention and treatment of disease in order to foster the normal growth and development of children. The use of antineoplastic drug therapy in infants, children, and adolescents with cancer presents many challenges to the pediatric oncologist who strives to maintain a balance between using antineoplastic drugs to their full efficacy while minimizing their short- and long-term toxicities.

Effects of Antineoplastic Drugs on Growth and Development

Pediatric clinicians need to understand the various effects of antineoplastic drug therapy on the different stages and milestones of growth and development during infancy and childhood. For example, the ototoxicity of cisplatin and carboplatin may affect language development, the neurotoxicity of vincristine may interfere with motor development, refractory nausea and emesis may lead to food aversion, and subtle neuropsychological sequelae associated with the use of methotrexate may require long-term follow-up in survivors of childhood leukemia. Appropriate assessment and intervention from pediatricians, psychologists, nurses, dietitians, and occupational therapists are all necessary to help children and their families cope with and overcome these acute and late complications of antineoplastic drug therapy.

Physiologic Processes during Growth and Development

Understanding how physiologic processes during infancy and childhood affect the pharmacokinetics and pharmacodynamics of drugs is equally important. As these physiologic processes mature in neonates, infants, and children, they significantly alter drug disposition (*see* Chapter 10).

Absorption is determined by gastric acidity, gastric emptying time, GI motility, pancreatic enzyme activity, and GI surface area. In children younger than 1 year, these factors may increase the absorption of orally administered drugs.

Total body water (TBW), albumin, and fat composition vary during infancy, childhood, and adolescence. TBW, extracellular fluid (ECF), blood volume, and fat composition do not approach adult levels until adolescence. TBW and ECF volumes are important compartments for drug distribution. They correlate with body surface area (BSA), which is commonly used to determine antineoplastic dosages. Since BSA is larger in relation to an infant's weight, dose calculation by BSA results in a larger dose per weight when compared to older children and adults. In spite of this, it is unwise to have generalized recommendations on dosage adjustment for infants and children since any rational rule should be based on the pharmacokinetic behavior of each individual drug. Protein binding is also lower during the first year of life; thus, an increased amount of unbound drug is available for interaction with its target(s) or receptor(s).

Drug **metabolism** and **excretion** generally are decreased during the first year of life, resulting in the delayed metabolic clearance and decreased biliary excretion of many drugs (e.g., vinca alkaloids, anthracyclines). Hepatic dysfunction also affects the metabolism of numerous drugs. Elevated alkaline phosphatase or elevated bilirubin serum concentrations generally correlate with compromised hepatic function. Drugs excreted via the kidneys can have limited clearance in young infants because of immature renal function and because the amount of cardiac output that reaches the kidneys is only 5% compared to 25% in an older child or adult.

Genetic polymorphisms that affect drug metabolism and/or elimination have been identified because of their differing frequency in ethnic or racial groups (see Chapter 11). One well-described example is a **polymorphism** that affects N-acetyltransferase activity. The activity of this enzyme affects the elimination of isoniazid. For example, patients with the slow-acetylator phenotype are at higher risk for neurotoxicity (Weber & Hein, 1985) because they do not efficiently modify the parent drug to make it more water soluble and, hence, to facilitate renal clearance. A more poignant example has been the discovery of mercaptopurine therapy intolerance and heterozygosity at the thiopurine S-methyltransferase (TPMT) gene locus. Children with TPMT deficiency (two mutant alleles) or heterozygous for TPMT (one mutant allele) can exhibit mild-to-profound intolerance to mercaptopurine or thioguanine (Relling et al., 1999). In addition, when TPMT-deficient patients receive cranial radiotherapy and antimetabolite therapy, they suffer a higher incidence of secondary brain tumors. Many lessons regarding drug metabolism and disposition and their relationship to drug efficacy and toxicity remain to be learned. In fact, what has traditionally been known as idiosyncratic drug reactions most likely represent the interaction of one or several polymorphisms that affect drug metabolism and excretion.

Disposition of Antineoplastic Drugs in Children

Generally, there is a lack of data concerning the disposition of most antineoplastic drugs in infants and young children. However, guidelines are available for cytarabine, doxorubicin, etoposide, mercaptopurine, methotrexate, teniposide, and vincristine. The caveat for most of these recommendations is that only a small number of infants were included in the studies used to formulate these recommendations (McLeod et al., 1992). In addition, not all studies included analysis of plasma protein binding, systemic clearance of unbound drug, and other relevant factors. The available pharmacokinetic studies reported that cytarabine, etoposide, mercaptopurine, and teniposide may be dosed using BSA criteria in children who are less than 2 years of age. For methotrexate, although there is a reduced clearance in infants, the lack of increased toxicity obviates the need to adjust the drug dose. In contrast, there is evidence of increased toxicity with vincristine, doxorubicin, and dactinomycin, requiring dose adjustment by weight rather than BSA for both infants and children less than 2 years of age and those with a BSA less than 0.5 m^2. Excess toxicity with dactinomycin was reported in the second National Wilms' Tumor Study; in subsequent studies, excess toxicity was eliminated by using weight rather than BSA for dose calculation (D'Angio, 1987).

Intrathecal Therapy

The importance of age-related anatomical differences was demonstrated in studies of intrathecal therapy in children by Bleyer (1977). There is no correlation between the BSA and volume of cerebrospinal fluid (CSF) in children. The CSF volume reaches adult levels by 4–6 years of age, while BSA reaches adult values by 16–18 years of age. The dosing of intrathecal chemotherapy (methotrexate, cytarabine, or a combination of methotrexate, cytarabine, and hydrocortisone) is based solely on age.

Renal Toxicity

Ifosfamide, and less frequently cyclophosphamide, can cause renal tubular injury manifested as Fanconi syndrome, metabolic acidosis, hypokalemia, hypomagnesemia, proteinuria, and rickets (Cachat & Guignard, 1996). The chronic nature of these injuries may interfere with normal growth and development and, thus, requires close follow-up and appropriate intervention (e.g., counseling, psychotherapy). Cisplatin and less frequently carboplatin can cause glomerular injury manifested as acute or chronic decreased glomerular filtration rate (Cachat & Guignard, 1996). Pediatric patients who are either less than 3 years of age or receiving a cumulative dose of ifosfamide greater than 45 grams/m^2 appear to be at particular risk for nephrotoxicity (Loebstein et al., 1999; Raney et al., 1994).

The use of ifosfamide in pediatric patients with pre-existing renal abnormalities should only be contemplated if the potential benefit of use clearly outweighs the risk of further nephrotoxicity. There are case reports documenting the reversibility of ifosfamide nephrotoxic injury in some patients; however, the long-term outlook for most patients is unknown. Several antineoplastic drugs (carboplatin, cisplatin, cyclophosphamide, ifosfamide, methotrexate) require prehydration to achieve adequate renal perfusion, urine filtration, and bladder flow and, consequently, to avoid delayed renal excretion and associated bladder toxicity.

Cardiotoxicity

The heart is another organ at risk of early and late toxicity associated with pediatric antineoplastic drug therapy. Anthracyclines have been used to treat various pediatric cancers. However, the cumulative and peak dose of these drugs can result in restrictive or dilated cardiomyopathy. Children are at high risk because the degree of cardiomyopathy depends on the amount of somatic growth remaining and the duration of survival. The late form of congestive heart failure in survivors of childhood cancer is not entirely related to the total dose received (Grenier & Lipshultz, 1998).

Neurotoxicity

Antineoplastic drug therapy carries with it the risk of neurotoxicity. Several antineoplastic drugs produce neurotoxic effects that need to be considered prior to therapy (Table 12-1).

Myelotoxicity and Infection

The use of high-dose therapy in children commonly results in myelosuppression requiring blood product support. Management of infectious diseases is also important in the pediatric population. Advances in the care and support of the neutropenic and febrile patient have improved the survival of children (Zinner, 1998). Prophylactic antibiotics are commonly used for pediatric patients receiving immunosuppressive therapy to prevent pneumococcal pneumonia or PCP. Oral antifungal agents are also used in most patients with acute myelocytic leukemia (AML) who experience prolonged neutropenia while receiving therapy. (*See* Chapter 14 for additional information.)

Proactive Pharmacologic Intervention

Newer drugs. The use of drugs (e.g., amifostine, leucovorin, mesna) that modify the ADRs of antineoplastic drugs and the availability of hematopoietic growth factors (e.g., filgrastim, sargramostim) have allowed the use of the maximally tolerated doses of many antineoplastic drugs and the development of more dose-intensive protocols.

Emetogenic potential and antiemetics.
Emesis is a major concern with the use of many antineoplastic drugs. Fortunately, significant progress has been made in making it less of a problem. Table 12-2 summarizes the emetogenic potential of many currently used antineoplastics. Table 12-3 provides information on the most commonly used antiemetics including their ADRs.

Antineoplastic drug therapy-associated **nausea and vomiting** are two of the most

TABLE 12-1
Neurotoxicities of Antineoplastic Drug Therapy[a]

AFFECTED AREA	SIGNS AND SYMPTOMS	ANTINEOPLASTIC DRUG(S)
Autonomic Nervous System	Abdominal pain, bladder incontinency/atony, constipation/ileus	Vinblastine, vincristine
Cerebellum	Ataxic tremor, diplopia, horizontal nystagmus, loss of coordination	Cytarabine
Cerebrum	Confusion, level of consciousness, memory loss, mental status changes, seizures	Asparaginase, carboplatin, cisplatin, ifosfamide
	Seizures	Methotrexate
Cranial Nerves		
Abducens, oculomotor, trochlear	Alterations in color vision, diplopia, nystagmus, papilledema	Carboplatin, cisplatin, cyclophosphamide
Auditory	Hearing loss, tinnitus	Cisplatin
Facial	Alterations in taste, facial palsies	Carboplatin, cisplatin, vincristine
Glossopharyngeal	Alterations in taste, dysphagia	Cyclophosphamide
Optic	Loss of vision, papilledema	Carboplatin, cisplatin
Trigeminal	Jaw pain	Vincristine
Vagus	Dysphagia, dysphonia, hoarseness	Vincristine
Meninges	Loss of vision, meningismus, paralysis	Vincristine
Peripheral Nerves		
Sensory	Decreased deep tendon reflexes, decreased sensation, jaw pain, numbness, paresthesia of hands and feet	Carboplatin, cisplatin, cytarabine, etoposide, paclitaxel, vinblastine, vincristine
Motor	Foot drop, muscle weakness	Paclitaxel, vinblastine, vincristine

[a] Adapted from Meehand, J. I., & Johnson, B. L., *The neurotoxicity of antineoplastic agents*, 1992, and *Current issues in cancer nursing practice updates*, 1(8), 2–9.

distressing ADRs experienced by oncology patients (Coates et al., 1983). In addition to patient discomfort, nausea and vomiting can lead to dehydration, electrolyte imbalances, increased toxicity of the antineoplastic drugs, anorexia, weight loss, and noncompliance with treatment. The control of antineoplastic drug therapy-associated nausea and vomiting has improved vastly during the 1990s. The advent of the serotonin antagonists as antiemetics accounts for much of this improvement. However, the control of antineoplastic drug therapy-associated nausea and vomiting remains more of an art than a science. Anti-

(Continued on page 500)

TABLE 12-2
Emetogenic Potential of Antineoplastic Drugs[a]

HIGH EMETOGENIC POTENTIAL (>80% INCIDENCE)	MODERATE EMETOGENIC POTENTIAL (25%–80% INCIDENCE)	LOW EMETOGENIC POTENTIAL (0%–25% INCIDENCE)	VERY LOW OR NO EMETOGENIC POTENTIAL (0% INCIDENCE)
Busulfan (>4 mg/kg/day—BMT dose)	Carboplatin	Bleomycin	Cyclophosphamide (oral)
Carmustine (>15 mg/kg—BMT dose)	Cyclophosphamide (600–999 mg/m^2)	Cyclophosphamide (<600 mg/m^2)	Etoposide (<100 mg/m^2)
Cisplatin	Dactinomycin	Cytarabine (<500 mg/m^2)	Hydroxyurea
Cyclophosphamide (>1000 mg/m^2)	Daunorubicin (>30 mg/m^2)	Daunorubicin (<30 mg/m^2)	Mercaptopurine
Cyclophosphamide (>60 mg/kg—BMT dose)	Doxorubicin (>30 mg/m^2)	Doxorubicin (<30 mg/m^2)	Methotrexate (20–40 mg/m^2)
Cytarabine (>500 mg/m^2)	Fluorouracil (>1000 mg/m^2)	Etoposide (100–300 mg/m^2)	Thioguanine
Dacarbazine	Idarubicin	Fluorouracil (<1000 mg/m^2)	Vinblastine
Etoposide (60 mg/kg—BMT dose)	Ifosfamide	Intrathecals	Vincristine
Mechlorethamine	Lomustine	Methotrexate (<1000 mg/m^2)	
Melphalan (60 mg/m^2 IV—BMT dose)	Methotrexate (>1000 mg/m^2)	Paclitaxel	
	Mitoxantrone	Teniposide	
	Procarbazine	Topotecan	

[a] BMT = bone marrow transplant.

TABLE 12-3
Antiemetics[a]

GENERIC (*TRADE*) NAMES [CLASSIFICATION]	USUAL PEDIATRIC ANTIEMETIC DOSAGE AND ADMINISTRATION	ADRs	COMMENTS
Chlorpromazine (*Thorazine®*) [Phenothiazine]	0.5–1 mg/kg every 6 hr PO/IV/IM as indicated.	Agitation, blurred vision, dry mouth, EPS,[b] hypotension, sedation, tachycardia, urinary retention	
Dexamethasone (*Decadron®*) [Corticosteroid]	10 mg/m² as loading dose, then 5 mg/m² PO/IV every 6 hr as indicated. The total duration of therapy for this indication generally should not exceed 5 days beyond antineoplastic pharmacotherapy.	Fluid retention, hyperglycemia, increased appetite, insomnia, mood swing	Wide variety of dosing for adults in literature suggests lower doses may also be effective. Not used in patients with acute lymphoblastic leukemia.
Dolasetron (*Anzemet®*) [Serotonin antagonist]	1.8 mg/kg/day IV or PO 30 min before the administration of antineoplastic pharmacotherapy. **Note:** Not approved by the FDA or HPB for use among children or adolescents.	Diarrhea, dizziness, fatigue, elevated liver transaminases, headache	
Dronabinol (*Marinol®*) [Cannabinoid]	5–15 mg/m² PO 1–3 hr before the administration of antineoplastic pharmacotherapy. May repeat every 2–6 hr as needed.	Depression, dizziness, dry mouth, hallucinations, mood changes, sedation	
Droperidol (*Inapsine®*) [Butyrophenone]	0.05–0.06 mg/kg IV every 6 hr as indicated. **Note:** Not approved for this indication by the FDA or HPB for use among children or adolescents.	Constipation, EPS,[b] hypotension, sedation	Use only for children > 2 years of age. Use only if other therapies ineffective.
Granisetron (*Kytril®*) [Serotonin antagonist]	10–40 µg/kg/day IV or 1 mg PO twice a day.	Diarrhea, fever, headache, somnolence	Studies suggest larger doses may be needed in children.
Lorazepam (*Ativan®*) [Benzodiazepine]	0.02–0.04 mg/kg PO/IV every 6 hr as needed. **Note:** Not approved for this indication by the FDA or HPB for use among children or adolescents.	Antegrade amnesia, blurred vision, dizziness, hypotension, sedation	Effective for anticipatory nausea; start with lower doses.
Metoclopramide (*Reglan®*) [Substituted benzamide]	1–2 mg/kg IV 30 min pre-antineoplastic drug; then every 2–4 hr as indicated. **Note:** Not approved by the FDA or HPB for this indication for use among children or adolescents.	Agitation, anxiety, depression, diarrhea, EPS[b] (more common in adolescent boys), sedation	May treat concurrently with diphenhydramine 1 mg/kg.
Ondansetron (*Zofran®*) [Serotonin antagonist]	0.15 mg/kg PO/IV prior to and 4 and 8 hr following the first dose as indicated. Available in oral disintegrating tablet (ODT) (*see* Chapter 14).	Constipation, diarrhea, headache, transient increases in liver transaminases	Single daily dose of 0.45 mg/kg effective in adults, but data lacking in children. In adults, also effective to adjust dose related to emetogenicity of therapy, but data lacking in children.
Prochlorperazine (*Compazine®*) [Phenothiazine]	>10 kg: 2.5 mg/dose PO or rectal. May repeat two or three times per day, as indicated. IV use **not** recommended in children.	Agitation, blurred vision, dry mouth, EPS,[b] hypotension, sedation, tachycardia, urinary retention	
Promethazine (*Phenergan®*) [Phenothiazine]	0.25–0.5 mg/kg every 4–6 hr PO/IV or rectal.	Agitation, blurred vision, dry mouth, EPS,[b] hypotension, sedation, tachycardia, urinary retention	Oral form well tolerated for treatment of delayed nausea in home setting.
Scopolamine (*Transderm Scop®*, *Transderm-V®*) [Anticholinergic]	One patch behind ear, approximately 12 hr before the administration of antineoplastic therapy; change every 3 days as indicated. Fixed dose patch **not** recommended for small children. **Note:** Not approved by the FDA or HPB for use among children.	Dizziness, dry mouth, fixed pupil, hypotension	Best if applied at least 12 hr prior to chemotherapy. May ameliorate EPS[b] of phenothiazines.

[a] *See* Chapter 14 for additional information.
[b] Extrapyramidal syndrome.

emetic efficacy has significant interpatient and intrapatient variability. Well-designed, randomized, controlled trials in the pediatric population have not been carried out. Although serotonin antagonists clearly benefit children, the optimal schedule, in regard to both efficacy and cost, of these drugs is yet to be determined. Unfortunately, few drugs seem to be effective for delayed-onset antineoplastic drug therapy-associated nausea and vomiting.

The following guidelines can assist pediatric healthcare professionals in minimizing the antineoplastic drug therapy-associated nausea and vomiting among the children in their care.

- Antiemetics should be scheduled and administered prophylactically. Breakthrough nausea and vomiting are difficult to treat.
- Serotonin antagonists (e.g., dolasetron, granisetron, ondansetron) are the drugs of first choice because they generally have minimal adverse effects. However, these drugs must be used judiciously due to their high cost.
- The antiemetic schedule should be planned considering the degree of emetogenicity and patterns of emesis of the particular antineoplastic drug therapy regimen. Data exist in the adult population to support varying the dose of serotonin antagonist used to match the emetogenicity of the antineoplastic drug therapy (Hesketh et al., 1995).
- The oral form of a serotonin antagonist provides a cost-effective method of using this class of drug. The oral form is less expensive and its use may decrease the need for additional IV supplies. Ondansetron now comes in an oral disintegrating tablet (ODT), eliminating the child's need to swallow a tablet or syrup when he or she may be nauseated.
- Delayed-onset emesis may have a different mechanism of action than acute emesis. Serotonin antagonists lose efficacy several days following antineoplastic drug therapy. Other pharmacologic and nonpharmacologic methods should be implemented to treat delayed-onset vomiting.
- Antiemetics should be started early for patients who experience anticipatory nausea and vomiting. Lorazepam often is effective in this situation.
- Noxious stimuli (e.g., strong smells from foods or cleaning materials, vomiting roommate) should be eliminated or minimized.
- Nonpharmacologic methods to control nausea (e.g., hypnosis, distraction, massage, exercise) should be attempted.
- The intake of small, frequent meals should be encouraged, as tolerated.
- Other possible contributors to a patient's nausea should be examined (metabolic abnormalities, constipation, the use of other drugs [e.g., antibiotics and opiate analgesics], parenteral nutrition, increased intracranial pressure).

Follow-up. Antineoplastic drug therapy is often a long-term process, but the appropriate follow-up should continue, in many instances, for years. Long-term ADRs are of particular interest to pediatric clinicians due to the high cure rate and long-term survival of most patients. The possible effects on growth, development, and reproduction and the risk of permanent damage to the heart and kidneys and the risk of second malignancies are of great concern. One objective of current clinical research is to cure the pediatric patient with the least morbidity possible by modifying toxic antineoplastic drug therapies so that the child survives into adulthood with the best quality of life possible. Table 12-4 provides guidelines for follow-up after completion of a course of antineoplastic drug therapy.

Therapeutic Drug Monitoring

Drug levels are monitored for methotrexate to avoid toxicity and to assess the need for increased hydration or continued rescue with leucovorin. As more is learned about the pharmacokinetics of antineoplastic drugs and their relationship to efficacy and toxicity, the use of pharmacokinetically guided dosing, including therapeutic drug monitoring, may become more common. Individualized antineoplastic

TABLE 12-4
Guidelines for Long-Term Follow-Up after Antineoplastic Therapy[a]

ANTINEOPLASTIC DRUG	TEST/EXAM	BASELINE, THEN AS NEEDED	YEARLY	EVERY 2 YEARS	AS NEEDED
Anthracyclines: Daunorubicin, Doxorubicin, Idarubicin, Mitoxantrone	Echocardiogram			x	
	ECG				x
	CXR				x
Bleomycin	PFTs, CXR			x	
Carmustine	PFTs, CXR			x	
	Creatinine, uric acid	x			
	CBCD		x		
	Male endocrine[b]	x			
	Female endocrine[c] if amenorrheic				x
Chlorambucil	Male endocrine[b]	x			
	Female endocrine[c] if amenorrheic				x
Cisplatin	Audiogram	x			
	Creatinine, magnesium, potassium			x	
Cyclophosphamide	Uric acid		x		
	CBCD		x		
	Echocardiogram	With high dose only			
	Male endocrine[b]	x			
	Female endocrine[c] if amenorrheic				x
Etoposide	CBCD		x	x	
Ifosfamide	Uric acid		x		
	Electrolytes, calcium, phosphate, magnesium	x			
Intrathecal therapy	School performance		x		
Lomustine	Creatinine, uric acid	x			
	CBCD		x		
	Male endocrine[b]	x			
	Female endocrine[c] if amenorrheic				x
Mechlorethamine	CBCD		x		
Melphalan	PFTs, CXR			x	
Methotrexate	LFTs	x			
	Creatinine, uric acid	x			
	School performance		x		
Steroids	Plot growth		x		
	Ophthalmology	x			
	If osteoporosis, growth suppression, or aseptic necrosis is suspected, x-ray site				x
Teniposide	CBCD		x	x	

[a] CBCD = complete blood count and differential, CXR = chest radiograph, LFTs = liver function (enzyme levels) tests, PFTs = pulmonary function tests.
[b] Male (age 14 or older): FSH, LH, testosterone.
[c] Female if amenorrheic: FSH, LH, estradiol.

drug therapy for childhood acute lymphocytic leukemia has been demonstrated to be superior to conventional therapy (Evans et al., 1998). (See Chapters 10 and 14 for additional discussion of therapeutic drug monitoring.)

Guidelines for Use

These guidelines are provided because the reconstitution, administration, and disposal of many antineoplastic drugs have been associated with local (e.g., dermatological and corneal damage) and systemic (e.g., hepatocellular damage) toxicity among healthcare, housekeeping, and other workers who have been exposed to these drugs in their occupational settings.[3] Carcinogenic and mutagenic effects also have been reported among occupationally exposed men and women in addition to teratogenic effects among their off-

---

3. These guidelines apply to both ambulatory and nonambulatory pediatric patient care settings. Following these guidelines will not totally eliminate all exposure and risk (e.g., accidental spills). However, if followed, occupational exposure to antineoplastic drugs should be reduced to the lowest level possible. Occupational expo-

spring.[4] Occupational exposure to the antineoplastic drugs occurs most frequently when antineoplastic drugs are being reconstituted, intravenous equipment is being primed for drug delivery, antineoplastic drugs are administered to patients, and unused drugs and used administration equipment are disposed of. For example, cyclophosphamide has been found in the urine of pharmacy technicians and nurses involved with drug preparation, delivery, and administration. Although direct skin contact with antineoplastic drugs related to inadvertent spills or splashes has been identified as a major route of occupational exposure, exposure also may occur as a result of inhaling aerosolized drug product.[5] For example, concentrations of fluorouracil (up to 90 ng/m^3) were found in room air when the drug was prepared without the use of a laminar airflow hood.

The nature and severity of health consequences related to occupational exposure to antineoplastic drugs result from several interacting factors. These factors include the toxicity of the antineoplastic drug involved in the exposure and the nature of the exposure (ingestion, inhalation, direct skin contact). They also include the general health status of the exposed person (e.g., pregnancy, disease state, drugs being taken), the extent of exposure, and other related factors (e.g., time elapsed between exposure and the implementation of decontamination or emergency care).

These guidelines, when properly followed, limit the exposure of workers to the antineoplastic drugs and, consequently, to their potentially toxic effects. However, no set of guidelines can eliminate all risk for accidental occupational exposure. Therefore, healthcare and other workers (e.g., housekeeping staff) must also be advised of and prepared to follow necessary courses of action (proper decontamination, assessment and evaluation of the effects of occupational exposure, appropriate medical intervention) in the event that occupational exposure does occur.[6]

Reconstituting and Preparing Antineoplastic Drugs for Transport

All antineoplastic drugs are designated as class II biologicals. Thus, they require reconstitution and preparation in a class II biological safety cabinet before delivery and administration to patients.[7] This cabinet should vent to the outside environment and its blower should be left on 24 hours a day, 7 days a week. It should be serviced regularly according to the manufacturer's recommendations. The biological safety cabinet should be located in a centralized area of the hospital or other specially designated and equipped area to decrease the risk for occupational exposure. These areas also should be designed to minimize interruptions that may result in drug errors or contamination. In addition, personal activities (eating, drinking, smoking, applying cosmetics) should be **strictly prohibited**.

All antineoplastic drugs should be prepared by specially trained pharmacists according to manufacturer's guidelines for reconstitution and administration with attention to the following:

- Prepare antineoplastic drugs using aseptic technique.

---

sure may involve different situations (preparation, stocking, delivery, administration, disposal, as well as custodial cleaning of the rooms and areas where these activities occur) and types of workers (physicians, nurses, patient care assistants, pharmacists, pharmacy technicians, housekeepers) in a variety of healthcare settings.

4. *See* Chapter 2 for additional related discussion.

5. Note that these types of exposures, including aerosolization, splattering, and spraying, typically are associated with breaking open drug ampules, transferring the drug by means of syringes and needles or filter straws, withdrawing needles from drug vials, and expelling air from drug-filled syringes.

6. *See also* Chapter 8 for additional information.

7. Horizontal airflow work benches provide an aseptic environment for the preparation of antineoplastic drugs. However, these units provide a flow of filtered air originating at the back of the work space and exiting toward the employee using the unit. Thus, they increase the likelihood of drug exposure to both the preparer and other personnel in the room. Horizontal biological safety cabinets should **not** be used to prepare antineoplastic drugs.

- Protect the work surface with a plastic absorbent pad and replace the pad each day or each shift when drug preparation is completed. In the event of contamination, change the pad immediately.
- Wear disposable closed-front gowns made of lint-free low permeability fabric (Kaycel®, Tyvek®, Saranex®-laminated Tyvek) with long sleeves and elastic or knit closed cuffs during antineoplastic drug preparation.
- Use disposable surgical latex unpowdered gloves when reconstituting and preparing antineoplastic drugs for administration. Change the gloves hourly or immediately if they become contaminated, torn, or punctured.
- Wear a thermoplastic (Plexiglas™) face shield or goggles and use a powered air-purifying respirator (approved by the National Institute for Occupational Safety and Health [NIOSH]) if a biologic safety cabinet is not available.
- Use an aerosol protection device (Cyto-Guard®) to avoid inadvertent exposure to aerosolized drug particles during drug reconstitution or preparation for intravenous delivery.
- Before withdrawing antineoplastic drugs supplied in ampules, tap down the liquid drug from the stem to the base of the ampule before it is broken open.
- When reconstituting antineoplastic drugs supplied in vials, ensure that the powdered drug is "tapped down" from the top and sides of the vial before the diluent is added. This tapping will help to assure that all of the drug is mixed into solution. To avoid drug leakage, vent the vial with a large-gauge needle and use luer-lock fittings. Wrap a sterile gauze around the neck of the vial before inserting the needle and keep the gauze in place for needle withdrawal. Expel air from syringes and inject the drug into the intravenous delivery systems while within the biological safety cabinet.
- Prior to the addition of the drug, attach and prime intravenous tubing and drug administration sets while within the biological safety cabinet.
- Once reconstituted, label the antineoplastic drug delivery equipment (e.g., intravenous infusion device, syringe) according to current regulations and institutional policies and procedures. The label should provide a clear and distinctive antineoplastic drug warning and also note the vesicant properties of the drug.
- After reconstitution and preparation for administration is completed, transport antineoplastic drugs in a container of impervious packing material marked with a distinctive warning label. Personnel responsible for drug transport must be knowledgeable of procedures to follow in the event of drug spillage.

Administering Antineoplastic Drugs

Antineoplastic drugs should be administered by specially trained physicians and nurses who are designated as qualified by current certification guidelines and regulations. Table 12-5 provides guidelines to minimize errors. Before administering antineoplastic drugs, these physicians and nurses should:

- Ensure the accuracy of the prescriber's order for antineoplastic drug therapy in relation to drug name, dose, frequency, and route of administration.
- Ensure that informed consent has been obtained and that any questions have been answered to the satisfaction of the child or adolescent and his or her parents.
- Ensure that appropriate laboratory tests (e.g., hematology, renal function) (see Table 12-6) have been performed and that the results obtained are within acceptable limits.
- Ensure that measures to minimize expected ADRs (e.g., anxiety, nausea, vomiting) associated with antineoplastic pharmacotherapy have been implemented.
- Protect themselves from inadvertent oc-

TABLE 12-5
Strategies to Minimize Errors in Antineoplastic Drug Therapy

- Check the date of the last time that antineoplastic drug therapy was administered and ensure that the patient is correctly scheduled at the correct time for a subsequent dose (i.e., in relation to the current course of antineoplastic drug therapy).
- Ensure that all appropriate laboratory test results are within acceptable limits. If the laboratory tests are performed at an outside facility, ensure that the results are properly recorded.
- Use preprinted antineoplastic drug therapy orders (fill in the blanks), whenever possible.
- If using paper with multiple copies, check to see that all copies are legible. Ensure that key figures such as decimal points are legible on the last copy.
- All orders must include the drug dose, route, dilution, rate, frequency, and date to be administered; protocol week number, cycle number, etc., whether or not patient is enrolled in study (some protocols use investigational agents, available only to those patients on study); pre- and posthydration requirements as necessary; and premedication/reaction medications, as necessary.
- Use generic names, not trade names or abbreviations, for antineoplastic drugs.
- Spell out units rather than "u" (which can be confused for a zero).
- Never trail a whole number with a decimal point followed by a zero (e.g., write 12 not 12.0).
- For numbers less than one, write dose with a decimal point preceded by zero (e.g., 0.12 not .12).
- Use consistent notation in expressing quantifiable units (e.g., if using 1.2 grams, do not change to 1200 mg elsewhere in order).
- Ensure that all antineoplastic drug orders are written by oncology staff and cosigned (one signature should be that of an attending physician).
- Double-check all antineoplastic drug orders (provider should confirm all points [laboratory values, patient weight, proper week in protocol]).
- If an antineoplastic drug is given only on selected days, make this explicit (e.g., write "Day 1 only").
- Include the total antineoplastic drug dose planned for treatment course (e.g., Cytarabine [150 mg/m^2/day] IV as continuous infusion x 3 days = 120 mg/24 hours IV as continuous infusion, with total dose = 360 mg/72 hours).
- Write and check all antineoplastic drug therapy orders in a quiet location, with minimal distractions.
- If writing preprinted orders, individualized roadmaps, or institutional protocols, involve nursing and pharmacy in the development process (nursing and pharmacy should review content to determine feasibility, internal consistency, and clarity of information).

---

cupational exposure to the antineoplastic drug by wearing disposable latex surgical gloves and a disposable gown made with lint-free, low permeability fabric with a closed front and long sleeves with elastic or knit cuffs.

- Protect work surfaces with a disposable absorbent pad. For example, a plastic-backed absorbent pad should be placed under the tubing during antineoplastic drug administration to absorb any leakage of drug or drug solution that may occur during administration.
- Ensure that all settings in which antineoplastic drugs are administered (i.e., home settings, hospital unit drug rooms, patient hospital rooms, physician's offices) have emergency skin and eye decontamination kits available and that relevant safety data sheets are available for guidance in the case of occupational exposure. These sheets also should be readily available in the workplace for all employees who work directly with, or have the potential for inadvertent contact with, antineoplastic drugs.
- Safely administer the antineoplastic drug according to manufacturer's guidelines and approved protocol procedures.
- In the event of accidental exposure, immediately remove contaminated gloves and gowns and discard according to current guidelines, wash the contaminated skin with soap and water, flood an eye that has been exposed to an antineoplastic drug with water or isotonic eye wash for at least 5 minutes, obtain medical evaluation as soon as possible after exposure, and document the incident appropriately.
- Document the administration of the antineoplastic drug according to hospital or other approved guidelines.
- Monitor pediatric patients who have received antineoplastic pharmacotherapy for the occurrence of any ADRs associated with their pharmacotherapy and document these in the patient's chart.
- Any ADRs also should be reported according to adverse drug reaction reporting procedures. (*See* Chapter 5.)

TABLE 12-6
Suggested Monitoring during Antineoplastic Drug Therapy Administration[a]

DRUG	PARAMETER
Amifostine	Electrolytes, particularly calcium; blood pressure (hypotension may be severe requiring saline boluses and placing patient in Trendelenberg position)
Asparaginase	Assess for anaphylaxis, urine/serum glucose, PT/aPTT, fibrinogen, amylase, lipase
Bleomycin	Blood pressure; assess for anaphylaxis; oral mucosa; PFTs
Busulfan	CBCD (expect prolonged nadir); LFTs; assess for seizures with high doses; PFTs
Carboplatin	CBCD (expect prolonged thrombocytopenia); renal function; electrolytes
Carmustine	CBCD (expect prolonged thrombocytopenia); assess administration site for signs of phlebitis; LFTs
Chlorambucil	CBCD; LFTs; PFTs; assess for seizures.
Cisplatin	CBCD; renal function; electrolytes: magnesium; hydration status; audiogram; assess administration site for ulceration.
Cladribine	CBCD; LFTs
Cyclophosphamide	CBCD; electrolytes, particularly sodium; urine output and presence of red blood cells; cardiac function with high doses
Cytarabine	CBCD; assess conjunctiva; neurological status; LFTs
Dacarbazine	CBCD; assess administration site for signs of phlebitis; LFTs
Dactinomycin	CBCD; assess administration site for ulceration; assess any prior radiation site for added toxicity.
Daunorubicin	CBCD; echocardiogram; LFTs; assess administration site for ulceration.
Dexamethasone	Urine/serum glucose; assess for GI distress.
Dexrazoxane	CBCD
Doxorubicin	CBCD; echocardiogram; LFTs; assess administration site for ulceration.
Etoposide	CBCD; blood pressure; assess for anaphylaxis; assess administration site for ulceration.
Filgrastim	CBCD
Fluorouracil	CBCD
Hydroxyurea	CBCD
Idarubicin	CBCD; echocardiogram; LFTs; assess administration site for ulceration.
Ifosfamide	CBCD; electrolytes, particularly potassium, carbon dioxide, phosphate, magnesium, urine for presence of red blood cells
Irinotecan	CBCD; LFTs
Isotretinoin	CBCD; LFTs, triglycerides, cholesterol
Leucovorin	Methotrexate level
Lomustine	CBCD; LFTs
Mechlorethamine	CBCD; assess administration site for ulceration.
Melphalan	CBCD
Mercaptopurine	CBCD
Methotrexate	CBCD; LFTs, methotrexate serum levels with high doses
Mitoxantrone	CBCD; echocardiogram; assess administration site for ulceration.
Prednisone	Urine/serum glucose; assess for GI distress.
Procarbazine	CBCD
Sargramostim	CBCD
Teniposide	CBCD; blood pressure; monitor for anaphylaxis; assess administration site for ulceration.
Thioguanine	CBCD; LFTs
Thiotepa	CBCD
Topotecan	CBCD; LFTs
Tretinoin	LFTs, triglycerides, cholesterol; pulmonary status
Vinblastine	CBCD; assess administration site for ulceration.
Vincristine	CBCD; bilirubin; bowel pattern; assess for paresthesias; assess administration site for ulceration.

[a] Frequency to be determined by drug dose, patient's baseline condition, and previous reaction to chemotherapy. CBCD = complete blood count and differential, LFTs = liver function (enzyme levels) tests, PFTs = pulmonary function tests, and PT/aPTT = prothrombin time/activated partial thromboplastin time.

Regardless of setting, all unused antineoplastic drugs and contaminated equipment should be treated as hazardous and disposed of according to current recommended guidelines. Any unused drug should be returned to the pharmacy for appropriate disposal. Administration sets and other administration equipment (e.g., needles and syringes) should be disposed of intact to prevent inadvertent contact (e.g., aerosolization, spills), and all contaminated needles and syringes should be disposed of in a leak-proof, puncture-proof sharps container, labeled with a distinctive warning label and placed in an appropriately labeled, sealable 4-mil polyethylene bag or a 2-mil polypropylene bag.

Patient Care following Antineoplastic Pharmacotherapy

Healthcare professionals and others who have direct contact with patients who have received antineoplastic pharmacotherapy within the previous 48 hours should wear unpowdered disposable surgical latex gloves and a disposable gown when providing direct personal pa-

TABLE 12-7
Recommended Care for Extravasated Vesicants[a]

ANTINEOPLASTIC DRUG	ANTIDOTE	LOCAL CARE	SPECIFIC PROCEDURE
Cisplatin[b]	1/6 or 1/3 M sodium thiosulfate	Neither heat nor cold proven effective	Mix 4–8 ml of 10% sodium thiosulfate with 6 ml of sterile water for a 1/6 or 1/3 M solution. Inject 2 ml into site for each 100 mg of cisplatin extravasated.
Dactinomycin	Unknown	Cold compresses	Apply immediately for 30–60 min, then periodically for 15 min, at least four times a day for 24–48 hr.
Daunorubicin	Use of topical dimethyl sulfoxide (DMSO) 50%–99% solution is controversial	Cold compresses	Apply immediately for 30–60 min, then periodically for 15 min, at least four times a day for 24–48 hr.
Doxorubicin			If dimethyl sulfoxide used, apply 1.5 ml to the site every 6 hr for 14 days. Allow to air dry; do not cover.
Etoposide[b] Teniposide[b] Vinblastine Vincristine[b]	Hyaluronidase	Warm compresses Elevation	Inject 150 units hyaluronidase with 1–3 ml saline into site. Apply compress for 30–60 min, then periodically for 15 min, at least four times a day for 24–48 hr. Elevate the extremity.
Idarubicin	Unknown	Cold compresses	Apply immediately for 30–60 min, then periodically for 15 min, at least four times a day for 24–48 hr.
Mechlorethamine	1/6 or 1/3 M sodium thiosulfate		Mix 4–8 ml of 10% sodium thiosulfate with 6 ml of sterile water for a 1/6 or 1/3 M solution. Inject 2 ml into site for each milligram of mechlorethamine extravasated.
Paclitaxel	Hyaluronidase	Cold compresses	Apply for 30–60 min, then periodically for 15 min, at least four times a day for 24–48 hr. Inject 150 units hyaluronidase with 1–3 ml saline into site.

[a] Adapted from Dorr, R. T., Pharmacologic management of vesicant chemotherapy extravasation (Table 6). In *Cancer chemotherapy handbook,* 2nd ed., (1994), R. T. Dorr & D. D. Hoff, Eds., Englewood Cliffs, NJ: Appleton & Lange, and *Cancer chemotherapy guidelines and recommendations for practice,* 2nd ed. (Table 11), M. Fishman & M. Mrozek-Orlowski, Eds., (1999), Oncology Nursing Press Inc.
[b] Treatment indicated only for large extravasations (half or more of the planned dose).

tient care or when handling body excretions (e.g., blood, stool, urine, vomitus) from patients. Linen contaminated with body excretions should be put in a specially marked laundry bag that is then placed in an impervious bag marked with a distinctive warning label.

Extravasation. If extravasation is suspected, stop the infusion, and withdraw residual drug, if possible. Then remove the intravenous needle, and administer local care (Table 12-7). Antineoplastic drugs for which extravasation is particularly serious are bleomycin, carboplatin, carmustine, dacarbazine, doxorubicin liposomonal, and ifosfamide.

Dosages. Common antineoplastic drug regimens used in the treatment of pediatric cancers are provided in Table 12-8. Information on dosing as well as indications and adverse reactions is available in Table 12-9 where ADRs are divided into common (frequency 21%–100%), occasional (frequency 5%–20%), and rare (frequency 1%–4%).

TABLE 12-8
Common Antineoplastic Drug Regimens

Acute Lymphoblastic Leukemia:
Prednisone or dexamethasone, vincristine, asparaginase ± daunomycin, and intrathecal therapy with methotrexate.

Non-Hodgkin's Lymphoma:
1. Cyclophosphamide, doxorubicin, vincristine, and prednisone (CHOP)
2. Teniposide and cytarabine (VM26/Ara-C)

Hodgkin's Disease:
1. Nitrogen mustard, vincristine, prednisone, and procarbazine (MOPP)
2. Doxorubicin (Adriamycin®), bleomycin, vinblastine, and dacarbazine (ABVD)
3. Bleomycin, etoposide, doxorubicin (Adriamycin), cyclophosphamide, vincristine, prednisone, and procarbazine (BEACOPP)

Neuroblastoma and Sarcomas:
Vincristine, doxorubicin (Adriamycin), and cyclophosphamide (VAdriaC)

Sarcomas and Germ Cell Tumors:
Vincristine, actinomycin-D, and cyclophosphamide (VAC)

Sarcomas:
1. Ifosfamide and etoposide (Ifos/VP).
2. Mesna, doxorubicin (Adriamycin), ifosfamide, and dacarbazine (MAID)

Acute Myeloid Leukemia: Induction
Daunomycin, cytarabine (Ara-C), and thioguanine (DAT)

Solid Tumors:
Ifosfamide, carboplatin, and etoposide (ICE)

TABLE 12-9
Antineoplastic Drug Dosing for Children and Adolescents

DRUG TRADE AND OTHER NAMES [CLASS AND TYPE]	INDICATIONS	USUAL PEDIATRIC DOSAGE AND ADMINISTRATION[a]	DOSAGE FORMS[b]	ADRs[c]	CAUTIONS AND COMMENTS[d]	REFERENCES[e]
Amifostine *Ethyol®* [Cytoprotector, reactive species antagonist]	Chemoprotection and radioprotection after infusion of high doses of cisplatin, cyclophosphamide, or ifosfamide **Note:** Not approved by the FDA or HPB for pediatric use.	825 mg/m²/dose IV over 15 min at 30 min before and 3 hr after high doses of cisplatin, cyclophosphamide, or ifosfamide.	500-mg vials (anhydrous); reconstitute in 9.7 ml of 0.9% sodium chloride to 50 mg/ml.	**Common:** Hypotension, nausea, peripheral sensory neuropathies, vomiting. **Occasional:** Decreased renal function, diarrhea, increased alkaline phosphatase, myelosuppression. **Rare:** Agitation, alopecia, confusion, depression, hallucinations, pruritus, rash.	Contraindications include hypersensitivity to amifostine, other aminothiols, and mannitol. Patients should be adequately hydrated **prior** to receiving amifostine. Monitor blood pressure during infusion. Administer antiemetics (e.g., dexamethasone, dolasetron) prior to and during IV infusion.	Glover 1988 Shaw 1988
Amsacrine *AMSA P-D®*, m-AMSA [Acridine dye]	Refractory leukemia **Note:** Not approved by the FDA or HPB for pediatric use.	120 mg/m² IV over 1–2 hr in 500 ml of D_5W for 3–5 days.	1.5-ml ampules (75 mg); mix with 13.5 ml of L-lactic acid diluent provided by the manufacturer and further dilute in 500 ml of dextrose injection **prior** to administration. Not compatible with sodium chloride solutions.	**Common:** Flushing, hyperkalemia with tumor lysis, hypotension, mucositis, myelosuppression (anemia, leukopenia, thrombocytopenia), nausea, phlebitis and local pain, vomiting. **Occasional:** Dizziness, hypocalcemia with multiple dosing, sleepiness, sneezing. **Rare:** Chills, hiccups.	Use with caution if patient has received prior anthracyclines; may potentiate cardiotoxicity. Acute dysrhythmias are associated with hypokalemia.	Steuber 1996
Arsenic Trioxide [Miscellaneous, trivalent inorganic arsenical]	Acute promyelocytic leukemia **Note:** Not approved by the FDA or HPB for pediatric use.	0.15 mg/kg/day PO for 25 days; repeat cycle after 10–14 days of rest.	Inorganic arsenical in 10-ml ampules (from NCI and PolaRx Biopharmaceuticals, Inc.)	**Common:** Abdominal pain, anorexia, fluid retention (pleura and pericardium) associated with leukocytosis, flushing with IV infusion, nausea, vomiting. **Occasional:** Acute hemolysis; elevated bilirubin, liver enzymes, and serum creatinine; fatigue; headache; lightheadedness; muscle weakness; myalgia. **Rare:** Agitation, ataxia or dysmetria; confusion or hallucinations, hearing loss, paresthesias, QT prolongation, sensory loss. **Note:** At doses greater than 0.2 mg/kg/day, flaccid paralysis, renal failure, severe exfoliative or ulcerative dermatitis.	Induction with cytarabine, daunorubicin, and tretinoin, followed by consolidation with arsenic trioxide and tretinoin plus daunorubicin. Maintenance is randomized to observation or tretinoin every other week for 1 year.	Soignet 1998

[a] *See* Chapter 8 for specific information regarding IV administration including IV push, continuous infusion, and intermittent infusion.
[b] *See* Chapter 8 for additional specific information regarding dilution and compatibilities.
[c] *See also* Table 12-1 for neurotoxicities, Table 12-2 for emetogenic potential, and Chapter 5.
[d] *See also* text, Table 12-4 for long-term follow-up, and Table 12-6 for monitoring guidelines.
[e] Only the first author and year of publication are listed in the table. For complete citations, *see* References.

TABLE 12-9 continued

DRUG TRADE AND OTHER NAMES [CLASS AND TYPE]	INDICATIONS	USUAL PEDIATRIC DOSAGE AND ADMINISTRATION[a]	DOSAGE FORMS[b]	ADRs[c]	CAUTIONS AND COMMENTS[d]	REFER-ENCES[e]
Asparaginase *Elspar®, Kidrolase®* [Enzyme]	Leukemia Lymphoma	6000–10,000 IU/m^2 IM three times a week. **High-dose therapy:** 25,000 IU/m^2/week IM for 9–20 weeks. **Note:** Can also be administered by intermittent IV infusion.	Powder, 10,000 units/vial; reconstitute in 2 ml of 0.9% normal saline (5000 IU/ml) and use within 8 hr. Filter any precipitate with a 5-μm filter. Store at less than 8°C before use.	**Common:** Decreased synthesis of albumin, fibrinogen, and other clotting factors; hyperammonemia, local allergic reactions. **Occasional:** Abnormal liver function tests, hyperglycemia, rash. **Rare:** Anorexia, CNS ischemic attacks, convulsions, edema, hemorrhage pancreatitis, renal complications, thrombosis. **Note:** For high doses, the incidence of ADRs may vary. Pediatric patients exhibiting a positive skin reaction may be desensitized according to a prescribed schedule. A negative skin test does **not** preclude the possibility of an allergic reaction.	Because of allergic reactions, an intradermal skin test should be performed prior to the initial dose and when therapy is reinitiated after an interval of 1 week or more. Due to the risk of anaphylactic shock, have available epinephrine 1:10,000 (0.1 ml/10 kg SC) and diphenhydramine and hydrocortisone (1 mg/kg IV).	Evans 1982 Kucuk 1985 Land 1972 Muller 1998 Zubrod 1970
Azacitidine [Antimetabolite, pyrimidine analog]	Refractory leukemia (AML) **Note:** Not approved by the FDA or HPB for pediatric use, but it may be used in the treatment of refractory leukemia.	100 mg/m^2 IV every 8 hr for 5 days **or** 150–200 mg/m^2/day IV as a continuous infusion for 5 days.	Investigational use only. Prepare fresh before use in Ringer's lactate and dispose after 8 hr if not used.	**Common:** Diarrhea, nausea, phlebitis, severe myelosuppression, vomiting. **Occasional:** Lethargy, muscle pain, rash, stomatitis, transient fever, weakness. **Rare:** Azotemia, coma, hepatotoxicity.		Hakami 1987
Bleomycin *Blenoxane®* [Natural product, antibiotic]	Germ cell tumors Lymphoma	10–20 units/m^2/week (0.25–0.5 unit/kg) IV, IM, SC.	15 units (sterile powder); reconstitute with 0.9% sodium chloride or a sterile water solution to provide 3–15 units/ml, stable for 24 hr at room temperature. Use within 24 hr of reconstitution and discard unused portion. There may be a loss of potency when diluted in dextrose-containing IV solutions.	**Common:** Anorexia, hyperpigmentation, nausea, skin rash, skin tenderness, vomiting. **Occasional:** Interstitial pneumonitis. **Rare:** Anaphylactoid reaction with severe fever and hypotension, leading to renal failure or death (very rare); pulmonary fibrosis.	Pulmonary toxicity **potentiated** by pulmonary radiation or exposure to high oxygen concentration. Do pulmonary function tests during therapy and at 1 year after completion.	Carter & Blum 1974, 1976 Comis 1992 Yagoda 1972
Busulfan *Myleran®* [Alkylating agent, alkyl sulfonate]	Bone marrow transplant (BMT) Chronic myeloid leukemia (CML)	1 mg/kg PO every 6 hr for 4 days. **CML:** 0.06–0.12 mg/kg/day PO, titrate to a WBC of 20,000/mm^3.	Tablet: 2 mg scored	**Common:** Hyperuricemia (proportional to disease burden), myelosuppression (pancytopenia). **Occasional:** Alopecia, blurred vision, cheilosis, dizziness, dryness of skin and mucous membranes, fatigue, glossitis, gynecomastia (mild),		Galton 1958 Murphy 1992

TABLE 12-9 continued

DRUG *TRADE* AND OTHER NAMES [CLASS AND TYPE]	INDICATIONS	USUAL PEDIATRIC DOSAGE AND ADMINISTRATION[a]	DOSAGE FORMS[b]	ADRs[c]	CAUTIONS AND COMMENTS[d]	REFER- ENCES[e]
Busulfan *continued*				hepatic dysfunction and cholestatic jaundice, intermittent muscle twitching, loss of consciousness, melanoderma, myoclonic and generalized tonic-clonic seizures, rashes, urticaria. **Rare:** Anorexia, diarrhea, hemorrhagic cystitis, nausea, veno-occlusive disease, vomiting.		
Carboplatin CBDCA, *Paraplatin*® [Alkylating agent, metal salt]	Bone marrow transplant (BMT) Germ cell tumors Neuroblastoma	400–600 mg/m²/day IV for 2 days every 28 days. **BMT:** 300–725 mg/m²/day by continuous infusion or 1 hr push. **Note:** Prehydration is required.	Lyophilized powder: 50, 150, 450 mg; store at room temperature (RT) away from light. Reconstitute with 5, 15, or 45 ml of sterile water (5% dextrose or 0.9% sodium chloride) to 10 mg/ml. May further dilute to 0.5–2 mg/ml with 5% dextrose or 0.9% sodium chloride; stable at RT for 8 hr and under refrigeration for 24 hr.	**Common:** Myelosuppression, nausea, vomiting. **Occasional:** Electrolyte disturbances. **Rare:** Hepatotoxicity, metallic taste, neuropathy, ototoxicity, peripheral renal toxicity, secondary leukemia.	Avoid the use of needles or IV administration sets that contain aluminum parts. Aluminum can react with carboplatin, resulting in a precipitate and reduced carboplatin potency.	Canetta 1988 Foster 1985 Gaynon 1994
Carmustine BCNU, *BiCNU*®, *Gliadel Wafer*® [Alkylating agent, nitrosourea]	Brain tumors Hodgkin's disease Lymphoma	150–200 mg/m² IV (single dose) every 4–6 weeks.	100 mg of dried powder with 3 ml of dehydrated absolute alcohol; reconstitute with 27 ml of sterile water for injection (3.3-mg/ml solution with 10% alcohol). May be diluted with 0.9% saline or 5% dextrose solution for IV administration over 1–2 hr.	**Common:** Myelosuppression, nausea, transaminase elevation, vomiting. **Occasional:** Anorexia, diarrhea, dysphagia, esophagitis. **Rare:** Ataxia, dizziness, loss of equilibrium, thrombophlebitis.	Do not give by intravenous push. Give last if several drugs are to be given through peripheral line. Infusions longer than 2 hr not recommended due to incompatibility with IV tubing. Delayed pulmonary toxicity (i.e., pulmonary fibrosis) has been reported several years after the termination of carmustine use and has resulted in **death**. The risk appears highest for patients treated with carmustine during childhood.	Mitchell 1986 O'Driscoll 1990
Chlorambucil *Leukeran*® [Alkylating agent, nitrogen mustard]	Hodgkin's disease Non-Hodgkin's lymphoma (rarely used in children)	4.5 mg/m²/day PO for 3–6 weeks.	Tablets: 2 mg	**Common:** Myelosuppression. **Occasional:** Abdominal pain, anorexia, diarrhea, nausea, rash, vomiting. **Rare:** Agitation, ataxia, confusion, elevated transaminases, flaccid	Use in prepubertal and pubertal boys carries a risk of sterility.	Alberts 1979 Miller 1959 Palmer 1984

(Continued)

Footnotes are on page 507.

TABLE 12-9 continued

DRUG TRADE AND OTHER NAMES [CLASS AND TYPE]	INDICATIONS	USUAL PEDIATRIC DOSAGE AND ADMINISTRATION[a]	DOSAGE FORMS[b]	ADRs[c]	CAUTIONS AND COMMENTS[d]	REFER- ENCES[e]
Chlorambucil continued				paralysis, focal or generalized seizures, interstitial pneumonitis or pulmonary fibrosis, mucositis, muscular twitching, peripheral neuropathy, secondary malignancy, Stevens-Johnson syndrome, toxic epidermal necrolysis, tremor.		
Cisplatin CDDP, *Platinol-AQ*® [Alkylating agent, metal salt]	Brain tumors Germ cell tumors Neuroblastoma Osteosarcoma	50–200 mg/m² IV over 4–6 hr every 3–4 weeks. **Germ cell tumors:** Standard dose: 20 mg/m²/day IV for 5 days. High dose: 40 mg/m²/day IV for 5 days. **Note:** Prehydration is required.	Aqueous solution (1 mg/ml) in 50- and 100-ml vials; store away from light. Also 10- and 50-mg vials; reconstitute by adding 10 and 50 ml of sterile water, respectively. If not used within 6 hr, protect from light; stable for 20 hr at room temperature. Avoid contact with aluminum because this causes a loss of potency. May further dilute with 0.9% sodium chloride to maintain stability.	**Common:** Anorexia, high frequency hearing loss, hypomagnesemia, myelosuppression, nausea, nephrotoxicity, tinnitus, vomiting. **Occasional:** Electrolyte disturbances, metallic taste. **Rare:** Anaphylactic reaction, liver toxicity, peripheral neuropathy, secondary malignancy, seizures.	Dose adjustment necessary if Cr Cl <60 ml/min. Vesicant if large volume extravasates. Nausea/emesis may last 1 week or longer. May interact with aluminum in needles and IV sets, forming a black precipitate.	Brock 1991, 1992 Loehrer 1984 Meyer 1994 Schaefer 1985
Cladribine 2-Chlorodeoxy-adenosine, *Leustatin*® [Antimetabolite, purine analog]	Acute myeloid leukemia (AML) **Note:** Not approved by the FDA or HPB for pediatric use. Phase I studies for the treatment of AML in combination with other agents are ongoing.	8 mg/m²/day IV for 5 days every 4 weeks or until count recovery for two courses.	Preservative-free solution with 10 ml (1 mg/ml); refrigerate. Stable for 24 hr at room temperature; use within 8 hr is recommended due to the lack of preservatives. Loss of efficacy if diluted in 5% dextrose.	**Common:** Damage to nerve tissue (high dose), fatigue, fever, increased risk of infection, myelosuppression, nausea, rash. **Occasional:** Anorexia, arthralgia, breathing problems, constipation, cough, diarrhea, dizziness, headache, hepatotoxicity, injection site reactions, insomnia, myalgia, nephrotoxicity (high dose), vomiting.	Used in combination with idarubicin to treat AML.	Santana 1991 Saven 1993
Cyclophosphamide CTX, *Cytoxan*®, *Neosar*® [Alkylating agent, nitrogen mustard]	Bone marrow transplant (BMT) Leukemia Neuroblastoma Retinoblastoma Sarcomas Wilms' tumor	250–1800 mg/m²/day IV for 1–4 days every 3–4 weeks. **Maintenance:** 100–300 mg/m² PO twice weekly every 3–4 weeks. **BMT:** 50–100 mg/kg/dose IV for two to four doses (total dose 60–200 mg/kg); use ideal body weight for dosing. **Note:** Prehydration is required.	Tablets: 25 and 50 mg Injectable: White powder with sodium chloride in vials of 100, 200, 500, 1000, 2000 mg; stable at room temperature. Reconstitute with sterile water to 20 mg/ml. Use within 6 hr since no preservatives are recommended in the diluent. Discard solution after 24 hr.	**Common:** Alopecia, anorexia, gonadal dysfunction/sterility, immunosuppression, myelosuppression, nausea, vomiting. **Occasional:** Hemorrhagic cystitis, metallic taste, inappropriate ADH secretion. **Rare:** Bladder fibrosis, dysrhythmias and myocardial necrosis (high dose), pulmonary fibrosis, secondary malignancy, transient blurred vision.	IV push may cause fleeting oropharyngeal sensation.	Gershwin 1974 Moore 1991 Stillwell 1988

TABLE 12-9 continued

DRUG TRADE AND OTHER NAMES [CLASS AND TYPE]	INDICATIONS	USUAL PEDIATRIC DOSAGE AND ADMINISTRATION[a]	DOSAGE FORMS[b]	ADRs[c]	CAUTIONS AND COMMENTS[d]	REFER- ENCES[e]
Cyclosporine *Sandimmune®* [Immuno- suppressive] See also Chapter 14.	Modulation of multidrug resistance in acute myeloid leukemia (AML) and solid tumors. Investigational use only. **Note:** Not approved by the FDA or HPB for this indication for use among children or adolescents.	10 mg/kg IV over 2 hr as loading dose, then 30 mg/kg/day with AML pharmacotherapy (etoposide 60 mg/m^2, mitoxantrone 6 mg/m^2).	5-ml ampule (50 mg/ml) in a polyoxyethyl- ated castor oil base for IV use. Stable for 24 hr in glass when diluted 1:20 in 5% dextrose or 0.9% sodium chloride.	**Common:** Elevated bilirubin, gum hyperplasia, hirsutism, hypertension, hypomagnesemia, reversible renal dysfunction with short-term use, tremor. **Occasional:** Burning palmar and plantar paresthesia, confusion, diarrhea, headache, nausea, somnolence, vomiting. **Rare:** Acute respiratory distress, blood pressure changes and tachycardia, dyspnea, facial flushing, hypersensitivity reactions with anaphylaxis, sneezing.	Continuously observe pediatric patients for at least 30 min following the initiation of infusion and at frequent intervals thereafter because of the possibility of hypersensitivity to the castor oil vehicle present in the injectable formulation of cyclosporine. Subject to many clinically significant drug interactions; see Chapter 6.	Dahl 2000 Lum 1992
Cytarabine ara-C, *Cytosar-U®*, Cytosine Arabinoside [Antimetabolite, pyrimidine analog]	Leukemia Lymphoma	**Standard dose:** 100–200 mg/m^2 IV every 12 hr or as a continuous infusion for 5–7 days. **High dose:** 1000–3000 mg/m^2 IV every 12 hr for 7 days. **Intrathecal dose:** Age dependent; see specific protocol. Used in combination with methotrexate and hydrocortisone in some acute lymphocytic leukemia (ALL) protocols.	Freeze-dried powder in vials of 100, 500, 1000, 2000 mg. Stable at room temperature for at least 2 years. May reconstitute with 10 ml of sterile water or bacteriostatic water, except for intrathecal administration. Reconstituted drug should be used within 8 hr at room temperature or within 6 days if refrigerated at 2–8°C.	**IV ADRs** **Common:** Alopecia, anorexia, conjunctivitis, diarrhea, myelosuppression, nausea, stomatitis, vomiting. **Occasional:** Flulike symptoms with fever. **Rare:** Bleeding, cerebellar dysfunction, encephalopathy, gonadal dysfunction, hepatotoxicity, pneumonitis, pulmonary capillary leak, rash, veno-occlusive disease. **Intrathecal ADRs** **Occasional:** Convulsions, fever, headache, learning disability, nausea, pleocytosis, vomiting. **Rare:** Ataxia; CNS deterioration (progressive), convulsions, leukoencephalopathy, meningismus, myelosuppression, paraplegia, rash, somnolence.	Administer artificial tears or dexamethasone eye drops with high doses.	Baker 1991 Barnett 1985 Lass 1982
Dacarbazine DIC, *DTIC-Dome®*, Imidazole Carboxamide [Alkylating agent, triazene]	Hodgkin's disease Lymphoma Malignant melanoma Neuroblastoma Soft tissue sarcoma	250 mg/m^2/day IV for 5 days every 3–4 weeks. **Neuroblastoma:** 800–900 mg/m^2 IV as a single dose.	Powder: Vials of 100, 200 mg. Protect from light and refrigerate at 2–8°C. Reconstitute by adding 9.9 ml (for the 100-mg vial) or 19.7 ml (for the 200-mg vial) of sterile water for injection. The resultant 10-mg/ml solution can be further diluted	**Common:** Anorexia, myelosuppression, nausea, pain and tissue necrosis with extravasation, vomiting. **Occasional:** Alopecia; blurred vision; confusion; flulike syndrome with fever, myalgia, and malaise; headache; lethargy; rashes; seizures;		Carter 1976 Gottlieb 1976

(Continued)

Footnotes are on page 507.

TABLE 12-9 continued

DRUG TRADE AND OTHER NAMES [CLASS AND TYPE]	INDICATIONS	USUAL PEDIATRIC DOSAGE AND ADMINISTRATION[a]	DOSAGE FORMS[b]	ADRs[c]	CAUTIONS AND COMMENTS[d]	REFERENCES[e]
Dacarbazine *continued*			with 0.9% sodium chloride or 5% dextrose in a 250-ml volume for infusion over 15–30 min.	transient elevation of transaminases. **Rare:** Diarrhea, hepatic vein thrombosis with hepatocellular necrosis (extremely rare), intractable vomiting, photosensitivity reactions.		
Dactinomycin act-D, Actinomycin D, *Cosmegen*® [Antibiotic]	Sarcoma Wilms' tumor	15 µg/kg/day IV (maximum dose 0.45 mg) daily for 5 days every 3–6 weeks.	Lyophilized powder: Vials of 500 µg with 20 mg of mannitol; store at room temperature. Reconstitute by adding 1.1 ml of sterile water without preservative to make a 0.5-mg/ml solution. Use within 24 hr and store away from light.	**Common:** Alopecia, diarrhea (severe), immunosuppression, local ulceration with extravasation, myelosuppression, nausea, vomiting. **Rare:** Cheilitis, dysphagia, esophagitis, mucosal ulceration, pharyngitis. **Note:** Incidence is reportedly increased when administered to infants. Several ADRs may be delayed in onset and may not become apparent until 2–5 days after a course of dactinomycin and may not become maximal until after 7–14 days.	Extremely corrosive to soft tissue. Administer only IV. Avoid extravasation which may result in pain, ulceration, and necrosis of the affected soft tissue. Daily platelet and white blood cell counts are recommended to detect severe myelosuppression.	Frei 1974
Daunorubicin *Cerubidine*®, Daunomycin, DNR, Rubidomycin [Natural product, antibiotic]	Leukemia Sarcoma	25–45 mg/m²/day IV daily for 3–6 days. If younger than 2 years or if BSA <0.5 m², may need to adjust dose to 1 mg/kg **or** consult protocol. **Dose adjustment:** T. bili 1.2–3 mg/dl, 50% dose; T. bili >3 mg/dl, 25% dose.	Lyophilized powder: 20-mg vial. Stable up to 2 years at room temperature if shielded from light. When reconstituted in sterile water, stable for 48 hr if shielded from light and refrigerated at 2–8°C.	**Common:** Alopecia, cardiac dysrhythmias (rarely clinically significant), local ulceration if extravasated, myelosuppression, nausea, pink or red color in urine, vomiting, worsens ADRs due to radiation. Also, associated with hyperuricemia due to rapid lysis of leukemic cells; prevent or minimize by allopurinol pretreatment and monitoring of blood uric acid levels. **Occasional:** Cardiomyopathy (cumulative dose dependent), hepatotoxicity, mucositis, stomatitis. **Rare:** Allergic reactions, anaphylaxis, rash, secondary malignancy. **Note:** Both immediate and delayed myocardial toxicity, including fatal congestive heart failure, has been noted, particularly among infants and children. Incidence increases for both infants	Extremely corrosive to soft tissue. Administer by a rapidly flowing IV solution; avoid extravasation, which may result in pain, ulceration, and necrosis of the affected soft tissue.	Matthews 1972 Van Hoff 1984

TABLE 12-9 continued

DRUG TRADE AND OTHER NAMES [CLASS AND TYPE]	INDICATIONS	USUAL PEDIATRIC DOSAGE AND ADMINISTRATION[a]	DOSAGE FORMS[b]	ADRs[c]	CAUTIONS AND COMMENTS[d]	REFER-ENCES[e]
Dauno-rubicin *continued*				and children up to 2 years of age who have received a total cumulative dose exceeding 10 mg/kg and children older than 2 years who have received a total cumulative dose exceeding 300 mg/m². Delayed toxicity may be independent of dose. Other factors that may increase the risk for myocardial toxicity include pre-existing cardiac disease, previous daunorubicin therapy, and thoracic irradiation. Obtain a baseline ECG prior to each course. The incidence of ADRs may vary with high doses.		
Dexa-methasone *Decadron*® [Hormone, corticosteroid]	Acute lymphocytic leukemia (ALL) Brain tumors (used for palliative management)	**ALL:** 6 mg/m²/day PO for 28 days. **Brain tumors:** 2–4 mg/kg/day IV in divided doses; use slow tapering schedule.	Tablets: 0.25, 0.5, 0.75, 1.5, 4, 6 mg Elixir: 0.5 mg/ml Injectable solution: 1, 10, 20 mg/ml	**Common:** Acne, Cushing's syndrome, hyperphagia, immunosuppression, personality changes, pituitary-adrenal axis suppression. **Occasional:** Gastritis, hyperglycemia, muscle weakness, poor wound healing, upset stomach. **Rare:** Aseptic necrosis of the femoral head, cataracts, electrolyte imbalance, GI bleeding, growth retardation, hypertension, increased intraocular pressure, osteopenia, pancreatitis, peptic ulcer, striae.		Gutin 1975
Dexrazoxane ICRF-187, *Zinecard*® [Cytoprotector, reactive species agonist]	Cardioprotective, used with anthracycline therapy **Note:** Not approved by the FDA or HPB for pediatric use.	10 mg of dexrazoxane IV for every 1 mg of doxorubicin; administer within 30 min prior to doxorubicin pharmacotherapy.	Lyophilized powder: 500 mg; reconstitute with 50 ml of 0.167 M sodium lactate injection to 10 mg/ml. Stable for 6 hr at room temperature. May dilute further to 1.3–5 mg/ml with 0.9% sodium chloride or 5% dextrose solution.	**Common:** Myelosuppression and may exacerbate myelosuppression from anthracyclines. **Occasional:** Constipation, headache, pain with injection, phlebitis.		Vogel 1987
Docetaxel *Taxotere*® [Natural product, microtubule stabilizer]	Solid tumors refractory to other conventional pharmacotherapy	150–185 mg/m²/dose IV over 1 hr every 3 weeks; requires filgrastim support.	Injection concentrate: 40 mg of anhydrous drug to be diluted in 250 ml of either 0.9% sodium chloride or 5% dextrose solution to 0.3–0.9 mg/ml.	**Common:** Alopecia, asthenia, diarrhea (mild), fatigue, mucositis (mild), myalgia, myelosuppression, nausea, vomiting. **Occasional:** Conjunctivitis; fluid retention	Completed phase I study in children with refractory solid tumors. Treat with dexamethasone 8 mg PO, twice a day for 5 days starting 1 day	Seibel 1999

(Continued)

Footnotes are on page 507.

TABLE 12-9 continued

DRUG *TRADE* AND OTHER NAMES [CLASS AND TYPE]	INDICATIONS	USUAL PEDIATRIC DOSAGE AND ADMINISTRATION[a]	DOSAGE FORMS[b]	ADRs[c]	CAUTIONS AND COMMENTS[d]	REFER- ENCES[e]
Docetaxel *continued*				with repeated courses; increases in transaminases, alkaline phosphatase, and bilirubin. **Rare:** Diarrhea (severe), hypersensitivity reaction, hypotension.	before docetaxel. Use with caution if bilirubin is above upper limit of normal since neutropenia will be more profound. **Deaths,** due primarily to sepsis, have occurred in a significant minority of patients. Monitor patients for neutropenia and discontinue docetaxel if neutrophil counts fall below 1500/mm^3.	
Doxorubicin ADR, *Adriamycin*®, Hydroxydauno- rubicin, *Rubex*® [Natural product, antibiotic]	Leukemia Lymphoma Sarcomas	45–75 mg/m^2/dose IV every 21 days; 20–30 mg/m^2 weekly; 45–90 mg/m^2 single dose. If younger than 2 years or if BSA <0.5 m^2, may need to adjust dose or consult protocol. **Dose adjustment:** T. bili 1.2–3 mg/dl, 50% dose; T. bili >3 mg/dl, 25% dose.	Freeze-dried powder: vials of 10, 20, 50, 100, 150 mg Solution (2 mg/ml): Multidose vials of 5, 10, 25, 100 ml Dried powder may be stored at room temperature. Powder reconstituted in 0.9% sodium chloride (to 2 mg/ml) should be refrigerated and protected from light and exposure to aluminum.	**Common:** Alopecia (generally complete and reversible), cardiac dysrhythmias (rarely clinically significant), immunosuppression, local ulceration if extravasated, myelosuppression, nausea and vomiting (acute and may be severe), pink or red color to urine, worsens ADRs due to radiation. **Occasional:** Cardiomyopathy (cumulative and dose dependent), hepatotoxicity, mucositis, stomatitis. **Rare:** Allergic reactions, anaphylaxis, rash, secondary malignancy. **Note:** Incidence of ADRs may vary with high doses. Use of dexrazoxane may reduce the incidence of cardiomyopathy.	IV infusion over 5 min or more in a well-established line. **Vesicant;** avoid extravasation and exposure to mucosa, skin, or conjunctiva.	Carter & Blum 1974 Lipshultz 1991 Rosenfeld 1992
Doxorubicin Liposomal *Doxil*® [Natural product, antibiotic]	Leukemia Lymphoma Sarcomas **Note:** Not approved by the FDA or HPB for pediatric use.	60 mg/m^2/dose IV every 4 weeks.	Liposomal formulation: Dilute in 250 ml of 5% dextrose solution for injection.	**Common:** Alopecia, cardiac dysrhythmias (rarely clinically significant), immunosuppression, local ulceration if extravasated, myelosuppression, nausea, pink or red color to urine, vomiting, worsens ADRs due to radiation. **Occasional:** Cardiomyopathy (cumulative and dose dependent), hepatotoxicity, mucositis, palmar-plantar erythrodysesthesia, stomatitis. **Rare:** Allergic reactions, anaphylaxis, rash, secondary malignancy.	Completed phase I study. Do not substitute doxorubicin liposomal for doxorubicin. Pharmacokinetic differences between these formulations may result in modified therapeutic response and severe ADRs. Use with dexrazoxane as a premedication has not been investigated in children.	Harney 1999

CHAPTER 12: PEDIATRIC ANTINEOPLASTIC DRUG THERAPY

TABLE 12-9 continued

DRUG TRADE AND OTHER NAMES [CLASS AND TYPE]	INDICATIONS	USUAL PEDIATRIC DOSAGE AND ADMINISTRATION[a]	DOSAGE FORMS[b]	ADRs[c]	CAUTIONS AND COMMENTS[d]	REFERENCES[e]
Etoposide *Etopophos®*, *VePesid®*, VP-16 [Natural product, topoisomerase II inhibitor]	Bone marrow transplant (BMT) Brain tumors Germ cell tumors Leukemia Lymphoma Neuroblastoma Sarcoma Wilms' tumor	60–300 mg/m²/day IV for 1–5 days every 3 weeks. 50 mg/m² PO every day for 21-day cycles. **BMT:** 40–60 mg/kg IV. Administer by slow IV infusion over 30–60 min to avoid hypotension that has occurred following rapid IV administration.	Capsule: 50 mg (pink) Multiple-dose sterile vial: 20 mg/ml; dilute in 0.9% sodium chloride or 5% dextrose solution. Stable at room temperature for 48 hr at 0.4 mg/ml. At higher concentrations, stability is highly unpredictable.	**Common:** Myelosuppression, nausea, vomiting. **Occasional:** Alopecia, diarrhea, increased damage due to radiation. **Rare:** Anaphylaxis, hypotension, peripheral neuropathy, secondary malignancy, skin rash, stomatitis.	Injectable formulation may contain polysorbate 80 which has caused a life-threatening syndrome (ascites, hepatic and renal failure, pulmonary dysfunction, thrombocytopenia) in premature neonates.	Fleming 1989 O'Dwyer 1998
Filgrastim G-CSF, *Neupogen®* [Biologic agent, granulocyte colony-stimulating factor]	Postmyelosuppressive pharmacotherapy (reduces neutrophil nadir and recovery time)	5–10 µg/kg/day SC for 10–14 days.	Clear solution (300 µg/ml) in vials of 1 or 1.6 ml. Vials are single use since they do not contain preservatives. When stored at 2–8°C, solution is stable for 24 months. Do not use if exposed to freezing temperatures, discolored, or contains particulate matter. Do not shake or freeze.	**Occasional:** Increased alkaline phosphatase, lactate dehydrogenase, and uric acid; local irritation at the injection site; medullary bone pain; thrombocytopenia. **Rare:** Allergic reactions, alopecia, cutaneous vasculitis, fever (low grade), exacerbation of pre-existing skin rashes, subclinical splenomegaly.	Obtain complete blood and platelet counts before initiating therapy (i.e., at baseline) and then twice weekly to monitor neutrophil count and avoid leukocytosis.	Hartmann 1995 Laver 1998
Fludarabine FAMP, *Fludara®* [Antimetabolite, purine analog]	Refractory leukemia (AML) used with cytarabine, filgrastim, and idarubicin (FLAG-IDA regimen). **Note:** Not approved by the FDA or HPB for pediatric use.	30 mg/m²/day IV for 5 days at 28-day intervals.	Powder for injection: Vial of 50 mg; dilute in 2 ml of sterile water to provide a solution of 25 mg/ml. Dilute in 100 or 125 ml of 5% dextrose or 0.9% sodium chloride solution.	**Common:** Immunosuppression, myelosuppression, nausea, vomiting. **Occasional:** Allergic pneumonitis, diarrhea, edema, fatigue, mucositis, paresthesias, rash, somnolence, twitching of extremities. **Rare:** Abnormal renal or liver function test, potentially fatal autoimmune hemolytic anemia, visual disturbances (at higher than recommended doses).	Completed phase II study.	Leahey 1997
Fluorouracil *Adrucil®*, 5-Fluorouracil, 5-FU [Antimetabolite, pyrimidine analog]	Hepatoblastoma Nasopharyngeal carcinoma	500 mg/m² IV as a single dose or divided over 5 days. 800–1200 mg/m² IV by continuous infusion for 24–120 hr.	Clear, yellow aqueous solution: 500 mg/10 ml, light sensitive; store at room temperature. Precipitates commonly from solution at lower temperatures; dissolve by heating. Solution must be cooled to room temperature before administration.	**Common:** Alopecia, anorexia, myelosuppression, nausea, vomiting. **Occasional:** Diarrhea (mild to moderate), esophagitis, headache, hyperpigmentation, immunosuppression, partial loss of nails, proctitis, rash, visual disturbances. **Rare:** Cardiotoxicity, cerebellar ataxia, dysphagia, hypotension, palmar-plantar erythrodysesthesia, severe diarrhea and stomatitis with erythema and ulceration of the oral cavity.		Balis 1990 Mertens 1997

Footnotes are on page 507.

TABLE 12-9 continued

DRUG *TRADE* AND OTHER NAMES [CLASS AND TYPE]	INDICATIONS	USUAL PEDIATRIC DOSAGE AND ADMINISTRATION[a]	DOSAGE FORMS[b]	ADRs[c]	CAUTIONS AND COMMENTS[d]	REFER- ENCES[e]
Hydroxyurea *Hydrea®*, *Mylocel®*) [Miscellaneous, substituted urea]	Chronic myeloid leuke- mia (CML)	800–2000 mg/m² PO as a single or divided dose every third day.	Capsules: 200, 300, 400, 500 mg Tablet: 1000 mg	**Common:** Myelosup- pression (leukopenia). **Occasional:** Facial erythema, maculo- papular rash, pruritus. **Rare:** Alopecia, chills and malaise, dizziness, fever, hallucinations and convulsions, headache. Potential human carcin- ogen; secondary leuke- mias have been reported.		Creutzig 1996
Idarubicin 4-Demethoxy- dauno-rubicin, IDA, *Idamycin®* [Natural product, antibiotic]	Acute myeloid leukemia (AML) **Note:** Not ap- proved by the FDA or HPB for pediatric use.	12 mg/m²/day IV for 4 days every 3–4 weeks. If younger than 2 years or if BSA <0.5 m², may need to adjust dose **or** consult protocol. **Dose adjustment:** T. bili 1.2–3 mg/dl, 50% dose; T. bili >3 mg/dl, 25% dose.	Sterile lyophilized powder for injection: Vials of 5 and 10 mg. Reconstitute with 5 and 10 ml, respec- tively, of 0.9% sodium chloride to 1 mg/ml. Reconstituted drug is stable for 7 days if re- frigerated or 3 days at room temperature.	**Common:** Alopecia, cardiac dysrhythmias (rarely clinically signifi- cant), immunosuppres- sion, local ulceration if extravasated, myelosup- pression, nausea, pink or red color to urine, vomiting, worsens ADRs due to radiation. **Occasional:** Cardiomyopathy (cumu- lative dose dependent), hepatotoxicity, muco- sitis, stomatitis. **Rare:** Allergic reac- tions, anaphylaxis, rash, secondary malignancy.	Used in combina- tion with cladribine, or to substitute other anthracyclines for AML therapy. Use with dexrazo- xane as a premedi- cation has not been investigated in children.	Bern- stein 1997 Neuen- dank 1997
Ifosfamide *Ifex®*, IFOS [Alkylating agent, nitrogen mustard]	Germ cell tu- mors Osteosarcoma Sarcoma	1.5–2.4 grams/m²/day IV for 5 days. Doses >2.4 grams/m² admin- ister over a longer infu- sion period 2 or 3 days/ week. **Note:** Prehydration is required.	Vials: 1, 3 grams with- out preservative; re- constitute with sterile water to 50 mg/ml. All reconstituted solutions should be used or dis- carded within 24 hr.	**Common:** Alopecia, anorexia; dysrhythmias, ECG changes, myelo- suppression, nausea, vomiting. **Occasional:** Confu- sion, Fanconi's renal syndrome, hemorrhagic cystitis, inappropriate ADH secretion, myocar- dial necrosis, seizures, somnolence, weakness. **Rare:** Acute renal fail- ure, bladder fibrosis, encephalopathy, periph- eral neuropathy, pulmo- nary fibrosis, secondary malignancy. **Note:** Patients <3 years and who receive cumulative doses >45– 72 grams/m² are at high risk of nephrotoxicity.	High-dose use is investigational. Rule out renal abnormalities in patient before using. Obtain a urinalysis prior to each dose to monitor for urotoxic ADRs, particularly hemorrhagic cysti- tis. (Prophylactic use of mesna is gen- erally recommended to reduce the inci- dence.)	Pratt 1989, 1996
Irinotecan *Camptosar®*, CPT-11 [Natural product, topoisomerase I inhibitor]	Sarcoma **Note:** Not ap- proved by the FDA or HPB for pediatric use.	20 mg/m²/day IV over 1 hr for 5 days. Diarrhea may be severe; administer antidiarrheal drugs concurrently.	Single-dose vials: 40 and 100 mg (20-mg/ml solution); dilute in 5% dextrose (preferred) or 0.9% sodium chloride to 0.12–2.8 mg/ml prior to administration. Stable for 6 hr at	**Common:** Alopecia, anorexia, chills, diarrhea (early), fever, headache, myelosuppression (neutropenia), nausea (early mild), vomiting. **Occasional:** Diarrhea (late), elevated trans- aminases, rash and	Up-front window study in high-risk children with newly diagnosed meta- static rhabdomyo- sarcoma.	Stewart 1996

CHAPTER 12: PEDIATRIC ANTINEOPLASTIC DRUG THERAPY

TABLE 12-9 continued

DRUG TRADE AND OTHER NAMES [CLASS AND TYPE]	INDICATIONS	USUAL PEDIATRIC DOSAGE AND ADMINISTRATION[a]	DOSAGE FORMS[b]	ADRs[c]	CAUTIONS AND COMMENTS[d]	REFER-ENCES[e]
Irinotecan *continued*			room temperature and 24 hr under refrigeration.	flushing during infusion. **Note:** Early diarrhea is very common (within 24 hr) and should be treated with an anticholinergic agent such as atropine at 0.01 mg/kg IV every 4–6 hr. Late diarrhea may be treated with loperamide at usually recommended doses until child is diarrhea free for 12 hr.		
Isotretinoin 13-*cis*-Retinoic Acid, 13-cRA [Vitamin A derivative]	Neuro-blastoma Investigational drug **Note:** Not approved by the FDA or HPB for pediatric use.	160 mg/m^2/day PO for 2 weeks per month for 6 months.	Soft gelatin capsules: 10, 20, 40 mg	**Common:** Cheilitis, dry mucosa, dry skin. **Occasional:** Conjunctivitis; fatigue; headache; musculoskeletal pain; nausea; rash; serum elevations of triglycerides, cholesterol, and transaminases; vomiting. **Rare:** Anemia, changes in skin pigmentation, dizziness, fever, leukopenia, nonspecific GI complaints, pseudotumor-cerebri, retinoic acid syndrome (hyperleukocytosis, hypotension, pulmonary infiltrates, respiratory distress, skeletal hyperostosis). **Note:** Isotretinoin is a known human teratogen; *see* Chapter 2.	Used for high-risk children with metastatic neuroblastoma as post-transplant biological therapy.	Villablanca 1995
Leucovorin Calcium *Wellcovorin*® [Vitamin derivative]	Methotrexate rescue	5–150 mg/m^2 PO or IV after therapy with methotrexate or fluorouracil. Refer to protocol for rescue dose. Usual dose is 10 mg/m^2 (PO/IV) at 18–24 hr after the end of methotrexate infusion, then every 6 hr for 24–72 hr. If toxic levels of methotrexate persist, administer 10–100 mg/m^2 (IV/PO) every 3–6 hr with vigorous hydration until level drops below toxic threshold. For levels >20 μM after 48 hr, must give 100 mg/m^2 IV every 3 hr, and monitor methotrexate serum, BUN, and creatinine levels.	Tablets: 5, 10, 15, 25 mg Injection: Vials of 50, 100, 350 mg; dilute to 10 mg/ml in sterile water for injection. For doses greater than 10 mg/m^2, dilute with sterile water for injection, not bacteriostatic water which contains benzyl alcohol.	**Rare:** Allergic sensitization, pernicious anemia, rash.		Goorin 1995

Footnotes are on page 507.

TABLE 12-9 continued

DRUG TRADE AND OTHER NAMES [CLASS AND TYPE]	INDICATIONS	USUAL PEDIATRIC DOSAGE AND ADMINISTRATION[a]	DOSAGE FORMS[b]	ADRs[c]	CAUTIONS AND COMMENTS[d]	REFERENCES[e]
Lomustine CCNU, *CeeNU*® [Alkylating agent, nitrosourea]	Brain tumors Hodgkin's disease Lymphoma	75–150 mg/m²/dose PO every 4–6 weeks. **Note:** Dose is not repeated until leukocytes and platelets have returned to acceptable levels.	Capsules: 10, 40, 100 mg; store at 15–30°C.	**Common:** Anorexia, myelosuppression, nausea, vomiting. **Occasional:** Alopecia, elevated transaminases. **Rare:** Pulmonary fibrosis or infiltrates, renal failure with cumulative dosing, stomatitis. (Very rare neurologic reactions such as disorientation, lethargy, ataxia, and dysarthria have been reported.)		Geyer 1988 Jenkin 1987
Mechlorethamine *Mustargen*®, Nitrogen Mustard [Alkylating agent, nitrogen mustard]	Hodgkin's disease	6 mg/m²/dose IV on days 1 and 8 every 28 days.	Powder: 10-mg vial; reconstitute in vial with 10 ml of sterile water or 0.9% sodium chloride. Only give IV since it is too toxic for IM or SC administration.	**Common:** Moderate nausea and vomiting, myelosuppression. **Occasional:** Maculopapular eruption, severe nausea and vomiting with anorexia and diarrhea. **Rare:** Alopecia, fever, jaundice, metallic taste, neurotoxicity with high doses, peptic ulcers, tinnitus.	**Vesicant**	Hunger 1994 Weiner 1997
Melphalan *Alkeran*®, l-PAM [Alkylating agent, nitrogen mustard]	Bone marrow transplant (BMT) (leukemia) Neuroblastoma Sarcoma	10–35 mg/m²/dose IV every 3–4 weeks. 4–20 mg/m²/day PO for 1–21 days. **BMT:** 70–140 mg IV as a single dose. Administer by IV infusion over 15–30 min.	Tablets: 2 mg Vials: 50 mg of drug and diluent containing alcohol (0.52 ml), propylene glycol, and sodium citrate	**Common:** Myelosuppression, phlebitis, and skin necrosis with extravasation. **Occasional:** Diarrhea, maculopapular and urticarial rashes, nausea, stomatitis, vomiting. **Rare:** Anaphylaxis, hemolytic anemia, hepatic venoocclusive disease, pulmonary fibrosis, vasculitis. **Note:** Secondary leukemias have been reported; known human teratogen (*see* Chapter 2).		Adamson 1995 Belasco 1987 Chan 1997
Mercaptopurine 6-Mercaptopurine, 6-MP, *Purinethol*® [Antimetabolite, purine analog]	Leukemia **Note:** IV use is investigational.	50–75 mg/m²/day PO or 1000 mg/m² IV by continuous infusion over 6–24 hr.	Tablets: 50 mg; store at 15–30°C away from light. IV preparation: Under study, available from the NCI.	**Common:** Myelosuppression. **Occasional:** Anorexia, diarrhea, mucositis, nausea, vomiting. **Rare:** Anaphylactic reaction, hepatic fibrosis, hyperbilirubinemia, urticaria. **Note:** Concurrent administration of allopurinol will necessitate a mercaptopurine dosage reduction of 65%–75% in order to avoid severe toxicity (*see* Chapter 6).	Monitor patients for thiopurine *S*-methyltransferase (TPMT) genotype since standard doses can be **fatal** for TPMT-deficient patients. Heterozygous patients are also at high risk for toxicity at standard doses. *See* Chapter 11. When given as a single daily dose, give with clear fluids at bedtime; otherwise, considerable variation in bioavailability occurs.	Bostrom 1993

CHAPTER 12: PEDIATRIC ANTINEOPLASTIC DRUG THERAPY

TABLE 12-9 continued

DRUG TRADE AND OTHER NAMES [CLASS AND TYPE]	INDICATIONS	USUAL PEDIATRIC DOSAGE AND ADMINISTRATION[a]	DOSAGE FORMS[b]	ADRs[c]	CAUTIONS AND COMMENTS[d]	REFER-ENCES[e]
Mesna *Mesnex*®, Sodium 2-Mercapto-ethanesulfonate [Cytoprotector, reactive species antagonist]	Hemorrhagic cystitis prophylaxis, co-administered with cyclophosphamide or ifosfamide **Note:** Not approved by the FDA or HPB for pediatric use.	Usually 20% of cyclophosphamide or ifosfamide dose IV push over 15 min, at 15 min prior to dose of chemotherapy, then at 3, 6, and 9 hr after chemotherapy with adequate hydration in the 24 hr after each dose. **Note:** The injectable solution can be administered orally to patients with poor veins, usually as 40% of cyclophosphamide or ifosfamide dose at time 0 and then at 4 and 8 hr after chemotherapy with adequate hydration in the 24 hr after each dose.	Ampules (100 mg/ml): 200, 400, 1000 mg. Store at 15–30°C. Dilute to 20 mg/ml with 5% dextrose and 5% dextrose in 0.45% sodium chloride or lactated Ringer's. Use within 6 hr of mixing. Compatible with ifosfamide.	**Common:** Bad taste with oral use. **Occasional:** Nausea, stomach pain, vomiting. **Rare:** Allergy; diarrhea; fatigue; headache; pain in arms, legs, and joints; rash; transient hypotension. **Note:** Generally well tolerated at recommended dosages.		Skinner 1995
Methotrexate Amethopterin, *Mexate*®, MTX [Antimetabolite, antifolate]	Leukemia Lymphoma Osteosarcoma (high dose)	**Standard dose:** 7.5–30 mg/m² IV, IM, or SC weekly or biweekly. **Intermediate dose:** 1–5 grams/m² IV with push and continuous infusion for 24 hr. Needs leucovorin rescue and monitoring of methotrexate serum levels. **High dose:** 10–12 grams/m² IV over 4–6 hr. Needs leucovorin rescue and monitoring of methotrexate serum levels. **Intrathecal dose** (for CNS prophylaxis in acute lymphoblastic leukemia): Dose adjusted to age. See specific protocols. **Note:** Prehydration is required.	Tablets: 2.5 mg Injection: 25 mg/ml with benzyl alcohol in 0.9% sodium chloride Preservative-free powder: 20, 25, 50, 1000 mg; store at 15–30°C and protect from light. Reconstitute as recommended by the manufacturer.	**Common:** Transaminase elevations. **Occasional:** Anorexia, diarrhea, learning disability, mucositis, myelosuppression, nausea, photosensitivity, stomatitis, vomiting. **Rare:** Allergic reactions, alopecia, blurred vision, CNS deterioration (progressive), dizziness, folliculitis, hyperpigmentation, leukoencephalopathy, liver damage, lung damage, malaise, osteoporosis, renal toxicity, seizures. **Intrathecal ADRs** **Occasional:** Convulsions, fever, headache, learning disability, nausea, pleocytosis, vomiting. **Rare:** Ataxia, CNS deterioration (progressive), convulsions, leukoencephalopathy, meningismus, myelosuppression, paresis, rash, somnolence. **Note:** The incidence of ADRs may vary for high doses.	Use preservative-free methotrexate for intrathecal therapy. Pleural or peritoneal effusions may result in decreased elimination and severe toxicity after IV, intrathecal, or oral dosages. If used in this setting, monitor levels closely to avoid toxicity.	Matherly 1996 Treon 1996
Methylprednisolone [Hormone, corticosteroid]	Leukemia Lymphoma (used for palliative management)	40 mg/m²/day PO or IV (maximum dose 60 mg).	Tablets: 4, 16 mg Ampules: 1 ml (40 mg/ml in acetate form) Ampules with 40, 125, 500, 1000 mg (succinate)	**Common:** Acne, Cushing's syndrome, hyperphagia, immunosuppression, personality changes, pituitary-adrenal axis suppression. **Occasional:** Gastritis, hyperglycemia, muscle		Bleyer 1991 Ryalls 1992

(Continued)

Footnotes are on page 507.

TABLE 12-9 continued

DRUG TRADE AND OTHER NAMES [CLASS AND TYPE]	INDICATIONS	USUAL PEDIATRIC DOSAGE AND ADMINISTRATION[a]	DOSAGE FORMS[b]	ADRs[c]	CAUTIONS AND COMMENTS[d]	REFER- ENCES[e]
Methyl- prednisolone *continued*				weakness, poor wound healing, upset stomach. **Rare:** Aseptic necrosis of the femoral head, cataracts, electrolyte imbalance, GI bleeding, growth retardation, hypertension, increased intraocular pressure, osteopenia, pancreatitis, peptic ulcer, striae.		
Mitoxantrone DHAD, DHAQ, Dihydroxyanthra-cenedione, *Novantrone*® [Natural product, antibiotic]	Leukemia (AML)	10 mg/m^2/day IV for 3–5 days. Do **not** administer if baseline neutrophil counts are below 1500/mm^3.	2-mg/ml dark blue sterile solution in 20- and 25-mg vials. Reconstitute with 50 ml of 5% dextrose or 0.9% sodium chloride; maintains potency for 7 days. Administer over >3 min in a volume >50 ml of 5% dextrose or 0.9% normal saline.	**Common:** Alopecia, blue–green color to urine, cardiac dysrhythmias (not clinically significant), immunosuppression, local ulceration if extravasated, nausea, myelosuppression, vomiting, worsens ADRs due to radiation. **Occasional:** Cardiomyopathy (cumulative dosing), hepatotoxicity, mucositis, stomatitis. **Rare:** Allergic reactions, anaphylaxis, rash, secondary malignancy.	**Vesicant.** Cardiomyopathy is especially problematic in patients pretreated with doxorubicin.	Behar 1992
Paclitaxel *Taxol*® [Natural product, microtubule stabilizer]	Leukemia Sarcoma **Note:** Not approved by the FDA or HPB for this indication for use among children or adolescents.	175–300 mg/m^2 IV by continuous infusion for 3 or 24 hr every 3 weeks. **Note:** Pretreat all patients with oral dexamethasone 20 mg 12 hr before dose, cimetidine 300 mg 30–60 min before dose, and diphenhydramine 1 mg/kg IV 30–60 min before dose. Do **not** administer if baseline neutrophil counts are below 1500/mm^3.	Vials: 6 mg/ml; dilute in 0.9% sodium chloride, 5% dextrose, or Ringer's solution to 0.3–1.2 mg/ml.	**Common:** Alopecia, myalgia and arthralgia, myelosuppression, nausea, sensory neuropathy, vomiting. **Occasional:** Abnormal ECG; diarrhea (mild); **potentially fatal** hypersensitivity reactions with dyspnea, hypotension, bronchospasm, urticaria, and rash; mucositis. **Rare:** Seizures. **Note:** At high doses severe neurotoxicity seen in children. This toxicity may be due to the high ethanol content (~50%) of the injectable formulation.	Completed phase I study. No active phase II studies.	Hurwitz 1993
Pegaspargase *Oncaspar*® [Enzyme, asparaginase derivative]	Leukemia Lymphoma (as part of a selected multiple-drug regimen)	2500 IU/m^2/dose IM every 1–2 weeks.	Solution: 750 IU/ml	See **Asparaginase**.	See **Asparaginase**.	
Prednisolone [Hormone, corticosteroid]	Leukemia (used for palliative management)	40 mg/m^2/day PO (maximum dose 60 mg).	Oral liquid solution in sodium phosphate form: 5 mg/ml in a 120-ml bottle (*Pediapred*®) or	**Common:** Acne, Cushing's syndrome, hyperphagia, immunosuppression, personality changes, pituitary-adrenal axis suppression.		Jones 1972

CHAPTER 12: PEDIATRIC ANTINEOPLASTIC DRUG THERAPY

TABLE 12-9 continued

DRUG TRADE AND OTHER NAMES [CLASS AND TYPE]	INDICATIONS	USUAL PEDIATRIC DOSAGE AND ADMINISTRATION[a]	DOSAGE FORMS[b]	ADRs[c]	CAUTIONS AND COMMENTS[d]	REFER-ENCES[e]
Prednisolone *continued*			3-mg/ml solution (Prelone®)	**Occasional:** Gastritis, hyperglycemia, muscle weakness, poor wound healing, upset stomach. **Rare:** Aseptic necrosis of the femoral head, cataracts, electrolyte imbalance, GI bleeding, growth retardation, hypertension, increased intraocular pressure, osteopenia, pancreatitis, peptic ulcer, striae.		
Prednisone *Deltasone®*, PRED [Hormone, corticosteroid]	Leukemia (used for palliative management)	40 mg/m²/day PO for 28 days (maximum dose 60 mg); other regimens use same dose daily for 7–14 days.	Tablets: 2.5, 5, 10, 20 mg Oral liquid solution: 5 mg/ml in a 120-ml bottle	**Common:** Acne, Cushing's syndrome, hyperphagia, immunosuppression, personality changes, pituitary-adrenal axis suppression. **Occasional:** Gastritis, hyperglycemia, muscle weakness, poor wound healing, upset stomach. **Rare:** Aseptic necrosis of the femoral head, cataracts, electrolyte imbalance, GI bleeding, growth retardation, hypertension, increased intraocular pressure, osteopenia, pancreatitis, peptic ulcer, striae.		Leikin 1968 Wolff 1967
Procarbazine *Matulane®*, PCZ [Miscellaneous, methylhydrazine derivative]	Brain tumors Hodgkin's disease Neuroblastoma	50–200 mg/m²/day PO for 10–14 days.	Capsules: 50 mg; do **not** open.	**Common:** Myelosuppression, severe nausea and vomiting. **Occasional:** Abdominal pain, anorexia, diarrhea and constipation, dryness of the mouth, dysphagia, stomatitis. **Rare:** CNS reactions such as paresthesias, neuropathies, and confusion; dyserythropoeisis, hemolysis.		Lange 1978
Rituximab *Rituxan®* [Biological agent, monoclonal antibody]	Post-transplant lymphoproliferative disease, CD20 positive **Note:** Not approved by the FDA or HPB for pediatric use.	375 mg/m²/dose IV weekly for 4 weeks. Requires premedication with acetaminophen 650 mg and diphenhydramine 25 mg PO. Withhold antihypertensives. Infuse IV slowly as per protocol to avoid ADRs.	Solution: 10 mg/ml; dilute to 1–4 mg/ml. **Potentially fatal** infusion-related events can occur.	**Common:** B cell depletion, infusion-related hypersensitivity (resolves with interrupting the infusion or slowing the rate). **Occasional:** Dizziness, myalgia, nausea, pruritus, rash, urticaria, vomiting. **Rare:** Angioedema (severe), dysrhythmias and angina, bronchospasm, chest pain, edema and postural hypotension, tachycardia.	Very limited experience in children. Currently under investigation for the treatment of post-transplant lymphoproliferative disease. Not active in non-Hodgkin's lymphoma (NHL) clinical trials due to the rare incidence of mature B-cell NHL in children.	Leget 1998

Footnotes are on page 507.

TABLE 12-9 continued

DRUG TRADE AND OTHER NAMES [CLASS AND TYPE]	INDICATIONS	USUAL PEDIATRIC DOSAGE AND ADMINISTRATION[a]	DOSAGE FORMS[b]	ADRs[c]	CAUTIONS AND COMMENTS[d]	REFER-ENCES[e]
Sargramostim GM-CSF, *Leukine*®, Granulocyte Macrophage Colony-stimulating Factor [Biologic agent]	Post bone marrow transplant (BMT) for delayed engraftment. Myelodysplastic syndrome	50–100 μg/m²/day SC for 10–14 days. Post BMT for engraftment delay: 250 μg/m²/day.	Lyophilized powder: Vials of 250 or 500 μg; store at 2–8°C. Discard after 6 hr at room temperature (lack of preservatives).	**Common:** Bone, back, or leg pain; mild local reaction at injection site. **Occasional:** Acute hypersensitivity reaction, asthenia, chills, fever, headache, malaise, myalgia, nausea, pruritus, rash, vomiting. **Rare:** Fluid retention, pericarditis, venous thrombosis.		Hann 1995
Teniposide VM-26, *Vumon*® [Podophyllotoxin derivative, topoisomerase II inhibitor]	Leukemia	130–250 mg/m²/day IV for 2 or 3 days every 3 weeks. **Note:** To avoid the risk of hypotension or other ADRs, administer by IV infusion over 30–60 min. Frequently monitor the patency of the venous access device because occlusion has occurred during infusion.	Vials: 10 mg/ml with dehydrated alcohol and polyoxyl 35 castor oil; dilute with 0.9% sodium chloride or 5% dextrose solution to 0.1, 0.2, 0.4, or 1 mg/ml.	**Common:** Diarrhea, mucositis, myelosuppression, nausea, vomiting. **Occasional:** Alopecia. **Rare:** Hypersensitivity reactions characterized by anaphylaxislike signs (fever, chills, tachycardia, flushing, bronchospasm, dyspnea, blood pressure changes); hypertensive reactions with cardiac failure, rash, and fever; secondary acute myeloid leukemia; transient hypotension, associated with somnolence and metabolic acidosis. **Note:** Patients with both Down's syndrome and leukemia may be particularly sensitive to the myelosuppressive effects of teniposide chemotherapy. Initial dosages should be reduced by 50% for these patients and then adjusted as indicated by clinical response, including degree of myelosuppression and mucositis.	Schedule may be related to secondary leukemia. Vesicant if large volume extravasates.	Dahl 1987
Thioguanine *Tabloid*®, 6-TG, 6-Thioguanine [Antimetabolite, purine analog]	Leukemia (AML)	75–100 mg/m²/day PO for 5–7 days.	Tablets: 40 mg	**Common:** Myelosuppression. **Occasional:** Anorexia, diarrhea, mucositis, nausea, vomiting. **Rare:** Anaphylactic reactions, hepatic fibrosis, hyperbilirubinemia, urticaria.		Hann 1997 Moreno 1977
Thiotepa Triethylenethiophosphoramide [Alkylating agent, ethylenimine derivative]	Bone marrow transplant (BMT)	200 mg/m²/dose IV for 2 or 3 days. Administer high doses over 2 hr.	Vials: 15 mg; reconstitute with 1.5 ml of sterile water for injection to make a 10-mg/ml solution. Store at 2–8°C and protect from light.	**Common:** Anorexia, gonadal dysfunction or infertility, mucositis and esophagitis (high doses), myelosuppression, nausea, vomiting.		Kletzel 1998 Przepiorka 1995

CHAPTER 12: PEDIATRIC ANTINEOPLASTIC DRUG THERAPY

TABLE 12-9 continued

DRUG TRADE AND OTHER NAMES [CLASS AND TYPE]	INDICATIONS	USUAL PEDIATRIC DOSAGE AND ADMINISTRATION[a]	DOSAGE FORMS[b]	ADRs[c]	CAUTIONS AND COMMENTS[d]	REFERENCES[e]
Thiotepa *continued*			Further dilute with 0.9% sodium chloride, 5% dextrose, dextrose and sodium chloride, Ringer's or lactated Ringer's solution. Use within 8 hr of mixing.	**Occasional:** Confusion, dizziness, headache, hyperpigmentation of the skin, inappropriate behavior (at high doses), increased bilirubin, increased liver transaminases, pain at the injection site, somnolence. **Rare:** Febrile reaction, hives, skin rash.		
Topotecan *Hycamtin*® [Camptothecin derivative, topoisomerase I inhibitor]	Sarcomas **Note:** Not approved by the FDA or HPB for use for this indication among children or adolescents.	2.4 mg/m²/day IV for 5 days every 3 weeks. **Note:** Monitor pediatric patients for neutropenia and withhold therapy if neutrophil counts are below 1500/mm³.	Lyophilized powder: Vials of 4 mg with 48 mg of mannitol and 20 mg of tartaric acid. The pH is adjusted to 3 and the solution is diluted to 1 mg/ml in 4 ml of sterile water for injection, then further diluted to 10–500 µg/ml with 0.9% sodium chloride or to 6.7–330 µg/ml in 5% dextrose. Drug diluted to 20–100 µg/ml is stable at room temperature for 24 hr.	**Common:** Alopecia, myelosuppression. **Occasional:** Asthenia, diarrhea; elevated serum transaminases, alkaline phosphatase, and bilirubin; flulike symptoms; headache; mucositis; nausea; rash; vomiting. **Rare:** Abdominal pain, microscopic hematuria, rigors.	Up-front window study in high-risk children with intermediate-risk rhabdomyosarcoma. Phase II study in refractory acute leukemia.	Blaney 1998 Nitschke 1998
Trastuzumab *Herceptin*® [Biological agent, monoclonal antibody]	Osteosarcoma with HER2 antigen overexpression	Loading dose: 4 mg/kg, then 2 mg/kg/week IV for 6 months. **Note:** Administer by IV infusion only. Do **not** administer by IV bolus or push.	Preservative-free lyophilized powder: Vials of 440 mg **Note:** Do not admix with other drugs or solutions. Do not use dextrose solutions	**Common:** Asthenia, chills (mild to moderate), fever, nausea, pain, vomiting and headaches (during first infusion). **Occasional:** Angioedema, back pain, bronchospasm, chest pain, diarrhea, dyspnea and cough, hypotension, pruritus, rash, urticaria. **Note:** Adults treated with anthracyclines and trastuzumab suffer from cardiac dysfunction. The potential effect in children is unknown.	First pediatric study not open.	
Tretinoin all-*trans*-Retinoic Acid, ATRA, t-RNA, *Vesanoid*® [Vitamin A derivative, differentiation inducing agent]	Acute promyelocytic leukemia	45 mg/m²/day PO divided in two doses 6 hr apart. **Note:** Administer with meals to increase bioavailability.	Capsules: 10 mg soft gelatin	**Common:** Cheilitis, dry mucosa and skin. **Occasional:** Conjunctivitis; elevated serum levels of triglycerides, cholesterol, and transaminases; fatigue; headache; musculoskeletal pain; nausea; rash; vomiting. **Rare:** Anemia; changes in skin pigmentation; dizziness; leukopenia; nonspecific GI complaints; pseudotumor-cerebri; retinoic acid syndrome (fever,		Fenaux 1998

(Continued)

Footnotes are on page 507.

TABLE 12-9 continued

DRUG TRADE AND OTHER NAMES [CLASS AND TYPE]	INDICATIONS	USUAL PEDIATRIC DOSAGE AND ADMINISTRATION[a]	DOSAGE FORMS[b]	ADRs[c]	CAUTIONS AND COMMENTS[d]	REFER- ENCES[e]
Tretinoin *continued*				hyperleukocytosis, hypotension, pulmonary infiltrates, respiratory distress, skeletal hyperostosis). **Note:** Tretinoin is a known human teratogen; *see* Isotretinoin in Chapter 2.		
Vinblastine *Velban®*, VLB, Vincaleuko-blastine Sulfate [Natural product, mitotic inhibitor]	Hodgkin's disease Histiocytosis	3.5–6 mg/m^2/week IV for 3–6 weeks. **Dose adjustment:** T. bili >3 mg/dl, 50% dose. **Note:** For IV use only; intrathecal administration has resulted in **death**.	Solution: 1 mg/ml Sterile powder: Vials of 10 mg; reconstitute with 0.9% sodium chloride with or without preservative is recommended. Light sensitive; protect from light. If the diluent contains a preservative, the drug may be stable at 2–8°C for 28 days.	**Common:** Hair loss, local ulceration if extravasated, loss of deep tendon reflexes, myelosuppression, nausea, vomiting and anorexia. **Occasional** (less common than with vincristine): Constipation, jaw pain, peripheral neuropathies and clumsiness, weakness. **Rare:** Abdominal pain with paralytic ileus; hemorrhagic enterocolitis; dysfunction of the autonomic nervous system manifested by urinary retention; eighth cranial nerve damage manifested by dizziness, nystagmus, vertigo, and hearing loss; headache; orthostatic hypotension; sinus tachycardia; stomatitis; tender parotid glands.	Vesicant	Khan 1994 Skapek 1998
Vincristine *Oncovin®*, VCR [Natural product, mitotic inhibitor]	Leukemia Lymphoma Sarcoma	1–1.5 mg/m^2/week IV (maximum dose 2 mg) for 3–6 weeks. **Dose adjustment:** T. bili >3 mg/dl, 50% dose. **Note:** For IV use only; intrathecal administration has resulted in **death**.	Solutions: 1 mg/ml in vials of 1, 2, or 5 ml; refrigerate and protect from light.	**Common:** Hair loss, local ulceration if extravasated, loss of deep tendon reflexes. **Occasional:** Constipation, jaw pain, peripheral neuropathy and clumsiness, weakness. **Rare:** CNS depression, inappropriate ADH secretion, myelosuppression, paralytic ileus, ptosis, seizures, vocal cord paralysis.	Vesicant	Crom 1994

Summary

The successes of pediatric oncology are a tribute to the sacrifice and cooperation of children and their families over the last four decades. The revolution in genomic sciences holds great promise for the nearly 20% of children who have not benefited from multi-drug antineoplastic therapy, in particular those who suffer from CNS neoplasms. The ongoing challenge for clinician-scientists will be to choose wisely from the large number of new drugs in development that target abnormal signal transduction pathways in cancer cells. And to translate the knowledge derived from pharmacogenomics and the molecular taxonomy of cancer into rational therapeutic strategies (Brown & Botstein, 1999; Evans & Relling, 1999; Scherf et al., 2000).

References

Adamson, P. C., Balis, F. M. , Belasco, J. E., et al. (1995). A phase I trial of amifostine (WR-2721) and melphalan in children with refractory cancer. *Cancer Research, 55*(18), 4069–4072.

Alberts, D. S., Chang, S. Y., Chen, H. S., et al. (1979). Pharmacokinetics and metabolism of chlorambucil in man: A preliminary report. *Cancer Treatment Reviews, 6*(Suppl), 9–17.

Baker, W. J., Royer, G. L., & Weiss, R. B. (1991). Cytarabine and neurologic toxicity. *Journal of Clinical Oncology, 9*, 679–693.

Balis, F. M., Gillespie, A., Belasco, J., et al. (1990). Phase II trial of sequential methotrexate and 5-fluorouracil with leucovorin in children with sarcomas. *Investigational New Drugs, 8*, 181.

Barnett, M. J., Richards, M. A., Ganesan, T. S., et al. (1985). Central nervous system toxicity of high-dose cytosine arabinoside. *Seminars in Oncology, 12*(2 Suppl 3), 227–232.

Behar, C., Bertrand, Y., Rubie, H., et al. (1992). Mitoxantrone and high dose Ara-C for the treatment of ANLL in childhood: A pilot study of the EORTC CLCG (EORTC 58 872). *Leukemia, 6*(Suppl 2), 63–65.

Belasco, J. B., Mitchell, C. D., Rohrbaugh, T., et al. (1987). IV melphalan in children. *Cancer Treatment Reports, 71*(12), 1277–1278.

Bernstein, L., Abshire, T. C., Pollock, B. H., et al. (1997). Idarubicin and cytosine arabinoside re-induction therapy for children with multiple recurrent or refractory acute lymphoblastic leukemia: A Pediatric Oncology Group study. *Journal of Pediatric Hematology/Oncology, 19*(1), 68–72.

Blaney, S. M., Needle, M. N., Gillespie, A., et al. (1998). Phase II trial of topotecan administered as 72-hour continuous infusion in children with refractory solid tumors: A collaborative Pediatric Branch, National Cancer Institute, and Children's Cancer Group Study. *Clinical Cancer Research, 4*(2), 357–360.

Bleyer, W. A. (1977). Current status of intrathecal chemotherapy for human meningeal neoplasms. *National Cancer Institute Monograph, 46*, 171–178

Bleyer, W. A., Sather, H. N., Nickerson, H. J., et al. (1991). Monthly pulses of vincristine and prednisone prevent bone marrow and testicular relapse in low-risk childhood acute lymphoblastic leukemia: A report of the CCG-161 study by the Children's Cancer Study Group. *Clinical Oncology, 9*(6), 1012–1021.

Bostrom, B., & Erdmann, G. (1993). Cellular pharmacology of 6-mercaptopurine in acute lymphoblastic leukemia. *American Journal of Pediatric Hematology-Oncology, 15*(1), 80–86.

Brock, P. R., Koliouskas, D. E., Barratt, T. M., et al. (1991). Partial reversibility of cisplatin nephrotoxicity in children. *The Journal of Pediatrics, 118*(4), 531–534.

Brock, P. R., Yeomans, E. C., Bellman, S. C., et al. (1992). Cisplatin therapy in infants: Short and long-term morbidity. *British Journal of Cancer, 18*(Suppl), S36–40.

Brown, P. O., & Botstein, D. (1999). Exploring the new world of the genome with DNA microarrays. *Nature Genetics, 21*(1 Suppl), 33–37.

Cachat, F., & Guignard, J. P. (1996). The kidney in children under chemotherapy. *Revue Medicale de la Suisse Romande, 116*(12), 985–993.

Canetta, R., Bragman, K., Smaldone, L., et al. (1988). Carboplatin: Current status and future prospects. *Cancer Treatment Reviews, 15*(Suppl B), 17–32.

Carter, S. K. (1976). Proceedings of the sixth new drug seminar. *DTIC-Cancer Treatment Reports, 60*, 123–214.

Carter, S. K., & Blum, R. H. (1974). New chemotherapeutic agents—Bleomycin and adriamycin. *CA: Cancer Journal for Clinicians, 24*(6), 322–331.

Carter, S. K., & Blum, R. H. (1976). Current status of American studies with bleomycin. *Progress in Biochemical Pharmacology, 11*, 158–171.

Chan, K. W., Petropoulos, D., Choroszy, M., et al. (1997). High-dose sequential chemotherapy and autologous stem cell reinfusion in advanced pediatric solid tumors. *Bone Marrow Transplant, 20*(12), 1039–1043.

Coates, A., Abraham, S., Kaye, S. B., et al. (1983). On the receiving end–Patient perception of the side-effects of cancer chemotherapy. *European Journal of Cancer and Clinical Oncology, 19*, 203–208.

Comis, R. L. (1992). Bleomycin pulmonary toxicity: Current status and future directions. [Review]. *Seminars in Oncology, 19*(2 Suppl 5), 64–70.

Controlling occupational exposure to hazardous drugs. Occupational Safety and Health Administration (1996). *American Journal of Health-System Pharmacists, 53,* 1669–1685.

Creutzig, U., Ritter, J., Zimmermann, M., et al. (1996). Prognosis of children with chronic myeloid leukemia: A retrospective analysis of 75 patients. *Klinische Padiatroe, 208*(4), 236–241.

Crom, W. R., de Graaf, S. S., Synold, T., et al. (1994). Pharmacokinetics of vincristine in children and adolescents with acute lymphocytic leukemia. *The Journal of Pediatrics, 125*(4), 642–649.

Dahl, G. V., Lacayo, N. J., Brophy, N., et al. (2000). Mitoxantrone, etoposide, and cyclosporine therapy in pediatric patients with recurrent or refractory acute myeloid leukemia. *Journal of Clinical Oncology, 18*(9), 1867–1895.

Dahl, G. V., Rivera, G. K., Look, A. T., et al. (1987). Teniposide plus cytarabine improves outcome in childhood acute lymphoblastic leukemia presenting with a leukocyte count greater than or equal to 100 × 10(9)/L. *Journal of Clinical Oncology, 5*(7), 1015–1021.

D'Angio, G. J. (1987). Unexpected toxicity encountered in the National Wilms' Tumor Study. *Cancer Treatment Reports, 71*(10), 993.

Evans, W. E., & Relling, M. V. (1999). Pharmacogenomics: Translating functional genomics into rational therapeutics. *Science, 286,* 487–491.

Evans, W. E., Relling, M. V., Rodman, J. H., et al. (1998). Conventional compared with individualized chemotherapy for childhood acute lymphoblastic leukemia. *New England Journal of Medicine, 338,* 499–505.

Evans, W. E., Tsiatis, A., Rivera, G., et al. (1982). Anaphylactoid reactions to Escherichia coli and Erwinia asparaginase in children with leukemia and lymphoma. *Cancer, 49*(7), 1378–1383.

Fenaux, P., & De Botton, S. (1998). Retinoic acid syndrome. Recognition, prevention and management. *Drug Safety, 18*(4), 273–279.

Fleming, R. A., Miller, A. A., & Stewart, C. F. (1989). Etoposide: An update. *Clinical Pharmacy, 8,* 274–293.

Foster, B. J., Clagett-Carr, K., Leyland-Jones, B., et al. (1985). Results of NCI-sponsored phase I trials with carboplatin. *Cancer Treatment Reviews, 12*(Suppl A), 43–49.

Frei, E. (1974). The clinical use of actinomycin. *Cancer Chemotherapy Reports, 58,* 49–54.

Galton, D. A. G., Till, M., & Wiltshaw, E. (1958). Busulfan: Summary of clinical practice results. *Annals of the New York Academy of Sciences, 68,* 967–973.

Gaynon, P. S. (1994). Carboplatin in pediatric malignancies. *Seminars in Oncology, 21*(5 Suppl 12), 65–76.

Gershwin, M. E., Goetzl, E. J., & Steinberg, A. D. (1974). Cyclophosphamide: Use in practice. *Annals of Internal Medicine, 80*(4), 531–540.

Geyer, J. R., Pendergrass, T. W., Milstein, J. M., et al. (1988). Eight drugs in one day chemotherapy in children with brain tumors: A critical toxicity appraisal. *Clinical Oncology, 6*(6), 996–1000.

Glover, D., Fox, K. R., Weiler, C., et al. (1988). Clinical trials of WR-2721 prior to alkylating agent chemotherapy and radiotherapy. *Pharmacology and Therapeutics, 39*(1–3), 3–7.

Goorin, A., Strother, D., Poplack, D., et al. (1995). Safety and efficacy of l-leucovorin rescue following high-dose methotrexate for osteosarcoma. *Medical and Pediatric Oncology, 24*(6), 362–367.

Gottlieb, J., Benjamin, R. S., & Baker, L. H. (1976). Role of DTIC (NSC-45388) in the chemotherapy of sarcomas. *Cancer Treatment Reports, 60,* 199–203.

Grenier, M. A., & Lipshultz, S. E. (1998). Epidemiology of anthracycline cardiotoxicity in children and adults. *Seminars in Oncology, 25*(4 Suppl 10), 72–85.

Gutin, P. H. (1975). Corticosteroid therapy in patients with cerebral tumors: Benefits, mechanisms, problems, and practicalities. *Seminars in Oncology, 2,* 49–56.

Hakami, N., Look, A. T., Steuber, P. C., et al. (1987). Combined etoposide and 5-azacitidine in children and adolescents with refractory or relapsed acute nonlymphocytic leukemia: A Pediatric Oncology Group study. *Journal of Clinical Oncology, 5*(7), 1022–1025.

Hann, I. M. (1995). Haemopoietic growth factors and childhood cancer. *European Journal of Cancer, 31A*(9), 1476–1478.

Hann, I. M., Stevens, R. F., Goldstone, A. H., et al. (1997). Randomized comparison of DAT versus ADE as induction chemotherapy in children and younger adults with acute myeloid leukemia. Results of the Medical Research Council's 10th AML trial (MRC AML10). Adult and Childhood Leukaemia Working Parties of the Medical Research Council. *Blood, 89*(7), 2311–2318.

Harney, E., Cochrane, D., Marina, N., et al. (1999). Phase I trial of pegylated liposomal doxorubicin (Doxil) in children with solid tumors. *Proceedings American Society of Clinical Oncology, 18,* #2146a, p. 556a.

Hartmann, O. (1995). New strategies for the application of high-dose chemotherapy with haematopoietic support in paediatric solid tumours. *Annals of Oncology, 6*(Suppl 4), 1316.

Hesketh, P. J., Beck, T., Uhlenhopp, M., et al. (1995). Adjusting the dose of intravenous ondansetron plus dexamethasone to the emetogenic potential of the chemotherapy regimen. *Journal of Clinical Oncology, 13*(8), 2117–2122.

Hunger, S. P., Link, M. P., & Donaldson, S. S. (1994). ABVD/MOPP and low-dose involved-field radiotherapy in pediatric Hodgkin's disease: The Stanford experience. *Journal of Clinical Oncology, 12*(10), 2160–2166.

Hurwitz, C. A., Relling, M. V., Weitman, S. D., et al.

(1993). Phase I trial of paclitaxel in children with refractory solid tumors: A Pediatric Oncology Group study. *Journal of Clinical Oncology, 11*(12), 2324–2329.

Jenkin, R. D., Boesel, C., Ertel, I., et al. (1987). Brain-stem tumors in childhood: A prospective randomized trial of irradiation with and without adjuvant CCNU, VCR, and prednisone. A report of the Children's Cancer Study Group. *Journal of Neurosurgery, 66*(2), 227–233.

Jones, B., Cuttner, J., Levy, R. N., et al. (1972). Daunorubicin (NSC-83142) versus daunorubicin plus prednisone (NSC-10023) versus daunorubicin plus vincristine (NSC-67574) plus prednisone in advanced childhood acute lymphocytic leukemia. *Cancer Chemotherapy Reports, 56*(6), 729–737.

Khan, S. P., Gilchrist, G. S., Arndt, C. A., et al. (1994). Vancouver hybrid: Preliminary experience in the treatment of Hodgkin's disease in childhood and adolescence. *Mayo Clinic Proceedings, 69*(10), 949–954.

Kletzel, M., Abella, E. M., Sandler, E. S., et al. (1998). Thiotepa and cyclophosphamide with stem cell rescue for consolidation therapy for children with high-risk neuroblastoma: A phase I/II study of the Pediatric Blood and Marrow Transplant Consortium. *Journal of Pediatric Hematology/Oncology, 20*(1), 49–54.

Kucuk, O., Kwan, H. C., Gunnar, W., et al. (1985). Thromboembolic complications associated with L-asparaginase therapy. *Cancer, 55,* 702–706.

Land, V. J., Sutow, W. W., Fernback, D. J., et al. (1972). Toxicity of L-asparaginase in children with advanced leukemia. *Cancer, 30,* 339–347.

Lange, B., Littman, P., Schnaufer, L., et al. (1978). Treatment of advanced Hodgkin's disease in pediatric patients. *Cancer, 42*(3), 1141–1145.

Lass, J. H. (1982). Topical corticosteroid therapy for corneal toxicity from systemically administered cytarabine. *American Journal of Ophthalmology, 94,* 617–621.

Laszlo, J. (1995). *The cure of childhood leukemia: Into the age of miracles.* Piscataway, NJ: Rutgers University Press.

Laver, J., Amylon, M., Desai, S., et al. (1998). Randomized trial of r-mctHu granulocyte colony stimulating factor in an intensive treatment for T-cell leukemia and advanced-stage lymphoblastic lymphoma of childhood: A Pediatric Oncology Group pilot study. *Journal of Clinical Oncology, 16*(2), 522.

Leahey, A., Kelly, K., Rorke, L. B., et al. (1997). A phase I/II study of idarubicin (Ida) with continuous infusion fludarabine (F-ara-A) and cytarabine (ara-C) for refractory or recurrent pediatric acute myeloid leukemia (AML). *Journal of Pediatric Hematology/Oncology, 19*(4), 304–308.

Leget, G. A., & Czuczman, M. S. (1998). Use of rituximab, the new FDA-approved antibody. *Current Opinion in Oncology, 10*(6), 548–551.

Leikin, S. L., Brubaker, C., Hartmann, J. R., et al. (1968). Varying prednisone dosage in remission induction of previously untreated childhood leukemia. *Cancer, 21*(3), 346–351.

Lipshultz, S. E., Colan, S. D., & Gelber, R. D. (1991). Late cardiac effects of doxorubicin therapy for acute lymphocytic leukemia in childhood. *New England Journal of Medicine, 324,* 808–815.

Loebstein, R., Atanackovic, G., Bishai, R., et al. (1999). Risk factors for long-term outcome of ifosfamide-induced nephrotoxicity in children. *Journal of Clinical Pharmacology, 39*(5), 454–461.

Loehrer, P. J., & Einhorn, L. H. (1984). Drugs five years later. Cisplatin. *Annals of Internal Medicine, 100*(5), 704–713.

Lum, B. L., Kaubisch, S., Yahanda, A. M., et al. (1992). Alteration of etoposide pharmacokinetics and pharmacodynamics by cyclosporine in a phase I trial to modulate multidrug resistance. *Journal of Clinical Oncology, 10*(10), 1635–1642.

Matherly, L. H., & Taub, J. W. (1996). Methotrexate pharmacology and resistance in childhood acute lymphoblastic leukemia. *Leukemia and Lymphoma, 21*(5–6), 359–368.

Matthews, R. N., & Colebatch, J. H. (1972). Daunorubicin: Results in childhood leukemia. *Archives of Disease in Childhood, 47,* 272–277.

McLeod, H. L., Relling, M. V., Crom, W. R., et al. (1992). Disposition of antineoplastic agents in the very young child. *British Journal of Cancer, 66*(Suppl 18), 23–29.

Mertens, R., Granzen, B., Lassay, L., et al. (1997). Nasopharyngeal carcinoma in childhood and adolescence: Concept and preliminary results of the cooperative GPOH study NPC-91. Gesellschaft fur Pädiatrische Onkologie und Hamatologie. *Cancer, 80*(5), 951.

Meyer, K. B., & Madias, N. E. (1994). Cisplatin nephrotoxicity. *Mineral and Electrolyte Metabolism, 20*(4), 201–213.

Miller, M. (1959). The use of chlorambucil: A critical study. *New England Journal of Medicine, 261,* 525–528.

Mitchell, E. P., & Schein, P. S. (1986). Contributions of nitrosoureas to cancer treatment. *Cancer Treatment Reports, 70*(1), 31–41.

Moore, M. J. (1991). Clinical pharmacokinetics of cyclophosphamide. *Clinical Pharmacokinetics, 20*(3), 194–208.

Moreno, H., Castleberry, R. P., & McCann, W. P. (1977). Cytosine arabinoside and 6-thioguanine in the treatment of childhood acute myeloblastic leukemia. *Cancer, 40*(3), 998–1004.

Muller, H. J., & Boos, J. (1998). Use of L-asparaginase in childhood ALL. *Critical Reviews in Oncology/Hematology, 28*(2), 97–113.

Murphy, C. P., Harden, E. A., & Thompson, J. M. (1992). Generalized seizures secondary to high-dose busulfan therapy. *Annals of Pharmacotherapy, 26*(1), 30–31.

Neuendank, A., Hartmann, R., Buhrer, C., et al. (1997). Acute toxicity and effectiveness of idarubicin in childhood acute lymphoblastic leukemia. *European Journal of Haematology, 58*(5), 326–332.

Nitschke, R., Parkhurst, J., Sullivan, J., et al. (1998). Topotecan in pediatric patients with recurrent and progressive solid tumors: A Pediatric Oncology Group phase II study. *Journal of Pediatric Hematology/Oncology, 20*(4), 315–318.

Occupational Safety & Health Administration (1999, May 4). Office of Occupational Medicine: Hazardous Drugs/Antineoplastic Drugs.

Occupational Safety & Health Administration (2000, January 31). Technical Links: OSHA Technical Manual. (http://www.osha-slc.gov/dts/osta/otm/otm_vi/otm_vi_2.html).

O'Driscoll, B., Hasleton, P., Taylor, P., et al. (1990). Active lung fibrosis up to 17 years after chemotherapy with carmustine (BCNU) in childhood. *New England Journal of Medicine, 323*, 378–382.

O'Dwyer, P. J., Leyland-Jones, B., Alonso, M. T., et al. (1998). Etoposide, current status of an active anticancer drug. *New England Journal of Medicine, 312*, 692–700.

Palmer, R. G., & Denman, A. M. (1984). Malignancies induced by chlorambucil. *Cancer Treatment Reviews, 11*, 121–129.

Pratt, C. B., Douglass, E. C., Etcubanas, E. L., et al. (1989). Ifosfamide in pediatric malignant solid tumors. *Cancer Chemotherapy and Pharmacology, 24*(Suppl 1), S24–27.

Pratt, C. B., Luo, X., Fang, L., et al. (1996). Response of pediatric malignant solid tumors following ifosfamide or ifosfamide/carboplatin/etoposide: A single hospital experience. *Medical and Pediatric Oncology, 27*(3), 145–148.

Przepiorka, D., Madden, T., Ippoliti, C., et al. (1995). Dosing of thioTEPA for myeloablative therapy. *Cancer Chemotherapy and Pharmacology, 37*(1–2), 155–160.

Raney, B., Ensign, L. G., Foreman, J., et al. (1994). Renal toxicity of ifosfamide in pilot regimens of the intergroup rhabdomyosarcoma study for patients with gross residual tumor. *American Journal of Pediatric Hematology-Oncology, 16*(4), 286–295.

Relling, M. V., Hancock, M. L., Rivera, G. K., et al. (1999). Mercaptopurine therapy intolerance and heterozygosity at the thiopurine S-methyltransferase gene locus. *Journal of the National Cancer Institute, 91*, 2001–2008.

Rosenfeld, C. S., Weosberg, S. R., & York, R. M. (1992). Prevention of Adriamycin cardiomyopathy with dexrazoxane (ADR-529, ICRF-187). *Proceedings of the American Society of Clinical Oncology, 11*, 62.

Ryalls, M. R., Pinkerton, C. R., Meller, S. T., et al. (1992). High-dose methylprednisolone sodium succinate as a single agent in relapsed childhood acute lymphoblastic leukaemia. *Medical and Pediatric Oncology, 20*(2), 119–123.

Santana, V. M., Mirro, J. Jr., Harwood, F. C., et al. (1991). A phase I clinical trial of 2-chlorodeoxyadenosine in pediatric patients with acute leukemia. *Journal of Clinical Oncology, 9*(3), 416–422.

Saven, A., Kawasaki, H., Carrera, C. J., et al. (1993). 2-Chlorodeoxyadenosine dose escalation in nonhematologic malignancies. *Journal of Clinical Oncology, 11*(4), 671–678.

Schaefer, S. D., Post, J. D., Close, L. G., et al. (1985). Ototoxicity of low- and moderate-dose cisplatin. *Cancer, 56*, 1934–1939.

Scherf, U., Ross, D. T., Waltham, M., et al. (2000). A gene expression database for the molecular pharmacology of cancer. *Nature Genetics, 24*(3), 236–244.

SEER Data, NCI. http://rex.nci.nih.gov/NCI_Pub_Interface/raterisk/rates31.html

Seibel, N. L., Blaney, S. M., O'Brien, M., et al. (1999). Phase I trial of docetaxel with filgrastim support in pediatric patients with refractory solid tumors: A collaborative Pediatric Oncology Branch, National Cancer Institute and Children's Cancer Group trial. *Clinical Cancer Research, 5*(4), 733–737.

Shaw, L. M., Glover, D., Turrisi, A., et al. (1988). Pharmacokinetics of WR-2721. *Pharmacology and Therapeutics, 39*(1–3), 195–201.

Skapek, S. X., Hawk, B. J., Hoffer, F. A., et al. (1998). Combination chemotherapy using vinblastine and methotrexate for the treatment of progressive desmoid tumor in children. *Journal of Clinical Oncology, 16*(9), 3021–3027.

Skinner, R. (1995). Strategies to prevent nephrotoxicity of anticancer drugs. *Current Opinion in Oncology, 7*(4), 310–315.

Soignet, S. L., Maslak, P., Wang, Z. G., et al. (1998). Complete remission after treatment of acute promyelocytic leukemia with arsenic trioxide. *New England Journal of Medicine, 339*(19), 1341–1348.

Steuber, C. P., Krischer, J., Holbrook, T., et al. (1996). Therapy of refractory or recurrent childhood acute myeloid leukemia using amsacrine and etoposide with or without azacitidine: A Pediatric Oncology Group randomized phase II study. *Journal of Clinical Oncology, 14*(5), 1521–1525.

Stewart, C. F., Zamboni, W. C., Crom, W. R., et al. (1996). Topoisomerase I interactive drugs in children with cancer. *Investigational New Drugs, 14*(1), 37–47.

Stillwell, T. J., & Benson, R. C. Jr. (1988). Cyclophosphamide-induced hemorrhagic cystitis. A review of 100 patients. *Cancer, 61*(3), 451–457.

Treon, S. P., & Chabner, B. A. (1996). Concepts in use of high-dose methotrexate therapy. *Clinical Chemistry, 42*(8 Pt 2), 1322–1329.

Van Hoff, D. (1984). Use of daunorubicin in patients with solid tumors. *Seminars in Oncology, 11*(4, Suppl 3), 23–27.

Villablanca, J. G., Khan, A. A., Avramis, V. I., et al. (1995). Phase I trial of 13-cis-retinoic acid in children with neuroblastoma following bone marrow transplantation. *Journal of Clinical Oncology, 13*(4), 894–901.

Vogel, C., Gorowski, E., & Davila, E. (1987). Phase I clinical trial and pharmacokinetics of weekly ICRF-187 (NSC 169780) infusion in patients with solid tumors. *Investigational New Drugs, 5*, 187–198.

Weber, W. W., & Hein, D. W. (1985). N-Acetylation pharmacogenetics. *Pharmacological Reviews, 37*(1), 25–69.

Weiner, M. A., Leventhal, B., Brecher, M. L., et al. (1997). Randomized study of intensive MOPP-ABVD with or without low-dose total-nodal radiation therapy in the treatment of stages IIB, IIIA2, IIIB, and IV Hodgkin's disease in pediatric patients: A Pediatric Oncology Group study. *Journal of Clinical Oncology, 15*(8), 2769–2779.

Wolff, J. A., Brubaker, C. A., Murphy, M. L., et al. (1967). Prednisone therapy of acute childhood leukemia: Prognosis and duration of response in 330 treated patients. *The Journal of Pediatrics, 70*(4), 626–631.

Yaffe, S. J., & Aranda, J. V. (1992). Introduction and historical perspective. In S. J. Yaffe and J. V. Aranda, Eds., *Pediatric pharmacology: Therapeutic principles in practice,* 2nd ed., pp. 3–9. Philadelphia: Saunders.

Yagoda, A., Mukherji, B., Young, C., et al. (1972). Bleomycin, an antitumor antibiotic. Clinical experience in 274 patients. *Annals of Internal Medicine, 77*(6), 861–870.

Zinner, S. H. (1998). Relevant aspects in the Infectious Diseases Society of America (IDSA) guidelines for the use of antimicrobial agents in neutropenic patients with unexplained fever. *International Journal of Hematology, 68*(Suppl 1), S31–34.

Zubrod, C. G. (1970). The clinical toxicities of L-asparaginase in treatment of leukemia and lymphoma. *Pediatrics, 45*(4), 555–559.

13

Drug Dosing for Neonates

Robert P. Lemke

Much has changed in neonatal pharmacotherapeutics since the first edition of this handbook, which was published more than 20 years ago. At that time, fewer drugs were available for use in neonatal intensive care units and the pharmacological basis for recommending drug dosages for neonates was less well developed. Many early neonatal drug dosing regimens were based on rudimentary knowledge of the neonate's greater relative total body water and immature renal function. Currently, drug level measurements (therapeutic drug monitoring) and drug dose response trials form the cornerstones for most recommendations regarding neonatal drug dosing. The application of the knowledge gleaned from the recent explosion in neonatal research has resulted in many changes in neonatal drug dosing. For example, some of the "old standbys" have fallen into disuse, whereas the dosages of other drugs have been modified significantly or they are being administered in novel ways. In addition, new drugs and new drug groups (e.g., lung surfactants) are being developed rapidly.

Although necessity has mandated an expansion of this chapter and Table 13-1, the volume of neonatal drug research has encouraged an emphasis on the inclusion of drugs that are FDA or HPB approved. For this reason, some obscure, experimental, or infrequently used drugs are not included (for information regarding such drugs, readers are referred to the earlier editions of this text). Thus, this chapter is not all inclusive but focuses on current empirically validated approaches to neonatal drug therapy with attention to the most common clinical implications for managing drug therapy for neonates. For example, only the more common or serious adverse drug reactions (ADRs) are mentioned. (For additional information concerning adverse drug reactions, *see* Chapter 5.) With these considerations in mind, this chapter has been modified and revised to reflect optimal neonatal drug dosing while maintaining the practical use of this chapter in the modern neonatal intensive care unit, which was the hallmark of the previous editions of this handbook.

TABLE 13-1
Recommended Drug Dosing for Neonates

DRUG (*TRADE* AND OTHER NAMES)	INDICATION(S)	USUAL NEONATAL DOSAGE[a] AND ADMINISTRATION[b]	CONTRAINDICATIONS, ADRs, AND COMMENTS[c]
Acetaminophen (*Atasol*®, Paracetamol, *Tempra*®, *Tylenol*®)	Fever Pain	5–10 mg/kg PO or rectal every 4 hr as needed.	**Contraindications:** Hypersensitivity to acetaminophen and severe hepatic dysfunction. **ADRs:** Toxicity may occur at recommended dosages; overdosage may cause significant hepatotoxicity. *See* Chapters 4 and 5. **Note:** Does not possess significant anti-inflammatory activity.
Acetazolamide (*Diamox*®)	Drug-induced edema and edema due to congestive heart failure **Note:** Not beneficial with posthemorrhagic hydrocephalus	5 mg/kg/day PO or IV in three divided doses.	**Contraindications:** Hyperchloremic acidosis, hypersensitivity to acetazolamide, hypokalemia, hyponatremia, and severe hepatic or renal impairment. **ADRs:** Anorexia, diarrhea, hearing dysfunction, metabolic acidosis, vomiting. **Comments:** Monitor serum electrolytes.
Acyclovir (*Zovirax*®)	Mucosal and cutaneous herpes simplex virus (HSV-1 and HSV-2) infections and varicella-zoster (shingles) infections in immunocompromised neonates	**Premature** (<33 weeks gestation): 10 mg/kg IV every 12 hr. **Term:** 10 mg/kg IV every 8 hr for 7–10 days. **With renal or hepatic dysfunction:** SCr 70–109 μmol/liter: 10 mg/kg IV every 12 hr. SCr 110–130 μmol/liter: 10 mg/kg IV every 24 hr. SCr >130 μmol/liter or urine output <1 ml/kg/hr: 5 mg/kg IV every 24 hr. **With renal failure receiving peritoneal dialysis:** 5 mg/kg IV every 24 hr. **With renal or hepatic failure receiving exchange transfusions:** 5 mg/kg IV every 48 hr. **Note:** Administer by IV infusion over at least 60 min. *Maximum concentration:* 10 mg/ml.	**ADRs:** Inflammation or phlebitis at the injection site, nausea, thrombocytosis, and vomiting. Encephalopathic reactions (agitation, coma, lethargy, seizures) have been noted in ~1% of patients receiving IV acyclovir. **Comments:** Transient elevations in blood urea nitrogen and serum creatinine may occur, particularly following rapid IV infusion.
Adenosine (*Adenocard*®)	Supraventricular tachycardia	50 μg/kg rapid IV push via patent central venous access device. May double and repeat this dose until desired clinical response is achieved. Follow each dose with a rapid saline flush. **Note:** Appropriate cardiac monitoring is required during administration.	**Contraindications:** AV block (second or third degree), hypersensitivity to adenosine, sick sinus syndrome, and symptomatic bradycardia. **ADRs:** Dyspnea and facial flushing. **Comments:** Associated with transient heart block (first, second, or third degree); does not convert atrial flutter, atrial fibrillation, or ventricular tachycardia to normal sinus rhythm. **Note:** Methylxanthines antagonize the action of adenosine.
Albumin (Normal Human Serum)	Hypoproteinemia Hypovolemia	10–20 ml/kg IV of 5% solution as needed according to individual clinical response.	**Contraindications:** Congestive heart failure and hypernatremia. **ADRs:** Hypersensitivity reactions (chills, fever, nausea, rash) and protein overload. **Note:** Rapid albumin infusion may result in vascular overload.

[a] Usual dosages recommended for neonates are listed. Individual dosage requirements may vary because of variability in maturity, genetics, organ function, and concomitant medical disorders and drug therapy. Thus careful monitoring of drug serum concentrations and individual clinical response is imperative to ensure optimal drug therapy. The usual dosages and related information have been derived from several sources, including the previous editions of this text, current product monographs, the references listed at the end of this chapter, and extensive clinical experience. For additional information on drug interactions, *see* Chapter 6; for detailed information regarding neonatal vaccines, *see* Chapter 9; and for information on pharmacokinetics and pharmacogenetics, *see* Chapters 10 and 11, respectively.

[b] For information on the initial dilution and compatibilities of IV drugs, *see* Chapter 8.

[c] For additional information on ADRs, *see* Chapter 5.

TABLE 13-1 continued

DRUG (TRADE AND OTHER NAMES)	INDICATION(S)	USUAL NEONATAL DOSAGE[a] AND ADMINISTRATION[b]	CONTRAINDICATIONS, ADRs, AND COMMENTS[c]
Albuterol (Salbutamol, Ventolin®)	Severe bronchospasm	5–10 µg/kg IV over 10 min followed by 0.2 µg/kg/min; increase dosage by 0.1-µg/kg increments according to individual clinical response. *Maximum:* 10 µg/kg/min. **Note:** Dilute injectable solution by at least 50% prior to administration. **Inhalation:** With metered-dose inhaler and spacer, 200–600 µg every 4 hr as required.	**Contraindications:** Cardiac tachydysrhythmias and hypersensitivity to albuterol. **ADRs:** Fine muscle tremor, hypokalemia, insomnia, tachycardia, and vomiting. **Comments:** Administration by inhalation is associated with fewer ADRs. Drug delivery, however, is extremely variable. **Note:** Monitor potassium serum, blood pressure, ECG, and heart rate during IV infusion.
Alprostadil (Prostaglandin E_1, Prostin VR®)	Temporary maintenance of patency in neonates dependent upon a patent ductus arteriosus. **Note:** For optimal therapeutic benefit, initiate within 96 hr after birth.	0.1 µg/kg/min as continuous IV infusion into a large vein until the desired effect on the ductus arteriosus is achieved; then decrease to lowest dosage possible that maintains patency (generally, 0.01–0.05 µg/kg/min).	**Contraindications:** Asplenia, cyanosis associated with persistent fetal circulation, hypersensitivity to alprostadil, polysplenia, and total anomalous pulmonary venous return below the diaphragm. **ADRs:** Apnea, bradycardia, fever, flushing, and hypotension. **Comments:** Apnea occurs in ~10% of neonates receiving alprostadil. Neonates <2 kg are at particular risk. **Note:** Monitor ECG, oxygenation status, respiratory status, and temperature during infusion. Blood pressure should be monitored by umbilical artery catheter or by a Doppler transducer. Immediately reduce the infusion rate if a significant decrease in arterial blood pressure is noted.
Amikacin (Amikin®)	Gram-negative bacterial infections resistant to other aminoglycosides **Note:** Ensure that appropriate culture and sensitivity tests have been performed and that the organism is sensitive to amikacin.	**0–7 days of age** <800 grams: 10 mg/kg IV every 36 hr. 800–1500 grams: 10 mg/kg IV every 24 hr. 1501–2000 grams: 7.5 mg/kg IV every 18 hr. >2000 grams: 7.5 mg/kg IV every 12 hr. **>7 days of age** (dosed according to postconceptual age [PCA], which is gestational age in weeks at birth plus postnatal age in weeks) PCA <27 weeks: 7.5 mg/kg IV every 36 hr. PCA 27–30 weeks: 7.5 mg/kg IV every 24 hr. PCA 31–34 weeks: 7.5 mg/kg IV every 18 hr. PCA 35–38 weeks: 7.5 mg/kg IV every 12 hr. PCA >38 weeks: 7.5 mg/kg IV every 8 hr. **Note:** Reduce dosage for neonates who have renal dysfunction.	**ADRs:** Nephrotoxicity and ototoxicity. **Comments:** Clinical experience during the neonatal period is limited. Individualize dose and dosing interval based on serum concentrations; peak target serum concentration is 15–20 µg/ml and trough 3–5 µg/ml. **Note:** Continuous use >10 days is associated with a significant increase in the frequency and severity of ADRs.
Aminocaproic Acid (Amicar®)	Hemorrhage associated with overactivity of the fibrinolytic system	100 mg/kg IV, then 20–30 mg/kg IV at hourly intervals until bleeding is managed (generally ~ eight hourly intervals are required).	**Contraindications:** Active intravascular clotting processes. **ADRs:** Generally well tolerated; may cause diarrhea, malaise, nasal stuffiness, and nausea. **Comments:** Therapeutic plasma levels = ~130 µg/ml.
Aminophylline (Theophylline Ethylenediamine)	Apnea Bradycardia Bronchospasm Preparation for extubation Diuresis	6 mg/kg IV over 20–30 min, then 1–3 mg/kg IV every 12 hr over 20–30 min **or** 1–3 mg/kg PO. If preferred, may administer 0.15 mg/kg/hr IV. Administer with an electronic infusion control device. *Maximum:* 3 mg/kg IV or PO every 8 hr. **Note:** Aminophylline contains 85% anhydrous theophylline.	**ADRs:** CNS reactions (insomnia, irritability, seizures), GI disturbances, and tachycardia. **Comments:** Consider withholding if apical heart rate is consistently >180 beats/min. Individualize dose and dosing interval based on theophylline serum concentration (therapeutic serum concentration 10–20 µg/ml [55–110 µmol/liter]. Mild diuretic action; clinically significant drug interactions common (*see* Chapter 6).

Footnotes are on page 532.

TABLE 13-1 continued

DRUG (TRADE AND OTHER NAMES)	INDICATION(S)	USUAL NEONATAL DOSAGE[a] AND ADMINISTRATION[b]	CONTRAINDICATIONS, ADRs, AND COMMENTS[c]
Amoxicillin (Amoxil®)	**Susceptible gram-positive or gram-negative bacteria** **Bacterial endocarditis infections** **Note:** Ensure that appropriate culture and sensitivity tests have been performed and that the organism is sensitive to amoxicillin.	20–40 mg/kg/day PO in three divided doses every 8 hr.	**Contraindications:** Hypersensitivity to amoxicillin and to other penicillins. **ADRs:** Abdominal cramps, cutaneous reactions, diarrhea, hypersensitivity reactions, interstitial nephritis, pancytopenia, pseudomembranous colitis, and urticaria.
Amphotericin B (Fungizone®)	**Severe systemic infection or meningitis** caused by susceptible fungi	0.1 mg/kg/day IV as a single daily dose over 2–4 hr; gradually increase by increments of 0.25 mg/kg/day to a maximum of 0.5–1 mg/kg/day **or** 1.5 mg/kg every other day according to individual clinical response.	**Contraindications:** Hypersensitivity to amphotericin B. **ADRs:** Fever, flushing, maculopapular rash, malaise, renal dysfunction, and thrombocytopenia. **Comments:** Indicated only for neonates with a confirmed diagnosis of a progressive and potentially fatal fungal infection susceptible to amphotericin B; **not** indicated for neonates who only have a positive skin or serologic test for fungal infection. **Note:** After initial test dose, monitor vital signs closely and observe for ADRs. Measure blood urea nitrogen and serum creatinine every other day while increasing dosage and at least weekly thereafter. Monitor potassium and magnesium serum concentrations, hematologic status, and hepatic function weekly. Consider discontinuing if hepatic dysfunction is significant.
Ampicillin (Ampicin®)	**Meningitis** caused by susceptible bacteria **Neonatal sepsis**	**0–7 days of age ≤2 kg:** 50 mg/kg IV every 12 hr. **>7 days of age ≤ 2 kg:** 50 mg/kg IV every 8 hr. **0–7 days of age >2 kg:** 50 mg/kg IV every 8 hr. **>7 days of age >2 kg:** 50 mg/kg IV every 6 hr.	**Contraindications:** Hypersensitivity to any penicillin or cephalosporin. **ADRs:** Diarrhea, hypersensitivity reactions, infection, and skin rash. **Note:** Stable for 1 hr after mixing with IV solutions. Normal saline solutions are preferred for admixtures because ampicillin degrades rapidly in dextrose solutions. Oral ampicillin is **not** indicated for neonates.
	Other infections (pneumonia, urinary tract infections). **Note:** Ensure that appropriate culture and sensitivity tests have been performed and that the organism is sensitive to ampicillin.	**0–7 days of age ≤2 kg:** 25 mg/kg IV every 12 hr. **>7 days of age ≤2 kg:** 25 mg/kg IV every 8 hr. **0–7 days of age >2 kg:** 25 mg/kg IV every 8 hr. **>7 days of age >2 kg:** 25 mg/kg IV every 6 hr.	
Atropine	**Bradycardia** caused by vagal stimulation **Nonemergency endotracheal intubation** **Reversal of neuromuscular blockade**	0.01 mg/kg endotracheal, IM, or IV as needed according to individual clinical response, at 20-min intervals. *Minimum:* 0.1 mg/dose. *Maximum:* 0.4 mg/dose.	**Contraindications:** Glaucoma and pyloric stenosis or pyloric obstruction. **ADRs:** Dry mouth, flushing, hyperthermia, tachycardia, and urinary retention. **Note:** Administer by rapid IV push to avoid paradoxical bradycardia, which has been associated with slow IV injection.
Beractant [Surfactant, Bovine] (Survanta®)	**Neonatal respiratory distress syndrome** (RDS) prophylaxis or treatment (rescue)	**At birth:** 100 mg/kg (4 ml/kg) in four divided doses intratracheally through a number 5 French end-hole catheter over 2–3 sec with ventilation between each dose. May repeat 100-mg/kg dose every 6 hr up to four times during the first 48 hr of life. **For intratracheal use only.** The catheter tip should be positioned above the neonate's carina to evenly distribute the drug throughout the lungs. Do **not** directly administer into a mainstem bronchus.	**ADRs:** Bradycardia (transient) and decreased oxygen saturation. **Comments:** Monitor heart rate, skin color, chest expansion, transcutaneous oxygen saturation, and placement of endotracheal tube continuously. Decrease dose if heart rate slows, neonate becomes agitated, skin color becomes dusky, oxygen saturation decreases by more than 15%, or drug backs up in the endotracheal tube. After administration, check endotracheal tube position in the trachea by

TABLE 13-1 *continued*

DRUG (*TRADE AND OTHER NAMES*)	INDICATION(S)	USUAL NEONATAL DOSAGE[a] AND ADMINISTRATION[b]	CONTRAINDICATIONS, ADRs, AND COMMENTS[c]
Beractant *continued*		**Note:** Prior to administration, warm the vial by allowing to stand at room temperature for at least 20 min or holding the vial in the hand for 8 min. Do **not** use artificial warming methods (microwave). Begin warming before birth. Do **not** shake or filter the suspension. If settling has occurred during storage, redisperse by gently swirling the vial.	listening for equal breath sounds and monitor arterial blood gases. Use an arterial catheter for arterial blood gas sampling. Use of surfactant has been shown to reduce the need for ECMO. Rapid administration leads to improved lung function compared to slower administration.
Caffeine Citrate (*Cafcit®*)	**Apnea** of prematurity	**Loading dose:** 10–20 mg/kg IV or PO. **Maintenance:** 5–10 mg/kg IV or PO every 24 hr (first maintenance dose administered 24 hr after initial loading dose). **Note:** Usual recommended dosages are for citrate salt, **not** caffeine base. Caffeine citrate contains 50% caffeine. Thus, the usual recommended dosages listed are twice as high as those calculated for caffeine base.	**ADRs:** Generally well tolerated. Cardiovascular, GI, or neurologic toxicity (at caffeine serum concentrations >50 µg/ml). Sodium benzoate present in some injectable caffeine formulations may cause kernicterus. **Comments:** Therapeutic serum concentrations for caffeine citrate = 5–25 µg/ml. Preterm neonates metabolize theophylline to caffeine. Caffeine readily crosses the placenta. Obtain baseline serum concentrations of caffeine.
Calcium Chloride	**Hypocalcemia** **Hyperkalemia** (antagonist to cardiac effect) **Cardiac resuscitation**	**Initial:** 10–20 mg/kg IV over 30 min. **Maintenance:** 3–10 mg/kg/hr IV. 20 mg/kg (0.2 ml of 10% solution/kg) IV every 10 min. Administer slowly; rapid administration may lead to hypotension and cardiac arrest.	**Contraindications:** Hypercalcemia, hypercalciuria, and severe cardiac or renal dysfunction. **ADRs:** Bradycardia, cardiac dysrhythmias, drowsiness, flushing, hypotension, increased potential for digoxin toxicity for neonates receiving digoxin, nausea, phlebitis at injection site, vasodilation, and vomiting. **Comments:** Monitor total calcium serum concentration (target range = 2.1–2.5 mmol/l [4.5–5.2 mEq/liter]). (1 gram of calcium chloride = 270 mg [13.5 mEq] of elemental calcium.) **Note:** Avoid extravasation during IV infusion because calcium deposition, severe tissue necrosis, and sloughing may occur. Be particularly cautious when using scalp veins.
Calcium Gluconate	**Hypocalcemia** **Hypokalemia** (antagonist to cardiac effect of hypokalemia)	**Initial:** 100 mg/kg IV over 30 min. **Maintenance:** 10 mg/kg/hr IV. **Note:** Discontinue if heart rate <100 beats/min. Avoid administering via the umbilical artery because the solution is hypertonic and can cause major complications involving the large vessels. Also avoid using scalp veins because of potential tissue necrosis associated with extravasation. Available as a 10% solution that contains 9 mg/ml (0.45 mEq/ml) of elemental calcium.	**Contraindications:** Hypercalcemia, hypercalciuria, and severe cardiac or renal dysfunction. **ADRs:** Hypercalcemia. **Comments:** Monitor ECG and apical heart rate for bradycardia after administration. **Note:** Intermittent administration of an equivalent dose may be used to avoid incompatibilities with other injectable drugs (sodium bicarbonate).
Captopril (*Capoten®*)	**Mild-to-moderate hypertension** **Congestive heart failure** **Intractable edema**	0.05–0.1 mg/kg PO every 6–8 hr. *Maximum:* 6 mg/kg/day. **Note:** Reduce dosage or increase dosing interval for neonates who have renal dysfunction.	**Contraindications:** Fixed renovascular obstruction and hypersensitivity to captopril. **ADRs:** Acute reversible renal failure, hyperaldosteronism, hyperkalemia, hypotension, metabolic acidosis, neutropenia, proteinuria, rash, tachycardia, seizures. **Comments:** A 25-mg tablet dissolved in 25 ml of distilled water is stable for 14 days at 4°C and for 7 days at room temperature (22°C).

Footnotes are on page 532.

TABLE 13-1 continued

DRUG (TRADE AND OTHER NAMES)	INDICATION(S)	USUAL NEONATAL DOSAGE[a] AND ADMINISTRATION[b]	CONTRAINDICATIONS, ADRs, AND COMMENTS[c]
Cefazolin (Ancef®, Kefzol®)	**Infections** caused by gram-positive bacteria (*Staphylococcus aureus*) **Infection prophylaxis** during cardiac surgery **Note:** Ensure that appropriate culture and sensitivity tests have been performed and that the organism is sensitive to cefazolin.	**≤2 kg:** 40 mg/kg/day IV in two divided doses every 12 hr. **0–7 days of age >2 kg:** 40 mg/kg/day IV in two divided doses every 12 hr. **>7 days of age >2 kg:** 60 mg/kg/day IV in three divided doses every 8 hr. **Note:** Reduce dosage or increase dosing interval for neonates who have renal dysfunction.	**Contraindications:** Hypersensitivity to cefazolin or to other cephalosporins or penicillins. **ADRs:** Allergic reactions (pruritus), eosinophilia, false-positive Coomb's test, fever, increased aspartate transaminase serum concentration, neutropenia, serum sickness, thrombophlebitis, and urticaria.
Cefotaxime (Claforan®)	**Neonatal meningitis** caused by susceptible bacteria **Note:** Ensure that appropriate culture and sensitivity tests have been performed and that the organism is sensitive to cefotaxime.	**≤2 kg:** 100 mg/kg/day IV in two divided doses every 12 hr. **0–7 days of age >2 kg:** 100 mg/kg/day IV in two divided doses every 12 hr. **>7 days of age >2 kg:** 150 mg/kg/day IV in three divided doses every 8 hr.	**Contraindications:** Hypersensitivity to cefotaxime or to other cephalosporins or penicillins. **ADRs:** Diarrhea, eosinophilia, granulocytopenia, leukopenia, nausea, phlebitis, rash, and vomiting.
Ceftazidime (Ceptaz®, Tazidime®)	**Infections** caused by susceptible gram-negative bacteria (particularly *Pseudomonas aeruginosa*) **Note:** Ensure that appropriate culture and sensitivity tests have been performed and that the organism is sensitive to ceftazidime.	**≤2 kg:** 100 mg/kg/day IV in two divided doses every 12 hr. **0–7 days of age >2 kg:** 100 mg/kg/day IV in two divided doses every 12 hr. **>7 days of age >2 kg:** 150 mg/kg/day IV in three divided doses every 8 hr.	**Contraindications:** Hypersensitivity to ceftazidime or to other cephalosporins or penicillins. **ADRs:** Diarrhea, eosinophilia, increases in hepatic enzyme concentrations, pain at injection site, and skin reactions.
Ceftriaxone (Rocephin®)	**Meningitis or other infections** caused by susceptible gram-negative bacteria (particularly *Enterobacteriaceae* resistant to multiple antibiotics) **Note:** Ensure that appropriate culture and sensitivity tests have been performed and that the organism is sensitive to ceftriaxone.	**≤2 kg:** 50 mg/kg/day IV as a single daily dose. **0–7 days of age >2 kg:** 50 mg/kg/day IV as a single daily dose. **>7 days of age >2 kg:** 75 mg/kg/day IV as a single daily dose. **Note:** Decrease dosage for neonates who have combined hepatic and renal dysfunction.	**Contraindications:** Hypersensitivity to ceftriaxone or to other cephalosporins or penicillins. **ADRs:** Diarrhea, elevations in renal and hepatic enzymes, eosinophilia, irritability, leukopenia, pain and phlebitis at injection site, and thrombocytosis. **Comments:** Jaundiced neonates may be at increased risk for kernicterus.
Chloral Hydrate	Sedation	20–30 mg/kg PO every 8 hr as needed according to individual clinical response. *Maximum:* 1 gram/day.	**Contraindications:** Hypersensitivity to chloral hydrate and severe hepatic or renal dysfunction. **ADRs:** Gastric irritation, nausea, paradoxical excitement, and vomiting. **Comments:** Avoid repeated dosing because of accumulation of metabolites (trichloroethanol and trichloroacetic acid).
Chloramphenicol (Chloromycetin®)	**Infection** caused by susceptible gram-positive or gram-negative bacteria Use only when less toxic antibiotics are unavailable or ineffective. **Note:** Ensure that appropriate culture and sensitivity tests have been performed and that the organism is sensitive to chloramphenicol.	**<36 weeks gestation ≤2 kg:** 25 mg/kg/day IV as a single daily dose. **≤7 days of age >2 kg:** 25 mg/day as a single daily dose. **>7 days of age >2 kg:** 50 mg/kg/day IV in two divided doses. **Note:** Decrease dosage for neonates who have hepatic failure or renal dysfunction.	**Contraindications:** Hypersensitivity to chloramphenicol. **ADRs:** Irreversible aplastic anemia (more commonly associated with oral chloramphenicol) and vomiting; gray baby syndrome (a potentially fatal reaction characterized by abdominal distention, cyanosis, and vasomotor collapse) has been described in premature neonates and is related to excessive dosage. To avoid the gray baby syndrome, maintain chloramphenicol blood concentrations at <25 µg/ml. **Comments:** Monitor white blood cell count closely.
Chlorpromazine (Largactil®, Thorazine®)	**Agitation** associated with the neonatal opiate analgesic-withdrawal syndrome	2–3 mg/kg/day IV or PO in four divided doses every 6 hr. **Note:** Monitor closely, particularly when administered IV.	**Contraindications:** Coma, hypersensitivity to chlorpromazine, severe CNS depression, and subcortical brain damage. **ADRs:** Hypotension, hypothermia, rigidity, and tremor.

TABLE 13-1 continued

DRUG (TRADE AND OTHER NAMES)	INDICATION(S)	USUAL NEONATAL DOSAGE[a] AND ADMINISTRATION[b]	CONTRAINDICATIONS, ADRs, AND COMMENTS[c]
Clindamycin (*Dalacin C®*)	**Infections** caused by susceptible staphylococci, streptococci, and selected anaerobic bacteria **Note:** Ensure that appropriate culture and sensitivity tests have been performed and that the organism is sensitive to clindamycin.	**<1200 grams:** 5 mg/kg IM or IV every 12 hr. **0–7 days of age 1200–2000 grams:** 5 mg/kg IM or IV every 12 hr. **>7 days of age 1200–2000 grams:** 5 mg/kg IM or IV every 8 hr **0–7 days of age >2000 grams:** 5 mg/kg IM or IV every 8 hr. **>7 days of age >2000 grams:** 5 mg/kg IM or IV every 6 hr.	**Contraindications:** Hepatic dysfunction, hypersensitivity to clindamycin, and previous history of pseudomembranous colitis. **ADRs:** Generally well tolerated; may cause diarrhea and maculopapular skin rashes. **Comments:** Monitor for changes in stool frequency.
Cloxacillin (*Tegopen®*)	**Infections** caused by susceptible gram-positive bacteria **Note:** Ensure that appropriate culture and sensitivity tests have been performed and that the organism is sensitive to cloxacillin.	**0–7 days of age ≤2 kg:** 50 mg/kg/day IM, IV, or PO in two divided doses every 12 hr. **>7 days of age ≤2 kg:** 75 mg/kg/day IM, IV, or PO in three divided doses every 8 hr. **0–7 days of age >2 kg:** 75 mg/kg/day IM, IV, or PO in three divided doses every 8 hr. **>7 days of age >2 kg:** 100 mg/kg/day IM, IV, or PO in four divided doses every 6 hr.	**Contraindications:** Hypersensitivity to cloxacillin or to any other penicillins. **ADRs:** Generally well tolerated; may cause GI irritation (diarrhea, nausea, vomiting) and hypersensitivity reactions (both immediate and delayed). **Comments:** For optimal absorption, administer each oral dose on an empty stomach.
Colfosceril Palmitate [Synthetic Lung Surfactant] (*Exosurf Neonatal®*)	**Neonatal respiratory distress syndrome** (RDS) prophylaxis or treatment (rescue)	**Prophylaxis ≤1.1 kg:** 5 ml/kg intratracheally via endotracheal tube immediately after birth. **Treatment (rescue) for ventilated neonates:** 5 ml/kg intratracheally via endotracheal tube 2–24 hr after birth and 12 hr later. **Note:** Administer through special endotracheal tube adapter supplied with the product. Do **not** interrupt mechanical ventilation for administration.	**ADRs:** Apnea, decreased oxygen saturation, and reflux of colfosceril. **Comments:** Monitor arterial blood gases (use arterial catheter for arterial blood gas sampling). Continuously monitor heart rate, skin color, chest expansion, transcutaneous oxygen saturation, and patency of endotracheal tube during administration. Decrease dose if heart rate slows, neonate becomes agitated, skin color becomes dusky, oxygen saturation decreases by more than 15%, or drug backs up in the endotracheal tube. After administration, assure correct placement of endotracheal tube by auscultating for equal breath sounds. **Note:** More rapid administration associated with improved subsequent lung function.

Co-trimoxazole, see **Trimethoprim–Sulfamethoxazole**

Cyclopentolate (*Cyclogyl®*)	**Mydriasis** for examination of fundi oculi	One drop of 0.5% or 1% ophthalmic solution in each eye 0.5 hr prior to ophthalmic examination. **Note:** Gently occlude the lacrimal duct when instilling eye drops to prevent or minimize systemic absorption (*see* Chapter 1).	**Contraindications:** Angle-closure glaucoma. **ADRs:** May be absorbed systemically via the nasolacrimal duct and cause abdominal distention. **Comments:** Causes paralysis of the ciliary muscle.
Dexamethasone (*Decadron®*)	**Oxygen and ventilator weaning** for neonates with bronchopulmonary dysplasia	0.25 mg/kg IV or PO every 12 hr. Gradually reduce dosage over 7–10 days while weaning off oxygen and ventilation. Some centers use prolonged tapering courses of up to 42 days. **Note:** Each dose of the oral tablets may be crushed and administered with feedings	**Contraindications:** Administration of live virus vaccines and systemic fungal infections. **ADRs:** Hypernatremia, hypokalemia, impaired wound healing, and muscle weakness. **Comments:** Tailor duration of therapy to clinical response. Long-term use has the potential to impair and mask the normal response to infection, interfere with growth, and has been associated with an increased risk of cerebral palsy.
	Subglottic stenosis or inflammation	0.5–1 mg/kg/dose IV or PO. *Maximum:* Three doses/day.	
Dextrose 10% in Sterile Water for Injection	**Hypoglycemia prophylaxis** during first 48 hr of life	8–10 mg/kg/min IV. **Note:** 1 ml of dextrose 10% in sterile water for injection = 100 mg dextrose.	**Comments:** Dose is calculated based on neonate's nutritional requirements; try to provide 10–12 grams/kg/day; in premature and low-birth-weight neonates, may cause hyperglycemia, osmotic diuresis, and glucosuria; if so, reduce amount of dextrose.

Footnotes are on page 532.

TABLE 13-1 continued

DRUG (TRADE AND OTHER NAMES)	INDICATION(S)	USUAL NEONATAL DOSAGE[a] AND ADMINISTRATION[b]	CONTRAINDICATIONS, ADRs, AND COMMENTS[c]
Dextrose 25%–50% in Sterile Water for Injection	Hypoglycemia	0.5–1 gram/kg/dose by rapid IV push, then 5 mg/kg/min by continuous IV infusion. Titrate rate of infusion to blood glucose concentration.	**Comments:** Irritating to veins; dilute with sterile water for injection to a concentration of 25% or less. IV dextrose solutions in concentrations less than 12.5% may be administered via a peripheral vein. However, concentrations greater than 12.5% should be infused via a central venous access device. Oral dextrose solutions in concentrations greater than 15% can cause diarrhea because of their associated osmotic effect. **Note:** Close monitoring of glucose blood concentrations is essential to avoid hyperglycemia.
Diazepam (Valium®)	Second-line agent for convulsions (status epilepticus)	0.1–0.2 mg/kg/dose by slow IV push. Repeat, as needed, every 10 min for three doses according to individual clinical response. *Maximum:* 0.5 mg/kg/dose. **Note:** The injectable formulation contains sodium benzoate that displaces bilirubin from albumin and thus should **not** be used with high bilirubin concentrations and low reserve albumin binding capacities.	**Contraindications:** Coma, hypersensitivity to diazepam, myasthenia gravis, and shock. **ADRs:** CNS depression, hypotension, and respiratory depression (also may cause apnea, particularly when administered IV too rapidly). **Comments:** The injectable formulation is incompatible with many other drugs and tends to precipitate when diluted. **Note:** Overdosages may be treated with flumazenil.
Diazoxide (Hyperstat® Proglycem®)	Profound or prolonged hypoglycemia unresponsive to dextrose infusions and other therapy Idiopathic hypoglycemia of infancy	8–15 mg/kg/day PO in two or three equally divided doses every 8–12 hr.	**Contraindications:** Hypersensitivity to diazoxide or to thiazide diuretics. **ADRs:** Hirsutism, hyperbilirubinemia, hyperglycemia, hypotension, and thrombocytopenia. **Comments:** Frequently ineffective in primary persistent hyperinsulinism in neonates.
Digoxin (Lanoxin®)	Congestive heart failure Certain dysrhythmias (re-entrant supraventricular tachycardia, atrial flutter)	**<2.7 kg:** Digitalizing dose, 15 µg/kg IV. Maintenance dosage is based on lean body weight and is administered IV every 24 hr: Weight — Dosage 0.8–1 kg — 4 µg/kg/day 1.1–1.4 kg — 5 µg/kg/day 1.5–1.8 kg — 6 µg/kg/day 1.9–2.4 kg — 7 µg/kg/day 2.5–2.7 kg — 8 µg/kg/day **Term >2.7 kg:** Total digitalizing dose 20–30 µg/kg IV Usually administer 1/2 of digitalizing dose IV immediately, 1/4 of dose IV after 6–8 hr, and the last 1/4 of dose IV 6–8 hr later. **Maintenance:** Administer 1/4 of total digitalizing dose daily IV or PO in two divided doses twice daily, starting 12 hr after the last digitalizing dose. **Note:** IM injection is extremely painful and is **not** recommended.	**Contraindications:** Ventricular fibrillation. **ADRs:** Bradycardia (if apical heart rate is <100 beats/min, withhold dose). Do not administer in conjunction with calcium because this combination may potentiate bradycardia. **Comments:** Routine monitoring of digoxin serum concentrations is not necessary. However, a trough concentration should be drawn if toxicity is suspected. Therapeutic serum trough concentrations for adults generally are 0.8–2 ng/ml (1–2.5 nmol/liter), but neonates may require and tolerate higher concentrations. Differences in bioavailability among the elixir, injectable, and tablet forms should be taken into consideration when planning a change in dosage form (see Chapters 1 and 10). Use for dysrhythmias should only be undertaken after consultation with a pediatric cardiologist. **Note:** Life-threatening overdosages may be treated with digoxin immune fab.
Digoxin Immune Fab (Digibind®)	Life-threatening digoxin overdosage	38 mg (contents of one reconstituted vial) by IV infusion over 30 min. **Note:** Infuse the reconstituted digoxin immune fab solution IV through a 0.22-µm membrane filter to ensure that no undissolved particulate matter is inadvertently administered.	**ADRs:** Generally well tolerated; may cause hypersensitivity reactions or hypokalemia. **Comments:** Each vial (38 mg of digoxin immune fab) binds approximately 0.5 mg of digoxin or digitoxin. Once administered, digoxin immune fab interferes with digitalis immunoassays. Therefore, monitor clinical response (including parameters such as ECG) rather than digoxin serum concentrations until the digoxin immune fab fragments (and digoxin complex) are eliminated.

TABLE 13-1 continued

DRUG (TRADE AND OTHER NAMES)	INDICATION(S)	USUAL NEONATAL DOSAGE[a] AND ADMINISTRATION[b]	CONTRAINDICATIONS, ADRs, AND COMMENTS[c]
Dobutamine (*Dobutrex®*)	Refractory congestive heart failure and shock	1–2 μg/kg/min IV; increase dosage to a **maximum** of 7.5–20 μg/kg/min according to individual clinical response.	**Contraindications:** Hypersensitivity to dobutamine, idiopathic hypertrophic subaortic stenosis, and pheochromocytoma. **ADRs:** Cardiac dysrhythmias (including tachycardia), dyspnea, hypotension (at low dosages), nausea, palpitations, vasoconstriction (at high dosages), and vomiting. **Comments:** Monitor blood pressure, ECG, oxygenation status, and urine output. Use separate IV tubing to obtain blood samples and to administer other drugs so that dobutamine infusion is not interrupted. **Note:** Derivative of isoproterenol.
Dopamine (*Intropin®*)	Low cardiac output due to myocardial failure	2–20 μg/kg/min as a continuous IV infusion. **Note:** To prepare IV solution, add 6 mg to 100 ml of dextrose 5% in water to yield 60 μg/ml (1 ml/kg/hr = 1 μg/kg/min). Do **not** admix with alkaline diluents.	**Contraindications:** Pheochromocytoma. **ADRs:** Cardiac dysrhythmias (including ventricular tachycardia), increased pulmonary vascular resistance (at dosages >10 μg/kg/min), vasoconstriction (at dosages >20 μg/kg/min), and vomiting. Peripheral extravasation may result in local ischemia and ulceration or gangrene with resultant loss of effected extremity. **Comments:** Monitor blood pressure, ECG, oxygenation status, and urine output. Closely monitor injection site for any signs of extravasation. If extravasation occurs, immediately (or within 12 hr) inject phentolamine 0.1 mg/kg SC into five sites near area of extravasation; change needle before each injection.
Epinephrine (1:1000 and 1:10,000) (Adrenaline, *Adrenalin®*)	Cardiac arrest	10 μg/kg (0.01 ml/kg of 1:1000 solution or 0.1 ml/kg of 1:10,000 solution) endotracheally via endotracheal tube, IV, or SC. Dilute, if necessary, with normal saline.	**ADRs:** Cardiac dysrhythmias, coldness of extremities, dizziness, hypertension, tachycardia, and tremor. **Comments:** Monitor blood pressure, ECG, and oxygenation status. **Note:** Compatible with D$_5$W. To prepare solution, add 6 ml of 1:1000 (1-mg/ml) solution to 100 ml 5% dextrose and water to yield 60 μg/ml (1 μg/kg/min = 1 ml/kg/hr). Do **not** dilute with alkaline solutions. Protect solution from exposure to light. **Note:** Endotracheal and IV doses usually are administered in the presence of a physician experienced with administering endotracheal epinephrine to neonates. Intracardiac doses also should be administered by a physician experienced with the intracardiac administration of epinephrine to neonates. Avoid extravasation because of associated tissue damage. If extravasation occurs, immediately (or within 12 hr) inject phentolamine 0.1 mg/kg SC into five sites near area of extravasation; change needle before each injection.
	Hypotension	**Infusion:** 0.05–1 μg/kg/min using an electronic infusion control device. Titrate dosage to desired clinical response.	
Epinephrine (1:200 long-acting suspension) (Adrenaline)	**Hypoglycemia** unresponsive to dextrose infusion	0.025–0.05 mg/kg (0.005–0.01 ml/kg) SC every 6–8 hr as needed for hypoglycemia.	**ADRs:** Blanching of injection site, coldness of extremities, tachycardia, and tremor. **Comments:** Inhibits the secretion of insulin and stimulates the conversion of glycogen to glucose.

Footnotes are on page 532.

TABLE 13-1 continued

DRUG (TRADE AND OTHER NAMES)	INDICATION(S)	USUAL NEONATAL DOSAGE[a] AND ADMINISTRATION[b]	CONTRAINDICATIONS, ADRs, AND COMMENTS[c]
Ergocalciferol (*Drisdol*®, Vitamin D_2)	Dietary supplementation for low-birth-weight, premature, and breast-fed term neonates	**Breast- or formula-fed premature or term <2 kg:** 750 units/day PO. **Breast-fed term:** 500 units/day PO. **Note:** 1 µg of ergocalciferol = 40 units	**Contraindications:** Hypercalcemia and vitamin D toxicity. **ADRs:** Hypercalcemia. **Comments:** Monitor calcium serum concentration (normal range 1.75–3 mmol/liter). **Note:** Oral ingestion of vitamin D is limited by the small size of the neonatal stomach, which corresponds to the neonate's weight.
Erythromycin (*EES*®, *EryPed*®)	Infections caused by *Chlamydia*	**0–7 days of age ≤2 kg:** 20 mg/kg/day PO in two divided doses every 12 hr. **>7 days ≤2 kg:** 30 mg/kg/day PO in three divided doses every 8 hr. **0–7 days of age >2 kg:** 20 mg/kg/day PO in two divided doses every 12 hr. **>7 days >2 kg:** 30–40 mg/kg/day PO in three divided doses every 8 hr.	**Contraindications:** Cisapride administration and hypersensitivity to erythromycin. **ADRs:** Abdominal cramps, GI distress, intrahepatic cholestasis (at high dosages), rash, and thrombophlebitis. **Comments:** Use oral erythromycin cautiously with hepatic dysfunction.
	Mycoplasma gonococcal ophthalmia neonatorum prophylaxis	Apply one dose of ophthalmic ointment (0.5%) within 1 hr after birth. A new tube of ophthalmic ointment should be used to assure sterility and prevent cross-infection.	
Ethacrynic Acid (*Edecrin*®, Ethacrynate Sodium)	Fluid overload (edema) (refractory to furosemide)	**Premature:** 1 mg/kg/day IV or as a single oral daily dose. *Maximum:* 4 mg/kg/day IV or PO. **Term:** 2 mg/kg/day IV or PO in two divided doses every 12 hr. *Maximum:* 6 mg/kg/day IV or PO. **Note:** Clinical experience with oral ethacrynic acid is limited; titrate dosage carefully.	**Contraindications:** Anuria, hypersensitivity to ethacrynic acid, and hypotension. **ADRs:** Anorexia, diarrhea, fluid and electrolyte imbalance (hypokalemia, hyponatremia), GI bleeding, nausea, ototoxicity, thrombophlebitis, and vomiting. **Comments:** Monitor blood pressure and pulse. Also monitor potassium serum concentration when used concomitantly with digoxin. Hypokalemia enhances digoxin toxicity. **Note:** Risk of ototoxicity is increased with rapid IV infusion and when used concurrently with aminoglycosides.
Fat Emulsions (*Intralipid*®, 10%, 20%, 30%)	Energy source (nutritional)	0.25–4 grams/kg/day by continuous IV infusion over 24 hr.	**Contraindications:** Acute myocardial infarction, severe hepatic dysfunction, and shock. **ADRs:** Chills, cyanosis, fever, headache, nausea, and vomiting. **Comments:** Small for gestational age and very-low-birth-weight neonates eliminate IV fat emulsion more slowly than term neonates. Therefore, they are at significantly increased risk for developing hyperlipidemia.
Fentanyl	Pain and agitation during invasive procedures (bronchoscopy, mechanical ventilation, patent ductus arteriosus ligation)	2–5 µg/kg IV as a single dose or 3–10 µg/kg/hr by continuous IV infusion. **Note:** Reduce dosage when neonate is receiving other CNS depressants.	**Contraindications:** Acute asthmatic attack, acute respiratory depression, hypersensitivity to fentanyl or to other opiate analgesics, and upper airway obstruction. **ADRs:** Apnea, bradycardia, hypotension, muscular rigidity, nausea, respiratory depression, and vomiting. **Comments:** Monitor blood pressure, heart rate, and respiratory status. The neonate should be ventilated or ventilation equipment and appropriately trained emergency personnel should be readily available because of the risk for respiratory depression. The appropriate antagonist for the treatment of respiratory depression associated with fentanyl overdosage is naloxone (0.1 mg/kg IV repeated as needed according to individual clinical response).

TABLE 13-1 continued

DRUG (*TRADE AND OTHER NAMES*)	INDICATION(S)	USUAL NEONATAL DOSAGE[a] AND ADMINISTRATION[b]	CONTRAINDICATIONS, ADRs, AND COMMENTS[c]
Ferrous Sulfate (Iron)	Iron-deficiency anemia prophylaxis or treatment (when reticulocyte count exceeds 2%)	**Prophylaxis:** 1–2 mg/kg/day elemental iron PO **Treatment:** 2–6 mg/kg/day elemental iron PO as a single daily dose or two divided doses. **Note:** 5 mg of ferrous sulfate = 1 mg of elemental iron	**Contraindications:** Primary hemochromatosis. **Comments:** May cause mild GI upset. For optimal absorption, administer with water or juice on an empty stomach at least 30 min prior to feeding. Do **not** administer with milk.
Filgrastim (Human Granulocyte Colony-Stimulating Factor, *Neupogen*®)	**Congenital neutropenia** (autoimmune neutropenia) **Neutropenia associated with extreme prematurity**	5 µg/kg SC twice daily; adjust dosage based upon individual clinical course and absolute neutrophil count.	**Contraindications:** Hypersensitivity to filgrastim or to *E. coli*-derived proteins. **ADRs:** Generally well tolerated; may cause abdominal pain, generalized musculoskeletal pain, mild-to-moderate bone pain, palpable splenomegaly, and thrombocytopenia. **Comments:** Complete blood and platelet counts should be performed twice weekly in leukocytosis. Once stabilized, these tests may be performed monthly.
Flucytosine (*Ancobon*®, 5-Fluorocytosine)	Severe fungal infections	**<1.5 kg:** 10–100 mg/kg/day IV or PO in four divided doses every 6 hr. **≥1.5 kg:** 50–150 mg/kg/day IV or PO in four divided doses every 6 hr. **Note:** Injectable formulation available for emergency use only. Modify dosage and dosing interval with renal dysfunction (use 12-hr interval for moderate dysfunction and 24–48-hr interval for severe dysfunction) to maintain serum concentration at 25 µg/ml). Therapeutic plasma concentrations in adults reportedly are 50–100 µg/ml.	**ADRs:** GI problems (anorexia, bowel perforation [rare], diarrhea, nausea, vomiting), and hypoplasia of bone marrow (agranulocytosis [rare], anemia, leukopenia, pancytopenia, thrombocytopenia). **Comments:** Perform hematologic, renal, and hepatic function tests, including frequent determinations of serum alkaline phosphatase, AST, and ALT, prior to and at frequent intervals during therapy. Should only be used in combination with amphotericin B because of the rapid development of resistance when used alone and in lower dosages (≤100 mg/kg/day). The normal peak serum concentration is 25–100 µg/ml 2 hr after a dose. Administer cautiously with bone marrow depression or impaired renal function. Monitor for the development of resistance in originally susceptible strains of *Candida* and *Cryptococcus*.
Flumazenil (*Anexate*®, *Romazicon*®)	Benzodiazepine overdosage	0.01 mg/kg IV over 30 sec; may repeat initial dose at 60-sec intervals until a cumulative dosage of 1 mg is reached.	**Contraindications:** Hypersensitivity to flumazenil or to the benzodiazepines. **ADRs:** Generally well tolerated; may cause nausea and vomiting. **Comments:** Because of the short half-life (~1 hr), repeated doses may be required.
Folic Acid (Pteroylglutamic acid)	Dietary supplementation for parenteral nutrition **Folic acid deficiency Megaloblastic anemia**	15 µg/kg/day PO or administered as a single dose IM once a week.	**ADRs:** Relatively nontoxic, allergic-type reactions with pruritus have been reported (rare). **Comments:** May obscure symptoms of pernicious anemia related to cyanocobalamin deficiency.
Furosemide (Frusemide, *Lasix*®)	**Bronchopulmonary dysplasia (BPD) Congestive heart failure**	**Premature:** 1–2 mg/kg IV or PO every 6 hr. **Term:** 1–2 mg/kg IV or PO every 6 hr. *Maximum:* 6 mg/kg/dose IV or PO.	**Contraindications:** Hepatic coma, hypersensitivity to furosemide, hypotension, hypovolemia, jaundice, and renal failure. **ADRs:** Dehydration, hypocalcemia, hypokalemia, hyponatremia, hypovolemia, metabolic alkalosis, and ototoxicity. **Comments:** Monitor fluid and electrolyte status. Do not administer to a jaundiced neonate with hemolytic disease because it may displace bilirubin from albumin. Does not prevent decreased urine output associated with indomethacin administration. Studies on *(Continued)*

Footnotes are on page 532.

TABLE 13-1 continued

DRUG (TRADE AND OTHER NAMES)	INDICATION(S)	USUAL NEONATAL DOSAGE[a] AND ADMINISTRATION[b]	CONTRAINDICATIONS, ADRs, AND COMMENTS[c]
Furosemide *continued*			inhalational administration suggest effective alternative route in infants with BPD. **Note:** The risk of ototoxicity is increased when used concurrently with aminoglycoside antibiotics. Prolonged use may cause hypercalciuria, osteopenia, and renal stones.
Ganciclovir (*Cytovene®*)	Congenital cytomegalovirus retinitis	2.5–5 mg/kg IV every 12 hr. **Note:** Reduce dosage for neonates who have renal dysfunctionn.	**Contraindications:** Hypersensitivity to acyclovir or to ganciclovir. **ADRs:** Commonly causes neutropenia and thrombocytopenia; may cause anemia, chills, fever, rash, somnolence, tremor, and vomiting. Rapid IV administration is associated with an increased incidence of ADRs. **Comments:** Avoid IM and SC injections because of associated tissue necrosis, which may be severe. Monitor white blood cell counts and platelets daily or every other day.
Gentamicin (*Garamycin®*)	Infections caused by susceptible gram-positive or gram-negative bacteria **Note:** Ensure that appropriate culture and sensitivity tests have been performed and that the organism is sensitive to gentamicin.	**0–7 days of age <800 grams:** 3.5 mg/kg every 36 hr. **0–7 days of age 800–1500 grams:** 3 mg/kg every 24 hr. **0–7 days of age 1501–2000 grams:** 2.5 mg/kg every 18 hr. **0–7 days of age >2000 grams:** 2.5 mg/kg every 12 hr. **>7 days of age** (dosed according to postconceptual age [PCA], which is gestational age in weeks at birth plus postnatal age in weeks): PCA <27 weeks: 3 mg/kg every 36 hr. PCA 27–30 weeks: 2.5 mg/kg every 24 hr. PCA 31–34 weeks: 2.5 mg/kg every 18 hr. PCA 35–38 weeks: 2.5 mg/kg every 12 hr. PCA >38 weeks: 2.5 mg/kg every 8 hr. **Note:** Reduce dosage for neonates who have renal dysfunction.	**Contraindications:** Hypersensitivity to gentamicin. **ADRs:** Nephrotoxicity, ototoxicity, tremor, and vomiting. **Comments:** Individualize the dosage and dosing interval based on serum concentrations to achieve trough concentrations ≤1.5 mg/liter and peak concentrations ≤10 mg/liter. Do **not** administer for longer than 10 days. Avoid concomitant use of other nephrotoxic or ototoxic drugs (furosemide).
Glucagon	Prolonged hypoglycemia unresponsive to dextrose infusion	0.3 mg IM, IV, or SC. Repeat dose once or twice at 30-min intervals as needed according to individual clinical response *Maximum:* 1 mg/dose. **Note:** 1 mg = 1 unit of glucagon.	**Contraindications:** Hypersensitivity to glucagon and pheochromocytoma. **ADRs:** Hypokalemia, nausea, and vomiting. **Comments:** Monitor glucose blood concentration.
Glycerin	Constipation	Administer only a small portion of a glycerin rectal suppository as needed for constipation.	**ADRs:** Diarrhea and rectal irritation. **Comments:** Cautiously insert the small portion of the rectal suppository to avoid intestinal perforation.
Heparin	Occlusion prophylaxis for umbilical arterial or central venous catheter	To prepare flush solution for umbilical arterial or central venous catheter, add 300 units of heparin to 30 ml of normal saline (or 2/3 dextrose and 1/3 saline solution).	**Contraindications:** Active bleeding from a local lesion (ulcer), 4 hr following major surgery, hemophilia, hypersensitivity to heparin, recent neurosurgery, severe hepatic dysfunction, and shock. **ADRs:** Bleeding.
	Hypercoagulability	50 units/kg followed by 10–25 units/kg/hr by continuous IV infusion to maintain activated partial thromboplastin time (aPTT) 1.5–2 times control. **Note:** Repeated bolus (IV push) administration is not recommended because of associated difficulty maintaining aPTT in the therapeutic range.	
Hyaluronidase (*Wydase®*)	Extravasation of vesicant drugs and solutions	Reconstitute 150-unit vial with 1 ml of normal (0.9%) saline for injection. Withdraw 0.1 ml of the reconstituted solution and dilute with 0.9 ml normal saline	**Contraindications:** Hypersensitivity to hyaluronidase. **ADRs:** Dizziness, hypotension, nausea, urticaria, and vomiting.

TABLE 13-1 continued

DRUG (TRADE AND OTHER NAMES)	INDICATION(S)	USUAL NEONATAL DOSAGE[a] AND ADMINISTRATION[b]	CONTRAINDICATIONS, ADRs, AND COMMENTS[c]
Hyaluronidase *continued*		to yield 1 ml containing 15 units of hyaluronidase. Using a dry sterile needle for each injection, administer five 0.2-ml injections intradermally or subcutaneously into the leading edge of the extravasation site. Administer within 1 hr of diagnosis of extravasation.	**Comments:** Do **not** administer for extravasation of dopamine or other alpha adrenergic agonists (epinephrine).
Hydralazine *(Apresoline®)*	Hypertension	0.1–0.5 mg/kg IV every 3–6 hr, as needed for blood pressure control. Gradually increase the dosage every 2–3 days according to individual clinical response M *Maximum:* 2 mg/kg IV every 6 hr **or** 0.2–0.75 mg/kg PO every 6–12 hr. **Note:** Reduce dosage for neonates who have renal dysfunction. **Note:** An oral dose twice the effective IV dose may be required because of significant loss of orally administered hydralazine from hepatic first-pass metabolism.	**Contraindications:** Cor pulmonale, hypersensitivity to hydralazine, myocardial insufficiency due to mechanical obstruction, systemic lupus erythematosus, and thyrotoxicosis. **ADRs:** Diarrhea, nausea, palpitations, tachycardia, and vomiting. **Comments:** Reduce the dosage when used concomitantly with other antihypertensive drugs. Tachyphylaxis occurs with continued use.
Hydro-chlorothiazide *(HydroDIURIL®)*	Edema	3 mg/kg/day PO in two divided doses every 12 hr.	**Contraindications:** Anuria and hypersensitivity to hydrochlorothiazide or to other thiazide diuretics. **ADRs:** Anorexia, dizziness, hyperglycemia, hyperuricemia, hypokalemia, and nausea. **Comments:** Monitor blood pressure, serum electrolytes, and serum creatinine. When compared with furosemide (*Lasix®*), hydrochlorothiazide does not promote calcium loss in the urine.
Hydrocortisone *(Cortisol)*	Acute adrenal insufficiency Congenital adrenal hyperplasia thrombocytopenia Other conditions responsive to corticosteroids Shock	2.5 mg/kg IM, IV, or PO every 6 hr. 25 mg/kg IV.	**Contraindications:** Administration of live virus vaccines, hypersensitivity to hydrocortisone, and systemic fungal infections. **ADRs:** Glucose intolerance, hypokalemia, hyponatremia, vomiting, and weight gain. **Comments:** May mask signs of infection.
Immune Globulin (Human) *(WinRho SDF®)*	**Suspected sepsis** (particularly *Group B Streptococcus*) **Neutropenia** (leukocyte count below 3000) during first few days of life **Hemolytic jaundice**	500–750 mg/kg IV as a one-time dose at least 12 hr after birth. Initiate infusion at a rate of 0.02 ml/kg/min and, if tolerated, increase to a maximum of 0.08 ml/kg/min.	**Contraindications:** Hypersensitivity to immune globulin. **ADRs:** Chills, fever, malaise, and vomiting. **Comments:** An aseptic meningitis syndrome has been reported in relation to IV immune globulin use. Signs and symptoms include drowsiness, headache, nausea, nuchal rigidity, photophobia, and vomiting. Discontinuation results in remission of the syndrome with no sequelae. May reduce immune hemolysis by binding to and blocking antigen. Prophylactic administration to prevent future infections in premature infants controversial.
Indomethacin *(Indocid®, Indocin®)*	**Nonsurgical closure of patent ductus arteriosus** in premature neonates	**0–7 days of age:** 0.2 mg/kg IV, then 0.1 mg/kg IV 12 hr later, and 0.1 mg/kg IV 36 hr after the initial dose. **>7 days:** 0.2 mg/kg IV, then 0.2 mg/kg IV 12 hr later, and 0.2 mg/kg IV 36 hr after the initial dose.	**Contraindications:** Hypersensitivity to indomethacin or to other NSAIDs. **ADRs:** Bowel perforation and nephrotoxicity (oliguria with elevated blood urea nitrogen and serum creatinine). **Comments:** Withhold in the presence of poor renal function or necrotizing enterocolitis. Monitor urine output, blood urea nitrogen, serum creatinine, and platelet count. Use in prevention of intraventricular hemorrhage with improved long-term outcomes is promising and under investigation. Prolonged (5–7 days) low-dose administration has no advantage over shorter courses.

Footnotes are on page 532.

TABLE 13-1 continued

DRUG (TRADE AND OTHER NAMES)	INDICATION(S)	USUAL NEONATAL DOSAGE[a] AND ADMINISTRATION[b]	CONTRAINDICATIONS, ADRs, AND COMMENTS[c]
Insulin (Regular) Human	Glucose intolerance (hyperglycemia)	0.01–0.02 unit/kg/hr as a continuous IV infusion; adjust dosage according to individual clinical response.	**Contraindications:** Hypoglycemia. **Comments:** Monitor blood glucose concentration carefully. May cause hypoglycemia. Onset of action is rapid, generally occurring within 30 min and lasting for up to 8 hr. **Note:** When used for hyperkalemia, use dextrose infusion to avoid hypoglycemic reactions.
	Hyperkalemia	0.01–0.02 unit/kg/hr IV with at least 1–2 ml/kg/hr of $D_{10}W$; adjust dosage according to individual clinical response.	
Isoproterenol (Isoprenaline, *Isuprel®*)	Bradycardia Cardiac arrest Shock	0.05–0.5 µg/kg/min by continuous IV infusion using an electronic infusion control device; increase dosage by increments of 0.1 µg/kg/min every 5–10 min until desired clinical response is achieved or signs and symptoms of toxicity are observed. **Note:** To prepare IV solution, dilute 0.6 mg isoproterenol in 100 ml of D_5W to yield 6 µg/ml (1 ml/kg/hr = 0.1 µg/kg/min).	**Contraindications:** Coronary insufficiency, digitalis toxicity, hypersensitivity to isoproterenol, and tachydysrhythmias. **ADRs:** Hypotension, tachycardia and other cardiac dysrhythmias, and vomiting. **Comments:** Monitor blood pressure, ECG, oxygenation, and urine output. Do **not** administer concomitantly with epinephrine, but may alternate with epinephrine at 1-hr intervals.
Lidocaine (*Xylocaine®*)	Persistent ventricular dysrhythmias Dysrhythmias associated with digitalis toxicity	0.5–1 mg/kg IV over 5 min. Immediately after initial dose, 10–50 µg/kg/min by continuous IV infusion using an electronic infusion control device. **Note:** To prepare IV solution, add 120 mg lidocaine to 100 ml of D_5W to yield 1200 µg/ml (20 µg/kg/min = 1 ml/kg/hr).	**Contraindications:** Complete heart block (lidocaine suppresses ventricular pacemakers, resulting in ventricular standstill) and hypersensitivity to lidocaine or to other amide-type local anesthetics. **ADRs:** Agitation, bradycardia, convulsions, disorientation, dissociation, drowsiness, hearing loss, hypotension, muscle twitching, and respiratory arrest. May cause CNS depression, myocardial depression, and seizures at serum concentrations exceeding 5 µg/ml (therapeutic range = 1.5–5 µg/ml). **Comments:** Monitor blood pressure, ECG, serum concentrations, and respirations.
Lorazepam (*Ativan®*)	Status epilepticus	0.05 mg/kg IV over 5 min. May repeat dose, if needed, at 10–15-min intervals according to individual clinical response. **Note:** Injectable formulation contains benzyl alcohol, polyethylene glycol, and propylene glycol.	**Contraindications:** Hypersensitivity to lorazepam or to other benzodiazepines and myasthenia gravis. **ADRs:** Clonic movements and drowsiness. **Comments:** Avoid intra-arterial injection because of arteriospasm and resultant gangrene. Antidote for overdosage is flumazenil.
Magnesium Sulfate	Hypomagnesemia	25–50 mg/kg IM or IV every 8–12 hr. *Maximum:* 1 gram/day. **Note:** Reduce dosage for neonates who have renal dysfunction. **Note:** To prepare IV solution, dilute 50% (500 mg/ml) magnesium sulfate solution to 5% (50 mg/ml).	**Contraindications:** Heart block, hypermagnesemia, and renal dysfunction (severe). **ADRs:** Bradycardia, hypotension, and respiratory depression. **Comments:** Monitor blood pressure, ECG, and respirations during administration; monitor serum concentration daily. **Note:** Do **not** administer magnesium sulfate in conjunction with calcium gluconate or sodium bicarbonate. Intravenous calcium gluconate may be used as an antidote, if necessary.
Medium Chain Triglyceride Oil (*M.C.T. Oil®*)	Suspected inadequate oral fat intake	0.5 mg/kg PO every 3–6 hr with feedings; increase the dosage gradually to avoid associated diarrhea.	**Contraindications:** Advanced hepatic cirrhosis and encephalopathy. **ADRs:** GI problems (abdominal distention, diarrhea). **Comments:** Provides 7.6 calories/ml; does **not** contain essential fatty acids.
Meperidine (*Demerol®*, Pethidine)	Moderate-to-severe pain	0.5–1 mg/kg IV every 4–6 hr as needed for pain. **Note:** Some injectable formulations contain sulfites; sulfites have been associated with hypersensitivity reactions among some patients.	**Contraindications:** Acute asthma attack, acute respiratory depression, hypersensitivity to meperidine or to other opiate analgesics, and upper airway obstruction. **ADRs:** Bradycardia, hypotension, respiratory depression, shocklike syndrome, and tachycardia.

TABLE 13-1 continued

DRUG (TRADE AND OTHER NAMES)	INDICATION(S)	USUAL NEONATAL DOSAGE[a] AND ADMINISTRATION[b]	CONTRAINDICATIONS, ADRs, AND COMMENTS[c]
Metronidazole (*Flagyl®*)	**Infections** caused by *Trichomonas*, anaerobic organisms (*Bacteroides*), or other susceptible organisms	**0–7 days of age ≤2 kg:** 10 mg/kg IV or PO every 24 hr. **0–7 days of age >2 kg:** 5–7.5 mg/kg IV or PO every 12 hr. **>7 days of age ≤2 kg:** 7.5 mg/kg IV or PO every 12 hr. **>7 days of age >2 kg:** 15 mg/kg IV or PO every 12 hr.	**Contraindications:** Hepatic dysfunction and hypersensitivity to metronidazole or to other nitroimidazole derivatives. **ADRs:** Darkened urine, eosinophilia, leukopenia, and rash.
Midazolam (*Versed®*)	**Sedation prior to and during short diagnostic procedures** (endoscopy) **Sedation for intubated, mechanically ventilated neonates in intensive care**	0.2–1 µg/kg/min by continuous IV infusion with an electronic infusion control device. **Note:** Bolus (IV push) administration has been associated with myoclonic movements in neonates.	**Contraindications:** Acute pulmonary insufficiency, coma, hypersensitivity to midazolam or to other benzodiazepines, myasthenia gravis, and shock. **ADRs:** Decreased mean arterial pressure, hypotension, and increased pulse and respiratory rates. **Comments:** The immediate availability of oxygen, other appropriate drugs, and trained personnel and equipment necessary for resuscitation and support of ventilation and cardiac function should be ensured **prior** to the use of IV midazolam. Continuously monitor for early signs of hypoventilation or apnea that may lead to hypoxia and cardiac arrest unless effective countermeasures are taken. Limited experience as second-line anticonvulsant for refractory seizures (administer as continuous infusion). **Note:** Flumazenil is a specific antidote for midazolam overdosage.
Morphine	**Moderate-to-severe pain**	0.05–0.1 mg/kg IV every 4–6 hr, as needed according to individual clinical response. If preferred, 0.1–0.2 mg/kg IV push followed by 5–15 µg/kg/hr IV.	**Contraindications:** Acute asthma attack, acute respiratory depression, hypersensitivity to morphine or to other opiate analgesics, and upper airway obstruction. **ADRs:** Bradycardia, CNS and respiratory depression, and hypotension. **Comments:** Monitor for CNS and respiratory depression. **Note:** Naloxone is a specific antidote for morphine overdosage.
Naloxone (*Narcan®*)	**Respiratory depression at birth** associated with maternal opiate analgesic use **Reversal of opiate analgesic overdosage**	0.1 mg/kg IV; may repeat initial dose every 2–3 min and, if needed, every 20–60 min according to individual clinical response. **Note:** If IV administration is not feasible, may be administered by IM or SC injection or via endotracheal tube.	**ADRs:** May precipitate acute neonatal opiate analgesic-withdrawal syndrome. **Comments:** Short duration of action (~1–2 hr). Monitor individual clinical response for 24–48 hr after commencing naloxone, particularly when respiratory depression at birth or reversal of opiate analgesic overdose involves long-acting opiate analgesics (e.g., methadone).
Neostigmine (*Prostigmin®*)	**Reversal of nondepolarizing neuromuscular blockade**	0.02–0.08 mg/kg/dose IV. **Note:** Prior to use, administer atropine 0.02 mg/kg to prevent the severe vagal reaction associated with neostigmine.	**Contraindications:** Bronchial asthma, hypersensitivity to neostigmine, and mechanical obstruction of the intestinal or urinary tracts. **ADRs:** Diarrhea, increased salivation, miosis, muscle cramps, nausea, and vomiting. **Comments:** Does **not** antagonize (and may actually prolong) the phase I block of depolarizing muscle relaxants (e.g., succinylcholine).

Footnotes are on page 532.

TABLE 13-1 continued

DRUG (TRADE AND OTHER NAMES)	INDICATION(S)	USUAL NEONATAL DOSAGE[a] AND ADMINISTRATION[b]	CONTRAINDICATIONS, ADRs, AND COMMENTS[c]
Nitroglycerin (Glyceryl Trinitrate)	Pulmonary hypertension	0.25 µg/kg/min; increase the initial dose by 0.25–0.5 µg/kg/min at 3–5-min intervals as indicated by individual clinical response. Therapeutic response is generally obtained at doses <5 µg/kg/min. **Note:** Injectable formulations may contain alcohol and/or propylene glycol.	**Contraindications:** Hypersensitivity to nitroglycerin or to other nitrates, hypotension, hypovolemia, pericardial tamponade, and severe anemia. **ADRs:** Headache, which occurs in ~50% of patients and generally resolves with continued administration. **Comments:** Continuously monitor blood pressure and heart rate during IV administration.
Norepinephrine (Levarterenol, Levophed®)	Shock unresponsive to fluid volume replacement	0.05–0.1 µg/kg/min using an electronic infusion control device. Titrate dose to desired clinical response. **Note:** Injectable formulation may contain sodium metabisulfite, which may cause allergic-type reactions among susceptible neonates.	**Contraindications:** Hypotension associated with blood volume deficit and vascular thrombosis. **ADRs:** Anxiety, bradycardia, ischemic injury, and respiratory difficulty. **Comments:** Monitor infusion frequently for inadvertent free flow of solution. Inspect injection site for signs of extravasation (edema, inflammation, local tissue necrosis). If extravasation occurs, immediately (or within 12 hr) inject phentolamine 0.1 mg/kg SC into five sites near area of extravasation; change needle before each injection.
Nystatin (Mycostatin®)	Prophylaxis or treatment of *Candida* infection involving the oral cavity or esophagus	100,000 units topically four times daily applied to the tongue with a cotton swab or dropper.	**ADRs:** GI distress, including diarrhea.
Pancuronium	Facilitation of intubation, mechanical ventilation, and anesthesia	0.1 mg/kg IV; repeat as needed to maintain muscle relaxation. Individualize dose according to response. Paralysis exceeding 4 hr is suggestive of excessive dosing. **Note:** Decrease the initial dose by approximately 33% when succinylcholine is used for intubation.	**Contraindications:** Hypersensitivity to pancuronium or to bromides and tachycardia. **ADRs:** Hypotension, paralysis, and tachycardia (usually rare at recommended dosages). Several formulations of pancuronium (Pavulon®) contain benzyl alcohol. Prolonged administration may lead to sensorineural hearing loss and muscle weakness. **Comments:** To reverse action, administer atropine 0.02 mg/kg IV followed by neostigmine 0.08 mg/kg IV in three divided doses 1–2 min apart.
Paraldehyde (Paracetaldehyde)	Convulsions or status epilepticus refractory to conventional pharmacotherapy	0.15–0.3 ml/kg PO or rectal every 6 hr as needed to control seizures. **Oral or rectal administration:** Dilute paraldehyde 1:10 with mineral oil or normal saline to prevent or minimize associated mucosal irritation. **Note:** Only use freshly prepared oral or rectal solutions (appropriately discard unused solutions). The use of decomposed paraldehyde has been associated with severe corrosion of mucous membranes and metabolic acidosis. When preparing solutions, use glass rather than plastic syringes. Avoid contact with skin, eyes, and clothing.	**Contraindications:** Gastric ulcer and severe hepatic impairment. **ADRs:** Gastric irritation (with oral use) and respiratory depression. **Comments:** Although paraldehyde may be administered IM, it is **not** recommended because it is associated with a high incidence of sterile abscesses. **Note:** An injectable form is available in Canada, but it is not readily available in the United States (see Chapter 8).
Penicillin G	Meningitis caused by susceptible bacteria	**0–7 days of age ≤2 kg:** 100,000 units/kg/day IM, IV, or SC in two divided doses every 12 hr. **>7 days of age ≤2 kg:** 150,000 units/kg/day IM, IV, or PO in three divided doses every 8 hr.	**Contraindications:** Hypersensitivity to penicillin G or to other penicillins. **ADRs:** Diarrhea, hemolytic anemia, hypersensitivity reactions, *Candida* infection, and rash.

CHAPTER 13: DRUG DOSING FOR NEONATES

TABLE 13-1 *continued*

DRUG (*TRADE* AND OTHER NAMES)	INDICATION(S)	USUAL NEONATAL DOSAGE[a] AND ADMINISTRATION[b]	CONTRAINDICATIONS, ADRs, AND COMMENTS[c]
Penicillin G *continued*		**0–7 days of age >2 kg:** 150,000 units/kg/day IM, IV, or PO in three divided doses every 8 hr **>7 days of age >2 kg:** 200,000 units/kg/day IM, IV, or PO in four divided doses every 6 hr.	
	Other infections caused by susceptible gram-positive or gram-negative bacteria **Note:** Ensure that appropriate culture and sensitivity tests have been performed and that the organism is sensitive to penicillin G.	**0–7 days of age ≤2 kg:** 50,000 units/kg/day IM, IV, or PO in two divided doses every 12 hr. **>7 days of age ≤2 kg:** 75,000 units/kg/day IM, IV, or PO in three divided doses every 8 hr. **0–7 days of age >2 kg:** 75,000 units/kg/day IM, IV, or PO in three divided doses every 8 hr. **>7 days of age >2 kg:** 100,000 units/kg/day IM, IV, or PO in four divided doses every 6 hr. **Note:** Reduce dosage for neonates who have renal dysfunction.	
Penicillin G Benzathine (*Bicillin L-A®*)	**Congenital syphilis** **Note:** Ensure that appropriate culture and sensitivity tests have been performed and that the organism is sensitive to penicillin G benzathine.	50,000 units/kg IM as a single dose.	**Contraindications:** Hypersensitivity to penicillin G benzathine or to other penicillins. **ADRs:** Diarrhea, hemolytic anemia, hypersensitivity reactions, *Candida* infection, and rash.
Pethidine, see Meperidine			
Phenobarbital	**Opiate analgesic-withdrawal seizures**	**Initial:** 5–20 mg/kg by slow IV push (can repeat once if neonate remains symptomatic), followed by 10–12 mg/kg/day IV in two divided doses for 48 hr if seizures continue. **Maintenance:** 5 mg/kg/day IM, IV (slow-push), or PO in two divided doses every 12 hr.	**Contraindications:** Hepatic or renal dysfunction (severe), hypersensitivity to phenobarbital or to other barbiturates, porphyria, and respiratory dysfunction (severe). **ADRs:** Hypotension and respiratory depression. Therapeutic serum concentrations = 20–40 µg/liter; individualize dosage according to clinical response. **Note:** Does not control GI effects of withdrawal syndrome.
Phentolamine (*Regitine®*, *Rogitine®*)	**Prophylaxis or treatment of dermal necrosis and sloughing** after IV administration or extravasation of dobutamine, dopamine, epinephrine, or norepinephrine	0.1 mg/kg SC immediately into five sites near area of extravasation. **Note:** To prepare solution, dilute 1 ml of 5-mg/ml solution to 5 ml with normal saline or D₅W to yield 1-mg/ml solution.	**Contraindications:** Hypersensitivity to phentolamine, hypotension, and myocardial ischemia. **ADRs:** Diarrhea, flushing, hypotension, tachycardia (severe), and vomiting. **Comments:** Do not inject solution into an inflamed or infected area.
Phenytoin (*Dilantin®*, Diphenylhydantoin)	**Generalized tonic-clonic (grand mal) and partial (focal) seizures**	**Initial:** 10–20 mg/kg IV; may repeat once if seizures persist. **Maintenance:** 4–8 mg/kg/day IV in two or three divided doses, every 8–12 hr. **Note:** Inject IV slowly at a rate not exceeding 0.5–1 mg/min. Therapeutic serum concentrations = 10–20 µg/ml. Do not dilute with IV solutions; flush the IV tubing with normal saline for injection before and after IV administration.	**Contraindications:** Hypersensitivity to phenytoin or to other hydantoin anticonvulsants. **ADRs:** Blood dyscrasias, bradycardia, cardiovascular collapse, CNS depression, constipation, heart block, hypotension, intolerance to feedings (nausea), and skin rash. **Comments:** IV route is preferred because neonates absorb orally administered phenytoin erratically from the GI tract.

Footnotes are on page 532.

TABLE 13-1 continued

DRUG (TRADE AND OTHER NAMES)	INDICATION(S)	USUAL NEONATAL DOSAGE[a] AND ADMINISTRATION[b]	CONTRAINDICATIONS, ADRs, AND COMMENTS[c]
Piperacillin (Pipracil®)	**Infections** caused by susceptible bacteria (*Pseudomonas aeruginosa, Enterbacteriaceae*) **Note:** Ensure that appropriate culture and sensitivity tests have been performed and that the organism is sensitive to piperacillin.	**0–7 days of age ≤2 kg:** 100 mg/kg/day IV in two divided doses every 12 hr. **>7 days of age ≤2 kg:** 150 mg/kg/day IV in three divided doses every 8 hr. **0–7 days of age >2 kg:** 150 mg/kg/day IV in three divided doses every 8 hr. **>7 days of age >2 kg:** 200 mg/kg/day IV in four divided doses every 6 hr. **Note:** Reduce dosage for neonates who have renal dysfunction.	**Contraindications:** Hypersensitivity to penicillins or cephalosporins. **ADRs:** Blood dyscrasias; diarrhea; elevated blood urea nitrogen, serum creatinine, or hepatic enzymes; fever; interstitial nephritis (rare); lethargy; nausea; phlebitis at infusion site; pseudomembranous colitis (rare); and vomiting. **Note:** Always use in combination with an aminoglycoside.
Potassium Chloride	Hypokalemia	1–2 mmol/kg/day by continuous IV infusion at a rate not exceeding 1 mmol/kg/hr **or** PO in two or three divided doses every 8–12 hr. **Note:** Assure adequate renal function and urine output before administering. 1 mmol of potassium chloride = 1 mEq.	**Contraindications:** Hyperkalemia and significant renal dysfunction. **ADRs:** Cardiac dysrhythmias, GI irritation and vomiting with oral administration, hyperkalemia, and hypotension. **Comments:** Maintain serum concentration of 3.5–6 mmol/liter.
Prednisone	**Adrenal insufficiency** **Other conditions responsive to corticosteroids** **Hypoglycemia** unresponsive to dextrose infusion	2 mg/kg/day PO as a single daily dose or in four divided doses every 6 hr; adjust dosage according to individual clinical response.	**Contraindications:** Administration of live virus vaccines and systemic fungal infections. **ADRs:** Fluid and electrolyte disturbances (hypercalcemia, hypernatremia, hypokalemia, hypokalemic acidosis) and growth retardation. **Comments:** May mask signs of, or increase susceptibility to, infection.
Propranolol (Inderal®)	**Certain cardiac dysrhythmias** (supraventricular tachycardia, tachydysrhythmia associated with digoxin toxicity, ventricular tachycardia unresponsive to conventional therapy)	**Initial:** 0.01–0.03 mg/kg IV up to a maximum of 1 mg/dose IV. May repeat initial dose after 10 min, if needed, until dysrhythmia is controlled. **Maintenance:** 0.01–0.03 mg/kg IV up to a maximum of 1 mg/kg every 8 hr **or** 0.5–4 mg/kg/day PO in three or four divided doses every 6–8 hr. May increase dosage as required to control dysrhythmia.	**Contraindications:** Bronchospasm, cardiogenic shock, and congestive heart failure unrelated to indications. **ADRs:** Bradycardia, bronchoconstriction, congestive heart failure, and hypoglycemia. **Comments:** Monitor heart rate and blood pressure frequently after initial dose. Use atropine or isoproterenol as an antidote if bradycardia occurs. Action may be adversely affected by concurrent phenobarbital and cimetidine (see Chapter 6).
	Hypertension **Neonatal thyrotoxicosis** **Obstructive hypertrophic subaortic stenosis, spells associated with Tetralogy of Fallot**	0.25–1 mg/kg/day PO in two to four divided doses every 6–12 hr. *Maximum:* 4 mg/kg/day PO.	
Protamine Sulfate	Heparin overdosage	1 mg for each 100 units of heparin administered in preceding 4 hr. Administer by slow IV push over 1–3 min.	**Contraindications:** Hypersensitivity to protamine sulfate. **ADRs:** Bradycardia and hypotension from rapid IV administration. **Comments:** Monitor blood coagulation.
Pyridoxine (Vitamin B_6)	Pyridoxine-dependent seizures	25–50 mg IV; if seizures do not stop within 2–3 min, an additional 50–100 mg may be administered. **Note:** Some neonates may require 2–100 mg/day for life.	**Contraindications:** Hypersensitivity to pyridoxine. **ADRs:** Generally well tolerated and nontoxic. Headache, nausea, paresthesia, and somnolence. **Comments:** An EEG at the time of the first dose may facilitate evaluation of the efficacy of therapy and help confirm the diagnosis of pyridoxine-dependent seizures.
Ranitidine (Zantac®)	**Peptic ulcer disease** **Reflux esophagitis** **Short bowel syndrome**	1.25–2 mg/kg/day IV in two to four divided doses every 6–12 hr **or** 2.5–4 mg/kg/day PO in two divided doses every 12 hr. **Note:** Reduce dosage for neonates who have renal dysfunction.	**Contraindications:** Hypersensitivity to ranitidine. **ADRs:** Abdominal pain, arthralgia, cardiac dysrhythmias (bradycardia, tachycardia), constipation, diarrhea, headache (irritability), hepatotoxicity, insomnia (rare), nausea, and vomiting.

TABLE 13-1 continued

DRUG (TRADE AND OTHER NAMES)	INDICATION(S)	USUAL NEONATAL DOSAGE[a] AND ADMINISTRATION[b]	CONTRAINDICATIONS, ADRs, AND COMMENTS[c]
Salbutamol, see **Albuterol**			
Sodium Bicarbonate	Metabolic acidosis	1–3 mmol/kg immediately by continuous IV infusion **or** by IV push over 10 min. May be administered orally for chronic metabolic acidosis. *Maximum:* 8 mmol/kg/day. Dosage must be individualized according to acid–base status. **Note:** Hypertonic; prior to use, dilute with sterile water for injection to a concentration **not** exceeding 0.5 mmol/ml. 1 mEq sodium bicarbonate = 1 mmol of sodium bicarbonate. Each IV dose in milliequivalents can be estimated from: $HCO_3^- \text{ (mEq)} \approx \text{base deficit} \times \text{weight (kg)} \times 0.3 = (HCO_{3\ desired}^- - HCO_{3\ actual}^-) \times \text{weight (kg)} \times 0.3$.	**Contraindications:** Alkalosis and hypochloremia. **ADRs:** Alkalosis, edema, hypernatremia. **Comments:** Monitor serum bicarbonate, serum osmolarity, serum sodium, and body weight. Ensure adequate ventilation and oxygenation prior to initiating therapy. **Note:** IV admixture incompatibilities include calcium (precipitates) and epinephrine (epinephrine is partially inactivated).
Sodium Chloride	Hyponatremia prophylaxis Hyponatremia treatment	2 mmol/kg/day in 100 ml solution by continuous IV infusion **or** PO with feedings; higher dosages (8–10 mmol/kg/day) may be required for premature neonates. **Note:** Sodium replacement dosage equals sodium deficit (mmol/liter) $\times$ 0.6 $\times$ body weight (kg). 1 mEq = 1 mmol of sodium chloride. Sodium IV dose (in mEq) can be estimated from: $Na^+ \text{ (mEq)} \approx \text{sodium deficit} \times \text{weight (kg)} \times 0.6 = (Na^+_{\ desired} - Na^+_{\ actual}) \times \text{weight (kg)} \times 0.6$.	**Contraindications:** Hypernatremia. **ADRs:** Acidosis, hypernatremia, hypokalemia, and osmotic diuresis. **Comments:** Monitor sodium and potassium serum concentrations. **Note:** 3% sodium chloride contains 513 mmol of sodium/liter; 0.9% sodium chloride contains 154 mmol of sodium/liter.
Sodium Nitroprusside (Nitroprusside)	Insufficient cardiac output after cardiac surgery Refractory congestive heart failure	0.1–3 μg/kg/min by continuous IV infusion beginning with a low dosage and titrating to desired effect. **Note:** To prepare continuous IV infusion solution, dissolve 50 mg sodium nitroprusside in 3 ml D_5W without preservatives and then dilute further in 500 ml D_5W to yield 100 μg/ml. During infusion, protect infusion container from light using aluminum foil.	**Contraindications:** Arteriovenous shunt, coarctation of the aorta, hypovolemia, and insufficient cerebral perfusion. **ADRs:** Hypotension, muscular twitching, nausea, and sweating (particularly in presence of metabolic acidosis and convulsions). **Comments:** Measure arterial blood pressure and cardiac output during continuous IV infusion. Monitor thiocyanate blood concentration (nitroprusside toxicity generally occurs at blood concentrations >10 μg/ml).
Sodium Polystyrene Sulfonate (Kayexalate®)	Hyperkalemia	0.5–1 gram/kg PO or rectal every 6 hr. **Note:** Usually is administered rectally by the following procedure. Dilute in tap water initially and then further dilute with 10% methylcellulose, tap water, or other suitable suspending agent (3–4 ml of vehicle per gram of resin). Shake well before use. Administer high in sigmoid colon using tube. (Solution should be retained for 30–45 min.) Follow with a saline enema. **Note:** Avoid use of commercially available **liquid** formulations because of their preservative content.	**Contraindications:** Bowel obstruction, hypersensitivity to sodium polystyrene sulfonate, necrotizing enterocolitis, and serum potassium <5 mmol/liter. **ADRs:** Constipation, hypocalcemia, hypokalemia, and sodium retention. **Note:** 1 gram removes 1 mmol potassium ions in exchange for 1 mmol sodium ions. Monitor potassium serum concentration. Use with caution with concurrent digoxin because hypokalemia sensitizes the myocardium to digitalis glycosides.
Spironolactone (Aldactone®)	Ascites Congestive heart failure Edema Hyperaldosteronism	1–3 mg/kg/day PO in two divided doses every 12 hr (usually with feedings).	**Contraindications:** Hyperkalemia, hypersensitivity to spironolactone, and renal failure. **ADRs:** Cramping, diarrhea, drowsiness, hyperkalemia, lethargy, and nausea. **Comments:** Monitor serum electrolyte concentrations and body weight daily.

Footnotes are on page 532.

TABLE 13-1 *continued*

DRUG (*TRADE* AND OTHER NAMES)	INDICATION(S)	USUAL NEONATAL DOSAGE[a] AND ADMINISTRATION[b]	CONTRAINDICATIONS, ADRs, AND COMMENTS[c]
Succinylcholine (*Anectine®*, Suxamethonium)	Adjunct to general anesthesia Facilitation of tracheal intubation Skeletal muscle relaxation during mechanical ventilation or surgery	**Initial:** 1–2 mg/kg IV. **Maintenance:** 0.3–0.6 mg/kg IV every 5–10 min as needed according to individual clinical response. **Note:** Continuous IV infusion is **not** recommended because of the risk for malignant hyperthermia.	**Contraindications:** Hypersensitivity to succinylcholine, hyperkalemia, increased intracranial pressure, malignant hyperthermia, and skeletal muscle myopathies. **ADRs:** Bradycardia, fever, hypotension, increased salivation, muscle fasciculations, myoglobinemia, and postparalysis myalgias. **Comments:** Metabolized by plasma cholinesterase; neonates deficient in this enzyme exhibit markedly prolonged paralysis after small doses. **Note:** Onset of relaxation is often preceded by a short period of painful muscle fasciculation. To avoid this effect, fentanyl should be administered before succinylcholine. Premedicate with atropine 0.02 mg/kg IV to prevent vagally mediated bradycardia.
Sulfacetamide Sodium (*Sulamyd®*)	Conjunctivitis or superficial ocular infections caused by *Chlamydia, Staphylococci, Streptococci*, or other susceptible bacteria **Note:** Ensure that appropriate culture and sensitivity tests have been performed and that the organism is sensitive to sulfacetamide.	**Ophthalmic drops:** Instill one drop into each affected eye every 6 hr for 10 days. The ophthalmic drops are incompatible with silver preparations (silver nitrate). Nonsusceptible microorganisms, including fungi, may proliferate. **Ophthalmic ointment:** Apply a small amount of the sulfacetamide ophthalmic ointment to each affected eye every 6 hr for 10 days. **Note:** Ointment may retard corneal wound healing.	**Contraindications:** Hypersensitivity to sulfonamides.
Sulfamethoxazole, *see* **Trimethoprim–Sulfamethoxazole**			
Sulfisoxazole	None (use is **not** recommended)		**Comments:** Contraindicated during the immediate neonatal period (particularly in jaundiced neonates) because it can predispose the neonate to hyperbilirubinemia and resultant bilirubin encephalopathy; competitively interferes with bilirubin–albumin binding.
Theophylline (*Theolair®*)	Apnea Bradycardia Bronchospasm Preparation for extubation	**Initial:** 6 mg/kg IV over 20 min. **Maintenance:** 1–3 mg/kg every 8 hr beginning 8 hr after initial loading dose. **Note:** Marked differences in serum levels are commonly observed among patients receiving the same dosage. This variation is believed to be due to individual differences in rates of theophylline metabolism. These differences have been related to developmental differences (particularly among premature neonates), diet, concurrent disease states, and concurrent drug therapy. Thus, therapy must be carefully individualized and serum levels monitored.	**Contraindications:** Hypersensitivity to theophylline or to other xanthine derivatives, peptic ulcer, and uncontrolled cardiac dysrhythmias. **ADRs:** CNS and GI system disturbances, irritability, and tachycardia. Withhold dose if apical heart rate >180 beats/min. Individualize dose and dosing interval based on serum concentration; therapeutic range = 10–20 µg/ml (55–110 µmol/liter).
Tobramycin (*Tobrex®*)	**Infections** caused by *Pseudomonas aeruginosa* and other susceptible bacteria **Note:** Ensure that appropriate culture and sensitivity tests have been performed and that the organism is sensitive to tobramycin.	**0–4 weeks of age <1200 grams:** 2.5 mg/kg IV by slow intermittent infusion over 30 min every 18–24 hr. **0–4 weeks of age 1200–2000 grams:** 2.5 mg/kg IV by slow intermittent infusion over 30 min every 12–18 hr. **0–7 days of age >2000 grams:** 2.5 mg/kg IV by slow intermittent infusion over 30 min every 12 hr.	**Contraindications:** Hypersensitivity to tobramycin and to other aminoglycoside antibiotics. **ADRs:** Nephrotoxicity and ototoxicity. **Comments:** Individualize the dose and dosing interval based on serum concentrations to achieve trough concentrations ≤2 mg/liter and peak concentrations ≤12 mg/liter. Do **not** administer for longer than 10 days.

TABLE 13-1 continued

DRUG (TRADE AND OTHER NAMES)	INDICATION(S)	USUAL NEONATAL DOSAGE[a] AND ADMINISTRATION[b]	CONTRAINDICATIONS, ADRs, AND COMMENTS[c]
Tobramycin *continued*		>7 days of age >2000 grams: 2.5 mg/kg IV by slow intermittent infusion over 30 min every 8 hr.	Avoid concomitant use of other nephrotoxic or ototoxic drugs (e.g., furosemide).
Trimethoprim–Sulfamethoxazole (Co-trimoxazole) (trimethoprim [T] + sulfamethoxazole [S] in 1:5 combination) *(Bactrim®, Septra®)*	***Pneumocystis carinii* pneumonia or infections** caused by susceptible gram-positive or gram-negative bacteria **Note:** Ensure that appropriate culture and sensitivity tests have been performed and that the organism is sensitive to trimethoprim–sulfamethoxazole.	**0–7 days of age >1 kg:** 2.5 mg/kg T and 12.5 mg/kg S IV or PO every 48 hr. **>7 days of age >1 kg:** 5 mg/kg T and 25 mg/kg S IV or PO every 24 hr. **Note:** Reduce dosage or increase dosing interval for neonates who have renal dysfunction.	**Contraindications:** Hypersensitivity to trimethoprim or to sulfamethoxazole or to any other sulfonamides, blood dyscrasias, and severe hepatic or renal dysfunction. **ADRs:** Anorexia, jaundice in neonates with glucose 6-phosphate dehydrogenase deficiency, kernicterus, nausea, neutropenia (<1500 white blood cells/ml), and vomiting. **Comments:** Except for *Pneumocystis carinii* pneumonia, **not** generally antibiotic of first choice. General use for neonates is **not** approved by the FDA or HPB.
Vancomycin *(Vancocin®)*	**Infections** caused by methicillin-resistant *Staphylococcus aureus* or *S. epidermidis* **Necrotizing enterocolitis** caused by *Clostridium difficile*	**0–7 days of age <800 grams:** 20 mg/kg IV every 36 hr. **0–7 days of age 800–1500 grams:** 20 mg/kg IV every 24 hr. **0–7 days of age 1501–2000 grams:** 20 mg/kg IV every 18 hr. **0–7 days of age >2000 grams:** 15 mg/kg IV every 12 hr. **>7 days of age** (dosage is determined by postconceptual age [PCA], which is gestational age at birth plus postnatal age in weeks): PCA <27 weeks: 20 mg/kg IV every 36 hr. PCA 27–30 weeks: 20 mg/kg IV every 24 hr. PCA 31–34 weeks: 20 mg/kg IV every 18 hr. PCA 35–38 weeks: 15 mg/kg IV every 12 hr. PCA >38 weeks: 15 mg/kg IV every 8 hr. **Note:** Reduce dosage for neonates who have renal dysfunction.	**Contraindications:** Hypersensitivity to vancomycin. **ADRs:** Nephrotoxicity, ototoxicity, and skin rash or flushing ("red-neck" syndrome). **Comments:** Close clinical monitoring is recommended in order to detect dose-related and idiosyncratic toxicity. Adjust dosage based on serum concentrations measured twice weekly beginning 48 hr after initiating therapy. The target peak concentration (generally obtained 1 hr after end of infusion) is 25–40 µg/ml and the target trough concentration (generally obtained immediately before the next dose) is 5–10 µg/ml. **Note:** Some enterococci are developing resistance. Additive nephrotoxicity has been associated with concomitant use with other nephrotoxic drugs.
	Antibiotic-associated pseudomembranous colitis or staphylococcal enterocolitis **Note:** Ensure that appropriate culture and sensitivity tests have been performed and that the organism is sensitive to vancomycin.	40 mg/kg/day PO in three or four divided doses for 7–10 days. **Note:** Oral vancomycin is effective only for these indications; **not** effective for the treatment of other types of infections.	
Zidovudine (Azidothymidine, AZT, *Retrovir®*)	**HIV infection**	**Premature ≤2 weeks of age:** 1.5 mg/kg PO every 12 hr. **Premature >2 weeks of age:** 1.5 mg/kg PO every 8 hr. **Term:** 2 mg/kg PO every 6 hr.	**Contraindications:** Hypersensitivity to zidovudine. **ADRs:** Anemia, anorexia, fatigue, granulocytopenia, headache, myalgia, nausea, peripheral neuropathy, pruritus, and rash. **Comments:** Use with extreme caution with bone marrow suppression. Observe closely to detect and manage opportunistic infections associated with HIV infection. **Note:** A positive test for HIV-antibody in neonates younger than 15 months of age may represent passively acquired maternal antibodies and not an active antibody response to HIV infection. Auxiliary clinical assessment and related diagnostic tests may be required to confirm an HIV-positive diagnosis in this clinical situation.

Footnotes are on page 532

References[1]

Abadi, J. (1997). Acyclovir. *Pediatrics in Review, 18*(2), 70–71.

Alpay, F., Sarici, S. U., Okutan, V., et al. (1999). High-dose intravenous immunoglobulin therapy in neonatal immune haemolytic jaundice. *Acta Paediatrica, 88*(2), 216–219.

Anand, K. J., McIntosh, N., Lagercrantz, H., et al. (1999). Analgesia and sedation in preterm neonates who require ventilatory support: Results from the NOPAIN trial. Neonatal Outcome and Prolonged Analgesia in Neonates. *Archives of Pediatrics and Adolescent Medicine, 153*(4), 331–338.

Bailey, J. M., Miller, B. E., Kanter, K. R., et al. (1997). A comparison of the hemodynamic effects of amrinone and sodium nitroprusside in infants after cardiac surgery. *Anesthesia and Analgesia, 84*(2), 294–298.

Bakshi, F., Barzilay, Z., & Paret, G. (1998). Adenosine in the diagnosis and treatment of narrow complex tachycardia in the pediatric intensive care unit. *Heart and Lung, 27*(1), 47–50.

Bell, C., Simon, D., & Sovcik, J. (Eds.) (1999). *Formulary handbook from Children's Memorial Hospital*, 4th ed. Hudson, OH: Lexi-Comp.

Botha, J. H., du Preez, M. J., Miller, R., et al. (1998). Determination of population pharmacokinetic parameters for amikacin in neonates using mixed-effect models. *European Journal of Clinical Pharmacology, 53*(5), 337–341.

Brion, L. P., & Campbell, D. E. (1999). Furosemide in indomethacin-treated infants: Systematic review and meta-analysis. *Pediatric Nephrology, 13*(3), 212–218.

Bromiker, R., Adelman, C., Arad, I., et al. (1999). Safety of gentamicin administered by intravenous bolus in the nursery. *Clinical Pediatrics, 38*(7), 433–435.

Chang, A. C., Hanley, F. L., Wernovsky, G., et al. (1998). *Pediatric cardiac intensive care*. Baltimore, MD: Williams and Wilkins.

Chang, G. Y., Lueder, F., DiMichele, D., et al. (1997). Heparin and the risk of intraventricular hemorrhage in premature infants. *The Journal of Pediatrics, 131*, 362–366.

Chess, P. R., & D'Angio, C. T. (1998). Clonic movements following lorazepam administration in full-term infants. *Archives of Pediatrics and Adolescent Medicine, 152*(1), 98–99.

Cheung, P. Y., Tyebkhan, J. M., Peliowski, A., et al. (1999). Prolonged use of pancuronium bromide and sensorineural hearing loss in childhood survivors of congenital diaphragmatic hernia. *The Journal of Pediatrics, 135*(2 Pt 1), 233–239.

Chou, Y. H., & Yau, K. I. (1998). The use of prophylactic intravenous immunoglobulin therapy in very low birthweight infants. *Chang-Keng i Hsueh Tsa Chih, 21*(4), 371–376.

Coleman, D. M., Kelly, H. W., & McWilliams, B. C. (1996). Determinants of aerosolized albuterol delivery to mechanically ventilated infants. *Chest, 109*(6), 1607–1613.

Conroy, S. (1998). Unlicensed and off label drug use for paediatric patients. Optimal dosing schedules with gentamicin are needed for premature neonates. *British Medical Journal, 317*(7152), 204–205.

Davies, M. W., & Cartwright, D. W. (1998). Gentamicin dosage intervals in neonates: Longer dosage interval—less toxicity. *Journal of Paediatrics and Child Health, 34*(6), 577–580.

de Alba Romero, C., Gomez Castillo, E., Manzanares Secades, C., et al. (1998). Once daily gentamicin dosing in neonates. *Pediatric Infectious Disease Journal, 17*(12), 1169–1171.

Elibol, O., Alcelik, T., Yuksel, N., et al. (1997). The influence of drop size of cyclopentolate, phenylephrine and tropicamide on pupil dilatation and systemic side effects in infants. *Acta Ophthalmologica Scandinavica, 75*(2), 178–180.

Fanaroff, A. A., & Martin, R. J. (1997). *Neonatal-perinatal medicine: Diseases of the fetus and infant*, 6th ed. St. Louis, MO: C. V. Mosby.

Gappa, M., Gartner, M., Poets, C. F., et al. (1997). Effects of salbutamol delivery from a metered dose inhaler versus jet nebulizer on dynamic lung mechanics in very preterm infants with chronic lung disease. *Pediatric Pulmonology, 23*(6), 442–448.

Gross, G. J., Epstein, M. R., Walsh, E. P., et al. (1998). Characteristics, management, and midterm outcome in infants with atrioventricular nodal reentry tachycardia. *American Journal of Cardiology, 82*(8), 956–960.

Guidelines 2000 for Cardiopulmonary Resuscitation and Emergency Cardiovascular Care. Part 11: Neonatal Resuscitation. The American Heart Association in Collaboration with the International Liaison Committee on Resuscitation (2000). *Circulation, 102*(8 Suppl), I343–I357.

Halliday, H. L. (1996). Natural vs synthetic surfactants in neonatal respiratory distress syndrome. *Drugs, 51*(2), 226–237.

Heubi, J., & Bien, J. (1997). Acetaminophen use in children: More is not better. *The Journal of Pediatrics, 130*, 175–177.

International randomised controlled trial of acetazolamide and furosemide in posthaemorrhagic ventricular dilatation in infancy. International PHVD Drug Trial Group. (1998). *The Lancet, 352*(9126), 433–440.

---

1. These references are meant to provide the reader with some benchmarks only and are not intended to comprise a comprehensive reference list. For additional references to original or earlier citations, please refer to previous editions of this text.

Ishisaka, D. Y. (1996). Exogenous surfactant use in neonates. [Review]. *Annals of Pharmacotherapy, 30*(4), 389–398.

Jenson, H. B., & Pollock, B. H. (1998). The role of intravenous immunoglobulin for the prevention and treatment of neonatal sepsis. *Seminars in Perinatology, 22*(1), 50–63.

Kimberlin, D., Powell, D., Gruber, W., et al. (1996). Administration of oral acyclovir suppressive therapy after neonatal herpes simplex virus disease limited to the skin, eyes and mouth: Results of a phase I/II trial. *Pediatric Infectious Disease Journal, 15*(3), 247–254.

Krause, M. F., Schulte-Monting, J., & Hoehn, T. (1998). Rate of surfactant administration influences lung function and gas exchange in a surfactant-deficient rabbit model. *Pediatric Pulmonology, 25*(3), 196–204.

Laws, D. E., Morton, C., Weindling, M., et al. (1996). Systemic effects of screening for retinopathy of prematurity. *British Journal of Ophthalmology, 80*(5), 425–428.

Lee, T. C., Charles, B. G., Harte, G. J., et al. (1999). Population pharmacokinetic modeling in very premature infants receiving midazolam during mechanical ventilation: Midazolam neonatal pharmacokinetics. *Anesthesiology, 90*(2), 451–457.

Libenson, M. H., Kaye, E. M., Rosman, N. P., et al. (1999). Acetazolamide and furosemide for posthemorrhagic hydrocephalus of the newborn. *Pediatric Neurology, 20*(3), 185–191.

Lochan, S. R., Adeniyi-Jones, S., Assadi, F. K., et al. (1998). Coadministration of theophylline enhances diuretic response to furosemide in infants during extracorporeal membrane oxygenation: A randomized controlled pilot study. *The Journal of Pediatrics, 133*(1), 86–89.

Lotze, A., Mitchell, B. R., Bulas, D. I., et al. (1998). Multicenter study of surfactant (beractant) use in the treatment of term infants with severe respiratory failure. Survanta in Term Infants Study Group. *The Journal of Pediatrics, 132*(1), 40–47.

Lowry, J. A., Jarrett, R. V., Wasserman, G., et al. (2001). Theophylline toxicokinetics in premature newborns. *Archives of Pediatric and Adolescent Medicine, 155*, 934–939.

Luedtke, S. A., Kuhn, R. J., & McCaffrey, F. M. (1997). Pharmacologic management of supraventricular tachycardias in children. Part 1: Wolff-Parkinson-White and atrioventricular nodal reentry. *Annals of Pharmacotherapy, 31*(10), 1227–1243.

Lundergan, F. S., Glasscock, G. F., Kim, E. H., et al. (1999). Once-daily gentamicin dosing in newborn infants. *Pediatrics, 103*(6 Pt 1), 1228–1234.

Maggioni, A., Orzalesi, M., & Mimouni, F. (1998). Intravenous correction of neonatal hypomagnesemia. *The Journal of Pediatrics, 132,* 652–655.

McSherry, G. D., Shapiro, D. E., Coombs, R. W., et al. (1999). The effects of zidovudine in the subset of infants infected with human immunodeficiency virus type-1 (Pediatric AIDS Clinical Trials Group Protocol 076). *The Journal of Pediatrics, 134*(6), 717–724.

Ment, L. R., Vohr, B., Oh, W., et al. (1996). Neurodevelopmental outcome at 36 months' corrected age of preterm infants in the Multicenter Indomethacin Intraventricular Hemorrhage Prevention Trial. *Pediatrics, 98*(4 Pt 1), 714–718.

Mofenson, L. M. (1999). Short-course zidovudine for prevention of perinatal infection. *The Lancet, 353*(9155), 766–767.

Murphy, J. E., Austin, M. L., & Frye, R. F. (1998). Evaluation of gentamicin pharmacokinetics and dosing protocols in 195 neonates. *American Journal of Health-System Pharmacists, 55*(21), 2280–2288.

Neonatal drug withdrawal. (1998). American Academy of Pediatrics Committee on Drugs. *Pediatrics, 101*(6), 1079–1088.

Newton, N., Leonard, C., Piecuch, R., et al. (1999). Neurodevelopmental outcome of prematurely born children treated with recombinant erythropoietin in infancy. *Journal of Perinatology, 19,* 403–406.

Ohki, Y., Nako, Y., Koizumi, T., et al. (1997). The effect of aerosolized furosemide in infants with chronic lung disease. *Acta Paediatrica, 86*(6), 656–660.

O'Shea, T. M., Kothadia, J. M., Klinepeter, K. L., et al. (1999). Randomized placebo-controlled trial of a 42-day tapering course of dexamethasone to reduce the duration of ventilator dependency in very low birth weight infants: Outcome of study participants at 1-year adjusted age. *Pediatrics, 104*(1 Pt 1), 15–21.

Padbury, J. (1998). Neonatal dopamine pharmacodynamics: Lessons from the bedside. *The Journal of Pediatrics, 133,* 719–720.

Papile, L. A., Tyson, J. E., Stoll, B. J., et al. (1998). A multicenter trial of two dexamethasone regimens in ventilator-dependent premature infants. *New England Journal of Medicine, 338*(16), 1112–1118.

Peng, C. C., Chen, M. R., Hou, C. J., et al. (1998). Atrial flutter in the neonate and early infancy. *Japanese Heart Journal, 39*(3), 287–295.

Peter, G. (Ed.). (1997). *Red book: Report of the Committee of Infectious Diseases,* 24th ed. Elk Grove Village, IL: American Academy of Pediatrics.

Pfammatter, J. P., & Stocker, F. P. (1998). Reentrant supraventricular tachycardia in infancy: Current role of prophylactic digoxin treatment. *European Journal of Pediatrics, 157*(2), 101–106.

Prabhu, V. G., Keszler, M., & Dhanireddy, R. (1997). Pulmonary function changes after nebulised and intravenous frusemide in ventilated premature infants. *Archives of Disease in Childhood—Fetal and Neonatal Edition, 77*(1), F32–F35.

Prabhu, V. G., Keszler, M., & Dhanireddy, R. (1998). Dose-dependent evaluation of the effects of nebulized furosemide on pulmonary function in ventilated preterm infants. *Journal of Perinatology, 18*(5), 357–360.

Rabalais, G. P., Samiec, T. D., Bryant, K. K., et al. (1996). Invasive candidiasis in infants weighing more than 2500 grams at birth admitted to a neonatal intensive care unit. *Pediatric Infectious Disease Journal, 15*(4), 348–352.

Reiter, P. D., Makhlouf, R., & Stiles, A. D. (1998). Comparison of 6-hour infusion versus bolus furosemide in premature infants. *Pharmacotherapy, 18*(1), 63–68.

Rivera-Penera, T., Gugig, R., Davis, J., et al. (1997). Outcome of acetaminophen overdose in pediatric patients contributing to hepatotoxicity. *The Journal of Pediatrics, 130,* 300–304.

Rohrer, T., Rinaldi, D., Bubl, R., et al. (1999). Combined treatment with zidovudine, lamivudine, nelfinavir and ganciclovir in an infant with human immunodeficiency virus type 1 infection and cytomegalovirus encephalitis: Case report and review of the literature. *Pediatric Infectious Disease Journal, 18*(4), 382–386.

Scott, C., Riggs, W., Ling, E., et al. (1999). Morphine pharmacokinetics and pain assessment in premature newborns. *The Journal of Pediatrics, 135,* 423–429.

Seri, I., Abbasi, S., Wood, D., et al. (1998). Regional hemodynamic effects of dopamine in the sick premature infant. *The Journal of Pediatrics, 133,* 728–734.

Shaffer, N., Chuachoowong, R., Mock, P. A., et al. (1999). Short-course zidovudine for perinatal HIV-1 transmission in Bangkok, Thailand: A randomised controlled trial. Bangkok Collaborative Perinatal HIV Transmission Study Group. *The Lancet, 353*(9155), 773–780.

Shannon, K., Keith, J., Mentzer, W., et al. (1995). Recombinant human erythropoietin stimulates erythropoiesis and reduces erythrocyte transfusions in very low birthweight infants. *Pediatrics, 95,* 1–8.

Sherwood, M. C., Lau, K. C., & Sholler, G. F. (1998). Adenosine in the management of supraventricular tachycardia in children. *Journal of Paediatrics and Child Health, 34*(1), 53–56.

Sheth, R. D., Buckley, D. J., Gutierrez, A. R., et al. (1996). Midazolam in the treatment of refractory neonatal seizures. *Clinical Neuropharmacology, 19*(2), 165–170.

Shorter, N. A., Liu, J. Y., Mooney, D. P., et al. (1999). Indomethacin-associated bowel perforations: A study of possible risk factors. *Journal of Pediatric Surgery, 34*(3), 442–444.

Sreenan, C., & Osiovich, H. (1999). Myeloid colony-stimulating factors: Use in the newborn. *Archives of Pediatrics and Adolescent Medicine, 153*(9), 984–988.

Subhani, M., Sridhar, S., & DeCristofaro, J. (2001). Phentolamine use in a neonate for the prevention of dermal necrosis caused by dopamine: A case report. *Journal of Perinatology, 21,* 324–326.

Tammela, O., Ojala, R., Iivainen, T., et al. (1999). Short versus prolonged indomethacin therapy for patent ductus arteriosus in preterm infants. *The Journal of Pediatrics, 134*(5), 552–557.

Thomson, A. H., Kerr, S., & Wright, S. (1996). Population pharmacokinetics of caffeine in neonates and young infants. *Therapeutic Drug Monitoring, 18*(3), 245–253.

Thureen, P. J., Reiter, P. D., Gresores, A., et al. (1999). Once- versus twice-daily gentamicin dosing in neonates 34 weeks' gestation: Cost-effectiveness analyses. *Pediatrics, 103*(3), 594–598.

Touati, G., Poggi-Travert, F., Ogier de Baulny, H., et al. (1998). Long-term treatment of persistent hyperinsulinaemic hypoglycaemia of infancy with diazoxide: A retrospective review of 77 cases and analysis of efficacy-predicting criteria. *European Journal of Pediatrics, 157*(8), 628–633.

van Lingen, R. A., Deinum, J. T., Quak, J. M., et al. (1999). Pharmacokinetics and metabolism of rectally administered paracetamol in preterm neonates. *Archives of Disease in Childhood—Fetal and Neonatal Edition, 80*(1), F59–F63.

Waisman, D., Weintraub, Z., Rotschild, A., et al. (1999). Myoclonic movements in very low birth weight premature infants associated with midazolam intravenous bolus administration. *Pediatrics, 104*(3 Pt 1), 579.

Walti, H., & Monset-Couchard, M. (1998). A risk-benefit assessment of natural and synthetic exogenous surfactants in the management of neonatal respiratory distress syndrome. *Drug Safety, 18*(5), 321–337.

Weindling, S. N., Saul, J. P., & Walsh, E. P. (1996). Efficacy and risks of medical therapy for supraventricular tachycardia in neonates and infants. *American Heart Journal, 131*(1), 66–72.

Williams, G. D., Bratton, S. L., Riley, E. C., et al. (1999). Efficacy of epsilon-aminocaproic acid in children undergoing cardiac surgery. *Journal of Cardiothoracic and Vascular Anesthesia, 13*(3), 304–308.

Yeung, M., Downe, L., & Coughtrey, H. (1999). Gentamicin doses and dose intervals in neonatal intensive care. [Letter]. *Journal of Paediatrics and Child Health, 35*(4), 411–412.

14

Drug Dosing for Infants, Children, and Adolescents

Louis A. Pagliaro and Ann Marie Pagliaro

Over twenty-five years ago when we began work on the first edition of this text, drug dosages for infants and children were usually determined by age and weight. Pediatric patients were often thought of as "small adults" and were dosed accordingly. Adolescents were generally considered to be "almost adult" and, thus, were generally given adult dosages usually based on the lowest recommended dosage. None of these dosing methods was ideal and calculations for infants and children that were based on body surface area (BSA) generally became preferred. This parameter, based on both height and weight, better reflected the physiologic changes that occurred during infancy and childhood, which, in turn, influence drug pharmacodynamics.

Although the science of clinical pharmacokinetics (see Chapter 10) evolved significantly during this period,[1] most new drugs approved by the FDA or HPB for pediatric use still did not have specific recommended dosages for infants, children, and adolescents. In fact, although the current expressed attitude and formal guidelines from the FDA demonstrate increasing concern with prescription drug use and testing among children and adolescents,[2] an overwhelming majority of new drugs currently released for use in Canada and the United States provide no specific pe-

---

1. For example, with the development of increasingly valid and reliable analytical methods over the past three decades, it is now possible to measure the concentration of many drugs in body fluids. Therapeutic drug monitoring (TDM) (Table 14-3) has increased the accuracy of pediatric dosing and has provided a means for individualizing optimal drug therapy for infants, children, and adolescents while minimizing adverse drug reactions (ADRs) and toxicity, particularly for pediatric patients who have cardiac, hepatic, or renal dysfunction (Table 14-2). However, TDM is only available for a limited number of drugs. Thus, in most cases, dosing decisions must be made in accordance with clinical experience and individual patient response. The importance of appropriately monitoring pediatric patients during all aspects of drug therapy (e.g., initiation, short term, long term, discontinuation, and for some drugs, for several months following the completion of a course of drug therapy) cannot be overemphasized.

2. In this regard, the 107th Congress of the United States enacted the "Best Pharmaceuticals for Children Act" on January 3, 2001. This act encourages "pediatric studies of drugs," established an "Office of Pediatric Therapeutics" within the FDA, facilitates the dissemination of pediatric drug information, and promulgated the use of a "toll-free number in labeling" to report observed ADRs occurring among pediatric patients.

diatric dosing or pharmacokinetic data in their official labeling.

Pediatric drug dosing is complicated by the continuous change in body weight, composition, and organ function as the infant, child, and adolescent grows and matures (see Chapters 10 and 11 for related discussion). These changes,[3] such as alterations in the relative weight and function of various organs and in fluid volumes and their maintenance, may significantly affect the absorption, distribution, metabolism, and elimination of various drugs and the likelihood of subtherapeutic response, adverse drug reactions (ADRs), and toxicity. Consequently, long-term pharmacotherapy (e.g., anticonvulsant drug therapy for the symptomatic management of seizure disorders) should be re-evaluated periodically. In addition, pediatric clinicians should be aware of, and be alert for, the possibility of ADRs peculiar to the pediatric patient, particularly those reactions that may adversely affect mental (e.g., cognition, learning, and memory impairment associated with sedative-hypnotic therapy and consequent impact on scholastic performance) and physical development (e.g., growth retardation associated with systemic corticosteroid pharmacotherapy; precocious puberty associated with androgen and anabolic steroid use) (see Chapter 5 for additional discussion and details).

Drug Dosages for Infants, Children, and Adolescents

In order to help pediatric clinicians provide optimal drug therapy for their patients, clinically important drug data have been analyzed and synthesized for presentation in Table 14-1, with attention to the indications for use of a particular drug; recommended dosages for infants, children, and adolescents; available dosage forms; and contraindications, ADRs, and comments, including other related clinical information and suggestions for therapeutic monitoring. These data were compiled from several sources including the previous edition of *Problems in Pediatric Drug Therapy*, recently published pediatric clinical research, official drug monographs, and more than 60 years of combined academic and clinical experience.

Some drugs listed in Table 14-1 are not officially approved by the FDA or HPB for pediatric use or, if approved, they are not indicated for the treatment of a particular listed condition for infants, children, and adolescents. Although not officially approved for pediatric use, many of these drugs have made important contributions to pediatric health and are, therefore, included in this table.[4] Pediatric clinicians should regard the use of these drugs with particular caution because widespread clinical experience may be limited. Thus, untoward ADRs or unreported drug interactions may occur. However, these drugs may also provide significant therapeutic benefit to the pediatric patient. Therefore, use is attendant with a requirement for a commensurate degree of careful attention to baseline assessment, prior to the initiation of pharmacotherapy, and monitoring during the course of pharmacotherapy, for both therapeutic and toxic effects.

Recommended dosages and routes of administration are provided in the "Usual Pediatric Dosage and Administration" column. The formulations available for pediatric patients and their storage and disposal are provided in the "Dosage Forms" column. For details regarding approaches and proper techniques for administering the various dosage forms to pediatric patients, see Chapter 1. In addition to Chapter 1, also see Chapter 8 for additional details regarding the intravenous administration of a particular drug (e.g., maximal rate of infusion, minimal concentration for infusion, and compatibility with intravenous solutions or other intravenous drugs). Contraindications, ADRs, and other clinical information are provided in the "Contraindications, ADRs, and Comments" column. For further information

---

3. These changes are relatively greatest during the neonatal period. Thus, neonatal dosing is discussed in its own separate chapter (see Chapter 13).

4. These drugs are clearly identified in the "Indications" column by the following, or similar, note: "Not approved by the FDA or HPB for infants, children, or adolescents."

regarding the ADRs and toxicity associated with a particular drug when used for pediatric patients, see Chapter 5. For further information regarding the management of pediatric poisoning and drug overdosages, see Chapter 4. For further information regarding drug interactions, see Chapter 6.

Although Table 14-1 is comprehensive,[5] providing drug data for more than 600 drugs, the antineoplastic drugs are not included in this table because of the wide variation in dosage protocols used for the treatment of pediatric cancers. Pediatric clinicians who require dosing information for antineoplastic drugs are referred to Chapter 12. In addition, vaccines and related drugs are generally discussed separately in Chapter 9. Neonatologists and others who are interested in drug dosing recommendations for neonates are referred to Chapter 13.

This chapter provides pediatric clinicians and students with accurate and authoritative data for the prescription and management of pediatric drug therapy[6] emphasizing current approved FDA and HPB guidelines when used alone as monopharmacotherapy or as adjunctive pharmacotherapy in combination with other drugs. However, as noted previously, "off-label" indications, when supported by both relevant pediatric clinical practice experience and experimental research data, also are included.

Each drug entry in Table 14-1 is clearly and concisely written to reflect only essential and important data that are commonly required by prescribing pediatric clinicians and others involved with the professional management of optimal drug therapy for infants, children, and adolescents. Drug entries are organized by generic name in alphabetical order.[7]

As previously noted, the drugs included in Table 14-1 are referred to by their USAN names. However, pediatric clinicians who use brand or trade names may access needed information by consulting the Index located at the end of this text. All of the dosages included in Table 14-1 are average dosages derived, using population-based statistical models, from data obtained from sample groups of research subjects (both healthy volunteers and patients) and are, therefore, approximate estimates. In all cases, variability in individual patient response may necessitate alterations in drug dose or frequency of dosing. Accepted guidelines for the use of each drug, including drug information centers, current manufacturer patient and product package inserts, or other authoritative references, should be consulted whenever there is further question about a particular use or dosage of a drug.[8] For detailed discussion of teratogenic and fetotoxic drugs, see Chapter 2, and for detailed discussion regarding drugs excreted in breast milk, see Chapter 3. Finally, for further information regarding abusable psychotropic drug use among children and adolescents, see Chapter 7.

It is hoped that the information presented in this chapter will better enable pediatric clinicians and students, as they strive to significantly improve drug therapy for their pediatric patients, to provide maximal pharmacotherapeutic benefits with minimal adverse and toxic effects.

---

5. Note that all drugs used in pediatric clinical practice are not included. However, every attempt has been made (with the input and assistance of the Pediatric Advisory Committee) to ensure that the major drugs of current clinical interest have been included. For information regarding drugs that have been used earlier to treat specific medical disorders and which are now seldom used, please refer to the previous editions of *Problems in Pediatric Drug Therapy*.

6. Because this is a specialized pediatric drug therapy text, drugs that are exclusively, or primarily, used for adult patients (e.g., drugs for the treatment of erectile dysfunction, Alzheimer's disease, Parkinson's disease) are not included.

7. The generic names used in this chapter (and, consistently, throughout this text) are those that have been officially designated by the United States Adopted Names (USAN) Council. International drug names, such as those used by the British Pharmacopeia (British Adopted Names [BAN]), are cross-referenced for convenience. Major brand/trade names for products available in Canada and the United States also are provided.

8. Readers have a professional responsibility to seek and obtain clarification whenever presented information seems unclear or incomplete.

TABLE 14-1
Recommended Drug Dosing for Infants, Children, and Adolescents

DRUG (TRADE AND OTHER NAMES)	INDICATION(S)	USUAL PEDIATRIC DOSAGE AND ADMINISTRATION[a]	DOSAGE FORMS	CONTRAINDICATIONS, ADRs, AND COMMENTS[b]
Abacavir (*Ziagen®*)	**HIV infection** (in combination with other antiretroviral pharmacotherapy) **Note:** Available data suggest that abacavir in combination with both lamivudine and zidovudine provides additional antiretroviral activity (reduced viral load). **Note:** Not approved by the FDA or HPB for children or adolescents. **Note:** Patients who are receiving abacavir may continue to develop opportunistic infections and other complications associated with HIV infection. Abacavir pharmacotherapy does not reduce the risk for HIV transmission to others.	**Children:** 8 mg/kg/day PO in two divided doses. *Maximum:* 600 mg/day PO. **Adolescents:** 600 mg/day PO in two divided doses.	Solutions, oral: 20 mg/ml (strawberry–banana flavored; contains saccharin sodium and sorbitol) Tablets, oral: 300 mg	**Contraindications:** Hypersensitivity to abacavir. Note that hypersensitivity reactions to abacavir reportedly occur more frequently among children (up to 5%) and may be fatal. A patient warning card summarizing the signs and symptoms of the hypersensitivity reaction associated with abacavir should be provided by the dispensing pharmacist to both the patient and the patient's parent or guardian. **ADRs:** Generally fairly well tolerated. Commonly causes nausea. May cause abdominal pain, anorexia, cough, diarrhea, fatigue, headache, insomnia, malaise, and vomiting. **Comments:** Patients should be advised that clinical experience with abacavir is limited and, thus, its long-term effects, both in terms of therapeutic efficacy and toxicity, are unknown.
Acetaminophen (*Abenol®, Atasol®,* Paracetamol, *Pediatrix®, Tempra®, Tylenol®*)	**Fever**	**Infants, children, and adolescents:** 40–90 mg/kg/day PO in four to six divided doses as indicated by response. *Maximum:* 90 mg/kg/day PO **or** 3 grams/day PO, whichever is less.	Caplets, oral: 160, 325, 500, 650 mg Capsules, oral: 325, 500 mg Capsules, oral sprinkle: 80, 160 mg Drops, oral (supplied with graduated dropper): 80 mg/ml (fruit and grape flavored) Elixirs, oral: 120, 160, 325 mg/5 ml (cherry and grape flavored) Solutions, oral: 50, 80, 100 mg/5 ml (berry and fruit flavored) Suppositories, rectal: 80, 120, 125, 300, 325, 650 mg Tablets, oral: 160, 325, 500, 650 mg Tablets, oral chewable: 80, 100 mg (bubble gum, grape, and fruit flavored) **Note:** Widely available in combination products.	**Contraindications:** Hypersensitivity to acetaminophen. **ADRs:** Generally well tolerated. Avoid acetaminophen pharmacotherapy for adolescents who chronically consume alcohol because of the increased risk for hepatotoxicity. *See* Chapter 5. **Comments:** To avoid unnecessary exposure to alcohol and associated gastric irritation, preferentially select alcohol-free oral dosage formulations. Note that most acetaminophen pediatric elixir products have been reformulated to be alcohol free.
	Pain	**Infants, children, and adolescents:** 40–60 mg/kg/day PO or rectal in four to six divided doses. *Maximum:* 65 mg/kg/day **or** 3 grams/day, whichever is less.		
Acetazolamide (*Diamox®*)	**Absence (petit mal) seizures** **Note:** For short-term use **only** because	**Children and adolescents:** 8–30 mg/kg/day PO in three or four divided doses.	Capsule, oral sustained release: 500 mg Injectable, IM, IV: 500 mg/vial	**Contraindications:** Adrenocortical insufficiency; cirrhosis; hyperchloremic acidosis; hypersensitivity to acetazolamide,

[a]Usual dosages recommended for infants, children, and adolescents are listed in this table. Individual infant, child, and adolescent dosage requirements may vary because of variability in maturity, genetics, organ function, and concomitant medical disorders and drug therapy. Thus, careful monitoring of drug serum concentrations and individual clinical response is imperative to ensure optimal drug therapy. For related information regarding pharmacokinetics and pharmacogenetics, *see* Chapters 10 and 11.

[b]For information on the initial dilution and compatibilities of IV drugs, *see* Chapter 8. For additional information regarding ADRs associated with specific drugs, *see* Chapter 5. For information regarding clinically significant drug interactions, *see* Chapter 6.

TABLE 14-1 continued

DRUG (TRADE AND OTHER NAMES)	INDICATION(S)	USUAL PEDIATRIC DOSAGE AND ADMINISTRATION[a]	DOSAGE FORMS	CONTRAINDICATIONS, ADRs, AND COMMENTS[b]
Acetazolamide *continued*	tolerance develops to the anticonvulsant actions of acetazolamide.		Tablets, oral: 125, 250 mg	sulfonamides, or thiazides; hypokalemia; hyponatremia; and marked hepatic or renal dysfunction. **ADRs:** May cause anorexia, dizziness, drowsiness, photosensitivity, or rash (including various forms of erythema multiforme). **Comments:** IV injection is preferred when injectable therapy is required. IM injection is painful.
	Drug-induced edema	**Children and adolescents:** 5 mg/kg/day PO or IV as a single morning dose every other day.		
	Glaucoma	**Children:** 15–30 mg/kg/day PO in three or four divided doses. *Maximum:* 1000 mg/day PO. **Adolescents:** 250–1000 mg/day PO. For dosages exceeding 250 mg/day, administer in four divided doses. **Note:** May be dosed twice daily if sustained-release capsules are used.		
Acetylcholine (Miochol-E®)	**Miosis of the iris** (generally in the context of cataract surgery, and only after delivery of the lens; iridectomy; or penetrating keratoplasty) **Note:** Not approved by the FDA or HPB for intraocular use in children or adolescents.	**Children:** Instill 0.5 ml into the anterior chamber of the affected eye(s). *Maximum:* 2 ml/dose. **Adolescents:** Instill 1–2 ml into the anterior chamber of the affected eye(s). **Note:** Sterile technique is required for opening and instilling the solution. In order to help to ensure the use of sterile products, any unused solution should be safely and appropriately discarded after use. DIRECTIONS FOR USE 1. Inspect the Univial in the unopened blister. Diluent must be in upper chamber. 2. Peel open the blister. 3. Aseptically transfer Univial to sterile field. Maintain sterility of outer container during preparation of the drug solution for intraocular administration. 4. Immediately before use, turn the plunger-stopper a quarter turn and press to force the diluent and center plug into the lower chamber. 5. Gently shake the Univial to dissolve the drug. 6. Using a dry sterile needle (18–20 gauge) and syringe, withdraw all of the drug solution from the Univial. **Prior to intraocular instillation of the acetylcholine solution, replace the needle with an appropriate atraumatic cannaulae for intraocular irrigation.** 7. After the drug has been instilled, appropriately discard the Univial and any unused drug solution.	Ophthalmic solution, two-chamber vial (Univial®): 10 mg/ml after reconstitution with diluent provided with product. *See* accompanying directions. **Note:** For intraocular use only. **Note:** Safely store Univial blister packages between 4 and 25°C. Do not freeze.	**Contraindications:** None identified. **ADRs:** Generally well tolerated. May cause corneal clouding, decompensation, or edema. If absorbed systemically, may cause bradycardia, breathing difficulty, flushing, hypotension, or sweating. **Comments:** Gas sterilization of the Univial may result in damage to the vial and resultant loss of sterility and, thus, should be avoided.
Acetylcysteine (N-Acetylcysteine, Mucomyst®, Parvolex®) **Note:** *See also* Chapter 4.	**Acetaminophen overdosage** **Note:** If possible, initiate within 24 hr following acetaminophen overdosage; most effective when administered within 8 hr of overdosage.	**Infants, children, and adolescents:** 150 mg/kg IV in 200 ml dextrose 5% in sterile water for injection over 15 min; follow with 50 mg/kg in 500 ml dextrose 5% in sterile water for injection over 4 hr; then follow with 100 mg/kg in 1000 ml dextrose 5% in sterile water for injection over the next 16 hr. **Alternatively, infants, children, and adolescents:** Initially, 140 mg/kg PO as loading dose. Follow with 17	Solution, injectable: 20% **Note:** To prepare solution for oral administration, dilute the 20% injectable solution with cola or another soft drink to yield a 5% solution. Oral solutions should be freshly prepared and administered within 1 hr of preparation.	**Contraindications:** None when used to treat acetaminophen overdosage. **ADRs:** May cause a generalized urticaria (rare). May also aggravate vomiting associated with acetaminophen overdosage.

(Continued)

Footnotes are on page 558.

TABLE 14-1 continued

DRUG (TRADE AND OTHER NAMES)	INDICATION(S)	USUAL PEDIATRIC DOSAGE AND ADMINISTRATION[a]	DOSAGE FORMS	CONTRAINDICATIONS, ADRs, AND COMMENTS[b]
Acetylcysteine *continued*		maintenance doses of 70 mg/kg PO at 4-hr intervals. **Note:** If oral loading dose or any oral maintenance dose is vomited within 1 hr of administration, repeat that dose.		
Acetylsalicylic Acid, *see* **Aspirin**				
Acyclovir (*Avirax*®, *Zovirax*®)	**Genital herpes simplex**	**Adolescents:** *Initial episode,* 1000 mg/day PO in five divided doses for 10 days. *Chronic suppressive pharmacotherapy,* 400–1000 mg/day PO in two to five divided doses **or** 800 mg/day PO in two divided doses. *Recurrence,* 1000 mg/day PO in five divided doses **or** 1600 mg/day PO in two divided doses. **Note:** Daily therapy may be required for up to 1 year. *Topical:* Apply ointment liberally to affected area(s) six times daily (approximately every 3 hr while awake) for 7 days. **Note:** Apply ointment with finger cot or glove to avoid cross-infection with herpes simplex virus.	Capsule, oral: 200 mg Injectables, IV: 500, 1000 mg/vial Ointment, topical: 5% Suspension, oral: 200 mg/5 ml; shake well before use. Tablets, oral: 200, 400, 800 mg **Note:** Oral doses may be administered with food to avoid associated nausea and vomiting. **Note:** The injectable solution contains no preservatives. Therefore, after opening, any unused solution should be appropriately and safely discarded.	**Contraindications:** Hypersensitivity to acyclovir. **ADRs:** May cause diarrhea, headache, malaise, nausea, and vomiting. IV acyclovir also is associated with encephalopathy, local irritation at infusion site, and renal tubular damage. *See* Chapter 5. **Comments:** Maintain adequate hydration.
	Genital herpes simplex among immunocompromised children and adolescents	**Children:** 30 mg/kg/day IV in three divided doses, every 8 hr, for 7 days. **Adolescents:** 15 mg/kg/day IV in three divided doses, every 8 hr, for 7 days.		
	Herpes simplex encephalitis	**Infants:** 30 mg/kg/day IV in three divided doses, every 8 hr, for 10 days. **Children:** 60 mg/kg/day IV in three divided doses, every 8 hr, for 10 days. **Adolescents:** 30 mg/kg/day IV in three divided doses, every 8 hr, for 10 days.		
	Herpes zoster	**Children (>2 years) and adolescents:** 3200 mg/day PO in six divided doses, every 4 hr, for 7–10 days.		
	Varicella zoster (chickenpox)	**Children (≥2 years and ≤40 kg):** 80 mg/kg/day PO in four divided doses, every 6 hr, for 5 days. **Children (>40 kg) and adolescents:** 3200 mg/day PO in four divided doses, every 6 hr, for 5 days. **Note:** Initiate within 24 hr of initial signs and symptoms of chickenpox.		
	Varicella zoster (chickenpox) among immunocompromised infants, children, and adolescents	**Infants:** 30 mg/kg/day IV in three divided doses, every 8 hr, for 7 days. **Children:** 60 mg/kg/day IV in three divided doses, every 8 hr, for 7 days.		

TABLE 14-1 *continued*

DRUG (*TRADE* AND OTHER NAMES)	INDICATION(S)	USUAL PEDIATRIC DOSAGE AND ADMINISTRATION[a]	DOSAGE FORMS	CONTRAINDICATIONS, ADRs, AND COMMENTS[b]
Acyclovir *continued*		**Adolescents:** 30 mg/kg/day IV in three divided doses, every 8 hr, for 7 days. **Note:** For IV use, infuse slowly IV over at least 1 hr to prevent precipitation in the renal tubules and kidney damage. Do **not** exceed infusion concentration of 10 mg/ml. Reduce dosage for pediatric patients who have renal dysfunction (*see* Table 14-2).		
Adenosine (*Adenocard®*)	**Supraventricular tachycardia** **Note:** Appropriate vagal maneuvers (e.g., valsalva maneuver) should be attempted **prior** to initiating adenosine. **Note:** Not approved by the FDA or HPB for use in infants or children.	**Children and adolescents:** Initial dose, 0.08 mg/kg/dose by rapid IV injection. If not effective within 1–2 min, increase dose to 0.15 mg/kg/dose. *Maximum:* 0.25 mg/kg/dose **or** 12 mg/dose, whichever is less. **Note:** Because of its short half-life of elimination (<10 sec), adenosine must be injected IV by rapid IV injection over 1–2 sec in order to ensure that it reaches its site of action in sufficient quantity to elicit the desired therapeutic effect.	Injectable, IV: 25 mg/ml **Note:** Also available as 3 mg/ml (in single-dose vials and prefilled syringes [supplied with a 22-gauge needle]). **Note:** Do not refrigerate because crystallization may occur.	**Contraindications:** Hypersensitivity to adenosine, and patients who do not have a functioning pacemaker and also have the following conditions: AV block (second and third degree); bradycardia (symptomatic); and sick sinus syndrome. **ADRs:** May cause bradycardia, bronchoconstriction, chest pain/pressure, dyspnea, facial flushing, headache, lightheadedness, and nausea. **Comments:** Adenosine pharmacotherapy should be accompanied by appropriate cardiac monitoring.

Adrenaline, *see* **Epinephrine**

Adrenocorticotropic Hormone, *see* **Corticotropin**

Albumin (normal human serum), *see* **Chapter 13**

Albuterol (*Proventil®, Salbutamol, Ventolin®, Volmax®*)	**Asthma** **Note:** When albuterol is used regularly, on a daily basis, concurrent corticosteroid pharmacotherapy is generally recommended.	**Note:** For children and adolescents, the albuterol dosage is usually determined by age, dosage form, and method of administration, as follows. **Children (≥4 years) and adolescents, powder for inhalation:** 200 or 400 µg/dose by inhalation device (e.g., Rotahaler®). Repeat every 4–6 hr as indicated by response. **Children (≥4 years) and adolescents, solution for inhalation by metered-dose inhaler:** 100 or 200 µg/dose by metered-dose inhaler. Repeat every 4–6 hr as indicated by response. **Children (≥2 years) and adolescents, solution for inhalation:** 0.1–0.3 mg/kg/dose by nebulizer. Repeat every 6–8 hr as indicated by response. **Note:** Each dose must be diluted with sterile normal saline to a total volume of 3 ml before administration by nebulizer. *Maximum:* 2.5 mg/dose of inhalation solution by nebulizer. **Children and adolescents, injectable:** 8 µg/kg/dose IM	Injectable, IM: 0.5 mg/ml Injectables, IV: 0.05, 1 mg/ml **Note:** The 1-mg/ml albuterol injectable is for IV infusion and requires dilution **before** administration. Powders, inhalation (capsules for use with inhalation device): 200, 400 µg (contains lactose) Solutions, inhalation: 1 mg/ml (0.1%), 5 mg/ml (0.5%) Solutions, inhalation (metered-dose inhaler): 90, 100 µg/actuation Solution, oral: 0.4 mg/ml Syrup, oral: 2 mg/5 ml (strawberry flavored) Tablets, oral: 2, 4 mg Tablets, oral extended release: 4, 8 mg **Note:** Albuterol oral formulations are **not** recommended for the treatment of acute or severe bronchospasms because of their slow onset of action.	**Contraindications:** Angina, hypersensitivity to albuterol, and tachydysrhythmias. **ADRs:** May cause metabolic changes including hyperglycemia and hypokalemia. *See* Chapter 5. **Comments:** Albuterol IV pharmacotherapy requires intensive care unit (ICU) monitoring. Use of inhaler attachments may significantly enhance drug delivery and pulmonary absorption (*see* Chapter 1).

(Continued)

Footnotes are on page 558.

TABLE 14-1 continued

DRUG (TRADE AND OTHER NAMES)	INDICATION(S)	USUAL PEDIATRIC DOSAGE AND ADMINISTRATION[a]	DOSAGE FORMS	CONTRAINDICATIONS, ADRs, AND COMMENTS[b]
Albuterol *continued*		every 4 hr as indicated by response **or** 4 μg/kg/dose IV over 5 min. Repeat IV dose after 15 min if required. *Maximum:* 500 μg/dose IM and 2000 μg/day IM; 250 μg/dose IV and 1000 μg/day IV. **Note:** Albuterol injectable pharmacotherapy for this indication is not approved by the HPB for children. **Children (≥6 years) and adolescents, oral tablets, solution, or syrup:** Initially, 6 or 8 mg/day PO, in three or four divided doses. *Maximum:* 24 mg/day PO. **Note:** When replacing nonextended-release oral formulations with the oral extended-release tablets, the same total oral daily dosage is used, but the dosing interval is twice daily, every 12 hr.		
Alcohol, *see* **Chapters 4 and 7**				
Alglucerase *(Ceredase®)*	Replacement pharmacotherapy in Gaucher's disease, types I, II, and III	**Children and adolescents:** Initially, 60 units/kg/dose IV by infusion over 1–2 hr. Subsequently, dosage must be individualized according to signs and symptoms and clinical response. Typically, doses are repeated once weekly to once monthly. **Note:** Prior to IV infusion, alglucerase injectable solution must be diluted with 0.9% sodium chloride for injection to a final volume of up to 200 ml. The use of an in-line particulate filter is recommended for IV infusion of alglucerase.	Solutions, IV: 50, 400 units/5 ml (contains 1% human albumin); do **not** shake. **Note:** Store refrigerated at 2–8°C. **Note:** Not generally available in Canada.	**Contraindications:** None identified. Hypersensitivity to alglucerase has generally been handled successfully by pretreatment with antihistamines and reducing the rate of IV infusion. **ADRs:** Generally well tolerated. May cause abdominal discomfort, chills, fever, nausea, and vomiting. **Comments:** Alglucerase is derived from pooled human placental tissue and contains low levels of chorionic gonadotropin. A case of precocious puberty has been associated with alglucerase and, thus, alglucerase should be used with caution among pediatric patients with androgen-dependent carcinomas (*see* Chorionic Gonadotropin).
Allopurinol *(Zyloprim®)*	Hyperuricemia	**Children and adolescents:** 10 mg/kg/day PO in three divided doses **or** 300 mg/m²/day PO in three divided doses, every 8 hr. *Maximum:* 600 mg/day PO. **Note:** Reduce dosage for pediatric patients who have renal dysfunction; *see* Table 14-2.	Tablets, oral: 100, 200, 300 mg	**Contraindications:** Hypersensitivity to allopurinol. **ADRs:** Generally well tolerated. May cause skin rashes, which may be followed by a severe, delayed hypersensitivity reaction. Thus, patients should be closely monitored for skin rashes. Some pediatric clinicians recommend the discontinuation of allopurinol at the first sign of a skin rash, as a preventative measure. **Comments:** Monitor serum and urine uric acid levels and adjust allopurinol pharmacotherapy accordingly.

TABLE 14-1 continued

DRUG (TRADE AND OTHER NAMES)	INDICATION(S)	USUAL PEDIATRIC DOSAGE AND ADMINISTRATION[a]	DOSAGE FORMS	CONTRAINDICATIONS, ADRs, AND COMMENTS[b]
Alprostadil, see Chapter 13				
Alteplase (*Cathflo Activase*®)	Restoration of function of central venous access devices (as assessed by the ability to withdraw blood from the device) **Note:** Not indicated for catheter dysfunction caused by nonthrombus factors (e.g., catheter misplacement or malposition, drug or nutritional precipitates within the catheter lumen, mechanical failure of the device).	**Children (≥2 years and ≥10–<30 kg):** Using a 1-mg/ml concentration of alteplase, instill 110% of the internal lumen volume of the catheter into the catheter. After 30 min, assess catheter function by attempting to withdraw blood. *If the catheter is functional:* Aspirate 4–5 ml of blood to remove alteplase and any residual clot; and then gently irrigate the catheter with normal saline. *If catheter is **not** functional:* Wait an additional 90 min and recheck for catheter function by attempting to withdraw blood. If function still has not been restored, instill one additional dose of alteplase into the catheter. *Maximum*: 2 mg/catheter instillation. **Children (≥30 kg) and adolescents:** Instill 2 mg (2 ml of reconstituted alteplase solution) into the occluded catheter. After 30 min, assess catheter function by attempting to withdraw blood. *If the catheter is functional:* Aspirate 4–5 ml of blood to remove alteplase and any residual clot; and then gently irrigate the catheter with normal saline. *If catheter is **not** functional:* Wait an additional 90 min and recheck for catheter function by attempting to withdraw blood. If function still has not been restored, instill one additional dose of alteplase into the catheter. *Maximum*: 2 mg/intracatheter instillation.	Powder for reconstitution, for intracatheter instillation: 2 mg/vial **Note:** Store refrigerated at 2–8°C (36–46°F). **Note:** Reconstitute immediately before use with 2.2 ml of sterile water for injection (**without** preservatives) to yield 1 mg/ml. Gently swirl vial to dissolve powder; do **not** shake. **Note:** Not generally available in Canada for this indication.	**Contraindications:** Hypersensitivity to alteplase. **ADRs:** May cause GI bleeding, sepsis, and venous thrombosis.
Aluminum Hydroxide (*Alu-Cap*®, *Alu-Tab*®, *Amphojel*®)	Gastric hyperacidity	**Infants, children, and adolescents:** 40 mg/kg/dose PO after meals and 30 min before bedtime. *Maximum:* 1500 mg/dose PO.	Capsules, oral: 400, 500 mg Suspensions, oral: 320 mg/5 ml (flavorless), 450 mg/5 ml (peppermint flavored), 600 mg/5 ml (flavorless), 675 mg/5 ml (creamsicle flavored); shake well before use. Tablets, oral: 300, 500, 600 mg	**Contraindications:** None identified. **ADRs:** Generally well tolerated. May cause constipation. See Chapter 5. **Comments:** High-dosage aluminum hydroxide pharmacotherapy has been associated with a worsening of dialysis osteomalacia among patients undergoing renal dialysis.
	Hyperphosphatemia	**Children and adolescents:** 50–150 mg/kg/day PO in four divided doses, every 6 hr.		
Amantadine (*Symmetrel*®)	Viral infection	**Children (1–9 years):** 5 mg/kg/day PO as a single dose or as two divided doses. *Maximum:* 150 mg/day PO. **Children (>9 years) and adolescents:** 200 mg/day PO as a single dose or as two divided doses.	Capsule, oral: 100 mg Syrup, oral: 50 mg/5 ml (raspberry flavored)	**Contraindications:** Hypersensitivity to amantadine. **ADRs:** *See* Chapter 5. **Comments:** Continue prophylactic amantadine pharmacotherapy for at least 10 days following exposure; continue for 2 days after resolution of signs and symptoms.

(Continued)

Footnotes are on page 558.

TABLE 14-1 continued

DRUG (TRADE AND OTHER NAMES)	INDICATION(S)	USUAL PEDIATRIC DOSAGE AND ADMINISTRATION[a]	DOSAGE FORMS	CONTRAINDICATIONS, ADRs, AND COMMENTS[b]
Amantadine *continued*		**Note:** Dividing the daily dosage may reduce associated CNS ADRs. **Note:** Reduce dosage for pediatric patients who have renal dysfunction; see Table 14-2.		
Amethopterin, *see* **Methotrexate**				
Amifostine, *see* **Chapter 12**				
Amikacin *(Amikin®)*	Gram-negative bacterial infections **Note:** Ensure that appropriate culture and sensitivity tests have been performed and that the organism is sensitive to amikacin. **Note:** Short-term therapy (≤14 days) is generally recommended in order to minimize possible drug accumulation and resultant toxicity.	**Infants, children, and adolescents:** 15 mg/kg/day IM or IV in three divided doses, every 8 hr. *Maximum:* 1.5 grams/day IM or IV. **Note:** Reduce dosage for pediatric patients who have renal dysfunction; see Table 14-2.	Injectables, IM, IV: 50 (pediatric), 250 mg/ml **Note:** Amikacin injectables contain sodium bisulfite or sodium metabisulfite. Sulfites may cause hypersensitivity reactions among susceptible patients, particularly those who have a history of asthma. These reactions include life-threatening anaphylaxis and less severe asthmatic episodes.	**Contraindications:** Hypersensitivity to amikacin or to other aminoglycosides. **ADRs:** May cause ototoxicity (high-frequency hearing loss) or nephrotoxicity, particularly with high dosages, prolonged use, and renal dysfunction. *See* Chapter 5. **Comments:** Monitor renal function. Therapeutic drug monitoring is recommended; see Table 14-3.
Aminocaproic Acid *(Amicar®)*	Potentially life-threatening hemorrhage resulting from an overactivity of the fibrinolytic system	**Adolescents:** Initially, 5 grams by IV infusion or PO; then 1-gram doses at hourly intervals to achieve and maintain plasma levels of 0.13 mg/ml (concentration generally required for the inhibition of fibrinolysis). *Maximum:* 30 grams/24 hr. **Note:** Rapid IV infusion may result in bradycardia or hypotension and, thus, should be avoided.	Injectable, IV: 250 mg/ml (contains benzyl alcohol as a preservative) Syrup, oral: 250 mg/ml (raspberry flavored, contains sorbitol) Tablet, oral: 500 mg	**Contraindications:** Active intravascular clotting, disseminated intravascular coagulation (DIC), and hematuria of upper urinary tract origin. **ADRs:** Generally well tolerated. May cause cramps, diarrhea, dizziness, headache, malaise, myopathy, nasal stuffiness, skin rash, and tinnitus. **Comments:** Use should be accompanied by tests designed to determine the amount of fibrinolysis present. Therapeutic drug monitoring is recommended; see Table 14-3.
	Subarachnoid hemorrhage	**Adolescents:** 36 grams/day by continuous IV infusion. **Note:** Generally administered as 18 grams in 400 ml of 5% dextrose and water for injection every 12 hr for 10 days. Then replace with oral aminocaproic acid pharmacotherapy (3 grams every 2 hr) until surgery is performed. If surgery is not performed within 21 days, dosage should be reduced over the following week and then discontinued (2 grams every 2 hr for 3 days, followed by 1 gram every 2 hr for 3 days, and then discontinued). **Note:** Reduce dosage for pediatric patients who have renal dysfunction; see Table 14-2.		

Aminophylline (Theophylline Ethylenediamine), *see* **Theophylline**

5-Aminosalicylic Acid, *see* **Mesalamine**

TABLE 14-1 continued

DRUG (TRADE AND OTHER NAMES)	INDICATION(S)	USUAL PEDIATRIC DOSAGE AND ADMINISTRATION[a]	DOSAGE FORMS	CONTRAINDICATIONS, ADRs, AND COMMENTS[b]
Amiodarone (Cordarone®, Pacerone®)	**Ventricular dysrhythmias,** potentially life threatening (ventricular fibrillation and recurrent, unstable ventricular tachycardia) **Note:** Because of its extreme potential for toxicity, amiodarone pharmacotherapy should be reserved for those patients who are refractory to other less toxic antidysrhythmics. Pediatric patients should be hospitalized and closely observed until the cardiac dysrhythmia is corrected. **Note:** Not approved by the FDA or HPB for children.	**Children and adolescents:** Initially, 10–20 mg/kg/day PO as a single daily dose or as two divided doses, every 12 hr, for 1–2 weeks, until initial therapeutic response is achieved. Then, 3–5 mg/kg/day PO as a single daily dose for several weeks. **Note: Avoid** administration with grapefruit juice; grapefruit juice can significantly increase amiodarone serum concentrations.	Tablet, oral: 200 mg	**Contraindications:** Hypersensitivity to amiodarone, AV block (second or third degree), and sinus bradycardia (marked). **ADRs:** Amiodarone is highly toxic and has been associated with ADRs affecting several major body organ systems. The most severe and potentially fatal reactions include dysrhythmogenic reactions (heart block, ventricular fibrillation), hepatitis, and interstitial pneumonitis, which is fatal in approximately 10% of patients. *See* Chapter 5. **Comments:** Amiodarone and its active metabolite have a long half-life of elimination (1–2 months). Amiodarone's long half-life of elimination contributes to its involvement in drug interactions. Amiodarone can inhibit the production of cytochrome P-450 drug-metabolizing enzymes and, consequently, significantly increase the therapeutic and toxic effects of a number of different drugs (*see* Chapter 6). Therapeutic drug monitoring is recommended; *see* Table 14-3. Monitor thyroid function. Monitor hepatic function upon initiation of therapy and at regular intervals, particularly with high maintenance dosages. **Note:** Plasticizers (e.g., di-[2-ethylhexyl]phthalate [DEHP]) reportedly can leach out of IV tubing when amiodarone is administered intravenously. Concerns have been raised regarding DEHP exposure risk for adverse effects on male reproductive tract development during fetal development or among neonates, infants, and children ≤3 years of age.
Amitriptyline (Elavil®)	**Depression,** particularly endogenous depression **Note:** The sedative action has been found to be of benefit for depressed patients who also exhibit signs and symptoms of anxiety.	**Adolescents:** Initially, 50–75 mg/day PO in two or three divided doses. *Maximum:* 150 mg/day PO. *Maintenance:* Use the lowest effective dose. Many adolescents can be maintained with once daily dosing at bedtime for convenience and to improve compliance. Bedtime dosing also takes advantage of amitriptyline's sedative effects, which otherwise may result in daytime drowsiness.	Tablets, oral: 10, 25, 50, 75 mg	**Contraindications:** Acute congestive heart failure, acute recovery phase following myocardial infarction, MAOI pharmacotherapy (concurrent or within 14 days), hypersensitivity to amitriptyline or to other tricyclic antidepressants, and narrow-angle glaucoma. **ADRs:** May cause a variety of ADRs affecting several major body systems including anticholinergic effects (e.g., blurred vision, confusion, constipation, drowsiness, dry mouth, mydriasis, and urinary retention), bone marrow *(Continued)*

Footnotes are on page 558.

TABLE 14-1 *continued*

DRUG (*TRADE* AND OTHER NAMES)	INDICATION(S)	USUAL PEDIATRIC DOSAGE AND ADMINISTRATION[a]	DOSAGE FORMS	CONTRAINDICATIONS, ADRs, AND COMMENTS[b]
Amitriptyline *continued*				suppression (including agranulocytosis and thrombocytopenia), quinidinelike effects on the cardiovascular system, and behavioral effects (including agitation, anxiety, hallucinations, insomnia, nightmares, and restlessness). The anticholinergic effects are the most commonly encountered and can be largely controlled or mitigated by dosing the entire daily dosage as a single bedtime dose (when warranted by the clinical condition of the patient). **Comments:** Amitriptyline use can precipitate seizures and it should, therefore, be used with particular caution and careful monitoring among patients who have a history of seizure disorder. **Note:** All depressed patients should be evaluated for suicide risk and any risk should be appropriately dealt with.
Ammonium Chloride	Urinary acidification	**Children and adolescents:** 30 mg/kg/dose PO every 4–6 hr. *Maximum:* 6 grams/day PO. **Note:** Monitor urinary pH and adjust dosage as necessary according to response.	Tablet, oral: 500 mg Tablet, oral enteric coated: 500 mg **Note:** 75 mEq = 4 grams	**Contraindications:** Severe hepatic or renal dysfunction. **ADRs:** Generally well tolerated. May cause metabolic acidosis, particularly with overdosage. May cause gastric irritation, nausea, and vomiting. **Comments:** Monitor urinary pH.
Amoxicillin (*Amoxil®, Trimox®, Wymox®*)	Bacterial infection **Note:** Ensure that appropriate culture and sensitivity tests are performed and that the organism is sensitive to amoxicillin.	**Infants (≥3 months), children, and adolescents:** 20–40 mg/kg/day PO in three divided doses, every 8 hr. *Maximum:* 2 grams/day PO.	Capsules, oral: 250, 500 mg Drops, oral: 50 mg/ml (bubble gum flavored) Suspensions, oral (powder for reconstitution): 125, 250 mg/5 ml (after reconstitution) (bubble gum or strawberry flavored); shake well before use. Tablets, oral: 500, 875 mg Tablets, oral chewable: 125, 250 mg (cherry flavored)	**Contraindications:** Hypersensitivity to amoxicillin or to other penicillins. **ADRs:** *See* Chapter 5. **Comments:** Amoxicillin pharmacotherapy generally is associated with significantly less diarrhea than ampicillin pharmacotherapy.
	Gonorrhea **Note:** Probenecid is often used adjunctively with amoxicillin pharmacotherapy to decrease the renal elimination of amoxicillin and to promote its therapeutic effect (*see* Probenecid).	**Children (>2 years):** 50 mg/kg PO as a single dose (as adjunctive pharmacotherapy with probenecid, 25 mg/kg). *Maximum:* 2 grams/dose PO. **Adolescents:** 3 grams PO as a single dose. **Note:** Reduce dosage for pediatric patients who have renal dysfunction; see Table 14-2.		
Amoxicillin (A) and Potassium Clavulanate (PC) (*Augmentin®, Clavulin®*)	Bacterial infection/ Otitis media **Note:** Ensure that appropriate culture and sensitivity tests are performed and that the organism is sensitive to amoxicillin and potassium clavulanate.	**Infants (<3 months):** Amoxicillin 30 mg/kg/day PO in two divided doses, every 12 hr. **Infants (≥3 months), children, and adolescents:** Amoxicillin 20–40 mg/kg/day PO in three divided doses, every 8 hr. *Maximum:* Amoxicillin, 1.5 grams/day PO.	Suspension, oral (amounts of amoxicillin, clavulanic acid, and potassium per 5 ml after reconstitution follow) Tablets, oral (amounts of amoxicillin, clavulanic acid, and potassium per oral tablet follow)	**Contraindications:** Hypersensitivity to amoxicillin or to other penicillins, infectious mononucleosis, and previous history of drug-related jaundice or hepatic dysfunction. **ADRs:** *See* "Amoxicillin" in Chapter 5. **Comments:** Consider alternative pharmacotherapy for patients who

CHAPTER 14: DRUG DOSING FOR INFANTS, CHILDREN, AND ADOLESCENTS

TABLE 14-1 continued

DRUG (TRADE AND OTHER NAMES)	INDICATION(S)	USUAL PEDIATRIC DOSAGE AND ADMINISTRATION[a]	DOSAGE FORMS	CONTRAINDICATIONS, ADRs, AND COMMENTS[b]
Amoxicillin (A) and Potassium Clavulanate (PC) *continued*		**Note:** Use of a slightly higher total daily dosage (25–45 mg/kg/day PO) in two divided doses, every 12 hr, has been recommended for those pediatric patients for whom diarrhea has been a troublesome ADR. **Note:** Reduce dosage for pediatric patients who have hepatic or renal (see Table 14-2) dysfunction. **Note:** Administration with food increases GI absorption and decreases associated GI ADRs.	Tablets, oral chewable (amounts of amoxicillin, clavulanic acid, and potassium per oral chewable tablet follow) **Note:** *Augmentin* chewable tablets and oral suspension contain saccharin. Shake oral suspension well before use.	have a glomerular filtration rate <35 ml/min/1.73 m² because of differential effect of renal failure on amoxicillin and potassium clavulanate elimination. **Note:** Duration of therapy for active otitis media is generally recommended to be 10 days.

Suspension, oral

AMOXICILLIN (mg)	CLAVULANIC ACID (mg)	POTASSIUM (mEq)	
125	31.25	0.16	(banana flavored)
200	28.5	0.14	(orange–raspberry flavored)
250	62.5	0.32	(orange flavored)
400	57	0.29	(orange–raspberry flavored)

Tablets, oral

AMOXICILLIN (mg)	CLAVULANIC ACID (mg)	POTASSIUM (mEq)
250	125	0.63
500	125	0.63
875	125	0.63

Tablets, oral chewable

AMOXICILLIN (mg)	CLAVULANIC ACID (mg)	POTASSIUM (mEq)	
125	31.25	0.16	(lemon–lime flavored)
200	28.5	0.14	(cherry–banana flavored)
250	62.5	0.32	(lemon–lime flavored)
400	57	0.29	(cherry–banana flavored)

DRUG	INDICATION(S)	USUAL PEDIATRIC DOSAGE AND ADMINISTRATION	DOSAGE FORMS	CONTRAINDICATIONS, ADRs, AND COMMENTS
Amphetamines, mixed *(Adderall®)*	**Attention-deficit/ hyperactivity disorder** (A-D/HD) **Note:** When clinically feasible, occasionally interrupt therapy in order to determine continued need. **Narcolepsy** **Note:** Narcolepsy seldom occurs among children.	**Children (3–5 years):** Initially, 2.5 mg/day PO as a single morning dose. Increase the daily dosage at weekly intervals by 2.5 mg, according to response. Larger maintenance dosages may be administered daily as two divided doses (upon awakening in the morning and 4–6 hr later). **Children (≥6 years):** Initially, 5 mg/day PO as a single morning dose. Increase the daily dosage at weekly intervals by 5 mg, according to response. Larger maintenance doses may be administered daily as two divided doses (upon awakening in the morning and 4–6 hr later). **Note:** Oral, extended-release formulations are administered as a single morning dose. **Children (≥6 years):** Initially, 5 mg/day PO as a single morning dose. Increase the daily dosage at weekly intervals by 5 mg, according to response.	Tablets, oral: 5, 10, 20, 30 mg (see following for composition). Capsules, oral, extended release *(Adderall XR®)*: 10, 20, 30 mg	**Contraindications:** Agitation, amphetamine or other abusable psychotropic abuse (history of), hypertension, hyperthyroidism, hypersensitivity to amphetamines, psychosis, and MAOI therapy (concurrent or within 14 days). **ADRs:** May cause anorexia, constipation, dizziness, diarrhea, dysphoria, dry mouth, euphoria, exacerbation of motor and phonic tics, exacerbation of Tourette's syndrome, hypertension, insomnia, psychosis (rare), restlessness, tachycardia, and weight loss. **Comments:** Amphetamines have a high abuse potential and are capable of producing both addiction and habituation. **Note:** Mixed amphetamines pharmacotherapy generally is of most therapeutic benefit for the treatment of A-D/HD when used in combination with appropriate educational, family, and psychological interventions. *(Continued)*

Footnotes are on page 558.

TABLE 14-1 continued

DRUG (*TRADE* AND OTHER NAMES)	INDICATION(S)	USUAL PEDIATRIC DOSAGE AND ADMINISTRATION[a]	DOSAGE FORMS	CONTRAINDICATIONS, ADRs, AND COMMENTS[b]
Amphetamines, mixed *continued*		Larger maintenance dosages may be administered daily in two or three divided doses (upon awakening in the morning and 4–6 hr later). **Adolescents:** Initially, 10 mg/day PO as a single morning dose. Increase the daily dosage at weekly intervals by 10 mg, according to response. Larger maintenance dosages may be administered daily in two or three divided doses (upon awakening in the morning and 4–6 hr later). **Note:** Avoid late evening doses because of associated insomnia.		

EACH *ADDERALL* TABLET CONTAINS	5 mg	10 mg	20 mg	30 mg
amphetamine aspartate	1.25 mg	2.5 mg	5 mg	7.5 mg
amphetamine sulfate	1.25 mg	2.5 mg	5 mg	7.5 mg
dextroamphetamine saccharate	1.25 mg	2.5 mg	5 mg	7.5 mg
dextroamphetamine sulfate	1.25 mg	2.5 mg	5 mg	7.5 mg
Total amphetamine base equivalence	3.13 mg	6.3 mg	12.6 mg	18.8 mg

DRUG (*TRADE* AND OTHER NAMES)	INDICATION(S)	USUAL PEDIATRIC DOSAGE AND ADMINISTRATION[a]	DOSAGE FORMS	CONTRAINDICATIONS, ADRs, AND COMMENTS[b]
Amphotericin B *(Fungizone®)* **Note:** *See also* Amphotericin B Liposome.	Systemic fungal infections **Note:** Amphotericin B pharmacotherapy commonly is associated with severe toxicity. Thus, its use is generally reserved for hospitalized patients with disseminated fungal (mycotic) infections that are progressive and potentially fatal or that are refractory to less toxic pharmacotherapy. **Note:** Ensure that appropriate culture and sensitivity tests are performed and that the organism is sensitive to amphotericin B. **Note:** Not approved by the FDA or HPB for infants or children.	**Infants, children, and adolescents:** Initially, 0.25 mg/kg/day by slow IV infusion over 6 hr. Increase dosage, as indicated by response, to a maximum of 1 mg/kg/day **or,** if dosed on alternate days (every other day), then to a maximum of 1.5 mg/kg/dose.	Injectable, IV (powder for reconstitution): 50 mg/vial **Note:** Dilute amphotericin B injectable with nonbacteriostatic sterile water for injection to 0.1 mg/ml prior to administration.	**Contraindications:** Hypersensitivity to amphotericin B. **ADRs:** May cause anemia (reversible), anorexia, diarrhea, fever, headache, hypokalemia, nausea, pain (generalized), renal dysfunction, thrombophlebitis, and vomiting during infusion. *See* Chapter 5.
Amphotericin B Liposome *(AmBisome®)* **Note:** *See also* Amphotericin B.	Systemic fungal infections: *Aspergillus, Candida,* and *Cryptococcus* Visceral leishmaniasis	**Infants, children, and adolescents:** 3–5 mg/kg/day by slow IV infusion over 120 min. **Note:** An IV infusion control device should be used for administration. Do not use an in-line filter. **Infants, children, and adolescents, immunocompromised:** 4 mg/kg/dose by slow IV infusion over 120 min. Administer doses on days 1, 2, 3, 4, 5, 10, 17, 24, 31, and 38.	Injectable, IV (powder for reconstitution): 50 mg/vial after reconstitution with sterile water for injection. **Note:** For IV use only. Do not reconstitute with saline solutions or admix with other drugs.	**Contraindications:** Hypersensitivity to amphotericin B. **ADRs:** The ADR profile for amphotericin B liposome is similar to that for amphotericin B, except for a significantly reduced incidence. *See* Chapter 5.

CHAPTER 14: DRUG DOSING FOR INFANTS, CHILDREN, AND ADOLESCENTS

TABLE 14-1 continued

DRUG (TRADE AND OTHER NAMES)	INDICATION(S)	USUAL PEDIATRIC DOSAGE AND ADMINISTRATION[a]	DOSAGE FORMS	CONTRAINDICATIONS, ADRs, AND COMMENTS[b]
Amphotericin B Liposome *continued*		**Infants, children, and adolescents, nonimmunocompromised:** 3 mg/kg/dose by slow IV infusion over 120 min. Administer doses on days 1, 2, 3, 4, 5, 14, and 21. May repeat the course of amphotericin B liposome pharmacotherapy, if required.		
Ampicillin (Omnipen®, Principen®, Totacillin®)	**Bacterial meningitis** (generally due to *Haemophilus influenzae, Neisseria meningitidis,* or *Streptococcus pneumoniae*) **Note:** Ensure that appropriate culture and sensitivity tests are performed and that the organism is sensitive to ampicillin.	**Children and adolescents:** 200–300 mg/kg/day IV in six divided doses, every 4 hr. *Maximum:* 12 grams/day IV. **Note:** Reduce dosage for pediatric patients who have renal dysfunction; *see* Table 14-2.	Capsules, oral: 250, 500 mg Drops, oral: 100 mg/ml Injectables, IM, IV: 125, 250, 500 mg/vial; 1, 2 grams/vial; contain 3 mEq of sodium per gram of ampicillin. Suspensions, oral (powder for reconstitution): 125, 250 mg, 500 mg/5 ml (after reconstitution); shake well before use.	**Contraindications:** Hypersensitivity to ampicillin, to other penicillins, or to cephalosporins. **ADRs:** *See* Chapter 5. **Comments:** Monitor pediatric patients for diarrhea and treat appropriately.
	Bacterial infections, other than meningitis infections **Note:** Ensure that appropriate culture and sensitivity tests are performed and that the organism is sensitive to ampicillin.	**Children and adolescents:** 50–100 mg/kg/day IM, IV, or PO in six divided doses, every 4 hr. *Maximum:* 3 grams/day PO. **Note:** Reduce dosage for pediatric patients who have renal dysfunction; *see* Table 14-2.		
	Bacterial endocarditis, prophylaxis for patients at moderate risk or for whom ampicillin oral pharmacotherapy is not feasible.	**Children and adolescents:** 50 mg/kg IM or IV as a single dose 30 min prior to procedure (e.g., dental surgery). *Maximum:* 20 grams/dose IM or IV.		
Amprenavir, oral capsules (Agenerase® Oral Capsules) **Note:** Amprenavir is formulated for use as oral capsules and oral solution. These two formulations differ significantly in relation to both dosage and toxicity and are **not** interchangeable on a milligram-per-milligram basis. **Note:** *See also* Amprenavir, oral solution.	**HIV-1 infection,** in combination with other antiretroviral drugs **Note:** Data regarding efficacy and toxicity of long-term amprenavir pharmacotherapy are not available. **Note:** Patients who are receiving amprenavir pharmacotherapy may continue to develop opportunistic infections and other complications associated with HIV infection. Amprenavir pharmacotherapy does not reduce the risk for HIV transmission to others.	**Children (≥4 years) and adolescents (13–16 years and <50 kg):** *Oral capsules,* 40 mg/kg/day PO in two divided doses **or** 45 mg/kg/day PO in three divided doses. *Maximum, Oral capsules:* 2400 mg/day PO. **Adolescents (13–16 years and ≥50 kg or >16 years):** *Oral capsules,* 2400 mg/day PO in two divided doses. **Note:** Administration with a high fat meal may decrease GI absorption. **Note:** The amprenavir dosage may require reduction for pediatric patients who have renal dysfunction.	Capsules, oral: 50, 150 mg; contain small amounts of propylene glycol (19 and 57 mg, respectively). **Note:** Amprenavir oral capsules are formulated with a large amount of vitamin E (109 international units of vitamin E/capsule). Thus, vitamin E supplementation is usually unnecessary.	**Contraindications:** Hypersensitivity to amprenavir or to the sulfonamides and concurrent pharmacotherapy with any of the following drugs: amiodarone, bepridil, diazepam, dihydroergotamine, disulfiram, ergotamine, flurazepam, lidocaine, lovastatin, metronidazole, midazolam, pimozide, quinidine, rifampin, sildenafil, simvastatin, triazolam, and tricyclic antidepressants. **ADRs:** May cause abdominal pain, diarrhea, nausea, paresthesias, rash, and vomiting. **Note:** Amprenavir associated rash is generally delayed in onset (mean onset is 10 days), maculopapular, mild to moderate, and sometimes accompanied by pruritus. In ~4% of patients who developed a rash, the rash progressed into severe, life-threatening reactions (e.g., Stevens-Johnson syndrome). *(Continued)*

Footnotes are on page 558.

TABLE 14-1 continued

DRUG (TRADE AND OTHER NAMES)	INDICATION(S)	USUAL PEDIATRIC DOSAGE AND ADMINISTRATION[a]	DOSAGE FORMS	CONTRAINDICATIONS, ADRs, AND COMMENTS[b]
Amprenavir, oral capsules *continued*				**Comments:** The clinical use of protease inhibitors such as amprenavir has been associated with spontaneous bleeding among patients who had hemophilia, redistribution of body fat among some patients and a "cushingoid" appearance, and possible development of resistance or cross-resistance to the various protease inhibitors.
Amprenavir, oral solution *(Agenerase® Oral Solution)* **Note:** Amprenavir is formulated for use as oral capsules and oral solution. These two formulations differ significantly in relation to both dosage and toxicity and are **not** interchangeable on a milligram-per-milligram basis. **Note:** See also Amprenavir, oral capsules.	HIV-1 infection, in combination with other antiretroviral drugs **Note:** Data regarding efficacy and toxicity of long-term amprenavir pharmacotherapy are not available. **Note:** Patients who are receiving amprenavir pharmacotherapy may continue to develop opportunistic infections and other complications associated with HIV infection. Amprenavir pharmacotherapy does not reduce the risk for HIV transmission to others.	**Children (≥4 years) and adolescents (13–16 years and <50 kg):** *Oral solution*, 45 mg/kg/day PO in two divided doses **or** 51 mg/kg/day PO in three divided doses. *Maximum, Oral solution:* 2800 mg/day PO. **Adolescents (13–16 years and ≥50 kg or >16 years):** *Oral solution*, 2800 mg/day PO in two divided doses. **Note:** Administration with a high fat meal may decrease GI absorption. **Note:** The amprenavir dosage may require reduction for pediatric patients who have hepatic dysfunction.	Solution, oral: 15 mg/ml (grape bubble gum–peppermint flavored); store at controlled room temperature (25°C [77°F]). **Note:** The oral solution contains saccharin sodium. It also contains a large amount of propylene glycol (550 mg/ml) and is, thus, **contraindicated** for infants and children younger than 4 years. **Note:** Amprenavir is formulated with a large amount of vitamin E (6 international units of vitamin E/ml of oral amprenavir solution). Thus, vitamin E supplementation is usually unnecessary.	**Contraindications:** Hypersensitivity to amprenavir or to the sulfonamides and concurrent pharmacotherapy with any of the following drugs: amiodarone, bepridil, diazepam, dihydroergotamine, disulfiram, ergotamine, flurazepam, lidocaine, lovastatin, midazolam, metronidazole, pimozide, quinidine, rifampin, sildenafil, simvastatin, triazolam, and tricyclic antidepressants. In addition, amprenavir oral solution is contraindicated for infants and children younger than 4 years and those who have hepatic or renal failure. **ADRs:** May cause abdominal pain, diarrhea, nausea, paresthesias, rash, and vomiting. **Note:** Amprenavir-associated rash is generally delayed in onset (mean onset is 10 days), maculopapular, mild to moderate, and sometimes accompanied by pruritus. In ~4% of patients who developed a rash, the rash progressed into severe, life-threatening reactions (e.g., Stevens-Johnson syndrome). **Comments:** The clinical use of protease inhibitors such as amprenavir has been associated with spontaneous bleeding among patients who had hemophilia, redistribution of body fat among some patients and a "cushingoid" appearance, and possible development of resistance or cross-resistance to the various protease inhibitors.
Amyl Nitrite, *see* **Chapter 4**				
Anethol-trithion *(Anethole Trithione, Sialor®)*	Xerostomia, drug induced	**Adolescents:** 50 mg/day PO in two divided doses, morning and evening. Dosage may be increased after 7 days, if indicated, to 75 mg/day PO in three divided doses before meals. *Maximum:* 75 mg/day PO. **Note:** Reduce dosage for pediatric patients who have severe renal dysfunction.	Tablet, oral: 25 mg **Note:** Not generally available in the United States.	**Contraindications:** Bile duct obstruction, biliary tract obstruction, cirrhosis, hypersensitivity to anetholtrithion, and jaundice. **ADRs:** Generally well tolerated. May cause soft stools and impart a yellow color to the urine.

TABLE 14-1 continued

DRUG (TRADE AND OTHER NAMES)	INDICATION(S)	USUAL PEDIATRIC DOSAGE AND ADMINISTRATION[a]	DOSAGE FORMS	CONTRAINDICATIONS, ADRs, AND COMMENTS[b]
Antihemophilic Factor VIII (Recombinant) (Kogenate®, Recombinate®)	Hemophilia A, prophylaxis or management of bleeding episode	**Infants, children, and adolescents:** 10–50 international units/kg IV according to need and response. **Alternatively,** the following formula may be used to determine appropriate dosage: $$\text{Dosage required (international units)} = \frac{\text{body weight (kg)} \times \text{desired \% factor VIII increase}}{(2\%/\text{international units/kg})}$$	Injectable, IV: 100 international units/ml **Note:** Antihemophilic factor VIII injectable is for IV use only. The product must be administered within 3 hr after reconstitution. Do not refrigerate after reconstitution.	**Contraindications:** Hypersensitivity to bovine, hamster, or mouse protein. **ADRs:** Generally well tolerated. May cause minor burning, erythema, and pruritus at the injection site. **Comments:** When available, serial determinations of antihemophilic factor plasma concentrations can be used to guide dosage.
Anthrax vaccine, adsorbed **Note:** Anthrax vaccine, adsorbed, has been developed and produced under the auspices of the U.S. government military, Department of Defense. Available data are very limited. For additional or updated information, consult the following website: http://www.usamriid.army.mil or call 1-877-438-8222.	**Pre-exposure prophylaxis** against anthrax infection related to bioterrorist attack **Note:** Not approved by the FDA or HPB for use in infants, children, and adolescents. **Postexposure treatment** to prevent or minimize morbidity and mortality in the event of a bioterrorist attack	**Adolescents:** Initially, a series of six vaccine doses should be administered subcutaneously at 1, 2, 4, 26, 52, and 78 weeks. Subsequently, a single booster dose is required annually. **Note:** Healthy subcutaneous tissue over the deltoid muscle of the upper arm is generally recommended for subcutaneous injection. **Adolescents:** Initially, first administer appropriate antibiotic (e.g., ciprofloxacin) for 30 days, then follow with three doses of anthrax vaccine, adsorbed, injected subcutaneously at 0, 2, and 4 weeks.	Injectable solution, SC: Aluminum hydroxide adsorbed cell-free anthrax vaccine. Store refrigerated at 2–8°C (36–46°F). Do not freeze.	**Contraindications:** Active infection with anthrax, depressed immune response, hypersensitivity to anthrax vaccine or any of its components, positive HIV status, and a previous history of cutaneous (skin) anthrax. **ADRs:** Commonly causes chills, fatigue, fever, headache, itching, joint pain, malaise, muscle aches, nausea, pain, redness, and swelling at the injection site that generally resolve within a few days following vaccination. May also commonly cause a "lump" at the injection site that may persist for a few weeks. **Note:** Anthrax vaccine, adsorbed, does not contain whole or live anthrax bacteria; thus, it cannot cause infection with anthrax disease. **Comments:** Following exposure to anthrax, it is recommended that all individuals receive appropriate antibiotic (e.g., ciprofloxacin) pharmacotherapy even if they have been previously immunized with the anthrax vaccine, adsorbed. **Note:** Anthrax vaccine, adsorbed, is a newly developed vaccine that has only been recently released for public use. Available clinical data are extremely limited. For additional information, contact the manufacturer, BioPort Corp, at (517) 327-1500.
Antivenin (Crotalidae) Polyvalent (Crotalid Serum Antivenin)	Snake bite (to neutralize the venoms of pit vipers native to Central, North, and South America, including bushmaster, moccasins, and rattlesnakes)	**Children and adolescents:** | DEGREE OF ENVENOMATION	ASSOCIATED SIGNS AND SYMPTOMS	DOSAGE	 |---|---|---| | Minimal	Local swelling No systemic manifestations Normal laboratory findings	Initially, 20–40 ml (two to four vials) of antivenin IV			**Contraindications:** None. **Comments:** Typical **local** signs and symptoms of envenomation include ecchymosis, pain, skin discoloration, and swelling. Typical **systemic** signs and symptoms of envenomation include faintness, hypotension, *(Continued)*

Footnotes are on page 558.

TABLE 14-1 *continued*

DRUG (*TRADE* AND OTHER NAMES)	INDICATION(S)	USUAL PEDIATRIC DOSAGE AND ADMINISTRATION[a]		DOSAGE FORMS	CONTRAINDICATIONS, ADRs, AND COMMENTS[b]
Antivenin (Crotalidae) Polyvalent (Crotalid Serum Antivenin) *continued*		**DEGREE OF ENVENOMATION**	**ASSOCIATED SIGNS AND SYMPTOMS** / **DOSAGE**	Injectable, IV: 10 ml of pure concentrated serum/vial after reconstitution. **Note:** Antivenin polyvalent is supplied with both a vial of diluent and a vial of normal horse serum (1 to 10 strength) for sensitivity testing prior to use of the antivenin. **Note:** Store at room temperature below 37°C (99°F). Do not freeze.	muscle fasciculations, nausea, prolonged bleeding and clotting times, sweating, and weakness.
		Moderate	Swelling progressing beyond bite site / One or more manifestations / Abnormal laboratory findings (e.g., decreased hematocrit or platelets) — Initially, 50–90 ml (five to nine vials) of antivenin IV		
		Severe	Marked local response / Severe systemic manifestations / Significant alterations in laboratory findings — Initially, 100–150 ml (10–15 vials) of antivenin IV		
		Note: If swelling progresses, systemic signs and symptoms increase, or new signs and symptoms appear, then administer an additional 10–50 ml (one to five vials) of antivenin IV.			
Arsenic Trioxide, *see* **Chapter 12**					
Ascorbic Acid (Vitamin C)	Dietary supplement	**Infants, children, and adolescents:** 60 mg/day PO as a single daily dose.		Caplet, oral: 500 mg Capsule, oral extended release: 500 mg Lozenge, oral: 60 mg (grape, lemon, and orange flavored) Solutions, oral: 35, 50 mg/0.6 ml, 100 mg/ml (supplied with dropper) (contains 5% alcohol) Syrup, oral: 500 mg/5 ml Tablets, oral: 25, 50, 100, 250, 500 mg; 1 gram Tablets, oral chewable: 100, 250, 500 mg (orange flavored)	**Contraindications:** None identified. **ADRs:** Generally well tolerated. *See* Chapter 5.
	Urinary acidification **Note:** Although often used for this indication, efficacy is questionable. Ammonium chloride is generally a better choice for urinary acidification.	**Children and adolescents:** 2000–4000 mg/day PO in four divided doses, every 6 hr.			
	Scurvy, prophylaxis	**Infants:** 30 mg/day PO as a single daily dose. **Children and adolescents:** 75 mg/day PO as a single daily dose.			
	Scurvy, treatment	**Infants:** 300 mg/day PO as a single daily dose. **Children and adolescents:** 1 gram/day PO as a single daily dose.			
Asparaginase, *see* **Chapter 12**					
Aspirin (Acetylsalicylic Acid, *Aspergum®*, *Easprin®*, *Ecotrin®*, *ZORprin®*)	Fever/Pain, mild to moderate **Note:** Not recommended as an antipyretic for infants, children,	**Children and adolescents:** 40–90 mg/kg/day PO in four to six divided doses every 4–6 hr, according to response. *Maximum:* **Children,** 2.4 grams/day PO; **adolescents,** 3.6 grams/day PO.		Caplets, oral: 325, 500 mg Caplets, oral enteric coated: 325, 500 mg Gum, oral chewable: 228, 325 mg (orange or cherry flavored)	**Contraindications:** Hypersensitivity to aspirin, to other salicylates, or to other non-steroidal anti-inflammatory drugs (NSAIDs). **ADRs:** *See* Chapter 5.

TABLE 14-1 continued

DRUG (TRADE AND OTHER NAMES)	INDICATION(S)	USUAL PEDIATRIC DOSAGE AND ADMINISTRATION[a]	DOSAGE FORMS	CONTRAINDICATIONS, ADRs, AND COMMENTS[b]
Aspirin *continued*	or adolescents who have viral infections (e.g., chickenpox, influenza) because of association with Reye's syndrome. Acetaminophen is generally used in these pediatric patients as the preferred antipyretic.		Suppositories, rectal: 60, 120, 200, 300, 600 mg Tablets, oral: 325, 500, 650, 975 mg Tablet, oral chewable: 80 mg (orange flavored) Tablets, oral enteric coated: 81, 165, 325, 500, 650 mg Tablets, oral extended release: 81, 650, 800, 975 mg **Note:** Aspirin rectal suppositories should be stored under refrigeration.	**Comments:** Therapeutic drug monitoring is recommended, particularly when higher dosages are required. *See* Table 14-3. Monitor mental status and hepatic function during long-term aspirin pharmacotherapy.
	Juvenile rheumatoid arthritis	**Children and adolescents:** 80–130 mg/kg/day PO in three or four divided doses, every 6 or 8 hr. *Maximum:* 6 grams/day PO.		
	Rheumatic fever, acute	**Children and adolescents:** Initially, 100 mg/kg/day PO in three divided doses, every 8 hr, for 2 weeks. Then 75 mg/kg/day PO in three divided doses, every 8 hr, for 4–6 additional weeks. *Maximum:* 6 grams/day PO.		
	Kawasaki disease (mucocutaneous lymph node syndrome)	**Children and adolescents:** Initially, 100–150 mg/kg/day PO in four divided doses, every 6 hr, for 36 hr or until acute fever has resolved. Then 5–10 mg/kg/day PO as a single daily dose every morning for 2 months or until platelet count and erythrocyte sedimentation rate are normal. *Maximum:* 150 mg/kg/day PO.		
Atenolol *(Tenormin®)*	**Hypertension,** mild to moderate **Note:** May be used alone, but usually used in combination with other antihypertensive drugs (e.g., thiazide diuretics). **Note:** Not approved by the FDA or HPB for infants or children.	**Children and adolescents:** 1–2 mg/kg PO as a single daily dose. *Maximum:* 2 mg/kg/day PO. **Note:** Decrease dosage for pediatric patients who have renal dysfunction; *see* Table 14-2.	Tablets, oral: 50, 100 mg	**Contraindications:** AV block (second or third degree), bradycardia, cardiogenic shock, congestive heart failure, hypersensitivity to atenolol, hypotension, metabolic acidosis, pheochromocytoma, and sick sinus syndrome. **ADRs:** *See* Chapter 5.
Atovaquone *(Mepron®)*	***Pneumocystis carinii* pneumonia** (PCP), mild to moderate, among patients who are intolerant to trimethoprim–sulfamethoxazole pharmacotherapy **Note:** Not approved by the FDA or HPB for this indication for adolescents.	**Adolescents:** 1500 mg/day PO in two divided doses with food for 21 consecutive days. **Note:** Food significantly enhances GI absorption.	Suspension, oral: 750 mg/5 ml (tutti frutti flavored); shake well before measuring each dose. **Note:** Contains saccharin sodium. **Note:** Store between 15 and 25°C. Do **not** freeze.	**Contraindications:** Hypersensitivity to atovaquone. **ADRs:** May cause cough, diarrhea, fever, headache, nausea, rash, and vomiting. Anemia, hyperglycemia, and hyponatremia also have been associated with atovaquone pharmacotherapy.

Footnotes are on page 558.

TABLE 14-1 continued

DRUG (TRADE AND OTHER NAMES)	INDICATION(S)	USUAL PEDIATRIC DOSAGE AND ADMINISTRATION[a]	DOSAGE FORMS	CONTRAINDICATIONS, ADRs, AND COMMENTS[b]
Atracurium	Facilitation of mechanical ventilation	**Infants and children (≤2 years):** Initially, 0.3–0.4 mg/kg IV. **Children (>2 years) and adolescents:** Initially, 0.4–0.5 mg/kg IV, then 0.06–0.1 mg/kg IV every 20–45 min. **Alternatively:** After initial dose of 0.4–0.5 mg/kg IV, 5–10 µg/kg/min by continuous IV infusion. **Note:** Adjust dosage according to response to peripheral nerve stimulation.	Injectable, IV: 10 mg/ml (contains benzyl alcohol) **Note:** For IV use only. IM use may cause tissue irritation.	**Contraindications:** Hypersensitivity to atracurium. **ADRs:** Generally well tolerated. May cause skin flushing. *See* Chapter 5. **Comments:** Reduce dosage for patients who are receiving inhalation anesthetics. Have anticholinesterases immediately available to reverse atracurium's effects, if necessary.
Atropine, ophthalmic (*Atropine-1®, Atropine-Care®, Atropisol®, Isopto Atropine®*)	Cycloplegic refraction for eye examination	**Children:** One or two drops of 0.5% ophthalmic solution instilled into the eye(s) twice daily for 1–3 days before the eye examination. **Adolescents:** One or two drops of 1% ophthalmic solution instilled into the eye(s) as a single dose 1 hr before the eye examination.	Ointment, ophthalmic: 1% Solutions, ophthalmic: 0.5%, 1%, 2% **Note:** Atropine ophthalmic ointment and solution are for ophthalmic use only. **Note:** In order to minimize cross-infection when both eyes require atropine ophthalmic pharmacotherapy, ensure that separate containers are dispensed for each eye.	**Contraindications:** Glaucoma, hypersensitivity to atropine or to other belladonna alkaloids, and synechiae (adhesions between the iris and the lens). **ADRs:** Generally well tolerated. May cause blurred vision, drowsiness, and sensitivity to light. Children with Down's syndrome or organic brain damage may demonstrate a hyperreactive response to ophthalmic atropine. **Comments:** Systemic absorption and resultant ADRs can be minimized by appropriate use of nasolacrimal occlusion (*see* Chapter 1).
	Ureitis (inflammation of the intraocular structures)	**Children:** One or two drops of 0.5% ophthalmic solution instilled into the affected eye(s) two or three times daily. **Alternatively**, 0.3 cm 1% ophthalmic ointment applied to center of conjunctival sac of affected eye(s) two or three times daily, as indicated by response. **Adolescents:** One or two drops of 1% ophthalmic solution instilled into the affected eye(s) two to four times daily, as indicated by response. **Alternatively**, 0.5 cm 1% ophthalmic ointment applied to center of conjunctival sac of affected eye(s) two or three times daily, as indicated by response. **Note:** Patients with heavily pigmented irides may require higher dosages (e.g., use of 1% or 2% ophthalmic solutions instead of 0.5% or 1% ophthalmic solutions).		
Atropine, systemic (dl-Hyoscyamine) **Note:** *See also* Chapter 4.	Inhibition of salivation and excessive respiratory secretions during surgery	**Infants, children, and adolescents:** 0.01–0.02 mg/kg/dose IM or PO 30–60 min before surgery (minimal dose, 0.15 mg). Repeat dose every 4–6 hr as indicated by response. *Maximum:* 0.6 mg/dose IM or PO.	Injectables, IM, IV, SC: 0.05, 0.1, 0.3, 0.4, 0.5, 0.8, 1 mg/ml Tablet, oral: 0.4 mg	**Contraindications:** GI obstruction, glaucoma, hypersensitivity to atropine or to other belladonna alkaloids, obstructive uropathy, paralytic ileus, and tachycardia. **ADRs:** *See* Chapter 5.
	AV block due to increased vagal tone (e.g., digoxin intoxication)/ Bradycardia and syncope due to hyperactive carotid sinus reflex (i.e., sinus bradycardia)/	**Children:** 0.01–0.03 mg/kg/dose IV, intraosseous, or endotracheal (by endotracheal tube instillation). Repeat dose every 5–30 min as indicated by response. *Maximum:* 0.04 mg/kg/dose **or** 1 mg, whichever is less, endotracheal, intraosseous, or IV.		

TABLE 14-1 continued

DRUG (TRADE AND OTHER NAMES)	INDICATION(S)	USUAL PEDIATRIC DOSAGE AND ADMINISTRATION[a]	DOSAGE FORMS	CONTRAINDICATIONS, ADRs, AND COMMENTS[b]
Atropine, systemic *continued*	**Cardiovascular collapse** due to choline ester overdosage. **Note:** IV atropine pharmacotherapy for the management of cardiovascular collapse requires external cardiac massage to help to distribute the drug. **Note:** Not approved by the HPB for infants or children.	**Adolescents:** 0.01–0.03 mg/kg/dose IV, intraosseous, or endotracheal (by endotracheal tube instillation). Repeat dose every 5–30 min as indicated by response. *Maximum:* 0.04 mg/kg/dose **or** 2 mg, whichever is less, endotracheal, intraosseous, or IV. **Note:** *See* Chapter 1, for details regarding intraosseous drug administration.		

Atropine and Diphenoxylate, *see* **Diphenoxylate and Atropine**

Azacitidine, *see* **Chapter 12**

Azathioprine *(Imuran®)*	**Renal transplantation**	**Children and adolescents:** Initially (starting the day of transplantation or 1–3 days before), 3–5 mg/kg/day IV or PO as a single dose. Then (generally within 1–4 days following transplantation), start maintenance dosage of 1–3 mg/kg/day PO as a single daily dose. **Note:** Reduce dosage for pediatric patients who have renal dysfunction; *see* Table 14-2.	Tablet, oral: 50 mg (contains povidone) Injectable, IV: 100 mg/vial	**Contraindications:** Hypersensitivity to azathioprine. **ADRs:** May cause anorexia, bone marrow depression, diarrhea, hepatotoxicity, infection, nausea, rash, serum sickness, and vomiting. **Comments:** Regular monitoring of hematologic function (i.e., complete blood counts) and hepatic function (i.e., serum alkaline phosphatase, aminotransferase, and bilirubin concentrations) is required. Concurrent azathioprine and allopurinol pharmacotherapy necessitates a 75% dosage reduction for azathioprine (*see* Chapter 6). **Note:** Monitor patients for TPMT genotype because standard doses can be **fatal** for TPMT-deficient patients (*see* Chapter 11).
Azelastine, nasal *(Astelin®)*	**Seasonal allergic rhinitis/Nasal pruritus**	**Children (≥5 years):** One spray in each nostril twice daily. **Adolescents:** Two sprays in each nostril twice daily. **Note:** If the azelastine pump unit has not been used for more than 2 or 3 days, it may require repriming before use with two sprays or until a fine mist is obtained.	Spray, intranasal: 137 µg/metered-dose pump spray **Note:** For intranasal use only. Avoid spraying in the eyes. **Note:** Store at controlled room temperature between 20 and 25°C (68–77° F). Do **not** freeze. **Note:** Not generally available in Canada.	**Contraindications:** Hypersensitivity to azelastine. **ADRs:** Generally well tolerated. Intranasal use has been associated with a bitter aftertaste, myalgia, somnolence, and weight gain.

Azidothymidine, *see* **Zidovudine**

Azithromycin *(Zithromax®)*	**Otitis media,** acute, caused by *Haemophilus influenzae, moraxella, catarrhalis,* or *Streptococcus pneumoniae/* **Pneumonia,** community acquired,	**Infants (≥6 months), children, and adolescents:** Initially, 10 mg/kg/day PO as a single dose on day 1. Follow by 5 mg/kg/day PO as a single dose on days 2, 3, 4, and 5. *Maximum:* 500 mg/day PO on day 1; 250 mg/day PO on days 2, 3, 4, and 5.	Capsule, oral: 250 mg Injectable, IV: 500 mg/vial (100 mg/ml after reconstitution)	**Contraindications:** Hypersensitivity to azithromycin, erythromycin, or other macrolide antibiotics. **ADRs:** Generally well tolerated. May cause abdominal pain,

(Continued)

Footnotes are on page 558.

TABLE 14-1 continued

DRUG (TRADE AND OTHER NAMES)	INDICATION(S)	USUAL PEDIATRIC DOSAGE AND ADMINISTRATION[a]	DOSAGE FORMS	CONTRAINDICATIONS, ADRs, AND COMMENTS[b]
Azithromycin *continued*	caused by *H. influenzae, Chlamydia pneumoniae, Mycoplasma pneumoniae,* or *S. pneumoniae*.	**Note:** Administer on an empty stomach 1 hr before or 2 hr after meals.	Powder, oral (single-dose packets): 1000 mg (powder for reconstitution) (banana and cherry flavored). Suspensions, oral: 100, 200 mg/5 ml (after reconstitution) (cherry flavored); shake well before use. Tablets, oral: 250, 600 mg **Note:** Mix the contents of each single-dose packet of azithromycin with 60 ml of water just prior to ingestion. Follow with an additional 60 ml of water to ensure that the total dose is ingested.	diarrhea, nausea, and vomiting. *See* Chapter 5.
	Pharyngitis/ Tonsillitis **Note:** Ensure that appropriate culture and sensitivity tests are performed and that the organism is sensitive to azithromycin.	**Children (≥2 years) and adolescents:** 12 mg/kg/day PO as a single dose for 5 consecutive days. *Maximum:* 500 mg/day.		
Azthreonam, *see* Aztreonam				
Aztreonam (*Azactam®*)	**Bacterial infection among patients with cystic fibrosis**	**Infants, children, and adolescents:** 200 mg/kg/day IV in four divided doses, every 6 hr. *Maximum:* 8 grams/day IV.	Injectables, IM, IV: 500 mg/vial; 1, 2 grams/vial **Note:** Not generally available in Canada.	**Contraindications:** Hypersensitivity to aztreonam. **ADRs:** *See* Chapter 5.
	Bacterial infections, mild to moderate	**Infants, children, and adolescents:** 90 mg/kg/day IV in three divided doses, every 8 hr. *Maximum:* 3 grams/day IV.		
	Bacterial infections, severe **Note:** Ensure that appropriate culture and sensitivity tests are performed and that the organism is sensitive to aztreonam.	**Infants, children, and adolescents:** 120–200 mg/kg/day IV in four divided doses, every 6 hr. *Maximum:* 8 grams/day IV. **Note:** Reduce dosage for pediatric patients who have renal (*see* Table 14-2) or hepatic dysfunction.		
Bacitracin (*Baciguent®, Bacitin®*)	**Infections** associated with minor external burns, cuts, or wounds (prevention and treatment)	**Children and adolescents:** Apply ointment liberally to affected area once daily or more often as indicated. **Note:** Application site should be appropriately cleaned with soap and warm water prior to applying ointment. Following application, the site may be covered with a Band-aid® or sterile dry surgical gauze dressing.	Ointment, topical: 500 units/gram **Note:** For topical use only. Avoid contact with the eyes.	**Contraindications:** Hypersensitivity to bacitracin. **ADRs:** Generally well tolerated. May cause sensitization or overgrowth of nonsusceptible organisms (e.g., *Candida*) at site of application. **Comments:** Discontinue if sensitization or overgrowth of nonsusceptible organisms occurs.
Baclofen (*Lioresal®*)	**Spasticity associated with sclerosis** **Note:** Not approved by the FDA or HPB for children.	**Children:** 5–15 mg/day PO in three divided doses. Increase the dosage gradually, over a 2-week period, to the maximal dosage, as indicated by response. *Maximum:* 30 mg/day PO. **Adolescents:** 15–30 mg/day PO in three divided doses. Increase the dosage gradually, over a 2-week period, to the maximal dosage, as indicated by response. *Maximum:* 80 mg/day PO.	Tablets, oral: 10, 20 mg **Note:** Baclofen also is available as a formulation for intrathecal injection via an intrathecal catheter attached to an implanted infusion pump with an injection port.	**Contraindications:** Hypersensitivity to baclofen. **ADRs:** May cause blurred vision, confusion, dizziness, drowsiness, dysuria, fatigue, headache, hypotension, insomnia, lethargy, nausea, vomiting, and weakness. May aggravate seizure and psychotic disorders. Pediatric patients with these concomitant disorders must be carefully monitored for seizures and psychotic behavior.

CHAPTER 14: DRUG DOSING FOR INFANTS, CHILDREN, AND ADOLESCENTS

TABLE 14-1 continued

DRUG (TRADE AND OTHER NAMES)	INDICATION(S)	USUAL PEDIATRIC DOSAGE AND ADMINISTRATION[a]	DOSAGE FORMS	CONTRAINDICATIONS, ADRs, AND COMMENTS[b]
Baclofen *continued*				**Comments:** Excessive dosages may result in deterioration of clinical condition. Chronic long-term use may result in tolerance. Abrupt discontinuation of chronic long-term use may result in hallucinations or seizures.
Basiliximab (*Simulect®*)	Renal transplantation, prophylaxis of acute organ rejection (in combination with cyclosporine and corticosteroid-based immunosuppression) **Note:** Approved by the FDA but not by the HPB for this indication in children.	**Children (<35 kg):** 10 mg IV as a single dose within 2 hr **prior** to renal transplantation surgery. An additional 10 mg IV should be administered 4 days after transplantation. **Children (≥35 kg) and adolescents:** 20 mg IV as a single dose within 2 hr **prior** to renal transplantation surgery. An additional 20 mg IV should be administered 4 days after transplantation. **Note:** Reconstituted basiliximab may be administered by a bolus IV injection or diluted to a volume ≥50 ml with NS or D₅W and administered as an IV infusion over 20–30 min.	Injectable, IV: 20 mg/vial (4 mg/ml after reconstitution with 5 ml of sterile water for injection) **Note:** Store vials of injectable powder refrigerated at 2–8°C; reconstitute immediately before use. **Note:** Do **not** shake (to avoid foaming). Do **not** admix with other drugs or solutions.	**Contraindications:** Hypersensitivity to basiliximab or to mouse proteins. **ADRs:** Generally well tolerated. Type and incidence of ADRs is essentially the same as seen with placebo in controlled clinical trials. Can induce hypersensitivity reactions (*see* Contraindications).
Beclomethasone, nasal (*Beconase®, Beconase AQ®, Vancenase AQ®, Vancenase Pockethaler®*) **Note:** *See also* Beclomethasone, pulmonary.	Symptomatic relief of perennial or seasonal rhinitis	**Children (6–12 years):** One metered-dose nasal spray (42 µg) in each nostril three times daily. **Adolescents:** One metered-dose nasal spray (42 µg) in each nostril two to four times daily. **Alternative dosage for children (≥6 years) and adolescents:** One or two double-strength metered-dose nasal sprays (84 µg) in each nostril once daily. **Note:** Dosing schedule depends on patient age and formulation strength (42 µg versus 84 µg/actuation).	Suspensions, metered-dose manual pump nasal spray: 42, 84 µg/spray; shake well before use. **Note:** Generally avoid prescription of the double-strength product (84 µg/actuation) for children. **Note:** Some beclomethasone metered-dose units (e.g., *Beconase AQ, Vancenase AQ*) use a manual pump mechanism that requires priming with four to six actuations prior to first use and after periods of nonuse generally exceeding 5 days.	**Contraindications:** Hypersensitivity to beclomethasone; tuberculosis (history); and untreated bacterial, fungal, or viral infections, particularly of the mouth, nasal sinuses, nose, and respiratory tract. **ADRs:** Generally well tolerated. May cause loss of, or alteration in, smell and taste. May also cause local ADRs, including dryness and irritation of the mouth, nose, and throat. Systemic ADRs may affect several body systems. *See* Chapter 5.
Beclomethasone, pulmonary (*Vanceril®*) **Note:** *See also* Beclomethasone, nasal.	Asthma prophylaxis **Note:** Not indicated for the management of acute asthmatic attacks (acute bronchospasm).	**Children (3–5 years):** *Metered-dose inhaler (MDI),* one actuation of MDI aerosol (42 µg) two or three times daily. *Maximum:* Three actuations (126 µg)/day by MDI. **Children (≥6 years):** *Metered-dose inhaler (MDI),* one or two actuations of MDI aerosol (42 or 84 µg) three or four times daily. *Maximum:* 10 actuations (420 µg)/day by MDI. **Adolescents:** *Metered-dose inhaler (MDI),* two actuations (84 µg) of MDI aerosol three or four times daily.	Solutions, metered-dose inhalers (MDIs): 42, 84 µg/actuation; shake well before use. **Note:** For pulmonary inhalation only. **Note:** Generally avoid prescription of the double-strength product (84 µg/actuation) for children.	**Contraindications:** Hypersensitivity to beclomethasone; status asthmaticus; tuberculosis (history); and untreated bacterial, fungal, or viral infections, particularly of the respiratory tract. **ADRs:** May cause loss of, or alteration in, smell and taste. May also cause local ADRs, including dryness and irritation of the mouth and throat. Systemic ADRs may affect several body systems. *See* Chapter 5. **Comments:** Pulmonary beclomethasone pharmacotherapy while able to provide intended pharmacologic response *(Continued)*

Footnotes are on page 558.

TABLE 14-1 continued

DRUG (TRADE AND OTHER NAMES)	INDICATION(S)	USUAL PEDIATRIC DOSAGE AND ADMINISTRATION[a]	DOSAGE FORMS	CONTRAINDICATIONS, ADRs, AND COMMENTS[b]
Beclo-methasone, pulmonary *continued*		*Maximum*: 20 actuations of MDI aerosol (840 µg)/day. **Alternative dosage for children (≥6 years) and adolescents:** *Metered-dose inhaler,* four actuations (168 µg) of MDI aerosol twice daily (336 µg/day). *Maximum:* **Children (≥6 years),** five actuations of MDI aerosol twice daily (420 µg/day); **adolescents,** 10 actuations of MDI aerosol twice daily (840 µg/day). **Note:** Dosing schedule depends on patient's age and strength of MDI formulation (42 µg/actuation versus 84 µg/actuation). **Note:** Rinse mouth after use in order to avoid local ADRs and to reduce ingestion of drug and unnecessary systemic absorption and associated ADRs.		(prevention of asthma attacks), may not be able to provide sufficient corticosteroid to prevent adrenal insufficiency among pediatric patients whose systemic corticosteroid pharmacotherapy was replaced with beclomethasone pulmonary pharmacotherapy.
Benzocaine, anesthetic lubricant *(Americaine Anesthetic Lubricant®)* **Note:** *See also* Benzocaine, otic, and Benzocaine, topical.	Local anesthesia (anesthetic lubricant to obtund pharyngeal and tracheal reflexes and diminish associated pain and discomfort) **Note:** For use with endoscopic tubes, intratracheal catheters, laryngoscopes, nasogastric tubes, proctoscopes, sigmoidoscopes, urinary catheters, and vaginal specula.	**Children and adolescents:** Apply an even coating to exterior surface of tube or instrument immediately prior to use.	Gel, topical: 20% (contains polyethylene glycol)	**Contraindications:** Hypersensitivity to benzocaine. **ADRs:** Generally well tolerated. May cause local irritation.
Benzocaine, otic *(Americaine Otic®)* **Note:** *See also* Benzocaine, anesthetic lubricant, and Benzocaine, topical.	Otitis externa/ Otitis media/ Swimmer's ear, acute (provides temporary relief of acute pain and pruritus) **Note:** Benzocaine otic products should **not** be used if ear discharge is present or if the tympanic membrane is ruptured.	**Children and adolescents:** Instill 4 or 5 drops of otic solution into external ear canal of affected ear(s). May repeat several times per day, generally every 1–2 hr, as indicated by response.	Solution, otic: 20% (contains glycerin and polyethylene glycol) **Note:** For instillation into the external ear canal only. **Note:** Commonly available in combination otic products.	**Contraindications:** Hypersensitivity to benzocaine. **ADRs:** Generally well tolerated. May cause local irritation.
Benzocaine, topical *(Americaine®, Anbesol®, Babee Teetbing®,* ethyl aminobenzoate, *Orajel Mouth-Aid®, Orabase Gel®)* **Note:** *See also* Benzocaine, anesthetic lubricant, and Benzocaine, otic.	Mouth irritation, minor (e.g., canker sores, cold sores, fever blisters, orthodontic brace pain, teething pain, and toothaches), temporary relief **Note:** For temporary use only, **not** for prolonged use.	**Infants, children, and adolescents:** Apply a small amount to the affected area. May repeat up to four times daily, as needed.	Gels, topical (gums and oral mucous membranes): 6.4%, 7.5% (*Anbesol Baby®*, grape flavored), 20% Solutions, topical (gums and oral mucous membranes): 6.5%, 20% **Note:** Concentrated benzocaine topical gels and solutions (20% formulations) are	**Contraindications:** Hypersensitivity to benzocaine. **ADRs:** May cause local effects, including a sensation of burning or stinging, pruritus, and tenderness at application site. Rarely causes methemoglobinemia with related respiratory distress and cyanosis; risk is highest for infants and pediatric patients who have glucose-6-phosphate dehydrogenase deficiency.

TABLE 14-1 continued

DRUG (TRADE AND OTHER NAMES)	INDICATION(S)	USUAL PEDIATRIC DOSAGE AND ADMINISTRATION[a]	DOSAGE FORMS	CONTRAINDICATIONS, ADRs, AND COMMENTS[b]
Benzocaine, topical *continued*		not generally recommended for infants or children. **Note:** For topical use only (application to gums and oral mucous membranes). Avoid contact with eyes. **Note:** Benzocaine topical products may contain flammable ingredients (e.g., alcohol). Caution patients and their parents to avoid use near open fire or flame. Caution tobacco smokers to avoid smoking after topical application of benzocaine until product has dried.		**Comments:** The application of topical benzocaine to affected sites in the oral cavity may impair swallowing and increase risk for aspiration. Generally, food should **not** be ingested for 1 hr following oral use. Children should be instructed to refrain from chewing gum.
Benzoyl Peroxide *(Benoxyl®, Brevoxyl®, Clearasil Maximum Strength®, Desquam-X®, Fostex®, Neutrogena Acne Mask®, PanOxyl®, Persa-Gel®)*	**Acne vulgaris**, mild to moderate **Note:** Benzoyl peroxide topical products are often used as part of a multimodal therapeutic regimen that includes retinoic acid products and systemic antibiotics. **Note:** Not approved by the FDA or HPB for children.	**Adolescents:** Apply a small amount topically to affected areas once or twice daily. **Note:** Because of variability in formulations, read and follow additional manufacturer's directions (e.g., cleansers are generally applied with water, worked into a lather, and then thoroughly rinsed; creams and lotions may be applied and left on the skin for a specified period).	Cleansers (bar or liquid), topical: 4%, 5%, 8%, 10% Creams, topical: 5%, 10% Gels, topical: 2.5%, 4%, 5%, 6%, 10%, 20% Lotions, topical: 5%, 5.5%, 10%; shake well before use. Mask, topical: 5% **Note:** All benzoyl peroxide topical products are for **external use only**. Avoid contact with eyes or mucous membranes.	**Contraindications:** Hypersensitivity to benzoyl peroxide. **ADRs:** May cause local reactions, including excessive drying, erythema, and peeling of skin at application site. Allergic contact dermatitis (sensitization) occurs in ~1% of patients. **Comments:** May bleach bed linens, carpeting, clothing, furniture fabric, or hair.
Beractant, see Chapter 13				
Betaine *(Cystadane®)*	**Homocystinuria** **Note:** Often used concomitantly with cyanocobalamin, folic acid, and pyridoxine pharmacotherapy.	**Infants and children (<3 years):** Initially, 100 mg/kg/day PO as a single dose or in two divided doses. Gradually increase dosage, as indicated by homocysteine plasma concentration, in increments of 100 mg/kg at weekly intervals until plasma homocysteine is undetectable. **Children (≥3 years) and adolescents:** 6 grams/day PO in two divided doses. Gradually increase dosage, as indicated by homocysteine plasma concentration, by increments of 100 mg/kg at weekly intervals until plasma homocysteine is undetectable. *Maximum:* 20 grams/day PO. **Note:** Each dose of betaine oral powder should be prepared immediately before use. Dissolve each dose in 125–200 ml of juice, milk, or water, or mix in a small amount of compatible food.	Powder, oral (for dilution or mixing with food prior to ingestion): Supplied in a plastic bottle with a polystyrene measuring scoop. One level scoop (1.7 ml) will contain 1 gram of anhydrous betaine powder. **Note:** Safely store plastic bottle of betaine oral powder at room temperature and always tightly replace cap following each use.	**Contraindications:** None currently identified. **ADRs:** Generally well tolerated. May occasionally cause diarrhea and nausea. **Comments:** Monitor homocysteine plasma concentrations. Therapeutic response (reduced homocysteine plasma concentrations) generally occurs within 1 week and is optimal within 1 month.

Footnotes are on page 558.

TABLE 14-1 continued

DRUG (TRADE AND OTHER NAMES)	INDICATION(S)	USUAL PEDIATRIC DOSAGE AND ADMINISTRATION[a]	DOSAGE FORMS	CONTRAINDICATIONS, ADRs, AND COMMENTS[b]
Betamethasone, injectable (*Betaject®, Celestone Soluspan®*) *Note: See also* Betamethasone, oral.	**Adrenocortical insufficiency**, primary or secondary/ **Allergic conditions**, severe and incapacitating/ **Autoimmune hemolytic anemia/ Exfoliative dermatitis/Juvenile rheumatoid arthritis**	**Children and adolescents:** 0.5–9 mg/day IM, intra-articular, or intralesional. **Note:** Dosage and route of injectable betamethasone administration are guided by indication for use, general health of patient, and response. Generally, ⅓ to ½ of the oral daily dose is administered IM twice daily, every 12 hr. Intra-articular and intralesional administration is generally used for short-term adjunctive pharmacotherapy and is administered at intervals of 3–14 days.	Injectable suspension, IM, intra-articular, or intralesional: 6 mg/ml (3 mg betamethasone sodium phosphate for rapid onset of action and 3 mg betamethasone acetate for sustained action). **Note:** Safely store protected from light between 2 and 30°C; shake well before use. **Note: Not** for IV use.	**Contraindications:** Systemic fungal infections. **ADRs:** May cause a variety of systemic ADRs (*see* Chapter 5). **Comments:** To discontinue high dosage or long-term therapy, gradually reduce the dosage in order to avoid HPA axis suppression.
Betamethasone, oral (*Celestone®*) *Note: See also* Betamethasone, injectable.	**Adrenocortical insufficiency**, primary or secondary/ **Allergic conditions**, severe and incapacitating/ **Autoimmune hemolytic anemia/ Exfoliative dermatitis/Juvenile rheumatoid arthritis**	**Children and adolescents:** Initially, 0.6–7.2 mg/day PO. Adjust dosage according to indication for use, patient's general health, and response.	Syrup, oral: 0.6 mg/5 ml (cherry–orange flavored; contains alcohol) Tablet, oral: 0.6 mg **Note:** Not generally available in Canada. **Note:** Also is available in combination topical formulations.	**Contraindications:** Systemic fungal infections. **ADRs:** May cause a variety of systemic ADRs (*see* Chapter 5). **Comments:** To discontinue high dosage or long-term therapy, gradually reduce the dosage in order to avoid associated HPA axis suppression, which may occur with abrupt discontinuation.
Betamethasone, topical (*Celestoderm®, Celestoderm-V®, Diprolene®, Luxiq®*)	**Dermatoses**, corticosteroid responsive (to provide relief of inflammation and pruritus) **Note: Not** indicated for the treatment of diaper dermatoses among infants and toddlers. **Psoriasis of the scalp**, moderate to severe **Note:** Not approved by the FDA or HPB for this indication for children	**Children and adolescents:** Apply topical product sparingly to affected area once or twice daily. *Maximum*: Do **not** exceed 50 grams (or 50 ml)/week and do **not** exceed 2 consecutive weeks of use. Excessive use increases potential risk for associated hypothalamic-pituitary-adrenal (HPA) axis suppression and related sequelae. **Note:** Do **not** cover treated areas with an occlusive dressing or with tight-fitting diapers or plastic pants. Covering treated sites may increase systemic absorption and associated ADRs (*see* Chapter 1). **Adolescents:** Apply to affected area(s) of scalp twice daily, morning and evening, according to the following instructions: Invert can containing betamethasone foam (*Luxiq*) and dispense a small amount onto a clean saucer or other cool surface (do **not** dispense directly onto hands because foam will begin to melt immediately upon skin contact). Using the fingertips, take a small amount of foam and gently massage into affected area(s) on scalp until the foam disappears. Repeat until all affected area(s) have been treated.	Creams, topical: 0.05%, 0.1% Foam, topical: 0.12% (contains 60% alcohol; supplied in a 100-gram aluminum can under pressure; do **not** incinerate or puncture can and do **not** expose can to temperatures exceeding 49°C [120°F]). Gel, topical: 0.05% Lotion, topical: 0.05% Ointments, topical: 0.05%, 0.1% **Note:** Betamethasone topical products are for external topical use only. They are **not** for ophthalmic or other use.	**Contraindications:** Herpes simplex, superficial fungal or yeast infections, tuberculosis of the skin, vaccinia, and varicella. **ADRs:** Generally well tolerated. May cause local ADRs, including folliculitis, irritation, and a sensation of stinging at the application site. Application of topical betamethasone to large areas of denuded or inflamed skin may result in HPA axis suppression and the associated potential for the development of glucocorticosteroid insufficiency upon discontinuation of betamethasone pharmacotherapy. When compared to older children and adolescents, infants and young children, because of their higher ratio of skin surface area to body mass, are at relatively greater risk for the development of HPA axis suppression. **Note:** *See* Chapter 5 for systemic ADRs.

TABLE 14-1 continued

DRUG (*TRADE* AND OTHER NAMES)	INDICATION(S)	USUAL PEDIATRIC DOSAGE AND ADMINISTRATION[a]	DOSAGE FORMS	CONTRAINDICATIONS, ADRs, AND COMMENTS[b]
Bethanechol (*Duvoid*®, *Myotonachol*®, *Urecholine*®)	**Gastroesophageal reflux** **Note:** Not approved by the FDA or HPB for this indication.	**Children and adolescents:** 0.1–0.2 mg/kg/dose PO three or four times daily, 30 min **prior** to meals. *Maximum:* 100 mg/day PO. **Note:** Administer each oral dose on an empty stomach. Administration with food may cause nausea and vomiting.	Injectable, SC: 5 mg/ml **Note:** For SC use only. Do **not** administer IM or IV. Tablets, oral: 5, 10, 25, 50 mg	**Contraindications:** Asthma, bradycardia (marked), coronary artery disease, epilepsy, hypersensitivity to bethanechol, hyperthyroidism, hypotension, peptic ulcer, and vasomotor instability. (*See also* ADRs.) **ADRs:** Generally well tolerated when administered orally at recommended dosages. May cause abdominal discomfort, flushing of the skin, salivation (excessive), and sweating (excessive). Higher dosages have been associated with asthmatic attacks, headache, hypotension, malaise, and nausea. Because bethanechol stimulates the parasympathetic nervous system and, consequently, increases the tone of related muscles, it should **not** be used for pediatric patients who have mechanical obstruction within the GI or urinary tracts or when the integrity of the GI or bladder walls is in doubt. **Note:** Atropine is a specific antidote for bethanechol overdosage. Whenever bethanechol is administered subcutaneously for children and adolescents, ensure that a syringe containing a dose of atropine (0.01 mg/kg or 0.4 mg, whichever is less) is available for the emergency treatment of bethanechol overdosage.
	Urinary retention (acute postoperative and as a result of neurogenic atony of the urinary bladder)	**Children and adolescents:** *Oral pharmacotherapy*, 0.6 mg/kg/day PO in three or four divided doses every 6 or 8 hr. *Maximum:* 50 mg/dose PO; 200 mg/day PO. *Subcutaneous pharmacotherapy*, 0.15–0.2 mg/kg/day SC in three or four divided doses every 6 or 8 hr. *Maximum:* 10 mg/dose SC. **Note:** Injectable pharmacotherapy is **not** generally recommended.		
Bioallethrin and Piperonyl Butoxide in a fixed-ratio combination (*PARA*®)	**Head lice** (*Pediculus capitis*) and their nits, infestation	**Infants, children, and adolescents:** Apply shampoo to wet hair and rub well into scalp. Leave on scalp for 5 min, then rinse thoroughly. Repeat. When hair is dry, comb hair with a fine tooth comb to remove dead lice and their nits. **Note:** Treatment should be repeated in 7 days in order to reduce the risk for re-infestation.	Shampoo: 1.1% bioallethrin and 4.4% piperonyl butoxide **Note:** For external use only. Avoid contact with eyes.	**Contraindications:** Hypersensitivity to bioallethrin or to other synthetic or natural pyrethrins/pyrethroids. **ADRs:** Generally well tolerated. Avoid contact with eyes; may cause minor eye irritation. **Comments:** To minimize potential for re-infestation, all family and household members should be treated and all clothing and bedding dry cleaned, washed in very hot water, or treated with an appropriate domestic insecticide spray.
Bisacodyl (*Dulcolax*®)	**Constipation,** occasional **Note:** Generally indicated for short-term use not exceeding 7 consecutive days.	**Children:** 0.3 mg/kg/day PO, in a single dose. *Maximum:* Children (<6 years), 5 mg/day PO; children (≥6 years), 15 mg/day PO.	Solution, rectal enema: 10 mg/30 ml in a single-dose squeeze bottle with prelubricated tip; shake well before use. Suppositories, rectal: 5, 10 mg Tablet, oral enteric coated: 5 mg (contains tartrazine)	**Contradictions:** Acute surgical abdomen, appendicitis, dehydration (severe), gastroenteritis, hypersensitivity to bisacodyl, intestinal obstruction, and rectal bleeding. **ADRs:** Generally well tolerated. May cause some abdominal discomfort and diarrhea. *See* Chapter 5.
	Bowel preparation for diagnostic procedure or surgery	**Children (<6 years):** 15-ml enema (5 mg) rectal 15–60 min before laxative effect is required.		

(Continued)

TABLE 14-1 *continued*

DRUG (*TRADE* AND OTHER NAMES)	INDICATION(S)	USUAL PEDIATRIC DOSAGE AND ADMINISTRATION[a]	DOSAGE FORMS	CONTRAINDICATIONS, ADRs, AND COMMENTS[b]
Bisacodyl *continued*		**Children (≥6 years) and adolescents:** 10-mg suppository or 30-ml enema (10 mg) rectal 15–60 min before laxative effect is required. **Note:** Combination oral and rectal bisacodyl pharmacotherapy is indicated for most bowel preparations.	**Note:** Do not break, crush, or divide bisacodyl oral enteric-coated tablets and do **not** administer with milk or antacids. Advise children and adolescents not to chew enteric-coated tablets. **Note:** If rectal suppository appears to be soft, hold it within its foil wrapper under cold water for 1 or 2 min to harden it. The rectal suppository may be lubricated with water or a water-soluble lubricant to facilitate insertion.	**Comments:** Therapeutic effect generally occurs within 6–12 hr if the oral dose is ingested before bedtime or within 6 hr if the oral dose is ingested before breakfast.
Bismuth Subsalicylate (*Pepto-Bismol®, Pink Bismuth®*)	Diarrhea/ Indigestion	**Children (3–6 years):** Initially, 87 mg PO. Repeat dose at 0.5–1-hr intervals as indicated by response. *Maximum:* Eight doses (698 mg)/24 hr PO. **Children (>6–9 years):** Initially, 174 mg PO. Repeat dose at 0.5–1-hr intervals as indicated by response. *Maximum:* Eight doses (1392 mg)/24 hr PO. **Children (>9 years):** Initially, 262 mg PO. Repeat dose at 0.5–1-hr intervals as indicated by response. *Maximum:* Eight doses (2096 mg)/24 hr PO. **Adolescents:** Initially, 524 mg PO. Repeat dose at 0.5–1-hr intervals as indicated by response. *Maximum:* Eight doses (4192 mg)/24 hr PO.	Caplet, oral: 262 mg Suspensions, oral: 130 mg/15 ml, 262 mg/15 ml, 524 mg/15 ml; shake well before use. Tablet, oral chewable: 262 mg (cherry flavored) **Note:** Each dose of the bismuth subsalicylate oral caplets should be swallowed whole. Each dose of the oral chewable tablets may be chewed, dissolved in the mouth, or swallowed whole.	**Contraindications:** Hypersensitivity to salicylates. **ADRs:** Generally well tolerated. **Comments:** Contains nonaspirin salicylates. Children and adolescents who have a viral infection (e.g., chickenpox or influenza) should **not** be treated with bismuth subsalicylate because of the risk for Reye's syndrome, which is usually associated with aspirin. **Note:** Bismuth subsalicylate pharmacotherapy has been associated with a harmless, temporary darkening of the tongue and/or stool.
Bleomycin, *see* **Chapter 12**				
Botulinum Toxin Type A (*Botox®*)	Blepharospasm associated with dystonia	**Adolescents:** Initially, 1.25–2.5 units (0.05–0.1 ml) IM into both the medial and lateral pretarsal orbicularis oculi of the upper lid and into the lateral pretorsal orbicularis oculi of the lower lid. **Note:** Therapeutic effects should last ~3 months. The initial dose may be repeated, as needed, indefinitely. If the therapeutic effects last ≤2 months, then the dosage may be increased. *Maximum, single dose:* 5 units/injection/site. *Maximum, cumulative dosage:* 200 units/2 months.	Injectable, IM: 100 units/vial (vacuum dried) **Note:** Reconstitute botulinum toxin injectable with 1–8 ml of preservative-free, sterile normal saline for injection. Botulinum toxin is denatured by frothing associated with severe agitation of the vial. Therefore, gently inject the diluent into the vial and do **not** shake to mix. Reconstituted botulinum toxin is stable for 4 hr, if refrigerated between 2 and 8°C. Safely and appropriately discard any unused reconstituted solution after 4 hr.	**Contraindications:** Amyotrophic lateral sclerosis, Eaton-Lambert syndrome, hypersensitivity to botulinum toxin, infection at the intended IM injection site, myasthenia gravis, and peripheral neuromuscular dysfunction. **ADRs:** Commonly causes dysphagia (generally mild, but rarely has been associated with aspiration, pneumonia, and death), focal weakness (an expected pharmacological action of botulinum toxin), and pain associated with localized response to IM injections(s).
	Dynamic equinus foot deformity associated with spasticity among pediatric patients with cerebral palsy	**Children (≥2 years):** Initially, 4 units/kg IM in two divided doses. When therapeutic benefit diminishes, dosage may be repeated, but not more frequently than every 2 months.		

TABLE 14-1 continued

DRUG (TRADE AND OTHER NAMES)	INDICATION(S)	USUAL PEDIATRIC DOSAGE AND ADMINISTRATION[a]	DOSAGE FORMS	CONTRAINDICATIONS, ADRs, AND COMMENTS[b]
Botulinum Toxin Type A *continued*		*Maximum*: 200 units/single dose. **Note:** Generally administered intramuscularly into the medial and lateral heads of the gastrocnemius muscle of the affected lower limb(s). **Note:** Therapeutic benefit usually lasts, on average, ~3 months.	**Note:** For IM use **only**. **Note:** Store vials containing vacuum-dried botulinum toxin in a freezer $\leq -5°C$.	
	Strabismus **Note:** Botulinum toxin creates a temporary paralysis of the injected muscles of the eye, which generally begins within 2 days after injection; increases in intensity over the first week following the injection; and lasts for up to 6 weeks. Resolution of paralysis generally follows a similar time frame in reverse.	**Note:** Prior to the injection of botulinum toxin for the treatment of strabismus, it is recommended that the affected eye be prepared by instilling several drops of a local anesthetic and an ocular decongestant several minutes before the injection. *Maximum, single dose*: 25 units per IM injection site. **Adolescents:** Initial dosage is determined by specific type of strabismus, as follows. Note that the recommended volume of botulinum toxin type A injected for the treatment of strabismus is 0.05–0.15 ml per muscle site.		**Note:** Inducing paralysis in one or more extraocular muscles may produce partial disorientation, double vision, or past-pointing. Covering the affected eye may alleviate these effects. In addition, extraocular muscles adjacent to the injection site may be affected by the botulinum toxin type A resulting in ptosis or vertical deviation, particularly when higher doses are injected. The incidence rates for these ADRs are ~16% for ptosis and ~17% for vertical deviation.

Botulinum Toxin Type A Dosage per Strabismus Site

TYPE OF STRABISMUS	DOSAGE
Vertical muscles and horizontal strabismus of less than 20 prism diopters	1.25–2.5 units in any one ocular muscle site
Horizontal strabismus of 20 prism diopters to 50 prism diopters	2.5–5 units in any one ocular muscle site
Persistent (1 month or longer duration) VI nerve palsy of the eye	1.25–2.5 units in the medial rectus muscle of the eye

DRUG	INDICATION(S)	USUAL PEDIATRIC DOSAGE AND ADMINISTRATION	DOSAGE FORMS	CONTRAINDICATIONS, ADRs, AND COMMENTS
	Note: Botulinum toxin type A is intended for injection into extraocular muscles using the electrical activity recorded from the tip of the injection needle as a guide to placement within the target muscle. Injection without surgical exposure or electromyographic guidance should **not** be attempted. Physicians should be familiar with electromyographic techniques.	Subsequent dosage is determined by response and the following recommendations. *Note that subsequent injections of botulinum toxin should not be administered until the effects of the initial or previous dose have dissipated as evidenced by substantial function in the injected and adjacent muscles of the eye.* *Recommendations*: • Re-examine patients 7–14 days after each injection to monitor response. • Patients who have adequate paralysis of the target muscle, but who may require subsequent injections, should receive a dose comparable to the initial dose. • Patients who have incomplete paralysis of the target muscle may require a subsequent dose increased by up to twofold of the initial dose.		
Brompheniramine (*Dimetane®*, *Dimetapp Allergy®*, Parabromdylamine)	**Allergic rhinitis**, perennial and seasonal	**Children and adolescents:** 0.35–0.5 mg/kg/day PO in three or four divided doses. *Maximum:* Children, 12 mg/day PO; adolescents, 24 mg/day PO.	Capsule, oral: 4 mg Tablet, oral: 4 mg **Note:** Commonly found in combination cough and cold products often with a decongestant.	**Contraindications:** Acute status asthmaticus, hypersensitivity to brompheniramine, narrow-angle glaucoma, peptic ulcer, and urinary retention. **ADRs:** May cause blurred vision and drowsiness.

Footnotes are on page 558.

TABLE 14-1 continued

DRUG (TRADE AND OTHER NAMES)	INDICATION(S)	USUAL PEDIATRIC DOSAGE AND ADMINISTRATION[a]	DOSAGE FORMS	CONTRAINDICATIONS, ADRs, AND COMMENTS[b]
Budesonide, nasal (*Rhinocort Aqua®, Rhinocort Turbuhaler®*) **Note**: See also Budesonide, pulmonary.	**Rhinitis**, perennial or seasonal **Nasal polyps**, treatment and prevention (after polypectomy)	**Children (≥6 years) and adolescents:** *Nasal solution*, 256 µg/day intranasal. Daily dosage may be administered either once daily in the morning or divided into two doses, morning and evening. **Children (≥6 years) and adolescents:** *Nasal solution*, 256 µg/day intranasal in two divided doses, morning and evening. **Note:** Divide each dose between left and right nostrils (64 µg in each nostril, morning and evening). *Nasal powder*, 400 µg/day intranasal once daily in the morning. **Note:** Divide daily dose between left and right nostrils (200 µg in each nostril).	Powder, metered-dose nasal inhaler: 100 µg/actuation *(Rhinocort Turbuhaler)*; shake well before use. Solution, metered-dose nasal inhaler: 32 µg/actuation, 64 µg/actuation *(Rhinocort Aqua)*; shake well before use. **Note:** For intranasal use only. The metered-dose nasal inhaler requires priming with four actuations prior to first use.	**Contraindications:** Hypersensitivity to budesonide; tuberculosis (history); and untreated infections, active (bacterial, fungal, or viral), particularly those in the nasal mucosa. **ADRs:** Generally well tolerated. May cause headache, nasal irritation (bleeding, crusting, drying), nausea, and sore throat.
Budesonide, pulmonary (*Pulmicort Nebuamp®, Pulmicort Turbuhaler®*) **Note:** See also Budesonide, nasal.	**Asthma**, chronic prophylactic management **Note: Not** indicated for the management of acute asthmatic attacks (acute bronchospasm).	**Infants (≥3 months) and children:** 250–500 µg by nebulizer inhalation twice daily. **Alternative:** Children (≥6 years), 200–400 µg/day by MDI in two divided doses. *Maximum:* 2000 µg/day by nebulizer inhalation. **Adolescents:** 500–1000 µg by nebulizer inhalation twice daily; **or**, initially, 400–2400 µg/day by MDI in two to four divided doses. *Maintenance*, 400–800 µg/day by MDI in two divided doses. *Maximum:* 4000 µg/day by nebulizer. **Note:** Rinse mouth after budesonide nebulizer inhalation or MDI use in order to help prevent associated candidiasis.	Powder for inhalation in metered-dose inhaler (MDI): 100, 200, 400 µg/actuation *(Pulmicort Turbuhaler)*. **Note:** Budesonide pulmonary products are for pulmonary inhalation only. The budesonide powder inhaler requires priming prior to first use. Do **not** shake the powder inhaler after loading. Solution for inhalation by nebulizer or respirator: 0.125, 0.25, 0.5 mg/ml in 2-ml ampules *(Pulmicort Nebuamp)*. **Note:** Budesonide pulmonary solutions are for inhalation only. The solution for inhalation should be administered by nebulizer with a compressed air or oxygen flow rate of 6–10 liters/min.	**Contraindications:** Hypersensitivity to budesonide; status asthmaticus; and untreated bacterial, fungal, or viral infections of the respiratory tract. **ADRs:** Generally well tolerated. May cause cough or hoarseness and loss of, or alteration in, smell and taste. May also cause dryness and irritation of the mouth, nose, and throat. Associated systemic ADRs may affect several body systems. **Comments:** The pulmonary inhalation of budesonide, while providing intended pharmacologic response (prevention of asthma attacks), may not provide sufficient corticosteroid to prevent adrenal insufficiency among pediatric patients whose systemic corticosteroid pharmacotherapy for the treatment of asthma was replaced with budesonide pulmonary pharmacotherapy.
Bumetanide (*Burinex®*)	**Edema/ Hypertension** **Note:** Not approved by the FDA or HPB for children or adolescents.	**Adolescents:** Initially, 0.5–1 mg/day IM, IV, or PO, as a single dose. May repeat dose, if required, at 2–3-hr intervals IM or IV (4–5-hr intervals PO), as indicated by response. *Maximum:* 10 mg/day IM, IV, or PO. **Note:** When feasible, the oral route is preferred.	Injectable, IM, IV: 0.25 mg/ml (contains benzyl alcohol as a preservative) Tablets, oral: 0.5, 1, 2, 5 mg	**Contraindications:** Anuria, hepatic coma, hypersensitivity to bumetanide or to other sulfonamide derivatives, and severe electrolyte depletion. **ADRs:** May cause deafness, dehydration, dizziness, and electrolyte imbalance. **Comments:** A potent diuretic. Carefully monitor fluid and electrolyte status.

TABLE 14-1 continued

DRUG (TRADE AND OTHER NAMES)	INDICATION(S)	USUAL PEDIATRIC DOSAGE AND ADMINISTRATION[a]	DOSAGE FORMS	CONTRAINDICATIONS, ADRs, AND COMMENTS[b]
Bupivacaine *(Marcaine®, Sensorcaine®)*	**Anesthesia**, local or regional (used to facilitate diagnostic, surgical, or other therapeutic procedures)	**Children (>2 years):** Initial dosage is determined by the type of anesthesia desired, as follows. In most clinical situations, a single dose of bupivacaine is sufficient. However, if necessary, the initial dose may be repeated up to once every 3 hr. *Maximum*: 175 mg/dose; 400 mg/day.	Solutions, injectable, local or regional: 0.25%, 0.5%, 0.75% **Note:** Protect solutions from light. Do **not** use if solutions are discolored pink, darker than light yellow, or contain a precipitate. **Note:** The 0.25% and 0.5% bupivacaine injectable solutions may contain sodium metabisulfite and are available with epinephrine (1:200,000). The 0.75% hyperbaric injectable solution is for spinal use **only**.	**Contraindications:** Hypersensitivity to bupivacaine or to other amide-type local anesthetics, intravenous regional anesthesia (leakage has resulted in **cardiac arrest and death**), and obstetrical paracervical block anesthesia (use of obstetrical paracervical block anesthesia has resulted in **fetal bradycardia and death**). **ADRs:** Generally well tolerated. High doses have been associated with cardiovascular depression and CNS stimulation (followed by drowsiness, unconsciousness, and respiratory arrest). **Comments:** Administration into the head and neck (e.g., dental, retrobulbar, and stellate ganglia blocks) have been associated with significant ADRs (e.g., confusion, convulsions, respiratory depression), even with low dosages. Patients must be carefully observed and monitored, particularly for adverse circulatory and respiratory changes.

Dosage for Type of Anesthesia (Children)

TYPE OF BLOCK	BUPIVACAINE CONCENTRATION	EACH DOSE (ml/kg)	EACH DOSE (mg/kg)
Caudal	0.25%	0.4–0.8	1–2
	0.5%	0.2–0.4	1–2
Dorsal (penile)	0.25% (without epinephrine)	0.1–0.2	0.3–0.5
	0.5% (without epinephrine)	0.06–0.1	0.3–0.5
Intercostal	0.25% (without epinephrine)	0.8–1.2	2–3
	0.5% (without epinephrine)	0.4–0.6	2–3
Local infiltration for hernia repair	0.25%	0.2–0.8	0.5–2
	0.5%	0.1–0.4	0.5–2
Lumbar epidural	0.25%	0.6–1	1.5–2.5
	0.5%	0.3–0.5	1.5–2.5

Adolescents: Initial dosage is determined by the type of anesthesia desired, as follows. In most clinical situations, a single dose of bupivacaine is sufficient. However, if necessary, the initial dose may be repeated up to once every 3 hr.
Maximum: 175 mg/dose; 400 mg/day.

Dosage for Type of Anesthesia (Adolescents)

TYPE OF BLOCK	BUPIVACAINE CONCENTRATION	EACH DOSE (in ml)	EACH DOSE (in mg)
Caudal	0.25%	15–30	37.5–75
	0.5%	15–30	75–150
Epidural	0.25%	10–20	25–50
	0.5%	10–20	50–100
	0.75%	10–20	75–150
Local infiltration	0.25%	up to 70	up to 175
Peripheral nerves	0.25%	5–60	12.5–150
	0.5%	5–30	25–150
Retrobulbar	0.75%	2–4	15–30
Sympathetic	0.25%	20–50	50–125

Busulfan, *see* **Chapter 12**

Footnotes are on page 558.

TABLE 14-1 continued

DRUG (*TRADE* AND OTHER NAMES)	INDICATION(S)	USUAL PEDIATRIC DOSAGE AND ADMINISTRATION[a]	DOSAGE FORMS	CONTRAINDICATIONS, ADRs, AND COMMENTS[b]
Butenafine (*Mentax®*)	**Tinea pedis** (athlete's foot), interdigital	**Adolescents:** Apply sufficient amount of cream to cover affected areas and immediately surrounding skin twice daily for 7 days.	Cream, topical: 1% **Note:** For external topical use only. Not for ophthalmic use or for use in the mouth, nose, or on other mucous membranes. **Note:** Not generally available in Canada.	**Contraindications:** Hypersensitivity to butenafine. **ADRs:** Generally well tolerated. May cause contact dermatitis, erythema, irritation, and itching at site of application.
	Tinea corporis (ringworm)/**Tinea cruris** (jock itch) **Note:** Generally effective against superficial dermatophytoses due to *Epidermophyton floccosum, Trichophyton mentagrophytes, T. rubrum,* and *T. tonsurans*.	**Adolescents:** Apply sufficient amount of cream to cover affected areas and immediately surrounding skin once daily for 14 days.		
Butoconazole (*Femstat-3®, Gynazole-1®*)	**Vulvovaginal candidiasis** (vaginal yeast infection)	**Adolescents:** One applicatorful of vaginal cream/day intravaginally at bedtime for 3–6 days. **Note:** *See* Chapter 1 for administration of vaginal cream.	Cream, vaginal: 2% (in 5-gram single-dose prefilled disposable applicator) (contains mineral oil that may weaken latex or rubber products, such as condoms or vaginal contraceptive diaphragms) **Note:** For vaginal use only. **Note:** Not generally available in Canada.	**Contraindications:** Hypersensitivity to butoconazole and pregnancy (first trimester). **ADRs:** Generally well tolerated. May cause vulvovaginal burning sensation, discharge, itching, and soreness. **Comments:** Recurrent vaginal infections among nonpregnant adolescents, particularly those that are difficult to treat, may be indicative of HIV infection.
Caffeine Citrate, *see* **Chapter 13**				
Calamine	**Temporary relief of itching** associated with minor skin irritation, including that related to mild hypersensitivity reactions to poison ivy, oak, and sumac	**Children and adolescents:** Apply topically to affected area(s) two or three times daily. **Note:** Affected skin sites should be gently cleaned with soap and warm water and dried carefully prior to each application.	Lotion, topical: 8%; shake well before use. **Note:** For external use only. Avoid contact with eyes.	**Contraindications:** Hypersensitivity to calamine. **ADRs:** May cause rash or skin irritation at site of topical application.
Calcitriol (*Calcijex®,* 1α,25-Dihydroxycholecalciferol, *Rocaltrol®*)	**Vitamin D deficiency**	**Infants, children, and adolescents:** Initially, 0.015–0.025 μg/kg/day PO as a single dose. Increase the dosage gradually to 0.5–1 μg/day PO according to response.	Capsules, oral: 0.25, 0.5 μg Injectables, IV: 1, 2 μg/ml Solution, oral: 1 μg/ml	**Contraindications:** Hypercalcemia, hypersensitivity to vitamin D, and hypervitaminosis D. **ADRs:** Generally well tolerated. *See* Chapter 5 **Comments:** Monitor calcium and phosphate serum concentrations.
Calcium	**Hypocalcemia**	**Infants, children, and adolescents:** 0.1–0.2 mmol elemental calcium/kg/hr IV. **Note:** Adjust infusion rate every 4 hr according to calcium and phosphate (PO_4) plasma concentrations. **Note:** The use of IV calcium is generally avoided in digitalized patients.	Elemental calcium content of various calcium salts: carbonate (40%) chloride (27%) citrate (21%) glubionate (6.5%) glucoheptonate (8%) gluconate (9%) lactate (13%) phosphate dibasic anhydrous (29%) phosphate dibasic dihydrate (23%) phosphate tribasic (40%) **Note:** For IV use only. Avoid extravasation,	**Contraindications:** Digitalis toxicity, hypercalcemia, hypercalciuria, hypervitaminosis D, renal dysfunction (severe), and ventricular fibrillation. **ADRs:** Generally well tolerated. Rapid IV administration may cause bradycardia, cardiac arrest, drowsiness, fainting, flushing, hypotension, nausea, sweating, and vomiting. **Comments:** ECG and heart rate must be continuously monitored during IV infusion.
	Calcium deficiency and hyperphosphatemia prophylaxis among patients with renal disease	**Infants:** 375 mg elemental calcium/day PO in three divided doses. **Children:** 750 mg elemental calcium/day PO in three divided doses.		

TABLE 14-1 continued

DRUG (TRADE AND OTHER NAMES)	INDICATION(S)	USUAL PEDIATRIC DOSAGE AND ADMINISTRATION[a]	DOSAGE FORMS	CONTRAINDICATIONS, ADRs, AND COMMENTS[b]
Calcium *continued*			which may result in skin necrosis and sloughing. **Note:** 1 gram of elemental calcium = 25 mmol of elemental calcium = 50 mEq of elemental calcium.	
Calcium Carbonate *(Alka-Mints®, Dicarbosil®, Maalox Antacid Caplets®, Mylanta Lozenges®, Tums®)*	Dyspepsia/ Gastroesophageal reflux/Peptic ulcer disease	**Children and adolescents:** Initially, 0.5–1.5 grams PO as a single dose. Repeat dose as indicated. **Note:** Tablets should be chewed thoroughly before swallowing.	Lozenges, oral: 600 mg (cherry creme and cool mint creme flavored) Tablets, oral: 500, 600, 650, 1000, 1250 mg Tablets, oral chewable: 350, 420, 500, 750, 850, 1000 mg (assorted flavors) **Note:** Calcium carbonate contains 40% calcium; 20 mEq/gram.	**Contraindications:** Calcium loss due to immobility, cardiac disease (severe), hypercalcemia, and ventricular fibrillation. **ADRs:** Generally well tolerated. May cause alkalosis, constipation, and hypercalcemia. *See* Chapter 5. **Comments:** Calcium obtained from dolomite, fossil or oyster shells, or bone meal contains varying significant amounts of lead. For chronic long-term pharmacotherapy, it is advised that a refined calcium carbonate product be used that generally contains lower amounts of lead.

Calcium Chloride, *see* Chapters 4 and 13
Calcium Citrate, *see* Chapter 13
Calcium Gluconate, *see* Chapter 13

DRUG (TRADE AND OTHER NAMES)	INDICATION(S)	USUAL PEDIATRIC DOSAGE AND ADMINISTRATION[a]	DOSAGE FORMS	CONTRAINDICATIONS, ADRs, AND COMMENTS[b]
Captopril *(Capoten®)*	Hypertension/ Congestive heart failure **Note:** Captopril pharmacotherapy is commonly used in combination with diuretic pharmacotherapy.	**Infants, children, and adolescents:** Initially, 0.2–0.3 mg/kg/day PO in two or three divided doses. Increase dosage to 0.5–6 mg/kg/day PO in two or three divided doses according to response. *Maximum:* 6 mg/kg/day PO **or** 450 mg/day PO, whichever is less. **Note:** Each dose should be administered 1 hr before meals in order to maximize GI absorption. **Note:** Reduce dosage for pediatric patients who have renal dysfunction; *see* Table 14-2.	Tablets, oral: 12.5, 25, 50, 100 mg	**Contraindications:** Hypersensitivity to captopril or to other angiotensin-converting enzyme (ACE) inhibitors. **ADRs:** May cause angioedema, angina pectoris, flushing, nausea, neutropenia, proteinuria, pruritus, rash, renal failure, and tachycardia. *See* Chapter 5. **Comments:** Monitor blood pressure because of potential hypotension, hematology because of potential neutropenia, and urinary protein because of potential proteinuria.
Carbamazepine *(Tegretol®)*	Generalized tonic-clonic (grand mal) seizures/Partial (focal) seizures/ Benign Rolandic epilepsy	**Infants, children, and adolescents:** Initially, 10 mg/kg/day PO as a single daily dose or as two divided doses; then 20–40 mg/kg/day PO in two or three divided doses, every 8 or 12 hr. **Note:** Reduce dosage for pediatric patients who have hepatic dysfunction. **Note:** Carbamazepine oral chewable tablets must be thoroughly chewed before swallowing, not swallowed whole; controlled-release tablets may be divided to adjust dosage or facilitate ingestion; administer with food or milk.	Suspension, oral: 100 mg/5 ml; shake well before use. Tablet, oral: 200 mg Tablets, oral chewable: 100, 200 mg Tablets, oral controlled release: 200, 400 mg	**Contraindications:** AV heart block, blood dyscrasias, hepatic dysfunction (severe), hypersensitivity to carbamazepine or to the tricyclic antidepressants (TCA), intermittent porphyria, and MAOI therapy (concurrent or within the previous 14 days). **ADRs:** May cause diplopia, dizziness, headache, and nausea. *See* Chapter 5. **Comments:** Monitor hepatic function upon initiation of therapy and periodically. Therapeutic drug monitoring is recommended; *see* Table 14-3. **Note:** Carbamazepine is a hepatic microsomal enzyme inducer and may, therefore, increase the hepatic metabolism of other drugs. *See* Chapter 6.

Footnotes are on page 558.

DRUG (TRADE AND OTHER NAMES)	INDICATION(S)	USUAL PEDIATRIC DOSAGE AND ADMINISTRATION[a]	DOSAGE FORMS	CONTRAINDICATIONS, ADRs, AND COMMENTS[b]
Carbamide Peroxide, for intra-oral use (*Gly-Oxide*®, *Orajel Perioseptic*®, *Proxigel*®, Urea Peroxide) **Note:** For topical intra-oral use only.	Relief of minor oral inflammation, including that associated with canker sores or denture irritation/**Aid to oral hygiene** for patients who wear orthodontic or dental appliances	**Children (>3 years) and adolescents:** Apply topical intra-oral gel or undiluted topical intra-oral solution to affected area in the oral cavity four times daily according to the following recommendations: *Topical intra-oral gel*: Gently massage a small amount into the affected oral site. Advise children and adolescents to avoid drinking liquids or rinsing the mouth for 5 min after topical application. *Topical intra-oral solution*: Either drip several drops onto the affected mucous membranes of the mouth and instruct the child or adolescent to expectorate after 2–3 min **or** drip ~10 drops on the tongue, mix with saliva in the mouth, swish the solution and saliva in the mouth for 2–3 min, and then expectorate.	Gel, topical intra-oral: 10% Solutions, topical: 10%, 15% **Note:** Carbamide peroxide 10% and 15% gel and solution products are for intra-oral topical use only. These products are **not** to be swallowed.	**Contraindications:** None identified. **ADRs:** Generally well tolerated.
Carbamide Peroxide, for otic use (*Auro Ear Drops*®, *Debrox Otic*®, *E.R.O Ear*®, *Molifene Ear Wax Removing Formula*®, *Murine Ear Drops*®, Urea Peroxide)	Ear wax removal	**Children and adolescents:** Instill 5–10 drops in affected ear(s) twice daily for up to 4 days. **Note:** Gently flush the external ear canal with warm water using a soft rubber bulb syringe to facilitate the removal of any remaining ear wax after treatment.	Solution, otic: 6.5% (generally also contains alcohol and glycerin) **Note:** For use in the external ear canal only.	**Contraindications:** Perforated or ruptured tympanic membrane. **ADRs:** Generally well tolerated.
Carbenicillin Indanyl Sodium (*Geocillin*®)	Acute and chronic bacterial infections of the lower and upper urinary tracts **Note:** Ensure that appropriate culture and sensitivity tests are performed and that the organism is sensitive to carbenicillin. **Note:** Not approved by the FDA or HPB for infants or children.	**Infants, children, and adolescents:** 30–50 mg/kg/day PO in four divided doses, every 6 hr. *Maximum:* 3 grams/day PO.	Tablet, oral: 500 mg (382 mg carbenicillin base and 118 mg indanyl sodium) **Note:** Tablets have a bitter taste.	**Contraindications:** Hypersensitivity to carbenicillin, other penicillins, or cephalosporins. **ADRs:** May cause diarrhea, flatulence, glossitis, nausea, and vomiting. *See* Chapter 5.
Carboplatin, *see* Chapter 12				
Carmustine, *see* Chapter 12				
Cascara Sagrada	Constipation	**Infants:** 1.25 ml/day PO at bedtime, as needed, for relief of constipation. **Children:** 2.5 ml/day PO at bedtime, as needed, for relief of constipation. **Adolescents:** 325 mg **or** 5 ml/day PO at bedtime, as needed, for relief of constipation.	Fluidextract, oral: contains ~18% alcohol Tablet, oral: 325 mg	**Contraindications:** Abdominal pain (undiagnosed), fecal impaction, hypersensitivity to cascara sagrada, intestinal obstruction, and signs and symptoms of appendicitis (e.g., nausea, vomiting). **ADRs:** May cause abdominal cramps, diarrhea, and flatulence. *See* Chapter 5. **Comments:** Onset of action generally occurs within 6–10 hr of administration.

TABLE 14-1 continued

DRUG (TRADE AND OTHER NAMES)	INDICATION(S)	USUAL PEDIATRIC DOSAGE AND ADMINISTRATION[a]	DOSAGE FORMS	CONTRAINDICATIONS, ADRs, AND COMMENTS[b]
Castor Oil	Colonic evacuation (prior to medical examination, radiology, or surgery) **Note:** Routine use for the treatment of constipation is not recommended. Other safer and more effective laxatives are available.	**Infants:** 1–5 ml/dose PO. **Children:** 5–15 ml/dose PO. **Adolescents:** 15–60 ml/dose PO. **Note:** Strength of castor oil formulations differ and, therefore, affect recommended dosage.	Capsule, oral liquid filled: 0.62 ml Emulsions, oral: 36.4%, 60%, 67%, 95% Liquids, oral: 95%, 100%	**Contraindications:** Acute surgical abdomen, appendicitis, fecal impaction, hypersensitivity to castor oil, and intestinal obstruction. **ADRs:** May cause abdominal cramps, diarrhea, and nausea. **Comments:** Usually effective within 2–6 hr; therefore, do not administer at bedtime.
Cefaclor (Ceclor®)	Bacterial infection **Note:** Ensure that appropriate culture and sensitivity tests are performed and that the organism is sensitive to cefaclor.	Infants, children, and adolescents: 20–40 mg/kg/day PO in two or three divided doses. *Maximum:* 2 grams/day PO. **Note:** Reduce dosage for pediatric patients who have renal dysfunction; see Table 14-2.	Capsules, oral: 250, 500 mg Suspensions, oral: 125, 250, 375 mg/5 ml (strawberry flavored); shake well before use.	**Contraindications:** Hypersensitivity to penicillins or cephalosporins. **ADRs:** See Chapter 5.
Cefadroxil (Duricef®)	Bacterial infection **Note:** Ensure that appropriate culture and sensitivity tests are performed and that the organism is sensitive to cefadroxil.	Infants, children, and adolescents: 30 mg/kg/day PO in two divided doses, every 12 hr. **Note:** Ingestion with food or milk may decrease associated GI irritation. **Note:** Reduce dosage for pediatric patients who have renal dysfunction; see Table 14-2.	Capsule, oral: 500 mg Suspensions, oral: 25, 50, 100 mg/ml; shake well before use. Tablet, oral: 1 gram	**Contraindications:** Hypersensitivity to penicillins or cephalosporins. **ADRs:** See Chapter 5.
Cefamandole (Mandol®)	Bacterial infections, mild to moderate	Infants, children, and adolescents: 50–100 mg/kg/day IM or IV in three or four divided doses, every 6 or 8 hr. *Maximum:* 2 grams/dose IM or IV; 6 grams/day IM or IV.	Injectables, IM, IV: 500 mg/vial; 1, 2 grams/vial	**Contraindications:** Hypersensitivity to cephalosporins or penicillins. **ADRs:** See Chapter 5.
	Bacterial infections, severe **Note:** Ensure that appropriate culture and sensitivity tests are performed and that the organism is sensitive to cefamandole.	Infants, children, and adolescents: 100–150 mg/kg/day IM or IV in four or six divided doses, every 4 or 6 hr. *Maximum:* 2 grams/dose IM or IV; 12 grams/day IM or IV. **Note:** Reduce dosage for pediatric patients who have renal dysfunction; see Table 14-2.		
Cefazolin (Ancef®, Kefzol®)	Bacterial infections, mild to moderate	Infants, children, and adolescents: 25–50 mg/kg/day IM or IV in three divided doses, every 8 hr. *Maximum:* 2 grams/day IM or IV.	Injectables, IM, IV: 500 mg/vial; 1 gram/vial	**Contraindications:** Hypersensitivity to cephalosporins or penicillins. **ADRs:** See Chapter 5.
	Bacterial infections, severe **Note:** Ensure that appropriate culture and sensitivity tests are performed and that the organism is sensitive to cefazolin.	Infants, children, and adolescents: 50–150 mg/kg/day IM or IV in three divided doses, every 8 hr. *Maximum:* 6 grams/day IM or IV. **Note:** Reduce dosage for pediatric patients who have renal dysfunction; see Table 14-2.		

Footnotes are on page 558.

TABLE 14-1 continued

DRUG (TRADE AND OTHER NAMES)	INDICATION(S)	USUAL PEDIATRIC DOSAGE AND ADMINISTRATION[a]	DOSAGE FORMS	CONTRAINDICATIONS, ADRs, AND COMMENTS[b]
Cefepime (*Maxipime®*)	Febrile neutropenia	**Infants (>2 months), children, and adolescents:** 150 mg/kg/day IV in three divided doses, every 8 hr, for 7–10 days. *Maximum:* 6 grams/day IV.	Injectables, IM, IV: 500 mg; 1, 2 grams **Note:** Safely store protected from light between 2 and 25°C (36–77°F).	**Contraindications:** Hypersensitivity to cefepime, cephalosporins, penicillins, or other beta-lactam antibiotics. **ADRs:** May cause diarrhea, headache, pain or inflammation at the injection site, nausea, phlebitis, and rash. *See* Chapter 5. **Comments:** Monitor patients for the development of pseudomembranous colitis. If observed, discontinue cefepime pharmacotherapy and initiate appropriate intervention as indicated.
	Bacterial infections **Note:** Ensure that appropriate culture and sensitivity tests are performed and that the organism is sensitive to cefepime.	**Infants, children, and adolescents:** 100 mg/kg/day IV in two divided doses, every 12 hr, for 7–10 days. *Maximum:* 6 grams/day IV. **Note:** Can be administered IM or IV; however, pediatric experience with IM administration is limited. **Note:** Reduce dosage for pediatric patients who have renal dysfunction; *see* Table 14-2.		
Cefixime (*Suprax®*)	Bacterial infections **Note:** Ensure that appropriate culture and sensitivity tests are performed and that the organism is sensitive to cefixime.	**Infants, children, and adolescents:** 8 mg/kg/day PO as a single daily dose or as two divided doses, every 12 hr. *Maximum:* 400 mg/day PO. **Note:** Reduce dosage for pediatric patients who have renal dysfunction; *see* Table 14-2.	Suspension, oral: 100 mg/5 ml (after reconstitution); shake well before use. Tablets, oral: 200, 400 mg	**Contraindications:** Hypersensitivity to cephalosporins or penicillins. **ADRs:** *See* Chapter 5.
	Gonorrhea, uncomplicated	**Children (<9 years or <45 kg):** 8–16 mg/kg/dose PO as a single one-time dose. **Children (≥9 years or ≥45 kg) and adolescents:** 400–800 mg/dose PO as a single one-time dose.		
Cefoperazone (*Cefobid®*)	Bacterial infections **Note:** Ensure that appropriate culture and sensitivity tests are performed and that the organism is sensitive to cefoperazone. **Note:** Not approved by the FDA or HPB for infants or children.	**Infants, children, and adolescents:** 100–150 mg/kg/day IM or IV in two or three divided doses, every 8 or 12 hr. *Maximum:* 10 grams/day IM or IV. **Note:** Reduce dosage for pediatric patients who have hepatic dysfunction.	Injectables, IM, IV: 1, 2 grams/vial	**Contraindications:** Hypersensitivity to cephalosporins or penicillins. **ADRs:** *See* Chapter 5. **Comments:** Avoid concurrent use of alcohol-containing products (e.g., cough elixirs) because of potential for the occurrence of a disulfiramlike reaction. May also cause a disulfiramlike reaction among children and adolescents who consume alcoholic beverages.
Cefotaxime (*Claforan®*)	Bacterial infections, mild to moderate	**Infants, children, and adolescents:** 100 mg/kg/day IM or IV in two or four divided doses, every 6 or 8 hr. *Maximum:* 6 grams/day IM or IV.	Injectables, IM, IV: 500 mg/vial; 1, 2 grams/vial	**Contraindications:** Hypersensitivity to cephalosporins or penicillins. **ADRs:** *See* Chapter 5.
	Bacterial infections, severe **Note:** Ensure that appropriate culture and sensitivity tests are performed and that the organism is sensitive to cefotaxime.	**Infants, children, and adolescents:** 150–200 mg/kg/day IM or IV in three or four divided doses, every 6 or 8 hr. *Maximum:* 8 grams/day IM or IV. **Note:** Reduce dosage for pediatric patients who have renal dysfunction; *see* Table 14-2.		
Cefoxitin (*Mefoxin®*)	Bacterial infections, mild to moderate	**Infants, children, and adolescents:** 80–100 mg/kg/day IM or IV in three or four divided doses, every 6 or 8 hr. IM injection is painful and,	Injectables, IM, IV: 1, 2 grams/vial	**Contraindications:** Hypersensitivity to cephalosporins or penicillins. **ADRs:** *See* Chapter 5.

TABLE 14-1 *continued*

DRUG (*TRADE* AND OTHER NAMES)	INDICATION(S)	USUAL PEDIATRIC DOSAGE AND ADMINISTRATION[a]	DOSAGE FORMS	CONTRAINDICATIONS, ADRs, AND COMMENTS[b]
Cefoxitin *continued*		therefore, generally is not recommended. *Maximum:* 4 grams/day IM or IV.		
	Bacterial infections, severe **Note:** Ensure that appropriate culture and sensitivity tests are performed and that the organism is sensitive to cefoxitin.	**Infants, children, and adolescents:** 80–160 mg/kg/day IM or IV in four or six divided doses, every 4 or 6 hr. IM injection is painful and, therefore, generally is not recommended. *Maximum:* 12 grams/day IM or IV. **Note:** Reduce dosage for pediatric patients who have renal dysfunction; *see* Table 14-2.		
Cefpodoxime Proxetil (*Vantin®*)	**Otitis media, acute, mild to moderate**	**Infants (≥2 months) and children:** 10 mg/kg/day PO in two divided doses, every 12 hr, for 5 days. *Maximum:* 400 mg/day PO.	Suspensions, oral: 50, 100 mg/5 ml (lemon creme flavored); shake well before use. Tablets, oral: 100, 200 mg	**Contraindications:** Hypersensitivity to cefpodoxime proxetil or to other cephalosporins. **ADRs:** May cause diaper rash or other skin rash, diarrhea, nausea, and vaginal fungal infections. *See* Chapter 5. **Comments:** Although the cefpodoxime proxetil oral suspension may be administered without regard to meals, the oral tablet should be administered with food in order to increase GI absorption. Monitor patients for the development of pseudomembranous colitis. If observed, discontinue cefpodoxime proxetil and initiate appropriate intervention, as indicated.
	Maxillary sinusitis, acute (mild to moderate)	**Infants (≥2 months) and children:** 10 mg/kg/day PO in two divided doses, every 12 hr, for 10 days. *Maximum:* 400 mg/day PO.		
	Pharyngitis/ Tonsillitis	**Infants (≥5 months):** 10 mg/kg/day PO in two divided doses, every 12 hr, for 5–10 days. **Adolescents:** 200 mg/day PO in two divided doses, every 12 hr, for 5–10 days.		
	Bacterial exacerbations of chronic bronchitis, acute	**Adolescents:** 400 mg/day PO in two divided doses, every 12 hr, for 10 days. **Note:** Reduce dosage for pediatric patients who have renal dysfunction; *see* Table 14-2.		
	Pneumonia, acute community acquired **Note:** Ensure that appropriate culture and sensitivity tests are performed and that the organism is sensitive to cefpodoxime proxetil.	**Adolescents:** 400 mg/day PO in two divided doses, every 12 hr, for 14 days.		
	Infections of the skin and related structures **Note:** Ensure that appropriate culture and sensitivity tests are performed and that the organism is sensitive to cefpodoxime proxetil.	**Adolescents:** 800 mg/day PO in two divided doses, every 12 hr, for 7–14 days.		
	Uncomplicated gonorrhea (adolescent boys and girls) and rectal gonorrhea (adolescent girls)	**Adolescents:** 200 mg PO as a single dose.		

(Continued)

Footnotes are on page 558.

TABLE 14-1 continued

DRUG (TRADE AND OTHER NAMES)	INDICATION(S)	USUAL PEDIATRIC DOSAGE AND ADMINISTRATION[a]	DOSAGE FORMS	CONTRAINDICATIONS, ADRs, AND COMMENTS[b]
Cefpodoxime Proxetil *continued*	Urinary tract infections, uncomplicated **Note:** Ensure that appropriate culture and sensitivity tests are performed and that the organism is sensitive to cefpodoxime proxetil.	**Adolescents:** 200 mg/day PO in two divided doses, every 12 hr, for 7 days.		
Cefprozil *(Cefzil®)*	Bacterial infections of the skin and skin structures caused by susceptible bacteria	**Children (≥2 years):** 20 mg/kg/day PO in a single dose. **Adolescents:** 500 mg/day PO in a single dose or in two divided doses, every 12 hr. *Maximum:* 1 gram/day PO.	Suspensions, oral (powder for reconstitution): 125 mg/5 ml, 250 mg/5 ml (after reconstitution) (bubble gum flavored); shake well before use. Tablets, oral: 250, 500 mg **Note:** Store at room temperature between 15 and 30°C. Protect from light and excessive humidity. Reconstituted suspension is stable for 14 days when stored in the refrigerator between 2 and 8°C (36–46°F).	**Contraindications:** Hypersensitivity to cefprozil or to other cephalosporins. **ADRs:** Generally well tolerated. May cause diarrhea, nausea, and vomiting. *See* Chapter 5.
	Pharyngitis/Tonsillitis caused by susceptible bacteria	**Infants (≥6 months) and children:** 15 mg/kg/day PO in two divided doses, every 12 hr. **Adolescents:** 500 mg/day PO in a single dose. *Maximum:* 1 gram/day PO.		
	Sinusitus (acute) caused by susceptible bacteria **Note:** Ensure that appropriate culture and sensitivity tests are performed and that the organism is sensitive to cefprozil	**Infants (≥6 months) and children:** 15 or 30 mg/kg/day PO in two divided doses, every 12 hr. **Adolescents:** 500 mg or 1 gram/day PO in two divided doses, every 12 hr. *Maximum:* 1 gram/24 hr. **Note:** Reduce dosage for pediatric patients who have renal dysfunction; *see* Table 14-2.		
Ceftazidime *(Ceptaz®, Fortaz®)*	Bacterial infections among patients with cystic fibrosis	**Infants, children, and adolescents:** 200 mg/kg/day IM or IV in three divided doses, every 8 hr. *Maximum:* 12 grams/day IM or IV.	Injectables, IM, IV: 500 mg/vial; 1, 2, 6 grams/vial	**Contraindications:** Hypersensitivity to ceftazidime, other cephalosporins, or penicillins. **ADRs:** *See* Chapter 5.
	Bacterial infections, mild to moderate	**Infants, children, and adolescents:** 75–100 mg/kg/day IM or IV in three divided doses, every 8 hr. *Maximum:* 3 grams/day IM or IV.		
	Bacterial infections, severe **Note:** Ensure that appropriate culture and sensitivity tests are performed and that the organism is sensitive to ceftazidime.	**Infants, children, and adolescents:** 125–150 mg/kg/day IM or IV in three divided doses, every 8 hr. *Maximum:* 6 grams/day IM or IV. **Note:** Reduce dosage for pediatric patients who have renal dysfunction; *see* Table 14-2.		
Ceftizoxime *(Cefizox®)*	Bacterial infections **Note:** Ensure that appropriate culture and sensitivity tests are performed and that the organism is sensitive to ceftizoxime.	**Infants, children, and adolescents:** 150–200 mg/kg/day IM or IV in two to four divided doses, every 6, 8, or 12 hr. *Maximum:* 12 grams/day IM or IV. **Note:** Reduce dosage for pediatric patients who have renal dysfunction; *see* Table 14-2.	Injectables, IM, IV: 1, 2 grams/vial	**Contraindications:** Hypersensitivity to ceftizoxime, other cephalosporins, or penicillins. **ADRs:** *See* Chapter 5.

TABLE 14-1 continued

DRUG (TRADE AND OTHER NAMES)	INDICATION(S)	USUAL PEDIATRIC DOSAGE AND ADMINISTRATION[a]	DOSAGE FORMS	CONTRAINDICATIONS, ADRs, AND COMMENTS[b]
Ceftriaxone (Rocephin®)	Bacterial infections, mild to moderate	**Infants, children, and adolescents.** 50–75 mg/kg/day IM or IV in two divided doses, every 12 hr. *Maximum:* 2 grams/day IM or IV.	Injectables, IM, IV: 250, 500 mg/vial; 1, 2 grams/vial	**Contraindications:** Hypersensitivity to ceftriaxone, other cephalosporins, or penicillins. **ADRs:** *See* Chapter 5.
	Bacterial infections, severe/ Bacterial meningitis	**Infants, children, and adolescents:** 80–100 mg/kg/day IM or IV in two divided doses, every 12 hr. *Maximum:* 2 grams/dose IM or IV; 4 grams/day IM or IV.		
	Gonorrhea, uncomplicated **Note:** Ensure that appropriate culture and sensitivity tests are performed and that the organism is sensitive to ceftriaxone.	**Infants, children, and adolescents:** 125 mg IM as a single dose for patients weighing less than 45 kg; 250 mg IM as a single dose for patients weighing 45 kg or more.		
Cefuroxime Axetil (Ceftin®)	Bacterial infections	**Infants, children, and adolescents:** 250–500 mg/day PO in two divided doses, every 12 hr. *Maximum:* 2 grams/day PO. **Note:** Reduce dosage for pediatric patients who have renal dysfunction; *see* Table 14-2.	Suspensions, oral: 125, 250 mg/5 ml (after reconstitution) (tutti-frutti flavored); shake well before use. Tablets, oral: 125, 250, 500 mg **Note:** Crushed tablets have a bitter taste.	**Contraindications:** Hypersensitivity to cephalosporins or penicillins. **ADRs:** *See* Chapter 5.
	Otitis media	**Infants and children (<2 years):** 250 mg/day PO in two divided doses, every 12 hr. **Children (≥2 years):** 500 mg/day PO in two divided doses, every 12 hr. **Note:** Reduce dosage for pediatric patients who have renal dysfunction; *see* Table 14-2.		
	Gonorrhea, uncomplicated **Note:** Ensure that appropriate culture and sensitivity tests are performed and that the organism is sensitive to cefuroxime axetil.	**Adolescents:** 1 gram PO as a single one-time dose.		
Celecoxib (Celebrex®)	Juvenile rheumatoid arthritis (refractory to conventional pharmacotherapy) **Note:** Not approved by the FDA or HPB for adolescents.	**Adolescents:** 200 mg/day PO in two divided doses. *Maximum:* 400 mg/day PO.	Capsules, oral: 100, 200 mg	**Contraindications:** Hepatic impairment (severe) and hypersensitivity to celecoxib, other NSAIDs, or sulfonamides. **ADRs:** May cause abdominal pain, diarrhea, dyspepsia, flatulence, and nausea. GI bleeding, perforation, and ulceration may occur rarely. **Comments:** Celecoxib has the potential to adversely affect renal function (reduce both renal blood flow and renal prostaglandin production), particularly among adolescents who have pre-existing renal impairment, are receiving diuretics or ACE inhibitors, or have heart failure.

Footnotes are on page 558.

TABLE 14-1 continued

DRUG (*TRADE* AND OTHER NAMES)	INDICATION(S)	USUAL PEDIATRIC DOSAGE AND ADMINISTRATION[a]	DOSAGE FORMS	CONTRAINDICATIONS, ADRs, AND COMMENTS[b]
Cephalexin (*Keflex®*)	Bacterial infections, mild to moderate **Note:** Ensure that appropriate culture and sensitivity tests are performed and that the organism is sensitive to cephalexin.	**Infants, children, and adolescents:** 25–50 mg/kg/day PO in four divided doses, every 6 hr. *Maximum:* 4 grams/day PO. **Note:** Reduce dosage for pediatric patients who have renal dysfunction; see Table 14-2.	Capsules, oral: 250, 500 mg; 1 gram Suspensions, oral: 25, 50, 100 mg/ml; shake well before use. Tablets, oral: 250, 500 mg	**Contraindications:** Hypersensitivity to cephalexin, other cephalosporins, or penicillins. **ADRs:** *See* Chapter 5.
Cephalothin (*Ceporacin®*)	Bacterial infections, mild to moderate	**Infants, children, and adolescents:** 80–100 mg/kg/day IM or IV in four divided doses, every 6 hr. *Maximum:* 4 grams/day IM or IV.	Injectables, IM, IV: 1, 2, 4, grams/vial **Note:** Not generally available in the United States.	**Contraindications:** Hypersensitivity to cephalothin, other cephalosporins, or penicillins. **ADRs:** *See* Chapter 5.
	Bacterial infections, severe **Note:** Ensure that appropriate culture and sensitivity tests are performed and that the organism is sensitive to cephalothin	**Infants, children, and adolescents:** 100–150 mg/kg/day IM or IV in four or six divided doses, every 4 or 6 hr. *Maximum:* 12 grams/day IM or IV. **Note:** Reduce dosage for pediatric patients who have renal dysfunction; see Table 14-2.		
Cetirizine (*Zyrtec®*)	Chronic urticaria/ Perennial allergic rhinitis/Seasonal allergic rhinitis **Note:** The same dosage is used for each indication.	**Children (2–5 years):** 2.5 mg/day PO as a single dose. *Maximum:* 5 mg/day PO. **Children (≥ 6 years) and adolescents:** 5 or 10 mg/day PO as a single dose. **Note:** Reduce dosage for pediatric patients who have renal (*see* Table 14-2) or hepatic dysfunction.	Syrup: 5 mg/5 ml (banana–grape flavored) Tablets, oral: 5, 10 mg	**Contraindications:** Hypersensitivity to cetirizine. **ADRs:** May cause abdominal pain, dry mouth, fatigue, and somnolence. **Comments:** May cause cognitive impairment and, therefore, adversely affect scholastic performance.
Charcoal, Activated (*Actidose®, CharcoAid®, Charcodote®, Liqui-Char®*) **Note:** *See also* Chapter 4.	Poisoning, acute **Note:** Activated charcoal is **not** indicated for caustic or corrosive poisoning ingestions. Not particularly effective for alcohol (ethanol), iron salts, or methanol poisonings.	**Children and adolescents:** 0.5–1 gram/kg/dose PO or by nasogastric tube every 4–6 hr. *Maximum:* **Children,** 25 grams/dose PO or by nasogastric tube; **adolescents,** 100 grams/dose PO or by nasogastric tube. **Note:** Administer a laxative with the initial dose and with every other dose thereafter, as needed.	Capsule, oral: 260 mg Suspensions, oral (in aqueous solution): 0.625 gram/5 ml, 1 gram/5 ml, 1.25 grams/5 ml; shake well before use. Suspensions, oral (in sorbitol): 0.625 gram/5 ml, 0.7 gram/5 ml, 1 gram/5 ml; shake well before use. Tablet, oral: 325 mg	**Contraindications:** None identified. **ADRs:** May cause constipation, diarrhea, and vomiting. **Comments:** *See* Chapter 4 for additional discussion of poisoning.
Chloral Hydrate	Sedation for diagnostic or surgical procedures **Note:** Most radiologic examinations may be performed without sedation. However, diagnostic examinations that require prolonged periods of immobility (e.g., tomography) usually require sedation.	**Infants, children, and adolescents:** 50–75 mg/kg/dose PO or rectal 20–45 min before procedure. *Maximum:* 1 gram/dose PO or rectal.	Capsules, oral: 250, 500 mg Suppositories, rectal: 325, 500, 650 mg Syrup, oral: 50 mg/ml **Note:** Chloral hydrate oral capsules may be administered rectally when chloral hydrate rectal suppositories are unavailable. To administer oral capsules rectally, moisten slightly with tap water and insert in the same manner as for the rectal suppository.	**Contraindications:** Cardiac dysfunction, gastritis, hepatic dysfunction (severe), hypersensitivity to chloral hydrate, and renal dysfunction (severe). **ADRs:** May cause diarrhea, flatulence, nausea, vomiting, and unpleasant taste. *See* Chapter 5. **Comments:** Neonates and children <6 years rarely require sedation unless they are developmentally disabled. **Note:** Monitor respiratory function.

CHAPTER 14: DRUG DOSING FOR INFANTS, CHILDREN, AND ADOLESCENTS

TABLE 14-1 continued

DRUG (TRADE AND OTHER NAMES)	INDICATION(S)	USUAL PEDIATRIC DOSAGE AND ADMINISTRATION[a]	DOSAGE FORMS	CONTRAINDICATIONS, ADRs, AND COMMENTS[b]
Chloral Hydrate *continued*	**Agitation/Insomnia** Note: Chloral hydrate pharmacotherapy for these indications has been largely replaced by benzodiazepine pharmacotherapy because of the higher therapeutic index associated with the benzodiazepines.	**Infants, children, and adolescents:** 25–50 mg/kg/dose PO or rectally 30 min before bedtime or as needed. *Maximum:* 1 gram/dose PO or rectal; 2 grams/day, PO or rectal.		
Chlorambucil, *see* **Chapter 12**				
Chloramphenicol (*Chloromycetin®*)	**Bacterial infections** Note: Do **not** use chloramphenicol for infants or for patients who have cystic fibrosis. **Bacterial meningitis** Note: Ensure that appropriate culture and sensitivity tests are performed and that the organism is sensitive to chloramphenicol.	**Children and adolescents:** 50–75 mg/kg/day IV or PO in four divided doses, every 6 hr. *Maximum:* 4 grams/day IV; 3 grams/day PO. **Children and adolescents:** 75–100 mg/kg/day IV or PO in four divided doses, every 6 hr. *Maximum:* 4 grams/day IV; 3 grams/day PO. Note: Reduce dosage for pediatric patients who have hepatic dysfunction.	Capsule, oral: 250 mg Injectable, IV: 1 gram/vial Suspension, oral: 30 mg/ml; shake well before use. Note: Not generally available in the United States.	**Contraindications:** Hypersensitivity to chloramphenicol. **ADRs:** May cause a variety of ADRs including serious and potentially fatal blood dyscrasias. *See* Chapter 5. **Comments:** Monitor for signs and symptoms of bone marrow suppression. Note that the "gray baby" syndrome associated with chloramphenicol occurs predominantly among neonates during the first 48 hr after birth, but it may occur among infants and young children up to 2 years of age. Related signs and symptoms of this syndrome include abdominal distention, blue-gray skin discoloration, cardiovascular collapse, failure to feed, hypothermia, irregular breathing, and vomiting. Therapeutic drug monitoring is recommended; *see* Table 14-3.
Chlordiazepoxide	**Anxiety disorders** (therapy exceeding 30 days is **not** generally recommended)	**Children (≥6 years):** 10–20 mg/day PO in two to four divided doses. *Maximum:* 30 mg/day. **Adolescents:** 20–75 mg/day PO in two or three divided doses.	Capsules, oral: 5, 10, 25 mg	**Contraindications:** Hypersensitivity to chlordiazepoxide or other benzodiazepines. **ADRs:** Generally well tolerated. May cause ataxia, confusion, and drowsiness. *See* Chapter 5. May adversely affect cognitive abilities, including learning and memory, and, thus, scholastic performance. **Comments:** Paradoxical reactions (e.g., excitement, rage) have been observed, particularly among aggressive or hyperactive children receiving chlordiazepoxide.
Chlorhexidine (*Betasept®, Dyna-hex Skin Cleanser®, Exidine Skin Cleanser®, Hibiclens®, Hibitane®*)	**Acne vulgaris**	**Adolescents:** Twice daily, morning and evening, wash affected areas for 10–15 sec with 5–10 ml of cleanser. Rinse thoroughly with warm water. Repeat procedure. Note: Take care to avoid contact with eyes. If contact with the eyes occurs, immediately rinse affected eye(s) with copious amounts of water.	Solution, topical cleanser: 2%, 4% (also contains 4% isopropyl alcohol). Note: For external use only. Avoid contact with eyes. Note: Store at controlled room temperature between 15 and 25°C. Do not freeze. Protect from excessive exposure to heat or light.	**Contraindications:** Hypersensitivity to chlorhexidine. **ADRs:** Generally well tolerated. May cause local contact irritation at application sites.

(Continued)

Footnotes are on page 558.

TABLE 14-1 continued

DRUG (TRADE AND OTHER NAMES)	INDICATION(S)	USUAL PEDIATRIC DOSAGE AND ADMINISTRATION[a]	DOSAGE FORMS	CONTRAINDICATIONS, ADRs, AND COMMENTS[b]
Chlorhexidine *continued*	**Minor burns and wounds**, used as an antiseptic cleanser for the prevention of infection	**Children and adolescents:** Thoroughly rinse affected burn or wound site with warm water. Apply undiluted chlorhexidine solution to burn or wound sites. Wash gently and rinse thoroughly with warm water. Dry with a sterile towel.		
	Preoperative skin preparation	**Children and adolescents:** Topically apply liberally to surgical skin site and swab for 2–3 min. Dry with a sterile towel. Repeat procedure.		
	Preoperative whole body shower	**Children and adolescents:** Wet scalp and body. Wash the hair thoroughly using ~30 ml of cleanser. Wash the body thoroughly using an additional 30 ml. Rinse the scalp and body. Repeat the procedure. Rinse the hair and body thoroughly and dry with a clean towel. Ensure that eye contact with chlorhexidine has been avoided or that the affected eye(s) has been thoroughly rinsed with water.		
Chloroquine *(Aralen®)*	**Malaria prophylaxis**, *Plasmodium falciparum, P. vivax, P. ovale*, and *P. malariae* **Note:** In areas with chloroquine-resistant malaria, doxycycline is generally recommended (*see* Doxycycline).	**Children and adolescents:** 5 mg chloroquine base/kg PO once a week beginning 1 or 2 weeks **before** potential exposure and continuing for 4–6 weeks after last exposure. *Maximum:* 300 mg chloroquine base/week.	Tablets, oral: 250 mg (phosphate) (150 mg base), 500 mg (phosphate) (300 mg base)	**Contraindications:** Hypersensitivity to chloroquine or to related aminoquinolines, porphyria, psoriasis, retinal dysfunction, and visual field changes. **ADRs:** Generally well tolerated. However, children are particularly sensitive to ADRs associated with chloroquine and related 4-aminoquinoline derivatives. Long-term or high-dosage pharmacotherapy may result in irreversible retinal damage. **Comments:** Ophthalmologic examinations (expert slit lamp, funduscopic, visual acuity, and visual field tests) are recommended upon initiation (to establish a baseline) and periodically during pharmacotherapy.
	Malaria treatment, *P. falciparum, P. vivax, P. ovale,* and *P. malariae* **Note:** Resistant strains of *P. falciparum* may require treatment with quinine.	**Children and adolescents:** Initial dose, 10 mg chloroquine base/kg PO; follow by 5 mg chloroquine base/kg/dose PO at 6, 24, and 48 hr after initial dose **or** 0.83 mg chloroquine base/kg/hr by continuous IV infusion for 24 hr. *Maximum initial dose:* 600 mg chloroquine base PO. *Maximum subsequent doses:* 300 mg chloroquine base/dose PO.		
Chlorothiazide *(Diuril®)*	**Edema/ Hypertension**	**Infants:** 10–30 mg/kg/day PO as a single dose or as two divided doses. *Maximum:* 375 mg/day PO. **Children:** 10–20 mg/kg/day PO as a single dose or as two divided doses. *Maximum:* 1 gram/day PO. **Adolescents:** 25 mg/kg/day PO as a single dose or as two divided doses. *Maximum:* 2 grams/day PO. **Note:** Reduce dosage for pediatric patients who have renal (*see* Table 14-2) or hepatic dysfunction.	Suspension, oral: 250 mg/5 ml; contains 0.5% alcohol; shake well before use. Tablets, oral: 250, 500 mg **Note:** Not generally available in Canada.	**Contraindications:** Anuria and hypersensitivity to chlorothiazide, other thiazide diuretics, or other sulfonamide derivatives. **ADRs:** ADRs may affect several body systems (*see* Chapter 5). **Comments:** Monitor blood pressure and fluid and electrolyte status.

TABLE 14-1 continued

DRUG (TRADE AND OTHER NAMES)	INDICATION(S)	USUAL PEDIATRIC DOSAGE AND ADMINISTRATION[a]	DOSAGE FORMS	CONTRAINDICATIONS, ADRs, AND COMMENTS[b]
Chlor-pheniramine (Chlo-Amine®, Chlor-Tripolon®)	**Allergic conditions** (e.g., conjunctivitis, hay fever, rhinitis)	**Children and adolescents:** 0.35 mg/kg/day PO in two to four divided doses, every 6–12 hr. *Maximum:* 12 mg/day PO. **Note:** Administer with food or milk.	Capsules, oral extended release: 8, 12 mg Syrup, oral: 2 mg/5 ml (some formulations contain 5% alcohol) Tablet, oral: 4 mg Tablet, oral chewable: 2 mg Tablets, oral extended release: 8, 12 mg **Note:** Widely available in combination cough and cold products.	**Contraindications:** Bladder neck obstruction, hypersensitivity to chlorpheniramine or to other related antihistamines, chronic obstructive pulmonary disease, and MAOI therapy (concurrent or within 14 days). **ADRs:** Generally well tolerated. May cause anorexia, dizziness, drowsiness, dry mouth, headache, and weakness. *See* Chapter 5. **Comments:** Young children may be more susceptible than older children, adolescents, and adults to ADRs associated with chlorpheniramine.
Chlor-promazine (Largactil®, Thorazine®)	**Nausea and vomiting**	**Infants (≥6 months), children, and adolescents:** 2 mg/kg/day IM or PO in four to six divided doses, every 4–6 hr **or** 4 mg/kg/day rectal in three or four divided doses, every 6 or 8 hr. *Maximum:* **Infants (≥6 months) and children (<5 years),** 40 mg/day IM; **children (≥5 years),** 75 mg/day IM.	Capsule, oral: 30 mg Drops, oral: 40 mg/ml (custard flavored); contains 17.5% alcohol. Injectable, IM, IV: 25 mg/ml Solutions, oral: 5, 20 mg/ml (peach flavored); contains 0.5% alcohol. Suppository, rectal: 25 mg Syrup, oral: 2 mg/ml (orange–custard flavored) Tablets, oral: 10, 25, 50, 100 mg	**Contraindications:** Blood dyscrasias, coma, hypersensitivity to chlorpromazine or to other phenothiazines, Reye's syndrome, and subcortical brain damage. **ADRs:** *See* Chapter 5. **Comments:** Monitor blood pressure during IV administration. Effects following IM administration may persist for up to 12 hr.
	Tetanus (adjunctive pharmacotherapy often in conjunction with barbiturate pharmacotherapy)	**Infants (≥6 months) and children:** 2 mg/kg/day IM or IV in three or four divided doses, every 6 or 8 hr. *Maximum:* Body weight ≤23 kg, 40 mg/day IM or IV; 23–46 kg, 75 mg/day IM or IV. **Note:** For IV use, dilute to at least 1 mg/ml and infuse at a rate of 0.5 mg/min. **Adolescents:** Initially, 100 mg/day IM or IV in four divided doses, every 6 hr. *Maximum:* 200 mg/day IM or IV. **Note:** For IV use, dilute to at least 1 mg/ml and infuse at a rate of 1 mg/min.		
	Severe behavioral problems (marked by combativeness and explosiveness) **Note:** Although also approved by the FDA for the short-term treatment of attention-deficit/hyperactivity disorder, we do **not** recommend the use of chlorpromazine for this indication because of its associated ADRs.	**Children:** Initially, 2 mg/kg/day IM or PO in four divided doses, every 6 hr, **or** 4 mg/kg/day rectal in three divided doses, every 8 hr. Adjust dosage according to response. *Maximum:* Children (<5 years), 40 mg/day IM; children (≥5 years), 75 mg/day IM.		

Footnotes are on page 558.

TABLE 14-1 continued

DRUG (TRADE AND OTHER NAMES)	INDICATION(S)	USUAL PEDIATRIC DOSAGE AND ADMINISTRATION[a]	DOSAGE FORMS	CONTRAINDICATIONS, ADRs, AND COMMENTS[b]
Cholestyr-amine (*Prevalite®, Questran®*)	Hypercholesterol-emia	**Children (≥10 years) and adolescents:** 240 mg dried resin/kg/day PO in three divided doses. Titrate dosage according to cholesterol plasma level. **Note:** Do **not** administer dry powder formulation without first mixing with water or compatible noncarbonated liquid. *Maximum:* 24 grams/day PO.	Chewable bar, oral: 4 grams dried resin/bar Powder, oral: 4 grams dried resin/9 grams powder **Note:** Always mix dry powder with water or other compatible noncarbonated liquid **prior** to use. Suspension, oral (requires addition of liquid) (*Prevalite*): single-dose packets and cans containing 231 grams. **Note:** 5.5 grams of *Prevalite* contains 4 grams of anhydrous cholestyramine resin.	**Contraindications:** Biliary tract obstruction (complete) and hypersensitivity to cholestyramine. **ADRs:** Generally well tolerated. May cause constipation. **Comments:** May alter GI absorption of other drugs. In order to avoid this possible drug interaction, concurrent oral pharmacotherapy should be administered at least 1 hr before or 4 hr after cholestyramine.
Chorionic Gonadotropin (*A.P.L.®, Choron®, Glukor®, Novarel®, Pregnyl®, Profasi®*)	Prepubertal cryptorchidism (not due to an anatomical obstruction) **Note:** Although testicular descent following chorionic gonadotropin pharmacotherapy generally is temporary, it helps to predict whether orchiopexy will be required in the future.	**Children (≥4 years):** 4000 units/dose IM three times per week (e.g., Monday, Wednesday, Friday) for 3 weeks. **Note:** Several different dosage schedules have been proposed and are in current use.	Injectable, IM: 5000 units/10 ml, 10,000 units/10 ml, 20,000 units/10 ml (after reconstitution with diluent provided with the product [bacteriostatic water for injection]) **Note:** Reconstituted chorionic gonadotropin should be refrigerated and is stable for up to 30 days. **Note:** Some formulations of chorionic gonadotropin contain 0.9%–2% benzyl alcohol. **Note:** For IM use only.	**Contraindications:** Androgen-dependent carcinoma, hypersensitivity to chorionic gonadotropin, and precocious puberty. **ADRs:** May cause edema, fatigue, gynecomastia, headache, irritability, mental depression, pain at the injection site, precocious puberty, and restlessness. **Comments:** Induces androgen secretion which in turn may cause sodium and fluid retention. Caution should be used, therefore, among patients (e.g., those with asthma, cardiac disease, epilepsy, migraine, or renal disease) in whom sodium and fluid retention may be problematic.
Ciclopirox (*Penlac Nail Lacquer®*) **Note:** *See also* Ciclopirox Olamine.	Fungal infections of the fingernail or toenail	**Children and adolescents:** Apply a small amount to all affected nails and immediately adjacent skin sites once daily at bedtime.	Solution, topical: 8% **Note:** For external use only. Avoid contact with eyes. **Note:** Not generally available in Canada.	**Contraindications:** Hypersensitivity to ciclopirox. **ADRs:** Generally well tolerated. May cause local irritation or a burning sensation. **Comments:** Pharmacotherapy may need to be continued for up to 1 year.
Ciclopirox Olamine (*Loprox®*) **Note:** *See also* Ciclopirox.	Fungal infections affecting the skin and related structures (e.g., cutaneous candidiasis and *Tinea* infections) **Note:** Ensure that appropriate culture and sensitivity tests are performed and that the organism is sensitive to ciclopirox.	**Children (≥10 years) and adolescents:** Topically apply and gently massage a small amount of cream or lotion into affected areas and surrounding skin sites twice daily, morning and evening, for a minimum of 30 days.	Cream, topical: 1% Lotion, topical: 1% **Note:** Cream and lotion are for external use only. Avoid contact with eyes. **Not** for vaginal application.	**Contraindications:** Hypersensitivity to ciclopirox. **ADRs:** Generally well tolerated. May cause local irritation or a burning sensation at the application site.
Cimetidine (*Tagamet®*)	Peptic ulcer, prophylaxis and treatment	**Children and adolescents:** 20–40 mg/kg/day IV or PO in four divided doses, every 6 hr. *Maximum:* 2400 mg/day IV or PO. **Note:** Reduce dosage for pediatric patients who have renal dysfunction; *see* Table 14-2.	Injectable, IV: 150 mg/ml Solution, oral: 300 mg/5 ml (bittersweet melon–pineapple flavored) Tablets, oral: 200, 300, 400, 600, 800 mg	**Contraindications:** Hypersensitivity to cimetidine. **ADRs:** May cause CNS depression, diarrhea, dizziness, and skin rash (including severe reactions such as epidermal necrolysis). *See* Chapter 5. **Comments:** May inhibit the hepatic metabolism of other drugs. *See* Chapter 6.

TABLE 14-1 *continued*

DRUG (*TRADE* AND OTHER NAMES)	INDICATION(S)	USUAL PEDIATRIC DOSAGE AND ADMINISTRATION[a]	DOSAGE FORMS	CONTRAINDICATIONS, ADRs, AND COMMENTS[b]
Ciprofloxacin (*Cipro*®)	**Bacterial infections** **Note:** Ensure that appropriate culture and sensitivity tests are performed and that the organism is sensitive to ciprofloxacin. **Note:** Not approved by the FDA or HPB for infants or children, except for exposure to *Bacillus anthracis* associated with a bioterrorist attack.	**Children and adolescents:** 20–30 mg/kg/day PO in two divided doses, every 12 hr. *Maximum:* 2 grams/day PO.	Tablets, oral: 100, 250, 500, 750 mg Suspension, oral: 500 mg/5 ml (after reconstitution); shake well before use.	**Contraindications:** Hypersensitivity to ciprofloxacin or other quinolone antibiotics. **ADRs:** Generally well tolerated. May cause diarrhea, nausea, and rash. *See* Chapter 5. **Comments:** Long-term therapy is not recommended for prepubertal children because of reported arthropathy associated with ciprofloxacin use among several species of immature animals.
Cisatracurium (*Nimbex*®)	**To facilitate nonemergency endotracheal intubation and to provide skeletal muscle relaxation** during surgery or mechanical ventilation (as an **adjunct** to general anesthesia) **Note:** Cisatracurium should **not** be administered unless personnel and facilities for resuscitation and life support (i.e., tracheal intubation, artificial ventilation, oxygen therapy), and a cisatracurium antagonist (e.g., edrophonium or neostigmine) are immediately available.	**Children (≥2 years):** 0.1 mg/kg IV over 5–10 sec (during either halothane or opiate anesthesia). **Adolescents:** Initially, 0.15 or 0.2 mg/kg IV. Maintenance, 0.03 mg/kg IV (to provide an additional ~20 min of neuromuscular blockade during prolonged surgical procedures). **Note:** To minimize associated patient distress, cisatracurium should **not** be administered prior to the induction of unconciousness. **Note:** It is recommended that a peripheral nerve stimulator be used to measure neuromuscular function during the administration of cisatracurium in order to monitor drug effect; determine the need for additional doses; and confirm recovery from neuromuscular blockade.	Injectable, IV: 2, 10 mg/ml **Note:** The 2-mg/ml injectable contains benzyl alcohol. **Note:** Store under refrigeration between 2 and 8°C (36–46°F). Do not freeze. Protect from light.	**Contraindications:** Hypersensitivity to cisatracurium, atracurium, or other bisbenzylisoquinolinium drugs. **ADRs:** Generally well tolerated. May cause bradycardia, bronchospasm, flushing, and hypotension. **Comments:** Not compatible with ketorolac tromethamine, propofol, or lactated Ringer's solution.

Cisplatin, *see* **Chapter 12**
Citrate of Magnesium, *see* **Magnesium Citrate**
Cladribine, *see* **Chapter 12**

Clarithromycin (*Biaxin*®, *Biaxin XL*®)	**Acute otitis media/ Pharyngitis** **Note:** Ensure that appropriate culture and sensitivity tests are performed and that the organism is sensitive to clarithromycin. *Mycobacterium avium* **complex (MAC) disease,** prevention/prophylaxis, treatment **Note:** When used	**Infants, children, and adolescents:** 15 mg/kg/day PO in two divided doses, every 12 hr. *Maximum:* 250 mg/dose PO. **Note:** Reduce dosage for pediatric patients who have renal dysfunction; *see* Table 14-2. **Children and adolescents:** 15 mg/kg/day PO in two divided doses. *Maximum:* 1000 mg/day PO. **Note:** If clinical improvement is noted when used for the treatment	Tablets, oral: 250, 500 mg Tablet, oral, extended release (*Biaxin XL*®): 500 mg Suspension, oral (after reconstitution): 125 mg/5 ml (fruit flavored); shake well before use. Do **not** refrigerate. **Note:** Clarithromycin extended-release tablets are not approved by the FDA or HPB for pediatric use.	**Contraindications:** Hypersensitivity to clarithromycin, erythromycin, or to other macrolide antibiotics. **ADRs:** Generally well tolerated. May cause abdominal pain, diarrhea, headache, nausea, and alteration in taste. *See* Chapter 5. **Comments:** May inhibit the hepatic metabolism of other drugs metabolized by the cytochrome P-450 3A4 isoenzyme. *See* Chapter 6. Concurrent use with cisapride or pimozide is generally considered to be contraindicated.

(Continued)

Footnotes are on page 558.

TABLE 14-1 continued

DRUG (TRADE AND OTHER NAMES)	INDICATION(S)	USUAL PEDIATRIC DOSAGE AND ADMINISTRATION[a]	DOSAGE FORMS	CONTRAINDICATIONS, ADRs, AND COMMENTS[b]
Clarithromycin *continued*	for the treatment of MAC, clarithromycin should be used in **combination** with other antimycobacterial drugs that are effective against MAC (e.g., ethambutol, rifampin).	of MAC among pediatric patients with AIDS, clarithromycin pharmacotherapy is generally recommended to continue for life.		
Clemastine (Antihist-1®, Dayhist-1®, Tavist®)	Allergic rhinitis (for symptomatic management)	**Children (≥6 years):** Initially, 1.34 mg/day PO in two divided doses, every 12 hr. *Maximum:* 4.02 mg/day PO. **Adolescents:** Initially, 2.68 mg/day PO in two divided doses, every 12 hr. *Maximum:* 8.04 mg/day PO.	Solution, oral: 0.67 mg/5 ml (citrus flavored, may contain up to 5.5% alcohol) Tablets, oral: 1.34, 2.68 mg **Note:** Not generally available in Canada.	**Contraindications:** Hypersensitivity to clemastine and MAOI therapy (concurrent or within 14 days). **ADRs:** May cause blurred vision, constipation, drowsiness, dry mouth, fatigue, sedation, and urinary retention. *See* Chapter 5.
	Mild allergic urticaria and angioedema (for symptomatic management)	**Children (≥6 years):** Initially, 2.68 mg/day PO in two divided doses, every 12 hr. *Maximum:* 4.02 mg/day PO. **Adolescents:** Initially, 2.68 mg/day PO as a single dose. Additional doses may be added as indicated by response. *Maximum:* 8.04 mg/day PO.		
	Rhinorrhea or sneezing associated with the common cold (for symptomatic management)	**Adolescents:** 2.68 mg/day PO in two divided doses, every 12 hr. *Maximum:* 8.04 mg/day PO.		
Clindamycin (Cleocin®, Dalacin C®)	Bacterial infections, mild to moderate	**Infants, children, and adolescents:** 15–25 mg/kg/day IM or IV in three or four divided doses, every 6 or 8 hr **or** 8–25 mg/kg/day PO in four divided doses, every 6 hr. *Maximum:* 1.2 grams/day (hydrochloride) PO; 1.87 grams/day (phosphate) IM or IV.	Capsules, oral (hydrochloride): 75, 150, 300 mg Injectable (phosphate): 150 mg/ml (contains benzyl alcohol) Suspension, oral (palmitate hydrochloride): 15 mg/ml (cherry flavored); shake well before use. **Note:** Reconstituted suspension is stable for 14 days at room temperature; do not refrigerate.	**Contraindications:** Hypersensitivity to clindamycin. **ADRs:** Generally well tolerated. May cause abdominal pain, diarrhea, and vomiting. *See* Chapter 5. **Comments:** Monitor for the development of pseudomembranous colitis.
	Bacterial infections, severe **Note:** Ensure that appropriate culture and sensitivity tests are performed and that the organism is sensitive to clindamycin.	**Infants, children, and adolescents:** 25–40 mg/kg/day IM or IV in three or four divided doses, every 6 or 8 hr. *Maximum:* 1.8 grams/day (hydrochloride) PO; 2.7 grams/day (phosphate) IM or IV.		
Clobazam (Frisium®)	Seizures (adjunctive pharmacotherapy)	**Infants and children (≤2 years):** Initially, 0.25 mg/kg/day PO as a single daily dose 30 min before bedtime **or** in two divided doses every 12 hr. Increase dosage at 5-day intervals to 0.5–1 mg/kg/day PO in two or three divided doses. **Children (>2 years) and adolescents:** 5–40 mg/day PO. *Maximum:* Initial dose, 5 mg/day	Tablet, oral: 10 mg **Note:** Not generally available in the United States.	**Contraindications:** Hypersensitivity to clobazam, myasthenia gravis, and narrow-angle glaucoma. **ADRs:** May cause confusion, dizziness, drowsiness, and fatigue. *See* Chapter 5. **Comments:** Abrupt discontinuation may precipitate seizures. Reduce dosage gradually to discontinue.

TABLE 14-1 continued

DRUG (TRADE AND OTHER NAMES)	INDICATION(S)	USUAL PEDIATRIC DOSAGE AND ADMINISTRATION[a]	DOSAGE FORMS	CONTRAINDICATIONS, ADRs, AND COMMENTS[b]
Clobazam *continued*		PO; maintenance dose, 40 mg/day PO **Note:** Reduce dosage for pediatric patients who have hepatic dysfunction.		
Clonazepam (Klonopin®, Rivotril®)	Seizures, akinetic, myoclonic/ Lennox-Gastaut syndrome	**Infants and children (≤30 kg):** Initially, 0.01–0.05 mg/kg/day PO in two or three divided doses. Increase dosage by either 0.05 mg/kg/day every 3 days or 0.25–0.5 mg/kg every 3 days, **whichever is less**, to 0.1–0.2 mg/kg/day in three divided doses. *Maximum:* 0.2 mg/kg/day PO. **Children (>30 kg) and adolescents:** Initially, 1.5 mg/day PO in three divided doses. Increase dosage by 0.5–1 mg/day every 3 days, as needed, according to response. *Maximum:* 20 mg/day PO. **Note:** Reduce dosage for pediatric patients who have hepatic dysfunction.	Tablets, oral: 0.5, 1, 2 mg	**Contraindications:** Hepatic impairment (severe), hypersensitivity to clonazepam or to other benzodiazepines, narrow-angle glaucoma, and respiratory insufficiency (severe). **ADRs:** Commonly causes alterations in behavior (aggressiveness, hyperactivity), CNS depression (drowsiness), and increased salivation. *See* Chapter 5. **Comments:** In cases of clonazepam overdosage, the use of the benzodiazepine antagonist, flumazenil, should be considered with extreme caution because antagonism of the benzodiazepine effects will also result in antagonism of seizure control and possible initiation of status epilepticus. Abrupt discontinuation of clonazepam may precipitate seizures. Discontinue by gradually reducing the dosage.
Clonidine (Catapres®, Dixarit®)	**Hypertension** **Note:** Not approved by the FDA or HPB for infants or children.	**Infants, children, and adolescents:** 0.005 mg/kg/day PO in two or three divided doses. Increase dosage until desired blood pressure is achieved. *Maximum:* 0.03 mg/kg/day PO up to 2.4 mg/day. **Note:** Reduce dosage for pediatric patients who have renal dysfunction.	Tablets, oral: 0.1, 0.2, 0.3 mg	**Contraindications:** Hypersensitivity to clonidine and functional impairment of the sinus node. **ADRs:** Commonly causes constipation, dizziness, drowsiness, dry mouth, and sedation. May also cause agitation, depression, headache, nausea, nervousness, palpitation, tachycardia, and vomiting. *See* Chapter 5. **Comments:** Abrupt discontinuation may result in hypertension. Discontinue by reducing the dosage gradually over 2–4 days to avoid sympathetic overactivity and consequent significant rise in blood pressure.
Clorazepate (GenXene®, Novo-Clopate®, Tranxene®)	Alcohol-withdrawal syndrome (used for the symptomatic management of the signs and symptoms of acute alcohol withdrawal and for the prevention of alcohol-withdrawal seizures)	**Adolescents:** *Day 1* (1st 24 hr), initially, 30 mg PO as a single dose; then an additional 30–60 mg PO in three divided doses. *Day 2* (2nd 24 hr), 45–90 mg/day PO in three divided doses. *Day 3* (3rd 24 hr), 22.5–45 mg/day PO in three divided doses. *Day 4* (4th 24 hr), 15–30 mg/day PO in three divided doses. *Subsequent days*, continue to reduce dosage, according to response, to	Tablets, oral: 3.75, 7.5, 11.25, 15, 22.5 mg	**Contraindications:** Hypersensitivity to clorazepate or to other benzodiazepines. **ADRs:** Commonly causes drowsiness. *See* "Benzodiazepines" in Chapter 5.

(Continued)

Footnotes are on page 558.

TABLE 14-1 continued

DRUG (TRADE AND OTHER NAMES)	INDICATION(S)	USUAL PEDIATRIC DOSAGE AND ADMINISTRATION[a]	DOSAGE FORMS	CONTRAINDICATIONS, ADRs, AND COMMENTS[b]
Clorazepate *continued*		7.5 mg/day PO. Then discontinue as soon as patient is stable. *Maximum:* 90 mg/day PO.		
	Partial seizures	**Children (≥9 years):** Initially, 15 mg/day PO in two divided doses. Increase daily dosage by ≤7.5 mg at weekly intervals according to response. *Maximum:* 60 mg/day PO. **Adolescents:** Initially, 22.5 mg/day PO in three divided doses. Increase daily dosage by ≤7.5 mg at weekly intervals according to response. *Maximum:* 90 mg/day PO.		
Clotrimazole *(Canesten®, Clotrimaderm®, Lotrimin®)*	Oropharyngeal candidiasis	**Children (>3 years) and adolescents:** Dissolve 10-mg lozenge in the mouth over 15–30 min. Repeat every 3 or 4 hr (five times daily) for 14 days.	Cream, topical: 1% Creams, vaginal: 1%, 2%, 10% Lotion, topical: 1%; shake well before use. Lozenge, topical oral: 10 mg (for topical oral use only) Solution, topical: 1% Tablets, vaginal: 100, 500 mg **Note:** Topical cream, lotion, and solution are for external topical use only. Avoid contact with eyes.	**Contraindications:** Hypersensitivity to clotrimazole. **ADRs:** Generally well tolerated. May cause local irritation or sensitization with topical application. Use of the oral lozenge has been associated with nausea and vomiting. **Comments:** Recurrent vaginal infections, particularly when difficult to treat among nonpregnant patients, may be indicative of HIV infection.
	Dermatophytoses *(Tinea* infections)/ **Cutaneous candidiasis/Superficial mycoses**	**Infants, children, and adolescents:** Apply topical cream, lotion, or solution sparingly to affected area twice daily. Application sites should be clean and dry before application of topical formulations. **Note:** Avoid contact with the eyes.		
	Diaper rash caused by *Candida albicans* **Note:** Ensure that diaper rash is due to *C. albicans* and not to another etiology (e.g., prolonged skin contact with soiled diapers).	**Infants:** Apply a thin coat of topical cream to affected and surrounding skin areas twice daily (morning and evening) at a diaper change. Application site should be clean and dry before application of clotrimazole topical cream.		
	Vulvovaginal candidiasis (e.g., moniliasis, vaginal yeast infection)	**Adolescents:** Insert 200 mg (two 100-mg vaginal tablets) intravaginally at bedtime for 3 consecutive nights **or** insert one applicatorful (~5 grams) of vaginal cream intravaginally at bedtime for 7–14 consecutive nights.		
Cloxacillin *(Apo-Cloxi®, Novo-Cloxi®, Nu-Cloxi®)*	Bacterial infections, mild to moderate **Note:** Ensure that appropriate culture and sensitivity tests are performed and that the organism is sensitive to cloxacillin.	**Children and adolescents:** 50–100 mg/kg/day PO in four divided doses, every 6 hr. *Maximum:* 4 grams/day PO. **Note:** Administer on an empty stomach.	Capsules, oral: 250, 500 mg Suspension, oral: 25 mg/ml (cherry flavored); shake well before use.	**Contraindications:** Hypersensitivity to cloxacillin, other penicillins, or cephalosporins. **ADRs:** *See* Chapter 5.

TABLE 14-1 continued

DRUG (TRADE AND OTHER NAMES)	INDICATION(S)	USUAL PEDIATRIC DOSAGE AND ADMINISTRATION[a]	DOSAGE FORMS	CONTRAINDICATIONS, ADRs, AND COMMENTS[b]
Clozapine (Clozaril®)	Childhood schizophrenia **Note:** Not approved by the FDA or HPB for children.	**Children (≥6 years):** Initially, 12.5 mg/day PO as a single dose for 2 days. If well tolerated, the dose may be increased to 25 mg/day PO as a single dose. Thereafter, increase dosage by 25 mg/day, according to response. General therapeutic range is 200–400 mg/day PO. *Maximum:* 600 mg/day PO. **Note:** The total daily dosage may be divided unevenly, with the larger dose administered at bedtime in order to avoid or take advantage of some of clozapine's ADRs (e.g., dizziness and drowsiness, respectively).	Tablets, oral: 25, 100 mg	**Contraindications:** Coma, epilepsy (uncontrolled), history of clozapine-induced agranulocytosis or granulocytopenia, hypersensitivity to clozapine, myeloproliferative disorders, and significant hepatic dysfunction. **ADRs:** May cause severe and potentially life-threatening ADRs, including agranulocytosis. May also cause constipation, dizziness, drowsiness, eosinophilia, fever, headache, hyperglycemia, myocarditis, neuroleptic malignant syndrome, orthostatic hypotension, pulmonary embolism, salivation, seizures, tachycardia, tardive dyskinesia (rare, particularly among children and adolescents), tremor, and weight gain. **Comments:** Because of the risk for potentially fatal agranulocytosis, pediatric patients must have baseline white blood cell and differential counts performed **prior** to the initiation of clozapine. Subsequently, white blood cell counts should be obtained every week for the first 6 months. If white blood cell counts have remained within the normal range for the first 6 months, then they may be obtained every 2 weeks for the remainder of clozapine pharmacotherapy. White blood cell counts also must be obtained at weekly intervals for the first month following the discontinuation of clozapine.
Codeine (Methylmorphine)	Cough	**Infants, children, and adolescents:** 1–1.5 mg/kg/day PO in six divided doses, every 4 hr as needed.	Injectables, IM: 30, 60 mg/ml Tablets, oral: 15, 30, 60 mg **Note:** Widely available in combination products for either cough or pain relief.	**Contraindications:** Acute asthma attack, acute respiratory depression, hypersensitivity to codeine or to other opiate analgesics, and upper airway obstruction. **ADRs:** See Chapter 5. **Comments:** Pain relief is approximately equivalent to that provided by the NSAIDs.
	Pain, mild to moderate	**Infants, children, and adolescents:** 3–6 mg/kg/day IM or PO divided every 4–6 hr as needed. *Maximum:* 1.5 mg/kg/dose **or** 60 mg/dose, whichever is less, IM or PO.		
Colfosceril, see Chapter 13				
Corticotropin (Adrenocorticotropic Hormone [ACTH]), H.P. Acthar®)	Infantile spasms **Note:** Corticosteroid pharmacotherapy is generally preferred over corticotropin pharmacotherapy for	**Infants:** 1.6–2.4 units/kg/day IM as a single dose **or** 150 units/m²/day IM as two divided doses during week 1; 75 units/m²/day IM as a single dose during week 2;	Injectables, IM: 25, 40, 80 units/ml	**Contraindications:** Congestive heart failure, hypertension, ocular herpes simplex, recent surgery, scleroderma, sensitivity to porcine proteins, and systemic fungal infections.

(Continued)

Footnotes are on page 558.

TABLE 14-1 continued

DRUG (TRADE AND OTHER NAMES)	INDICATION(S)	USUAL PEDIATRIC DOSAGE AND ADMINISTRATION[a]	DOSAGE FORMS	CONTRAINDICATIONS, ADRs, AND COMMENTS[b]
Corticotropin *continued*	the treatment of related, responsive disorders.	75 units/m^2/day IM every 2 days during week 3; then gradually reduce dosage over weeks 4–12. **Note:** Chronic long-term therapy is not recommended and may result in irreversible ADRs.		**ADRs:** *See* "Corticosteroids" in Chapter 5. **Comments:** Monitor urine for glucose. Avoid concurrent immunization with live virus vaccines.
Cortisone *(Cortone®)*	**Allergic conditions,** severe or incapacitating/ **Adrenocortical insufficiency,** primary or secondary/ **Autoimmune hemolytic anemia/ Exfoliative dermatitis/Juvenile rheumatoid arthritis**	**Children and adolescents:** 20–300 mg/day IM or PO. **Note:** Dosage and route of administration are guided by indication for use and response.	Suspension, injectable, IM: 50 mg/ml; shake well before use. Tablet, oral: 25 mg **Note:** Cortisone injectable suspension is for IM use only.	**Contraindications:** Hypersensitivity, live virus vaccination (concurrent), and systemic fungal infections. **ADRs:** May cause a variety of ADRs affecting most major body systems (*see* "Corticosteroids" in Chapter 5). **Comments:** Because of the ability of corticosteroids to affect growth and development, children and adolescents on long-term therapy should be monitored closely. **Note:** Gradually discontinue high-dosage or long-term therapy in order to avoid HPA axis suppression.

Co-Trimoxazole, *see* **Trimethoprim and Sulfamethoxazole**

Cromolyn Sodium *(Gastrocrom®, Intal®, Nalcrom®,* Sodium Cromoglycate)	Allergic rhinitis	**Children and adolescents:** 5.2 mg (one spray of nasal solution) in each nostril three or four times daily.	Capsule, oral *(Nalcrom)*: 100 mg Metered-dose inhaler: 800 μg/actuation Powder, inhalation capsule *(Intal)*: 20 mg Solution, nasal spray: 40 mg/ml (5.2 mg/spray) Solution, nebulizer: 10 mg/ml Solution, oral concentrate *(Gastrocrom)*: 10 mg/ml (flexible ampule)	**Contraindications:** Hypersensitivity to cromolyn sodium. **ADRs:** Inhalation pharmacotherapy may cause bronchospasm, cough, nasal congestion, and wheezing. Oral pharmacotherapy may cause headache, insomnia, joint pain, nausea, and skin rash. *See* Chapter 5. **Comments:** Clinical benefit may not be observed for 3 weeks; dosage may be doubled if no therapeutic benefit is observed after 6 weeks; reduce dosage to minimal effective dosage once patient is stabilized.
	Food allergy	**Children (≥2 years):** Initially, 400 mg/day PO in four divided doses, 15–20 min before meals. If therapeutic benefit is not achieved within 3 weeks, then the daily dosage may be doubled but should not exceed 40 mg/kg/day. **Note:** Once satisfactory results are obtained, the dosage should be reduced to the minimal effective dosage. **Adolescents:** Initially, 800 mg/day PO in four divided doses, 15–20 min before meals. **Note:** Once satisfactory results are obtained, the dosage should be reduced to the minimal effective dosage.		
	Chronic inflammatory bowel disease	**Children (≥2 years):** 400 mg/day PO in four divided doses, 15–20 min before meals. **Adolescents:** 800 mg/day PO in four divided doses, 15–20 min before meals. **Note:** To prevent relapse, it is recommended to continue maintenance pharmacotherapy indefinitely. **Note:** For optimal therapeutic benefit, dissolve the contents of each dose of the oral capsules *(Nalcrom)* in warm water **or** gently stir the contents of the flexible ampule *(Gastrocrom)* into a small amount of water, and		

TABLE 14-1 continued

DRUG (TRADE AND OTHER NAMES)	INDICATION(S)	USUAL PEDIATRIC DOSAGE AND ADMINISTRATION[a]	DOSAGE FORMS	CONTRAINDICATIONS, ADRs, AND COMMENTS[b]
Cromolyn Sodium *continued*		administer as an oral liquid (*see* Chapter 1). Do not mix oral concentrate solution *(Gastrocrom)* with food, fruit juice, or milk for administration.		
	Asthma prophylaxis	**Children and adolescents:** Inhalation capsules or nebulizer solution, 40–80 mg/day in three or four divided doses **or** metered-dose inhaler, 6400 µg/day in four divided doses (two actuations four times daily).		
Crotalid Serum Antivenin, *see* **Antivenin (Crotalidae) Polyvalent**				
Cyanocobalamin (*Ener-B®, Nascobal®,* Vitamin B$_{12}$)	Maintenance of hematologic remission following injectable cyanocobalamin pharmacotherapy for vitamin B$_{12}$ malabsorption **Note: Not** indicated for the treatment of pernicious anemia.	**Children and adolescents:** 0.5 mg intranasal gel by metered-dose pump once weekly.	Gel, nasal metered-dose pump *(Nascobal):* 0.5 mg/actuation Injectable: 1 mg/ml **Note:** The metered-dose pump formulation is for intranasal use only. A 0.4-mg/unit nasal gel formulation *(Ener-B)* also is available for nonprescription use. Tablets, oral: 50, 100, 250 µg	**Contraindications:** Hypersensitivity to cobalt or to cyanocobalamin. **ADRs:** Generally well tolerated. **Comments:** Folate and iron levels, hematocrit, reticulocyte count, and vitamin B$_{12}$ levels should be obtained prior to the initiation of therapy. Recommended Dietary Allowance (RDA) of cyanocobalamin: Infants (to 6 months) 0.3 µg/day Infants (6–12 months) 0.5 µg/day Children (1–3 years) 0.7 µg/day Children (4–6 years) 1 µg/day Children (7–10 years) 1.4 µg/day Children (>10 years) 2 µg/day Adolescents 2 µg/day
Cyclopentolate (*AK-Pentolate®, Cyclogyl®, Pentolair®*)	Mydriasis/ Cycloplegia in the context of diagnostic procedures	**Infants:** Instill one drop of 0.5% ophthalmic solution into eye(s). **Children and adolescents:** Instill one or two drops of 0.5%, 1%, or 2% ophthalmic solution into eye(s). **Note:** Patients with heavily pigmented irides (darker eyes) are more likely to require the higher strength ophthalmic solutions.	Solutions, ophthalmic: 0.5%, 1%, 2% **Note:** For ophthalmic use only.	**Contraindications:** Hypersensitivity to atropine, other belladonna alkaloids, or cyclopentolate; primary glaucoma; and synechiae (adhesions between the iris and the lens of the eye). **ADRs:** May cause local reactions including conjunctivitis, increased intraocular pressure, and transient stinging or burning of the eye(s). Systemic absorption is generally minimal, particularly with nasolacrimal occlusion during instillation of the ophthalmic solutions. (*See* Chapter 1). However, systemic anticholinergic effects can occur (*see* Chapter 5). Pediatric patients, particularly infants, should be observed for a minimum of 30 min following instillation because of the possibility of systemic effects.
Cyclophosphamide, *see* **Chapter 12**				
Cyclosporine (*Neoral®, Sandimmune®*)	Bone marrow transplant	**Children and adolescents:** 3 mg/kg/day IV in two divided doses, every 12 hr **or** 9 mg/kg/day PO in two divided doses, every 12 hr.	Capsules, oral: 25, 50, 100 mg Injectable, IV: 50 mg/ml Solution, oral: 100 mg/ml	**Contraindications:** Hypersensitivity to cyclosporine. **ADRs:** May cause hypertension, nephrotoxicity, and seizures. *(Continued)*

Footnotes are on page 558.

TABLE 14-1 continued

DRUG (TRADE AND OTHER NAMES)	INDICATION(S)	USUAL PEDIATRIC DOSAGE AND ADMINISTRATION[a]	DOSAGE FORMS	CONTRAINDICATIONS, ADRs, AND COMMENTS[b]
Cyclosporine *continued*	Heart transplant	**Children and adolescents:** Initially, 1 mg/kg/day continuous IV infusion. Adjust dosage to maintain serum concentration within the desired range.	*Note:* Cyclosporine dosage forms contain between 12% and 33% alcohol. *Note: Neoral* and *Sandimmune* differ in formulation and should **not** be used interchangeably.	**Comments:** Cyclosporine pharmacokinetics are highly variable; close monitoring of response and serum concentrations (*see* **Table 14-3**) are **required.** Administer on an empty stomach (1 hr before meals or 2–3 hr after meals). Cyclosporine oral solution may be diluted in a glass container with a compatible beverage (chocolate milk, milk, orange juice) at room temperature **immediately** before administration. The glass container should be "rinsed" with some additional beverage to ensure that the complete dose has been administered. Oral administration must be consistent (e.g., always on an empty stomach, always with suggested beverages). *Note:* In general, IV doses are ~1/3 of oral doses because of avoidance of hepatic first-pass effect.
	Kidney transplant	**Children and adolescents:** 8–10 mg/kg/day PO in two divided doses, every 12 hr.		
	Liver transplant	**Children and adolescents:** Initially, 3 mg/kg/day continuous IV infusion for 3 days; then 2 mg/kg/day IV in three divided doses, every 8 hr. *Note:* Reduce dosage for pediatric patients who have hepatic dysfunction. *Note:* Do **not** administer oral dosage forms with grapefruit juice as it may increase cyclosporine serum concentrations.		
Cyclosporine A, *see* **Chapter 12**				
Cyproheptadine *(Periactin®)*	Allergic conditions (e.g., conjunctivitis, rhinitis)	**Children (2–6 years):** 4–6 mg/day PO in two or three divided doses. *Maximum:* 12 mg/day PO. **Children (>6 years):** 8–12 mg/day PO in two or three divided doses. *Maximum:* 16 mg/day PO. **Adolescents:** 12 mg/day PO in three divided doses. *Maximum:* 32 mg/day PO.	Syrup, oral: 2 mg/5 ml (contains 5% alcohol) Tablet, oral: 4 mg	**Contraindications:** Angle-closure glaucoma, bladder neck obstruction, hypersensitivity to cyproheptadine, pyloroduodenal obstruction, stenosing peptic ulcer, and urinary retention. **ADRs:** Commonly causes drowsiness and somnolence. May cause various anticholinergic effects. **Comments:** May decrease mental alertness and, therefore, adversely affect academic performance.
	Promotion of weight gain	**Children (2–6 years):** 6 mg/day PO in three divided doses. *Maximum:* 8 mg/day PO. **Children (>6 years):** 6–8 mg/day PO in three or four divided doses. *Maximum:* 12 mg/day PO. **Adolescents:** 12 mg/day PO in three divided doses. *Maximum:* 20 mg/day PO.		
Cysteamine *(Cystagon®)*	Nephropathic cystinosis	**Children and adolescents:** Initially, ¼ of the recommended maintenance dosage (see following table) PO in four divided doses, every 6 hr. This dosage is gradually increased over 4–6 weeks in order to avoid or minimize intolerance to cysteamine.	Capsules, oral: 50, 150 mg (bitartrate) *Note:* Because of risk for aspiration, it is recommended that intact capsules not be administered to children younger than 6 years. Instead, the number of capsules	**Contraindications:** Hypersensitivity to cysteamine or to penicillamine. **ADRs:** May cause anorexia, diarrhea, fever, lethargy, rash, and vomiting. **Comments:** Optimally, the goal of therapy is to maintain leukocyte cystine levels less than

TABLE 14-1 continued

DRUG (TRADE AND OTHER NAMES)	INDICATION(S)	USUAL PEDIATRIC DOSAGE AND ADMINISTRATION[a]	DOSAGE FORMS	CONTRAINDICATIONS, ADRs, AND COMMENTS[b]
Cysteamine *continued*		**MAINTENANCE DOSAGE** — BODY WEIGHT (lb / kg) / FREE BASE mg/day PO: 0–10 / 0–4.5 / 400 11–20 / 4.6–9.1 / 600 21–30 / 9.2–13.6 / 800 31–40 / 13.7–18.2 / 1000 41–50 / 18.3–22.7 / 1200 51–70 / 22.8–31.8 / 1400 71–90 / 31.9–40.9 / 1600 91–110 / 41–50 / 1800 >110 / >50 / 2000 *Maximum:* 1.95 grams/m^2/day PO. Note that this dosage has been associated with a significant increase in both ADRs and the number of patients prematurely discontinuing therapy.	required for a particular dose should be opened and the contents mixed gently in a small amount of food immediately before administration with a meal.	1 nmol/½ cystine/mg protein measured at 5–6 hr after cysteamine administration.

Cytarabine, *see* **Chapter 12**

Dacarbazine, *see* **Chapter 12**

Dacliximab (Daclizumab, *Zenapax®*)	Adjunctive prophylaxis against acute organ rejection associated with renal transplant **Note:** Generally used in combination with one or more of the following drugs: azathioprine, corticosteroids, and cyclosporine. **Note:** Not approved by the FDA or HPB for children or adolescents.	**Children and adolescents:** Initially, 1 mg/kg by IV infusion within 24 hr **prior** to transplantation. Four additional doses should be administered at 14-day intervals following transplantation. **Note:** Should be administered IV over 15 min using a central or peripheral vein.	Injectable, IV: 5 mg/ml **Note:** Store under refrigeration between 2 and 8°C (36–46°F). Protect from light. Do **not** shake or freeze. **Note:** The dacliximab IV injectable must be further diluted with 50 ml of normal saline solution for injection (0.9% sodium chloride solution) **prior** to IV infusion.	**Contraindications:** Hypersensitivity to dacliximab or to mouse cell proteins. **ADRs:** Generally well tolerated. May cause acne, diarrhea, hypertension, lymphocele, pulmonary edema, tremor, and vomiting.

Daclizumab, *see* **Dacliximab**

Dactinomycin, *see* **Chapter 12**

Dalfopristin and Quinupristin, *see* **Quinupristin and Dalfopristin**

Danaparoid (*Orgaran-HIT®*)	Thrombosis, acute (associated with heparin-induced thrombocytopenia [HIT]) Heparin-induced thrombocytopenia (HIT), prophylaxis among patients who have a previous history of HIT. **Note:** Approved by the HPB but not by the FDA for these indications.	**Children and adolescents:** Initially, 30 units/kg IV push; then 1.2–4 units/kg/hr by IV infusion. **Note:** Expected plasma antifactor-Xa concentrations after the initial IV bolus dose should be within 400–700 units/liter. **Children and adolescents:** 20 units/kg/day SC in two divided doses, every 12 hr. **Note:** Reduce dosage for pediatric patients who have renal dysfunction.	Injectable, IV, SC: 750 anti-Xa units/ampule (0.6 ml) **Note:** For IV or SC use only. Do **not** administer IM. **Note:** Contains sodium sulfite. Sulfites may cause hypersensitivity reactions, including anaphylactic reactions, among susceptible patients, particularly patients who have asthma.	**Contraindications:** Active bleeding, bacterial endocarditis, blood clotting disorders, duodenal ulcer (active), gastric ulcer (active), hemorrhagic diathesis (severe), hemorrhagic stroke (acute phase), hypersensitivity to danaparoid, hypertension (severe, untreated), retinopathy (diabetic or hemorrhagic), surgery (involving the brain, ears, eyes, or spinal cord), and thrombocytopenia related to previous danaparoid pharmacotherapy. **ADRs:** May cause bleeding, hematoma at injection site, rash, and thrombocytopenia (rare).

(Continued)

Footnotes are on page 558.

TABLE 14-1 continued

DRUG (TRADE AND OTHER NAMES)	INDICATION(S)	USUAL PEDIATRIC DOSAGE AND ADMINISTRATION[a]	DOSAGE FORMS	CONTRAINDICATIONS, ADRs, AND COMMENTS[b]
Danaparoid *continued*				**Comments:** Whenever possible, exclude potential cross-reactivity to heparin before initiation of danaparoid pharmacotherapy. Baseline platelet count should be obtained prior to the initiation of danaparoid pharmacotherapy, every other day during the first week, twice weekly during weeks two and three, and once weekly thereafter. Danaparoid pharmacotherapy should be monitored by following anti-factor Xa plasma concentrations. Midinterval anti-factor Xa plasma concentrations >0.5 unit/ml should generally be avoided during postoperative prophylaxis of thromboembolism.
Dantrolene *(Dantrium®)*	Malignant hyperthermia, prophylaxis	**Children and adolescents:** 4–8 mg/kg/day PO in four divided doses 1–2 days prior to surgery. *Maximum:* 400 mg/day PO.	Capsules, oral: 25, 50, 100 mg Injectable, IV: 20 mg/vial	**Contraindications:** Active hepatic disease and obstructive pulmonary disease. **Note:** There are no absolute contraindications to dantrolene pharmacotherapy when used to treat malignant hyperthermia. **ADRs:** Commonly causes diarrhea, dizziness, drowsiness, drooling, enuresis, fatigue, lightheadedness, malaise, muscle weakness, nausea, and slurred speech. **Comments:** Long-term therapy for the treatment of chronic skeletal muscle spasticity has been associated with liver hepatotoxicity. Therefore, hepatic function tests are recommended before (baseline) and during dantrolene pharmacotherapy.
	Malignant hyperthermia, treatment	**Children and adolescents:** 1 mg/kg by IV push; repeat until symptoms subside or a maximal cumulative dosage of 10 mg/kg is reached. *Maximum:* Total dosage, 10 mg/kg/IV.		
	Malignant hyperthermia, postcrisis prophylaxis (to prevent relapse)	**Children and adolescents:** 4–8 mg/kg/day PO in four divided doses for 1–3 days following malignant hyperthermia crisis.		
	Chronic skeletal muscle spasticity **Note:** Not indicated for the treatment of skeletal muscle spasms associated with rheumatic disorders.	**Children (≥5 years) and adolescents:** Initially, 1 mg/kg/day PO in two divided doses. Increase the daily dosage by 0.5 mg/kg/day as indicated by response. *Maximum:* 12 mg/kg/day PO **or** 400 mg/day PO, whichever is less.		
Dapsone (Diaminodiphenylsulfone)	Leprosy **Note:** Not for use in pediatric patients who have dapsone-resistant leprosy.	**Children:** 1–2 mg/kg/day PO as a single dose. *Maximum:* 100 mg/day PO. **Adolescents:** 100 mg/day PO as a single dose. **Note:** In order to reduce secondary dapsone resistance, it is recommended that dapsone pharmacotherapy include combination therapy with one or more additional antileprosy drugs (e.g., rifampin) for a **minimum of 3 years** and that pharmacotherapy not be interrupted during this period	Tablets, oral: 25, 100 mg	**Contraindications:** Hypersensitivity to dapsone. **ADRs:** May cause abdominal pain, anorexia, headache, hemolysis, infectious mononucleosis-like syndrome, insomnia, lupus erythematosis, nausea, paresthesia, peripheral neuropathy, phototoxicity, psychosis, rash, vertigo, and vomiting. Use with particular caution for patients who have glucose-6-phosphate dehydrogenase deficiency because of increased risk for hemolysis. **Comments:** Periodic blood counts should be performed weekly for the first month of dapsone pharmacotherapy, then monthly for 6 months, and then every 6 months.

TABLE 14-1 continued

DRUG (*TRADE* AND OTHER NAMES)	INDICATION(S)	USUAL PEDIATRIC DOSAGE AND ADMINISTRATION[a]	DOSAGE FORMS	CONTRAINDICATIONS, ADRs, AND COMMENTS[b]
Daunorubicin, *see* **Chapter 12**				
Deferoxamine (*Desferal*®, Desferrioxamine) **Note:** *See also* Chapter 4.	Iron poisoning, acute	**Children and adolescents:** Initially, 90 mg/kg IM, then 45 mg/kg IM every 4–12 hr **or** initially, 15 mg/kg/hr IV for 4 hr, then 2–5 mg/kg/hr IV. **Note:** Recommended maximal IV infusion rate is 15 mg/kg/hr; rapid infusion may cause hypotension. However, infusions of 35 mg/kg/hr have been required for the treatment of severely poisoned adults. *Maximum:* 1 gram/dose IM; 120 mg/kg/day or 6 grams/day, whichever is less, IM or IV.	Injectables, IM, IV, SC: 500 mg/vial, 2 grams/vial **Note:** For SC infusion, a portable light-weight infusion pump is often used. The usual needle used is a 25- or 27-gauge wing-tipped needle, which is placed in the subcutaneous tissue of the anterior abdomen (*see* Chapter 1 for additional information regarding SC infusion).	**Contraindications:** Hypersensitivity to deferoxamine. **ADRs:** *See* Chapter 4. **Comments:** Patients suffering from iron intoxication reportedly experience a higher incidence of infections, particularly with *Yersinia enterocolitica* and *Y. pseudotuberculosis*. These infections are reportedly exacerbated by deferoxamine. Therefore, if patients develop abdominal pain, fever, or pharyngitis, perform appropriate culture and sensitivity tests. If infection is noted, begin appropriate antibiotic pharmacotherapy and withhold deferoxamine until the infection has been adequately treated.
	Beta thalassemia major (prevention and treatment of transfusional iron overload)	**Children and adolescents:** 25–60 mg/kg/day IV or SC over 10–12 hr. *Maximum:* 4 grams/dose IV or SC over 10–12 hr. **Note:** Deferoxamine dosage should be guided by ferritin serum concentrations and measures of 24-hr urinary iron excretion.		
Deltahydrocortisone, *see* **Prednisone**				
Desferrioxamine, *see* **Deferoxamine**				
Desloratadine (*Clarinex*®)	Rhinitis, perennial allergic/Urticaria, chronic idiopathic	**Adolescents:** 5 mg/day PO as a single dose. **Note:** Reduce dosage for pediatric patients who have hepatic or renal dysfunction.	Tablet, oral: 5 mg	**Contraindications:** Hypersensitivity to desloratadine or to loratadine. **ADRs:** May cause dizziness, dry mouth, fatigue, headache, myalgia, nausea, pharyngitis, and somnolence.
Desmopressin (*DDAVP*®, *Octostim*®, *Stimate*®)	Neurohypophyseal diabetes insipidus (vasopressin-sensitive central diabetes insipidus)	**Children and adolescents:** 5–20 μg/day intranasal as a single dose or as two divided doses **or** initially, 300 μg/day PO in three divided doses. *Maximum:* 40 μg/dose intranasal **or** 1.2 mg/day PO. **Note:** The oral dosage generally is 10–20 times the intranasal dosage.	Injectables, IM, IV, SC: 4, 15 μg/ml Solutions, metered-dose nasal spray: 10 μg/0.1 ml, 150 μg/0.1 ml Solution, nasal: 100 μg/ml Tablets, oral: 0.1, 0.2 mg **Note:** Desmopressin metered-dose nasal spray and nasal solution are for nasal use only.	**Contraindications:** Hypersensitivity to desmopressin and type II B (platelet type, pseudo) van Willebrand's disease. **ADRs:** Generally well tolerated. May cause abdominal pain, headache, and nasal discomfort, including nasal irritation and nosebleeds (epistaxis). **Comments:** For the treatment of diabetes insipidus, monitor for significant decreases in plasma osmolality and possible resultant seizures, particularly in young children. For the treatment of enuresis, use the lowest effective dosage for 4 weeks, then gradually reduce the dosage by 10 μg every month, if possible. Fluid intake should be carefully monitored and restricted, particularly for children, in order to prevent hyponatremia and water intoxication.
	Enuresis **Note:** For the management of nocturnal enuresis among pediatric patients who have normal ability to concentrate urine.	**Children and adolescents:** 20 μg (10 μg in each nostril) at bedtime for 7 days; may increase dosage every 7 days by 10-μg increments up to 30–40 μg/day. *Maximum:* 40 μg/dose intranasal. **Alternative for children (≥5 years) and adolescents:** Initially, 0.2 mg PO as a single dose 1 hr before bedtime. If nocturnal enuresis continues, dosage may be increased by 0.2 mg at 3-day intervals. *Maximum:* 0.6 mg/day PO. **Note:** For the treatment of nocturnal enuresis, desmopressin should be used in conjunction with appropriate nonpharmacologic interventions (e.g., bladder control exercises, counseling).		

Footnotes are on page 558.

TABLE 14-1 *continued*

DRUG (TRADE AND OTHER NAMES)	INDICATION(S)	USUAL PEDIATRIC DOSAGE AND ADMINISTRATION[a]	DOSAGE FORMS	CONTRAINDICATIONS, ADRs, AND COMMENTS[b]
Desoxyephedrine, *see* **Methamphetamine**				
Dexamethasone (Decadron®, Dexasone®) **Note:** *See also* Chapter 12.	Bacterial meningitis (adjunctive pharmacotherapy) **Note:** Not approved by the FDA or HPB for this indication for infants or children.	**Infants, children, and adolescents:** 0.6 mg/kg/day IV in four divided doses every 6 hr for the first 4 days of antibiotic pharmacotherapy. **Note:** For meningitis, administer first dose of dexamethasone **prior** to initiating antibiotic pharmacotherapy.	Injectables, IM, IV: 4, 10, 20, 24 mg/ml Solution, oral: 1 mg/ml **Note:** Dexamethasone injectables may contain sulfites. Sulfites may cause hypersensitivity reactions, including anaphylactic reactions, among susceptible patients, particularly patients who have asthma.	**Contraindications:** Concurrent live virus vaccination, hypersensitivity to dexamethasone, and systemic fungal infections. **ADRs:** See Chapter 5.
	Croup	**Infants and children:** 0.6 mg/kg IV as a single dose.		
Dexamphetamine, *see* **Dextroamphetamine**				
Dexrazoxane, *see* **Chapter 12**				
Dextroamphetamine (Dexamphetamine, Dexedrine®) **Note:** *See also* Amphetamines, mixed.	Attention-deficit/ hyperactivity disorder (A-D/HD)	**Children (3–5 years):** Initially, 2.5 mg/day PO as a single morning dose. Increase dose by 2.5 mg/day at weekly intervals as needed to achieve optimal therapeutic response. **Children (≥6 years) and adolescents:** Initially, 5 mg/day PO as a single morning dose. Increase dosage by 5 mg/day at weekly intervals as needed to produce optimal therapeutic response. *Maximum:* 40 mg/day PO. **Note:** "Drug holidays" on weekends and during summer vacation are recommended. Usually dosed once daily in the morning but, when administered in divided doses, additional doses may be given 4–6 hr apart; to avoid associated insomnia, do **not** administer after 6 pm.	Capsules, oral sustained release: 5, 10, 15 mg Tablets, oral: 5, 10 mg (contain tartrazine) **Note:** Tartrazine (FD&C yellow No. 5) has been associated with hypersensitivity reactions, including bronchial asthma, among susceptible patients, particularly those who are hypersensitive to aspirin.	**Contraindications:** Agitated states, history of drug abuse, hypersensitivity to dextroamphetamine, hypertension, and MAOI therapy (concurrent or within 14 days). **ADRs:** May cause anorexia, cardiac palpitation, headache, hypertension, growth retardation, insomnia, nervousness, seizures, tachycardia, and precipitation of Tourette's disorder.
	Narcolepsy	**Children (≥6 years):** Initially, 5 mg/day PO as a single morning dose. Increase dosage by 5 mg/day at weekly intervals as needed to produce optimal therapeutic response. **Adolescents:** Initially, 10 mg/day PO as a single morning dose. Increase dosage by 10 mg/day at weekly intervals as needed to produce optimal therapeutic response. *Maximum:* 60 mg/day PO.		
Dextromethorphan (Benylin DM®, Novahistex DM®, Triaminic Softchews Cough®)	Cough, nonproductive, hacking	**Infants, children, and adolescents:** 1 mg/kg/day PO in three or four divided doses, every 6 or 8 hr. *Maximum:* 120 mg/day PO. **Alternative for children (2–6 years):** Oral chewable tablet, 22.5–30 mg/day PO in three or four divided doses, every 6 or 8 hr.	Lozenge, oral: 5 mg Lozenge, oral chewable: 15 mg Syrups, oral: 2.5, 5, 7.5, 10, 15, 30 mg/5 ml (grape, orange, or raspberry flavored) Tablet, oral chewable: 7.5 mg (contains aspartame) (strawberry flavored)	**Contraindications:** Hypersensitivity to dextromethorphan. **ADRs:** Generally well tolerated. May cause dizziness, drowsiness, headache, nausea, and vomiting.

TABLE 14-1 continued

DRUG (TRADE AND OTHER NAMES)	INDICATION(S)	USUAL PEDIATRIC DOSAGE AND ADMINISTRATION[a]	DOSAGE FORMS	CONTRAINDICATIONS, ADRs, AND COMMENTS[b]
Dextromethorphan *continued*		**Alternative for children ($\geq$6 years):** Oral chewable tablet, 45–60 mg/day PO in three or four divided doses, every 6 or 8 hr. **Note:** Instruct children to either allow the oral chewable tablet to dissolve completely in the mouth or chew the tablet completely before swallowing.	**Note:** Widely available in combination cough and cold products. **Note:** Oral chewable tablets are fragile. Thus, blister packages should not be crushed or tablets pushed out. The blister packages must be peeled open carefully.	
Dextrose	Hypoglycemic coma	**Infants, children, and adolescents:** 0.5–1 gram/kg/dose IV followed by continuous IV infusion with 5%–10% dextrose and water.	Injectables, IV: 2.5%, 5%, 10%	**Contraindications:** Hyperglycemia. **ADRs:** Generally well tolerated. Rapid or excessive administration of dextrose by injection, particularly to infants with very low birth weight, may result in increased serum osmolality and possible intracranial hemorrhage. **Comments:** Monitor blood glucose levels.

Dextrose in Sterile Water for Injection, *see* **Chapter 13**

Diaphenylsulfone, *see* **Dopamine**

DRUG (TRADE AND OTHER NAMES)	INDICATION(S)	USUAL PEDIATRIC DOSAGE AND ADMINISTRATION[a]	DOSAGE FORMS	CONTRAINDICATIONS, ADRs, AND COMMENTS[b]
Diazepam (Diastat®, Diazemuls®, Valium®)	Anxiety before diagnostic procedure **Note:** Most radiologic examinations may be performed without sedation. However, pediatric patients undergoing examinations that require prolonged periods of immobility (e.g., tomography) benefit most from sedation.	**Children and adolescents:** 0.2–0.6 mg/kg/dose PO 30–90 min before diagnostic procedure **or** 0.1–0.4 mg/kg/dose IV immediately before or during procedure. *Maximum:* 10 mg/dose IV; 20 mg/dose PO. **Note:** IM injection is **not** recommended because of erratic absorption; administer by slow IV injection over at least 3 min unless patient is on a respirator.	Gels, rectal: 2.5, 5, 10, 15, 20 mg/unit (available in prefilled units with flexible, molded applicator tip and lubricating jelly) Injectable, IV: 5 mg/ml Solution, oral: 5 mg/ml Tablets, oral: 2, 5, 10 mg **Note:** The 15- and 20-mg rectal gel units are generally reserved for adult use. **Note:** Some injectable formulations (e.g., *Valium*) contain 10% alcohol and 40% propylene glycol.	**Contraindications:** Hypersensitivity to diazepam or other benzodiazepines. **ADRs:** *See* Chapter 5.
	Preoperative anxiety	**Children and adolescents:** 0.1–0.5 mg/kg/dose PO 30–90 min before surgery. *Maximum:* 20 mg/dose PO.		
	Status epilepticus	**Infants, children, and adolescents:** 0.1–0.3 mg/kg/dose IV; may repeat twice at 10–15-min intervals, as needed to manage acute seizures **or** 0.3–0.5 mg/kg/dose rectal as a single dose; may repeat rectal dose once, if required, after 4–12 hr. *Maximum:* **Infants and children (<5 years):** 5 mg/dose IV or rectal; **children ($\geq$5 years) and adolescents:** 10 mg/dose IV; 20 mg/dose rectal.		
Diazoxide, injectable (Hyperstat®) **Note:** *See also* Diazoxide, oral.	Acute hypertension	**Infants, children, and adolescents:** 1–5 mg/kg/dose IV every 5–15 min as needed to control blood pressure (up to four doses total). **Note:** Administer undiluted by rapid IV injection, over 30 sec or	Injectable, IV: 15 mg/ml **Note:** For IV use only. **Note:** The injectable formulation is **not** used to treat hypoglycemia.	**Contraindications:** Compensatory hypertension and hypersensitivity to diazoxide or thiazide diuretics. **ADRs:** May cause sodium and fluid retention. *See* Chapter 5. *(Continued)*

Footnotes are on page 558.

TABLE 14-1 *continued*

DRUG (TRADE AND OTHER NAMES)	INDICATION(S)	USUAL PEDIATRIC DOSAGE AND ADMINISTRATION[a]	DOSAGE FORMS	CONTRAINDICATIONS, ADRs, AND COMMENTS[b]
Diazoxide, injectable *continued*		less, into a peripheral vein with patient in a recumbent position. *Maximum:* 150 mg/dose. *Maximum total dosage:* 8 mg/kg or 600 mg, whichever is less.		**Comments:** A diuretic may be required to treat associated fluid and water retention and to prevent the associated development of congestive heart failure.
Diazoxide, oral *(Proglycem®)* **Note:** *See also* Diazoxide, injectable.	Hypoglycemia due to hyperinsulinism associated with extrapancreatic malignancy; islet cell adenoma or adenomatosis; islet cell hyperplasia; leucine sensitivity; and nesidioblastosis	**Infants:** Initially, 8 mg/kg/day PO in three divided doses, every 8 hr. If required, adjust dosage after 2–4 days based on blood glucose concentration and response. *Maximum:* 15 mg/kg/day PO. **Children and adolescents:** Initially, 3 mg/kg/day PO in three divided doses, every 8 hr. If required, adjust dosage after 2–4 days based on blood glucose concentration and response. *Maximum:* 8 mg/kg/day PO.	Capsules, oral: 50, 100 mg Suspension, oral: 50 mg/ml (chocolate–mint flavored); contains ~5% alcohol; shake well before use. **Note:** The oral formulations are **not** used to treat acute hypertension.	**Contraindications:** Functional hypoglycemia and hypersensitivity to diazoxide or to other thiazides. **ADRs:** Commonly causes fluid and electrolyte retention. May also cause hirsutism of the lanugo type, ketoacidosis, nonketotic hyperosmolar coma, tachycardia, and thrombocytopenia. *See* Chapter 5. **Comments:** Monitor blood or urine regularly for glucose and ketones.
Diclofenac, oral *(Arthrotec®, Cataflam®), Novo-Difenac-K®, Voltaren®)*	Juvenile rheumatoid arthritis (refractory to conventional pharmacotherapy) Analgesia/Primary dysmenorrhea	**Adolescents:** 100–225 mg/day PO in two to four divided doses. *Maximum:* 225 mg/day PO. **Adolescents:** Initially, 50–100 mg (regular tablets) PO as first dose. Then 150 mg/day PO in three divided doses. *Maximum:* 150 mg/day PO. **Note:** Reduce dosage for adolescents who have renal dysfunction.	Tablet, oral: 50 mg Tablets, oral delayed release: 25, 50, 75 mg Tablet, oral extended release: 100 mg Suppositories, rectal: 50, 100 mg **Note:** The delayed-release tablets should be dosed twice daily, every 12 hr. The extended-release tablets should be dosed once daily. **Note:** Although diclofenac oral extended-release tablets are available for once daily dosing, they are not generally recommended for adolescents because of the current lack of clinical data regarding their safety and efficacy among this age group.	**Contraindications:** Hypersensitivity to diclofenac or to other NSAIDs. **ADRs:** May cause abdominal cramps, constipation, diarrhea, dizziness, headache, nausea, rash, and vomiting. Rarely may cause erythema multiforme. *See also* "NSAIDs" in Chapter 5. **Comments:** Monitor for serious GI tract ulceration and bleeding, which may occur without warning among patients who are receiving long-term NSAID pharmacotherapy, including diclofenac. Monitor hepatic function upon initiation of therapy and periodically.
Diclofenac, ophthalmic *(Voltaren®)*	Postoperative inflammation following cataract extraction	**Children and adolescents:** Instill one drop in affected eye(s) four times daily, beginning 24 hr after cataract surgery and continuing throughout the entire first 2 weeks of the postoperative period.	Solution, ophthalmic: 0.1% **Note:** For ophthalmic use only.	**Contraindications:** Hypersensitivity to diclofenac or to other NSAIDs and concurrent use of hydrogel soft contact lenses. **ADRs:** May cause local ADRs including elevated intraocular pressure, keratitis, and transient burning and stinging upon instillation.
Dicloxacillin	Bacterial infection **Note:** Ensure that appropriate culture and sensitivity tests are performed and that the organism is sensitive to dicloxacillin.	**Infants, children, and adolescents:** 12–50 mg/kg/day PO in four divided doses, every 6 hr. **Note:** Administer on an empty stomach. *Maximum:* **Infants and children (<40 kg):** 2 grams/day PO; **children (≥40 kg):** 4 grams/day PO.	Capsules, oral: 125, 250, 500 mg Suspension, oral: 12.5 mg/ml; shake well before use. **Note:** Not generally available in Canada.	**Contraindications:** Hypersensitivity to dicloxacillin, other penicillins, or cephalosporins. **ADRs:** *See* Chapter 5.

TABLE 14-1 continued

DRUG (TRADE AND OTHER NAMES)	INDICATION(S)	USUAL PEDIATRIC DOSAGE AND ADMINISTRATION[a]	DOSAGE FORMS	CONTRAINDICATIONS, ADRs, AND COMMENTS[b]
Dicyclomine (*Antispas®, Bentyl®, Bentylol®,* Dicycloverine, *Di-Spaz®, Lomine®*)	Relief of GI tract smooth muscle spasms (as may occur, for example, with colitis, irritable bowel syndrome, and spastic colon)	**Infants (≥6 months) and children (<2 years):** 15–40 mg/day PO in three or four divided doses 15 min **before** a feeding. *Maximum:* 40 mg/day PO. **Note:** For infants and young children, dilute each dose with an equal volume of water prior to administration. **Children (≥2 years):** 30–40 mg/day PO in three or four divided doses. **Adolescents:** Initially, 30–80 mg/day PO. After 1 week, increase dosage according to response. *Maximum:* 160 mg/day PO.	Syrup, oral: 10 mg/5 ml (mixed fruit flavored) Tablets, oral: 10, 20 mg	**Contraindications:** Breast feeding, esophagitis, glaucoma, hypersensitivity to dicyclomine, infants younger than 6 months, intestinal atony, obstructive disease of the GI tract, obstructive uropathy, paralytic ileus, tachycardia, and ulcerative colitis (severe). **ADRs:** May cause blurred vision, dizziness, drowsiness, dry mouth, lightheadedness, nausea, nervousness, and weakness. *See also* "Anticholinergics" in Chapter 5.
Dicycloverine, *see* **Dicyclomine**				
Didanosine (Dideoxyinosine, *Videx®*)	HIV infection, advanced **Note:** Generally reserved for pediatric patients who are intolerant to zidovudine.	**Children and adolescents:** 100–300 mg/m²/day PO in three divided doses. **Note:** Administer on an empty stomach. Reduce dosage for pediatric patients who have renal dysfunction.	Powder (for reconstitution): 10 mg/ml (after reconstitution and dilution with a liquid antacid) Powder (for reconstitution in single-dose packets): 100, 167, 250, 375 mg Tablets, oral chewable: 25, 50, 100, 150 mg **Note:** The didanosine oral powder is initially reconstituted as a solution which is then immediately further diluted with a liquid antacid (e.g., *Maalox TC Suspension®* or *Mylanta Double Strength Liquid®*). Store under refrigeration between 2 and 8°C (36–46° F) and shake well before use.	**Contraindications:** Hypersensitivity to didanosine. **ADRs:** Commonly causes abdominal pain, chills, CNS depression, diarrhea, fever, headache, insomnia, leukopenia, nausea, peripheral neuropathy, pruritus, rash, and vomiting. **May cause potentially fatal pancreatitis.** *See* Chapter 5. **Comments:** Oral bioavailability is extremely variable. Didanosine is rapidly degraded at acidic pH. **Note:** Combination didanosine and stavudine pharmacotherapy for pregnant adolescents may result in fatal lactic acidosis.
Dideoxycytidine, *see* **Zalcitabine**				
Dideoxyinosine, *see* **Didanosine**				
Digoxin (*Lanoxin®*)	Congestive heart failure	*Digitalization:* See the following specific age-related dosage recommendations. Administer first dose immediately; second dose in 6 hr; and third dose in another 6 hr. **Infants and children (≤2 years):** 0.017 mg/kg/dose PO for three doses **or** 0.012 mg/kg/dose IV for three doses. **Children (>2 years) and adolescents:** 0.013 mg/kg/dose PO for three doses **or** 0.01 mg/kg/dose IV for three doses. *Maximum, digitalization:* 1-mg total dose IV or 1.5-mg total dose PO.	Capsules, oral: 0.05, 0.1, 0.2 mg Elixir, oral: 0.05 mg/ml (lime flavored; contains 10% alcohol) Injectables, IV: 0.05, 0.1, 0.25 mg/ml (contains 10% alcohol and propylene glycol) Tablets, oral: 0.125, 0.25 mg **Note:** IM injection is **not** recommended because of erratic and delayed absorption. Injectable formulations may contain alcohol and propylene glycol. Oral capsules have	**Contraindications:** Hypersensitivity to digoxin and ventricular fibrillation. **ADRs:** *See* Chapter 5. **Comments:** Begin maintenance dose 24 hr after first digitalization dose. Use with caution for patients who have hypokalemia. Therapeutic drug monitoring is recommended; *see* Table 14-3.

(Continued)

Footnotes are on page 558.

TABLE 14-1 continued

DRUG (TRADE AND OTHER NAMES)	INDICATION(S)	USUAL PEDIATRIC DOSAGE AND ADMINISTRATION[a]	DOSAGE FORMS	CONTRAINDICATIONS, ADRs, AND COMMENTS[b]
Digoxin *continued*		**Note:** Reduce dosage for pediatric patients who have renal dysfunction; *see* Table 14-2. *Maintenance:* **Infants and children (≤2 years):** 0.01–0.012 mg/kg/day PO as a single daily dose. **Children (>2 years) and adolescents:** 0.008–0.01 mg/kg/day PO as a single daily dose. *Maximum, maintenance:* 0.5 mg/day PO. **Note:** Reduce dosage for pediatric patients who have renal dysfunction; *see* Table 14-2.	greater bioavailability than do oral tablets; thus, the 0.1-mg oral capsule is equivalent to the 0.125-mg oral tablet and the 0.2-mg oral capsule is equivalent to the 0.25-mg oral tablet.	
Digoxin Immune Fab (ovine) *(Digibind®)* **Note:** *See also* Chapter 4.	Acute ingestion of unknown amount of digoxin	**Infants, children, and adolescents:** Dose of digoxin immune Fab (in number of 38-mg vials) = (digoxin serum concentration in ng/ml) × (patient weight in kg) ÷ (100). **Alternative for infants:** Initially, 190 mg IV (five vials). Monitor response and repeat dose, if needed. **Alternative for children:** Initially, 380 mg IV (10 vials). Monitor response and repeat dose, if needed. **Alternative for adolescents:** Initially, 760 mg IV (20 vials). Monitor response and repeat dose, if needed.	Injectable: 38 mg/vial **Note:** Generally administered as an IV infusion over 30 min through a 0.22-μm membrane filter. May be administered as a bolus IV injection if digitalis-induced cardiac arrest appears imminent.	**Contraindications:** None identified. **ADRs:** May cause hypokalemia; monitor potassium serum concentration. *See* Chapters 4 and 5. **Comments:** Carefully monitor clinical response and adjust dosage accordingly. **Note:** Standard immunoassay measurements of digoxin serum concentration following the administration of digoxin immune Fab will be clinically misleading until the Fab fragment is eliminated from the body.
	Acute ingestion of known amount of digoxin	**Infants, children, and adolescents:** Dose of digoxin immune Fab (in number of 38-mg vials) = (total digoxin body load in mg) ÷ (0.5 mg digoxin bound/vial).		
1α,25-Dihydroxycholecalciferol, *see* **Calcitriol**				
Dihydroergotamine *(Migranal®)*	Migraine headache, acute **Note:** Not indicated for the prophylactic management of migraine headache. **Note:** Not approved by the FDA or HPB for infants, children, or adolescents.	**Adolescents:** One spray of nasal solution (0.5 mg) into **each** nostril. After 15 min, an additional spray (0.5 mg) into **each** nostril for a total dosage of four sprays (2 mg). *Maximum:* 4 mg nasal spray solution over a 7-day period.	Solution, nasal spray: 4 mg/ml (in unit-dose kits with nasal spray applicator) **Note:** For intranasal use only. **Note:** The nasal spray applicator provided must be primed (squeezed four times) **prior** to use. Once the nasal spray applicator has been prepared, it should be discarded, together with any unused drug, after 8 hr.	**Contraindications:** Basilar or hemiplegic migraine, coronary artery disease, hepatic or renal impairment (severe), hypersensitivity to dihydroergotamine or other ergot alkaloids, other ergot alkaloid pharmacotherapy (concurrent or within 24 hr), serotonin agonist (e.g., sumatriptan) pharmacotherapy, and pregnancy. **ADRs:** May cause altered sense of taste, diarrhea, dizziness, nausea, pharyngitis, rhinitis, and vomiting. **Note:** Additional ADRs are associated with oral dihydroergotamine pharmacotherapy (*see* Chapter 5).

CHAPTER 14: DRUG DOSING FOR INFANTS, CHILDREN, AND ADOLESCENTS

TABLE 14-1 continued

DRUG (*TRADE* AND OTHER NAMES)	INDICATION(S)	USUAL PEDIATRIC DOSAGE AND ADMINISTRATION[a]	DOSAGE FORMS	CONTRAINDICATIONS, ADRs, AND COMMENTS[b]
Dihydro-tachysterol (*DHT®*, *Hytakerol®*, Vitamin D_2 Analog)	**Hypoparathyroidism** (to correct hypocalcemia)	**Infants and children:** Initially, 1–5 mg/day PO as a single dose. After 4 days, decrease dose to ¼ of initial dose, or continue with initial dose, based on response. *Maintenance:* 0.5–1.5 mg/day PO as a single dose. **Adolescents:** Initially, 0.75–2.5 mg/day PO as a single dose. After 4 days, decrease dose to ¼ of initial dose, or continue with initial dose, based on response. *Maintenance:* 0.2–1 mg/day PO as a single dose.	Capsule, oral: 0.125 mg (contains sesame oil) Solution, oral concentrate: 0.2 mg/ml (contains 20% alcohol) Tablets, oral: 0.125, 0.2, 0.4 mg **Note:** Store dihydrotachysterol dosage forms at controlled room temperature between 15 and 30°C in tightly closed, light-resistant containers.	**Contraindications:** Hypercalcemia, hypervitaminosis D, and renal failure. **ADRs:** Generally well tolerated. Too large a dose may result in hypercalcemia and associated effects. **Comments:** Monitor calcium and phosphate serum concentrations and renal function.
	Chronic renal failure (to suppress hyperparathyroidism and treat renal osteodystrophy) **Note:** Not approved by the FDA or HPB for the treatment of chronic renal failure for children or adolescents.	**Children and adolescents:** 0.1–0.5 mg/day PO.		
	Vitamin D-resistant rickets (familial hypophosphatemia) **Note:** Not approved by the FDA or HPB for the treatment of vitamin D-resistant rickets for children or adolescents.	**Children and adolescents:** Initially, 0.5–2 mg/day PO (until bone healing occurs). *Maintenance:* 0.2–1.5 mg/day PO. **Note:** Oral phosphate salts can be administered concurrently.		
Dimenhydrinate (*Dramamine®*, *Gravol®*)	**Allergic conditions/ Motion sickness**	**Children and adolescents:** 5 mg/kg/day IM, PO, or rectal in four divided doses, every 6 hr, as needed. *Maximum:* **Children (2–5 years),** 75 mg/day IM, PO, or rectal; **children (≥6 years),** 150 mg/day IM, PO, or rectal; **adolescents,** 300 mg/day IM, IV, PO, or rectal.	Injectable, IM, IV: 50 mg/ml Solutions, oral: 2.5, 3 mg/ml (cherry flavored); may contain 5% alcohol. Suppositories, rectal: 50, 100 mg Tablet, oral chewable: 50 mg Tablet, oral: 50 mg	**Contraindications:** Angle-closure glaucoma and hypersensitivity to dimenhydrinate. **ADRs:** May cause dizziness and drowsiness. *See* Chapter 5.
Dimercaprol (*BAL in Oil®*) **Note:** *See also* Chapter 4.	**Arsenic, gold, or mercury poisoning, severe** **Note:** Effective for acute mercury poisoning if administered within 2 hr of poisoning; not effective for the treatment of chronic mercury poisoning.	**Infants, children, and adolescents:** 3 mg/kg IM every 4 hr for 2 days, then four times daily for 1 day, then twice a day for 10 days.	Injectable, IM: 100 mg/ml (in peanut oil) **Note:** Not generally available in Canada.	**Contraindications:** Cadmium, iron, and selenium poisonings (the resultant complexes are nephrotoxic); hepatic or renal dysfunction; and hypersensitivity to peanuts. **ADRs:** Commonly associated with febrile reactions and hypertension among children (dose related). Feeling of constriction in chest, hands, or throat may occur (may be relieved by antihistamine pharmacotherapy), headache, nausea, nervousness, and vomiting. May also cause hemolysis among patients with *(Continued)*
	Arsenic or gold poisoning, mild	**Infants, children, and adolescents:** 2.5 mg/kg IM four times daily for 2 days, then twice a day for 1 day, then once daily for 10 days.		

Footnotes are on page 558.

TABLE 14-1 continued

DRUG (TRADE AND OTHER NAMES)	INDICATION(S)	USUAL PEDIATRIC DOSAGE AND ADMINISTRATION[a]	DOSAGE FORMS	CONTRAINDICATIONS, ADRs, AND COMMENTS[b]
Dimercaprol *continued*	Lead poisoning, severe (with signs and symptoms of encephalopathy or lead blood concentration >70 µg/dl)	**Infants, children, and adolescents:** 4 mg/kg IM every 4 hr for 5 days **or** 300 mg/m²/day in six divided doses every 4 hr for 3–5 days (may discontinue on day 3, if lead blood concentration <50 µg/dl).		glucose-6-phosphate dehydrogenase deficiency. **Comments:** *See* Chapter 4 for additional information.
	Lead poisoning, less severe	**Infants, children, and adolescents:** 4 mg/kg IM, then 3 mg/kg IM every 4 hr for 5–7 days. **Note:** For lead poisoning, administer first dose of dimercaprol alone. When adequate urine output has been established, administer subsequent doses of dimercaprol, with concomitant calcium disodium EDTA IM or by IV infusion. *See* Chapter 4.		
	Mercury poisoning, acute	**Infants, children, and adolescents:** Initial dose, 5 mg/kg IM; then 2.5 mg/kg IM once or twice daily for 10 days.		
Diphenhydramine, systemic *(AllerMax®, Benadryl®, Simply Sleep®)*	Allergic conditions	**Infants, children, and adolescents:** 5 mg/kg/day IM, IV, or PO in four divided doses every 6 hr. *Maximum:* 300 mg/day IM, IV, or PO.	Caplets, oral: 25, 50 mg Capsules, oral: 25, 50 mg Capsule, oral soft gel: 25 mg Elixir, oral: 12.5 mg/5 ml (cherry flavored) (contains 5%–15% alcohol) Injectables, IM, IV: 10, 50 mg/ml Solution, oral *(Children's Liquid Benadryl®):* 12.5 mg/5 ml (bubble gum flavored) Syrup, oral: 12.5 mg/5 ml (contains 5% alcohol) Tablets, oral: 25, 50 mg Tablet, oral chewable: 12.5 mg	**Contraindications:** Hypersensitivity to diphenhydramine. **ADRs:** Commonly causes drowsiness. Infants and young children may be more susceptible than older children, adolescents, and adults to ADRs. Excitation may also occur in young children. *See* Chapter 5.
	Anaphylaxis	**Infants, children, and adolescents:** 1–2 mg/kg/dose IV. *Maximum:* 50 mg/dose IV.		
	Insomnia	**Adolescents:** 25–50 mg/day PO as a single bedtime dose.		
Diphenhydramine, topical *(Benadryl®)*	**Itching** due to insect bites, mild cases of sunburn, poison oak, or poison ivy	**Children and adolescents:** Apply a small amount of topical cream to affected area(s) three or four times daily.	Cream, topical: 2% **Note:** For external use only. Avoid contact with eyes.	**Contraindications:** Extensive denuded or creeping skin lesions and skin rashes associated with either chickenpox or measles. **ADRs:** Generally well tolerated. May cause local irritation, particularly with prolonged use.
Diphenoxylate and Atropine *(Lomotil®, Lonox®)*	Diarrhea **Note:** Diphenoxylate and Atropine pharmacotherapy should **not** be used for pediatric patients who have either high fevers or blood in their stools. Nor should it be used when diarrhea is the result of poisoning until it has been determined that the poison has been	**Children (≥2 years):** Initially, 0.3 mg/kg/day PO in divided doses. *Maximum:* 2–5 years, 5 mg/day PO in two divided doses; 6–8 years, 7.5 mg/day PO in three divided doses; 9–12 years, 10 mg/day PO in four divided doses. **Adolescents:** Initially, 15–20 mg/day in three or four divided doses. *Maximum:* 20 mg/day PO.	Solution, oral: 2.5 mg diphenoxylate and 0.025 mg atropine/5 ml (may contain up to 15% alcohol) Tablet, oral: 2.5 mg diphenoxylate and 0.025 mg atropine.	**Contraindications:** Cirrhosis, hepatic coma, hypersensitivity to atropine or to diphenoxylate, infants and children less than 2 years, jaundice, pseudomembranous colitis, and ulcerative colitis. **ADRs:** May cause abdominal discomfort, blurred vision, dry mouth, euphoria, flushing, headache, lethargy, nausea, tachycardia, thirst, and urinary retention. (*See also* "Opiate Analgesics" and "Anticholinergics" in Chapter 5.)

TABLE 14-1 continued

DRUG (TRADE AND OTHER NAMES)	INDICATION(S)	USUAL PEDIATRIC DOSAGE AND ADMINISTRATION[a]	DOSAGE FORMS	CONTRAINDICATIONS, ADRs, AND COMMENTS[b]
Diphenoxylate and Atropine *continued*	sufficiently removed from the GI tract. (*See* Chapter 4.)	**Note:** Dosages are expressed in terms of amount of diphenoxylate.		**Comments:** Ensure that adequate attention is given to appropriate fluid and electrolyte replacement, particularly among infants and children with diarrhea.
Diphenylhydantoin, *see* **Phenytoin**				
Diphtheria Toxoid, *see* **Chapter 9**				
Disopyramide (*Norpace®, Rythmodan®*)	Ventricular tachy-dysrhythmias	**Children and adolescents:** 6–15 mg/kg/day PO in four divided doses, every 6 hr, **or** if using controlled-release capsules or tablets, 6–15 mg/kg/day PO in two divided doses, every 12 hr. **Note:** Reduce dosage for pediatric patients who have hepatic or renal dysfunction; *see* Table 14-2.	Capsules, oral: 100, 150 mg Capsules, oral controlled release: 100, 150 mg Tablet, oral controlled release: 250 mg **Note:** Regular and controlled-release oral formulations have different dosing intervals and cannot be used interchangeably.	**Contraindications:** Bronchospastic disorders, cardiogenic shock, congestive heart failure, electrolyte imbalance (severe), hepatic failure, hypersensitivity to disopyramide, hypotension (severe), and sinus node dysfunction (in the absence of a functioning artificial pacemaker). **ADRs:** Commonly causes anticholinergic effects, particularly dry mouth. *See* Chapter 5. **Comments:** Therapeutic drug monitoring is recommended; *see* Table 14-3.
Disulfiram (*Antabuse®*)	Adjunctive pharmacotherapy for the behavioral management of chronic alcoholism, alcohol abstinence **Note:** Disulfiram should be used in conjunction with appropriate psychotherapy and other treatment modalities. The patient should be fully informed and aware of the nature and purpose of disulfiram pharmacotherapy.	**Adolescents:** Initially, **after the patient has abstained from alcohol consumption for a minimum of 24 hr,** 250–500 mg/day PO as a single morning dose. After 2 weeks, the daily dosage may be reduced to a maintenance dosage of 125–250 mg/day PO. *Maximum:* 500 mg/day PO.	Tablets, oral: 250, 500 mg	**Contraindications:** Cerebral damage, cirrhosis, coronary artery disease, diabetes mellitus, epilepsy, hypersensitivity to disulfiram or other thiuram derivatives, myocardial disease (severe), nephritis, patients who are using alcohol or taking alcohol-containing products (e.g., elixirs), and metronidazole or paraldehyde pharmacotherapy (concurrent). **ADRs:** May cause acneiforme eruptions, drowsiness, garliclike aftertaste, headache, hepatitis, optic neuritis, peripheral neuritis, and polyneuritis. **Comments:** Before increasing disulfiram dosage or discontinuing disulfiram pharmacotherapy because of inadequate benefit, ensure that the patient has been compliant.
Divalproex Sodium, *see* **Valproic Acid**				
DMSA, *see* **Succimer**				
Dobutamine (*Dobutrex®*)	Cardiogenic shock **Note:** Not approved by the FDA or HPB for infants or children.	**Infants, children, and adolescents:** 0.5–20 µg/kg/min IV. *Maximum:* 40 µg/kg/min IV. **Note:** Avoid extravasation; administer via central vein, if possible.	Injectable, IV: 12.5 mg/ml **Note:** Contains sodium bisulfite. Sulfites may cause hypersensitivity reactions among susceptible patients, particularly those who have a history of asthma. These reactions include life-threatening anaphylaxis and less severe asthmatic episodes.	**Contraindications:** Hypersensitivity to dobutamine, idiopathic subaortic stenosis, and pheochromocytoma. **ADRs:** Commonly causes increased heart rate and blood pressure. May cause anxiety, fatigue, hypotension, nausea, and vomiting. **Comments:** Monitor ECG and blood pressure continuously during IV administration.
Docetaxel, *see* **Chapter 12**				

Footnotes are on page 558.

TABLE 14-1 continued

DRUG (TRADE AND OTHER NAMES)	INDICATION(S)	USUAL PEDIATRIC DOSAGE AND ADMINISTRATION[a]	DOSAGE FORMS	CONTRAINDICATIONS, ADRs, AND COMMENTS[b]
Docusate Calcium/ Potassium/ Sodium (Dioctyl [Calcium /Potassium/Sodium] Sulfosuccinate, *Colace*®)	Constipation **Note:** Regular use of docusate calcium, potassium, or sodium is **not** recommended.	**Children and adolescents:** 5 mg/kg/day PO as a single daily dose **or** 50–100 mg of oral docusate sodium drops mixed in enema solution rectal, as needed. *Maximum:* 240 mg/day PO. **Note:** Dilute each oral dose of docusate oral drops in 5–15 ml of nonessential beverage or food to mask bitter taste.	Calcium salt Capsules, oral: 50, 240 mg Potassium salt Capsules, oral: 100, 240 mg Sodium salt Capsule, oral: 100 mg Drops, oral: 10 mg/ml Syrup, oral: 4 mg/ml	**Contraindications:** Appendicitis, fecal impaction, hypersensitivity to docusates, intestinal obstruction, and mineral oil (concurrent use). **ADRs:** Generally well tolerated. May cause abdominal cramps. *See* Chapter 5. **Comments:** Requires 1–3 days for effect when given PO; adequate hydration is required for therapeutic effect.
Dolasetron (*Anzemet*®)	Prevention of nausea and vomiting associated with emetogenic antineoplastic pharmacotherapy	**Children (≥2 years):** 1.8 mg/kg/dose IV or PO as a single dose 30 min before administration of antineoplastic pharmacotherapy. *Maximum:* 100 mg IV or PO. **Adolescents:** 100 mg IV or PO as a single dose 30 min before antineoplastic administration.	Injectable, IV: 20 mg/ml Tablets, oral: 50, 100 mg **Note:** The dolasetron injectable formulation has been mixed with apple or apple–grape juice for oral administration for pediatric patients. The diluted product may be kept for up to 2 hr at room temperature before oral use.	**Contraindications:** Hypersensitivity to dolasetron. **ADRs:** May cause dizziness, fatigue, headache, and tachycardia. **Comments:** Dolasetron may cause ECG changes including prolongation of the PR and QT intervals and widening of the QRS complex. Although generally self-limiting and self-resolving with declining dolasetron blood concentrations, these effects can rarely lead to cardiac dysrhythmias or heart block. Dolasetron should, therefore, be used with caution for pediatric patients who have hypokalemia or hypomagnesemia, have congenital QT syndrome, and are receiving antidysrhythmic pharmacotherapy or cumulative high-dose anthracycline pharmacotherapy.
Domperidone (*Motilium*®)	Gastroesophageal reflux **Note:** Not approved by the FDA or HPB for infants or children.	**Infants, children, and adolescents:** 0.9–2.4 mg/kg/day PO in three or four divided doses. *Maximum:* 80 mg/day PO. **Note:** Administer 15–30 min before meals and before bedtime.	Tablet, oral: 10 mg	**Contraindications:** GI hemorrhage, hypersensitivity to domperidone, and mechanical obstruction of the GI tract. **ADRs:** Generally well tolerated. May cause abdominal cramps, dry mouth, headache, and rash. **Comments:** More severe ADRs (e.g., galactorrhea, gynecomastia, menstrual irregularities) are generally dose related and gradually resolve with a lowering of the dosage or the discontinuation of domperidone pharmacotherapy.
Dopamine (*Intropin*®)	Cardiogenic shock **Note:** Not approved by the FDA or HPB for infants or children. Inadequate renal perfusion **Note:** Not approved by the FDA or HPB for infants or children.	**Infants, children, and adolescents:** 5–25 µg/kg/min IV. *Maximum:* 25 µg/kg/min IV. **Note:** Avoid extravasation; administer via central vein if possible. **Infants, children, and adolescents:** 1–5 µg/kg/min IV. *Maximum:* 25 µg/kg/min IV.	Injectable, IV: 40 mg/ml **Note:** Contains sodium metabisulfite. Sulfites may cause allergic reactions in susceptible patients, particularly those with a history of asthma. **Note:** Not generally available in the United States.	**Contraindications:** Pheochromocytoma. **ADRs:** May cause anginal pain, dyspnea, ectopic heartbeats, headache, hypotension, nausea, palpitation, tachycardia, vasoconstriction, and vomiting. **Comments: Correct hypovolemia with appropriate volume expanders prior to initiating dopamine pharmacotherapy.** Monitor ECG, blood pressure, and urine output closely during administration.

TABLE 14-1 continued

DRUG (*TRADE* AND OTHER NAMES)	INDICATION(S)	USUAL PEDIATRIC DOSAGE AND ADMINISTRATION[a]	DOSAGE FORMS	CONTRAINDICATIONS, ADRs, AND COMMENTS[b]
Dornase Alfa (*Pulmozyme®*)	Cystic fibrosis (in conjunction with other standard therapies)	**Infants, children, and adolescents:** 2.5 mg/day by pulmonary inhalation via nebulizer. **Note:** Tight-fitting face mask (i.e., Pari-Baby®) may be used for infants and young children who are unable to use a nebulizer mouthpiece.	Solution, inhalation: 1 mg/ml in 2.5-ml ampule **Note:** For pulmonary inhalation only. **Note:** Store under refrigeration (2–8°C [36–46°F]) and protect from light.	**Contraindications:** Hypersensitivity to dornase alfa or to Chinese hamster ovary cell products. **ADRs:** May cause chest pain, conjunctivitis, cough, laryngitis, pharyngitis, rash, rhinitis, and voice alteration.
Doxapram, *see* **Chapter 13**				
Doxorubicin, *see* **Chapter 12**				
Doxycycline (*Doxychel®, Doxycin®, Vibramycin®, Vibra-Tabs®*)	Lyme disease, early stage	**Children (≥8 years) and adolescents:** 200 mg/day PO in two divided doses for 10–30 days.	Capsules, oral: 20, 50, 100 mg Powder, oral: 25 mg/5 ml after reconstitution (raspberry flavored; shake oral suspension well before use) Syrup, oral: 50 mg/5 ml (raspberry–apple flavored) Tablets, oral: 50, 100 mg	**Contraindications:** Breast feeding, children (< 8 years), hypersensitivity to doxycycline or to other tetracyclines, myasthenia gravis, and pregnancy. **ADRs:** *See* Chapter 5.
	Gonococcal infection	**Children (≥8 years) and adolescents:** 200 mg/day PO in two divided doses for 7 days.		
	Malaria prophylaxis (for short-term travel, less than 4 months, to endemic areas of chloroquine-resistant malaria)	**Children (≥8 years):** 2 mg/kg/day PO beginning 1 or 2 days prior to travel and continuing during travel to endemic area and for 4 weeks after leaving the endemic area. *Maximum:* 100 mg/day PO. **Adolescents:** 100 mg/day PO as a single dose beginning 1 or 2 days prior to travel and continuing during travel to endemic area and for 4 weeks after leaving the endemic area.		
	Syphilis	**Children (≥8 years) and adolescents:** 200 mg/day PO in two divided doses for 28 days. **Note:** Reduce dosage for pediatric patients who have hepatic or renal dysfunction.		
D-Penicillamine, *see* **Penicillamine**				
Dronabinol (*Marinol®*, Tetrahydrocannabinol)	Prevention of nausea and vomiting associated with antineoplastic pharmacotherapy (for use among pediatric patients who are refractory to conventional antiemetic pharmacotherapy)	**Children and adolescents:** Initially, 5 mg/m² PO as a single dose 1–3 hr before antineoplastic pharmacotherapy is begun. May repeat, as required, every 2–4 hr following antineoplastic pharmacotherapy for a total of four to six doses/day. If necessary (and in the absence of significant ADRs), dose may be increased in 2.5-mg/m² increments to 15 mg/m². *Maximum:* 15 mg/m²/dose.	Capsules, oral: 2.5, 5, 10 mg (contains sesame oil in soft gelatin capsules) **Note:** Store capsules at controlled room temperature between 8 and 15°C (46–59°F). Can also be stored in the refrigerator. Do **not** freeze.	**Contraindications:** Hypersensitivity to dronabinol, other cannabinoids, or sesame oil. **ADRs:** May cause abdominal pain, anxiety, confusion, dizziness, euphoria, hallucinations, paranoia, psychological dependence, somnolence, tachycardia, and vision difficulties. **Note:** May adversely affect short-term memory and, thus, academic performance.
Droperidol	Production of preoperative tranquilization and to reduce the incidence of nausea and vomiting during surgery	**Children (≥2 years):** 0.088–0.165 mg/kg IM as a single dose 30–60 min before the induction of general anesthesia. **Adolescents:** 2.5–10 mg IM or IV as a single dose 30–60 min before the induction of general anesthesia.	Injectable, IM, IV: 2.5 mg/ml **Note:** Store at controlled room temperature between 15 and 30°C protected from light.	**Contraindications:** Hypersensitivity to droperidol or to other butyrophenones, such as haloperidol. **ADRs:** May cause drowsiness, hypotension, and respiratory depression. Extrapyramidal signs and symptoms (e.g., akathisia,

(Continued)

Footnotes are on page 558.

TABLE 14-1 continued

DRUG (TRADE AND OTHER NAMES)	INDICATION(S)	USUAL PEDIATRIC DOSAGE AND ADMINISTRATION[a]	DOSAGE FORMS	CONTRAINDICATIONS, ADRs, AND COMMENTS[b]
Droperidol *continued*		**Note:** May need to reduce dosage for pediatric patients who have hepatic dysfunction.		dystonia, oculogyric crisis) may occur in ~1% of patients. **Note:** May cause QT interval prolongation and resultant torsades de pointes or sudden death, particularly at higher doses. Monitor for this ADR and consider alternative pharmacotherapy for patients who are at risk for cardiac dysrhythmias.
Econazole *(Ecostatin®, Spectazole®)*	Cutaneous candidiasis	**Children and adolescents:** Apply topically to affected skin site(s) twice daily, morning and evening.	Cream, topical: 1% **Note:** For external use only. Avoid contact with eyes.	**Contraindications:** Hypersensitivity to econazole. **ADRs:** May cause local irritation including burning sensation, erythema, itching, and stinging at application site. **Comments:** In order to reduce incidence of recurrence of cutaneous candidiasis and other fungal infections, it is generally recommended that treatment be continued for the following periods of time in relation to the type of infection being treated: *Tinea corporis, T. cruris, T. versicolor,* and cutaneous candidiasis, 2 weeks; *T. pedis,* 4 weeks.
	Cutaneous fungal infections: *Tinea corporis* (ring worm), *T. cruris* (jock itch), *T. pedis* (athlete's foot), and *T. versicolor*	**Children and adolescents:** Apply topically to affected skin site(s) once daily. **Note:** Affected skin site(s) should generally be washed with soap and warm water and then thoroughly dried before each application.		

Edetate Calcium Disodium, *see* **Chapter 4**

DRUG (TRADE AND OTHER NAMES)	INDICATION(S)	USUAL PEDIATRIC DOSAGE AND ADMINISTRATION[a]	DOSAGE FORMS	CONTRAINDICATIONS, ADRs, AND COMMENTS[b]
Edrophonium *(Enlon®, Tensilon®)*	Myasthenia gravis, suspected (diagnostic test)	**Infants, children, and adolescents:** 0.04 mg/kg/dose IV; after 1 min, may administer additional doses of 1 mg each at 1-min intervals. *Maximum:* **Children and adolescents <34 kg,** 1 mg IV (initial dose) and 5 mg IV (total dose); **children and adolescents ≥34 kg,** 2 mg IV (initial dose) and 10 mg IV (total dose).	Injectable, IV: 10 mg/ml **Note:** Contains sodium sulfite which may cause allergic reactions, particularly among patients with a history of asthma.	**Contraindications:** Hypersensitivity to edrophonium or to other anticholinesterases and mechanical obstruction of either the intestinal or urinary tract. **ADRs:** May cause cholinergic reactions including bradycardia, convulsions, difficulty breathing, diplopia, diarrhea, dysphagia, urinary incontinence, vomiting, and weakness. **Comments:** Atropine should be readily available for use as an antidote.
Efavirenz *(Sustiva®)*	HIV-1 infection **Note:** Efavirenz must always be used in combination with the most appropriate antiretroviral pharmacotherapy (e.g., nelfinavir) because of the rapid emergence of viral resistance when efavirenz is used as a single drug to treat HIV infection.	**Children (>3 years and ≥13 kg) and adolescents:** <table><tr><td>BODY WEIGHT</td><td>DOSAGE (mg/day/PO)</td></tr><tr><td>13–<15</td><td>200</td></tr><tr><td>15–<20</td><td>250</td></tr><tr><td>20–<25</td><td>300</td></tr><tr><td>25–<32.5</td><td>350</td></tr><tr><td>32.5–<40</td><td>400</td></tr><tr><td>≥40</td><td>600</td></tr></table> **Note:** Daily dosage is administered as a single oral dose, generally at bedtime, in order to improve ability to tolerate associated ADRs affecting the CNS.	Capsules, oral: 50, 100, 200 mg	**Contraindications:** Hypersensitivity to efavirenz, pregnancy, and concurrent use of cisapride, ergot derivatives, midazolam, or triazolam. **ADRs:** Commonly causes mild maculopapular rash that generally resolves with continued use. However, in ~4% of pediatric patients, a grade 4 rash (e.g., erythema multiforme) occurs necessitating discontinuation. May also cause abnormal dreams, dizziness, headache, impaired concentration, and insomnia. **Comments:** The long-term effects are unknown.

TABLE 14-1 continued

DRUG (TRADE AND OTHER NAMES)	INDICATION(S)	USUAL PEDIATRIC DOSAGE AND ADMINISTRATION[a]	DOSAGE FORMS	CONTRAINDICATIONS, ADRs, AND COMMENTS[b]
Enalapril (Vasotec®)	**Congestive heart failure** (often as combination pharmacotherapy with digoxin and/or a diuretic) **Note:** Not approved by the FDA or HPB for infants or children.	**Children and adolescents:** 0.1–0.5 mg/kg/day PO as a single dose. *Maximum:* 40 mg/day PO. **Note:** Initial dose should not exceed 1.25 mg PO.	Tablets, oral: 2.5, 5, 10, 20 mg	**Contraindications:** Hypersensitivity to enalapril or other angiotensin converting enzyme (ACE) inhibitors and pregnancy, second or third trimester. **ADRs:** May cause angioedema, blurred vision, dizziness, fever, headache, hypotension, myalgia, renal dysfunction, and urticaria. May also cause persistent nonproductive cough and hyperkalemia. See Chapter 5. **Comments:** Although rare, monitor for signs and symptoms of agranulocytosis and neutropenia.
	Hypertension, essential or renovascular (often as combination pharmacotherapy with thiazide diuretics) **Note:** Generally reserved for pediatric patients who have failed to respond to beta-adrenergic blockers and/or diuretics or who cannot tolerate their associated ADRs.	**Infants and children:** Initially, 0.08 mg/kg/day PO as a single dose. Adjust dosage according to blood pressure response. *Maximum:* 0.58 mg/kg/day PO **or** 40 mg/day PO, whichever is less. **Adolescents:** Initially, 2.5 mg (if receiving concurrent diuretic pharmacotherapy)/day PO as a single dose; **or** 5 mg (if not receiving concurrent diuretic pharmacotherapy)/day PO as a single dose. Adjust dosage according to blood pressure response. Higher dosages may be administered in two divided doses. *Maximum:* 40 mg/day PO. **Note:** Reduce dosage for pediatric patients who have renal dysfunction; see Table 14-2.		
Enoxaparin (Lovenox®)	**Prophylaxis against thromboembolic complications** (e.g., deep vein thrombosis) among patients undergoing orthopedic surgery **Note:** Not approved by the FDA or HPB for this indication for adolescents.	**Adolescents:** 60 mg/day SC in two divided doses, every 12 hr. **Note:** First dose is administered 12–24 hr following surgery and then continued for 7–14 days.	Injectable, SC: 100 mg/ml (contains 1.5% benzyl alcohol) Injectable, single-dose prefilled syringes: 30 mg/0.3 ml, 40 mg/0.4 ml, 60 mg/0.6 ml, 80 mg/0.8 ml, 100 mg/1 ml **Note:** For SC injection only. **Note:** 1 mg of enoxaparin = 100 international units (IU) of enoxaparin.	**Contraindications:** Bacterial endocarditis, blood clotting disorders, diabetic retinopathy, duodenal ulcer, gastric ulcer, hemorrhagic retinopathy, hypersensitivity to enoxaparin, hypertension (severe, untreated), IM injection of enoxaparin, and thrombocytopenia due to enoxaparin. **ADRs:** May cause bleeding. Hematomas at injection sites are relatively common (~5%–10% of patients). However, the incidence of major hemorrhage is low, particularly if the plasma antifactor Xa concentration remains below 2 IU/ml. **Comments:** Enoxaparin cannot be substituted (unit for unit) with unfractionated heparin or other low-molecular-weight heparins because of product differences in anti-Xa and anti-IIa actions, dosages, manufacturing processes, molecular weights, volumes of distribution, and units. **Note:** Measurements of hemoglobin concentration, platelet counts, and antifactor Xa concentrations are required prior to the initiation of enoxaparin pharmacotherapy and periodically during pharmacotherapy. With normal
	Deep vein thrombosis, treatment **Note:** Not approved by the FDA or HPB for this indication for children or adolescents.	**Children and adolescents:** 2 mg/kg/day SC in two divided doses, every 12 hr. *Maximum:* 180 mg/day SC. **Note:** When enoxaparin is used as the reference standard, antifactor Xa plasma concentrations should be <0.3 international units/ml **before** the initiation of enoxaparin pharmacotherapy and <1.7 IU/ml 3–4 hr **following** the initiation of enoxaparin pharmacotherapy. **Note:** Initiate oral anticoagulant (e.g., warfarin) pharmacotherapy as soon as possible. Enoxaparin pharmacotherapy should be continued for ~7 days or until therapeutic anticoagulant effect (i.e., INR of 2–3) has been achieved.		

(Continued)

Footnotes are on page 558.

TABLE 14-1 continued

DRUG (TRADE AND OTHER NAMES)	INDICATION(S)	USUAL PEDIATRIC DOSAGE AND ADMINISTRATION[a]	DOSAGE FORMS	CONTRAINDICATIONS, ADRs, AND COMMENTS[b]
Enoxaparin *continued*				prophylactic use, enoxaparin does not modify global traditional clotting tests such as activated partial thromboplastin time (aPTT), prothrombin time (PT), or thrombin clotting time (TT). Therefore, these tests are **not** of clinical value for monitoring enoxaparin pharmacotherapy.
Ephedrine	Bronchial asthma, mild **Note:** Not generally recommended as the drug of first choice.	**Children (2–6 years):** 2–3 mg/kg/day PO in four to six divided doses, every 4–6 hr. **Children (7–12 years):** 37.5–75 mg/day PO in six divided doses, every 4 hr. **Adolescents:** 75–150 mg/day PO in six divided doses, every 4 hr. *Maximum:* **Children,** 75 mg/day PO; **adolescents,** 150 mg/day PO.	Capsules, oral: 25, 50 mg Jellies, nasal: 0.6%, 1% Solutions, nasal spray: 0.25%, 0.5% Tablets, oral: 15, 30 mg **Note:** Widely available in combination cough and cold products.	**Contraindications:** Cardiac tachydysrhythmias, hypersensitivity to ephedrine, hypertension, narrow-angle glaucoma, and shock during general anesthesia with cyclopropane and halogenated hydrocarbons. **ADRs:** Generally well tolerated. May cause CNS stimulation including insomnia and nervousness. **Comments:** Tachyphylaxis has been associated with ephedrine nasal decongestant pharmacotherapy lasting longer than a few days.
	Nasal congestion **Note:** Not generally recommended as drug of first choice.	**Infants, children, and adolescents:** Apply nasal jelly or nasal spray solution topically to the nasal mucosa every 4–8 hr, as needed.		
Epinephrine (*Adrenalin®*, Adrenaline, *Bronkaid Mistometer®*, *EpiPen Jr. Auto-Injector®*, *Primatene Mist®*, *Sus-Phrine®*) **Note:** Various products are formulated for different routes of administration.	Anaphylaxis	**Infants, children, and adolescents:** 0.01 mg/kg/dose (minimum 0.1 mg/dose) SC every 10–20 min, as needed for up to three doses according to response. Then repeat dose every 2–4 hr, if required. *Maximum:* **Children,** 0.5 mg/dose SC; **adolescents,** 1 mg/dose SC. **Alternatively** (if necessitated by severe anaphylactic shock and resulting compromise of SC absorption): Initially, 0.05–0.1 mg/dose IV over 5–10 min. Follow by a continuous IV infusion of 0.1 µg/kg/min. *Maximum:* 0.25 mg/dose IV; 1.5 µg/kg/min IV.	Aerosol, inhalation: 0.35 mg epinephrine bitartrate (equivalent to 0.16 mg epinephrine base)/spray. Injectable, endotracheal tube instillation, inhalation, or SC: 1 mg/ml Injectables, IV: 0.1, 1, 5 mg/ml Injectable, IM: 0.5 mg/ml (1:2000). *EpiPen Jr. Auto-Injector®* delivers a 0.15-mg IM dose from a 2-ml single-use disposable injector. *EpiPen Auto-Injector®* delivers a 0.3-mg IM dose from a 2-ml single-use disposable injector. Solution, inhalation: 2.25% racemic epinephrine (equivalent to 1.13% epinephrine base) **Note:** Repeated SC injection has been associated with local necrosis at injection site. *See* Chapter 1 for details regarding SC injection site rotation. **Note:** Epinephrine is light sensitive. If the formulation is discolored (pinkish or darker than slightly yellow) or contains a precipitate, it should be appropriately discarded.	**Contraindications:** Cardiac tachydysrhythmias, general anesthesia with cyclopropane or halogenated hydrocarbons (e.g., halothane), hypersensitivity to epinephrine or to other sympathomimetic amines, hypertension, narrow-angle glaucoma, organic brain damage, organic heart disease, and shock (nonanaphylactic). **ADRs:** May cause dizziness, headache, insomnia, palpitation, and tremor. Syncope has occurred in children following the administration of epinephrine. *See* Chapter 5. **Comments:** Administration of epinephrine during labor may result in acceleration of fetal heart rate and prolonged uterine atony.
	Asthma, acute attacks	**Infants:** 0.05 mg SC every 20–30 min, as needed according to response. **Children and adolescents:** 0.01 mg/kg/dose SC, to a maximum of 0.5 mg/dose, every 20–30 min, as needed according to response **or** 0.5 mg/dose of racemic epinephrine for inhalation **or** 5 mg/dose L-epinephrine, diluted with sodium chloride 0.9% and given by nebulizer, as needed, to a maximum of every 3 hr.		
	Cardiac arrest	**Children and adolescents:** 0.01 mg/kg/dose (minimum 0.1 mg/dose) IV **or** 0.1 mg/kg/dose endotracheal (by endotracheal tube instillation), then 0.1 mg/kg/dose IV or		

TABLE 14-1 *continued*

DRUG (*TRADE* AND OTHER NAMES)	INDICATION(S)	USUAL PEDIATRIC DOSAGE AND ADMINISTRATION[a]	DOSAGE FORMS	CONTRAINDICATIONS, ADRs, AND COMMENTS[b]
Epinephrine *continued*		endotracheal (by endotracheal tube instillation). Dosage may be repeated at 5-min intervals during cardiac resuscitation according to response. *Maximum:* 1 mg/dose.	**Note:** Injectable formulations may contain sulfites which may cause allergic reactions in susceptible patients, particularly those with a history of asthma. However, this should **not** exclude the use of epinephrine in emergency situations. **Note:** IM injection into the vastus lateralis site (thigh) is recommended. Avoid dorsogluteal and ventrogluteal sites (buttocks) because of possible poor absorption. *See* Chapter 1 for IM injection site selection. **Note:** *Primatene Mist®* aerosol for inhalation contains 34% alcohol.	
	Croup	**Children:** 0.5 ml/dose of racemic epinephrine solution for inhalation **or** 5 mg/dose L-epinephrine, diluted with sodium chloride 0.9% and given by nebulizer, as needed, up to a maximum of every 1 hr.		
Epoetin Alfa (*Epogen®, Eprex®*, Erythropoietin, *Procrit®*)	Anemia associated with chronic renal failure	**Infants, children, and adolescents (on renal dialysis):** 50–150 units/kg/dose IV or SC three times a week. Increase the dosage by 25 units/kg if target hematocrit (30%–33%) is not achieved within 8 weeks. Decrease dosage by 25 units/kg if target hematocrit is exceeded. *Maximum:* 300 units/kg/dose.	Injectables, IV, SC: 2000, 3000, 4000, 10,000, 20,000, 40,000 units/vial (single dose, preservative free); do **not** shake vial. Shaking the vial may denature the epoetin alfa protein and cause it to become inactive. **Note:** Store refrigerated at 2–8°C. Do not freeze.	**Contraindications:** Anemia (severe, uncorrected), hypersensitivity to products derived from mammalian cells or to human albumin, and severe hypertension (uncontrolled). **ADRs:** Generally well tolerated. May cause arthralgia, diarrhea, dizziness, edema, fever, headache, hypertension, nausea, rash, and seizures. **Comments:** Monitor hematocrit and serum iron, particularly during periods of dosage adjustment. Many patients may require iron supplementation.
	Anemia associated with zidovudine pharmacotherapy among HIV-infected pediatric patients	**Children and adolescents:** Initially, 100 units/kg IV or SC three times per week for 8 weeks. If hematocrit does not improve, increase dosage by 50–100 units/kg three times a week, as needed, until target hematocrit (30%–33%) is achieved. *Maximum:* 300 units/kg/dose IV or SC. **Note:** Administer by slow IV injection over 1–5 min. If "flulike" symptoms are observed during IV injection, a slower rate of injection may be used. **Note:** The maximal volume for each SC injection is 1 ml. SC injection sites should be rotated (*see* Chapter 1).		

Epsom Salt, *see* **Magnesium Sulfate**
Ergocalciferol, *see* **Chapter 13**

TABLE 14-1 continued

DRUG (TRADE AND OTHER NAMES)	INDICATION(S)	USUAL PEDIATRIC DOSAGE AND ADMINISTRATION[a]	DOSAGE FORMS	CONTRAINDICATIONS, ADRs, AND COMMENTS[b]
Erythromycin (*E.E.S.®, E-Mycin®, Erybid®, Eryc®, EryPed®, Ery-Tab®, Erythrocin®*)	Bacterial infections **Note:** Ensure that appropriate culture and sensitivity tests are performed and that the organism is sensitive to erythromycin.	**Infants, children, and adolescents:** 30–50 mg/kg/day **base or ethylsuccinate** PO in four divided doses, every 6 hr. *Maximum:* 2 grams/day PO. **Or** 30–40 mg/kg/day **estolate** PO in two or three divided doses, every 8–12 hr. *Maximum:* 2 grams/day PO. **Or** 20–50 mg/kg/day **gluceptate** IV in four divided doses, every 6 hr, or by continuous IV infusion. *Maximum:* 4 grams/day IV. **Or** 20–40 mg/kg/day **lactobionate** IV in four divided doses, every 6 hr. *Maximum:* 4 grams/day IV. **Or** 20–40 mg/kg/day **stearate** PO in four divided doses, every 6 hr. *Maximum:* 2 grams/day PO.	**Erythromycin base:** Capsule, oral delayed release: 250 mg Tablets, oral: 250, 500 mg Tablets, oral enteric coated: 250, 333, 500 mg **Erythromycin estolate:** Capsule, oral: 250 mg Suspensions, oral: 125, 250 mg/5 ml (cherry or orange flavored); shake well before use. Tablets, oral: 250, 500 mg Tablet, oral chewable: 200 mg **Erythromycin ethylsuccinate:** Drops, oral: 100 mg/2.5 ml Suspension, oral granules for reconstitution: 200 mg/5 ml (after reconstitution) (cherry flavored); shake well before use. Suspensions, oral: 200, 400 mg/5 ml (banana, fruit, or orange flavored); shake well before use. **Erythromycin gluceptate:** Injectable, IV: 1 gram/vial **Note:** Minimal dilution of erythromycin gluceptate injectable formulation for IV use is 5 mg/ml. **Erythromycin lactobionate:** Injectables, IV: 500 mg/vial, 1 gram/vial **Note:** Minimal dilution of erythromycin lactobionate injectable formulation for IV use is 5 mg/ml. **Erythromycin stearate:** Tablets, oral: 125, 250, 500 mg	**Contraindications:** Hepatic dysfunction (severe) and hypersensitivity to erythromycin. **ADRs:** Hepatotoxicity is rare and has not been associated with any one particular ester or salt. May exacerbate the weakness associated with myasthenia gravis. *See* Chapter 5. **Comments:** Erythromycin may inhibit the hepatic metabolism of a number of drugs resulting in clinically significant drug interactions (*see* Chapter 6).
Erythromycin Ethylsuccinate (E) in combination with Sulfisoxazole (S) in a fixed 1:3 ratio (*Eryzole®, Pediazole®*)	Otitis media **Note:** Ensure that appropriate culture and sensitivity tests are performed and that the organism is sensitive to erythromycin and sulfisoxazole.	**Infants (≥2 months), children, and adolescents:** (50 mg E + 150 mg S)/kg/day PO in four divided doses, every 6 hr. *Maximum:* 2 grams E and 6 grams S/day PO.	Suspension, oral granules for reconstitution: 200 mg E + 600 mg S/ml (after reconstitution) (strawberry and strawberry–banana flavored); shake well before use.	**Contraindications:** Hypersensitivity to erythromycin ethylsuccinate or other forms of erythromycin and to sulfisoxazole or other sulfonamides. **ADRs:** *See* Chapter 5. **Comments:** Maintain adequate hydration. Use with caution for pediatric patients with renal dysfunction. *See* individual entries for erythromycin and sulfisoxazole for additional information.

Erythropoietin, *see* **Epoetin Alfa**
Eserine, *see* **Physostigmine**

TABLE 14-1 continued

DRUG (TRADE AND OTHER NAMES)	INDICATION(S)	USUAL PEDIATRIC DOSAGE AND ADMINISTRATION[a]	DOSAGE FORMS	CONTRAINDICATIONS, ADRs, AND COMMENTS[b]
Esmolol (Brevibloc®)	Supraventricular tachycardia **Note:** Not approved by the FDA or HPB for infants or children.	**Children and adolescents:** Initially, 500 µg/kg IV by rapid IV push over 1 min. Then 50 µg/kg/min IV over 4 min, as indicated by response. If adequate response is not achieved (after 5 min), increase the infusion rate to 100 µg/kg/min. When desired heart rate is achieved, reduce the IV infusion rate to the lowest effective dosage (generally 25–50 µg/kg/min) and infuse for up to 48 hr.	Injectable, IV: 10 mg/ml **Note:** Injectable formulation contains 25% propylene glycol. It is **not** intended for direct IV injection but must be diluted before use.	**Contraindications:** Congestive heart failure and hypersensitivity to esmolol or other beta-adrenergic blockers. **ADRs:** See Chapter 5. **Comments:** Esmolol and the other beta-adrenergic blockers are involved in a number of significant drug interactions (see Chapter 6).
Etanercept (Enbrel®)	Juvenile rheumatoid arthritis, polyarticular (refractory to conventional pharmacotherapy) **Note:** Not approved by the FDA for infants or children.	**Children (≥4 years) and adolescents:** 0.4 mg/kg SC twice weekly, 3 and 4 days apart (e.g., Monday and Thursday). *Maximum:* 25 mg/dose **and** 50 mg/week.	Injectable, SC (powder for reconstitution): 25 mg/ml (after reconstitution with bacteriostatic water for injection, which contains benzyl alcohol) **Note:** For SC use only. **Note:** Etanercept injectable powder for reconstitution and reconstituted solution should be stored under refrigeration between 2 and 8°C (36–46°F). Reconstituted solution should be used within 6 hr or discarded appropriately.	**Contraindications:** Hypersensitivity to etanercept and sepsis. **ADRs:** May cause abdominal pain, depression, gastric irritation, headache, infection, nausea, personality changes, and vomiting. Rarely causes aplastic anemia, multiple sclerosis, myelitis, optic neuritis, and pancytopenia.

Ethacrynate Sodium, see **Ethacrynic Acid**

DRUG (TRADE AND OTHER NAMES)	INDICATION(S)	USUAL PEDIATRIC DOSAGE AND ADMINISTRATION[a]	DOSAGE FORMS	CONTRAINDICATIONS, ADRs, AND COMMENTS[b]
Ethacrynic Acid (Edecrin®)	Fluid retention (edema) **Note:** IV ethacrynic acid pharmacotherapy is not approved by the FDA or HPB for children or adolescents.	**Children and adolescents:** Initially, 1 mg/kg/day PO as a single dose. Increase the dosage by 25-mg increments every 2 or 3 days until desired response is achieved **or** 2 mg/kg/day IV as a single dose; repeated IV doses are **not** recommended. *Maximum:* 3 mg/kg/day PO or 200 mg/day PO, whichever is less; 50 mg/dose IV.	Injectable, IV: 50 mg/vial Tablets, oral: 25, 50 mg	**Contraindications:** Anuria, electrolyte depletion (severe, uncorrected), hepatic coma, and hypersensitivity to ethacrynic acid. **ADRs:** See Chapter 5. **Comments:** Use with caution for pediatric patients with hepatic and severe cardiac dysfunction. Pediatric patients with renal dysfunction may be at increased risk for ototoxicity.
Ethambutol (Etibi®, Myambutol®)	Tuberculosis, pulmonary (ethambutol is used in **combination** with at least one other antitubercular drug) **Note:** Not recommended for pediatric patients who cannot cooperate with ophthalmic examinations. **Note:** Not approved by the FDA or HPB for infants or children.	**Children and adolescents:** 15–25 mg/kg/day PO as a single daily dose (preferred) **or** 50 mg/kg/dose PO twice weekly (until susceptibility to isoniazid and rifampin is confirmed). *Maximum:* 2.5 grams/day. **Note:** Ingestion with food or milk may decrease associated GI irritation. **Note:** Reduce dosage for pediatric patients who have renal dysfunction; see Table 14-2.	Tablets, oral: 100, 400 mg	**Contraindications:** Hypersensitivity to ethambutol and optic neuritis. **ADRs:** May cause anorexia, dermatitis, dizziness, fever, headache, malaise, mental confusion, peripheral neuritis, and vomiting. **Comments:** Optic neuritis has been associated with ethambutol pharmacotherapy, particularly with high-dose or long-term pharmacotherapy. Ophthalmic examination, including color vision testing, is recommended before and during ethambutol pharmacotherapy.

Ethanol, see **Alcohol**

Footnotes are on page 558.

TABLE 14-1 continued

DRUG (TRADE AND OTHER NAMES)	INDICATION(S)	USUAL PEDIATRIC DOSAGE AND ADMINISTRATION[a]	DOSAGE FORMS	CONTRAINDICATIONS, ADRs, AND COMMENTS[b]
Ethinyl Estradiol and Levonorgestrel *(Alesse®, Min-Ovral®, Triphasil®, Triquilar®)*	Conception control	**Adolescents:** 20 µg ethinyl estradiol and 100 µg levonorgestrel/day PO as a single dose (preferably after the evening meal or at bedtime) for 21 consecutive days; then a 7-day interval without ethinyl estradiol and levonorgestrel. The entire dosing cycle is repeated (3 weeks of ethinyl estradiol and levonorgestrel followed by 1 week off). **Note:** Dosage for the triphasic formulations *(Triphasil®, Triquilar®)* must be taken in the exact order indicated by the dispenser because the 21 "active" tablets do **not** all contain the same ratio of estrogen and progestin (for days 1–6, tablets contain 30 µg ethinyl estradiol and 50 µg levonorgestrel; days 7–11, tablets contain 40 µg ethinyl estradiol and 75 µg levonorgestrel; and days 12–21, tablets contain 30 µg ethinyl estradiol and 125 µg levonorgestrel).	**Tablets,** oral: 20 µg ethinyl estradiol and 100 µg levonorgestrel *(Alesse®)*; 30 µg ethinyl estradiol and 150 µg levonorgestrel *(Min-Ovral®)*; see "Dosage" for *Triphasil®* and *Triquilar®*). **Note:** Packages contain 21 "active" ethinyl estradiol and levonorgestrel tablets with or without an additional seven "inactive" tablets. The active and inactive tablets differ in color, and vary among various manufacturers' brands (e.g., pink and green; white and pink).	**Contraindications:** Cancers (estrogen dependent), cerebrovascular disorders, coronary artery disease, hepatic dysfunction, pregnancy, thromboembolic disorders, and vaginal bleeding (undiagnosed, abnormal). **ADRs:** May cause nausea and vomiting, particularly during the first cycle of use. *See* "Oral Contraceptives" in Chapter 5. **Comments:** Cigarette smoking significantly increases the risk for oral-contraceptive-related cardiovascular ADRs (e.g., myocardial infarction, thromboembolism) and resulting morbidity and mortality. **Note:** Patients should be advised that use of ethinyl estradiol and levonorgestrel does not provide protection against HIV infection or other sexually transmitted diseases.
Ethinyl Estradiol and Norethindrone *(Brevicon®, Ortho®, Select®, Synphasic®)*	Conception control	**Adolescents:** One tablet/day PO as a single dose at the same time each day for 21 consecutive days (3 weeks). Follow by 7 days (1 week) with either no tablets or a "reminder" (nonactive) tablet. Then repeat the entire cycle (3 weeks on active pharmacotherapy and 1 week off). **Note:** The amounts of ethinyl estradiol and norethindrone vary among the various single phase, biphasic, and triphasic formulations.	Tablets, oral: **Single-Phase Formulations,** 35 µg ethinyl estradiol and 500 µg norethindrone *(Brevicon 0.5/35®)*; *Ortho 0.5/35®)*; 35 µg ethinyl estradiol and 1000 µg norethindrone *(Brevicon 1/35®; Ortho 1/35®; Select 1/35®)*. **Biphasic Formulations,** 10 tablets containing 35 µg ethinyl estradiol and 500 µg norethindrone and 11 tablets containing 35 µg ethinyl estradiol and 1000 µg norethindrone *(Ortho 10/11®; Synphasic®)*. **Triphasic Formulations,** seven tablets containing 35 µg ethinyl estradiol and 500 µg norethindrone, seven tablets containing 35 µg ethinyl estradiol and 750 µg norethindrone, and seven tablets containing 35 µg ethinyl estradiol and 1000 µg norethindrone *(Ortho 7/7/7®)*.	**Contraindications:** Cancers (estrogen dependent), cerebrovascular disorders, coronary artery disease, hepatic dysfunction, pregnancy, thromboembolic disorders, and vaginal bleeding (undiagnosed, abnormal). **ADRs:** May cause nausea and vomiting, particularly during the first cycle of use. *See* "Oral Contraceptives" in Chapter 5. **Comments:** Cigarette smoking significantly increases the risk for oral-contraceptive-related cardiovascular ADRs (e.g., myocardial infarction, thromboembolism) and resulting morbidity and mortality. **Note:** Patients should be advised that use of ethinyl estradiol and norethindrone does not provide protection against HIV infection or other sexually transmitted diseases.

TABLE 14-1 continued

DRUG (TRADE AND OTHER NAMES)	INDICATION(S)	USUAL PEDIATRIC DOSAGE AND ADMINISTRATION[a]	DOSAGE FORMS	CONTRAINDICATIONS, ADRs, AND COMMENTS[b]
Ethionamide (*Trecator®*)	Tuberculosis (in combination with one or two other antitubercular drugs) **Note:** Generally limited to use for pediatric patients who cannot receive, or are resistant to, standard antitubercular pharmacotherapy (e.g., isoniazid and rifampin pharmacotherapy). **Note:** Resistance to ethionamide rapidly develops if used alone for the treatment of tuberculosis.	**Children:** 15 mg/kg/day PO as a single dose. *Maximum:* 1000 mg/day PO. **Adolescents:** 15–20 mg/kg/day PO as a single dose. *Maximum:* 1000 mg/day PO. **Note:** Each daily dose of ethionamide may be administered in two divided doses with a meal, if required, to avoid or minimize associated GI irritation.	Tablet, oral: 250 mg (sugar coated) **Note:** Not generally available in Canada.	**Contraindications:** Hypersensitivity to ethionamide and hepatic dysfunction (severe). **ADRs:** May cause abdominal pain, anorexia, depression, diarrhea, dizziness, drowsiness, excessive salivation, headache, metallic taste, nausea, peripheral neuritis, postural hypotension, restlessness, and vomiting. **Comments:** Concurrent pyridoxine pharmacotherapy has been recommended to avoid or minimize possible neurotoxic effects associated with ethionamide pharmacotherapy.
Ethosuximide (*Zarontin®*)	Absence (petit mal) seizures	**Infants and children (≤6 years):** Initially, 250 mg/day PO in two divided doses **or** 15 mg/kg/day PO as a single dose or as two divided doses. Increase the dosage gradually every 3 days as needed, according to response. *Maximum:* 1500 mg/day **or** 40 mg/kg/day, whichever is less. **Children (>6 years) and adolescents:** 20 mg/kg/day PO as a single dose or as two divided doses. *Maximum:* 1500 mg/day PO. **Note:** Gradually discontinue to avoid associated seizures or status epilepticus. Whenever feasible, reduce the dosage over several days before completely discontinuing.	Capsule, oral: 250 mg Syrup, oral: 50 mg/ml	**Contraindications:** Hypersensitivity to ethosuximide or other succinimides. **ADRs:** Associated with potentially **fatal** blood dyscrasias including agranulocytosis and aplastic anemia. Therefore, complete blood counts should be obtained before initiating ethosuximide pharmacotherapy and periodically during ethosuximide pharmacotherapy. Also has been associated with abdominal pain, cramps, diarrhea, loss of appetite, nausea, and vomiting (*see also* Chapter 5). **Note:** Therapeutic drug monitoring is recommended; *see* Table 14-3.

Ethyl Alcohol, *see* **Alcohol**
Ethyl Aminobenzoate, *see* **Benzocaine**
Etoposide, *see* **Chapter 12**

Factor IX (Human) (*Mononine®*) **Note:** *See also* Factor IX Complex.	**Bleeding related to factor IX deficiency** (Christmas disease, hemophilia B), prevention and control	**Infants, children, and adolescents:** 15–50 units/kg IV administered at a rate of 200 units (2 ml)/min. Dosage is guided by indication for use and response. *Maximum:* 75 units/kg/dose.	Injectable, IV (powder for reconstitution): 100 units/ml (after reconstitution with sterile water for injection [diluent provided]) **Note:** For IV use only.	**Contraindications:** Hypersensitivity to mouse protein. **ADRs:** May cause chills, disseminated intravascular coagulation, fever, flushing, headache, hives, lethargy, nausea, stinging at the injection site, and vomiting. **Comments:** Current technology cannot fully guarantee 100% prevention of viral infection transmission for factor IX (human) and other products derived from human plasma.
	Minor spontaneous hemorrhage prophylaxis for patients with factor IX deficiency	**Infants, children, and adolescents:** Initially, 30 units/kg IV by infusion. Repeat dose once in 24 hr, if required, according to response.		
	Major trauma or surgery hemorrhage prophylaxis for patients with factor IX deficiency	**Infants, children, and adolescents:** Initially, 75 units/kg IV administered at a rate of 100–200 units (1–2 ml)/min. Repeat dose every 18–30 hr for up to 10 days, depending upon measured factor IX concentrations.		

(Continued)

Footnotes are on page 558.

TABLE 14-1 continued

DRUG (TRADE AND OTHER NAMES)	INDICATION(S)	USUAL PEDIATRIC DOSAGE AND ADMINISTRATION[a]	DOSAGE FORMS	CONTRAINDICATIONS, ADRs, AND COMMENTS[b]
Factor IX (Human) *continued*		**Note:** Monitor patients during IV infusion for flushing, headache, or changes in blood pressure or pulse. If noted, stop the infusion until the signs and symptoms subside and resume infusion at a slower rate.		
Factor IX Complex (Bebulin VH Immuno®, Konyne 80®, Proplex T®) **Note:** *See also* Factor IX (Human)	Prevention of bleeding caused by factor IX deficiency associated with hemophilia B (Christmas disease)	**Infants, children, and adolescents:** 20–30 units/kg IV at an infusion rate of up to 100 units/min. This dosage is generally administered once or twice a week depending upon response. **Note:** Laboratory monitoring of factor IX plasma concentrations is required to guide dosage.	Injectable, IV (powder for reconstitution): 25 units of factor IX/ml (after reconstitution with sterile water for injection [diluent provided]). The injectable also contains variable amounts of coagulation factors II, VII, and X. **Note:** For IV use only. **Note:** Factor IX complex must be used within 3 hr of reconstitution. Any unused portion should be discarded appropriately. Do **not** refrigerate after reconstitution.	**Contraindications:** None identified. **ADRs:** May cause transient chills, fever, flushing, headache, and tingling, particularly with rapid IV infusion. **Comments:** Factor IX complex and other products derived from human plasma may contain infectious viruses (e.g., hepatitis A virus, parvovirus B19).
	Bleeding episodes among patients with hemophilia A (factor VIII deficiency) who have inhibitors to factor VIII	**Infants, children, and adolescents:** 75 units/kg IV. Dose may be repeated in 12 hr, if required, according to response.		
Famotidine (Pepcid®)	Gastroesophageal reflux disease (GERD) with or without esophagitis	**Children and adolescents:** 1–2 mg/kg/day PO as a single dose or as two divided doses. *Maximum:* 80 mg/day PO.	Injectable, IV: 10 mg/ml Suspension, oral: 40 mg/5 ml (after reconstitution) (cherry, banana, and mint flavored); shake well before use. Tablets, oral: 20, 40 mg Tablets, oral disintegrating: 20, 40 mg (mint flavored)	**Contraindications:** Hypersensitivity to famotidine or to other H_2-receptor antagonists. **ADRs:** Generally well tolerated. May cause headache. *See* Chapter 5.
	Peptic ulcer	**Children and adolescents:** 0.5–1 mg/kg/day PO or IV as a single dose at bedtime or as two divided doses. *Maximum:* 40 mg/day IV or PO. **Note:** Administer IV pharmacotherapy either by slow IV injection (IV push) over ≥2 min or IV infusion over 15 min. **Note:** Reduce dosage for pediatric patients who have renal dysfunction; *see* Table 14-2.		
Fat Emulsions, *see* **Chapter 13**				
Fenofibrate, microcoated (Lipidil Supra®) **Note:** *See also* Fenofibrate, micronized.	Hypercholesterolemia (Fredrickson classification types IIa and IIb mixed hyperlipidemia), adjunctive management with diet and other therapeutic measures (e.g., exercise) **Note:** Not approved by the FDA or HPB for this indication for children or adolescents. **Note: Not** indicated for the treatment of type I hyperlipoproteinemia.	**Children and adolescents:** 5 mg/kg/day PO in a single dose with a large meal. *Maximum:* 160 mg/day PO. **Note:** Administration with food significantly increases bioavailability and conversion to the active metabolite. **Note:** Monitor and adjust dosage according to lipid blood concentrations and response. **Note:** Reduce dosage for pediatric patients who have severe renal dysfunction (creatinine clearance <50 ml/min).	Tablets, oral: 100, 160 mg	**Contraindications:** Biliary cirrhosis, breast feeding, creatinine clearance <20 ml/min, gallbladder disease, hepatic dysfunction, hypersensitivity to fenofibrate or to other related fibrates, and pregnancy. **ADRs:** May cause a variety of ADRs including abdominal pain, arthralgia, constipation, fatigue, flatulence, nausea, pruritus, and rash. May rarely cause cholelithiasis, myositis, and rhabdomyolysis. **Comments:** Baseline liver function tests are generally recommended and should be repeated (every 3–12 months, as required).

TABLE 14-1 continued

DRUG (TRADE AND OTHER NAMES)	INDICATION(S)	USUAL PEDIATRIC DOSAGE AND ADMINISTRATION[a]	DOSAGE FORMS	CONTRAINDICATIONS, ADRs, AND COMMENTS[b]
Fenofibrate, micronized (*Gen-Fenofibrate Micro®, Lipidil Micro®, PMS-Fenofibrate Micro®, Tricor®*) **Note:** *See also* Fenofibrate, microcoated.	**Hypercholesterolemia** (Fredrickson classification types IIa and IIb mixed hyperlipidemia), adjunctive management with diet and other therapeutic measures (e.g., exercise) **Note:** Not approved by the FDA or HPB for this indication for children or adolescents. **Note: Not** indicated for the treatment of type I hyperlipoproteinemia	**Children and adolescents:** Initially, 67 mg/day PO as a single dose. *Maximum:* 200 mg/day PO. **Note:** Monitor and adjust dosage according to lipid blood concentrations and response. **Note:** Reduce dosage for pediatric patients who have severe renal dysfunction (creatinine clearance <50 ml/min).	Capsules, oral hard gelatin: 67, 134, 200 mg; protect from moisture.	**Contraindications:** Biliary cirrhosis, breast feeding, creatinine clearance <20 ml/min, gallbladder disease, hepatic dysfunction, hypersensitivity to fenofibrate or to other related fibrates, and pregnancy. **ADRs:** May cause a variety of ADRs including constipation, fatigue, flatulence, nausea, pruritus, and rash. May rarely cause cholelithiasis, myositis, and rhabdomyolysis. **Comments:** Baseline liver function tests are generally recommended and should be repeated (every 3–12 months, as required).
Fentanyl (*Actiq®, Duragesic®*)	**Pain** **Note:** Indicated primarily for pediatric patients during or immediately following surgery (e.g., to enhance anesthesia, to provide short-acting analgesia during anesthesia, and to provide analgesia immediately following surgery).	**Children (≥2 years) and adolescents:** Initially, 1–5 μg/kg/dose IV **or** 2–3 μg/kg/dose IM. The initial dose may be repeated in 30–60 min as indicated by response.	Injectable, IM, IV: 50 μg/ml Transmucosal lozenge on a stick (*Actiq*): 200, 400, 600, 800, 1200, 1600 μg Transdermal patch (*Duragesic*): 25 μg/hr per 10 cm² **Note:** The safety and efficacy of transdermal and transmucosal fentanyl pharmacotherapy for children have not been established and such therapy is **not** generally recommended.	**Contraindications:** Hypersensitivity to fentanyl or to other opiate analgesics. **ADRs:** Addicting and habituating; associated with bradycardia, respiratory depression, and skeletal and thoracic muscle rigidity. If untreated, these ADRs may result in respiratory arrest, circulatory depression, and cardiac arrest. *See* Chapter 5. **Comments:** Muscle rigidity, particularly involving the muscles of respiration, appears to be related to the rate by which fentanyl is injected IV. To avoid this ADR, administer by slow IV injection. IV fentanyl pharmacotherapy also has been associated with bradycardia, bronchospasm, euphoria, and miosis. Only inject fentanyl IV in the hospital setting where resuscitative equipment and adequately prepared personnel are readily available for emergency symptomatic medical support of body systems, including airway maintenance (intubation) and assisted or controlled respiration. The opiate antagonist, naloxone *(Narcan®)* also should be readily available for emergency use, if needed.
Ferrous Salts, *see* **Iron, oral**				
Fexofenadine (*Allegra®*)	**Seasonal allergic rhinitis,** relief of signs and symptoms (e.g., itchy, red eyes; lacrimation; rhinorrhea; sneezing)/**Urticaria,** chronic, idiopathic	**Children (≥6 years):** 60 mg/day PO in two divided doses. **Adolescents:** 120 mg/day PO in two divided doses.	Tablets, oral: 30, 60 mg	**Contraindications:** Hypersensitivity to fexofenadine. **ADRs:** Generally well tolerated. May cause drowsiness, headache, and nausea.
Filgrastim, *see* **Chapter 12**				

Footnotes are on page 558.

TABLE 14-1 continued

DRUG (TRADE AND OTHER NAMES)	INDICATION(S)	USUAL PEDIATRIC DOSAGE AND ADMINISTRATION[a]	DOSAGE FORMS	CONTRAINDICATIONS, ADRs, AND COMMENTS[b]
Flecainide (*Tambocor*®)	Life-threatening ventricular dysrhythmias **Note:** Not approved by the FDA or HPB for infants or children.	**Children and adolescents:** 2–6 mg/kg/day PO in two or three divided doses. *Maximum:* 400 mg/day PO. **Note:** Reduce dosage for pediatric patients who have hepatic or renal dysfunction.	Tablets, oral: 50, 100, 150 mg	**Contraindications:** Atrial fibrillation (chronic), cardiogenic shock, heart block, and hypersensitivity to flecainide. **ADRs:** *See* Chapter 5. **Comments:** Therapeutic drug monitoring is recommended; *see* Table 14-3.
Fluconazole (*Diflucan*®)	Cryptococcal meningitis, treatment	**Infants, children, and adolescents:** 6–12 mg/kg/day PO as a single daily dose. *Maximum:* 400 mg/day PO. **Note:** Usually continued for 10–12 weeks following the achievement of culture-negative cerebrospinal fluid.	Capsule, oral: 250 mg Solutions, oral: 125, 250 mg/5 ml Suspension, oral: 50 mg/5 ml (orange flavored); shake well before use. Tablets, oral: 50, 100 mg	**Contraindications:** Hypersensitivity to fluconazole. **ADRs:** Generally well tolerated. May cause diarrhea and vomiting. ADRs occur more frequently and tend to be more severe among HIV-positive patients. *See* Chapter 5. **Comments:** Monitor hepatic function and discontinue pharmacotherapy if signs and symptoms of hepatotoxicity are observed.
	Cryptococcal meningitis among patients with AIDS, prevention of recurrence	**Infants, children, and adolescents:** 6 mg/kg/day PO as a single dose. *Maximum:* 200 mg/day PO.		
	Esophageal candidiasis	**Infants, children, and adolescents:** 3–6 mg/kg/day PO as a single dose. *Maximum:* 200 mg/day PO. **Note:** Usually required for a minimum of 3 weeks, including at least 2 weeks following the resolution of signs and symptoms.		
	Oropharyngeal candidiasis	**Infants, children, and adolescents:** 3 mg/kg/day PO as a single dose. *Maximum:* 100 mg/day PO.		
	Systemic candidiasis	**Infants, children, and adolescents:** 6–12 mg/kg/day PO as a single daily dose. *Maximum:* 400 mg/day PO. **Note:** Usually required for a minimum of 4 weeks, including at least 2 weeks following the resolution of signs and symptoms. **Note:** Reduce dosage for pediatric patients who have renal dysfunction; *see* Table 14-2.		
Flucytosine (*Ancobon*®, 5-Fluorocytosine)	Fungal infections	**Children and adolescents:** 50–150 mg/kg/day PO in four divided doses, every 6 hr. **Note:** Reduce dosage for pediatric patients who have renal dysfunction; *see* Table 14-2.	Capsules, oral: 250, 500 mg **Note:** Not generally available in Canada.	**Contraindications:** Hypersensitivity to flucytosine. **ADRs:** *See* Chapter 5. **Comments:** Monitor hematologic, hepatic, and renal function. **Note:** Therapeutic drug monitoring is recommended; *see* Table 14-3.
Fludarabine, *see* Chapter 12				
Fludrocortisone (*Florinef*®)	Addison's disease (generally in combination with cortisone or hydrocortisone)	**Children and adolescents:** Initially, 0.05 mg/day PO as a single dose. *Maximum:* 0.2 mg/day PO.	Tablet, oral scored: 0.1 mg	**Contraindications:** Systemic fungal infections and recent smallpox vaccination. **ADRs:** Generally well tolerated. May cause significant sodium retention and related sequelae. *See* "Corticosteroids" in Chapter 5.

TABLE 14-1 continued

DRUG (TRADE AND OTHER NAMES)	INDICATION(S)	USUAL PEDIATRIC DOSAGE AND ADMINISTRATION[a]	DOSAGE FORMS	CONTRAINDICATIONS, ADRs, AND COMMENTS[b]
Fludro-cortisone *continued*	Salt-losing adrenogenital syndrome	**Infants, children, and adolescents:** Initially, 0.05–0.1 mg/day PO as a single dose. *Maximum:* 0.2 mg/day PO. **Note:** Lowest effective dosage should be used to minimize ADRs.		**Comments:** Monitor growth and development of infants and children receiving long-term therapy. Monitor patients for corticosteroid-related ADRs, including the signs and symptoms of Cushing's syndrome (edema, hypertension, excessive potassium excretion, weight gain).
Flumazenil *(Anexate®, Romazicon®)* **Note**: *See also* Chapter 4.	Benzodiazepine overdosage	**Children and adolescents:** 0.01 mg/kg/dose IV over 30 sec (rapid IV push). Repeat, as indicated by response. May follow initial dose with a continuous IV infusion of 0.005–0.01 mg/kg/hr until the patient responds or the maximal recommended dosage is reached. *Maximum:* **Children and adolescents (≤30 kg),** 2 mg IV (total dosage); **children and adolescents >30 kg),** 3 mg IV (total dosage).	Injectables, IV: 0.1 mg/ml **Note:** *See* Chapter 8.	**Contraindications:** Cyclic antidepressant overdosage, head injury (may precipitate seizures), hypersensitivity to flumazenil or to the benzodiazepines, and seizure disorders including epilepsy (may precipitate seizures). **ADRs:** Generally well tolerated. May cause agitation, anxiety, flushing, headache, hypertension, nausea, tachycardia, and vomiting. **Comments:** Excessive or rapid administration to pediatric patients who are addicted to benzodiazepines may induce the benzodiazepine-withdrawal syndrome. Cardiac dysrhythmias and seizures also have been observed, particularly among patients with epilepsy, hepatic dysfunction (severe), history of long-term benzodiazepine use, and mixed-drug overdosages.
Flunarizine *(Sibelium®)*	Migraine prophylaxis (to reduce frequency of occurrence) **Note:** Not indicated for the treatment of acute migraine attacks. **Note:** Not approved by the FDA or HPB for children or adolescents.	**Adolescents:** 5–10 mg/day PO as a single dose at bedtime. **Note:** Onset of maximal therapeutic benefit may require several weeks.	Capsule, oral: 5 mg **Note:** Not generally available in the United States.	**Contraindications:** Depression (history), extrapyramidal disorders (history), and hypersensitivity to flunarizine. **ADRs:** Commonly causes drowsiness and weight gain. May cause depression, extrapyramidal symptoms, and insomnia. **Comments:** Flunarizine primarily reduces the frequency of migraine attacks, not their severity or duration.
Flunisolide, nasal *(Nasalide®, Nasarel®, Rhinalar®)* **Note:** *See also* Flunisolide, pulmonary.	Allergic rhinitis, perennial and seasonal, refractory to conventional pharmacotherapy	**Children (≥6 years):** 150 µg/day by nasal spray (one spray in each nostril three times daily). **Adolescents:** 300 µg/day by nasal spray (two sprays in each nostril three times daily). **Note:** After the rhinitis is controlled, children and adolescents can often be maintained on 50 µg/day by nasal spray (one spray in each nostril once each day).	Solution, nasal spray: 25 µg/spray (supplied with a metered-pump device that does not contain fluorocarbons)	**Contraindications:** Bacterial, fungal, or viral infections; hypersensitivity to flunisolide; and tuberculosis. **ADRs:** Generally well tolerated. May cause an aftertaste and mild nasal burning or stinging. **Comments:** Several days are generally required before therapeutic benefit is observed. *See* Chapter 1 for proper nasal spray administration techniques.

Footnotes are on page 558.

TABLE 14-1 *continued*

DRUG (*TRADE* AND OTHER NAMES)	INDICATION(S)	USUAL PEDIATRIC DOSAGE AND ADMINISTRATION[a]	DOSAGE FORMS	CONTRAINDICATIONS, ADRs, AND COMMENTS[b]
Flunisolide, pulmonary (*AeroBid®*) **Note:** *See also* Flunisolide, nasal.	**Asthma,** steroid responsive and refractory to conventional bronchodilator pharmacotherapy **Note:** Not indicated for the treatment of acute asthma attacks (acute bronchospasm or status asthmaticus).	**Children (>6 years) and adolescents (≤15 years):** Two actuations (500 µg) of metered-dose inhaler aerosol twice daily. *Maximum:* Four actuations (1000 µg) of metered-dose inhaler aerosol daily. **Adolescents (>15 years):** Two to four actuations (500–1000 µg) of metered-dose inhaler aerosol daily.	Solution, metered-dose inhaler (*AeroBid-M®*): 250 µg/actuation (menthol flavored); pressurized. Do not incinerate, puncture, or store at temperatures ≥49°C (120°F).	**Contraindications:** Acute bronchospasm, hypersensitivity to flunisolide, and status asthmaticus. **ADRs:** May cause cough, hoarseness, sore throat, and wheezing. May mask signs and symptoms of infections, particularly of the respiratory tract. **Comments:** Of no benefit for the treatment of acute asthmatic attacks. Assess pituitary-adrenal function periodically during chronic long-term therapy. *See* Chapter 1 for proper metered-dose inhaler administration techniques.
Fluocinolone (*Fluoderm®, Fluonid®, Flurosyn®, Lidemol®, Synalar®*)	**Corticosteroid-responsive acute and chronic skin disorders** (to provide anti-allergenic, anti-inflammatory, and antipruritic actions)	**Infants, children, and adolescents:** Apply a small amount to the affected skin site(s) two to four times daily according to response. **Note:** Do **not** cover or in any way occlude treated skin sites (e.g., do not cover with occlusive dressings, diapers, or plastic pants). **Note:** Topical solution generally is the most appropriate formulation for use on hairy skin sites, including the scalp. (*See* Chapter 1.)	Cream, topical: 0.01%, 0.025%, 0.2% (*Synalar-HP®*) Gel, topical: 0.05% Oil, topical (*Derma-Smoothe/FS®*): 0.01% (contains mineral oil and peanut oil) Ointment, topical: 0.01%, 0.025% (contains coconut oil) Shampoo, topical (*FS Shampoo®*): 0.01% (supplied in 12-mg capsule with shampoo base to be prepared by pharmacist **prior** to dispensing) Solution, topical: 0.01% (contains propylene glycol as vehicle) **Note:** For external use only. Avoid contact with the eye(s).	**Contraindications:** Hypersensitivity to fluocinolone and untreated bacterial, fungal, tubercular, and viral skin infections. **ADRs:** Generally well tolerated. May cause the following local skin reactions at the site(s) of application: atrophy, burning sensation, dryness, hypertrichosis, irritation, itching, pigmentation changes, secondary infection, and telangiectasia. **Comments:** May result in systemic absorption and associated ADRs when applied over a large area of the body or when occlusive dressings are used. *See* "Corticosteroids" in Chapter 5.
Fluocinonide (*Fluonex®, Lidex®, Lyderm®, Topactin®, Topsyn®*)	**Corticosteroid-responsive acute and chronic skin disorders** (to provide anti-allergenic, anti-inflammatory, and antipruritic actions)	**Infants, children, and adolescents:** Apply a small amount to the affected skin site(s) two to four times daily according to response. **Note:** Do **not** cover or in any way occlude treated skin sites (e.g., do not cover with occlusive dressings, diapers, or plastic pants). **Note:** Topical solution generally is the most appropriate formulation for use on hairy skin sites, including the scalp. (*See* Chapter 1.)	Cream, topical: 0.05% Gel, topical: 0.05% Ointment, topical: 0.05% Solution, topical: 0.05% (may contain up to 35% alcohol [*Lidex*]) **Note:** For external use only. Avoid contact with eye(s).	**Contraindications:** Hypersensitivity to fluocinonide and untreated bacterial, fungal, tubercular, and viral skin infections. **ADRs:** Generally well tolerated. May cause the following local skin reactions at the site of application: atrophy, burning sensation, dryness, hypertrichosis, irritation, itching, pigmentation changes, secondary infection, and telangiectasia. **Comments:** May result in systemic absorption and associated ADRs when applied over a large area of the body or when occlusive dressings are used. *See* "Corticosteroids" in Chapter 5.

Fluoride, *see* **Sodium Fluoride**

5-Fluorocytosine, *see* **Flucytosine**

TABLE 14-1 continued

DRUG (TRADE AND OTHER NAMES)	INDICATION(S)	USUAL PEDIATRIC DOSAGE AND ADMINISTRATION[a]	DOSAGE FORMS	CONTRAINDICATIONS, ADRs, AND COMMENTS[b]
Fluoro-metholone (Flarex®, Fluor-Op®, FML®)	Treatment of allergic and other steroid-responsive inflammatory conditions of the eye (including the anterior segment of the eye, bulbar conjunctiva, and palpebral conjunctiva)	**Children (≥2 years) and adolescents:** Initially, instill one or two drops of ophthalmic suspension into the conjunctival sac of the affected eye(s) two to four times daily. Alternatively, a small amount (¼–½ inch) of ophthalmic ointment can be applied to the conjunctival sac of the affected eye(s) one to three times daily. Increase dosage as needed, according to response. *Maximum, ophthalmic drops:* two drops instilled into the conjunctival sac of the affected eye(s) every 2 hr while awake. *Maximum, ophthalmic ointment:* ½ inch of ophthalmic ointment applied to the conjunctival sac of the affected eye(s) every 4 hr while awake.	Ointment, ophthalmic: 0.1% Suspension, ophthalmic: 0.1%, 0.25% (supplied in plastic dropper bottles); shake well before use. **Note:** For ophthalmic use only. **Note:** In order to minimize cross-infection, ensure that separate containers are dispensed for each eye whenever both eyes require fluorometholone ophthalmic pharmacotherapy.	**Contraindications:** Fungal infections of the eye, hypersensitivity to fluorometholone, superficial herpes simplex keratitis (acute), tuberculosis of the eye, untreated purulent eye infections (acute), vaccinia, varicella, viral disease of the conjunctiva, and viral disease of the cornea. **ADRs:** May cause blurred vision, eye discomfort or pain, glaucoma, loss of visual acuity, and secondary ocular infections. **Comments:** Maintain the sterility of ophthalmic formulations with attention to correct administration to help to ensure optimal therapeutic benefit (see Chapter 1). Inadvertent contamination of ophthalmic drug product containers (e.g., multiple-dose plastic ophthalmic suspension bottles with droppers) has resulted in bacterial keratitis, subsequent eye damage, and blindness.
Fluorouracil, see Chapter 12				
Fluoxetine (Prozac®)	Depression **Note:** Not approved by the FDA or HPB for infants or children.	**Children:** 10 mg/day PO as a single morning dose. *Maximum:* 20 mg/day PO. **Adolescents:** 20 mg/day PO as a single morning dose. *Maximum:* 40 mg/day PO.	Capsules, oral: 10, 20 mg Solution, oral: 20 mg/5 ml (mint flavored)	**Contraindications:** Hypersensitivity to fluoxetine and MAOI therapy (concurrent or within 14 days). **ADRs:** May cause anxiety, anorexia, asthenia, dry mouth, insomnia, nausea, nervousness, rash, and sweating. May adversely affect cognitive abilities, including learning and memory, and hence, adversely affect academic performance. See Chapter 5. **Note:** All depressed patients should be evaluated for suicide risk and any risk should be appropriately dealt with.
	Bulimia nervosa/ Obsessive compulsive disorder	**Adolescents:** Initially, 20 mg/day PO as a single dose. Gradually increase dosage, as required, to 60 mg/day PO over 2–4 weeks in order to minimize associated ADRs.		
Fluoxymes-terone (Halotestin®)	Delayed puberty among boys	**Adolescents:** Initially, 2–6 mg/day PO as a single dose or three divided doses. Increase the dosage gradually according to response and laboratory analysis (see "Comments"). **Note:** Priapism is indicative of excessive dosage and that therapy should be temporarily discontinued and then resumed at a lower dosage. *Maximum:* 20 mg/day PO. **Note:** It is generally recommended that therapy be limited to 4–6 months.	Tablets, oral: 2, 5, 10 mg (contains FD&C yellow No. 5 [tartrazine]) **Note:** Not generally available in Canada.	**Contraindications:** Androgen-dependent cancers; cardiac, hepatic, or renal dysfunction (severe); cholestatic hepatitis; hypercalcemia; and hypersensitivity to fluoxymesterone. **ADRs:** May cause acne, anxiety, cholestatic hepatitis, edema, headache, nausea, premature termination of linear growth, and priapism. **Comments:** Skeletal maturation among prepubertal boys must be monitored by roentgenogram examination of the hand and wrist every 6 months to determine bone age and rate of bone maturation. Periodic liver *(Continued)*

Footnotes are on page 558.

TABLE 14-1 *continued*

DRUG (*TRADE* AND OTHER NAMES)	INDICATION(S)	USUAL PEDIATRIC DOSAGE AND ADMINISTRATION[a]	DOSAGE FORMS	CONTRAINDICATIONS, ADRs, AND COMMENTS[b]
Fluoxymesterone *continued*				function tests also are recommended because of the association of fluoxymesterone pharmacotherapy with hepatotoxicity.
Fluticasone, nasal (*Flonase®*)	Allergic rhinitis, seasonal and perennial **Note: Not** indicated for the relief of nonallergic rhinitis.	Children (≥4 years) and adolescents: 100 µg/day intranasal (one spray in each nostril). *Maximum*: 200 µg/day intranasal. **Note:** Several days of pharmacotherapy are generally required before therapeutic benefit is observed.	Solution, nasal spray (*Flonase*): 50 µg/ actuation by a specially designed metering, atomizing spray pump with nasal attachment **Note:** For intranasal use only.	**Contraindications:** Bacterial, fungal, or viral infections (untreated); hypersensitivity to fluticasone; and tuberculosis. **ADRs:** Generally well tolerated. May cause nasal irritation or nose bleeds (epistaxis). **Comments:** Optimal therapeutic response is dependent upon continuous prophylactic use.
Fluticasone, pulmonary (*Flovent®, Flovent Rotadisk®*)	Asthma attacks, acute, prophylaxis **Note**: **Not** indicated for the **relief** of acute bronchospasm. It is indicated for the **prevention** of acute bronchospasm.	Children (≥4 years): 100 or 200 µg/day by *Diskhaler®* or *Flovent Rotadisk* in two divided doses. Adolescents: 100–1000 µg/day by *Diskhaler* or *Flovent Rotadisk* in two divided doses. **Note:** Administered by a specially designed *Diskhaler* or *Flovent Rotadisk* device. See Chapter 1 for proper administration techniques.	Aerosols for inhalation by metered-dose inhaler (*Flovent*): 44, 110, 220 µg Powders, inhalation (*Flovent Rotadisk*): 50, 100, 250 µg **Note:** For pulmonary inhalation only.	**Contraindications:** Bacterial, fungal, or viral infections (untreated); hypersensitivity to fluticasone; and tuberculosis. **ADRs:** May cause headache, hoarseness, nasal congestion, respiratory infection, rhinitis, sinusitis, sore throat, and thrush. **Comments:** Of no benefit for the treatment of acute asthmatic attacks.
Folic Acid (Pteroylglutamic Acid)	Folic acid (folate) deficiency, prophylaxis	Children: 0.1 mg/day PO as a single dose. Adolescents: 0.2 mg/day PO as a single dose. *Maximum:* 1 mg/day PO (for pregnant adolescent girls, *see* "Comments")	Tablets, oral: 0.1, 0.4, 0.7, 1.5 mg **Note:** Available in multivitamin products, particularly prenatal formulations.	**Contraindications:** Pernicious anemia (folic acid is not effective for correcting the neurological sequelae associated with vitamin B_{12} megaloblastic anemias and may obscure diagnosis by facilitating hematologic remission). **ADRs:** Generally well tolerated. **Comments:** May obscure the diagnosis of pernicious anemia with the resultant progression of neurologic complications. For the treatment of pernicious anemia, cyanocobalamin should generally be administered concurrently with folic acid. Higher dosages than those recommended may be required for adolescent girls with a history of pregnancy complicated by neural tube defects (*see* Chapter 2).
	Folic acid (folate) deficiency, treatment	Children and adolescents: 0.25–1 mg/day PO as a single dose. *Maximum:* 5–15 mg/day PO (for pediatric patients with tropical sprue).		
Fomepizole (*Antizol®*) **Note:** *See also* Chapter 4.	Ethylene glycol poisoning (*see* "Comments") **Note:** Not approved by the FDA or HPB for children.	Children and adolescents: Initially, 15 mg/kg IV as a loading dose. Follow with four doses of 10 mg/kg/dose IV every 12 hr. Then 15 mg/kg/dose IV every 12 hr until ethylene glycol blood concentrations have been reduced to <20 mg/dl. **Note:** All doses should be administered by slow IV infusion over 30 min. **Note:** For patients requiring hemodialysis, see the following dosing recommendations.	Injectable, IV: 1 gram/ml **Note:** For IV use only. **Note:** Prior to administration, dilute in a minimum of 100 ml of 0.9% sodium chloride for injection or dextrose 5% in water for injection. Appropriately discard any unused diluted product after 24 hr.	**Contraindications:** Hypersensitivity to fomepizole or to other pyrazoles. **ADRs:** May cause abdominal pain, dizziness, headache, metallic taste, and nausea. **Comments:** Ethylene glycol poisoning frequently causes acute renal failure, hypocalcemia, and metabolic acidosis. These and other related sequelae require appropriate emergency medical management in addition to fomepizole pharmacotherapy

TABLE 14-1 continued

DRUG (TRADE AND OTHER NAMES)	INDICATION(S)	USUAL PEDIATRIC DOSAGE AND ADMINISTRATION[a]	DOSAGE FORMS	CONTRAINDICATIONS, ADRs, AND COMMENTS[b]
Fomepizole *continued*		**Fomepizole Dosing Recommendations for Patients Requiring Hemodialysis** Beginning hemodialysis, <6 hr since last dose: Do **not** administer dose. ≥6 hr since last dose: Administer next scheduled dose. During hemodialysis: Every 4 hr. Following completion of hemodialysis: <1 hr since last dose: Do **not** administer dose. 1–3 hr since last dose: Administer ½ of next scheduled dose. >3 hr since last dose: Administer next scheduled dose. Maintenance dosing off hemodialysis: Administer next scheduled dose 12 hr from last dose.		(e.g., calcium supplementation, fluid and electrolyte administration, hemodialysis, oxygen, and sodium bicarbonate administration). **Note:** The concurrent use of fomepizole and alcohol (ethanol) will decrease the rate of elimination of both drugs by ~50% because of fomepizole's mechanism of action (fomepizole competitively inhibits the metabolism of alcohol dehydrogenase).
Formoterol Fumarate *(Foradil®, Oxeze®)*	**Asthma,** long-term maintenance treatment (may be used concurrently with corticosteroid pharmacotherapy for patients with asthma who are experiencing breakthrough signs and symptoms) **Note:** Acute asthma (bronchospasms) should be managed with a short-acting β_2-adrenergic agonist (e.g., albuterol, terbutaline) and **not** the long-acting β_2-adrenergic agonist, formoterol fumarate.	**Children (≥5 years) and adolescents:** 24 µg/day by inhalation in two divided doses, every 12 hr. *Maximum:* 48 µg/day by inhalation.	Capsule, inhalation powder: 12 µg (for use only with provided *Aerolizer®* inhaler) **Note:** Each *Foradil* capsule contains 25 mg of lactose as a carrier. Powder, metered-dose inhaler *(Turbuhaler®)*: 6, 12 µg/metered-dose inhalation **Note:** *Turbuhaler* contains 600 µg of lactose per each metered dose. This amount of lactose usually does not adversely affect patients with lactose intolerance. **Note:** For inhalation use only.	**Contraindications:** Hypersensitivity to formoterol or to inhaled lactose and tachydysrhythmias. **ADRs:** May cause cramps, dizziness, headache, oropharyngeal irritation, palpitations, and tremor. **Comments:** Severity of asthma may fluctuate significantly during childhood and adolescence and, therefore, requires periodic reassessment and, as indicated, readjustment of formoterol and other concurrent pharmacotherapy.
Fosphenytoin *(Cerebyx®)* **Note:** *See also* Phenytoin.	**Status epilepticus** **Note:** Concomitant IV benzodiazepine pharmacotherapy is usually required to adequately control status epilepticus because the actions of phenytoin, the active metabolite, are not immediate. **Note:** Not approved by the FDA or HPB for children or adolescents.	**Children and adolescents:** Initial loading dose, 15–20 mg phenytoin sodium equivalents (PE)/kg IV administered at a rate of 100 mg PE/min. *Maintenance:* 4–6 PE/kg/day IM or IV as a single dose or in two divided doses. *Maximum:* 150 mg PE/min. **Note:** Replace IV fosphenytoin with oral phenytoin as soon as clinically feasible. **Note:** Blood pressure, ECG, and respiratory function should be monitored continuously during IV infusion and for 20 min following the infusion.	Injectable, IM, IV: 50 mg PE/ml **Note:** In order to prevent or minimize potential dosing errors, fosphenytoin is always prescribed and dispensed in phenytoin sodium equivalent (PE) units.	**Contraindications:** Adams-Stokes syndrome, hypersensitivity to fosphenytoin or to other hydantoins, AV block (second and third degree), sino-atrial block, and sinus bradycardia. **ADRs:** May cause ataxia, cardiovascular collapse, CNS depression, dizziness, headache, hypotension, nausea, nystagmus, paresthesia, pruritus, and somnolence. *See also* Chapter 5. **Comments:** Initial loading doses are guided by efficacy in controlling status epilepticus. Monitor blood pressure, ECG, and respirations. Maintenance doses are guided by therapeutic drug monitoring. Total phenytoin plasma concentrations should generally be between 40 and 80 µmol/liter (10–20 µg/ml). (*See* Table 14-3.)

Footnotes are on page 558.

TABLE 14-1 continued

DRUG (TRADE AND OTHER NAMES)	INDICATION(S)	USUAL PEDIATRIC DOSAGE AND ADMINISTRATION[a]	DOSAGE FORMS	CONTRAINDICATIONS, ADRs, AND COMMENTS[b]
Frusemide, see **Furosemide**				
Furazolidone (*Furoxone*®)	**Bacterial or protozoal diarrhea** caused by susceptible organisms **Note:** Ensure that appropriate culture and sensitivity tests are performed and that the organism is sensitive to furazolidone.	**Infants, children, and adolescents:** 5 mg/kg/day PO in four divided doses. *Maximum:* 8.8 mg/kg/day PO.	Solution, oral: 50 mg/15 ml (contains saccharin sodium) Tablet, oral scored: 100 mg (contains sucrose) **Note:** Not generally available in Canada.	**Contraindications:** Hypersensitivity to furazolidone and neonates. **ADRs:** May cause anal pruritus, brown discoloration of the urine, headache, malaise, nausea, and vomiting. **Comments:** Mild reversible hemolysis may occur among patients who are glucose-6-phosphate dehydrogenase deficient. Caution patients who drink alcohol to avoid alcohol use during furazolidone pharmacotherapy. A disulfiramlike reaction may occur if alcohol is consumed during therapy.
Furosemide (Frusemide, *Lasix*®)	Edema	**Infants, children, and adolescents:** 0.5–2 mg/kg/dose PO every 6–8 hr. Increase dosage to 3–6 mg/kg/dose every 6–8 hr, as needed, according to response **or** 0.5–1 mg/kg/dose IV every 2–8 hr. Increase dosage to 6 mg/kg/dose IV every 2–8 hr, as needed, according to response. **Note:** Inject IV no faster than 20 mg/min. *Maximum:* 6 mg/kg/dose PO or IV.	Injectable, IV: 10 mg/ml Solution, oral: 10 mg/ml Tablets, oral: 20, 40, 80 mg	**Contraindications:** Anuria, hypersensitivity to furosemide, and uncorrected electrolyte depletion (severe). **ADRs:** *See* Chapter 5. **Comments:** May potentiate ototoxicity and nephrotoxicity associated with other pharmacotherapy. Monitor fluid and electrolyte status.
Gabapentin (*Neurontin*®)	**Partial seizures,** adjunctive pharmacotherapy for pediatric patients who are refractory to standard monoanticonvulsant pharmacotherapy	**Children (≥3 years):** Initially, 5 mg/kg PO as a single dose at bedtime on day 1; 10 mg/kg PO in two divided doses on day 2; and 15 mg/kg PO in three divided doses on day 3. Thereafter, increase dosage by increments of 5 mg/kg/day as indicated by response. Dosage is generally increased to 25 mg/kg/day PO in three divided doses. *Maximum:* 50 mg/kg/day or 3600 mg/day, whichever is less. **Adolescents:** Initially, 300 mg PO as a single dose at bedtime on day 1; 600 mg PO in two divided doses on day 2; and 900 mg PO in three divided doses on day 3. Thereafter, increase dosage by increments of 300 mg/day as indicated by response. Dosage is generally increased to 1800 mg/day PO in three divided doses. *Maximum:* 3600 mg/day PO. **Note:** Reduce dosage for pediatric patients who have renal dysfunction, *see* Table 14-2.	Capsules, oral hard gelatin: 100, 300, 400 mg Solution, oral: 250 mg/5 ml (strawberry–anise flavored). Store refrigerated at 2–8°C (36–46°F). Tablets, oral film coated: 600, 800 mg	**Contraindications:** Hypersensitivity to gabapentin. **ADRs:** May cause amnesia, ataxia, back pain, blurred vision, depression, diplopia, dizziness, dry mouth, dysarthria, dyspepsia, edema, fatigue, nervousness, nystagmus, pruritus, somnolence, tremor, twitching, vomiting, and weight gain. **Comments:** To minimize the risk for withdrawal-precipitated seizures associated with the discontinuation of gabapentin, discontinue gradually by reducing the dosage over at least 1 week.

Gamma Benzene Hexachloride, see **Lindane**

TABLE 14-1 continued

DRUG (TRADE AND OTHER NAMES)	INDICATION(S)	USUAL PEDIATRIC DOSAGE AND ADMINISTRATION[a]	DOSAGE FORMS	CONTRAINDICATIONS, ADRs, AND COMMENTS[b]
Ganciclovir (*Cytovene®*)	Cytomegalovirus infection (retinitis) prophylaxis for retinal transplant patients	**Children and adolescents:** 5 mg/kg/day IV as a single dose.	Capsules, oral: 250, 500 mg Injectable, IV: 500 mg/vial **Note:** Oral pharmacotherapy is less efficacious than IV pharmacotherapy and is not recommended.	**Contraindications:** Hypersensitivity to acyclovir or ganciclovir. **ADRs:** May cause abdominal pain, anemia, chills, diarrhea, fever, infection, leukopenia, nausea, neuropathy, paresthesia, rash, sepsis, sweating, thrombocytopenia, and vomiting. *See* Chapter 5. **Comments:** Monitor white blood cell count for neutropenia. Granulocyte-colony-stimulating factors have been used to treat ganciclovir-induced neutropenia. Complete blood counts and platelet counts should be performed frequently.
	Cytomegalovirus infection (retinitis) among immunocompromised patients **Note:** May slow the progression of cytomegalovirus retinitis but does not cure it.	**Children and adolescents:** 10 mg/kg/day IV in two divided doses, every 12 hr. **Note:** Administer each dose by slow IV infusion over 1 hr. Do **not** administer by rapid IV injection. **Note:** Reduce dosage for pediatric patients who have renal dysfunction; *see* Table 14-2.		
Gentamicin (*Garamycin®*) **Note:** *See also* Gentamicin, ophthalmic, and Gentamicin, topical.	Bacterial infections	**Infants, children, and adolescents:** 6–7.5 mg/kg/day IM or IV in three divided doses, every 8 hr.	Injectables, IM, IV: 10, 40, 60, 80, 100 mg/ml **Note:** Some injectable formulations contain sodium bisulfite which may cause allergic reactions in susceptible patients, particularly those with a history of asthma.	**Contraindications:** Hypersensitivity to gentamicin or to other aminoglycoside antibiotics. **ADRs:** *See* Chapter 5. **Comments:** Monitor auditory, renal, and vestibular function. Therapeutic drug monitoring is recommended; *see* Table 14-3.
	Bacterial infections among pediatric patients with cystic fibrosis **Note:** Ensure that appropriate culture and sensitivity tests are performed and that the organism is sensitive to gentamicin.	**Infants, children, and adolescents:** 10 mg/kg/day IM or IV in three or four divided doses, every 6 or 8 hr. **Note:** A significant increase in auditory, renal, and vestibular toxicities is associated with therapy exceeding 10 days. **Note:** Reduce dosage for pediatric patients who have renal dysfunction; *see* Table 14-2.		
Gentamicin, ophthalmic (*Garamycin®, Genoptic®, Gentacidin®, Gentak®*)	Eye infections involving the conjunctiva or cornea, superficial **Note:** Ensure that appropriate culture and sensitivity tests are performed and that the organism is sensitive to gentamicin.	**Infants, children, and adolescents:** Apply ointment or instill two drops of solution to affected eye(s) two to four times daily. **Note:** *See* Chapter 1 for details regarding ophthalmic drug administration.	Ointment, ophthalmic: 3 mg/gram Solution, ophthalmic: 3 mg/ml **Note:** For ophthalmic use only. **Note:** In order to minimize cross-infections whenever both eyes require gentamicin ophthalmic pharmacotherapy, ensure that separate containers are dispensed for each eye.	**Contraindications:** Dendritic keratitis, fungal infections of the eye, and hypersensitivity to gentamicin or to other aminoglycosides. **ADRs:** Generally well tolerated. May cause local sensitivity reactions (e.g., burning, irritation, stinging, tearing). May result in the overgrowth of nonsusceptible organisms. **Comments:** Use of the ophthalmic ointment may retard or delay healing of the corneal epithelium.
Gentamicin, topical (*Garamycin®, G-myticin®*)	Skin infections, primary and secondary	**Infants, children, and adolescents:** Apply topical cream or ointment to affected areas topically three or four times daily. **Note:** Affected site should be clean and dry before application of cream or ointment.	Cream, topical: 0.1% Ointment, topical: 0.1% **Note:** For external use only. Avoid contact with eyes.	**Contraindications:** Hypersensitivity to gentamicin or to other aminoglycosides. **ADRs:** Generally well tolerated. However, long-term use may result in overgrowth of nonsusceptible organisms, particularly fungi. **Comments:** Deep cutaneous infections may require concomitant systemic antibiotic pharmacotherapy.

Footnotes are on page 558.

TABLE 14-1 continued

DRUG (TRADE AND OTHER NAMES)	INDICATION(S)	USUAL PEDIATRIC DOSAGE AND ADMINISTRATION[a]	DOSAGE FORMS	CONTRAINDICATIONS, ADRs, AND COMMENTS[b]
Gentian Violet	**Bacterial and fungal infections of the skin** caused by susceptible organisms **Note:** Bactericidal to gram-positive organisms and inhibits the growth of several fungi including *Candida, Epidermophyton, Torula,* and *Trichophyton.* However, because of staining, generally no longer used except when these organisms are resistant to conventional topical antibiotics and antifungals. **Note:** Ensure that appropriate culture and sensitivity tests are performed and that the organism is sensitive to gentian violet.	**Children and adolescents:** Apply topically to affected skin site(s) two or three times daily. Allow to dry after application. Skin site(s) should be washed gently with soap and warm water and dried thoroughly before application. **Note:** Protect hands with gloves and use a cotton-tipped applicator to apply in order to avoid staining fingers or hands during application.	Solutions, topical: 1%, 2% **Note:** For external use only. Avoid contact with the eyes. **Note:** Stains clothes and skin. Protect skin, clothes, and bedding from inadvertent spills or other contact during application.	**Contraindications:** Hypersensitivity to gentian violet. **ADRs:** Generally well tolerated. May cause dark purple colored staining of skin, clothing, or bed linen. May "tattoo" skin, particularly if applied to abraded or denuded skin site(s). **Comments:** Do **not** apply to ulcerative facial lesions.
Glucagon **Note:** *See also* Chapter 4.	**Hypoglycemia** among pediatric patients with diabetes mellitus	**Children (<5 years):** 0.5 mg/dose SC. **Children (≥5 years) and adolescents:** 1 mg/dose SC. May repeat dose in 5–20 min, as needed, according to response. *Maximum:* 1 mg/dose SC.	Injectable, SC: 1 mg/ml (after reconstitution with the supplied diluent) **Note:** 1 mg = 1 unit.	**Contraindications:** Adrenal insufficiency, hypersensitivity to glucagon, pheochromocytoma, and starvation. **ADRs:** Generally well tolerated. May cause hypokalemia, nausea, and vomiting. **Comments:** Administer glucose infusion while awaiting effect of SC glucagon. Monitor glucose serum concentration and adjust IV glucose dosage accordingly.
Glycerin *(Fleet Babylax®)*	Constipation	**Infants and children:** Gently insert one glycerin pediatric rectal suppository high in the rectum for retention for 15 min **or** gently insert the tip of the disposable plastic solution container in the rectum and slowly squeeze the unit until nearly all of the glycerin solution is instilled. A small amount of solution will remain in the disposable plastic applicator unit. **Adolescents:** Gently insert one adult glycerin rectal suppository high in the rectum for retention for 15 min.	Suppositories, rectal: 1.44, 1.8 grams (infants and children), 2.6, 2.65 grams (adults) Solution, rectal: 4 ml/disposable plastic applicator unit *(Fleet Babylax)*	**Contraindications:** Fecal impaction and intestinal obstruction. **ADRs:** Generally well tolerated. *See* Chapter 5. **Comments:** *See* Chapter 1 for proper techniques for rectal administration.

Glycerol Guaiacolate, *see* **Guaifenesin**

Glyceryl Guaiacolate Carbamate, *see* **Methocarbamol**

Glyceryl Trinitrate, *see* **Nitroglycerin**

TABLE 14-1 continued

DRUG (TRADE AND OTHER NAMES)	INDICATION(S)	USUAL PEDIATRIC DOSAGE AND ADMINISTRATION[a]	DOSAGE FORMS	CONTRAINDICATIONS, ADRs, AND COMMENTS[b]
Glycopyrrolate (Robinul®)	Reduction of bronchial, gastric, nasal, and oral secretions during surgery or treatment procedures **Note:** The choice of preoperative pharmacotherapy depends on the clinical condition of the pediatric patient, the type of anesthesia to be administered, the type of surgery or treatment procedure to be performed, and the duration of the surgery or procedure.	**Children and adolescents:** 0.005–0.01 mg/kg IM 45 min before surgery or treatment procedure. *Maximum:* 0.35 mg/dose IM.	Injectable, IM: 200 µg/ml Tablets, oral: 1, 2 mg **Note:** Oral formulations are not generally recommended for this indication.	**Contraindications:** Hypersensitivity, myasthenia gravis, narrow-angle glaucoma, obstruction of the GI or genitourinary tract, and tachycardia. **ADRs:** *See* Chapter 5.
Gold Sodium Thiomalate (Aurolate®, Myochrysine®, Sodium Aurothiomalate)	Juvenile rheumatoid arthritis (refractory to conventional pharmacotherapy)	**Children (≥6 years) and adolescents:** *Week 1:* 5 mg IM once. *Week 2:* 10 mg IM once. *Weeks 3–20:* 0.5–1 mg/kg IM once a week for 20 weeks followed by long-term gold sodium thiomalate pharmacotherapy. *Maximum:* 50 mg/dose IM. *Long-term pharmacotherapy:* 0.5–1 mg/kg IM every 2 weeks for 3 months; then 0.5–1 mg/kg IM every 3 weeks for 3 months; and then 0.5–1 mg/kg IM every 4 weeks for 3 months. *Maximum:* **Children,** 25 mg/dose IM; **adolescents,** 50 mg/dose IM. **Note:** Maintain patient in recumbent position during IM injection and for 10 min after the injection.	Injectables, IM: 10, 25, 50 mg/ml; contains ~50% gold. Store protected from light. Discard solutions that are darker than pale yellow. **Note:** For IM use only, preferably utilizing the gluteal muscle.	**Contraindications:** Agranulocytosis (history of), blood dyscrasias, diabetes, hepatic dysfunction, hypersensitivity to gold or to gold sodium thiomalate, hypertension (severe), pregnancy, renal dysfunction, and systemic lupus erythematosis. **ADRs:** May cause diarrhea, rash, and stomatitis. *See* Chapter 5. **Note:** ADRs primarily are associated with initial and cumulative dosages. Incidence and severity are generally greatest at **cumulative** dosages exceeding 800 mg. **Comments:** Monitor complete blood cell counts and renal function prior to and during therapy.

Gonadotropin, Chorionic, *see* **Chorionic Gonadotropin**

Granisetron (Kytril®)	Prevention of nausea and vomiting associated with emetogenic antineoplastic pharmacotherapy (including high-dose cisplatin and radiation therapy)	**Children and adolescents:** 40 µg/kg IV over 5 min 30 min before the initiation of antineoplastic pharmacotherapy **or** 1 mg/dose PO 1 hr before the initiation of antineoplastic pharmacotherapy and repeated 12 hr after antineoplastic pharmacotherapy has been completed. **Note:** Product labeling recommends an IV dose of 10 µg/kg; however, published clinical literature supports the use of 40 µg/kg.	Injectable, IV: 1 mg/ml (in single-use vials) Tablet, oral film coated: 1 mg	**Contraindications:** Hypersensitivity to granisetron. **ADRs:** Generally well tolerated. May cause abdominal pain, anorexia, constipation, and headache.
	Prevention of postoperative vomiting among pediatric patients undergoing general anesthesia	**Children and adolescents:** 40 µg/kg IV immediately after the induction of general anesthesia. **Note:** Administer IV over 5 min.		

(Continued)

Footnotes are on page 558.

PROBLEMS IN PEDIATRIC DRUG THERAPY

TABLE 14-1 *continued*

DRUG (*TRADE* AND OTHER NAMES)	INDICATION(S)	USUAL PEDIATRIC DOSAGE AND ADMINISTRATION[a]	DOSAGE FORMS	CONTRAINDICATIONS, ADRs, AND COMMENTS[b]
Granisetron *continued*	**Note:** Not approved by the FDA or HPB for these indications for children or adolescents.			
Griseofulvin (*Fulvicin®, Grifulvin V®, Grisactin®, Gris-PEG®*)	**Dermatophytoses** (e.g., *Tinea capitis, T. unguinum*) **Note:** Ensure that appropriate culture and sensitivity tests are performed and that the fungal organism is sensitive to griseofulvin.	**Children (>2 years) and adolescents:** 10–20 mg/kg/day microsize formulation PO in two divided doses. *Maximum:* Microsize formulation, 1 gram/day PO; ultramicrosize formulation, 660 mg/day PO. **Note:** Administer with fatty food to increase GI absorption. The ultramicrosize tablet formulation generally requires approximately half the dose needed for the oral microsize formulations.	Capsule, oral microsize: 250 mg Suspension, oral microsize: 25 mg/ml; shake well before use. Tablets, oral microsize: 125, 250, 500 mg Tablets, oral ultramicrosize: 125, 165, 250, 330 mg	**Contraindications:** Hypersensitivity to griseofulvin, hepatic failure, and porphyria. **ADRs:** Generally well tolerated. May cause headache and hypersensitivity or photosensitivity reactions. May potentiate the cardiovascular effects of alcohol (e.g., flush, tachycardia). Reportedly has caused breast enlargement and hyperpigmentation of the mammary areolae, nipples, and external genitalia among some children. *See* Chapter 5. **Comments:** The ultramicrosize formulation is ~1.5 times more efficiently absorbed from the GI tract than are the microsize formulations.
Guaifenesin (*Anti-Tuss®, Balminil®, Gee Gee®*, Glycerol Guaiacolate, *Robitussin®, Uni-Tussin®*)	**Facilitation of the expectoration of thick, viscous, respiratory secretions** **Note:** Not for treatment of chronic cough related to COPD (e.g., asthma) or smoking.	**Children (2–6 years):** 200–600 mg/day PO in four to six divided doses, every 4–6 hr. *Maximum:* 600 mg/day PO. **Children (>6 years):** 400–1200 mg/day PO in four to six divided doses, every 4–6 hr. *Maximum:* 1200 mg/day PO. **Adolescents:** 800–2400 mg/day PO in four to six divided doses, every 4–6 hr. *Maximum:* 2400 mg/day PO.	Caplet, oral sustained release: 600 mg Capsule, oral: 200 mg Capsule, oral sustained release: 300 mg Solutions, oral: 100 mg/5 ml, 200 mg/5 ml (alcohol free, contains saccharin sodium) Syrup, oral: 100 mg/5 ml (cherry or raspberry flavored) (contains 3.5% alcohol) Tablets, oral: 100, 200, 1200 mg Tablet, oral sustained release: 600 mg	**Contraindications:** Hypersensitivity to guaifenesin. **ADRs:** Generally well tolerated. May cause drowsiness, GI distress, headache, nausea, rash, and vomiting. **Comments:** For optimal therapeutic benefit, ensure that the patient is adequately hydrated.
Haemophilus Influenza Vaccine, *see* **Chapter 9**				
Haloperidol (*Haldol®, Peridol®*)	**Schizophrenia and other psychotic disorders** **Note:** Approved by the FDA, but not the HPB, for infants and children.	**Children (≥3 years and 15–40 kg):** Initially, 0.5 mg/day PO in two divided doses. Increase the daily dosage by 0.5 mg at 5–7-day intervals, as needed, until therapeutic benefit is achieved. There is little evidence of further improvement of signs and symptoms with dosages exceeding 6 mg/day PO. **Children and adolescents (>40 kg):** 0.05–0.15 mg/kg/day PO in two or three divided doses. Children and adolescents who have severe signs and symptoms may require higher dosages. *Maximum:* 6 mg/day PO.	Drops, oral: 2 mg/ml Injectable, IM (short-acting lactate): 5 mg/ml Injectables, IM (long-acting decanoate): 50, 100 mg/ml Solution, oral concentrate: 2 mg/ml (colorless, odorless, tasteless) Tablets, oral: 0.5, 1, 2, 5, 10, 20 mg **Note:** Safety and effectiveness of intramuscular formulations have not been established in children.	**Contraindications:** CNS depression (severe), coma, and hypersensitivity to haloperidol or to other butyrophenones. **ADRs:** May cause anemia, anxiety, bronchospasm, confusion, constipation, depression, diaphoresis, diarrhea, drowsiness, dry mouth, dyspepsia, ECG changes (e.g., tachycardia, prolongation of the QT interval), extrapyramidal reactions, gynecomastia, hepatic dysfunction, insomnia, jaundice, laryngospasms, leukocytosis, leukopenia, photosensitivity, tardive dyskinesia, and urinary retention. *See* Chapter 5.

TABLE 14-1 continued

DRUG (TRADE AND OTHER NAMES)	INDICATION(S)	USUAL PEDIATRIC DOSAGE AND ADMINISTRATION[a]	DOSAGE FORMS	CONTRAINDICATIONS, ADRs, AND COMMENTS[b]
Haloperidol *continued*	Tic disorders, including Tourette's disorder (Gilles de la Tourette's syndrome)/ **Severe behavior problems** among children (e.g., combativeness, explosive behavior, and hyperexcitability which cannot be accounted for by immediate provocation) **Note:** Indicated for children with behavioral disorders only after they have failed to respond to psychotherapy alone or in combination with nonantipsychotic pharmacotherapy.	**Children (≥3 years):** 0.05–0.075 mg/kg/day PO in two or three divided doses. *Maximum:* 6 mg/day PO. **Note:** After signs and symptoms have been adequately controlled, the dosage should be gradually reduced to the lowest effective maintenance dosage.		
Haloprogin (Halotex®)	Fungal infections (e.g., *Tinea pedis, T. cruris, T. corporis,* and *T. manuum*) affecting the skin and related structures **Note:** Not approved by the FDA for this indication for children.	**Children and adolescents:** Apply a small amount of cream **or** two to four drops of solution to affected skin site(s) twice daily for 2–3 weeks.	Cream, topical: 1% (in water-dispersible base) Solution, topical: 1%; contains 75% alcohol. **Note:** For external use only. Avoid contact with eyes. **Note:** Not generally available in Canada.	**Contraindications:** Hypersensitivity to haloprogin. **ADRs:** Generally well tolerated. May cause local burning sensation, irritation, and pruritus at the site of application.
Heparin (unfractionated)	Anticoagulation **Note:** Large doses are generally not administered for at least 4 hr postoperatively.	**Infants and children:** Initially, 75 units/kg by slow IV injection over 3–5 min, follow by 20–28 units/kg/hr by continuous IV infusion. **Adolescents:** Initially, 5000 units by slow IV injection over 3–5 min, follow by 30,000–40,000 units/ 24 hr by continuous IV infusion **or** 30,000–40,000 units/24 hr in two divided doses, every 12 hr, by SC injection.	Injectables, IV, SC: 1000, 10,000 units/ml **Note:** Do not inject IM.	**Contraindications:** Active bleeding (e.g., acute ulcer), bleeding disorders (e.g., Christmas disease, hemophilia), hepatic dysfunction (severe), hypersensitivity to heparin, neurosurgery (recent), spinal surgery (recent), shock, and thrombocytopenia purpura. **ADRs:** May cause bleeding. *See* Chapter 5. **Comments:** Adjust maintenance dosage to maintain activated partial thromboplastin time (aPTT) 1.5–2 times normal (control). Heparin overdosage may be treated with protamine sulfate as an antidote.
Hepatitis A Vaccine Inactivated (Avaxim®, Havrix®)	Hepatitis A infection, pre-exposure active immunization	**Children and adolescents:** *Initial primary immunization dose,* 720 enzyme-linked immunosorbent assay (ELISA) units of hepatitis A virus antigen (0.5 ml) IM as a single dose into the deltoid muscle site. *Booster,* repeat initial dose after 6–12 months to provide long-term immunity. **Note:** *Avaxim-Pediatric®* 80 antigen units (in-house reference) is equivalent to 720 ELISA units of *Havrix Junior®*.	Injectables, IM (suspension): 720 ELISA units of hepatitis A virus antigen/0.5 ml *(Havrix Junior)* in single-dose prefilled syringes; 1440 ELISA units of hepatitis A virus antigen/1 ml in single-dose prefilled syringes; shake well before use. 80 antigen units (in-house reference) of hepatitis A virus antigen/0.5 ml *(Avaxim-Pediatric®)*	**Contraindications:** Acute febrile illness and hypersensitivity to inactivated hepatitis A vaccine. **ADRs:** Generally well tolerated. May cause fever, headache, malaise, and pain or swelling at the IM injection site. **Comments:** *See also* Chapter 9.

(Continued)

Footnotes are on page 558.

TABLE 14-1 continued

DRUG (*TRADE* AND OTHER NAMES)	INDICATION(S)	USUAL PEDIATRIC DOSAGE AND ADMINISTRATION[a]	DOSAGE FORMS	CONTRAINDICATIONS, ADRs, AND COMMENTS[b]
Hepatitis A Vaccine Inactivated *continued*			in single-dose prefilled syringes; shake well before use. **Note:** For IM use only. Do **not** inject in gluteal muscles.	
Hepatitis A Vaccine, Inactivated, Purified *(Vaqta®)*	Hepatitis A infection, pre-exposure active immunization	**Children (≥2 years) and adolescents:** *Initial primary immunization dose,* 25 units (0.5 ml) IM as a single dose into the deltoid muscle site. *Booster,* 25 units (0.5 ml) IM as a single dose into the deltoid muscle 6–18 months after the primary immunization to maintain elevated titers of hepatitis A virus antibodies.	Injectables, IM (suspension): 25 units of hepatitis A virus protein/0.5 ml (pediatric/adolescent suspension dose) in single-use prefilled syringes (contains trace amounts of neomycin B sulfate); 50 units of hepatitis A virus protein/1 ml (adult suspension dose) in single-use prefilled syringes (contains trace amounts of neomycin B sulfate); shake well before use. **Note:** For IM use only.	**Contraindications:** Acute febrile illness and hypersensitivity to inactivated, purified, hepatitis A vaccine and neomycin. **ADRs:** Generally well tolerated. May cause fever, headache, and pain or swelling at the IM injection site. **Comments:** *See also* Chapter 9.
Hepatitis A Vaccine, Inactivated, Virosome-Formulated *(Epaxal Berna®)*	Hepatitis A infection, pre-exposure active immunization	**Children and adolescents:** *Initial primary immunization dose,* 0.5 ml IM as a single dose into the deltoid muscle site. *Booster,* 0.5 ml IM as a single dose into the deltoid muscle site 1 year after primary immunization to maintain elevated titers of hepatitis A virus antibodies.	Injectable, IM (suspension): ≥500 radioimmunoassay units of hepatitis A virus antigen/0.5 ml; shake well before use. Store protected from light and humidity under refrigeration between 2 and 8°C (36–46°F). Do not freeze. (Product should be appropriately and safely discarded if frozen.) **Note:** For IM injection only. **Note:** Not generally available in the United States.	**Contraindications:** Acute febrile illness and hypersensitivity to inactivated, virosome-formulated hepatitis A vaccine or to influenza vaccine. **ADRs:** Generally well tolerated. May cause fever, headache, malaise, and pain or swelling at the injection site. **Comments:** Pediatric patients who are vaccinated against hepatitis A infection should continue to avoid, whenever possible, infection with hepatitis A virus (e.g., wash hands before eating; avoid consumption of contaminated foods or water; avoid contact with contaminated feces). *See also* Chapter 9.
Hepatitis A Vaccine and Hepatitis B Vaccine *(Twinrix®)*	Hepatitis A and hepatitis B infection, pre-exposure active immunization	**Infants, children, and adolescents:** Primary vaccination, 0.5 ml IM as a single dose into the deltoid muscle site. Follow with a second dose 1 month later. A third dose may be required 6 months after the first dose. **Note:** A booster dose may be required after ~5 years.	Injectables, IM suspension: 360 ELISA units of hepatitis A and 10 µg of hepatitis B/0.5 ml *(Twinrix Junior®)* in single-use prefilled syringes (contains trace amounts of neomycin B sulfate); 720 ELISA units of hepatitis A and 20 µg of hepatitis B/1 ml *(Twinrix Adult®)* in single-use prefilled syringes (contains trace amounts of neomycin B sulfate); shake well before use. Store under refrigeration between 2 and 8°C. Do not freeze. (Product should be safely and appropriately discarded if frozen). **Note:** For IM use only.	**Contraindications:** Acute febrile illness and hypersensitivity to hepatitis A vaccine, hepatitis B vaccine, or to neomycin B sulfate. **ADRs:** Generally well tolerated. May cause fever, headache, malaise, and local pain or swelling at the injection site. **Comments:** *See also* Chapter 9.

TABLE 14-1 *continued*

DRUG (*TRADE* AND OTHER NAMES)	INDICATION(S)	USUAL PEDIATRIC DOSAGE AND ADMINISTRATION[a]	DOSAGE FORMS	CONTRAINDICATIONS, ADRs, AND COMMENTS[b]
Hepatitis B Immune Globulin, Human, *see* **Chapter 9**				
Hepatitis B Vaccine, *see* **Chapter 9**				
Hepatitis B Vaccine and Hepatitis A Vaccine, *see* **Hepatitis A Vaccine and Hepatitis B Vaccine**				
Hexachlorophane, *see* **Hexachlorophene**				
Hexachlorophene (Hexachlorophane, *pHisoHex®*)	Bacteriostatic topical skin cleanser for cleaning skin site(s) to prevent infection	**Infants, children, and adolescents:** Place a small amount (~5 ml) of emulsion onto the palm of a gloved hand and rub with other gloved hand and with a sufficient amount of warm water to work into a lather; topically apply to skin site(s) requiring cleansing and clean site(s) gently. Rinse cleansed site thoroughly with warm water and carefully dry with a sterile towel. **Note:** Repeated, regular use over several days results in cumulative antibacterial action. **Note:** Should not be generally used for routine bathing of infants because of concerns regarding potential for hexachlorophene toxicity (*see* "Comments").	Emulsion, topical: 3% (contains lanolin and petrolatum [*pHisoHex*]) **Note:** For external use only. Avoid contact with the eye(s). If contact with the eye(s) occurs, rinse eye(s) promptly and thoroughly with copious amounts of water.	**Contraindications:** Dermatitis of Letterer-Siwe's syndrome, hypersensitivity to hexachlorophene, lesions of ichthyosis congenita, premature infants, use on burned or denuded skin sites, and use on mucous membranes. **ADRs:** Generally well tolerated. May cause local skin irritation and photosensitivity. **Comments:** Avoid significant systemic absorption (as could occur if hexachlorophene were applied to large areas of abraded, burned, or denuded skin and not thoroughly removed with rinsing). Infants are particularly at risk because of their thin skin and proportionately large surface area. Signs and symptoms of systemic hexachlorophene toxicity associated with systemic skin absorption include anorexia, convulsions, hypertension, irritability, and death. The latter resulted in the removal of the hexachlorophene topical 6% product from the market several decades ago.
Histrelin (*Supprelin®*)	Precocious puberty, central idiopathic or neuropathic **Note:** Pharmacotherapy generally should not begin after 8 years of age for girls and 9.5 years of age for boys.	**Children (girls, 2–8 years; and boys, 2–9.5 years):** 10 µg/kg/day SC as a single dose. **Note:** Inject each dose at approximately the same time each day. Rotate injection sites for each injection (*see* Chapter 1). **Note:** Pharmacotherapy generally is required until the child reaches the appropriate age for puberty.	Injectables, SC: 120 µg/0.6 ml, 300 µg/0.6 ml, 600 µg/0.6 ml (available in 30-day kits with single-use vials and seven sterile disposable needles and syringes) **Note:** For SC use only. **Note:** Not generally available in Canada.	**Contraindications:** Hypersensitivity to histrelin and pregnancy. **ADRs:** Commonly causes a wide variety of ADRs affecting virtually every body system. May commonly cause local irritation at injection site, vaginal bleeding (usually a light menstrual flow occurring only once for a few days among girls within 1–3 weeks of initiating therapy), and vasodilation. Also may cause acne, anxiety, arthralgia, breast pain, cough, depression, edema, fatigue, headache, hearing loss, hypersensitivity reactions, hyperventilation, insomnia, leukorrhea, mood changes, muscle cramps, nervousness, nocturia, pharyngitis, pruritus, pyrexia, sweating, tachycardia, vaginal dryness or pain, and visual disturbances. **Comments:** Efficacy of pharmacotherapy should be monitored by means of standard *(Continued)*

Footnotes are on page 558.

TABLE 14-1 continued

DRUG (TRADE AND OTHER NAMES)	INDICATION(S)	USUAL PEDIATRIC DOSAGE AND ADMINISTRATION[a]	DOSAGE FORMS	CONTRAINDICATIONS, ADRs, AND COMMENTS[b]
Histrelin *continued*				gonodotropin-releasing hormone testing and by serial determinations of sex steroid concentrations. Decreases in leutenizing hormone, follicle-stimulating hormone, and sex steroid concentrations generally should be evident within 3 months.
Homatropine *(AK-Homatropine®, Isopto Homatropine®)*	Ocular refraction (to provide mydriasis and cycloplegia)	**Children:** Instill one or two drops of 2% solution in appropriate eye(s). Initial dose may be repeated after 5–10 min, if needed. **Adolescents:** Instill one or two drops of 2% or 5% solution in appropriate eye(s). Initial dose may be repeated after 5–10 min, if needed.	Solutions, ophthalmic: 2%, 5% (in disposable dropper containers) **Note:** For ophthalmic use only. **Note:** Generally only use the 2% solution for children. **Note:** In order to minimize cross-infection whenever both eyes require homatropine ophthalmic pharmacotherapy, ensure that separate containers are dispensed for each eye.	**Contraindications:** Glaucoma; hypersensitivity to homatropine, atropine, or other belladonna alkaloids; and synechiae (adhesions between the iris and the lens). **ADRs:** May cause the following local reactions: blepharoconjunctivitis, blurred vision, increased intraocular pressure, irritation, sensitivity to light, transient burning sensation, and vascular congestion. If significant amounts of homatropine are absorbed systemically by way of drainage through the nasolacrimal apparatus, then typical anticholinergic effects may be noted. *See* Chapter 5. *See also* Chapter 1 for information on minimizing systemic absorption of ophthalmic drugs and proper techniques for the instillation of ophthalmic drops.
	Uveitis	**Children:** Instill one or two drops of 2% solution in appropriate eye(s) every 3–4 hr. **Adolescents:** Instill one or two drops of 2% or 5% solution in appropriate eye(s) every 3–4 hr. **Note:** Higher doses (additional drops or higher concentration) may be required for pediatric patients with heavily pigmented irides.		
Human Growth Hormone, *see* **Somatropin**				
Hyaluronidase *(Wydase®)* **Note:** *See also* Chapter 13.	Hypodermoclysis (hyaluronidase is used to prepare IV drugs and solutions for administration by SC infusion and to facilitate their SC absorption when the IV route is contraindicated or cannot be used [e.g., when venous access cannot be established or maintained].)	**Infants and children (<3 years):** First, add 150 units (1 ml) of hyaluronidase solution to diluted drug solution (up to 200 ml) to be infused SC. Then insert needle SC with tip of needle lying free and movable between skin and muscle and begin hypodermoclysis. **Children (≥ 3 years) and adolescents:** Inject 150 units (1 ml) SC at the intended site of the hypodermoclysis infusion. Then insert the needle with the tip lying free and movable between the skin and muscle tissues and begin the infusion (up to 1000 ml of hypodermoclysis solution may be infused). **Note:** *See* Chapter 1 for discussion of drug administration by hypodermoclysis.	Injectable, SC, lyophilized powder (for reconstitution and mixture with IV drug): 150 units/ml (bovine origin) Injectable, SC solution: 150 units/ml **Note:** For SC use only. **Note:** Reconstitute lyophilized powder for SC injection with 1 ml of 0.9% sodium chloride for injection/150 units. **Note:** Not generally available in Canada.	**Contraindications:** Hypersensitivity to hyaluronidase and SC injection into or around acutely inflamed, cancerous, or infected tissue sites. **ADRs:** Generally well tolerated. May cause urticaria at SC infusion site. **Comments:** Hypodermoclysis should be preceded with a skin test for possible hypersensitivity to hyaluronidase; inject ~0.02 ml intradermally. A positive skin reaction is indicated by the appearance of a wheal within 5 min and its persistance for 20–30 min.
Hydralazine *(Apresoline®)*	Congestive heart failure/ Hypertension **Note:** Not approved by the FDA or HPB for infants or children.	**Children and adolescents:** Initially, 0.15–0.8 mg/kg/dose IV every 4–6 hr (or 1.5 µg/kg/min IV); then 0.7–7 mg/kg/day PO in four divided doses, every 6 hr. *Maximum:* 200 mg/day PO **or** 7.5 mg/kg/day PO, whichever is less. **Note:** Administer with food to increase bioavailability.	Injectable, IV: 20 mg/ml Tablets, oral: 10, 25, 50, 100 mg	**Contraindications:** Coronary artery disease, cor pulmonale, dissecting aneurysm of the aorta (acute), hypersensitivity to hydralazine, rheumatic heart disease, systemic lupus erythematosus, and tachycardia (severe). **ADRs:** *See* Chapter 5. **Comments:** Associated with the development of systemic lupus

CHAPTER 14: DRUG DOSING FOR INFANTS, CHILDREN, AND ADOLESCENTS

TABLE 14-1 *continued*

DRUG (*TRADE* AND OTHER NAMES)	INDICATION(S)	USUAL PEDIATRIC DOSAGE AND ADMINISTRATION[a]	DOSAGE FORMS	CONTRAINDICATIONS, ADRs, AND COMMENTS[b]
Hydralazine *continued*				erythematosus. The incidence of this syndrome appears to be dose related and occurs more frequently among patients who are slow acetylators versus fast acetylators of hydralazine. (*See* Chapter 11.) **Note:** Blood pressure and heart rate should be monitored every 5 min during IV administration.
Hydrochloro-thiazide (*Esidrix®, HydroDIURIL®, Microzide®, Oretic®*)	Edema/ Hypertension	**Infants, children, and adolescents:** 2–4 mg/kg/day PO in two divided doses, every 12 hr. *Maximum:* 200 mg/day PO.	Capsule, oral: 12.5 mg Solution, oral: 50 mg/5 ml Solution, oral concentrate: 100 mg/ml Tablets, oral: 25, 50, 100 mg	**Contraindications:** Anuria; hepatic coma; hypersensitivity to hydrochlorothiazide, other thiazides, or sulfonamides; and renal failure. **ADRs:** *See* Chapter 5. **Comments:** Monitor fluid and electrolyte status.
Hydro-cortisone (*A-Hydrocort®, Cortef®*, Cortisol, *Solu-Cortef®*) **Note:** *See also* Hydrocortisone, topical.	Anaphylaxis	**Children and adolescents:** 5–10 mg/kg IV.	Injectables, IM, IV: 100, 250, 500 mg/vial; 1 gram/vial (sodium succinate); contains benzyl alcohol. Suspension, oral: 10 mg/5 ml (cypionate); shake well before use. Tablets, oral: 5, 10, 20 mg	**Contraindications:** Adreno-cortical insufficiency (primary), congestive heart failure, fungal infections (systemic), hypertension, and osteoporosis. **ADRs:** Long-term therapy may retard bone growth among children. Alternate-day dosing, when clinically feasible, appears to minimize growth suppression. *See* Chapter 5. **Comments:** In congenital adrenal hyperplasia, administer one-half of the daily dose at bedtime to suppress morning ACTH surge. Normal endogenous cortisol production = 10 ± 3 mg/m²/day. **Note:** May need to triple the maintenance dosage during concurrent illness or other stressful event (e.g., surgery). *Discontinuing therapy:* Pediatric patients receiving therapy for ≥ 10 days, reduce dose by 50% every 48 hr until a dosage of 10 ± 3 mg/m²/day is achieved, then reduce dose by 50% every 10–14 days.
	Asthma, acute	**Children and adolescents:** 4–6 mg/kg/dose IV every 4–6 hr.		
	Hypoadrenalism, treatment	**Children and adolescents:** 20 mg/m²/day PO in three divided doses, every 8 hr **or** 12 mg/m²/day IV in four divided doses, every 6 hr. **Note:** Administer oral doses with food or milk to minimize associated GI irritation.		
	Hypoadrenalism, pre-operative prophylaxis or acute adrenal crisis	**Children and adolescents:** 100 mg/m² IV as a single dose, then 100 mg/m²/day IV in four divided doses, every 6 hr.		
Hydro-cortisone, topical (*Cort-Dome®, Cortizone®, Dermacort®, Hydrocort®, Hytone®*)	Dermatoses, corticosteroid responsive	**Infants, children, and adolescents:** Apply topical formulation sparingly to affected area(s) once or twice daily. **Note:** *See* Chapter 1 for details regarding proper techniques for topical administration.	Cream, topical: 1% Gel, topical: 1% Lotion, topical: 1% Ointment, topical: 1% Spray, topical: 1% **Note:** For external use only. Avoid contact with eyes.	**Contraindications:** Hypersensitivity to hydrocortisone. **ADRs:** Generally well tolerated. May cause local reactions including burning, dryness, erythema, and pruritus at the application site. *See* Chapter 5. **Comments:** Although systemic absorption and resultant toxicity in pediatric patients can occur with topical use, particularly long term or with an occlusive dressing, it is not as likely to occur as when high potency corticosteroids (e.g., fluocinolone) are used.

Footnotes are on page 558.

TABLE 14-1 continued

DRUG (TRADE AND OTHER NAMES)	INDICATION(S)	USUAL PEDIATRIC DOSAGE AND ADMINISTRATION[a]	DOSAGE FORMS	CONTRAINDICATIONS, ADRs, AND COMMENTS[b]
Hydrogen Peroxide	Prevention of local infection of external suture lines, minor abrasions, and minor superficial open wounds (used to cleanse and debride suture sites and minor abrasions and wounds, particularly when antibacterial detergent cleansers cannot be used because they are too irritating to the skin tissues)	**Children and adolescents:** Apply 1.5% or 3% solution liberally to external skin sites requiring cleansing. Rinse with sterile normal saline, if appropriate, and dry gently with a sterile towel.	Solutions, topical: 1.5%, 3% **Note:** Store at controlled room temperature between 15 and 30°C in tightly closed, light-resistant containers. **Note:** For external use only.	**Contraindications:** Application to closed body cavities, wounds, or abscesses. **ADRs:** Generally well tolerated. **Comments:** Hydrogen peroxide has weak antibacterial action and the effervescence associated with oxygen release when applied to a wound or other tissue site results in mechanical loosening of tissue debris and exudate.
Hydromorphone *(Dilaudid®)*	Pain, moderate to severe	**Adolescents:** 1–2 mg IM, IV (injected over at least 2–3 min), PO, or SC every 4–6 hr as indicated by response. Alternatively, 3-mg rectal suppository every 6–8 hr as indicated by response. **Note:** A reduced duration of effect may signify the development of tolerance to hydromorphone.	Injectables, IM, IV, SC: 1, 2, 4 mg/ml Suppository, rectal: 3 mg (in a cocoa butter base) Tablets, oral: 2, 4 mg	**Contraindications:** Hypersensitivity to hydromorphone or other opiate analgesics, increased intracranial pressure, and significant respiratory depression. **ADRs:** Addicting and habituating; may cause CNS, respiratory, and other ADRs similar to other opiate analgesics (*see* Chapter 5).
Hydroxychloroquine *(Plaquenil®)*	Juvenile rheumatoid arthritis (refractory to conventional pharmacotherapy) **Note:** Not approved by the FDA or HPB for infants or children.	**Children and adolescents:** 5–7 mg/kg/day PO as a single daily dose. *Maximum:* 400 mg/day (sulfate). **Note:** Administer tablets with food or milk to minimize associated GI irritation.	Tablet, oral: 200 mg (sulfate) **Note:** 200 mg sulfate = 155 mg base.	**Contraindications:** Hypersensitivity to hydroxychloroquine and long-term pediatric hydroxychloroquine pharmacotherapy because of possible irreversible retinal damage. **ADRs:** May cause anorexia, hypotension, nausea, pruritus, and retinal damage (irreversible). **Comments:** Measure glucose-6-phosphate dehydrogenase for possible deficiency prior to initiating therapy. Monitor for decreased visual acuity.
Hydroxyurea, *see* Chapter 12				
Hydroxyzine *(Atarax®, Vistaril®)*	Allergic conditions/Pruritus **Note:** Also approved in Canada by the HPB for the treatment of anxiety disorders and nausea and vomiting.	**Children and adolescents:** 2–4 mg/kg/day PO in three or four divided doses. *Maximum:* 400 mg/day PO. **Note:** IM administration is painful. Oral administration is recommended. Administer with food or milk to decrease associated GI irritation.	Capsules, oral: 10, 25, 50, 100 mg Injectable, IM: 50 mg/ml Suspension, oral: 25 mg/5 ml (lemon flavored); shake well before use. Syrup, oral: 10 mg/5 ml (vanilla flavored) Tablets, oral: 10, 25, 50, 100 mg	**Contraindications:** Narrow-angle glaucoma and obstruction of the GI or urinary tract. **ADRs:** *See* Chapter 5. **Comments:** May impair cognition, learning, and memory. Paradoxical effects (CNS excitation) may occasionally occur in young children.
Hyoscine, *see* Scopolamine				
Ibuprofen *(Advil®, Children's Motrin®, Motrin®, Nuprin®)*	Fever	**Infants, children, and adolescents:** 5–10 mg/kg/dose PO every 6 hr. *Maximum:* 200 mg/dose PO; 40 mg/kg/day PO.	Caplet (gelatin-coated tablet): 200 mg Drops, oral: 50 mg/1.25 ml (dye free) (fruit or grape flavored) Suspensions, oral: 100, 200 mg/5 ml (berry, fruit, and grape flavored); shake well before use. Tablets, oral: 100, 200, 300, 400, 600, 800 mg	**Contraindications:** Hypersensitivity to ibuprofen or to other nonsteroidal anti-inflammatory drugs (NSAIDs). **ADRs:** *See* Chapter 5.
	Juvenile rheumatoid arthritis **Note:** Not approved by the FDA or HPB for the treatment of juvenile rheumatoid arthritis.	**Children and adolescents:** 30–70 mg/kg/day PO in three or four divided doses. *Maximum:* 2.4 grams/day PO.		

CHAPTER 14: DRUG DOSING FOR INFANTS, CHILDREN, AND ADOLESCENTS

TABLE 14-1 continued

DRUG (TRADE AND OTHER NAMES)	INDICATION(S)	USUAL PEDIATRIC DOSAGE AND ADMINISTRATION[a]	DOSAGE FORMS	CONTRAINDICATIONS, ADRs, AND COMMENTS[b]
Ibuprofen *continued*	Migraine, mild to moderate	Adolescents: 200–400 mg/dose PO. Repeat dose at 4-hr intervals as needed, according to response. *Maximum:* 2.4 grams/day PO.	Tablets, oral chewable: 50, 100 mg (citrus, fruit, and grape flavored)	
	Pain, mild to moderate	Infants, children, and adolescents: 5–10 mg/kg/dose PO every 6–8 hr. *Maximum:* 40 mg/kg/day PO. **Note:** Administer with food or milk to minimize associated GI irritation.		
Idarubicin, *see* **Chapter 12**				
Ifosfamide, *see* **Chapter 12**				
Imiglucerase *(Cerezyme®)*	Gaucher's disease, type 1 (long-term enzyme replacement therapy)	Children and adolescents: 60 units/kg/dose IV every 2 weeks. **Note:** Administer by slow IV infusion over 1–2 hr (alternatively, the rate of infusion may be calculated at 0.5–1 unit/kg/min).	Injectables, IV: 200, 400 units/vial (lyophilized powder for reconstitution) **Note:** For IV use only. **Note:** Prior to injection, reconstitute lyophilized powder with 5.1 ml of sterile water for injection per 200 units and then dilute with 100–200 ml of 0.9% sodium chloride for injection **prior** to administration. Prepare immediately before use and appropriately and safely discard any unused drug. **Note:** Not generally available in Canada.	**Contraindications:** Hypersensitivity to imiglucerase. **ADRs:** Generally well tolerated. May cause burning sensation, pain, or pruritus at infusion site. **Comments:** Depending on the severity of the disease, dosages can range from 2.5 units/kg three times per week to 60 units/kg once every 2 weeks.
Imipenem–Cilastatin (in a 1:1 fixed combination) *(Primaxin®)*	Bacterial infections **Note:** Ensure that appropriate culture and sensitivity tests are performed and that the organism is sensitive to imipenem–cilastatin. **Note:** Not approved by the HPB for infants or children. **Note:** Not recommended for pediatric patients with meningitis or other CNS infections because of the risk for seizures.	Infants and children (≤3 years): 100 mg/kg/day IV in four divided doses, every 6 hr. Children (>3 years): 60 mg/kg/day IV in four divided doses, every 6 hr. *Maximum:* 2 grams/day IV. Adolescents: 1–2 grams/day IV by intermittent infusion in three or four divided doses, every 6 or 8 hr; **or** 1–1.5 grams/day IM in two divided doses, every 12 hr. *Maximum:* 50 mg/kg/day IV or 4 grams/day IV, whichever is less; 1500 mg/day IM. **Note:** IM route is generally limited for the treatment of mild-to-moderate infections. For severe or life-threatening infections, the IV route should be used. **Note:** Reduce dosage for pediatric patients who have renal dysfunction; *see* Table 14-2.	Injectables, IM: 500, 750 mg/vial (after reconstitution with 1% lidocaine solution [without epineprhine]) **Note:** Reconstituted imipenem–cilastatin injectable for IM use should be used within 1 hr of preparation. For IM use only; do **not** administer IV. Injectables, IV: 250, 500 mg/vial **Note:** Contain equal amounts of imipenem and cilastatin.	**Contraindications:** Hypersensitivity to imipenem or cilastatin. **ADRs:** May cause diarrhea, phlebitis at IV injection site, rash, and vomiting. *See* Chapter 5. **Comments:** Use with caution among patients with a history of allergy to penicillins because of possible cross-sensitivity.

Footnotes are on page 558.

TABLE 14-1 continued

DRUG (TRADE AND OTHER NAMES)	INDICATION(S)	USUAL PEDIATRIC DOSAGE AND ADMINISTRATION[a]	DOSAGE FORMS	CONTRAINDICATIONS, ADRs, AND COMMENTS[b]
Immune Globulin (*Gamimune N®, Gammagard S/D®, Iveegam®, Sandoglobin®, Venoglobulin-S®*) **Note:** See also Chapter 9.	Hypogammaglobulinemia (primary humoral immunodeficiency)	Children and adolescents: 100–200 mg/kg/dose IV once a month. *Maximum:* 400 mg/kg/dose IV once a month.	Injectables, IV: 0.5, 1, 2.5, 3, 5, 6, 10 grams/vial **Note:** For IV use only.	**Contraindications:** Hypersensitivity to immune globulin (human), patients with anti-IgA antibodies, and renal dysfunction. **ADRs:** Generally well tolerated. May cause chest pain, chills, dyspnea, faintness, fever, headache, malaise, nausea, and vomiting. **Comments:** Reportedly associated with severe renal dysfunction and resultant death. Monitor patients for signs and symptoms of renal dysfunction.
	Idiopathic thrombocytopenic purpura	Children and adolescents: 1 gram/kg/day IV as a single daily dose for 1–2 days **or** 400 mg/kg/day IV as a single daily dose for 5 consecutive days.		
	Prevention or reduction of opportunistic bacterial infections among HIV-positive pediatric patients	Children and adolescents: 400 mg/kg/dose IV once a month.		
	Kawasaki disease (in combination with aspirin pharmacotherapy)	Children and adolescents: 2 grams/kg IV as a one-time dose over 10–12 hr **or** 400 mg/kg/day IV as a single daily dose for 4 days. **Note:** The recommended IV infusion rate differs for the various formulations. See manufacturer's recommendations. Do **not** inject IM or SC.		
Indinavir (*Crixivan®*)	HIV infection (as adjunctive pharmacotherapy with other antiretroviral drugs [e.g., lamivudine; zidovudine]) **Note:** Not approved by the FDA or HPB for this indication for children or adolescents.	Children: 1500 mg/m^2/day PO in three divided doses, every 8 hr. Adolescents: 2400 mg/day PO in three divided doses, every 8 hr. **Note:** Administer 1 hr before or 2 hr after a meal with adequate liquid chaser (e.g., coffee, juice, skim milk, tea, water) to maximize absorption. Do **not** administer with food or meals, which may decrease absorption. **Note:** May need to reduce dosage by 25%–50% for pediatric patients who have hepatic dysfunction.	Capsules, oral: 200, 400 mg	**Contraindications:** Concurrent pharmacotherapy with cisapride, ergot derivatives, midazolam, or triazolam; hemolytic anemia; hypersensitivity to indinavir; and nephrolithiasis. **ADRs:** May cause abdominal pain, acid regurgitation, bleeding tendencies (particularly spontaneous bleeding among pediatric patients who have hemophilia), diarrhea, flank pain, headache, insomnia, nephrolithiasis, pruritus, rash, and taste perception changes. See Chapter 5. **Comments:** To reduce the incidence of nephrolithiasis, patients should drink at least 1.5 liters of water daily.
Indomethacin (*Indocid®, Indocin®*)	Juvenile rheumatoid arthritis (refractory to conventional pharmacotherapy) **Note:** Not approved by the FDA or HPB for children.	Adolescents: 1–3 mg/kg/day PO in three divided doses with meals. *Maximum:* 200 mg/day PO. **Note:** Administer with meals to minimize associated GI irritation.	Capsules, oral: 25, 50, 100 mg	**Contraindications:** Diverticulitis, gastritis, hypersensitivity to indomethacin or to other nonsteroidal anti-inflammatory drugs (NSAIDs), peptic ulcers, and ulcerative colitis. **ADRs:** See Chapter 5. **Comments:** Monitor hepatic function.
Infliximab (*Remicade®*)	Crohn's disease (refractory to conventional pharmacotherapy)	Children and adolescents: 5 mg/kg IV as a single dose. **Note:** For patients who have fistulizing disease, the initial 5 mg/kg dose may be repeated in 2 weeks and again in 6 weeks.	Injectable, IV (lyophilized powder for reconstitution): 10 mg/ml (after reconstitution with sterile water for injection)	**Contraindications:** Active, potentially life-threatening infections; congestive heart failure; hypersensitivity to infliximab or to murine proteins; and sepsis.

TABLE 14-1 continued

DRUG (TRADE AND OTHER NAMES)	INDICATION(S)	USUAL PEDIATRIC DOSAGE AND ADMINISTRATION[a]	DOSAGE FORMS	CONTRAINDICATIONS, ADRs, AND COMMENTS[b]
Infliximab *continued*	Juvenile rheumatoid arthritis (refractory to conventional pharmacotherapy) **Note:** Generally used in combination with methotrexate. **Note:** Not approved by the FDA for these indications for children or adolescents.	**Adolescents:** Initially, 3 mg/kg IV as a single dose. Repeat initial dose at 2 and 6 weeks. *Maintenance:* 3 mg/kg IV as a single dose, every 8 weeks. **Note:** Should be IV infused over at least 2 hr. Appropriately and safely dispose of any unused drug.	**Note:** Store under refrigeration between 2 and 8°C. Do not freeze. **Note:** For IV use only. After reconstitution, the solution should be further diluted, prior to use, to 250 ml with 0.9% sodium chloride for injection and infused within 3 hr. **Note:** Not generally available in Canada.	**ADRs:** May cause ADRs affecting most body systems, including potentially fatal reactions. Reported ADRs include abdominal pain, coughing, drug-induced lupus, dyspnea, fatigue, headache, infections (particularly of the upper respiratory tract, but including tuberculosis and other serious opportunistic infections), lymphoma or other malignancies, nausea, pruritus, rhinitis, sinusitis, and urticaria.
Influenza Virus Vaccine, *see* **Chapter 9**				
Insulin *(Humulin®, Iletin®, Novolin®)* **Note:** *See also* Insulin Glargine.	Insulin-dependent diabetes mellitus	*Initial dose: See* "Insulin Sliding Scale" *Maintenance dose:* **Children:** 0.5–1 unit/kg/day SC. Adjust dosage according to need, type of insulin used, and response. **Adolescents:** 1–1.5 units/kg/day SC. Adjust dosage according to need, type of insulin used, and response. **Note:** Insulin requirements frequently change during periods of illness or other stress. They also change during puberty, necessitating close monitoring of previously stabilized children. Adolescent girls often require more insulin than adolescent boys and the incidence of early morning (prebreakfast) hyperglycemia is increased among both adolescent boys and girls. Appropriate dosage adjustment is required. **Note:** Reduce dosage for pediatric patients who have renal dysfunction.	Injectable, SC, IV (regular): 100 units/ml Injectable suspension, SC: 100 units/ml **Note:** The various formulations are derived from beef, pork, combination beef and pork, and human (biosynthetic) sources. **Note:** Insulin (regular) is an aqueous solution that can be administered IV or SC. All other insulin injectables are formulated as suspensions for SC injection only. Carefully mix all suspensions before use. Note also that insulin (regular) is only compatible with insulin formulations that are available from the **same** manufacturer. Insulin (regular) is not compatible with insulin formulations available from other manufacturers and mixing insulin (regular) with these formulations is **not** recommended because of formulation differences (e.g., amounts and types of buffers and preservatives, amounts of excess protamine and zinc). Insulin formulations should be stored in a cold place (between 2 and 10°C) protected from heat and light, preferably in a refrigerator. They should not be frozen. If necessary, insulin formulations may be stored at room temperature for up to 1 month. Check expiration date prior to use.	**Contraindications:** Hypoglycemia and hypersensitivity to any of the components of the insulin formulation (e.g., beef, pork). **ADRs:** May cause dose-related hypoglycemia (glucagon is an antidote for severe hypoglycemia). *See* Chapter 5. **Comments:** Monitor blood glucose and urine glucose and acetone. Patients with diabetic ketoacidosis may be particularly sensitive to the effects of insulin and must be closely monitored (too rapid a decrease in blood glucose may result in cerebral edema). Pediatric patients with diabetic ketoacidosis require monitoring of serum glucose, phosphate, and potassium concentrations and pH. **Note:** Many different drugs can affect blood glucose levels (*see* Chapters 5 and 6). Commonly used drugs that can **decrease** blood glucose levels include angiotensin-converting enzyme inhibitors, disopyramide, fibrates, fluoxetine, monoamine oxidase inhibitors, propoxyphene, salicylates, and sulfonamides. Commonly used drugs that can **increase** blood glucose levels include corticosteroids, diuretics, estrogens, isoniazid, phenothiazines, progestogens, sympathomimetics, and thyroid hormones.

(Continued)

Footnotes are on page 558.

TABLE 14-1 continued

DRUG (TRADE AND OTHER NAMES)	INDICATION(S)	USUAL PEDIATRIC DOSAGE AND ADMINISTRATION[a]	DOSAGE FORMS	CONTRAINDICATIONS, ADRs, AND COMMENTS[b]
Insulin *continued*	**Diabetic ketoacidosis** **Note:** Common signs and symptoms of diabetic ketoacidosis include acetone breath, air hunger, anorexia, dim vision, drowsiness, dry flushed skin, nausea, rapid pulse, soft eyeballs, thirst, and vomiting. Urine will be positive for both acetone and glucose.	*Initial dose:* 0.1 unit (regular)/kg IV, then 0.1 unit (regular)/kg/hr IV by continuous infusion. Adjust dosage according to response, usually to maintain a rate of glucose **decline** between 50 and 100 mg/dl/hr. **Note: Only insulin (regular) should be administered IV.**	**Note:** Insulin (regular) can adsorb to plastic IV infusion sets, resulting in a loss of up to 60% of the IV insulin dose. **Note:** Various formulations (e.g., inhalation, which is still experimental) and devices (e.g., insulin "pens" [*Novolin Penfill®*]) are available to individualize therapy for children and adolescents). *See* Chapter 1 for additional information and discussion.	

Insulin Sliding Scale

Initial dose: 2–4 units SC four times daily, 30 min before meals and at bedtime

Insulin Dose (units/kg)

URINE GLUCOSE	URINE KETONES (−)	URINE KETONES (+)
0–½%	0	0
¾%	0.03–0.1	0.05–0.12
1%	0.07–0.2	0.1–0.25
2%	0.15–0.4	0.2–0.5

Pharmacodynamics of Various Insulin Formulations

INSULIN FORMULATION	USUAL TIME TO ONSET OF ACTION (hr)	USUAL TIME TO PEAK CONCENTRATION (TIME OF MAXIMAL EFFECT) (hr)	USUAL DURATION OF ACTION (hr)
Insulin (regular)	0.5–1	1–5	5–8
Insulin zinc [suspension], prompt	0.5–2	3–10	12–16
Insulin zinc [suspension]	1–3	6–15	18–24
Insulin [suspension], isophane	1–3	4–15	18–24
Insulin zinc [suspension], extended	3–8	8–30	30+

DRUG (TRADE AND OTHER NAMES)	INDICATION(S)	USUAL PEDIATRIC DOSAGE AND ADMINISTRATION[a]	DOSAGE FORMS	CONTRAINDICATIONS, ADRs, AND COMMENTS[b]
Insulin Glargine (*Lantus®*) **Note:** *See also* Insulin.	Insulin-dependent diabetes mellitus	*Changing from once-daily NPH human insulin or ultralente human insulin to insulin glargine*: **Children (≥6 years) and adolescents:** Initially, administer 100% of previously used daily dose of NPH or ultralente by SC injection once daily at bedtime. Adjust dosage according to response. *Changing from twice-daily NPH human insulin to insulin glargine*: **Children (≥6 years) and adolescents:** Initially, administer 80% of previously used daily dose of NPH by SC injection once daily at bedtime. Adjust dosage according to response.	Injectable solution, SC: 100 units/ml **Note:** For SC use only. **Note:** Insulin glargine should **not** be diluted or mixed with any other insulin or injectable solution prior to SC injection.	**Contraindications:** Hypersensitivity to insulin glargine. **ADRs:** *See* Insulin. **Comments:** *See* Insulin. **Note:** The pharmacodynamics of insulin glargine require that it be administered **only** by SC injection. After injection into the subcutaneous tissue, the acidic solution (pH 4) forms microprecipitates from which relatively constant amounts of insulin glargine are slowly released over a period of approximately 24 hr with no pronounced peak of action.
Interferon Alfa-2b (Recombinant) (*Intron® A*)	Hepatitis B, chronic	**Children and adolescents:** Initially, 3 million international units/m² SC three times a week for 1 week. Then 6 million international units/m² SC three times a week for at least 16 weeks.	Injectables, SC: 3, 5, 10, 18, 25, 50 million units/vial	**Contraindications:** Hypersensitivity to interferon alfa-2b (recombinant). **ADRs:** May cause abdominal pain, alopecia, depression, flulike signs and symptoms (e.g., asthenia,

TABLE 14-1 continued

DRUG (TRADE AND OTHER NAMES)	INDICATION(S)	USUAL PEDIATRIC DOSAGE AND ADMINISTRATION[a]	DOSAGE FORMS	CONTRAINDICATIONS, ADRs, AND COMMENTS[b]
Interferon Alfa-2b (Recombinant) *continued*		**Note:** Reduce dosage by 50% if either the platelet count is <50,000/mm³ or the granulocyte count is <750/mm³. Withhold dose if either the platelet count is <30,000/mm³ or the granulocyte count <500/mm³. Resume dosage when platelet and granulocyte counts return to normal or baseline values.		fever, headache, myalgia, rigors), nausea, and vomiting.
Iodoquinol (Diiodohydroxyquin, *Diodoquin®*, *Yodoxin®*)	**Intestinal amebiasis** **Note:** For the treatment of amebiasis, the Communicable Disease Center recommends that iodoquinol be used in combination with metronidazole.	**Children and adolescents:** 40 mg/kg/day PO in three divided doses, after meals, for 20 days. *Maximum:* 650 mg/dose PO; 1950 mg/day PO. **Note:** Avoid long-term use.	Tablets, oral: 210, 650 mg	**Contraindications:** Hepatic dysfunction and hypersensitivity to iodoquinol, iodine, or 8-hydroxyquinolines. **ADRs:** May cause abdominal cramps, chills, diarrhea, fever, headache, optic neuritis, nausea, pruritus, skin eruptions, vertigo, and vomiting. **Comments:** Long-term use of high dosages has been associated with optic neuritis and peripheral neuropathy.
Ipecac Syrup	**Poisoning, emergency treatment** (to induce vomiting) **Note:** Do not administer to unconscious patients or to patients who would otherwise be at significant risk for aspiration of vomitus.	**Infants (6–9 months):** 5 ml PO as a single dose. **Infants (>9 months):** 10 ml PO as a single dose. **Children:** 15 ml PO as a single dose. **Adolescents:** 30 ml PO as a single dose. **Note:** Repeat the dose for children and adolescents **once** if desired results are not achieved after 20 min. Do **not** repeat the dose for infants. **Note:** Administer with 10–20 ml/kg of water to a maximum of 240 ml of water.	Syrup, oral: 7% (contains 2% alcohol and 10% glycerin)	**Contraindications:** Absent gag reflex, coma, convulsions, poisoning with strong acids or alkalies, and unconsciousness. **ADRs:** Generally does not cause systemic toxicity. **Do not confuse ipecac fluidextract with ipecac syrup. Fatal dosing errors may result.** **Comments:** *See also* Chapter 4.
Ipratropium, nasal (*Atrovent Nasal Spray®*)	**Rhinorrhea associated with perennial rhinitis,** both allergic and nonallergic **Note: Not** indicated for other related signs and symptoms, such as nasal congestion, postnasal drip, and sneezing.	**Children (≥6 years) and adolescents:** Two sprays of 0.03% nasal solution (42 µg) per nostril two or three times daily. **Note:** Efficacy beyond 21 days has not been established.	Solution, nasal spray: 0.03% (supplied with metered-dose nasal spray pump that delivers 21 µg/spray) **Note:** For nasal instillation only. **Note:** Initial use of the metered-dose nasal pump requires priming with seven sprays. If the pump is used daily, no further priming is required. Solution, nasal spray: 0.06% (supplied with metered-dose nasal spray pump that delivers 42 µg/spray) **Note:** For nasal instillation only.	**Contraindications:** Hypersensitivity to atropine or to ipratropium. **ADRs:** Generally well tolerated. May cause epistaxis, nasal dryness, and pharyngitis. **Comments:** Ipratropium generally provides relief of rhinorrhea from the first day of use. Signs and symptoms of nasal rebound have not been associated with its use. **Note:** Two different concentrations are produced by the same manufacturer for two different indications. **Ensure correct concentration is selected and used for each specific indication.**
	Rhinorrhea associated with the common cold **Note: Not** indicated for the symptomatic management of other related signs and symptoms of the common cold, such as nasal congestion and sneezing.	**Children (≥5 years) and adolescents:** Two sprays of 0.06% nasal spray solution (84 µg) per nostril three or four times daily. **Note:** Efficacy beyond 4 days has not been established.		

Footnotes are on page 558.

TABLE 14-1 continued

DRUG (TRADE AND OTHER NAMES)	INDICATION(S)	USUAL PEDIATRIC DOSAGE AND ADMINISTRATION[a]	DOSAGE FORMS	CONTRAINDICATIONS, ADRs, AND COMMENTS[b]
Ipratropium, pulmonary (*Atrovent®*)	Chronic obstructive pulmonary disease, including asthma and chronic bronchitis **Note:** Acute bronchospasm and severe asthma attacks require concomitant β_2-adrenergic agonist pharmacotherapy (e.g., albuterol).	**Children ($\geq$5 years):** 125–250 µg/dose (inhalation solution) in 3 ml normal saline by nebulizer three or four times daily, every 6 or 8 hr, as needed, according to response. **Adolescents:** 250–500 µg/dose (inhalation solution) in 3 ml normal saline by nebulizer three or four times daily, every 6 or 8 hr, as needed, according to response **or** 40 µg (two actuations of metered-dose inhaler) three or four times daily, every 6 or 8 hr, as needed, according to response. *Maximum:* 2 mg/day inhalation solution; 160 µg/day metered-dose inhaler. **Note:** In severe, acute asthma, may administer once an hour, as needed, according to response.	Solutions, inhalation: 125 µg/ml (unit-dose vial); 250 µg/ml (bottle); contains benzalkonium chloride and disodium ethylenediaminetetraacetic acid (EDTA) as preservatives. These preservatives may cause bronchoconstriction in some patients with hyperreactive airways. Solution, metered-dose inhaler: 20 µg/actuation; inhaler contains soya lecithin and is **contraindicated** for pediatric patients who are hypersensitive to peanuts or soya beans; shake well before use. **Note:** Ipratropium metered-dose inhaler is for pulmonary inhalation only. **Note:** *See* Chapter 1 for metered-dose inhaler and nebulizer administration techniques.	**Contraindications:** Hypersensitivity to atropine or to ipratropium (*see also* "Dosage Forms"). **ADRs:** Generally well tolerated. May cause dizziness, dry mouth, headache, nervousness, tremor, and urinary retention. *See* Chapter 5.
Irbesartan (*Avapro®*)	Hypertension, essential **Note:** Generally reserved for pediatric patients who have failed to respond to more conventional beta-adrenergic blocker and/or diuretic pharmacotherapy.	**Children ($\geq$6 years):** 75 mg/day PO as a single dose. *Maximum:* 150 mg/day PO. **Adolescents:** 150 mg/day PO as a single dose. *Maximum:* 300 mg/day PO.	Tablets, oral: 75, 150, 300 mg	**Contraindications:** Hypersensitivity to irbesartan. **ADRs:** May cause diarrhea, fatigue, headache, hypotension, musculoskeletal pain, and syncope. **Comments:** Concurrent diuretic pharmacotherapy (e.g., hydrochlorothiazide) may be required to augment antihypertensive action of irbesartan.
Irinotecan, *see* **Chapter 12**				
Iron, oral **Note:** *See also* Iron Dextran, injectable.	Iron-deficiency anemia, treatment	**Children and adolescents:** 6 mg elemental iron/kg/day PO in three divided doses. *Maximum:* 150 mg/day (elemental iron) PO.	Elemental iron content: Ferrous carbonate, anhydrous (48%); ferrous fumarate (33%); ferrous gluconate (12%); ferrous succinate (33%); ferrous sulfate (20%); ferrous sulfate, dried (30%) **Note:** Elemental iron is available in a wide variety of oral formulations including, capsules, drops, elixirs, and syrups both as single ingredient products and multiple ingredient products (e.g., multiple vitamins with minerals). *Ferrous Fumarate (Feostat®):* Suspensions, oral: 45 mg/0.6 ml, 100 mg/5 ml	**Contraindications:** Hemochromatosis, hemosiderosis, and non-iron-deficiency anemia. **ADRs:** *See* Chapter 5. **Comments:** Prior to administration, dilute each dose of the oral iron drops or suspension in a small amount of water or juice and mix thoroughly. Administer oral tablets with 120–240 ml of water or juice. Administer 1 hr before or 2 hr after dairy products, eggs, tea, whole grain bread, or whole grain cereal. Absorption may be decreased by antacids and increased by ascorbic acid. Monitor iron and hemoglobin serum concentrations.
	Iron-deficiency anemia, prophylaxis	**Children and adolescents:** 0.5–2 mg elemental iron/kg/day PO as a single dose or as two or three divided doses. *Maximum:* 150 mg/day (elemental iron) PO.		

CHAPTER 14: DRUG DOSING FOR INFANTS, CHILDREN, AND ADOLESCENTS

TABLE 14-1 continued

DRUG (TRADE AND OTHER NAMES)	INDICATION(S)	USUAL PEDIATRIC DOSAGE AND ADMINISTRATION[a]	DOSAGE FORMS	CONTRAINDICATIONS, ADRs, AND COMMENTS[b]
Iron, oral *continued*			Tablets, oral: 200, 324, 325, 350 mg *Ferrous Gluconate (Fergon®):* Tablets, oral: 300, 320, 325 mg *Ferrous Sulfate (Fero-Gradumet®, Fer-In-Sol®, Mol-Iron®):* Capsules, oral extended release: 150, 250 mg Solutions, oral: 125 mg/ml; 90, 220, 300 mg/5 ml (may contain up to 5% alcohol) Tablets, oral: 195, 300, 325 mg Tablet, oral enteric coated: 325 mg Tablet, oral extended release: 525 mg	
Iron Dextran, injectable *(DexFerrum®, Dexiron®, INFeD®, Infufer®)* **Note:** *See also* Iron, oral.	Iron-deficiency anemia	**Infants (≥4 months), children, and adolescents:** Total required dose (mg elemental iron) = [patient's weight (kg) × desired increase in hemoglobin concentration (grams/dl) × 2.5] + (10 mg/kg). **Alternatively:** Total required dose (ml of 50-mg/ml formulation) = (patient's lean body weight [kg] × 0.0442) × (hemoglobin, normal − hemoglobin, observed [in grams/dl]) + 1 ml/5 kg (lean body weight, up to a maximum of 14 ml). Administer total required dose IM or IV divided over several days to avoid exceeding maximum daily dosage. *Maximum:* **Infants and children (<5 kg)**, 20 mg/day IM; **children (5–10 kg)**, 50 mg/day IM; **children (>10–50 kg)**, 100 mg/day IM; **children and adolescents (>50 kg)**, 250 mg/day IM **or** 100 mg/day IV.	Injectable, IM, IV: 50 mg (elemental iron)/ml	**Contraindications:** Hemochromatosis, hemosiderosis, and non-iron-deficiency anemia. **ADRs:** *See* Chapter 5. **Comments:** Administer test dose (25 mg IM) before initiating therapy. Oral iron pharmacotherapy is generally preferred. For IM therapy, inject each dose IM using Z-track technique (*see* Chapter 1). For IV therapy, inject IV at a rate **not** exceeding 50 mg/min.
Isoephedrine, *see* **Pseudoephedrine**				
Isoetharine *(Bronkometer®, Bronkosol®)*	Bronchial asthma/ Reversible bronchospasm associated with bronchitis **Note:** Not approved by the FDA for this indication for children or adolescents.	**Children (≥2 years) and adolescents:** Dosage and administration are generally determined by the method of administration as follows. *Hand-bulb Nebulizer:* Initially, three to seven inhalations/dose of undiluted 1% isoetharine solution. May repeat initial dose every 3–4 hr as indicated by response. *Maximum:* Five doses/day. *IPPB:* Initially, 0.25–1 ml/dose of 1% isoetharine solution diluted	Aerosol, inhalation: 340 µg/actuation (contains 30% alcohol [Bronkometer®]) Solutions, inhalation: 0.1%, 0.125%, 0.167%, 0.2%, 0.25%, 1% (May contain sulfites which are associated with hypersensitivity reactions, including anaphylactic reactions, among susceptible patients. Although	**Contraindications:** Hypersensitivity to isoetharine or to other sympathomimetic amines and tachycardia. **ADRs:** May cause anxiety, dizziness, headache, hyperactivity, hypertension, insomnia, nausea, palpitation, restlessness, shakiness, tachycardia, tension, tremor, vomiting, and weakness. **Comments:** Tolerance may occur with long-term use but is generally *(Continued)*

Footnotes are on page 558.

TABLE 14-1 continued

DRUG (TRADE AND OTHER NAMES)	INDICATION(S)	USUAL PEDIATRIC DOSAGE AND ADMINISTRATION[a]	DOSAGE FORMS	CONTRAINDICATIONS, ADRs, AND COMMENTS[b]
Isoetharine *continued*		1:3 with 0.9% sodium chloride solution for inhalation. Alternatively, either 2–4 ml of 0.125% isoetharine solution, 2.5 ml of 0.2% isoetharine solution, or 2 ml of 0.25% isoetharine solution may be used. May repeat initial dose every 3–4 hr as indicated by response. *Maximum:* Five doses/day. *Metered-Dose Aerosol:* Initially, one or two inhalations (340 or 680 µg). May repeat initial dose every 3–4 hr as indicated by response. *Maximum:* Five doses/day. *Oxygen Aerosolization:* Initially, 0.25–0.5 ml/dose of 1% isoetharine solution diluted 1:3 with 0.9% sodium chloride for inhalation. Alternatively, either 2–4 ml of 0.125% isoetharine solution, 2.5 ml of 0.2% isoetharine solution, or 2 ml of 0.25% isoetharine solution may be used. May repeat initial dose every 3–4 hr as indicated by response. *Maximum:* Five doses/day.	uncommon, these reactions appear to occur with a higher incidence among pediatric patients with asthma.) **Note:** For inhalation use only. **Note:** Protect from light. Appropriately and safely discard solutions that are discolored or that contain a precipitate. **Note:** Dilute isoetharine solution as required with 0.9% normal saline solution for inhalation only. **Note:** Not generally available in Canada.	ally reversible with temporary discontinuation. **Note:** Severe paradoxical bronchoconstriction has occurred after repeated excessive use. This paradoxical bronchoconstriction is unresponsive to further isoetharine use and requires the immediate discontinuation of isoetharine pharmacotherapy and supportive medical care as needed.
Isoniazid (*INH®*, Isonicotinic Acid Hydrazide)	Tuberculosis, treatment (as adjunct with other antitubercular drugs [e.g., pyrazinamide, rifampin])	**Children and adolescents:** 10–20 mg/kg/day PO as a single dose for 9 months **or** 10 mg/kg/day PO as a single dose for 2 months followed by 20–40 mg/kg PO twice weekly for 7 months. *Maximum:* Daily dosing, 300 mg/day PO. Twice weekly dosing: 900 mg/dose PO.	Syrup, oral: 50 mg/5 ml Tablets, oral: 50, 100 mg	**Contraindications:** Drug-induced hepatitis, hepatic disease (acute), and hypersensitivity to isoniazid. **ADRs:** See Chapter 5. **Note:** Patients who are slow acetylators of isoniazid are at increased risk for drug-induced lupus erythematosus (*see* Chapter 11). **Comments:** Monitor hepatic function periodically. Severe, even fatal, hepatic dysfunction has been associated with therapy. Pyridoxine supplementation recommended for breast-fed infants and for infants and children with nutritional deficiencies. For the treatment of tuberculosis, isoniazid should **not** be used alone. Isoniazid can inhibit the hepatic metabolism of other drugs (*see* Chapter 6).
	Tuberculosis, prophylaxis	**Children and adolescents:** 10–15 mg/kg/day PO as a single dose for 9 months. *Maximum:* 300 mg/day PO.		
Isoprenaline, *see* **Isoproterenol**				
Isoproterenol (Isoprenaline, *Isuprel®*, *Medihaler-Iso®*)	Asthma	**Children and adolescents:** 0.05 mg/kg inhalation solution diluted to 2–3 ml with normal saline for inhalation via nebulizer every 3–4 hr, as needed, according to response **or** metered-dose inhaler: one or two actuations every 4–6 hr, as needed, according to response. *Maximum:* Inhalation solution, 1.25 mg/dose.	Injectables, IV: 1:5000 (0.2 mg/ml), 1:50,000 (0.02 mg/ml); contain sodium metabisulfite or sodium sulfite which are associated with hypersensitivity reactions, including anaphylactic reactions, among susceptible patients. Although uncommon,	**Contraindications:** AV block caused by cardiac glycoside intoxication and ventricular tachydysrhythmias. **ADRs:** May cause anxiety, excitement, fear, insomnia, nervousness, restlessness, and tension. See Chapter 5. **Comments:** Excessive use may result in the loss of the therapeutic effectiveness of isoproterenol

CHAPTER 14: DRUG DOSING FOR INFANTS, CHILDREN, AND ADOLESCENTS

TABLE 14-1 continued

DRUG (TRADE AND OTHER NAMES)	INDICATION(S)	USUAL PEDIATRIC DOSAGE AND ADMINISTRATION[a]	DOSAGE FORMS	CONTRAINDICATIONS, ADRs, AND COMMENTS[b]
Isoproterenol *continued*	Bradycardia/Sinus arrest	**Children and adolescents:** Initially, 3 µg/kg IV or by endotracheal tube instillation; then 0.05–1 µg/kg/min IV. *Maximum:* 100 µg/dose IV. **Note:** Initiate at 0.05 µg/kg/min and increase by 0.1 µg/kg/min every 5–10 min, as needed, according to response. For bradycardia/sinus arrest, dosage depends on ventricular rate and use of cardiac pacemaker.	these reactions appear to occur with a higher incidence among pediatric patients who have asthma. Solutions, inhalation (for nebulization): 0.25%, 0.5%, 1% Solutions, metered-dose inhalers: 80 µg/actuation (0.2%) (sulfate [*Medihaler-Iso®*]); 125, 131 µg/actuation (0.25%) (hydrochloride [*Isuprel Mistometer®*])	(tachyphylaxis) and the need for alternative bronchodilator pharmacotherapy.
Isotretinoin *(Accutane®)* **Note:** See also Chapter 12.	Acne conglobata/ Inflammatory acne/Nodular acne, severe/ Recalcitrant acne **Note:** Should be reserved for patients who are unresponsive to conventional therapy. **Note:** Prescription is limited to certified prescribers who have attended a special CME program or read a specially prepared booklet and who sign a "Letter of Understanding." In addition, all prescriptions for *Accutane* must have a yellow "Accutane Qualification Sticker" attached to them, even prescriptions for boys.	**Adolescents:** Initially, 0.5 mg/kg/day PO in two divided doses for 2–4 weeks. *Maintenance:* 0.1–1 mg/kg/day PO in two divided doses. *Maximum:* 2 mg/kg/day PO. **Note:** Each dose should be ingested with food or milk to maximize absorption. **Note:** Dosage should be carefully individualized according to response. The usual duration of therapy is 12–20 weeks. A second course of therapy may be initiated, if required, after a minimum of 8 weeks has elapsed. **Note:** Do **not** initiate isotretinoin therapy for adolescent girls who are sexually active until pregnancy has been excluded and oral contraceptives have been used for at least 1 month.	Capsules, oral: 10, 20, 40 mg **Note:** Store protected from light between 15 and 30°C (59–86°F).	**Contraindications:** Hypersensitivity to isotretinoin and pregnancy. **Note:** Isotretinoin is a known human teratogen (*see* Chapter 2). **ADRs:** Commonly causes alopecia, cheilitis, conjunctivitis, desquamation, dry nose, dry skin, eye irritation, facial dermatitis, facial erythema, hypertriglyceridemia, joint pain, pruritus, and skin rash. May also cause acute pancreatitis, benign intercranial hypertension (pseudotumor cerebri), cataracts, corneal opacities, decreased night vision, depression, hearing impairment, hyperostosis, inflammatory bowel disease, neutropenia, psychosis, and suicide ideation. **Note:** Dermabrasion should generally be avoided during isotretinoin therapy and for a period of 6 months following therapy because of the risk for hypertrophic scarring in atypical areas. Likewise, wax epilation should generally be avoided during isotretinoin therapy and for a period of 6 months following therapy because of the risk for dermatitis. **Comments:** For adolescent girls, pregnancy tests are recommended each month during therapy and for the first month following discontinuation of isotretinoin therapy. All patients should receive both oral and written information regarding the proper use of isotretinoin and the toxicity associated with its use. Prior to the initiation of isotretinoin therapy, all patients should view a video specially prepared by the manufacturer (Roche) and read and sign a proscribed patient consent form.

Footnotes are on page 558.

TABLE 14-1 continued

DRUG (TRADE AND OTHER NAMES)	INDICATION(S)	USUAL PEDIATRIC DOSAGE AND ADMINISTRATION[a]	DOSAGE FORMS	CONTRAINDICATIONS, ADRs, AND COMMENTS[b]
Ketamine (Ketalar®)	**Dissociative anesthesia** for diagnostic and surgical procedures **Note:** Not indicated for surgery of the bronchial tree, larynx, or pharynx, unless appropriate muscle relaxants are used concomitantly.	**Children and adolescents:** Initially (induction of anesthesia), 1–4.5 mg/kg IV over 60 sec **or** 6.5–13 mg/kg IM. *Maintenance:* 50% of the full induction dose may be repeated as indicated for the maintenance of anesthesia. **Note:** Movement in response to stimulation, nystagmus, and vocalizations generally indicates lightening of anesthesia and, if additional time is required for completion of the surgery or the therapeutic procedure, the need for additional dose(s) of ketamine.	Injectables, IM, IV: 10, 50, 100 mg/ml **Note:** For IM or IV use only.	**Contraindications:** History of stroke, hypersensitivity to ketamine, and hypertension (severe). **ADRs:** Generally well tolerated. May cause a temporary increase in blood pressure and heart rate. Upon emergence from anesthesia, patients may experience confusion, excitement, hallucinations, psychosis, and vivid dreams.
Ketoconazole, oral systemic (Nizoral®)	**Fungal infections** (chromomycosis, chronic mucocutaneous candidiasis, coccidioidomycosis, histoplasmosis, paracoccidioidomycosis, and systemic candidiasis) **Note:** Penetrates the CNS poorly and, thus, is not indicated for the treatment of fungal infections of the CNS. **Note:** Ensure that appropriate culture and sensitivity tests are performed and that the organism is sensitive to ketoconazole.	**Children (>2 years) and adolescents:** 5–10 mg/kg/day PO as a single daily dose. *Maximum:* 400 mg/day PO. **Note:** Administer oral dosages once daily with a meal.	Tablet, oral: 200 mg **Note:** GI absorption is decreased in an alkaline environment; avoid concomitant use of antacids.	**Contraindications:** Hepatic dysfunction and hypersensitivity to ketoconazole. Concurrent cisapride, lovastatin, midazolam, pimozide, quinidine, simvastatin, and triazolam pharmacotherapy also is contraindicated. **ADRs:** See Chapter 5. **Comments:** Monitor hepatic and hematologic function, particularly with long-term pharmacotherapy. May inhibit the hepatic metabolism of other drugs (see Chapter 6).
Ketoconazole, topical cream (Nizoral Cream®) **Note:** See also Ketoconazole, topical shampoo.	**Seborrheic dermatitis caused by** *Pityrosporum ovale* **Topical fungal infections** **Note:** Ensure that appropriate culture and sensitivity tests are performed and that the organism is sensitive to ketoconazole.	**Children and adolescents:** Apply cream to affected area twice daily for 4 weeks. **Children and adolescents:** Apply cream to affected area and to surrounding areas once daily for 2–6 weeks according to the following guidelines: Cutaneous candidiasis, 2–3 weeks *Tinea corporis,* 3–4 weeks *T. cruris,* 2–4 weeks *T. pedis,* 4–6 weeks *T. versicolor,* 2–3 weeks	Cream, topical: 2% **Note:** For external use only. Avoid contact with eyes. **Note:** Contains sodium sulfite. Sulfites may cause hypersensitivity reactions.	**Contraindications:** Hypersensitivity to ketoconazole. **ADRs:** Generally well tolerated. May cause pruritus, skin irritation (severe), and stinging at the application site.
Ketoconazole, topical shampoo (Nizoral Shampoo®) **Note:** See also Ketoconazole, topical cream.	**Dandruff (Pityriasis capitis)/Seborrheic dermatitis, treatment** **Dandruff (Pityriasis capitis)/Seborrheic dermatitis, prophylaxis**	**Children and adolescents:** Apply 5–10 ml to wet scalp and work into a lather. Leave lather on hair for 5 min before rinsing thoroughly with warm water. Repeat twice a week for 2–4 weeks as indicated by response. **Children and adolescents:** Apply 5–10 ml to wet scalp and work into a lather. Leave lather on hair for 5 min before rinsing thoroughly with warm water.	Shampoo, topical: 2% **Note:** For external topical use only. Avoid contact with eyes.	**Contraindications:** Hypersensitivity to ketoconazole. **ADRs:** Generally well tolerated. May cause scalp and skin irritation.

TABLE 14-1 *continued*

DRUG (*TRADE* AND OTHER NAMES)	INDICATION(S)	USUAL PEDIATRIC DOSAGE AND ADMINISTRATION[a]	DOSAGE FORMS	CONTRAINDICATIONS, ADRs, AND COMMENTS[b]
Ketoconazole, topical shampoo *continued*	**Note:** Ensure that appropriate culture and sensitivity tests are performed and that the organism is sensitive to ketoconazole.	Repeat once every 1–2 weeks as indicated by response.		
Ketotifen (*Zaditen®*)	**Atopic asthma and dermatitis, mild** (prophylaxis) **Note:** Maximal benefit usually observed after 10 weeks of therapy. **Not** effective for the treatment of acute asthma.	**Infants (≥6 months) and children (<3 years):** 0.1 mg/kg/day PO in two divided doses, every 12 hr. **Children (≥3 years):** 2 mg/day PO in two divided doses, every 12 hr. **Note:** It is recommended to initiate ketotifen at half the usual dosage to avoid associated drowsiness.	Syrup, oral: 1 mg/5 ml; contains 2% alcohol (strawberry flavored) Tablet, oral: 1 mg **Note:** The syrup contains 4 grams of carbohydrate per 5 ml. **Note:** Not generally available in the United States.	**Contraindications:** Hypersensitivity to benzoates or ketotifen. **ADRs:** Generally well tolerated. May cause excitation, insomnia, irritability, sedation, and weight gain. **Comments:** Used as adjunctive pharmacotherapy to reduce the dosage requirements of concomitant anti-asthmatic drugs (e.g., beta-adrenergic agonists and theophylline).
Labetalol (*Normadyne®*, *Trandate®*)	**Hypertension, severe** **Note:** Generally reserved for the emergency treatment of severe hypertension among hospitalized patients. **Note:** Not approved by the FDA or HPB for infants or children.	**Children and adolescents:** Initially, 0.25–0.5 mg/kg IV followed by 0.4–1.5 mg/kg/hr IV. *Maximum:* 20 mg/dose IV; 3 mg/kg/hr IV; and 300 mg total cumulative dose. **Note:** Reduce dosage for pediatric patients who have hepatic dysfunction.	Injectable, IV: 5 mg/ml	**Contraindications:** Asthma, AV block, congestive heart failure, hypersensitivity to labetalol, hypoperfusion states, and sinus bradycardia. **ADRs:** Commonly causes dizziness and postural hypotension. May cause nausea, somnolence, tingling sensation of the scalp, and vomiting. *See* Chapter 5. **Comments:** Patient should be kept in a recumbent position during IV administration and blood pressure monitored. Hypotension and associated syncope are likely to occur for up to 3 hr following IV administration.
Lactobacillus Acidophilus (*Bacid®*, *Fermalac®*, *Kyo-Dophilus®*, *Lactinex®*, *Superdophilus®*)	**Diarrhea, mild** **Note:** May be of particular therapeutic benefit for pediatric patients who have **mild** diarrhea associated with oral antibiotic pharmacotherapy.	**Children:** Three capsules/day PO in three divided doses. **Adolescents:** Six capsules/day PO in three divided doses.	Capsules, oral enteric coated: 1 billion fully viable bacilli, lyophilized mixed cultures of *Lactobacillus acidophilus*, *L. bulgarious*, and *Streptococcus lactis*. **Note:** Store oral enteric-coated capsules under refrigeration.	**Contraindications:** Sensitivity to milk products. **ADRs:** Generally well tolerated. May cause increased intestinal flatulence, particularly at the beginning of therapy.
Lactulose (*Acilac®*, *Chronulac®*, *Duphalac®*, *Laxilose®*)	**Constipation**	**Children and adolescents:** 2.5–10 ml/day PO as a single daily dose or as three or four divided doses; double the dosage until stool is produced. *Maximum:* 90 ml/day PO.	Syrup, oral: 10 grams/15 ml (some syrup formulations are cola flavored)	**Contraindications:** Pediatric patients who require a low galactose diet. **ADRs:** May cause abdominal discomfort, belching, cramping, and flatulence. **Comments:** Excessive dosage may result in diarrhea and associated dehydration and hyponatremia.
Lamivudine (*Epivir®*, *Epivir-HBV®*, *Heptovir®*, *3TC®*)	**HIV infection** (generally in **combination** with other antiretroviral drugs such as zidovudine)	**Infants (≥3 months) and children:** 8 mg/kg/day PO in two divided doses. *Maximum:* 300 mg/day PO. **Adolescents:** 300 mg/day PO in two divided doses.	Solutions, oral: 5, 10 mg/ml (strawberry–banana flavored) Tablets, oral: 100, 150 mg	**Contraindications:** Hypersensitivity to lamivudine. **ADRs:** May cause cough, diarrhea, fatigue, fever, headache, malaise, nasal congestion, nausea, pancreatitis, and runny nose. *(Continued)*

Footnotes are on page 558.

TABLE 14-1 continued

DRUG (TRADE AND OTHER NAMES)	INDICATION(S)	USUAL PEDIATRIC DOSAGE AND ADMINISTRATION[a]	DOSAGE FORMS	CONTRAINDICATIONS, ADRs, AND COMMENTS[b]
Lamivudine *continued*	**Note:** Approved for this indication by the FDA but not HPB.			**Comments:** Fatal cases of lactic acidosis, hepatomegaly with steatosis, and pancreatitis with steatorrhea have been reported among HIV-positive pediatric patients receiving combination lamivudine pharmacotherapy.
	Hepatitis B, chronic **Note:** Long-term (>1 year) safety and efficacy of therapy have not been established.	**Children (≥2 years) and adolescents:** 3 mg/kg/day PO as a single dose. *Maximum:* 100 mg/day PO. **Note:** Reduce dosage for pediatric patients who have renal dysfunction; see Table 14-2.		
Lamotrigine *(Lamictal®)*	**Generalized seizures associated with Lennox-Gastaut syndrome** (generally used in combination with other anticonvulsants)	**Children (≥2 years and ≥17 kg [37 lb]):** *Addition of Lamotrigine to an Anticonvulsant Pharmacotherapeutic Regimen containing Valproic Acid:* *Initially (weeks 1 and 2):* 0.15 mg/kg/day PO as a single dose or as two divided doses. Round dose down to nearest 5 mg (lowest dose oral tablet available). If the initial calculated dose is between 2.5 and 5 mg, then administer 5 mg every **other** day for 2 weeks. *Follow by (weeks 3 and 4):* 0.3 mg/kg/day PO as a single dose or as two divided doses. Round dose down to the nearest 5 mg (lowest dose oral tablet size available). *Subsequently (period of final dosage adjustment):* Increase dosage at 1–2-week intervals by 0.3 mg/kg/day (always rounding down to the nearest 5 mg) according to response. *Maintenance:* 1–5 mg/kg/day PO as a single dose or as two divided doses. *Maximum:* 200 mg/day PO. **Children (≥2 years and ≥17 kg [37 lb]):** *Addition of Lamotrigine to an Anticonvulsant Pharmacotherapeutic Regimen containing an Enzyme-Inducing Anticonvulsant (i.e., carbamazepine, phenobarbital, phenytoin, or primidone)* **without** *Valproic Acid:* *Initially (weeks 1 and 2):* 0.6 mg/kg/day PO in two divided doses. Round dose down to nearest 5 mg (lowest dose oral tablet available). *Follow by (weeks 3 and 4):* 1.2 mg/kg/day PO in two divided doses. Round dose down to nearest 5 mg (lowest dose oral tablet size available). *Subsequently (period of final dosage adjustment):* Increase dosage at 1–2-week intervals by 1.2 mg/kg/day (always round down to the nearest 5 mg) according to response.	Tablets, oral: 25, 100, 150, 200 mg Tablets, oral chewable: 5, 25 mg **Note:** Chewable tablets may be swallowed whole, chewed, or dissolved in a small amount of water or a beverage for oral administration by an oral syringe or spoon.	**Contraindications:** Hypersensitivity to lamotrigine. **ADRs:** May cause pharyngitis (sore throat) or rash. **Note:** In up to 1% of pediatric patients, the rash may be severe, resulting in Stevens-Johnson syndrome, toxic dermal necrolysis, and death. Therefore, discontinue at the first sign of rash. Monitor for any related sequelae and treat appropriately. **Comments:** Dispensing errors involving *Lamictal* and other drugs, most commonly labetalol, *Lamisil®*, lamivudine, *Lomotil®*, and *Ludiomil®*, have been noted.

CHAPTER 14: DRUG DOSING FOR INFANTS, CHILDREN, AND ADOLESCENTS

TABLE 14-1 *continued*

DRUG (*TRADE* AND OTHER NAMES)	INDICATION(S)	USUAL PEDIATRIC DOSAGE AND ADMINISTRATION[a]	DOSAGE FORMS	CONTRAINDICATIONS, ADRs, AND COMMENTS[b]
Lamotrigine *continued*		*Maintenance:* 5–15 mg/kg/day PO in two divided doses. *Maximum:* 400 mg/day PO. **Adolescents:** *Addition of Lamotrigine to an Anticonvulsant Pharmacotherapeutic Regimen containing Valproic Acid:* *Initially (weeks 1 and 2):* 25 mg PO every **other** day. *Follow by (weeks 3 and 4):* 25 mg/day PO. *Subsequently (period of final dosage adjustment):* Increase dosage at 1–2-week intervals by 25–50 mg/day PO. *Maintenance:* 100–400 mg/day PO as a single dose or as two divided doses. **Adolescents:** *Addition of Lamotrigine to an Anticonvulsant Pharmacotherapeutic Regimen containing an Enzyme-Inducing Anticonvulsant (i.e., carbamazepine, phenobarbital, phenytoin, or primidone)* ***without*** *Valproic Acid:* *Initially (weeks 1 and 2):* 50 mg/day PO. *Follow by (weeks 3 and 4):* 100 mg/day PO in two divided doses. *Subsequently (period of final dosage adjustment):* Increase dosage at 1–2-week intervals by 100 mg/day according to response. *Maintenance:* 300–500 mg/day PO in two divided doses. **Note:** Reduce dosage for pediatric patients who have hepatic dysfunction.		
Leflunomide *(Arava®)*	**Juvenile rheumatoid arthritis** (refractory to conventional pharmacotherapy) **Note:** Not approved by the FDA or HPB for use in adolescents.	**Adolescents:** Loading dose, 100 mg/day PO as a single dose for 3 days. *Maintenance:* 10–20 mg/day PO as a single dose. **Note:** Reduce dosage for adolescents who have renal dysfunction.	Tablets, oral: 10, 20, 100 mg **Note:** Store at controlled room temperature between 15 and 30°C. Protect from light.	**Contraindications:** Bone marrow suppression, breast feeding, hepatic dysfunction, hypersensitivity to leflunomide, immunodeficiency (severe [e.g., AIDS]), and pregnancy. **ADRs:** May cause a variety of ADRs including abdominal pain, allergic reactions, alopecia, amblyopia, angina pectoris, back pain, diarrhea, dizziness, dyspepsia, elevated liver enzymes, headache, hypertension, nausea, palpitation, pruritus, rash, and weight loss. May also rarely cause bone marrow suppression, erythema multiforme, hepatitis (potentially **fatal**), and lymphoma. **Comments:** Monitor hepatic function prior to the initiation of therapy and monthly, thereafter, or as indicated by response.

Footnotes are on page 558.

PROBLEMS IN PEDIATRIC DRUG THERAPY

TABLE 14-1 *continued*

DRUG (*TRADE* AND OTHER NAMES)	INDICATION(S)	USUAL PEDIATRIC DOSAGE AND ADMINISTRATION[a]	DOSAGE FORMS	CONTRAINDICATIONS, ADRs, AND COMMENTS[b]
Lepirudin (*Refludan®*)	Anticoagulation among patients with heparin-induced thrombocytopenia (HIT) (in order to prevent further thromboembolic complications) **Note:** Not approved by the FDA or HPB for children or adolescents.	**Children and adolescents:** Initially, 0.4 mg/kg by rapid IV injection over 15–20 sec. Then, generally, 0.15 mg/kg/hr as a continuous IV infusion for 2–10 days. *Maximum*: Initial dose for rapid IV injection, 44 mg; initial continuous infusion rate, 16.5 mg/hr. **Note:** Reduce dosage for pediatric patients who have renal dysfunction; see Table 14-2.	Injectable, IV: 50 mg/vial **Note:** Reconstitute with 1 ml of 0.9% sodium chloride for injection or sterile water for injection. *For rapid IV injection*, a concentration of 5 mg/ml should be used. *For continuous IV infusion*, a concentration of either 0.2 mg/ml or 0.4 mg/ml should be used.	**Contraindications:** Hypersensitivity to lepirudin and aPTT >2.5. **ADRs:** Bleeding is the most common ADR. May also cause allergic reactions (e.g., angioedema, bronchospasm, pruritus, and rash), abnormal liver function tests, and multiorgan failure. **Comments:** Obtain baseline aPTT determination prior to initiating therapy. The first aPTT for monitoring therapy should be obtained 4 hr after the IV infusion is begun, and subsequently determined at least once daily for the entire course of therapy. The clinically desired ratio of the patient's aPTT to the aPTT for the median of the laboratory normal range is generally 1.5–2.5.
Leucovorin, *see* **Chapter 12**				
Leuprolide (*Lupron®, Lupron Depot®, Lupron Depot-PED®*) **Note:** Dosage and route of administration are different for the various products.	Central precocious puberty (with onset of secondary sexual characteristics among girls younger than 8 years or among boys younger than 9 years)	**Children (girls <11 years and boys <12 years):** *Initially, using Lupron®*, 50 µg/kg/day SC as a single dose. The dosage can then be titrated up, based on response, by 10 µg/kg/day. The optimally determined therapeutic dosage is then used as the maintenance dosage. *Maximum*: 100 µg/kg/day SC. **Alternatively:** Initially, using *Lupron Depot®* or *Lupron Depot-PED®*, dosage is based on the child's body weight (each dose is injected IM once monthly [once every 4 weeks]): ≤25 kg, 7.5 mg 25–37.5 kg, 11.25 mg >37.5 kg, 15 mg This dose can be titrated up, based on response, by 3.75 mg every 4 weeks. The final therapeutic dose is then used as the maintenance dose. *Maximum*: 15 mg/month IM.	Injectable, SC: 5 mg/ml (contains benzyl alcohol) (*Lupron®*) **Note:** For SC use only. **Note:** Store under refrigeration between 2 and 8°C. Supplied as individual multiple-dose vials or 14-day kits containing a vial of leuprolide, 14 syringes, and 28 alcohol pledgets. Injectables, IM suspension: 3.75, 7.5, 11.25, 15-mg prefilled dual-chamber syringes with diluent. When mixed with diluent supplied with prefilled syringe, the sterile lyophilized microspheres of leuprolide become a suspension that is suitable for once monthly IM injection. **Note:** For IM use only. **Note:** Prefilled dual-chamber syringes should be stored at controlled room temperature between 15 and 30°C. Do not freeze. Supplied as single-dose kits containing prefilled dual-chamber syringes, a 23-gauge needle, and two alcohol pledgets.	**Contraindications:** Hypersensitivity to leuprolide and pregnancy. **ADRs:** May initially cause exacerbation of the signs and symptoms of precocious puberty during the first few weeks. May cause a variety of ADRs including acne, general body pain, local reactions at the injection site (e.g., abscesses, rashes including erythema multiforme, seborrhea, and vaginal bleeding or discharge. **Comments:** Response should be monitored 1–2 months after the initiation of therapy with determination of gonadotropin-releasing hormone (GnRH) stimulation tests and sex steroid concentrations. Measurements of bone age for advancement should be performed every 6–12 months.
Levalbuterol (*R-Albuterol, Xopenex®*)	Bronchospasm associated with reversible obstructive airway disease (e.g., asthma)	**Children (>6 years):** 0.63 mg/dose by nebulization three times daily, every 6–8 hr. *Maximum*: 1.89 mg/day by nebulization.	Solutions, inhalational: 0.63, 1.25-mg/3-ml unit-dose vial. **Note:** Generally administered with a PARI LC Jet® nebulizer or PARI	**Contraindications:** Hypersensitivity to albuterol or to levalbuterol. **ADRs:** May cause anxiety, dizziness, dyspepsia, nervousness, and tremor.

TABLE 14-1 continued

DRUG (TRADE AND OTHER NAMES)	INDICATION(S)	USUAL PEDIATRIC DOSAGE AND ADMINISTRATION[a]	DOSAGE FORMS	CONTRAINDICATIONS, ADRs, AND COMMENTS[b]
Levalbuterol *continued*		**Adolescents:** Initially, 0.63 mg/dose by nebulization three times daily, every 6–8 hr. *Maximum:* 3.78 mg/day by nebulization.	LC Plus® nebulizer and the PARI Master® or Dura Neb 2000® compressor. **Note:** Not generally available in Canada.	**Comments:** Observe for paradoxical bronchospasm. If noted, discontinue levalbuterol pharmacotherapy immediately and initiate alternative pharmacotherapy. Monitor respiratory function.
Levarterenol, *see* **Norepinephrine**				
Levomepromazine, *see* **Methotrimeprazine**				
Levonorgestrel *(Plan B®)*	**Prevention of pregnancy** following unprotected vaginal intercourse **Note:** The use of levonorgestrel does not provide protection against the transmission of sexually transmitted diseases.	**Adolescents:** Initially, 0.75 mg PO (first tablet) within 72 hr of unprotected vaginal intercourse. Follow with 0.75 mg PO (second tablet) within 12 hr of initial dose.	Tablet, oral: 0.75 mg (available in individual two-tablet foil blister packages)	**Contraindications:** Abnormal vaginal bleeding, hypersensitivity to levonorgestrel, and pregnancy. **ADRs:** Commonly causes abdominal pain, breast tenderness, dizziness, fatigue, headache, nausea, and vomiting. **Comments:** Following use, adolescent girls should be counseled either to abstain from sexual intercourse or to use a standard method of contraception until the onset of their next normal menstrual cycle (usually within 2–3 weeks). If their menstrual cycle does not resume within 4 weeks, then they should revisit their pediatric healthcare provider and a pregnancy test should be administered.
Levonorgestrel and Ethinyl Estradiol Emergency Contraceptive Combination *(Preven®)*	**Prevention of pregnancy** following unprotected vaginal intercourse **Note:** The use of levonorgestrel and ethinyl estradiol contraceptive combination does not provide protection against the transmission of sexually transmitted diseases.	**Adolescents:** Initially, 0.5 mg levonorgestrel and 0.1 mg ethinyl estradiol (total, two tablets) PO within 72 hr of unprotected vaginal intercourse. Repeat dose once 12 hr after the initial dose. **Note:** A negative pregnancy test result should be obtained prior to the administration of the initial dose.	Tablet, oral: 0.25 mg (levonorgestrel) and 0.05 mg (ethinyl estradiol)	**Contraindications:** Cerebral vascular disease, coronary artery disease, estrogen-dependent cancers, hypersensitivity to levonorgestrel or to estradiol, pregnancy, and thromboembolic disorders including deep-vein thrombosis. **ADRs:** Commonly causes nausea. May cause vomiting. **Note:** If vomiting occurs within 1 hr of ingestion, the dose should generally be repeated. Advise patient (or her parent) to notify her prescriber if vomiting occurs. **Comments:** Following use, adolescent girls should be counseled either to abstain from sexual intercourse or to use a standard method of contraception until the onset of their next normal menstrual cycle. If their menstrual cycle does not resume within 4 weeks, then they should revisit their pediatric healthcare provider and a pregnancy test should be administered.
Levothyroxine *(Eltroxin®, Levotec®,* Sodium Levothyroxine, *Synthroid®)*	Hypothyroidism	**Infants (≤3 months):** 10–15 µg/kg/day PO as a single dose. **Infants (3–6 months):** 8–10 µg/kg/day PO as a single dose. **Infants (>6 months):** 6–8 µg/kg/day PO as a single dose. **Children (<6 years):** 4–6 µg/kg/day PO as a single dose.	Tablets, oral: 12.5, 25, 50, 75, 88, 100, 112, 125, 150, 175, 200, 300 µg **Note:** All marketed products are not bioequivalent. Therefore, **patients should remain on the**	**Contraindications:** Adrenal insufficiency (uncorrected), myocardial infarction (acute), and thyrotoxicosis (untreated). **ADRs:** *See* Chapter 5. **Comments:** Adjust maintenance dosage according to response and serum T_4 and TSH concentrations. *(Continued)*

Footnotes are on page 558.

TABLE 14-1 continued

DRUG (TRADE AND OTHER NAMES)	INDICATION(S)	USUAL PEDIATRIC DOSAGE AND ADMINISTRATION[a]	DOSAGE FORMS	CONTRAINDICATIONS, ADRs, AND COMMENTS[b]
Levothyroxine *continued*		**Children (≥6 years):** 3–5 μg/kg/day PO as a single dose. **Adolescents:** 2–3 μg/kg/day PO as a single dose. *Maximum:* 400 μg/day PO. **Note:** Administer on an empty stomach to increase GI absorption.	same product once stabilized.	
Lidocaine (Lignocaine, Xylocaine®, Xylocard®)	**Ventricular tachycardia/ Ventricular fibrillation** **Note:** These disorders generally are initially treated by means of cardioversion. **Note:** Not approved by the FDA or HPB for infants or children.	**Children and adolescents:** 1 mg/kg by endotracheal tube instillation **or** IV over at least 2 min. May repeat once, as indicated by response, and then follow by 10–50 μg/kg/min IV. *Maximum:* Total cumulative initial dose, 300 mg **or** 4.5 mg/kg IV, whichever is less. **Note:** May need to reduce dosage for pediatric patients who have congestive heart failure or hepatic dysfunction.	Injectables, IV: 10, 20 mg/ml **Note:** Higher dosage formulations (e.g., 100, 200 mg/ml) are available but are **only** to be used for the preparation of IV infusion solutions.	**Contraindications:** Adams-Stokes syndrome, AV block, hypersensitivity to lidocaine or to other amide-type local anesthetics, and intraventricular block. **ADRs:** *See* Chapter 5. **Comments:** Therapeutic drug monitoring is recommended; *see* Table 14-3. Constant ECG monitoring is required during IV administration. Resuscitative drugs and equipment should be readily available.
Lidocaine and Prilocaine, topical *(EMLA®)*	Dermal anesthesia, local (to minimize pain during insertion of venous access device or during SC or IM injection; also to minimize pain associated with superficial surgical procedures [e.g., split thickness skin graft harvesting] on intact skin)	**Infants (≥6 months), children, and adolescents:** Apply a thick layer to proposed venipuncture, injection, or surgical site and cover with occlusive dressing provided with product **or** apply a single disk/patch to site. *Maximum:* The maximal amount to be applied to any one site is determined by patient age, dosage and formulation of cream product, size of area of application, and length of contact time at site before removal. See following.	Cream, topical: 5% (lidocaine 25 mg and prilocaine 25 mg as a 1:1 oil/water emulsion; supplied in a 5-gram tube with two occlusive dressings (6 cm × 7 cm *[Tegaderm®]*). Disk/Patch, topical: 1 gram (as a single-dose unit containing 500 mg of lidocaine and 500 mg of prilocaine as a 1:1 oil/water emulsion) **Note:** The entire surface area of the disk/patch is ~40 cm^2; however, active contact surface area is ~10 cm^2.	**Contraindications:** Application sites (e.g., external ear canal, scalp vein sites) that would allow lidocaine and prilocaine to enter the middle ear; hypersensitivity to lidocaine, prilocaine, or other amide-type local anesthetics; infants <6 months; infants 6–12 months who are concurrently receiving methemoglobin-inducing drugs (e.g., sulfonamides); and methemoglobinemia, congenital or idiopathic. **ADRs:** Generally well tolerated. May cause local allergic reactions at the site of application (e.g., abnormal sensation, edema, and erythema) and systemic allergic reactions (e.g., angioedema, bronchospasm, and urticaria). **Comments:** In Canada, the HPB has approved *EMLA* for application directly on the genital mucosa and on leg ulcers. However, published pediatric data regarding therapeutic effects are limited. In addition, several studies have suggested an increased risk for systemic absorption and resultant lidocaine and prilocaine toxicity.

Maximal dosage, cream:

AGE	DOSAGE	SURFACE AREA	TIME
6–12 months	2 grams	20 cm^2	4 hr
1–6 years	10 grams	100 cm^2	4 hr
7–12 years	20 grams	200 cm^2	4 hr
≥ 13 years	40 grams	400 cm^2	4 hr

Maximum, disk/patch: **Infants (≥6 months) and children (≤6 years),** one disk/patch; **children (>6 years) and adolescents,** two disks/patches (applied concurrently at two different skin sites).
Note: The cream or disk/patch should remain in place for 1 hr before the planned venipuncture procedure or injection and at least 2 hr before the planned surgical procedure.
Note: *See* Chapter 1 for more detailed discussion of the application and removal of lidocaine and prilocaine occlusive dressings and disks/patches.

TABLE 14-1 continued

DRUG (TRADE AND OTHER NAMES)	INDICATION(S)	USUAL PEDIATRIC DOSAGE AND ADMINISTRATION[a]	DOSAGE FORMS	CONTRAINDICATIONS, ADRs, AND COMMENTS[b]
Lignocaine, *see* Lidocaine				
Lindane (Gamma Benzene Hexachloride, G-well®, Hexit®)	Infestations with crab lice *(Phthirus pubis)*, head lice *(Pediculus humanus capitis)*, scabies *(Sarcoptes scabiei)*, and their nits (eggs)	**Infants, children, and adolescents,** *cream or lotion:* Apply a sufficient amount to thoroughly cover, in a **thin** coat, affected areas. Allow to remain in contact for 8–12 hr, then bathe or shower thoroughly, washing all areas of application. Remaining lice nit shells can be removed with a nit comb, tweezers, or the fingers. Treatment may be repeated once in 4–7 days, if indicated. *Maximum:* **Infants and children (<6 years),** 1 ounce/treatment; **children (≥6 years) and adolescents,** 2 ounces/treatment. **Infants, children, and adolescents,** *Shampoo:* Apply sufficient shampoo (generally 15–60 ml) to dry hair to thoroughly saturate. Work into affected area for 4–5 min; then add a little water at a time to form a thick lather. Continue shampooing for an additional 4–5 min. Rinse thoroughly and briskly towel dry. Remaining nit shells can be removed with a nit comb, tweezers, or the fingers. Treatment may be repeated once in 7 days, if indicated. *Maximum:* **Infants and children (<6 years),** 1 ounce/treatment; **children (≥6 years) and adolescents,** 2 ounces/treatment. **Note:** Children should not be allowed to apply this drug without direct adult supervision.	Cream, topical: 1% Lotion, topical: 1%, shake well before use. Shampoo, topical: 1%; shake well before use. **Note:** All lindane topical formulations are for external use only. Avoid contact with eyes, mucous membranes, and urethral meatus (if contact occurs, rinse thoroughly with warm water). For eyelash infestation, apply white petrolatum.	**Contraindications:** Hypersensitivity to lindane and seizure disorders. Not to be used for the treatment of Norwegian (crusted) scabies because of possible increased absorption. **ADRs:** Ensure that all clothes and bedding have been thoroughly washed in hot water or dry cleaned and that the patient puts on clean clothes after treatment. Assess and treat, as required, all household or sexual contacts. May cause contact dermatitis, pruritus, or rash. **Comments:** Because of the potential for systematic absorption and resultant, although rare, toxicity (e.g., aplastic anemia, hematuria, seizures), the use of permethrin may be preferred for infants and young children, pediatric patients with pre-existing seizure disorders, and patients with severely excoriated skin or underlying skin disorders. Young children should be assisted when rinsing off the shampoo. Rubber pants or elasticized diapers may increase drug absorption by forming an occlusive barrier and, thus, should not be worn by infants while lindane is on the skin. Care should be taken to prevent oral ingestion of lindane by infants or children through thumbsucking or mouthing.
Linezolid (Zyvox®, Zyvoxam®)	Infections caused by susceptible organisms (generally restricted to complicated infections of the skin and related structures, community-acquired pneumonia, nosocomial pneumonia, and vancomycin-resistant *Enterococcus faecium* infections) **Note:** Ensure that appropriate culture and sensitivity tests are performed and that the organism is sensitive to linezolid. **Note:** Not approved by the FDA or HPB for children or adolescents.	**Children:** Although dosage recommendations are the same, recommendations for the duration of therapy vary in regard to the infection being treated, as follows. *Community-acquired pneumonia, nosocomial pneumonia, and complicated infections of the skin and related structures:* 2 mg/kg/day IV or PO in two divided doses, every 12 hr, for 10–14 days. *Vancomycin-resistant* Enterococcus faecium *infections:* 2 mg/kg/day IV or PO in two divided doses, every 12 hr, for 14–28 days. **Adolescents:** Although dosage recommendations are the same, recommendations for the duration of therapy vary in regard to the infection being treated, as follows.	Injectable, IV: 2 mg/ml (available in 100-, 200-, and 300-ml single-use plastic IV infusion bags) Tablets, oral: 400, 600 mg Suspension, oral: 100 mg/5 ml (after reconstitution) (orange flavored, contains aspartame) **Note:** Gently mix reconstituted suspension by inverting the bottle several times. Do not shake. **Note:** Store protected from light at controlled room temperature. **Note:** Injectable is for IV use only; infuse over 30–120 min.	**Contraindications:** Hypersensitivity to linezolid. **ADRs:** May cause abnormal results on liver function tests, diarrhea (including pseudomembranous colitis), headache, insomnia, myelosuppression, nausea, oral candidiasis, thrombocytopenia, tongue discoloration, and vomiting. **Comments:** Linezolid is a reversible nonselective inhibitor of monoamine oxidase. Therefore, it has the potential to interact with a variety of drugs, including adrenergic and serotonergic drugs. *See* Chapter 6. **Note:** Weekly complete blood counts are recommended.

(Continued)

Footnotes are on page 558.

TABLE 14-1 continued

DRUG (TRADE AND OTHER NAMES)	INDICATION(S)	USUAL PEDIATRIC DOSAGE AND ADMINISTRATION[a]	DOSAGE FORMS	CONTRAINDICATIONS, ADRs, AND COMMENTS[b]
Linezolid *continued*		*Community-acquired pneumonia, nosocomial pneumonia, and complicated infections of the skin and related structures:* 1200 mg/day PO in two divided doses, every 12 hr, for 10–14 days. *Vancomycin-resistant Enterococcus faecium infections:* 1200 mg/day PO in two divided doses, every 12 hr, for 14–28 days.		
Lisinopril *(Prinivil®, Zestril®)*	**Hypertension, essential** **Note:** Lisinopril pharmacotherapy is used alone or in combination with a thiazide diuretic. Severe hypertension usually requires combination pharmacotherapy. **Note:** Not approved for this indication by the FDA or HPB for children or adolescents.	**Adolescents:** Initially, 5 mg/day PO as a single dose. Increase dosage gradually according to response. *Maximum:* 40 mg/day PO. **Note:** Reduce dosage for pediatric patients who have renal dysfunction; see Table 14-2.	Tablets, oral: 2.5, 5, 10, 20, 30, 40 mg	**Contraindications:** Angioedema, angioneurotic edema (history), bilateral stenosis of the renal arteries, hypersensitivity to lisinopril, pregnancy, and systolic blood pressure <100 mmHg. **ADRs:** Generally well tolerated. May cause asthenia, cough, diarrhea, dizziness, fatigue, headache, hypotension, increased blood urea nitrogen, and rash. Rarely causes angioedema (0.1%, potentially fatal) and agranulocytosis. **Comments:** Monitor blood pressure and be alert for signs and symptoms of serious ADRs (agranulocytosis and angioedema). If serious ADRs are observed, discontinue lisinopril pharmacotherapy and initiate appropriate medical management. **Note:** Anaphylactic reactions, although rare, have been reported among patients receiving lisinopril, or other ACE inhibitor pharmacotherapy, and concomitant dialysis with high-flux membranes (e.g., polyacrylonitrile), hymenoptera desensitization, and low density lipoprotein apheresis with dextran sulfate.
Lithium *(Carbolith®, Eskalith CR®, Lithane®, Lithobid®)*	**Acute mania** associated with bipolar disorder and prevention of subsequent manic episodes	**Adolescents:** 30 mg/kg/day PO in three divided doses **or** initially 0.5–1.5 grams/m²/day PO in three divided doses. If necessary, increase the dosage, according to response, by 300 mg/dose to 60 mg/kg/day PO in three divided doses. **Note:** Adjust dosage according to daily lithium serum concentration and response.	Capsules, oral: 150, 300, 600 mg Liquid, oral: 8 mEq/5 ml (8 mEq of lithium is equivalent to 300 mg of lithium carbonate) Syrup, oral: 300 mg/5 ml (contains 0.3% alcohol) Tablets, oral extended release *(Eskalith CR, Lithobid):* 300, 450 mg Tablet, oral: 300 mg **Note:** 150 mg = 4 mEq.	**Contraindications:** Brain damage; breast feeding; cardiovascular dysfunction; dehydration; diuretic pharmacotherapy (concurrent); pregnancy; renal dysfunction; and sodium depletion, including that associated with severe debilitation, dehydration, diuretic pharmacotherapy, and medical disorders that require sodium restriction (e.g., congestive heart failure; hypertension). **ADRs:** Monitor lithium serum concentrations regularly, and maintain levels below 1.5 mmol/liter (1.5 mEq/liter) to avoid toxicity. Initially, lithium pharmacotherapy is frequently associated with GI irritation, muscle weakness, nausea, and vertigo. These ADRs usually resolve when therapy has been stabilized. Lithium has been associated with fatigue, nephrogenic diabetes insipidus, and signs and symptoms

CHAPTER 14: DRUG DOSING FOR INFANTS, CHILDREN, AND ADOLESCENTS

TABLE 14-1 *continued*

DRUG (*TRADE* AND OTHER NAMES)	INDICATION(S)	USUAL PEDIATRIC DOSAGE AND ADMINISTRATION[a]	DOSAGE FORMS	CONTRAINDICATIONS, ADRs, AND COMMENTS[b]
Lithium *continued*				of renal dysfunction (e.g., polyuria, polydipsia). Mild-to-moderate ADRs may occur at lithium serum concentrations of 1.5–2 mmol/liter (1.5–2 mEq/liter). *See* Chapter 5. Monitor thyroid function periodically as indicated. **Comments:** Therapeutic drug monitoring is recommended; *see* Table 14-3.
Lodoxamide (*Alomide®*)	Vernal conjunctivitis/Vernal keratitis/Vernal keratoconjunctivitis	**Children (>2 years):** Instill one or two drops in each affected eye four times daily for up to 3 months.	Solution, ophthalmic: 0.1% **Note:** For ophthalmic use only. **Note:** In order to minimize cross-infection whenever both eyes require lodoxamide ophthalmic pharmacotherapy, ensure that separate containers are dispensed for each eye.	**Contraindications:** Hypersensitivity to lodoxamide. **ADRs:** Generally well tolerated. Commonly causes local transient burning and stinging upon ophthalmic instillation. **Comments:** Several continuous days of use may be required before noticeable improvement is observed.
Lomustine, *see* Chapter 12				
Loperamide (*Imodium®, Loperacap®*)	Diarrhea **Note:** Not approved by the FDA or HPB for infants or children (<2 years).	**Infants and children (<2 years):** 0.25–0.5 mg/dose PO three times daily or as needed according to response. **Children (2–5 years):** 1 mg/dose PO three times daily or as needed according to response. **Children (>5 years) and adolescents:** 2 mg/dose PO two or three times daily or as needed according to response. *Maximum:* 2 mg/dose PO and 16 mg/day PO. **Note:** Following the first day of therapy, administer 0.1 mg/kg/dose only after loose stool is produced.	Caplet, oral: 2 mg Capsule, oral: 2 mg Solution, oral: 0.2 mg/ml Tablet, oral quick dissolve: 2 mg **Note:** Oral quick-dissolve tablets contain phenylalanine. **Note:** Oral quick-dissolve tablets may be administered without water. The tablet disintegrates within seconds of contact with the surface of the tongue and is simply swallowed with saliva.	**Contraindications:** Dysentery (acute), hypersensitivity to loperamide, pseudomembranous colitis (acute), and ulcerative colitis (acute). **ADRs:** Generally well tolerated. May cause constipation.
Loracarbef (*Lorabid®*)	Mild-to-moderate bacterial infections caused by susceptible organisms **Note:** Ensure that appropriate culture and sensitivity tests are performed and that the organism is sensitive to loracarbef.	**Infants (≥6 months) and children:** Recommendations for dosages and duration of therapy vary in regard to the infection being treated, as follows. *Impetigo:* 30 mg/kg/day PO in two divided doses, every 12 hr, for 7 days. *Maxillary sinusitis (acute)/Otitis media (acute):* 60 mg/kg/day PO in two divided doses, every 12 hr, for 10 days. **Note:** See "Comments." *Pharyngitis/Tonsillitis:* 30 mg/kg/day PO in two divided doses, every 12 hr, for 10 days. **Note:** Administer PO on an empty stomach, 1 hr before or 2 hr after meals, for maximal absorption. **Adolescents:** Recommended dosages and duration of therapy vary in regard to the infection being treated, as follows.	Capsules, oral: 200, 400 mg Suspensions, oral: 100 mg/5 ml, 200 mg/5 ml (after reconstitution; strawberry bubble gum flavored); shake well before use. **Note:** Store at controlled room temperature between 15 and 30°C. **Note:** Appropriately and safely discard any unused oral suspension after 14 days. **Note:** Not generally available in Canada.	**Contraindications:** Hypersensitivity to loracarbef, cephalosporins, or penicillins. **ADRs:** Generally well tolerated. May cause allergic reactions, anorexia, diarrhea, headache, nausea, rash, rhinitis, somnolence, and vomiting. **Comments:** It is generally recommended that the oral suspension be used for the treatment of acute otitis media among infants and children because it has been studied more in regard to the treatment of this type of infection in the pediatric age group and, when compared to the pharmacokinetics of the loracarbef oral capsules, the suspension reaches peak serum concentrations earlier and at a higher level.

(Continued)

Footnotes are on page 558.

TABLE 14-1 continued

DRUG (TRADE AND OTHER NAMES)	INDICATION(S)	USUAL PEDIATRIC DOSAGE AND ADMINISTRATION[a]	DOSAGE FORMS	CONTRAINDICATIONS, ADRs, AND COMMENTS[b]
Loracarbef *continued*		*Acute bronchitis, secondary bacterial infection:* 800 mg/day PO in two divided doses, every 12 hr, for 7 days. *Chronic bronchitis, acute bacterial exacerbation:* 400–800 mg/day PO in two divided doses, every 12 hr, for 7 days. *Cystitis, uncomplicated/Skin infections, uncomplicated:* 400 mg/day PO in two divided doses, every 12 hr, for 7 days. *Pharyngitis/Tonsillitis:* 400 mg/day PO in two divided doses, every 12 hr, for 10 days. *Pneumonia/Pyelonephritis, uncomplicated:* 800 mg/day PO in two divided doses, every 12 hr, for 14 days. *Sinusitis:* 800 mg/day PO in two divided doses, every 12 hr, for 10 days. **Note:** Administer on an empty stomach, 1 hr before or 2 hr after meals, for maximal absorption. **Note:** Reduce dosage for pediatric patients who have renal dysfunction; *see* Table 14-2.		
Loratadine *(Claritin®)*	Allergic rhinitis/ Chronic idiopathic urticaria	**Children (≥2 years and <30 kg):** 5 mg PO once daily. **Children (≥2 years and >30 kg) and adolescents:** 10 mg PO once daily. *Maximum:* 10 mg/day PO. **Note:** Reduce dosage for pediatric patients who have hepatic or renal dysfunction; *see* Table 14-2.	Syrup, oral: 5 mg/5 ml (peach flavored) Tablet, oral: 10 mg Tablet, oral rapid dissolve *(Claritin Reditabs®):* 10 mg (mint flavored) **Note:** Rapid-dissolve tablets may be administered without water. The tablet disintegrates within seconds of contact with the surface of the tongue and is simply swallowed with saliva.	**Contraindications:** Hypersensitivity to loratadine. **ADRs:** Generally well tolerated. May cause dry mouth, fatigue, headache, hyperkinesia, nausea, nervousness, rash, and sedation.
Lorazepam *(Ativan®, Novo-Lorazem®, Nu-Loraz®)*	Status epilepticus **Note:** Not approved by the FDA or HPB for infants or children.	**Children and adolescents:** 0.05 mg/kg/dose IV. May repeat dose once after 5 min, if required, to manage seizures. **Note:** IV infusion rate should **not** exceed 2 mg/min. *Maximum:* 4 mg/dose **and** 8 mg/12 hr period IV. **Note:** Reduce dosage for pediatric patients who have hepatic dysfunction.	Injectables, IV: 2, 4 mg/ml; contain benzyl alcohol, polyethylene glycol, and propylene glycol. **Note:** Other dosage formulations (e.g., sublingual tablets) are available but are not appropriate for the management of status epilepticus.	**Contraindications:** Hypersensitivity to lorazepam or other benzodiazepines. **ADRs:** May cause agitation, confusion, depression, disorientation, dizziness, drowsiness, fatigue, lethargy, leukopenia (rare), skin rash, sleep disturbance, and weakness. *See* Chapter 5. **Comments:** Monitor for respiratory depression.
Mafenide *(Sulfamylon®)*	**Burns,** second and third degree (topical antibacterial therapy as an adjunct to other pharmacotherapy)	**Infants (≥3 months), children, and adolescents:** Apply **cream** once or twice daily over the entire burn site after the site has been appropriately cleansed and debrided. A sterile gloved hand may be used to apply the cream evenly to a thickness of 1/16th inch.	Cream, topical: 8.5%; contains sodium metabisulfite. Solution, topical: 5% after reconstitution with sterile water for injection or sterile 0.9% sodium chloride irrigation solution.	**Contraindications:** Hypersensitivity to mafenide. **ADRs:** Generally well tolerated. May cause local reactions (e.g., burning sensation, erythema, itching, rash) at the site of application. Systemic absorption may result in metabolic or respiratory acidosis and hyperventilation.

TABLE 14-1 *continued*

DRUG (*TRADE* AND OTHER NAMES)	INDICATION(S)	USUAL PEDIATRIC DOSAGE AND ADMINISTRATION[a]	DOSAGE FORMS	CONTRAINDICATIONS, ADRs, AND COMMENTS[b]
Mafenide *continued*		**Note:** The burn site should be covered with cream at all times, except for daily cleansing and debriding of site, until healing is progressing well or the site is ready for skin grafts. **Infants (≥3 months), children, and adolescents:** Apply **solution** to burn or grafted site by first covering the site, using sterile technique, with one layer of fine mesh gauze. Cut an eight-ply burn dressing to the size of the burn or graft site and saturate the dressing with mafenide 5% solution using an irrigation syringe or irrigation tubing. Using the irrigation syringe, keep the gauze dressing wet by irrigating the dressing every 6–8 hr with solution. If irrigation tubing is used, the tubing should be placed over the burn dressing at the burn or graft site and then covered with another piece of eight-ply dressing. The irrigation tube dressing should be secured with a bolster dressing and wrapped appropriately to keep the dressing intact. Inject the mafenide topical solution into the tubing every 4 hr, or as needed, to keep the gauze dressing wet. Allow the burn or graft site dressing to remain undisturbed, except for bathing and irrigations for up to 5 days. Additional dressings may be required until grafts are complete. **Note:** Maceration of skin may occur from the wet dressing within 24 hr of application. Monitor skin sites carefully when dressings are removed for bathing. Mafenide is usually continued until autograft vascularization occurs and sites are healing well (usually by 5 days). **Note:** May require discontinuation if allergic reactions are noted. If acidosis occurs and becomes difficult to manage, particularly for patients who have pulmonary dysfunction, discontinue the dressing irrigations for 24–48 hr and reassess the patient for restoration of acid–base balance. Monitor sites for bacterial growth during interrupted mafenide pharmacotherapy and adjust therapy, as needed, according to response.	**Note:** Filter reconstituted solution through a 0.22-μm sterilizing-grade filter **prior** to use. The reconstituted solution can be stored at controlled room temperature between 25 and 30°C (77–86°F) and must be used within 48 hr of reconstitution. **Note:** For topical use only. **Note:** Not generally available in Canada.	**Comments:** Fatal hemolytic anemia with disseminated intravascular coagulation has been associated with the use of topical mafenide for a patient with glucose-6-phosphate dehydrogenase deficiency.

Footnotes are on page 558.

TABLE 14-1 continued

DRUG (TRADE AND OTHER NAMES)	INDICATION(S)	USUAL PEDIATRIC DOSAGE AND ADMINISTRATION[a]	DOSAGE FORMS	CONTRAINDICATIONS, ADRs, AND COMMENTS[b]
Magnesium Citrate (Citrate of Magnesia, Citro-Mag®, Evac-Q-Mag®)	Bowel preparation	**Children and adolescents:** 4 ml/kg/dose PO as a one-time dose. *Maximum:* 296 ml/dose.	Solution, oral: 5%	**Contraindications:** Hypermagnesemia and renal failure. **ADRs:** Generally well tolerated. See Chapter 5. **Comments:** Use with caution for pediatric patients who have renal dysfunction.
Magnesium Hydroxide (Milk of Magnesia, M.O.M.®)	Constipation	**Children and adolescents:** 0.5 ml/kg/dose PO as a one-time dose. *Maximum:* 60 ml/dose.	Suspensions, oral: 7%–8.5%; shake well before use. Tablets, oral: 300, 600 mg	**Contraindications:** Hypermagnesemia and renal failure. **ADRs:** Generally well tolerated. See Chapter 5. **Comments:** Use with caution for pediatric patients with renal dysfunction.
Magnesium Sulfate (Epsom Salt)	Hypomagnesemia **Note:** Not approved for this indication by the FDA or HPB for infants or children.	**Children and adolescents:** 2–5 grams IV according to response and magnesium serum concentration. Infuse over 3 hr.	Injectables, IM, IV: 10%, 12.5%, 25%, 50% (0.8, 1, 2, 4 mEq/ml)	**Contraindications:** Heart block, hypermagnesemia, myocardial damage, and renal failure. **ADRs:** May cause CNS depression, hypermagnesemia, hypotension, and respiratory depression. **Comments:** Use with caution for pediatric patients who have renal impairment. Maintain adequate urine output, and monitor magnesium serum concentration.
	Control of seizures associated with acute nephritis, eclampsia, or pre-eclampsia	**Children and adolescents:** 2–5 grams IV or 20–40 mg/kg IM. Adjust dosage according to response and magnesium serum concentrations. **Note:** IV infusion rate should not exceed 150 mg/min (1.5 ml of 10% solution/min).		
Mannitol (Osmitrol®)	Cerebral edema **Note:** Establish adequate renal function and urinary output prior to initiating therapy. See Test for oliguria.	**Children and adolescents:** 250–500 mg/kg/dose IV over 30–60 min. May increase the dose incrementally to 1 gram/kg/dose as needed, according to response. *Maximum:* 2 grams/kg/dose IV. **Test for oliguria:** 0.2 gram/kg IV over 3–10 min. *Maximum:* 1 gram/kg/dose IV.	Injectables, IV: 50, 100, 150, 200, 250 mg/ml **Osmolarity of Mannitol Solutions** % MANNITOL / mOsm/liter 5 / 275 10 / 550 15 / 825 20 / 1100 25 / 1375 **Note:** May crystallize at concentrations exceeding 20%.	**Contraindications:** Anuria, congestive heart failure (severe), dehydration (severe), intracranial bleeding (active), and pulmonary edema (severe). **ADRs:** May cause severe fluid and electrolyte imbalance. May also cause acidosis, blurred vision, dizziness, dryness of the mouth, fever, headache, tachycardia, and vomiting. **Comments:** Monitor fluid and electrolyte status, central venous pressure, and renal function during IV administration.

Measles Virus Vaccine, *see* **Chapter 9**

DRUG (TRADE AND OTHER NAMES)	INDICATION(S)	USUAL PEDIATRIC DOSAGE AND ADMINISTRATION	DOSAGE FORMS	CONTRAINDICATIONS, ADRs, AND COMMENTS
Mebendazole (Vermox®)	Enterobiasis (pinworm infestation)	**Children and adolescents:** 100 mg PO as a single dose. Repeat dose in 2 weeks.	Tablet, oral chewable: 100 mg **Note:** Chewable tablets may be chewed or crushed; crushed tablets may be mixed with food for ingestion.	**Contraindications:** Hypersensitivity to mebendazole. **ADRs:** Generally well tolerated. May cause transient abdominal pain and diarrhea.
	Ascariasis (roundworm infestation)/ Hookworm infestation	**Children and adolescents:** 200 mg/day PO in two divided doses for 3 days.		

Mechlorethamine, *see* **Chapter 12**

DRUG (TRADE AND OTHER NAMES)	INDICATION(S)	USUAL PEDIATRIC DOSAGE AND ADMINISTRATION	DOSAGE FORMS	CONTRAINDICATIONS, ADRs, AND COMMENTS
Meclizine (Antivert®, Bonamine®, Bonine®, Dizmiss®, Dramamine II®)	Nausea, vomiting, and vertigo, prophylactic and symptomatic management (generally used for patients who have labyrinthitis and other vestibular disturbances, Meniere's	**Children and adolescents:** See accompanying table.	Tablet, oral scored: 25 mg (raspberry flavored) **Note:** May be chewed, swallowed whole, or allowed to dissolve in the mouth before swallowing.	**Contraindications:** Hypersensitivity to meclizine. **ADRs:** May cause blurred vision, drowsiness, dry mouth, fatigue, and vomiting. Some children may display hyperexcitability.

TABLE 14-1 continued

DRUG (TRADE AND OTHER NAMES)	INDICATION(S)	USUAL PEDIATRIC DOSAGE AND ADMINISTRATION[a]	DOSAGE FORMS	CONTRAINDICATIONS, ADRs, AND COMMENTS[b]
Meclizine continued	syndrome, motion sickness, or radiation sickness)			

Meclizine Dosing Recommendations

INDICATION	CHILDREN	ADOLESCENTS
Labyrinthitis and other vestibular disturbances	12.5–50 mg/day PO in two divided doses, as indicated by response.	25–100 mg/day PO in two divided doses, as indicated by response.
Meniere's syndrome	12.5–50 mg/day PO in two divided doses, as indicated by response.	25–100 mg/day PO in two divided doses, as indicated by response.
Motion sickness	12.5–25 mg/day PO as a single dose. **Note:** For motion sickness associated with vehicular travel, administer initial dose 1 hr before departure and repeat once every 24 hr, as indicated by response.	25–50 mg/day PO as a single dose. **Note:** For motion sickness associated with vehicular travel, administer initial dose 1 hr before departure and repeat once every 24 hr, as indicated by response.
Radiation sickness	25 mg PO as a single dose 2–12 hr before each scheduled radiation treatment.	50 mg PO as a single dose 2–12 hr before each scheduled radiation treatment.

Medium Chain Triglyceride Oil, see Chapter 13

DRUG (TRADE AND OTHER NAMES)	INDICATION(S)	USUAL PEDIATRIC DOSAGE AND ADMINISTRATION[a]	DOSAGE FORMS	CONTRAINDICATIONS, ADRs, AND COMMENTS[b]
Medrysone (HMS®)	Allergic conjunctivitis/ Episcleritis/ Vernal conjunctivitis **Note:** Not approved by the FDA for children. **Note:** Not indicated for the treatment of iritis or uveitis.	**Children and adolescents:** Instill one drop of suspension into affected eye(s). Repeat up to every 4 hr, as indicated by response.	Suspension, ophthalmic: 1%; shake well before use. **Note:** For ophthalmic use only. **Note:** Not generally available in Canada. **Note:** In order to minimize cross-infection whenever both eyes require medrysone ophthalmic pharmacotherapy, ensure that separate containers are dispensed for each eye.	**Contraindications:** Dendrite keratitis, eye infections, and hypersensitivity to medrysone. **ADRs:** May cause cataracts, delayed ocular wound healing, exacerbation of ocular infections, glaucoma, local irritation of the eye, loss of visual acuity, and secondary ocular infections. **Comments:** See Chapter 1 for details regarding the administration of ophthalmic drugs.
Mefloquine (Lariam®)	Malaria prophylaxis against *Plasmodium falciparum* (including chloroquine-resistant strains) and *P. vivax*	**Infants (≥3 months and ≥5 kg) and children (≤20 kg):** 62.5 mg (1/4 tablet PO) once weekly, beginning 1 week before traveling and continuing during travel and for 4 weeks after leaving the endemic area. **Children (21–30 kg):** 125 mg (1/2 tablet) PO once weekly, beginning 1 week before traveling and continuing during travel and for 4 weeks after leaving the endemic area. **Children and adolescents (31–45 kg):** 187.5 mg (3/4 tablet) PO once weekly beginning 1 week before traveling and continuing during travel and for 4 weeks after leaving the endemic area. **Children and adolescents (>45 kg):** 250 mg (one tablet)	Tablet, oral: 250 mg **Note:** Tablets are cross-scored on both sides to facilitate breaking. Each dose of the mefloquine oral tablets may be crushed and suspended in a small amount of water, milk, or other beverage for ingestion.	**Contraindications:** Hypersensitivity to mefloquine and to related drugs (e.g., chloroquine, quinidine, quinine). **ADRs:** May cause abdominal pain, diarrhea, dizziness, headache, nausea, and vomiting. Incidence of ADRs is generally higher in children than adults. **Comments:** Periodic assessment of hepatic function is recommended during prolonged prophylactic therapy. **Note:** When mefloquine pharmacotherapy is administered for the treatment of severe acute malaria following an initial short-term course of intravenous quinine pharmacotherapy (*see* Quinine), an adverse drug interaction may occur, possibly resulting in significant prolongation of the QTc interval. This potential

(Continued)

Footnotes are on page 558.

TABLE 14-1 *continued*

DRUG (*TRADE* AND OTHER NAMES)	INDICATION(S)	USUAL PEDIATRIC DOSAGE AND ADMINISTRATION[a]	DOSAGE FORMS	CONTRAINDICATIONS, ADRs, AND COMMENTS[b]
Mefloquine *continued*		PO once weekly beginning 1 week before traveling and continuing during travel and for 4 weeks after leaving the endemic area.		adverse drug interaction can be prevented or minimized by delaying the administration of the first dose of mefloquine for at least 12 hr following the last dose of quinine.
	Malaria treatment, *P. falciparum* (including chloroquine-resistant strains) and *P. vivax* **Note:** Treatment of *P. vivax* malaria generally requires subsequent treatment with primaquine.	**Infants (≥3 months and ≥5 kg) and children and adolescents (≤45 kg):** 25 mg/kg PO as a single dose. **Children and adolescents (>45 kg):** 1250 mg PO as a single dose. *Maximum:* 1500 mg/dose PO. **Note:** Vomiting has an expected incidence of >10% among pediatric patients receiving mefloquine pharmacotherapy. When it occurs <30 min after ingestion of a dose, a second full dose should be administered. If vomiting occurs 30–60 min after a dose, an additional ½ dose should be administered. **Note:** Administer with food and a minimum of 240 ml (8 ounces) of water. **Note:** May need to reduce dosage for pediatric patients who have hepatic dysfunction.		

Melphalan, *see* **Chapter 12**

Meningococcal Vaccine, *see* **Chapter 9**

| **Meperidine** (*Demerol®*, Pethidine) | **Pain, moderate to severe** | **Children and adolescents:** 1–1.5 mg/kg/dose IM, IV, PO, or SC every 3–4 hr, as needed. *Maximum:* **Children,** 2 mg/kg/dose IM, IV, or SC to a maximum of 100 mg/dose; **adolescents,** 4 mg/kg/dose IM, IV, or SC to a maximum of 150 mg/dose. **Note:** Reduce dosage for pediatric patients who have renal dysfunction; *see* Table 14-2. | Injectables, IM, IV, SC: 10, 25, 50, 75, 100 mg/ml Syrup, oral: 50 mg/5 ml (banana flavored) Tablets, oral: 50, 100 mg | **Contraindications:** Coma, hypersensitivity to meperidine, MAOI therapy (concurrent or within 14 days), porphyria, and ritonavir pharmacotherapy (*see* Chapter 6). **ADRs:** Can produce addiction and habituation similar to that associated with morphine and other opiate analgesics. May cause cardiac arrest, circulatory depression, respiratory arrest, respiratory depression, and shock. *See* "Opiate Analgesics" in Chapter 5. |
| | **Preoperative or preprocedure anxiety and agitation** | **Children and adolescents:** 1–2 mg/kg/dose IM, PO, or SC 60 min before surgery or procedure. *Maximum:* **Children,** 2 mg/kg/dose IM, PO, or SC **or** 100 mg/dose, whichever is less; **adolescents,** 4 mg/kg/dose IM, PO, or SC **or** 150 mg/dose, whichever is less. | | **Comments:** The choice of preoperative or preprocedure pharmacotherapy depends on the clinical condition of the pediatric patient, the type of anesthesia to be administered, the type of surgery or procedure to be performed, and the length of the surgery or procedure. Oral administration generally is preferred. Absorption from IM injection sites may be variable; intragluteal injection is recommended. Naloxone is an effective antagonist in cases of meperidine overdosage. |

TABLE 14-1 continued

DRUG (TRADE AND OTHER NAMES)	INDICATION(S)	USUAL PEDIATRIC DOSAGE AND ADMINISTRATION[a]	DOSAGE FORMS	CONTRAINDICATIONS, ADRs, AND COMMENTS[b]
Mephenytoin (Phenantoin)	**Seizures** refractory to management with less toxic anticonvulsants (e.g., phenobarbital, phenytoin, and primidone) **Note:** Indicated for the management of focal, Jacksonian, psychomotor, and tonic-clonic seizures and is often used in combination with other anticonvulsants.	**Children:** Initially, 50–100 mg/day PO as a single dose. Increase daily dosage by 50 or 100 mg at weekly intervals according to response. *Maintenance:* 100–400 mg/day PO in three divided doses. **Adolescents:** Initially, 50–100 mg/day PO as a single dose. Increase daily dosage by 50 or 100 mg at weekly intervals according to response. *Maintenance:* 200–600 mg/day PO in three divided doses. *Maximum:* 900 mg/day PO.	Tablet, oral: 100 mg **Note:** Not generally available in Canada.	**Contraindications:** Hypersensitivity to mephenytoin or to other hydantoins. **ADRs:** Frequently causes drowsiness. May cause potentially fatal blood dyscrasias and a variety of mucocutaneous reactions, including erythema multiforme. *See* "Hydantoins" and "Phenytoin" in Chapter 5. **Comments:** As with all anticonvulsants, abrupt discontinuation may result in status epilepticus. **Note:** It is recommended that complete blood and platelet counts be obtained prior to the initiation of therapy, 2 weeks following the initiation of pharmacotherapy, and 2 weeks following the initiation of maintenance therapy. Blood and platelet counts should then be obtained every month for 1 year and then once every 3 months for the duration of therapy.
Mephobarbital (Methylphenobarbital)	**Sedation** **Note:** Benzodiazepine pharmacotherapy is generally preferred over mephobarbital or other barbiturate pharmacotherapy for this indication.	**Children:** 16–32 mg/dose PO. Initial dose may be repeated three or four times daily, as indicated by response. **Adolescents:** 32–100 mg/dose PO. Initial dose may be repeated three or four times daily, as indicated by response.	Tablets, oral: 32, 50, 100 mg **Note:** Not generally available in Canada.	**Contraindications:** Hypersensitivity to mephobarbital or to other barbiturates, blood dyscrasias, bronchopneumonia, nephritis, porphyria, pulmonary insufficiency, and renal insufficiency. **ADRs:** *See* "Barbiturates" in Chapter 5. **Comments:** Approximately 75% of mephobarbital is converted in the liver to phenobarbital. *See also* "Phenobarbital."
Meprobamate (Equanil®, Meprospan®, Miltown®, Novo-Mepro®)	**Anxiety disorders** **Note:** The benzodiazepines, because of their higher therapeutic index, are generally considered to be the drugs of first choice for anxiety disorders.	**Children (≥6 years):** 25 mg/kg/day PO in two or three divided doses **or** 200–600 mg/day PO in two or three divided doses **or** 400 mg extended-release capsules/day PO in two divided doses (in the morning and 30 min before bedtime). *Maximum:* 800 mg/day PO. **Adolescents:** 1200–1600 mg/day PO in three or four divided doses. *Maximum:* 2400 mg/day PO.	Capsules, oral extended release *(Meprospan):* 200, 400 mg Tablets, oral: 200, 400, 600 mg	**Contraindications:** Breast feeding (meprobamate breast milk concentration is 2–4 times that of the maternal blood concentration), hypersensitivity to meprobamate or related drugs (e.g., carisoprodol [Soma®]), and porphyria (acute intermittent). **ADRs:** May cause addiction and habituation. May cause hypersensitivity or idiosyncratic reactions (mild or severe) between the first and fourth doses. Other ADRs include adenopathy, ecchymosis eosinophilia, fever, fixed drug eruptions, leukopenia, nonthrombocytopenic purpura, peripheral edema, and petechia. *See* Chapter 5. **Note:** Monitor patients for TPMT genotype because standard doses can be **fatal** for TPMT-deficient patients (*see* Chapter 11).

Mercaptopurine, *see* **Chapter 12**

Footnotes are on page 558.

TABLE 14-1 continued

DRUG (TRADE AND OTHER NAMES)	INDICATION(S)	USUAL PEDIATRIC DOSAGE AND ADMINISTRATION[a]	DOSAGE FORMS	CONTRAINDICATIONS, ADRs, AND COMMENTS[b]
Meropenem (Merrem®)	**Infections** caused by susceptible organisms **Note:** Ensure that appropriate culture and sensitivity tests are performed and that the organism is sensitive to meropenem.	Pediatric dosage is determined by indication, age, and body weight of patient. *See* following table. **Note:** May be administered as either a rapid IV injection (5–20 ml) over 3–5 min or as an intermittent IV infusion over 15–30 min. **Note:** Reduce dosage for pediatric patients who have renal dysfunction; *see* Table 14-2.	Injectable, IV (powder for reconstitution): 50 mg/ml, after reconstitution with sterile water for injection. **Note:** For IV use only. After reconstitution, stable for up to 2 hr at controlled room temperature (between 15 and 30°C) and up to 12 hr under refrigeration (4°C).	**Contraindications:** Hypersensitivity to cephalosporins, meropenem, or penicillins and pseudomembranous colitis. **ADRs:** Generally well tolerated. May cause local reactions at the IV injection site (e.g., edema, inflammation, pain). May also cause systemic ADRs, including agitation, candidiasis, diarrhea, fever, headache, increased platelets, nausea, pruritus, rash, taste distortion, and urticaria. Rarely causes erythema multiforme.

Recommended Pediatric Meropenem Dosage

INFECTION	INFANTS (≥3 months) AND CHILDREN (≤ 50 kg) (*Maximum:* 1.5 grams/day IV)	CHILDREN (>50 kg) AND ADOLESCENTS (*Maximum:* 6 grams/day IV)
Gynecologic infections/Pelvic inflammatory disease	Data are unavailable.	1500 mg/day IV in three divided doses, every 8 hr.
Intra-abdominal infection (complicated)	60 mg/kg/day IV in three divided doses, every 8 hr.	3000 mg/day IV in three divided doses, every 8 hr.
Meningitis	120 mg/kg/day IV in three divided doses, every 8 hr.	6000 mg/day IV in three divided doses, every 8 hr.
Pneumonia, community acquired/ Infections of skin and skin structures (uncomplicated)	30–60 mg/kg/day IV in three divided doses, every 8 hr.	1500 mg/day IV in three divided doses, every 8 hr.
Pneumonia, nosocomial/Septicemia	Data are unavailable.	3000 mg/day IV in three divided doses, every 8 hr.
Urinary tract infections (complicated)	30 mg/kg/day IV in three divided doses, every 8 hr.	1500 mg/day IV in three divided doses, every 8 hr.

DRUG (TRADE AND OTHER NAMES)	INDICATION(S)	USUAL PEDIATRIC DOSAGE AND ADMINISTRATION[a]	DOSAGE FORMS	CONTRAINDICATIONS, ADRs, AND COMMENTS[b]
Mesalamine (5-Aminosalicylic Acid, *Asacol®, Mesasal®, Pentasa®, Rowasa®*)	**Ulcerative colitis,** mild to moderate (symptomatic management of acute phase and prevention of relapse) **Distal ulcerative colitis,** mild to moderate **Colitis/Proctitis/ Proctosigmoiditis**	**Children (≥2 years):** 500–1500 mg/day PO in one to three divided doses (500-mg tablet/dose). **Note:** Symptomatic relief generally occurs within 3–21 days of continuous therapy. **Adolescents:** 1000 mg (four extended-release capsules)/day PO in four divided doses. **Adolescents:** 4000 mg (60 ml)/day rectal as a single dose at bedtime. **Note:** Enema should be retained for ~8 hr. *See* Chapter 1 for discussion of the administration of rectal enemas.	Capsule, oral extended release: 250 mg Suspension, rectal enema: 4-grams/60-ml unit; shake well before use. Tablet, oral enteric coated: 500 mg **Note:** Mesalamine rectal enema suspension contains sodium metabisulfite. Sulfites have been associated with hypersensitivity reactions among susceptible patients. Although uncommon, they appear to occur with a higher incidence among pediatric patients who have asthma.	**Contraindications:** Duodenal ulcers, gastric ulcers, hemorrhagic diathesis, hepatic or renal impairment (severe), hypersensitivity to mesalamine or to salicylates, infants and children <2 years, pregnancy (last trimester), and urinary tract obstruction. **ADRs:** Generally well tolerated. May cause abdominal pain, diarrhea, headache, nausea, pruritus, and rash. **Comments:** Periodic urinalysis should be performed when long-term therapy is required. Mesalamine pharmacotherapy should be guided by clinical response and sigmoidoscopic findings. Abrupt discontinuation should be avoided.
Mesna, *see* Chapter 12				
Mesoridazine (Serentil®)	**Schizophrenia and other psychotic disorders** (unresponsive to other antipsychotics)	**Adolescents:** 75–400 mg/day PO in three or four divided doses **or** 25–200 mg/day IM. *Maximum:* 400 mg/day PO; 200 mg/day IM.	Concentrate, oral: 25 mg/ml; contains 0.61% alcohol (supplied with calibrated dropper) Injectable, IM: 25 mg/ml (ampule) Tablets, oral: 10, 25, 50, 100 mg	**Contraindications:** Blood dyscrasias, bone marrow depression, cardiovascular disorders, CNS depression (severe), coma, concurrent use of other drugs that prolong the QT interval (*see* Chapter 6), hepatic disease (severe), hypersensitivity to mesoridazine or

TABLE 14-1 continued

DRUG (TRADE AND OTHER NAMES)	INDICATION(S)	USUAL PEDIATRIC DOSAGE AND ADMINISTRATION[a]	DOSAGE FORMS	CONTRAINDICATIONS, ADRs, AND COMMENTS[b]
Mesoridazine *continued*			**Note:** Injectable formulation not available in Canada.	other phenothiazines, hypertension (severe), and hypotension (severe). **ADRs:** Anticholinergic effects (e.g., blurred vision, decreased GI motility, dry mouth, tachycardia, urinary retention), particularly when initiated or with high doses, drowsiness, QT interval prolongation, and sedation. *See* "Phenothiazines" in Chapter 5. **Note:** Baseline ECG and serum potassium are recommended **prior** to the initiation of mesoridazine pharmacotherapy.
Mesuximide, *see* **Methsuximide**				
Metaproterenol (*Alupent*®, Orciprenaline)	Asthma	**Children (≥6 years) and adolescents:** 1.2–1.6 mg/kg/day PO in three or four divided doses **or** 0.01–0.02 ml/kg of 5% inhalation solution diluted to 2–3 ml with normal saline for inhalation by hand-bulb nebulizer every 4–6 hr **or** 1.3–2 mg/dose (two or three actuations) by metered-dose inhaler every 3–4 hr, as needed, according to response. *Maximum:* 0.2 ml/dose (5% inhalation solution); 80 mg/day PO; 7.8 mg/day (12 actuations) metered-dose inhaler. **Note:** For maximal effect, wait at least 2 min before administering each additional metered-dose inhaler dose.	Solution, metered-dose inhaler: 0.65 mg/actuation Solution, inhalation: 5% Syrup, oral: 2 mg/ml Tablets, oral: 10, 20 mg	**Contraindications:** Hypersensitivity to metaproterenol or to other sympathomimetic amines and tachycardia. **ADRs:** May cause a bad taste, dizziness, headache, hypertension, nausea, palpitation, tachycardia, and tremor. *See* Chapter 5.
Metformin (*Apo-Metformin*®, *Glucophage*®, *Glycon*®, *Novo-Metformin*®, *Nu-Metformin*®)	Diabetes mellitus (Type II) **Note:** Approved by the FDA but not the HPB for children.	**Children (≥10 years):** Initially, 1000 mg/day PO in two divided doses. Increase daily dosage by 500-mg increments at weekly intervals according to glucose blood concentrations. *Maximum:* 2000 mg/day PO. **Adolescents:** 1500–2000 mg/day PO in three or four divided doses; **or** 1700–2550 mg/day PO in two or three divided doses. Adjust daily dosage according to glucose blood concentrations. *Maximum:* 2550 mg/day PO. **Note:** Each dose of metformin oral tablets should be ingested with food to decrease associated GI distress. **Note:** Reduce dosage for pediatric patients who have mild renal dysfunction (*see* Contraindications).	Tablets, oral: 500, 850, 1000 mg (may contain povidone) Tablet, oral extended release: 500 mg **Note:** Safety and efficacy of the use of metformin extended-release tablets for pediatric patients has not been established.	**Contraindications:** Alcoholism, cardiovascular collapse, CHF, diabetic ketoacidosis, dehydration (severe), hepatic dysfunction (severe), lactic acidosis, hypersensitivity to metformin, pregnancy, and renal dysfunction (moderate to severe). **ADRs:** Commonly causes abdominal bloating, anorexia, diarrhea, flatulence, nausea, and vomiting. These ADRs affecting the GI system generally resolve with continued metformin pharmacotherapy. May also cause lactic acidosis, which, although rare, is fatal in ~50% of cases. Lactic acidosis is generally associated with the accumulation of metformin among patients who have renal dysfunction. **Comments:** Encourage appropriate dietary management, exercise, and weight reduction as important adjuncts to metformin pharmacotherapy. **Note:** Assess renal function **prior** to initiating metformin pharmacotherapy and monitor renal function at least annually thereafter.

Footnotes are on page 558.

TABLE 14-1 continued

DRUG (TRADE AND OTHER NAMES)	INDICATION(S)	USUAL PEDIATRIC DOSAGE AND ADMINISTRATION[a]	DOSAGE FORMS	CONTRAINDICATIONS, ADRs, AND COMMENTS[b]
Methamphetamine (Desoxyephedrine, *Desoxyn®*)	Attention-deficit/Hyperactivity disorder	**Children (≥6 years) and adolescents:** Initially, 5–10 mg/day PO in two divided doses. Increase the daily dosage weekly by increments of 5 mg until optimal therapeutic benefit is achieved. The usual effective dosage is 20–25 mg/day. Avoid late afternoon or early evening doses because of associated insomnia. Once the optimal daily dosage has been established, it may be administered as a single daily dose with the extended-release tablet formulation.	Tablet, oral: 5 mg Tablets, oral extended release *(Desoxyn Gradumet®):* 5, 10, 15 mg **Note:** The 15-mg *Gradumet* tablets contain tartrazine (FD&C yellow No. 5) that has been associated with hypersensitivity reactions, including bronchial asthma, among susceptible patients. Pediatric patients who are hypersensitive to aspirin appear to be at particular risk. **Note:** The extended-release tablet is **not** indicated for the initiation of therapy and should be reserved for use when the optimal daily dosage is equal to or exceeds the dosage provided by the extended-release formulation.	**Contraindications:** Addiction and habituation to methamphetamine or other amphetamines; agitation; cardiac disease (symptomatic); hypersensitivity to amphetamine, methamphetamine, or sympathomimetic amines; hypertension (moderate to severe); hyperthyroidism; and MAOI therapy (concurrent or within 14 days) and phenothiazine therapy (see Chapter 6). **ADRs:** *See* "Amphetamines, mixed." *See also* Chapter 5.
Methenamine Hippurate *(Hiprex®, Urex®)*	Urinary tract infections **Note:** Ensure that appropriate culture and sensitivity tests are performed and that the organism is sensitive to methenamine hippurate.	**Children (≥6 years) and adolescents:** 1 or 2 grams/day PO in two divided doses, every 12 hr. *Maximum:* 2 grams/day PO.	Tablet, oral: 1 gram **Note:** *Hiprex®* contains tartrazine (FD&C yellow No. 5) which may cause hypersensitivity reactions, including bronchial asthma, among susceptible patients, particularly those who have a hypersensitivity to aspirin.	**Contraindications:** Dehydration (severe), hepatic or renal dysfunction (severe), and hypersensitivity to methenamine. **ADRs:** Generally well tolerated. *See* Chapter 5. **Comments:** Maintain urine pH at less than 5.5. Ascorbic acid may be used to acidify the urine.
Methenamine Mandelate *(Mandelamine®)*	Urinary tract infections **Note:** Ensure that appropriate culture and sensitivity tests are performed and that the organism is sensitive to methenamine mandelate.	**Children (<6 years):** 20 mg/kg/day PO in four divided doses, every 6 hr. *Maximum:* 1 gram/day PO. **Children (≥6 years) and adolescents:** 50 mg/kg/day PO in four divided doses, every 6 hr. *Maximum:* **Children (≥6 years),** 2 grams/day PO; **adolescents,** 4 grams/day PO.	Granules, oral: 1 gram/packet Suspension, oral: 100 mg/ml; shake well before use. Tablets, oral: 500 mg, 1 gram Tablets, oral enteric coated: 500 mg, 1 gram	**Contraindications:** Hypersensitivity to methenamine and renal insufficiency. **ADRs:** Generally well tolerated. *See* Chapter 5. **Comments:** Maintain urine pH at less than 5.5. Ascorbic acid may be used to acidify the urine.
Methimazole *(Tapazole®,* Thiamazole)	Hyperthyroidism	**Children and adolescents:** Initially, 0.4–0.7 mg/kg/day PO in three divided doses, every 8 hr; dose may be increased up to 1.5 mg/kg/day if no improvement occurs within 2–3 weeks. Maintenance, once the hyperthyroidism has been controlled, is usually 0.2 mg/kg/day PO in three divided doses, every 8 hr. *Maximum:* Initially, 30 mg/day PO; *maintenance,* 15 mg/day PO. **Note:** Reduce dosage for pediatric patients who have hepatic dysfunction.	Tablets, oral: 5, 10 mg	**Contraindications:** Breast feeding and hypersensitivity to methimazole. **ADRs:** May cause abnormal hair loss, blood dyscrasias, drowsiness, jaundice, lymphadenopathy, skin pigmentation, and skin rash. **Comments:** Leukopenia occurs in up to 10% of patients; monitor white blood cell count. Monitor also for signs and symptoms of agranulocytosis, hepatic dysfunction, and hypothyroidism.

TABLE 14-1 continued

DRUG (TRADE AND OTHER NAMES)	INDICATION(S)	USUAL PEDIATRIC DOSAGE AND ADMINISTRATION[a]	DOSAGE FORMS	CONTRAINDICATIONS, ADRs, AND COMMENTS[b]
Metho-carbamol (*Delaxin®*, Glyceryl Guaiacolate Carbamate, *Marbaxin®*, *Robaxin®*, *Robomol®*)	**Tetanus,** adjunctive supportive pharmacotherapy **Note:** Not approved by the HPB for this indication.	**Children:** Initially, 15 mg/kg IV. May repeat initial dose every 6 hr as needed, according to response. *Maximum:* 6 grams/dose IV. **Adolescents:** Initially, 2 or 4 grams (one or two vials) IV. An additional 2 grams (one vial) may be added to the IV infusion for a total initial dose of 6 grams (three vials). Initial dose may be repeated every 6 hr as indicated by response. *Maximum:* 6 grams/dose IV; 24 grams/day IV.	Tablets, oral: 500, 750 mg Injectable, IM, IV: 100 mg/0.5 ml in single-dose 10-ml vials; contains propylene glycol. **Note:** Injectable is for IM or IV use only. **Note:** Undiluted injectable may be administered directly into the vein at a maximal rate of 3 ml/min.	**Contraindications:** Hypersensitivity to methocarbamol. **ADRs:** Generally well tolerated. May cause dizziness, drowsiness, lightheadedness, and nausea. Caution is needed when injectable therapy is administered to patients who have epilepsy because of associated risk for seizures (generally not recommended for these patients). **Comments:** Generally, maintain patients in a recumbent position during and for 10–15 min following the IV infusion because of associated risk for CNS depression.
	Pain associated with skeletal muscle spasm (including back strain, myositis, and whiplash), adjunctive to other measures (e.g., physical therapy, rest)	**Adolescents:** Initially, 100 mg/kg/day PO in three or four divided doses. When pain relief is achieved, generally after 2 or 3 days, reduce dosage to 60 mg/kg/day PO in three or four divided doses. *Maximum: Initially,* 8 grams/day PO; *maintenance,* 4 grams/day PO.		
Methohexital (*Brevital®*, Methohexitone)	**Rapid induction of general anesthesia for short diagnostic, surgical, or therapeutic procedures** (often used for rapid induction of anesthesia prior to the use of other general anesthetics) **Note:** IV administration not approved by the FDA for children.	**Children and adolescents:** Induction, 1 mg/kg IV. Generally, a 1% solution is administered IV at a rate of ~0.2 ml/sec. **Note:** The induction dose generally provides anesthesia for 5–7 min. However, response is highly variable and dosage must be determined by response.	Injectable, IV: 500 mg/vial; 10 mg/ml (1%), after reconstitution with 50 ml of sterile water for injection; stable for 24 hr at room temperature. **Note:** The 1% solution can be administered IV or rectally. The initial **rectal** dose for induction is 25 mg/kg. **Note:** Not generally available in Canada.	**Contraindications:** Hepatic impairment (severe), hypersensitivity to methohexital or to other barbiturates, porphyria (latent or manifest), shock, and status asthmaticus. **ADRs:** May cause bronchospasm, dyspnea, emergence delirium, headache, hypotension, laryngospasm, and respiratory depression. Psychomotor seizures may occur, particularly among patients with temporal lobe epilepsy. Prolonged administration may result in heightened or cumulative ADRs. In addition, transient hypotension and resultant tachycardia may occur following induction of anesthesia with methohexital. Caution is required for patients who have anemia (severe), asthma, bronchitis (severe), congestive heart failure, hepatic impairment, hypertension (severe), hypotension, myocardial disease, obesity (extreme), and renal impairment. **Comments:** Maintenance of a patent airway and adequate ventilation must be ensured at all times during methohexital anesthesia.
	Maintenance of general anesthesia for longer diagnostic, surgical, or therapeutic procedures **Note:** *See also* ADRs.	**Children and adolescents:** 0.5–0.75 mg/kg of 1% solution by intermittent IV infusion. Adjust infusion rate according to response. Generally, intermittent infusion can be repeated every 4–7 min **or** 3 ml/min (one drop/sec) of 0.2% solution by continuous IV infusion. **Note:** Adjust IV infusion rate according to response. For longer procedures, it is generally recommended that the rate of infusion be gradually reduced because of concern for accumulation of methohexital in body tissues, and subsequent toxicity.		
Methohexitone, *see* **Methohexital**				
Methotrexate (Amethopterin, *Rheumatrex®*) **Note:** *See also* Chapter 12.	**Juvenile rheumatoid arthritis** (refractory to conventional pharmacotherapy)	**Children and adolescents:** 0.15–0.3 mg/kg/week IM or PO **or** 5 mg/m²/week IM or PO as a single weekly dose; may double the weekly dose after 6–8 weeks, if needed according to response.	Injectables, IM: 2.5, 25 mg/ml; 2, 25, 50, 100, 200, 250 mg/vial Tablet, oral: 2.5 mg	**Contraindications:** Blood dyscrasias, breast feeding, cirrhosis, hepatitis, hypersensitivity to methotrexate, immunodeficiency, and pregnancy. **ADRs:** *See* Chapter 5.

(Continued)

Footnotes are on page 558.

TABLE 14-1 continued

DRUG (TRADE AND OTHER NAMES)	INDICATION(S)	USUAL PEDIATRIC DOSAGE AND ADMINISTRATION[a]	DOSAGE FORMS	CONTRAINDICATIONS, ADRs, AND COMMENTS[b]
Methotrexate *continued*	Note: Not approved by the FDA or HPB for this indication for infants or children.	*Maximum:* 20 mg/week IM or PO. **Note:** Administer oral formulation on an empty stomach. **Note:** Reduce dosage for pediatric patients who have renal dysfunction; see Table 14-2.		**Comments:** Monitor hematologic, hepatic, and renal function periodically.
Methotrimeprazine (Levomepromazine, *Levoprome®*, *Novo-Meprazine®*, *Nozinan®*)	Schizophrenia and other psychotic disorders	**Children:** Initially, 0.25 mg/kg/day PO in two or three divided doses with meals **or** 0.065 mg/kg/day IM as a single dose. Increase the dosage gradually until desired therapeutic response is achieved. *Maximum:* 40 mg/day PO. **Adolescents:** Initially, 75 mg/day IM or PO in three divided doses. Increase the dosage gradually until desired therapeutic response is achieved. *Maximum:* 1000 mg/day PO. **Note:** Use only large healthy muscle sites for IM injection of methotrimeprazine. Replace methotrimeprazine injectable pharmacotherapy with oral pharmacotherapy as soon as feasible.	Drops, oral: 40 mg/ml; contains 16.5% alcohol (apricot flavored). Injectables, IM, IV: 20, 25 mg/ml Liquid, oral: 25 mg/5 ml; contains 2.5% alcohol (apricot flavored) Tablets, oral: 2, 5, 25, 50 mg **Note:** Injectable contains sodium metabisulfite or sodium sulfite which is associated with hypersensitivity reactions, including anaphylactic reactions among susceptible patients. Although uncommon, they appear to occur with a higher incidence among pediatric patients who have asthma. **Note:** IV route is **not** to be used for this indication. **Note:** Not generally available in the United States.	**Contraindications:** Antihypertensive pharmacotherapy (concurrent), blood dyscrasias, CNS depression (due to CNS depressant pharmacotherapy), coma, heart disease (severe), hepatic dysfunction (severe), hypersensitivity to methotrimeprazine or to other phenothiazines, hypotension (clinically significant), MAOI therapy (concurrent or within 14 days), and renal dysfunction (severe). **ADRs:** May cause constipation, drowsiness (initially), oversedation, postural hypotension, tachycardia, tardive dyskinesia and other extrapyramidal reactions, unexpected sudden death, and weight gain (long-term high-dose therapy). **Comments:** Determine the daily dosage according to the severity of signs and symptoms and adjust the dosage according to response.
Methsuximide (*Celontin®*, Mesuximide)	Absence (petit mal) seizures refractory to other pharmacotherapy	**Children:** Initially, 150 mg/day PO for 7 days. If necessary, increase the daily dosage by 150 mg at weekly intervals according to response. *Maximum:* 900 mg/day PO. **Adolescents:** Initially, 300 mg/day PO for 7 days. If necessary, increase the daily dosage by 300 mg at weekly intervals according to response. *Maximum:* 1200 mg/day PO.	Capsules, oral: 150, 300 mg	**Contraindications:** Hypersensitivity to methsuximide or other succinimides. **ADRs:** May cause abdominal pain, anorexia, ataxia, blurred vision, diarrhea, dizziness, drowsiness, headache, leukopenia, nausea, nervousness, pancytopenia, vomiting, and weight loss. May impair cognitive abilities, including learning and memory, and, thus, academic performance.
Methyldopa (*Aldomet®*, Methyldopate)	Hypertension	**Children and adolescents:** Initially, 10 mg/kg/day PO in three or four divided doses; gradually increase dosage over several days until desired effect is achieved; **or** 20–40 mg/kg/day IV over 30–60 min in four divided doses, every 6 hr. *Maximum:* 3 grams/day PO or 65 mg/kg/day PO, whichever is less; 1 gram/dose IV. **Note:** Reduce dosage for pediatric patients who have renal dysfunction; see Table 14-2.	Injectable, IV: 50 mg/ml (methyldopate) Suspension, oral: 50 mg/ml; contains 1% alcohol (orange–pineapple flavored); shake well before use. Tablets, oral: 125, 250, 500 mg **Note:** Injectable and suspension contain sodium bisulfite. Sulfites may cause hypersensitivity reactions, including anaphylactic reactions, among susceptible patients, particularly those with asthma.	**Contraindications:** Hepatic disease, hypersensitivity to methyldopa, and MAOI therapy (concurrent or within 14 days). **ADRs:** *See* Chapter 5. **Comments:** Monitor hepatic function periodically and whenever an unexplained fever occurs.

TABLE 14-1 continued

DRUG (*TRADE* AND OTHER NAMES)	INDICATION(S)	USUAL PEDIATRIC DOSAGE AND ADMINISTRATION[a]	DOSAGE FORMS	CONTRAINDICATIONS, ADRs, AND COMMENTS[b]
Methyldopate, *see* **Methyldopa**				
Methylene Blue (*Methblue 65®, Urolene Blue®*) **Note:** *See also* Chapter 4.	Methemoglobinemia	**Children and adolescents:** 1–2 mg/kg/dose IV over 5–10 min. May repeat IV dose after 1 hr if cyanosis and hypoxia persist; **or** 195 mg/day PO in three divided doses after meals with a glassful (240 ml, 8 ounces) of water. *Maximum:* Total IV dose, 7 mg/kg IV; 390 mg/day PO.	Injectable, IV: 10 mg/ml Tablet, oral: 65 mg	**Contraindications:** Glucose-6-phosphate dehydrogenase deficiency, hypersensitivity to methylene blue, and renal insufficiency. **ADRs:** May cause bladder irritation, diarrhea, fever, nausea, and vomiting. *See* Chapter 4. **Comments:** May discolor skin, stool, or urine blue–green.
Methylmorphine, *see* **Codeine**				
Methylphenidate (*Concerta®, Metadate®, Riphenidate®, Ritalin®, Ritalin-SR®*)	Attention-deficit/ hyperactivity disorder (A-D/HD)	**Children (≥6 years) and adolescents:** Initially, 5–10 mg/day PO in two divided doses. Increase the daily dosage weekly by 5–10 mg, as indicated by response, up to 60 mg/day PO in two divided doses (usually in the morning before breakfast and at noon). If preferred, 0.25–0.5 mg/kg/day PO in two divided doses. If significant ADRs are not observed, double the daily dosage each week to achieve an optimal dosage of 2 mg/kg/day PO. Dosages exceeding 60 mg/day are not recommended. **Note:** Dosing should generally coincide with periods of greatest academic and other behavioral difficulties. However, late afternoon dosing may result in insomnia. The oral osmotic controlled-release tablets have a 12-hr duration of action and can generally be dosed once daily in the morning. **Note:** If therapeutic benefit is not achieved over a 1-month period with appropriate dosage adjustments, discontinue pharmacotherapy and re-assess patient. *Maximum:* 60 mg/day or 2 mg/kg/day, whichever is less.	Tablets, oral: 5, 10, 20 mg Tablets, oral extended release (*Metadate, Ritalin-SR*): 10, 20 mg **Note:** Oral extended-release tablets have a duration of action of ~8 hr and are indicated for pediatric patients who have been managed with regular oral tablets and prefer 8-hr dosing. Tablets, oral osmotic controlled release (*Concerta*): 18, 36, 54 mg **Note:** Oral osmotic controlled-release tablets have a duration of action of ~12 hr and are indicated for pediatric patients who have been managed with regular oral tablets and prefer once daily dosing. **Note:** Oral extended-release and oral osmotic controlled-release tablets should not be chewed, crushed, or divided.	**Contraindications:** Agitation, angina, anxiety, heart disease (severe), hypersensitivity to methylphenidate, MAOI therapy (concurrent or within 14 days), tachycardia, thyrotoxicosis, and Tourette's disorder. **ADRs:** Caution is indicated for pediatric patients with seizure disorders or EEG abnormalities in the absence of seizures. Commonly causes insomnia, particularly if the last dose of the day is ingested in the late afternoon or early evening. The insomnia may be managed by reducing the dosage or by omitting the afternoon or evening dose. Anorexia (transient) and nervousness also are common. The latter may be managed by reducing the dosage. Other ADRs include addiction and habituation with long-term therapy, angina, anorexia, blurred vision, cardiac dysrhythmias (e.g., tachycardia), convulsions, dizziness, drowsiness, dyskinesia, headache, hypertension, insomnia, psychotic episodes (e.g., hallucinations, tics, or their exacerbation, and Tourette's disorder) that usually subside with discontinuation of pharmacotherapy, and rash. *See* Chapters 5 and 7.
Methylphenobarbital, *see* **Mephobarbital**				
Methylprednisolone Sodium Succinate (*A-Methapred®, Solu-Medrol®*) **Note:** *See also* Chapter 12.	Adjunctive pharmacotherapy for life-threatening medical conditions (e.g., severe shock). **Note:** Efficacy in the treatment of septic shock remains unsubstantiated and is controversial. Spinal cord injury, acute **Note:** Approved by the HPB but not FDA for this indication.	**Children and adolescents:** 20–30 mg/kg/dose IV over 30–60 min every 4–6 hr for up to 48 hr. *Maximum:* 1 gram/dose IV. **Children and adolescents:** 30 mg/kg/dose IV over 15 min. Withhold for 45 min, then resume with 5.4 mg/kg/hr by continuous IV infusion for the next 23 hr.	Injectables, IM, IV: 40, 125, 500 mg/vial; 1, 2 grams/vial **Note:** The recommended diluent, bacteriostatic water for injection, contains benzyl alcohol which has been associated with a potentially fatal "gasping syndrome" in premature neonates and young infants.	**Contraindications:** Cushing's syndrome, herpes simplex, hypercreatininemia, keratitis, peptic ulcer, psychosis (acute), tuberculosis (arrested), vaccinia, and varicella. **Note:** Contraindications generally do not apply when used for acute management of potentially life-threatening medical conditions. **ADRs:** *See* Chapter 5.

(Continued)

Footnotes are on page 558.

TABLE 14-1 continued

DRUG (TRADE AND OTHER NAMES)	INDICATION(S)	USUAL PEDIATRIC DOSAGE AND ADMINISTRATION[a]	DOSAGE FORMS	CONTRAINDICATIONS, ADRs, AND COMMENTS[b]
Methylprednisolone Sodium Succinate *continued*	Status asthmaticus	**Children and adolescents:** Initially, 1–4 mg/kg IV, then 2–8 mg/kg/day IV in four divided doses, every 6 hr, for 1–5 days. *Maximum:* 250 mg/dose IV.		
Metoclopramide (Reglan®)	Delayed gastric emptying associated with gastritis or surgical procedures	**Children (≤5 years):** 0.5 mg/kg/day PO in three divided doses 30 min before meals. **Children (≥6 years):** 7.5–15 mg/day PO in three divided doses 30 min before meals. **Adolescents:** 15–30 mg/day PO in three divided doses 30 min before meals.	Injectable, IM, IV: 5 mg/ml Solution, oral: 1 mg/ml (chocolate, custard, or fruit-berry flavored) Tablets, oral: 5, 10 mg	**Contraindications:** GI hemorrhage, obstruction, or perforation and hypersensitivity to metoclopramide. **ADRs:** Generally well tolerated. May cause diarrhea, dizziness, drowsiness, extrapyramidal reactions, fatigue, headache, insomnia, lassitude, and menstrual disorders. **Comments:** May alter GI absorption of concurrent oral pharmacotherapy; antagonized by anticholinergic drugs. **Note:** Extrapyramidal ADRs occur frequently among children when the daily dosage exceeds 0.5 mg/kg/day.
	Small bowel intubation, adjunctive pharmacotherapy	**Infants and children (<6 years):** 0.1 mg/kg IV as a single dose. **Children (≥6 years):** 5 mg IV as a single dose. **Adolescents:** 10 mg IV as a single dose. *Maximum:* 10 mg/dose IV. **Note:** Reduce dosage for pediatric patients who have renal dysfunction; see Table 14-2.		
Metronidazole (Flagyl®)	Amebiasis **Note:** The Centers for Disease Control and Prevention (CDC) recommends that metronidazole be combined with iodoquinol for the treatment of amebiasis.	**Children:** 35–50 mg/kg/day PO in three divided doses for 7–10 days. *Maximum:* 2.25 grams/day PO and 2 grams/dose PO. **Adolescents:** 2.25 grams/day PO in three divided doses for 5–7 days. **Note:** Administer with food. Reduce dosage for pediatric patients who have hepatic dysfunction.	Capsules, oral: 375, 500 mg Cream, vaginal: 10% (with applicator) Gel, vaginal: 0.75% (with applicator) Injectables, IV: 5 mg/ml; 500 mg/vial Insert, vaginal: 500 mg (with applicator) Tablets, oral: 250, 500 mg	**Contraindications:** Hypersensitivity to metronidazole and neurological disorders. **ADRs:** *See* Chapter 5. **Comments:** May cause darkening of the urine. May cause a disulfiramlike reaction in children and adolescents who concurrently consume alcohol.
	Bacterial vaginosis **Note:** Not approved by the FDA for this indication for infants or children.	**Adolescents:** One applicatorful of vaginal gel every night at bedtime for 5 consecutive nights. **Alternatively:** 2 grams PO as a single dose after a meal.		
	Giardiasis **Note:** Not approved by the FDA for the treatment of giardiasis among pediatric patients.	**Children:** 15–35 mg/kg/day PO in three divided doses for 5–7 days. *Maximum:* 750 mg/day PO. **Adolescents:** 750 mg/day PO in three divided doses for 5–7 days.		
	Anaerobic bacterial infections **Note:** Ensure that appropriate culture and sensitivity tests are performed and that the organism is sensitive to metronidazole. **Note:** Not approved by the FDA for the treatment of anaerobic infections among pediatric patients.	**Children and adolescents:** Initially, 15 mg/kg/dose by IV infusion over 1 hr. Then 7.5 mg/kg/dose by intermittent IV infusion every 6 hr for 7–10 days. *Maximum:* 4 grams/24 hr IV. **Note:** Infuse each IV dose over 1 hr.		

CHAPTER 14: DRUG DOSING FOR INFANTS, CHILDREN, AND ADOLESCENTS

TABLE 14-1 *continued*

DRUG (*TRADE* AND OTHER NAMES)	INDICATION(S)	USUAL PEDIATRIC DOSAGE AND ADMINISTRATION[a]	DOSAGE FORMS	CONTRAINDICATIONS, ADRs, AND COMMENTS[b]
Metronidazole *continued*	**Trichomonas vaginalis** **Note:** Not approved by the FDA for the treatment of trichomonas vaginalis for pediatric patients.	**Children:** 15 mg/kg/day PO in three divided doses for 7 days. *Maximum:* 750 mg/day PO. **Adolescents:** 2 grams PO as a single dose after a meal. *Maximum:* 2.25 grams/day PO; 2 grams/dose PO. **Alternatively:** 500 mg vaginal (one applicatorful of vaginal cream or one vaginal insert) every night for 10–20 consecutive nights. **Note:** Vaginal administration may be considered obsolete when oral therapy is clinically feasible and generally preferred.		
Mexiletine (*Mexitil*®)	**Ventricular dysrhythmias** (e.g., ventricular tachycardia) **Note:** Not approved by the FDA or HPB for infants or children.	**Children and adolescents:** Initially, 6–8 mg/kg PO, follow with 6–16 mg/kg/day PO in three or four divided doses. *Maximum:* 1200 mg/day PO. **Note:** Administer with food to decrease associated GI irritation. **Note:** Reduce dosage for pediatric patients who have renal (*see* Table 14-2) and/or hepatic dysfunction.	Capsules, oral: 150, 200, 250 mg	**Contraindications:** AV block (second or third degree, in the absence of a pacemaker), cardiogenic shock, and hypersensitivity to mexiletine or to amide-type local anesthetics. **ADRs:** *See* Chapter 5. **Comments:** Patients should be hospitalized during initial therapy. Therapeutic drug monitoring is recommended; *see* Table 14-3.
Miconazole (*Desenex Prescription Strength*®, *Lotrimin*®, *Micatin*®, *Monazole*®, *Monistat*®)	**Cutaneous candidiasis/ Dermatophytoses/ Mycoses,** superficial (e.g., *Tinea corporis, T. cruris, T. pedis, T. versicolor*) **Vulvovaginal candidiasis** (e.g., moniliasis, vaginal yeast infection)	**Children (≥2 years) and adolescents:** Apply topical formulation sparingly to affected external areas twice daily, morning and evening. Apply formulation to clean and dry areas only. Continue for 2–4 weeks. **Adolescents:** <table><tr><th>DAILY BEDTIME VAGINAL DOSAGE</th><th>REQUIRED NUMBER OF CONSECUTIVE DAYS OF THERAPY</th></tr><tr><td>5 gram applicatorful of vaginal cream</td><td>7 days</td></tr><tr><td>100-mg vaginal suppository</td><td>7 days</td></tr><tr><td>200-mg vaginal suppository</td><td>3 days</td></tr><tr><td>400-mg vaginal ovule</td><td>3 days</td></tr><tr><td>1200-mg vaginal ovule</td><td>1 day</td></tr></table> **Note:** Individual courses of miconazole pharmacotherapy may be repeated if the patient remains symptomatic and appropriate culture and sensitivity tests confirm that the organism is sensitive to miconazole.	Cream, topical: 2% Cream, vaginal: 2% Ovules, vaginal: 400, 1200 mg (with applicator) Powder, topical: 2% Powder, topical aerosol: 2% Solution, topical aerosol: 2% Suppositories, vaginal: 100, 200 mg (with applicator) Tincture, topical: 2%; contains benzyl alcohol and isopropyl alcohol. **Note:** Topical formulations are for external use only. Avoid contact with eyes. Vaginal formulations are for vaginal use only.	**Contraindications:** Hypersensitivity to miconazole. **ADRs:** Generally well tolerated. May cause vulvovaginal burning, itching, irritation, and rash. **Comments:** Discontinue if signs and symptoms of local irritation occur. **Note:** Intravaginal use of miconazole has resulted in systemic drug interactions with heparin and warfarin and resultant increased prothrombin time.

Footnotes are on page 558.

TABLE 14-1 continued

DRUG (*TRADE* AND OTHER NAMES)	INDICATION(S)	USUAL PEDIATRIC DOSAGE AND ADMINISTRATION[a]	DOSAGE FORMS	CONTRAINDICATIONS, ADRs, AND COMMENTS[b]
Midazolam (*Versed*®)	**Premedication for diagnostic, endoscopic, or therapeutic procedures** (to provide sedation, anxiolysis, and amnesia)	**Infants (≥6 months) and children (<6 years):** 0.5 mg/kg PO as a single dose 20 min prior to procedure. *Maximum*: 1 mg/kg PO **or** 20 mg PO, whichever is less. **Children (≥6 years) and adolescents:** 0.25 mg/kg PO as a single dose 30–60 min prior to procedure. *Maximum*: 1 mg/kg PO **or** 20 mg PO, whichever is less.	Injectables, IM, IV: 1, 5 mg/ml; contain 1% benzyl alcohol. Syrup, oral: 2 mg/ml (cherry flavored); supplied with press-in bottle adaptor, single-use graduated oral dispensers (oral syringes; *see* Chapter 1), and tip caps. **Note:** Do **not** dispense to patient. Not intended for home use. For hospital or ambulatory care setting use only. **Note:** Benzyl alcohol, which is found in the injectable formulation, is associated with a potentially fatal "gasping syndrome" among premature neonates and young infants.	**Contraindications:** Hypersensitivity to midazolam or to other benzodiazepines. **ADRs:** *See* Chapter 5. **Comments:** IV administration has been associated with respiratory arrest. Ensure that the patient is appropriately monitored and that oxygen, the benzodiazepine antagonist flumazenil, resuscitative equipment, and trained personnel are readily available. **Note:** Frequent assessment of levels of pain and sedation is recommended at regular intervals during IV administration. **Note:** Continuously monitor pediatric patients during IV administration of midazolam with attention to early signs of hypoventilation and apnea. Pulse oximetry should be used and vital signs should continue to be monitored throughout the recovery period.
	Premedication for anesthesia or therapeutic procedures (e.g., insertion of central venous access device) (to provide sedation, anxiolysis, and amnesia).	**Infants (≥6 months), children, and adolescents:** 0.1 mg/kg IM as a single dose 5–15 min prior to anesthesia or procedure. *Maximum*: 0.5 mg/kg/dose IM **not to exceed** 10 mg/total dose IM.		
	Premedication for anesthesia and therapeutic procedures (e.g., endoscopy), both prior to, and during (to provide sedation, anxiolysis, and amnesia)	**Infants (≥6 months) and children (<6 years):** Initially, 0.05–0.1 mg/kg IV 5–10 min prior to anesthesia or procedure. Administer subsequent doses as indicated by response. *Maximum*: 0.6 mg/kg total dose IV **or** 6 mg/total dose IV, whichever is less. **Children (≥6 years):** Initially, 0.025–0.05 mg/kg IV 5–10 min prior to anesthesia or procedure. Administer subsequent doses, as indicated by response. *Maximum*: 0.4 mg/kg total dose IV **or** 10 mg/total dose IV, whichever is less. **Note:** Children, as a group, generally require higher dosages of midazolam than do adolescents. **Adolescents:** Initially, 1–2.5 mg IV; titrate slowly to the desired effect (e.g., initiation of slurred speech). Administer each subsequent dose after at least a 5-min interval, as indicated by response. *Maximum*: 2.5 mg/initial dose IV and 5 mg/total dose IV. **Note:** Initial IV dose should be administered by IV injection over 2–3 min.		
	Sedation (in critical care settings, such as pediatric intensive care units)	**Infants, children, and adolescents:** Initially, 0.05–0.2 mg/kg IV as a single dose administered over 2–3 min. May be followed by a continuous IV infusion of 1–2 µg/kg/min to maintain the desired response. **Note:** In order to maintain desired response, the rate of IV infusion can be adjusted or additional doses can be administered.		

TABLE 14-1 continued

DRUG (TRADE AND OTHER NAMES)	INDICATION(S)	USUAL PEDIATRIC DOSAGE AND ADMINISTRATION[a]	DOSAGE FORMS	CONTRAINDICATIONS, ADRs, AND COMMENTS[b]
Midazolam *continued*		**Note:** Reduce dosage for pediatric patients who are receiving opiate analgesics, sedative-hypnotics, or other CNS depressants. **Note:** Reduce dosage for pediatric patients who have renal (*see* Table 14-2) and/or hepatic dysfunction.		
Milk of Magnesia, *see* **Magnesium Hydroxide**				
Milrinone *(Primacor®)*	**Congestive heart failure,** severe/ **Decompensated heart failure,** acute **Note:** Not approved by the FDA or HPB for children or adolescents. **Note:** For short-term use only, generally 2 or 3 days. Often used in patients who are already receiving digoxin and diuretics.	**Children and adolescents:** *Initial loading dose,* 50 µg/kg by slow IV injection or infusion (diluted in 5% dextrose and water solution or normal saline solution) over 10 min. *Maintenance:* 0.5–0.75 µg/kg/min as a continuous IV infusion. Monitor patients carefully and adjust dosage according to response. *Maximum:* 1.13 mg/kg/day IV. **Note:** Reduce dosage for pediatric patients who have renal dysfunction; *see* Table 14-2.	Injectables, IV: 200 µg/ml (in Pre-mix Flexible Containers® with foil overwrap); 1 mg/ml (single-use vials) **Note:** For IV use only.	**Contraindications:** Hypersensitivity to milrinone or to amrinone, hypertrophic subaortic stenosis, myocardial infarction (acute and severe), obstructive aortic or pulmonic valvular disease, and ventricular dysrhythmias. **ADRs:** May cause angina pectoris, headache, hypokalemia, hypotension, thrombocytopenia, and ventricular dysrhythmias (in 2% of patients), including ventricular fibrillation (~0.2% of patients). **Comments:** Younger pediatric patients appear to eliminate milrinone at a significantly faster rate than adults. **Note:** Monitor blood pressure, ECG (continuous), fluid and electrolytes, heart rate, and renal function.
Mineral Oil *(Kondremul®, Milkinol®)*	**Constipation** **Note:** Not recommended for chronic or long-term use because of ADRs and availability of suitable therapeutic alternatives.	**Children (≥6 years) and adolescents:** 0.5–1 ml/kg/day PO as a single dose. *Maximum:* 45 ml/dose PO. **Alternatively:** Children (≥2 years), 30–60 ml/day rectal as a single dose; adolescents, 60–120 ml/day rectal as a single dose. **Note:** Avoid administering oral mineral oil emulsion or liquid within 2 hr of a meal because mineral oil may interfere with the GI absorption of nutrients and vitamins, particularly fat-soluble vitamins (A, D, E, and K).	Emulsion, oral: 50% Liquid, oral: 100% Oil, rectal: 100% Suspensions, rectal: 2.75, 4.75 ml/5 ml	**Contraindications:** Dysphagia (oral administration of mineral oil). **ADRs:** *See* Chapter 5. **Comments:** Inadvertent aspiration of oral dosage forms may result in lipoid pneumonitis.
Minocycline *(Minocin®)*	**Infections** caused by susceptible organisms **Note:** Ensure that appropriate culture and sensitivity tests are performed and that the organism is sensitive to minocycline.	**Children (≥8 years):** Initially, 4 mg/kg IV or PO, then 2 mg/kg IV or PO every 12 hr. **Adolescents:** Initially, 200 mg IV or PO, then 100 mg IV or PO every 12 hr. **Note:** Replace IV with oral therapy as soon as clinically feasible.	Capsules, oral: 50, 100 mg Injectable, IV: 100 mg/vial Suspension, oral: 50 mg/5 ml (custard flavored); contains 5% alcohol; shake well before use.	**Contraindications:** Hypersensitivity to minocycline or to other tetracyclines. **ADRs:** *See* Chapter 5. **Comments:** The use of tetracyclines during the second and third trimesters of pregnancy, infancy, and childhood (up to 8 years) may result in permanent yellow–gray–brown discoloration of the teeth.
Minoxidil *(Loniten®)*	**Hypertension,** severe	**Children:** Initially, 0.1–0.2 mg/kg/day PO as a single daily dose or as two divided doses, then gradually increase the dosage at intervals of at least 3 days to 0.25–1 mg/kg/day in two to four	Tablets, oral: 2.5, 10 mg	**Contraindications:** Hypersensitivity to minoxidil, pheochromocytoma, and pulmonary hypertension associated with mitral stenosis. **ADRs:** *See* Chapter 5. *(Continued)*

Footnotes are on page 558.

TABLE 14-1 continued

DRUG (TRADE AND OTHER NAMES)	INDICATION(S)	USUAL PEDIATRIC DOSAGE AND ADMINISTRATION[a]	DOSAGE FORMS	CONTRAINDICATIONS, ADRs, AND COMMENTS[b]
Minoxidil *continued*		divided doses to achieve desired blood pressure. *Maximum:* 2 mg/kg/day PO or 50 mg/day PO, whichever is less. **Adolescents:** Initially, 5 mg/day PO in two divided doses, then gradually increase dosage at intervals of at least 3 days according to response. *Maximum:* 100 mg/day PO.		**Comments:** Concurrent use of a diuretic may be necessary to treat associated sodium and water retention and to prevent possible congestive heart failure. Concurrent use of a ß-adrenergic blocker may be required to prevent tachycardia. Monitor for pericardial effusion.
Mithramycin, *see* **Plicamycin**				
Mitoxantrone, *see* **Chapter 12**				
Mivacurium *(Mivacron®)*	Adjunctive therapy with general anesthesia for the facilitation of nonemergency tracheal intubation/Skeletal muscle relaxation during surgery **Note:** Provides neuromuscular blockade.	**Children (≥2 years):** Initial rapid IV injection after patient is unconscious, 0.2 mg/kg IV over 30 sec. Continuous IV infusion upon spontaneous recovery from the initial rapid IV injection (after ~15 min), 14 µg/kg/min. *Maximum* continuous IV infusion rate: 30 µg/kg/min. **Adolescents:** Initial rapid IV injection after patient is unconscious, 0.15 mg/kg IV over 15 sec. Continuous IV infusion upon spontaneous recovery from the initial rapid IV injection (after ~15–20 min), 10 µg/kg/min. *Maximum* continuous IV infusion rate: 20 µg/kg/min. **Note:** Onset and recovery of neuromuscular blockade occur more rapidly among children than adolescents. Children, therefore, generally require a larger dose (on a milligram-per-kilogram basis), than do adolescents. **Note:** Do not inject initial rapid IV dose until patient is unconscious (see also "Comments")	Injectable, IV: 2 mg/ml (multiple-dose vial contains benzyl alcohol) **Note:** For IV use only.	**Contraindications:** Hypersensitivity to mivacurium or to histamine, homozygotes for atypical plasma cholinesterase, myasthenia gravis, and myasthenic (Eaton-Lambert) syndrome. **ADRs:** Generally well tolerated. Commonly causes transient dose-related cutaneous flushing of the chest, face, or neck. **Comments:** Patients should be continuously monitored during administration with a peripheral nerve stimulator to evaluate response, determine the need for additional doses, and measure the adequacy of spontaneous recovery or anticholinesterase (e.g., neostigmine) antagonism (in the event that an antagonist is needed). Additional doses should not be administered before there is a definite response to T_1 or to the first twitch. If no response is elicited, the infusion should be discontinued until a response returns.
Mixed Amphetamines, *see* **Amphetamines, mixed**				
Mometasone Furoate Monohydrate *(Nasonex®)*	Seasonal and perennial allergic rhinitis, prophylaxis and treatment of signs and symptoms	**Children (≥3 years) and adolescents:** Two actuations of nasal spray (100 µg) in each nostril once daily. **Note:** Initiate therapy 2–4 weeks prior to the beginning of the pollen season as prophylaxis for pediatric patients with a known seasonal allergy.	Solution, (metered-dose nasal spray pump): 50 µg/actuation; shake well before use. **Note:** Metered-dose nasal spray pump is for intranasal use only. **Note:** Initial use of the metered-dose nasal spray pump requires priming with 10 sprays. **Note:** Safely store between 2 and 25° C (36–77° F) and protect from light.	**Contraindications:** Hypersensitivity to mometasone furoate monohydrate. **ADRs:** Generally well tolerated. May cause dyspepsia, headache, nasal ulcers, and nausea. **Comments:** Take care not to inadvertently spray into the eyes.

TABLE 14-1 continued

DRUG (TRADE AND OTHER NAMES)	INDICATION(S)	USUAL PEDIATRIC DOSAGE AND ADMINISTRATION[a]	DOSAGE FORMS	CONTRAINDICATIONS, ADRs, AND COMMENTS[b]
Montelukast (Singulair®)	**Asthma,** chronic **Note:** Not indicated for the relief of an acute asthma attack.	**Children (2–5 years):** 4 mg PO once daily in the evening. **Children (≥6 years):** 5 mg PO once daily in the evening. **Adolescents:** 10 mg PO once daily in the evening.	Tablets, chewable: 4, 5 mg (cherry flavored) Tablet, oral: 10 mg	**Contraindications:** Hypersensitivity to montelukast. **ADRs:** Generally well tolerated. May cause headache. See Chapter 5. **Comments:** Montelukast in combination with corticosteroid inhalation therapy (e.g., beclomethasone) may result in increased therapeutic benefit.
Morphine (Duramorph®, Morphitec®, M.O.S.®, MS Contin®, Oramorph SR®)	**Acute pain, moderate to severe**	**Children:** 0.1–0.2 mg/kg IM or SC **or** 0.05–0.1 mg/kg IV slowly over 4–5 min **or** 0.15–0.3 mg/kg PO or rectal. Repeat the initial dose every 4 hr, as needed, according to response.	Capsules, oral: 15, 30 mg Capsules, oral extended release: 20, 50, 100 mg Injectables, IM, IV, SC: 0.5, 1, 2, 3, 4, 5, 8, 10, 15, 25, 30, 50 mg/ml Solutions, oral: 5, 10, 20 mg/5 ml Solutions, oral concentrate with calibrated dropper (M.O.S., M.O.S. SR, Roxanol® concentrated oral solution): 20, 50 mg/ml (unflavored) Suppositories, rectal (RMS®): 5, 10, 20, 30 mg Syrups, oral: 1, 5, 10, 20 mg/ml (orange flavored), contains 5% alcohol; unflavored, alcohol free. Tablets, oral: 5, 10, 15, 20, 25, 30, 35, 40, 50, 60 mg Tablets, oral extended release (MS Contin, Oramorph SR): 15, 30, 60, 100, 200 mg	**Contraindications:** Alcoholism (acute); biliary tract surgery or biliary or renal colic (morphine causes smooth muscle spasms); CNS depression (severe); heart failure secondary to chronic lung disease; hypersensitivity to morphine, other opiate analgesics, or any component of the morphine formulation (e.g., Rapiject® syringes contain sodium metabisulfite, which may cause hypersensitivity reactions among susceptible pediatric patients, particularly those who have a history of asthma); hypotension (severe); MAOI therapy (concurrent or within 14 days); obstructive pulmonary disease or cor pulmonale; and respiratory depression characterized by hypoxia. **ADRs:** May cause cardiac arrest, circulatory depression, constipation, depression, dizziness, lightheadedness, nausea, respiratory arrest, sedation, shock, sweating, and vomiting. See "Opiate Analgesics" in Chapters 5 and 7. **Comments:** For pediatric patients for whom injectable therapy is being replaced with oral, the ratio of IM dose to oral dose is approximately 1 to 2.5.
	Chronic pain, moderate to severe	**Children:** Initially, 0.2–0.4 mg/kg PO or rectal every 4–6 hr, as needed **or** 0.1–0.2 mg/kg SC every 4 hr, as needed **or** 0.05–0.1 mg/kg IV every 4 hr, as needed. Inject IV slowly over 3–5 min **or** 0.01–0.04 mg/kg/hr by continuous IV or SC infusion. Increase infusion rate every 8 hr as needed in increments not exceeding 25%. **Maximum:** 15 mg/dose IM, IV, or SC. No predetermined dose limits for palliative care. **Note:** Individualize dose according to pain relief and ADRs. Continuous IV or SC infusion preferred for the management of pain requiring frequent or high-dose morphine.		
	Pain associated with vaso-occlusive crisis in sickle cell disease	**Children and adolescents:** Initially, 0.15 mg/kg IV over 5 min followed by 0.04 mg/kg/hr IV; increase infusion rate every 8 hr by 0.02-mg/kg/hr increments, up to a maximum of 0.1 mg/kg/hr. **Maximum:** Initial morphine, 7.5 mg/dose IV; maintenance, 0.1 mg/kg/hr IV. **Note:** Reduce dosage for pediatric patients who have renal dysfunction; see Table 14-2.		
Mumps Virus Vaccine, see Chapter 9				
Mupirocin, nasal (Bactroban Nasal®) **Note:** See also Mupirocin, topical.	**Eradication of nasal colonization with methicillin-resistant Staphylococcus aureus** in adolescent patients and healthcare workers/volunteers **Note:** Mupirocin, pharmacotherapy for this indication is usually part of a comprehensive infec-	**Adolescents:** Apply ~½ tubeful of 2% nasal ointment into one nostril and the remaining ointment into the other nostril twice daily, morning and evening, for 5 days. **Note:** Each tube delivers approximately 0.5 gram of ointment (~0.25 gram/nostril when dosed as directed).	Ointment, nasal: 2% (in 1-gram single-use tubes) **Note:** For intranasal use only. **Note:** Not generally available in Canada.	**Contraindications:** Hypersensitivity to mupirocin. **ADRs:** Generally well tolerated. May cause cough, headache, pharyngitis, rhinitis, and taste perversion. **Comments:** Do not apply other nasal formulations concurrently with mupirocin nasal ointment.

(Continued)

TABLE 14-1 continued

DRUG (TRADE AND OTHER NAMES)	INDICATION(S)	USUAL PEDIATRIC DOSAGE AND ADMINISTRATION[a]	DOSAGE FORMS	CONTRAINDICATIONS, ADRs, AND COMMENTS[b]
Mupirocin, nasal *continued*	tion control program aimed at reducing the risk of infection among patients at high risk for methicillin-resistant *S. aureus* infections during institutional outbreaks with this pathogen.			
Mupirocin, topical (Bactroban®) **Note:** See also Mupirocin, nasal.	**Impetigo** due to *Staphylococcus aureus* or *Streptococcus pyogenes*	**Infants, children, and adolescents:** Apply a small amount of the cream or ointment to affected areas three times daily for 10 days. **Note:** If desired, the area being treated may be covered with a protective gauze dressing.	Cream, topical: 2% Ointment, topical: 2% **Note:** For topical external use only and not for ophthalmic use. Avoid contact with eyes.	**Contraindications:** Hypersensitivity to mupirocin. **ADRs:** Generally well tolerated. May cause headache, local burning or stinging sensation, nausea, and rash. **Comments:** When appropriately prescribed, reportedly as efficacious as systemically administered antibiotics for the treatment of impetigo.
Muromonab-CD3 (Orthoclone OKT3®)	**Renal allograph rejection, acute/ Steroid-resistant cardiac and hepatic allograph rejection, acute** **Note:** Not approved by the HPB for children. **Note:** Pretransplantation antiviral prophylaxis may prevent infection from the grafted organ or blood products while the pediatric patient is immunosuppressed and, thus, reduce the morbidity associated with herpes viruses (e.g., cytomegalovirus [CMV], Epstein-Barr virus [EBV], and herpes simplex virus [HSV]).	**Infants and children (<30 kg):** 2.5 mg/day as a single rapid IV injection over less than 1 min. Continue therapy for 10–14 days. **Children (≥30 kg) and adolescents:** 5 mg/day as a single rapid IV injection over less than 1 min. Continue therapy for 10–14 days.	Injectable, IV: 1 mg/ml **Note:** For IV use only. **Note:** Open ampule immediately before use. After drug is withdrawn, appropriately discard any remaining solution safely and appropriately. **Note:** Withdraw solution from ampule using a low protein-binding 0.2- or 0.22-μm filter. Replace filter needle with a dry, sterile needle for a single rapid IV injection. **Note:** Do not freeze or shake injectable solution.	**Contraindications:** Antimouse antibody titers ≥ 1:1000, breast feeding, heart failure (uncompensated), hypersensitivity to muromonab-CD3 or to other drugs of murine origin, hypertension (uncontrolled), pregnancy, and seizure disorders. **ADRs:** May cause a variety of ADRs affecting several body systems including anaphylaxis (if occurs, usually does so within the first 10 min following initial IV injection), asthenia, chest pain, chills, diarrhea, dyspnea, edema, fever, headache, herpes virus infections, hypertension, leukopenia, nausea, neck stiffness, pruritus, pyrexia, rigors, rash, tachycardia, tremor, vomiting, and wheezing. **Comments:** A serious potentially fatal cardiovascular and CNS reaction (referred to as the Cytokine release syndrome) can occur, generally during the first 2 days (often beginning within the first 30–60 min of the IV injection). Signs and symptoms of this reaction include blindness, cardiac arrest, cardiovascular collapse, cerebral edema, cerebral herniation, coma, paralysis, pulmonary edema, respiratory arrest, seizures, and shock. Pretreatment with methylprednisolone (8 mg/kg) 1–4 hr before administration of the first dose of muromonab-CD3 may significantly reduce incidence and severity of associated signs and symptoms. Carefully monitor fluid status prior to and during therapy. **Note:** Therapeutic drug monitoring is recommended; see Table 14-3.

TABLE 14-1 continued

DRUG (*TRADE* AND OTHER NAMES)	INDICATION(S)	USUAL PEDIATRIC DOSAGE AND ADMINISTRATION[a]	DOSAGE FORMS	CONTRAINDICATIONS, ADRs, AND COMMENTS[b]
Nabumetone (*Relafen*®)	Juvenile rheumatoid arthritis (refractory to conventional pharmacotherapy) **Note:** Not approved by the FDA or HPB for children or adolescents.	**Children (>8 years):** Initially, 500 mg/kg/day PO as a single daily dose. Increase dosage gradually, as indicated by response, at intervals ≥7 days. *Maximum:* 1000 mg/day PO. **Adolescents:** Initially, 1 gram/day PO as a single daily dose. Increase dosage gradually, as indicated by response, at intervals ≥7 days. *Maximum:* 2 grams/day PO.	Tablets, oral: 500, 750 mg **Note:** Store and dispense tablets in a light-resistant container.	**Contraindications:** GI bleeding; hepatic dysfunction (severe), hypersensitivity to nabumetone or to other NSAIDs, and peptic ulceration. **ADRs:** May cause abdominal pain, diarrhea, dizziness, dyspepsia, edema, headache, insomnia, pruritus, rash, and tinnitus. See Chapter 5. **Comments:** Monitor for signs and symptoms of GI bleeding or peptic ulceration. Monitor hepatic and renal function periodically for pediatric patients on long-term nabumetone pharmacotherapy.
N-Acetylcysteine, *see* **Acetylcysteine**				
Nadolol (*Corgard*®)	Hypertension **Note:** Not approved by the FDA or HPB for infants or children.	**Children and adolescents:** Initially, 1 mg/kg/day PO as a single daily dose. Increase dosage by 1 mg/kg/day every 3 or 4 days, according to response, to a maximum of 4 mg/kg/day. *Maximum:* Initially, 40 mg/day PO; maintenance, 320 mg/day PO. **Note:** Reduce dosage for pediatric patients who have renal dysfunction; *see* Table 14-2.	Tablets, oral: 20, 40, 80, 120, 160 mg	**Contraindications:** Allergic rhinitis, AV block, bronchospasm, cardiogenic shock, chronic obstructive pulmonary disease (severe), congestive heart failure, ether anesthesia, and sinus bradycardia. **ADRs:** May cause AV block, bradycardia, bronchospasm (severe), congestive heart failure, dizziness, fatigue, and hypotension. See Chapter 5.
Nafcillin (*Nallpen*®, *Unipen*®)	Bacterial infection, mild to moderate **Note:** Ensure that appropriate culture and sensitivity tests are performed and that the organism is sensitive to nafcillin.	**Infants, children, and adolescents:** 50–100 mg/kg/day IM, IV, or PO in four divided doses, every 6 hr. *Maximum:* 12 grams/day PO. **Note:** Reduce dosage for pediatric patients with hepatic dysfunction.	Capsule, oral: 250 mg Injectables, IM, IV (*Nallpen in Iso-osmotic Dextrose Injection*): 20 mg/ml (frozen; for IV infusion after thawing; in 2% or 3.6% dextrose); 500 mg/vial; 1, 2 grams/vial Tablet, oral: 500 mg **Note:** Not generally available in Canada.	**Contraindications:** Hypersensitivity to cephalosporins, to nafcillin, or to other penicillins. **ADRs:** See Chapter 5.
Nalbuphine (*Nubain*®)	Pain, moderate to severe **Note:** Not approved by the FDA or HPB for children or adolescents.	**Children:** 0.1–0.2 mg/kg/dose IM, IV, or SC. Initial dose may be repeated every 3–6 hr as indicated by response. *Maximum:* 20 mg/dose; 160 mg/day. **Adolescents:** 10–20 mg/kg/dose IM, IV, or SC. Initial dose may be repeated every 3–6 hr as indicated by response. *Maximum:* 20 mg/dose IM, IV or SC; 160 mg/day IM, IV, or SC. **Note:** Reduce dosage for pediatric patients who have significant hepatic or renal dysfunction.	Injectables, IM, IV, SC: 10, 20 mg/ml	**Contraindications:** Hypersensitivity to nalbuphine and opiate addiction (may precipitate acute opiate-withdrawal syndrome). **ADRs:** Frequently causes sedation. See "Opiate Analgesics" in Chapter 5. **Comments:** Monitor for signs and symptoms of respiratory depression.
Naloxone (*Narcan*®) **Note:** *See also* Chapter 4.	Opiate analgesic overdosage, known or suspected	**Infants:** 0.01 mg/kg endotracheal (by endotracheal tube instillation) or IV. If therapeutic response is not achieved, a subsequent dose of 0.1 mg/kg may be administered and repeated at 2–3-min intervals, as required.	Injectables, IM, IV, SC: 0.02 (neonatal formulation), 0.4 mg/ml; 1 mg/ml (child and adolescent formulation)	**Contraindications:** Hypersensitivity to naloxone. **ADRs:** Although naloxone, in the absence of other drugs, exhibits no direct pharmacologic action, abrupt reversal of opiate analgesic overdosage may result in *(Continued)*

Footnotes are on page 558.

TABLE 14-1 continued

DRUG (TRADE AND OTHER NAMES)	INDICATION(S)	USUAL PEDIATRIC DOSAGE AND ADMINISTRATION[a]	DOSAGE FORMS	CONTRAINDICATIONS, ADRs, AND COMMENTS[b]
Naloxone *continued*		**Children (<20 kg or <5 years):** 0.1 mg/kg endotracheal (by endotracheal tube instillation) or IV. If therapeutic response is not achieved, a subsequent dose of 0.1 mg/kg may be administered and repeated at 2–3-min intervals, as required. **Children (≥20 kg or ≥5 years) and adolescents:** 2 mg/dose endotracheal (by endotracheal tube instillation) or IV; repeat as needed at 2–3-min intervals. **Note:** IV infusion is generally initiated for opiate overdosage involving long-acting opiates (e.g., methadone). The infusion rate for infants, children, and adolescents should be adjusted according to individual patient factors and clinical response. **Note:** Although naloxone can be administered IM, IV, or SC, the most rapid onset of action (<2 min) is achieved with IV administration and this route is recommended in emergency situations.		cardiac arrest, increased blood pressure, nausea, sweating, tachycardia, tremor, and vomiting. *See* Chapter 4 for additional discussion. **Comments:** May precipitate the opiate analgesic-withdrawal syndrome among infants, children, and adolescents addicted to opiate analgesics. **Note:** Ensure that patient is appropriately monitored following successful therapeutic response and that repeat doses are administered at hourly intervals (half-life of naloxone) as required, particularly when overdosage or poisoning has involved opiate analgesics with long half-lives (e.g., methadone).
Naphazoline, nasal *(Privine®)*	Nasal congestion associated with allergies, common cold, and sinusitis (provision of temporary relief that is often followed by rebound congestion)	**Children (6–12 years):** Instill one drop or instruct child to sniff one spray of the 0.05% nasal solution into the affected nostril(s) every 6 hr as indicated by response. **Adolescents:** Instill one or two drops or instruct adolescent to sniff one or two sprays of the 0.05% nasal solution into the affected nostril(s) every 4–6 hr as indicated by response.	Solution, nasal: 0.05% (available as both drops and spray) **Note:** Most products contain benzalkonium chloride. **Note:** For nasal use only.	**Contraindications:** Hypersensitivity to naphazoline. **ADRs:** Generally well tolerated. May cause local irritation or sneezing. Systemic absorption may result in bradycardia, dizziness, drowsiness, nausea, nervousness, sweating, and weakness. **Comments:** Avoid prolonged use (in excess of 5 days). *See* Chapter 1 for recommended techniques for intranasal drug administration.
Naphazoline, ophthalmic *(AK-Con®, Allerest® Eye Drops, Clear Eyes®, Vasoclear®, Vasocon®)*	Ocular congestion, hyperemia, itching, and minor eye irritation **Note:** Not effective for the treatment of delayed hypersensitivity reactions (e.g., contact dermatoconjunctivitis).	**Infants and children:** Instill one or two drops of the 0.012%, 0.02%, or 0.03% ophthalmic solution into the conjunctival sac of the affected eye(s) every 4–6 hr as indicated by response. **Adolescents:** Instill one or two drops of the 0.1% ophthalmic solution into the conjunctival sac of the affected eye(s) every 4–6 hr as indicated by response.	Solutions, ophthalmic: 0.012%, 0.02%, 0.03%, 0.1% (supplied in plastic squeeze dropper bottle) **Note:** Most products contain benzalkonium chloride. **Note:** For ophthalmic use only. **Note:** In order to minimize cross-infection when both eyes require naphazoline ophthalmic pharmacotherapy, ensure that separate containers are dispensed for each eye.	**Contraindications:** Angle-closure glaucoma and hypersensitivity to naphazoline. **ADRs:** Generally well tolerated. May cause blurred vision and local irritation. Systemic absorption may result in bradycardia, dizziness, drowsiness, nausea, nervousness, sweating, and weakness. *See* Chapter 1 for recommended techniques to use to avoid or minimize systemic absorption of ophthalmic drops. **Comments:** Avoid prolonged use (in excess of 5 days).
Naproxen Sodium *(Anaprox®, Naprosyn®, Naxen®, Synflex®)*	Juvenile rheumatoid arthritis	**Children (≥2 years) and adolescents:** 10–20 mg/kg/day PO in two divided doses. *Maximum:* 1 gram/day PO. **Note:** Administer with food or milk.	Suppository, rectal: 500 mg (base) Suspension, oral: 25 mg/ml (orange flavored) (base); shake gently before use.	**Contraindications:** Hepatic disease (active), hypersensitivity to naproxen or to other NSAIDs, inflammatory disease of the GI tract, peptic ulcers (active), and renal dysfunction (severe).

CHAPTER 14: DRUG DOSING FOR INFANTS, CHILDREN, AND ADOLESCENTS

TABLE 14-1 continued

DRUG (TRADE AND OTHER NAMES)	INDICATION(S)	USUAL PEDIATRIC DOSAGE AND ADMINISTRATION[a]	DOSAGE FORMS	CONTRAINDICATIONS, ADRs, AND COMMENTS[b]
Naproxen Sodium *continued*	**Dysmenorrhea/Pain associated with dental extraction or skeletal trauma**	**Adolescents:** Initial dose, 500 mg PO, then 250 mg PO every 6–8 hr, as needed for pain. *Maximum:* 1250 mg/day PO. **Note:** Reduce dosage for pediatric patients who have renal dysfunction; see Table 14-2.	Tablets, oral: 125, 250, 375, 500 mg (base) Tablets, oral enteric coated: 250, 375, 500 mg (base) Tablet, oral sustained release: 750 mg (base) Tablets, oral: 275, 550 mg (naproxen sodium) **Note:** 250 mg naproxen base = 275 mg naproxen sodium. **Note:** Dosages are listed in terms of naproxen base.	**ADRs:** *See* Chapter 5.
Naratriptan (*Amerge®*)	**Migraine headache**	**Adolescents:** Not recommended, *see* "Comments."	Tablets, oral: 1, 2.5 mg	**Comments:** Studies of single-dose therapy for adolescents have not demonstrated better results than those obtained in comparative placebo studies. Therefore, the use of naratriptan for this age group is not recommended.
Nedocromil, ophthalmic (*Alocril®*) **Note:** *See also* Nedocromil, pulmonary.	**Allergic conjunctivitis,** prophylaxis and treatment (relief of itching)	**Children (≥3 years):** Instill one or two drops of 2% ophthalmic solution in each eye twice daily. **Note:** Therapy should be generally continued throughout the pollen season or until exposure to the offending allergen is over.	Solution, ophthalmic: 2% (in disposable dropper container) **Note:** For ophthalmic use only. **Note:** In order to minimize possible cross-contamination and infections, ensure that separate containers of nedocromil ophthalmic solution are dispensed for each eye.	**Contraindications:** Hypersensitivity to nedocromil. **ADRs:** Commonly causes headache, nasal congestion, ocular irritation (burning or stinging sensation), and unpleasant taste. May cause asthma, conjunctivitis, photophobia, and rhinitis.
Nedocromil, pulmonary (*Tilade®*) **Note:** *See also* Nedocromil, ophthalmic.	**Asthma,** chronic (mild or moderate) **Note:** Not indicated for the relief of an acute asthma attack (bronchospasm).	**Children (≥6 years) and adolescents:** Two actuations of a metered-dose inhaler (3.5 mg) four times daily at regularly spaced intervals.	Solution, metered-dose inhaler: 1.75 mg/actuation; shake well before use. **Note:** For pulmonary inhalation only. **Note:** Initial use of inhaler requires priming with three actuations.	**Contraindications:** Hypersensitivity to nedocromil. **ADRs:** Generally well tolerated. May cause a bad taste, headache, and nausea. **Comments:** Take care not to inadvertently spray solution into the eyes.
Nelfinavir (*Viracept®*)	**HIV infection** (in combination with reverse transcriptase inhibitor nucleoside analogs)	**Children (≥2 years) and adolescents:** 75–90 mg/kg/day PO in three divided doses with food or a light snack *Maximum:* 2250 mg/day PO. **Note:** The powder may be mixed with a small amount of water or other beverage. Acidic beverages (e.g., apple juice, orange juice) may contribute to a bitter taste and should not be used.	Powder, oral: 50 mg/gram (available in 144-gram multiple-use bottle with scoop) **Note:** Each level scoopful of powder contains 50 mg of nelfinavir. **Note:** Each gram of oral powder contains 11.2 mg of phenylalanine. Tablet, oral: 250 mg	**Contraindications:** Hypersensitivity to nelfinavir. **ADRs:** Generally well tolerated. *See* Chapter 5. **Comments:** Rifampin decreases nelfinavir plasma concentrations by more than 80%. Nelfinavir significantly decreases both ethinyl estradiol and norethindrone plasma levels. Concurrent use may result in contraception failure.
Neomycin (*Mycifradin®*, *Neo-Fradin®*)	**Hepatic coma,** adjunctive pharmacotherapy/**Intestinal bacterial infections** **Note:** Ensure that	**Children and adolescents:** 50–150 mg/kg/day PO in three or four divided doses, every 6 or 8 hr. *Maximum:* 12 grams/day PO. **Note:** For hepatic coma, therapy is generally required for 5–6 days. If	Solution, oral: 25 mg/ml (cherry flavored) Tablet, oral: 500 mg **Note:** Not generally available in Canada.	**Contraindications:** Hypersensitivity to neomycin or to other aminoglycosides, inflammatory or ulcerative GI disease (because of potential for increased neomycin absorption), and intestinal obstruction. *(Continued)*

Footnotes are on page 558.

TABLE 14-1 continued

DRUG (TRADE AND OTHER NAMES)	INDICATION(S)	USUAL PEDIATRIC DOSAGE AND ADMINISTRATION[a]	DOSAGE FORMS	CONTRAINDICATIONS, ADRs, AND COMMENTS[b]
Neomycin *continued*	appropriate culture and sensitivity tests are performed and that the organism is sensitive to neomycin.	less toxic drugs cannot be used to treat residual chronic hepatic insufficiency, then neomycin may be continued with a reduced maximal daily dose of 4 grams/day PO.		**ADRs:** May cause diarrhea, nausea, and vomiting. Systemic toxicity may occur with high dosages or prolonged pharmacotherapy. *See* Chapter 5. **Comments:** Poorly absorbed (<5%) from the GI tract.
	Preoperative preparation of the bowel, adjunctive pharmacotherapy **Note:** Often used in combination with erythromycin or metronidazole.	**Children and adolescents:** 100 mg/kg/dose PO immediately following a cathartic. Repeat dose every 4 hr for 24 hr. *Maximum:* 1 gram/dose PO; 6 grams/day PO.		
Neostigmine *(Prostigmin®)*	**Reversal of nondepolarizing neuromuscular blockade following surgery** (usually as adjunctive therapy with atropine)	**Infants, children, and adolescents:** 0.02–0.08 mg/kg/dose IV. *Maximum:* 2.5 mg/dose IV. **Note:** Reduce dosage for pediatric patients who have renal dysfunction; *see* Table 14-2.	Injectables, IM, IV: 0.25, 0.5, 1 mg/ml (1:4000, 1:2000, 1:1000) (methylsulfate salt) Tablet, oral: 15 mg (bromide salt)	**Contraindications:** Asthma, hypersensitivity to neostigmine, and intestinal or urinary tract obstruction. **ADRs:** Generally well tolerated. May cause bradycardia, dyspnea, skin rash, or weakness. **Comments:** Oral dosage requirements are approximately 30 times the dosage requirements for the injectable because the oral tablets are very poorly absorbed from the GI tract (<3%). Pediatric patients who are hypersensitive to bromides may develop an acneiform rash during oral neostigmine bromide therapy. Generally, neostigmine bromide is **not** recommended for these patients.
	Myasthenia gravis, diagnostic test **Note:** Patients with myasthenia gravis demonstrate a significant increase in muscle strength in response to neostigmine.	**Children and adolescents:** 0.04 mg/kg/dose IM as a one-time dose. **Note:** For the diagnostic test, neostigmine should be preceded by atropine (0.011 mg/kg IV, if administered concomitantly; **or** 0.011 mg IM 30 min prior to the administration of neostigmine) to prevent or minimize the adverse muscarinic effects associated with neostigmine.		
	Myasthenia gravis, treatment	**Children and adolescents:** 0.01–0.04 mg/kg/dose IM, IV, or SC every 2 or 3 hr **or** 2 mg/kg/day PO in six divided doses, every 4 hr. *Maximum:* 10 mg/day IM, IV, or SC; 15 mg/dose PO. **Note:** Reduce dosage for pediatric patients who have renal dysfunction; *see* Table 14-2. **Note:** Neostigmine dosage requirements for myasthenia gravis may vary daily depending on the physical and psychological stresses associated with the disease.		
Netilmicin *(Netromycin®)*	**Bacterial infections** **Note:** Ensure that appropriate culture and sensitivity tests are performed and that the organism is sensitive to netilmicin.	**Infants, children, and adolescents:** 3–7.5 mg/kg/day IM or IV in three divided doses, every 8 hr. **Note:** Reduce dosage for pediatric patients who have renal dysfunction; *see* Table 14-2.	Injectables, IM, IV: 10, 25, 50, 100 mg/ml; contains sodium metabisulfite, which is associated with hypersensitivity reactions, including anaphylactic reactions, among susceptible patients. Although uncommon, these reactions appear to occur with a higher incidence among pediatric patients who have asthma. **Note:** Not generally available in the United States.	**Contraindications:** Hypersensitivity to netilmicin or to other aminoglycosides. **ADRs:** *See* Chapter 5. **Comments:** Some pediatric patients (e.g., children with cystic fibrosis) may require higher dosages or more frequent dosing depending on blood concentrations. Therapeutic drug monitoring is recommended; *see* Table 14-3.

TABLE 14-1 *continued*

DRUG (*TRADE* AND OTHER NAMES)	INDICATION(S)	USUAL PEDIATRIC DOSAGE AND ADMINISTRATION[a]	DOSAGE FORMS	CONTRAINDICATIONS, ADRs, AND COMMENTS[b]
Nevirapine (*Viramune®*)	HIV-1 infection and AIDS (as adjunctive pharmacotherapy with other antiretroviral pharmacotherapy)	**Infants (≥2 months) and children (<8 years):** Initially, 4 mg/kg/day PO in a single daily dose for 2 weeks. Follow by 14 mg/kg/day PO in two divided doses. *Maximum:* 400 mg/day PO. **Children (≥8 years) and adolescents:** Initially, 4 mg/kg/day PO in a single daily dose for 2 weeks. Then, 8 mg/kg/day PO in two divided doses. *Maximum:* 400 mg/day PO.	Suspension, oral: 50 mg/5 ml; shake well before use. Tablet, oral: 200 mg	**Contraindications:** Hypersensitivity to nevirapine. **ADRs:** May cause alteration in liver function tests, fever, granulocytopenia, headache, hepatotoxicity, nausea, and rash. Associated with fatal hepatotoxicity and severe, life-threatening skin reactions, including the Stevens-Johnson syndrome and toxic epidermal necrolysis. **Comments:** Monitor hepatic function upon initiation of therapy and at regular intervals.
Nicotine (*Habitrol®*, *Nicoderm®*, *Nicorette®*, *Nicotrol NS®*, *Prostep®*)	Nicotine-withdrawal syndrome associated with the cessation of tobacco smoking **Note:** Not approved by the FDA or HPB for children.	**Adolescents:** Dosage must be prescribed according to tobacco smoking history, signs and symptoms of nicotine withdrawal, the dosage form prescribed (chewing gum, nasal spray, transdermal drug delivery system), and response. The level of nicotine addiction may be assessed using the Fragerström nicotine tolerance scale. Chewing Gum: Instruct patients to chew one piece of gum for up to 30 min when they have a desire to smoke tobacco and not to drink beverages or ingest other liquids (e.g., soup) while chewing the gum. Advise patients not to swallow gum and to discard chewed gum appropriately, to prevent access by children or pets. Nicotine chewing gum therapy may require 6 months for optimal benefit. Discontinue when patients demonstrate an ability to maintain abstinence from tobacco smoking. Decrease the dosage and discontinue use over 1–2 weeks. Advise abstinent patients to carry gum with them for up to 3 months to use when they have a sudden overpowering urge to smoke tobacco. Nasal Spray: Instruct patients to administer each dose of spray (e.g., *Nicotrol NS*) into the nostril(s) with the head tilted slightly backward. Caution them **not** to sniff, swallow, or inhale through the nose as the spray is being administered. One dose is defined as 1 mg of nicotine (one 0.5-mg spray in each nostril). Discontinue gradually (e.g., reduce the dosage of one spray in each nostril to one spray in a single nostril). Some patients may be able to simply discontinue without gradually reducing the dosage.	Chewing gums, buccal (e.g., *Nicorette*): 2, 4 mg (mint flavored) Solution, nasal spray (e.g., *Nicotrol NS*): 10 mg/ml **Note:** The nicotine nasal spray is supplied in a glass container capped with a metered spray pump and child-resistant cap. Each metered-dose spray contains approximately 0.5 mg of nicotine. The unit delivers approximately 200 sprays. Transdermal drug delivery systems (TDDSs) (e.g., *Nicotrol*), 16 hr: 5, 10, 15 mg/hr. Transdermal drug delivery systems (TDDSs) (e.g., *Habitrol*, *Nicoderm*), 24 hr **Note:** Some TDDSs are available in some states and provinces without a prescription.	**Contraindications:** Angina pectoris (severe or worsening), breast feeding, cardiac disease (severe), children, dysrhythmias (life threatening), myocardial infarction (immediately post-myocardial infarction), nonsmokers, peptic ulcer disease (active), pregnancy, skin disorders (generalized, for transdermal nicotine delivery system), and temporomandibular joint disease (active, for nicotine chewing gum). **ADRs:** ADRs include both local and systemic reactions. The local reactions generally are related to the dosage formulation. The systemic reactions are related to the pharmacologic actions of nicotine. **Local ADRs:** *Chewing Gum Formulation*, jaw muscle ache and traumatic injury to the oral tissues, teeth, and jaw related to the mechanical chewing of the gum formulations. Eructation (belching) secondary to air swallowing also may occur. These ADRs may be minimized by advising patients to modify their chewing techniques. Small (aphthous) ulcers on the mucous membranes of the mouth and inflammation of the gums (gingivitis), tongue (glossitis), pharynx (pharyngitis), and mouth (stomatitis), as well as changes in taste perception, can occur among smokers who have ceased tobacco smoking with or without the chewing gum formulation. *Transdermal Drug Delivery System Formulation*, generally associated with local skin irritation, most commonly a redness (erythema) and itching of the skin (pruritus) at the application site, which may be severe. Generally these ADRs are usually insignifi-

(Continued)

Footnotes are on page 558.

TABLE 14-1 *continued*

DRUG (*TRADE* AND OTHER NAMES)	INDICATION(S)	USUAL PEDIATRIC DOSAGE AND ADMINISTRATION[a]	DOSAGE FORMS	CONTRAINDICATIONS, ADRs, AND COMMENTS[b]
Nicotine *continued*		Transdermal Drug Delivery Systems 16- and 24-hr: Apply one 16- or 24-hr TDDS depending on pharmacotherapeutic need once per day upon awakening to a nonhairy, clean, and dry skin site on the upper arm or the hip. Rotate application sites daily. TDDS application sites should not be reused for at least 1 week. Generally, the active TDDS should not be worn for longer than 16–24 hr daily. Instruct patients to avoid unnecessary contact with the active system and to wash their hands only with water after applying the system. After removal, each TDDS should be folded over and placed in its original pouch for appropriate disposal. The used system should be immediately disposed of to prevent inadvertent access by children or pets. Used TDDSs generally contain, on average, over 50% of their initial drug content (enough nicotine to cause serious, even fatal, poisoning if accidentally ingested by small children or pets). If ADRs are experienced, particularly those affecting the cardiovascular system, the dose should be reduced or the transdermal therapy discontinued. Discourage use beyond 12 weeks by patients who cease smoking because long-term use of nicotine by any method is addicting and habituating and otherwise harmful. Discontinue nicotine pharmacotherapy for patients who continue to smoke.		cant and resolve within an hour of removal of the system. Some cases of local redness of the skin (erythema) may resolve within 24 hr. **Systemic ADRs:** Chest pains, fainting (syncope), headache, hypertension, insomnia, irritability, nausea, palpitation, salivation (excessive), tachycardia (tachydysrhythmias), and vomiting. Excessive weight gain has been associated with smoking cessation among smokers. This weight gain is thought to be caused by a combination of the discontinuation of the oral habit of tobacco smoking and its replacement with an increased ingestion of food. It also may be associated with reduced GI motility in the absence of nicotine. Monitor patients for weight gain. A weight maintenance program may be indicated. **Comments:** Nicotine is addicting and habituating. Patients can become addicted to nicotine chewing gum, nasal spray, or transdermal drug delivery systems. Transdermal pharmacotherapy has a lower abuse potential probably because it has a much slower rate of absorption, produces more consistent nicotine blood concentrations, maintains lower blood levels of nicotine, and requires less frequent use (once daily application). Advise patients to follow the instructions for use and gradually discontinue according to their individual planned schedule. **Nicotine pharmacotherapy should not exceed 12 weeks.**
Nifedipine *(Adalat CC®, Adalat XL®, Procardia XL®)*	Hypertension, refractory to less toxic antihypertensives **Note:** Not approved by the FDA or HPB for infants or children.	**Children and adolescents:** 0.5 mg/kg/day PO in two divided doses, every 12 hr; then increase dosage gradually as needed to 1–1.5 mg/kg/day PO in two divided doses, every 12 hr. *Maximum:* 120 mg/day (oral extended-release tablets); 80 mg/day (oral prolonged-action tablets).	Tablets, oral extended release: 20, 30, 60, 90 mg Tablets, oral prolonged action (Canada only): 10, 20 mg **Note:** Although still available, short-acting dosage forms (oral liquid-filled capsules) should **not** be used because of concerns regarding potential severe hypotension and cardiovascular toxicity (e.g., myocardial infarction and stroke) associated with their use.	**Contraindications:** Cardiovascular shock, hypersensitivity to nifedipine, lactation, and pregnancy. **ADRs:** *See* Chapter 5.

CHAPTER 14: DRUG DOSING FOR INFANTS, CHILDREN, AND ADOLESCENTS

TABLE 14-1 continued

DRUG (*TRADE* AND OTHER NAMES)	INDICATION(S)	USUAL PEDIATRIC DOSAGE AND ADMINISTRATION[a]	DOSAGE FORMS	CONTRAINDICATIONS, ADRs, AND COMMENTS[b]
Nitrazepam (*Mogadon*®, *Nitrazadon*®)	Myoclonic seizures	**Children (≤30 kg):** 0.2–1 mg/kg/day PO in three divided doses. *Maximum:* 40 mg/day PO. **Note:** Begin with lower dosages (e.g., 0.2 mg/kg/day PO) and monitor response. Higher dosages may be required for children who are refractory to anticonvulsant pharmacotherapy. However, higher dosages are commonly associated with excessive drowsiness.	Tablets, oral: 5, 10 mg **Note:** Tablets may be chewed, dissolved in liquid, or swallowed whole. **Note:** Not generally available in the United States.	**Contraindications:** Hepatic or respiratory dysfunction (severe), hypersensitivity to nitrazepam or other benzodiazepines, and myasthenia gravis. **ADRs:** Commonly causes ataxia, dizziness, drowsiness, falling, fatigue, lethargy, lightheadedness, mental confusion, and staggering gait. *See* Chapter 5. **Comments:** Long-term use may result in addiction and habituation. Abrupt discontinuation of long-term therapy has been associated with the benzodiazepine-withdrawal syndrome (including seizures). Gradually reduce the dosage when pharmacotherapy is being discontinued.
Nitrofurantoin (*MacroBID*®, *Macrodantin*®)	Urinary tract infections, prophylaxis **Note:** Long-term (≥6 months) prophylactic therapy is **not** recommended because of the risk for chronic pulmonary reactions. *See* "Comments."	**Infants (≥1 month), children, and adolescents:** 1–2 mg/kg/day PO as a single daily dose at bedtime or as two divided doses. *Maximum:* 100 mg/dose PO.	Capsules, oral: 25, 50, 100 mg **Note:** Administer with food or milk to decrease associated GI irritation.	**Contraindications:** Anuria, hypersensitivity to nitrofurantoin, infants (≤1 month), oliguria, and pregnancy. **ADRs:** Generally well tolerated. May cause flatulence, headache, and nausea. *See* Chapter 5. **Comments:** Acute, subacute, and chronic pulmonary reactions (e.g., diffuse interstitial pneumonitis or pulmonary fibrosis) can occur, particularly with long-term pharmacotherapy of 6 months or longer. These rare reactions can occur insidiously and may be fatal. **Note:** Periodically monitor hepatic function among patients receiving long-term therapy.
	Urinary tract infections, treatment **Note:** Ensure that appropriate culture and sensitivity tests have been performed and that the organism is sensitive to nitrofurantoin.	**Infants (≥1 month), children, and adolescents:** 5–7 mg/kg/day PO in four divided doses, every 6 hr. *Maximum:* 400 mg/day PO. **Note:** Reduce dosage for pediatric patients who have renal dysfunction; *see* Table 14-2.		
Nitrogen Mustard, *see* **Mechlorethamine**				
Nitroglycerin (Glyceryl Trinitrate)	Hypertension, severe/Hypertensive emergencies, perioperatively **Note:** Not approved by the FDA or HPB for infants or children.	**Children and adolescents:** Initially, 0.5 μg/kg/min by continuous IV infusion. Adjust dosage at 5-min intervals according to response. *Maximum:* Initial dose, 5 μg/min IV. **Note:** Adjust dosage according to blood pressure and heart rate.	Injectables, IV: 0.5, 0.8, 5, 10 mg/ml; contains alcohol and propylene glycol.	**Contraindications:** Anemia (severe), cerebral hemorrhage, constrictive pericarditis, glaucoma, head trauma, hypotension, hypersensitivity to nitroglycerin or to organic nitrates, myocardial infarction, and pericardial tamponade. **ADRs:** *See* Chapter 5. **Comments:** Continuously monitor blood pressure and heart rate during IV administration.
Nitroprusside, *see* **Sodium Nitroprusside**				
Noradrenaline, *see* **Norepinephrine**				
Norepinephrine (Levarterenol, *Levophed*®, Noradrenaline)	Restoration and maintenance of blood pressure in conditions of acute hypotension or shock, such as those that may occur in the context of blood transfusion reactions,	**Children and adolescents:** Initially, 0.05–0.1 μg/kg/min by continuous IV infusion. Adjust subsequent dosage according to blood pressure. **Note:** Ensure that blood volume deficits have been corrected **before** initiating pharmacotherapy.	Injectable, IV: 1 mg/ml **Note:** For IV use only (*see* "Comments"). **Note:** 1 mg norepinephrine = 2 mg norepinephrine bitartrate. The dosage formulation (*Levophed*), although containing	**Contraindications:** Cyclopropane anesthesia, halothane anesthesia, MAOI therapy (concurrent or within 14 days), and thrombosis. **ADRs:** May cause anxiety, bradycardia, headache (transient), hypertension, and respiratory difficulties.

(Continued)

Footnotes are on page 558.

TABLE 14-1 continued

DRUG (*TRADE* AND OTHER NAMES)	INDICATION(S)	USUAL PEDIATRIC DOSAGE AND ADMINISTRATION[a]	DOSAGE FORMS	CONTRAINDICATIONS, ADRs, AND COMMENTS[b]
Norepineph-rine *continued*	ADRs, myocardial infarction, hemorrhage, pheochromocytomectomy, septicemia, surgery, or trauma. **Note:** Not approved by the FDA or HPB for infants or children.		norepinephrine bitartrate, lists its concentration in terms of norepinephrine equivalents. **Note:** Injectable contains sodium metabisulfite, which is associated with hypersensitivity reactions, including anaphylactic reactions, among susceptible patients. Although uncommon, these reactions appear to occur with a higher incidence among pediatric patients who have asthma.	**Comments:** Extravasation may result in severe tissue sloughing; monitor patency of IV infusion frequently and treat immediately with phentolamine.

Norethindrone and Ethinyl Estradiol, *see* **Ethinyl Estradiol and Norethindrone**

Nortriptyline (*Aventyl®, Pamelor®*)	Endogenous depression	**Adolescents:** 30–50 mg daily PO in three or four divided doses. *Maximum:* 150 mg/day PO.	Capsules, oral: 10, 25, 50, 75 mg Solution, oral: 10 mg/5 ml; contains 4% alcohol. **Note:** Capsules contain sodium bisulfite. Sulfites may cause hypersensitivity reactions, including anaphylactic reactions, among susceptible patients, particularly those with asthma.	**Contraindications:** Hypersensitivity to nortriptyline or to other tricyclic antidepressants (TCAs); MAOI therapy (concurrent or within 14 days); and myocardial infarction, including acute recovery phase. **ADRs:** ADRs include those that are common to the tricyclic antidepressants. *See* Chapter 5. **Comments:** Caution is indicated for pediatric patients who have histories of urinary retention, cardiovascular disorders, bipolar disorder, psychotic disorders, seizure disorders, hypothyroidism, or who require electroconvulsive therapy. May interact with anticholinergics (e.g., atropine) or other drugs that produce anticholinergic actions (e.g., phenothiazines). *See* Chapter 6. **Note:** All depressed patients should be evaluated for suicide risk and any risk should be appropriately dealt with.
Nystatin (*Candistatin®, Mycostatin®, Nilstat®*)	Cutaneous and mucocutaneous mycotic infections caused by *Candida* (monilia) species	**Infants, children, and adolescents:** Apply topical cream or ointment liberally to affected area(s) twice daily.	Cream, topical: 100,000 units/gram Creams, vaginal: 25,000, 100,000 units/gram (with applicator) Suspension, topical oral: 100,000 units/ml (with calibrated dropper) (cherry flavored); may contain <1% alcohol; shake well before use. Tablet, oral: 500,000 units (contains tartrazine) Tablet, vaginal: 100,000 units (with applicator) Troche, topical oral: 200,000 units **Note:** Topical cream and ointment are for external use only. Avoid contact with eyes.	**Contraindications:** Hypersensitivity to nystatin. **ADRs:** Generally well tolerated. Oral therapy may cause diarrhea, nausea, and vomiting. *See* Chapter 5. **Comments:** Not absorbed across mucous membranes in the mouth and is poorly absorbed from the GI tract.
	Intestinal moniliasis	**Infants, children, and adolescents:** 400,000 units/day PO in four divided doses, every 6 hr.		
	Oral candidiasis (thrush)	**Infants, children, and adolescents:** 400,000 units/day (topical oral suspension or troche) topically to oral mucosa in four divided doses, every 6 hr. **Note:** Instruct patient to retain suspension or troche in mouth as long as possible before swallowing.		
	Vulvovaginal candidiasis	**Adolescents:** 100,000 units of vaginal cream or tablet vaginally once daily at bedtime for 14 days.		

CHAPTER 14: DRUG DOSING FOR INFANTS, CHILDREN, AND ADOLESCENTS

TABLE 14-1 continued

DRUG (TRADE AND OTHER NAMES)	INDICATION(S)	USUAL PEDIATRIC DOSAGE AND ADMINISTRATION[a]	DOSAGE FORMS	CONTRAINDICATIONS, ADRs, AND COMMENTS[b]
Octreotide (Sandostatin®)	**Gigantism** (usually as a result of a pituitary adenoma but may be associated with excess growth hormone secretion from other tumors such as macroadenoma or optic glioma)	**Children and adolescents:** Initially, 50 μg/dose SC once or twice daily. Dosage is then adjusted according to response. Usual dosage is 300 μg/day SC in three divided doses. *Maximum:* 1500 μg/day SC. **Note:** Significant reduction in growth hormone concentrations and clinical improvement of signs and symptoms should be noted within 3 months. (*See* "Comments.")	Injectables, IV, SC: 0.05, 0.1, 0.2, 0.5, 1 mg/ml	**Contraindications:** Hypersensitivity to octreotide. **ADRs:** May cause a variety of ADRs affecting several body systems, including abdominal pain, anemia, backache, bruising, congestive heart failure, diarrhea, dizziness, fatigue, fat malabsorption, headache, hyperglycemia, hypertension, hypothyroidism, joint pain, nausea, pain at injection site, palpitation, pancreatitis, pruritus, rash, reduction in vitamin B_{12} blood concentrations, rash, sinus bradycardia, and weakness. **Comments:** Growth hormone concentrations must be measured at 1-hr intervals for the first 8 hr of therapy to provide an indication of response and to guide dosage adjustments. Therapeutic benefit is generally associated with growth hormone concentrations <5 ng/ml.
Omeprazole (Losec®, Prilosec®)	**Refractory reflux esophagitis, treatment**	**Children and adolescents:** 20 mg/day PO as a single dose. *Maximum:* 40 mg/day PO.	Capsules, oral delayed release: 10, 20, 40 mg Tablets, oral delayed release: 10, 20 mg **Note:** The oral delayed-release capsule may be opened and the intact pellets administered in a small amount (5 ml) of an acidic beverage (pH <5.3). Stir pellets into the beverage immediately prior to ingestion.	**Contraindications:** Hypersensitivity to omeprazole. **ADRs:** Generally well tolerated. May cause abdominal pain, diarrhea, dizziness, flatulence, and headache. **Comments:** Omeprazole pharmacotherapy may alleviate (or mask) some of the signs and symptoms of gastric carcinoma, and thus confound diagnosis.
	Refractory reflux esophagitis, prophylaxis **Note:** Not approved by the FDA or HPB for these indications for infants or children.	**Children and adolescents:** 10 mg/day PO as a single dose. *Maximum:* 20 mg/day PO.		
Ondansetron (Zofran®)	**Prophylaxis of nausea and vomiting** associated with emetogenic antineoplastic pharmacotherapy	**Children (≥4 years) and adolescents:** 0.15 mg/kg/dose IV prior to and 4 and 8 hr following the administration of emetogenic antineoplastic pharmacotherapy; **or** 2 mg/dose PO for body surface area <0.6 m^2, 4 mg/dose PO for body surface area 0.6–1.2 m^2, and 8 mg/dose PO for body surface area >1.2 m^2, prior to and 4 and 8 hr following the administration of an emetogenic antineoplastic. *Maximum:* 8 mg/dose IV or PO. **Note:** First dose is generally administered 30 min prior to the administration of the emetogenic drug. **Note:** Reduce dosage for pediatric patients who have hepatic dysfunction.	Injectable, IV: 2 mg/ml Solution, oral: 4 mg/5 ml (strawberry flavored) Tablets, oral: 4, 8 mg Tablets, oral disintegrating (Zofran ODT®): 4, 8 mg (strawberry flavored); contain aspartame.	**Contraindications:** Hypersensitivity to ondansetron. **ADRs:** May cause agitation, anxiety, constipation, diarrhea, drowsiness, fever, headache, and sedation.

Orciprenaline, *see* **Metaproterenol**

Footnotes are on page 558.

TABLE 14-1 continued

DRUG (TRADE AND OTHER NAMES)	INDICATION(S)	USUAL PEDIATRIC DOSAGE AND ADMINISTRATION[a]	DOSAGE FORMS	CONTRAINDICATIONS, ADRs, AND COMMENTS[b]
Orlistat (Xenical®)	**Obesity** among patients who have a body mass index (BMI) ≥ 30 kg/m^2 **Note:** Generally reserved for use among obese patients who have one or more of the following cardiovascular risk factors: diabetes, excess visceral fat, dyslipidemia, and hypertension. **Note:** Optimal benefit requires use of orlistat in conjunction with an appropriate diet and exercise program. **Note:** Not approved by the FDA or HPB for children or adolescents.	**Adolescents:** 360 mg/day PO in three divided doses, with each main meal. **Note:** Can be administered during or up to 1 hr after the main meal.	Capsule, oral: 120 mg **Note:** Adolescents and their parents should be encouraged to contact the manufacturer at the toll-free number provided in order to enroll in and take advantage of the free "*Xenical* Body Wellness Support Program" offered by the manufacturer.	**Contraindications:** Cholestasis, hypersensitivity to orlistat, and malabsorption syndrome (chronic). **ADRs:** Generally well tolerated. Commonly causes GI ADRs when dietary fat intake exceeds 30% of total caloric intake. ADRs are directly related to the amount of dietary fat ingested and include abdominal pain, diarrhea (e.g., liquid or soft stools), fecal urgency, flatulence, and oily spotting. **Comments:** The absorption of fat-soluble vitamins may be affected by orlistat pharmacotherapy. Advise patients to take a multiple-vitamin supplement that contains fat-soluble vitamins and beta-carotene to ensure adequate nutrition is maintained. The vitamin supplement, and other required oral pharmacotherapy, generally should be ingested 2 hr before or after the ingestion of orlistat, or at bedtime, in order to minimize possible interference with absorption. **Note:** BMI can be calculated by simply dividing the total body weight in kilograms (kg) by height in meters squared (m^2).
Oseltamivir (Tamiflu®)	**Influenza infection, uncomplicated** **Note:** For maximal therapeutic benefit, initiate within 2 days of the onset of the signs and symptoms of influenza. **Note:** Approved by the FDA but not by the HPB for children.	**Children:** Dosing for children is based on body weight. *See* accompanying table. **Oseltamivir Dosing for Children**	BODY WEIGHT	RECOMMENDED DOSAGE		---	---		≤ 15 kg	60 mg/day PO in two divided doses		>15–23 kg	90 mg/day PO in two divided doses		>23–40 kg	120 mg/day PO in two divided doses		>40 kg	150 mg/day PO in two divided doses	*Maximum:* 150 mg/day PO. **Adolescents:** 150 mg/day PO in two divided doses for 5 days. **Note:** Reduce dosage for pediatric patients who have severe renal dysfunction (reduce the daily dosage by 50% if creatinine clearance is <30 ml/min).	Capsule, oral: 75 mg Suspension, oral: 12 mg/ml (tutti-frutti flavored); shake well before use. **Note:** Suspension should be constituted by pharmacist **prior** to dispensing to the patient. The oral suspension should be used within 10 days of preparation and any remaining suspension safely and appropriately discarded.	**Contraindications:** Hypersensitivity to oseltamivir. **ADRs:** Generally well tolerated. May cause abdominal pain, diarrhea, insomnia, nausea, and vomiting. **Comments:** Available data suggest that annual influenza vaccination should still be performed. Oseltamivir does not appear to impair humoral antibody response.

CHAPTER 14: DRUG DOSING FOR INFANTS, CHILDREN, AND ADOLESCENTS

TABLE 14-1 continued

DRUG (TRADE AND OTHER NAMES)	INDICATION(S)	USUAL PEDIATRIC DOSAGE AND ADMINISTRATION[a]	DOSAGE FORMS	CONTRAINDICATIONS, ADRs, AND COMMENTS[b]
Oseltamivir *continued*	Influenza prophylaxis (during community outbreak) **Note:** Not approved by the FDA or HPB for infants or children.	**Children and adolescents:** Dosage is based on body weight. See accompanying table. **Oseltamivir Dosing for Children and Adolescents: Community Influenza Outbreak** **BODY WEIGHT** / **RECOMMENDED DOSAGE** ≤15 kg / 30 mg/day PO in a single dose >15–23 kg / 45 mg/day PO in a single dose >23–40 kg / 60 mg/day PO in a single dose >40 kg / 75 mg/day PO in a single dose **Note:** For the prophylaxis of influenza during a community outbreak, oseltamivir can be safely administered on a daily basis for up to 6 weeks.		
Oxacillin	Bacterial infections, mild to moderate Bacterial infections, severe **Note:** Ensure that appropriate culture and sensitivity tests are performed and that the organism is sensitive to oxacillin.	**Infants, children, and adolescents:** 50–100 mg/kg/day PO in four divided doses, every 6 hr. *Maximum:* 3 grams/day PO. **Infants, children, and adolescents:** 150–200 mg/kg/day IM or IV in four to six divided doses, every 4–6 hr. *Maximum:* 12 grams/day IM or IV.	Capsules, oral: 250, 500 mg Injectables, IM, IV: 250, 500 mg/vial; 1, 2, 4, 10 grams/vial Solution, oral: 50 mg/ml **Note:** Not generally available in Canada.	**Contraindications:** Hypersensitivity to oxacillin or to other penicillins. **ADRs:** *See* Chapter 5.
Oxcarbazepine *(Trileptal®)*	Seizures, partial (used as adjunctive therapy generally in combination with carbamazepine or phenytoin, however, oxcarbazepine monotherapy also has been found to be efficacious)	**Children (≥4 years) and adolescents:** Initially, 8–10 mg/kg/day PO in two divided doses. Increase dosage gradually over 2 weeks according to response. **Note:** Dosages of 6–51 mg/kg/day (median: 31.4 mg/kg/day) have been required for the management of partial seizures for some pediatric patients. Generally, these dosages have been well tolerated. *Maximum:* Initial dosage, 600 mg/day PO. *Maintenance:* The recommended maintenance dosage is determined by body weight. *See* accompanying table:	Tablets, oral: 150, 300, 600 mg **Note:** Not generally available in Canada.	**Contraindications:** Hypersensitivity to oxcarbazepine or to carbamazepine. **ADRs:** May cause abdominal pain, abnormal vision, ataxia, diplopia, dizziness, dyspepsia, fatigue, headache, hyponatremia, nausea, rash, somnolence, tremor, and vomiting. **Comments:** Monitor patients for hyponatremia. **Note:** Oxcarbazepine can induce CYP 3A4 and inhibit CYP 2C19.

(Continued)

Footnotes are on page 558.

TABLE 14-1 *continued*

DRUG (*TRADE* AND OTHER NAMES)	INDICATION(S)	USUAL PEDIATRIC DOSAGE AND ADMINISTRATION[a]	DOSAGE FORMS	CONTRAINDICATIONS, ADRs, AND COMMENTS[b]
Oxcarbazepine *continued*		**Recommended Oxcarbazepine Maintenance Dosages for Children and Adolescents**		
		BODY WEIGHT / **RECOMMENDED DOSAGE**		
		20–29 kg / 900 mg/day PO in two divided doses		
		>29–39 kg / 1200 mg/day PO in two divided doses		
		>39 kg / 1800 mg/day PO in two divided doses		
		Note: Maximal maintenance dosage is 1800 mg/day PO.		
Oxybutynin (*Ditropan®*)	Neurogenic bladder	**Children (<5 years):** 0.5 mg/kg/day PO in four divided doses. **Children (≥5 years):** 10 mg/day PO in two divided doses. *Maximum:* 20 mg/day PO (5 mg/dose PO) in four divided doses.	Syrup, oral: 1 mg/ml Tablet, oral: 5 mg	**Contraindications:** Glaucoma, hypersensitivity to oxybutynin, megacolon, myasthenia gravis, and obstruction of the GI tract. **ADRs:** *See* "Anticholinergics" in Chapter 5. **Comments:** May cause heat prostration (fever and heat stroke as a result of inability to regulate body temperature [decreased perspiration] in hot climatic or environmental conditions).
	Nocturnal enuresis **Note: Not** approved by the FDA or HPB for infants or children younger than 5 years.	**Children:** 5 mg/day PO as a single daily dose 30 min before bedtime.		
Oxymetazoline, nasal (*Afrin Children's Nose Drops®, Afrin Nasal Solution®, Allerest 12 Hr Nasal Solution®, Dristan Long Lasting Nasal Mist/Solution®, Sinarest 12 Hr Nasal Solution®*)	Nasal congestion **Note:** For short-term use (generally not to exceed 5 days). Rebound nasal congestion can occur upon discontinuation.	**Children (2–5 years):** Instill two or three drops of 0.025% nasal solution in affected nostril(s) twice daily, morning and evening. **Children (>5 years) and adolescents:** Instill two or three drops of 0.05% nasal solution, or instruct child or adolescent to sniff spray, in affected nostril(s) twice daily, morning and evening.	Solution, nasal: 0.025%, 0.05% (available in both dropper and spray bottles) **Note:** For intranasal use only.	**Contraindications:** Hypersensitivity to oxymetazoline or to other sympathomimetic amines. **ADRs:** Generally well tolerated. May cause local irritation of mucous membranes of the nasal passages (e.g., burning sensation, drying of nasal mucosa). **Comments:** *See* Chapter 1 for recommended techniques for administering nasal drops and sprays to pediatric patients and for minimizing systemic absorption.
Oxymetazoline, ophthalmic (*Ocu Clear® Eye Drops, Visine L. R.® Eye Drops*)	Eye irritation and redness, minor **Note:** For short-term use (generally not to exceed 3 days). Rebound hyperemia can occur upon discontinuation.	**Children (≥6 years) and adolescents:** Instill one or two drops of 0.025% ophthalmic solution in affected eye(s) every 6 hr, as needed according to response.	Solution, ophthalmic: 0.025% **Note:** For ophthalmic use only. **Note:** Safely and appropriately discard cloudy or discolored solution. **Note:** In order to minimize cross-infections whenever both eyes require oxymetazoline ophthalmic pharmacotherapy, ensure that separate containers are dispensed for each eye.	**Contraindications:** Glaucoma and hypersensitivity to oxymetazoline. **ADRs:** Generally well tolerated. May cause local irritation (e.g., burning sensation, irritation, blurring of vision) and increased intraocular pressure. **Comments:** *See* Chapter 1 for recommended techniques for administering ophthalmic drops and for minimizing systemic absorption.

Paclitaxel, *see* **Chapter 12**

TABLE 14-1 continued

DRUG (TRADE AND OTHER NAMES)	INDICATION(S)	USUAL PEDIATRIC DOSAGE AND ADMINISTRATION[a]	DOSAGE FORMS	CONTRAINDICATIONS, ADRs, AND COMMENTS[b]
Palivizumab (*Synagis*®)	Respiratory syncytial virus (RSV) infection, prophylaxis (provision of passive immunity) **Note:** Efficacy is limited. Reduces the number of hospitalizations of high-risk patients for severe, RSV-associated, lower respiratory tract infections by ~55%. **Note:** Generally reserved for infants and children (<2 years) who have chronic lung disease (e.g., bronchopulmonary dysplasia; cystic fibrosis), congenital heart disease, a history of premature birth (gestational age ≤35 weeks), or immunodeficiency.	**Infants and children (≤2 years):** Initially, 15 mg/kg/dose IM prior to the RSV season. Administer each subsequent dose prophylactically at monthly intervals during the RSV season (generally from the beginning of November to the end of April). **Note:** Divide dosages exceeding 1 ml total volume of reconstituted solution so that no more than 1 ml is injected into any one site. The vastus lateralis IM injection site is recommended. *See* Chapter 1 for recommended IM injection sites and techniques for administering IM injections for infants and children.	Injectable, IM: 100 mg/ml (after reconstitution) (in single-use vials) **Note:** For IM use only. **Note:** Reconstitute by slowly injecting 1 ml of sterile water for injection into single-dose vial and gently swirling for ~30 sec to ensure dissolution without foaming. Do **not** shake. Before use, allow reconstituted solution to stand at room temperature for 20 min until clear or slightly opalescent. Safely and appropriately discard any unused reconstituted solution after 6 hr. **Note:** Not generally available in Canada.	**Contraindications:** Congenital heart disease and hypersensitivity to palivizumab or to murine protein. **ADRs:** Generally well tolerated. May cause cough, pain at injection site, pharyngitis, rhinitis, and rash.
Pancreatin (*Donnazyme*®, *Entozyme*®, *Hi-Vegi-Lip*®, *Pancrezyme*®)	Steatorrhea associated with pancreatic enzyme deficiency **Note:** Although not generally able to provide total management of steatorrhea, usually reduces steatorrhea significantly.	**Children and adolescents:** Initially, one or two tablets PO with each meal and snack. Adjust dosage according to response in regard to the management of steatorrhea. **Note:** Pancreatin microtablets should be swallowed whole and not chewed. Instruct children and adolescents to ingest each dose with a full glass (240 ml) of fruit juice or water.	Microtablets, oral enteric coated: 300, 500, 2400, 7200 mg **Note:** Microtablets contain varying amounts of amylase (12,500–180,000 units), lipase (1000–22,500 units), and protease (12,500–180,000 units) depending on manufacturer. **Note:** Instruct pediatric patients not to chew or crush microtablets. Caution patients not to ingest microtablets with antacids or foods or beverages that are highly alkaline (have a pH >5.5) because the protective enteric coating may be dissolved. **Note:** Not generally available in Canada.	**Contraindications:** Hypersensitivity to pancreatin or to pork products (some pancreatin formulations are derived from porcine sources) and pancreatitis (acute). **ADRs:** Generally well tolerated. May cause GI distress (e.g., cramps, diarrhea, nausea) and perianal irritation. **Comments:** Do not use pancreatin products interchangeably. Pancreatin products differ in enzyme content.
Pancrelipase (*Cotazym*®, *Pancrease*®, *Ultrase*®, *Viokase*®, *Zymase*®)	Steatorrhea associated with pancreatic enzyme deficiency **Note:** Although not generally able to provide total management of steatorrhea, usually reduces steatorrhea significantly.	**Infants (≥6 months):** 2000 units of lipase/dose PO with each meal. **Children (1–6 years):** 4000–8000 units of lipase/dose PO with each meal and snack. **Children (>6 years):** 4000–16,000 units of lipase/dose PO with each meal and snack. **Adolescents:** 4000–48,000 units of lipase/dose PO with each meal and snack.	Capsules, oral: 8000, 10,000, 12,000, 20,000, 25,000 units lipase Microcapsules, oral: 12,000, 25,000 units lipase Microtablets, oral: 10,000, 16,000 units lipase Tablets, oral: 8000, 10,000, 11,000, 16,000 units lipase	**Contraindications:** Hypersensitivity to pancrelipase or to pork products and pancreatitis (acute). **ADRs:** Generally well tolerated. May cause GI distress (e.g., cramps, diarrhea, nausea). **Comments:** Do not use pancrelipase products interchangeably. Pancrelipase products differ in enzyme content.

(Continued)

Footnotes are on page 558.

TABLE 14-1 continued

DRUG (TRADE AND OTHER NAMES)	INDICATION(S)	USUAL PEDIATRIC DOSAGE AND ADMINISTRATION[a]	DOSAGE FORMS	CONTRAINDICATIONS, ADRs, AND COMMENTS[b]
Pancrelipase *continued*		*Maximum:* 88,000 units of lipase/dose PO. **Note:** Adjust dosage according to response with attention to management of steatorrhea. **Note:** Each oral dose of pancrelipase microcapsules and microtablets should be swallowed whole and not chewed. Instruct children and adolescents to ingest each dose with a full glass (240 ml) of fruit juice or water.	**Note:** All products also contain varying amounts of amylase (24,000–75,000 units) and protease (24,000–75,000 units) depending on manufacturer. **Note:** Do not take with antacids or foods or beverages that are highly alkaline (have a pH >5.5) because the protective enteric coating may be dissolved.	
Pancuronium Bromide	Facilitation of endotracheal intubation in patients with status epilepticus/ Facilitation of mechanical ventilation **Note:** Succinylcholine is generally administered **prior** to pancuronium bromide to facilitate endotracheal intubation.	**Infants, children, and adolescents:** Initially, 40–100 µg/kg/dose IV; then 10–20 µg/kg/dose IV every 30–60 min, as needed according to response. **Note:** Reduce dosage for pediatric patients who have renal dysfunction. If succinylcholine is used for endotracheal intubation, decrease initial pancuronium dose by 33%. Reduce dosage for pediatric patients who have hepatic dysfunction.	Injectables, IV: 1, 2 mg/ml; contains benzyl alcohol.	**Contraindications:** Hypersensitivity to bromides or to pancuronium. **ADRs:** May cause excessive salivation, slightly elevated blood pressure and pulse, and sweating. **Comments:** Nondepolarizing neuromuscular blockers, such as pancuronium bromide, may cause respiratory paralysis. This action may be antagonized by cholinesterase inhibitors.

Parabromdylamine, *see* **Brompheniramine**

Paracetamol, *see* **Acetaminophen**

Paraldehyde	Status epilepticus/ Seizures refractory to conventional anticonvulsants **Note:** Paraldehyde pharmacotherapy is generally considered to be obsolete being replaced with newer and safer pharmacotherapy, such as diazepam. However, paraldehyde pharmacotherapy may still be of clinical usefulness in rare situations where the patient cannot tolerate, or is refractory to, the preferred safer pharmacotherapy.	**Children:** 200–400 mg/kg/dose (0.2–0.4 ml undiluted/kg/dose) prepared as a 30%–50% solution in cottonseed oil, olive oil, or normal saline rectally every 4–8 hr, as needed **or** 100–150 mg/kg (2–3 ml of 5% solution/kg) IV over 15–20 min, followed by 20 mg/kg/hr (0.4 ml of 5% solution/kg/hr) as a continuous IV infusion. **Note:** Reduce dosage for pediatric patients who have hepatic or renal dysfunction. Only use glass or hard plastic syringes and administration sets (avoid the use of polyvinylchloride [PVC] syringes and administration sets) for paraldehyde administration. Rectal administration is preferred. IV therapy only is recommended for emergency situations.	Injectable, IV: 1 gram/ml (Canada only) Solution, oral or rectal: 1 gram/ml **Note:** Injectable is not commercially available in the United States and must be freshly prepared under sterile conditions in the pharmacy department of a hospital prior to use. Avoid getting solution on the clothing, in the eyes, or on the skin because of associated contact dermatitis.	**Contraindications:** Chronic obstructive lung disease (e.g., asthma), gastroenteritis, and hepatic insufficiency (severe). **ADRs:** Commonly causes erythematous rash and gastric irritation. May also cause metabolic acidosis. Prolonged use may result in addiction and habituation. *See* Chapter 5.
Paromomycin *(Humatin®)*	Hepatic coma, adjunctive pharmacotherapy Intestinal amebiasis **Note:** Not effective for the treatment of extraintestinal amebiasis.	**Adolescents:** 4 grams/day PO in four divided doses for 5 or 6 days. **Children and adolescents:** 25–35 mg/kg/day PO in three divided doses with meals for 5–10 days. *Maximum:* 3 grams/day PO.	Capsules, oral: 250 mg **Note:** Not generally available in the United States.	**Contraindications:** Hypersensitivity to paromomycin or to other aminoglycosides, intestinal obstruction, and ulcerative colitis. **ADRs:** Generally well tolerated. May cause diarrhea, nausea, and vomiting, particularly when dosage exceeds 3 grams/day. **Comments:** Generally is not absorbed from the GI tract; therefore, systemic toxicity (e.g., eighth cranial nerve damage and renal damage) are only encountered rarely.

TABLE 14-1 continued

DRUG (TRADE AND OTHER NAMES)	INDICATION(S)	USUAL PEDIATRIC DOSAGE AND ADMINISTRATION[a]	DOSAGE FORMS	CONTRAINDICATIONS, ADRs, AND COMMENTS[b]
Paroxetine (Paxil®)	Depression/ Generalized anxiety disorder/ Obsessive-compulsive disorder/Panic disorder, with or without agoraphobia/ Post-traumatic stress disorder/ Social anxiety disorder **Note:** Not approved by the FDA or HPB for children or adolescents.	**Adolescents:** Initially, 10 mg/day PO as a single morning dose. Increase dosage by increments of 10 mg/day at weekly intervals. Adjust dosage according to response. *Maximum:* 60 mg/day PO.	Suspension, oral: 10 mg/15 ml (orange flavored); shake well before use Tablets, oral: 10, 20, 30, 40 mg Tablets, oral controlled release *(Paxil CR):* 12.5, 25 mg **Note:** Controlled-release formulation is not recommended for adolescents because of the lack of available clinical data regarding its use with this age group.	**Contraindications:** Hypersensitivity to paroxetine or to other selective serotonin reuptake inhibitors (SSRIs) and MAOI therapy (concurrent or within 14 days). **ADRs:** *See* Chapter 5. **Comments:** Paroxetine and other SSRIs are involved in clinically significant drug interactions primarily involving protein binding and inhibition of hepatic microsomal enzyme systems. For a comprehensive discussion, *see* "Selected Serotonin Reuptake Inhibitors," in Chapter 6. **Note:** All depressed patients should be evaluated for suicide risk and any risk should be appropriately dealt with.
Pemirolast (Alamast®)	Allergic conjunctivitis (treatment of itching of the eye[s])	**Children (≥ 3 years) and adolescents:** One or two drops pemirolast ophthalmic solution in affected eye(s) four times daily. **Note:** May require up to 4 weeks of pharmacotherapy to achieve maximal benefit.	Solution, ophthalmic: 0.1% (supplied in a 10-ml polyethylene bottle with a controlled dropper tip) **Note:** For ophthalmic use only. **Note:** Not generally available in Canada.	**Contraindications:** Hypersensitivity to pemirolast. **ADRs:** May cause cold- and flulike signs and symptoms, eye discomfort, headache, and rhinitis.
Pemoline (Cylert®)	Attention-deficit/ hyperactivity disorder (A-D/HD) **Note:** Not considered the drug of first choice for the symptomatic management of A-D/HD because of its association with life-threatening hepatic failure. *See* "Note" with ADRs.	**Children (≥6 years) and adolescents:** Initially, 37.5 mg/day PO as a single dose each morning. Increase the daily dosage weekly by 18.75-mg increments until optimal therapeutic response is achieved. Most patients benefit from daily dosages between 56.25 and 75 mg. Therapeutic response is gradual. Significant benefit may not be observed until the third or fourth week. *Maintenance:* 0.5–3 mg/kg/day PO as a single daily dose or as two divided doses. *Maximum:* 3 mg/kg/day PO **or** 112.5 mg/day PO, whichever is less.	Tablets, oral: 18.75, 37.5, 75 mg Tablet, oral chewable: 37.5 mg **Note:** Not generally available in Canada.	**Contraindications:** Hepatic dysfunction and hypersensitivity to pemoline. **ADRs:** Has been associated with insomnia prior to the achievement of an optimal therapeutic dosage. The insomnia usually remits with continued therapy or with a reduction in dosage. It also has been associated with anorexia and weight loss during the first weeks. Patients generally regain their lost weight within 3–6 months. Also may cause convulsions; depression (mild); dizziness; drowsiness; dyskinetic movements of the tongue, lips, face, and extremities; hallucinations; irritability (increased); nystagmus; and skin rashes. *See* Chapter 5. **Note:** Therapy over several months has been associated with hepatic dysfunction and abnormal changes in liver function tests. These abnormal changes in liver function are thought to be associated with a delayed hypersensitivity reaction and appear to be reversible upon discontinuation. Jaundice also has been reported. It also has been associated with potentially fatal acute hepatic failure, which may occur *(Continued)*

Footnotes are on page 558.

TABLE 14-1 continued

DRUG (TRADE AND OTHER NAMES)	INDICATION(S)	USUAL PEDIATRIC DOSAGE AND ADMINISTRATION[a]	DOSAGE FORMS	CONTRAINDICATIONS, ADRs, AND COMMENTS[b]
Pemoline *continued*				suddenly or following years of therapy and may require a liver transplant. **Comments:** Monitor for signs and symptoms of hepatotoxicity (change in liver enzymes, dark amber urine, fatigue, jaundice, nausea). If signs and symptoms are noted, immediately discontinue pemoline. **Note:** Whenever possible, occasionally interrupt long-term therapy to determine if there is a recurrence of the signs and symptoms of A-D/HD. Evaluate these signs and symptoms in order to determine if they are sufficient to necessitate continuation of pharmacotherapy.
Penicillamine (*Cuprimine®*, *Depen®*, D-Penicillamine) **Note**: *See also* Chapter 4.	Arsenic poisoning	**Children and adolescents:** 100 mg/kg/day PO in four divided doses, every 6 hr, for 5 days. *Maximum:* 2 grams/day PO.	Capsules, oral: 125, 250 mg Tablet, oral: 250 mg **Note:** Administer at least 1 hr before or 2 hr after a meal. Ensure adequate fluid intake.	**Contraindications:** Blood dyscrasias, hypersensitivity to penicillamine, pharmacotherapy (concurrent) with nephrotoxic drugs, pregnancy (except for the treatment of Wilson's disease), and renal insufficiency. **ADRs:** Causes many ADRs, including several that are potentially fatal. Thus, close monitoring is essential. ADRs include anorexia, bone marrow depression, diarrhea, dyspepsia, ecchymoses, glomerulonephritis, hepatic impairment, hypogeusia, intra-alveolar hemorrhage, lymphadenopathy, pemphigus, and thrombocytopenia. *See* Chapter 5. **Comments:** Check for allergy to penicillins or cephalosporins prior to administration. Monitor blood counts and hepatic function. Administer on an empty stomach. Do not co-administer penicillamine with any other drugs. The use of antimalarial, antineoplastic, gold, or phenylbutazone pharmacotherapy is contraindicated during penicillamine pharmacotherapy. Treatment of cystinuria should be adjusted to limit cystine urinary excretion to 100–200 mg/day (100 mg/day in patients with associated stone formation or pain). Treatment for lead poisoning should continue until the lead blood levels remain below 40 μg/dl for 2 consecutive months. For Wilson's disease, adjust dosage according to copper urinary concentration. Pyridoxine supplementation may be required, particularly for patients with Wilson's disease (if a multivitamin supplement is used, ensure that it does not contain copper).
	Cystinuria	**Children and adolescents:** 30 mg/kg/day PO in four divided doses, every 6 hr. *Maximum:* 2 grams/day PO.		
	Juvenile rheumatoid arthritis refractory to conventional pharmacotherapy	**Children and adolescents:** Initially, 3–5 mg/kg/day PO as a single daily dose; increase dosage at 2–3-month intervals to a maximum of 15 mg/kg/day PO; large dosages may be administered in two or three divided doses. *Maximum:* Initially, 250 mg/day PO; maintenance, 1 gram/day PO.		
	Lead poisoning	**Children and adolescents:** 30–40 mg/kg/day PO in four divided doses, every 6 hr. *Maximum:* 2 grams/day PO.		
	Wilson's disease	**Infants (<6 months):** 250 mg/day PO as a single daily dose. **Infants (≥6 months) and children:** 500–750 mg/day in two or three divided doses. **Adolescents:** 1 gram/day PO in four divided doses. *Maximum:* 2 grams/day PO.		

CHAPTER 14: DRUG DOSING FOR INFANTS, CHILDREN, AND ADOLESCENTS

TABLE 14-1 continued

DRUG (TRADE AND OTHER NAMES)	INDICATION(S)	USUAL PEDIATRIC DOSAGE AND ADMINISTRATION[a]	DOSAGE FORMS	CONTRAINDICATIONS, ADRs, AND COMMENTS[b]
Penicillin G	**Bacterial infections** **Note:** Ensure that appropriate culture and sensitivity tests are performed and that the organism is sensitive to penicillin G.	**Children and adolescents:** 25–50 mg/kg/day PO in three or four divided doses, every 6–8 hr, **or** 25,000–400,000 units/kg/day IM or IV in six divided doses, every 4 hr. *Maximum:* 3 grams/day PO; 24 million units/day IM or IV. **Note:** Reduce dosage for pediatric patients who have renal dysfunction; see Table 14-2.	**Potassium salt** Injectables, IM, IV: 200,000, 500,000, 1 million, 5 million, 10 million, 20 million units/vial Solutions, oral: 40,000, 80,000 units/ml Tablets, oral: 240, 250, 500 mg **Sodium salt** Injectable, IM, IV: 5 million units/vial **Note:** Penicillin G potassium: 1 mg = 1355–1595 units. Penicillin G sodium: 1 mg = 1420–1667 units.	**Contraindications:** Hypersensitivity to penicillin G or to other penicillins. **ADRs:** See Chapter 5.
Penicillin G Benzathine, see Chapter 13				
Penicillin G Procaine *(Wycillin®)*	**Bacterial infections** **Note:** Ensure that appropriate culture and sensitivity tests are performed and that the organism is sensitive to penicillin G procaine.	**Infants, children, and adolescents:** 25,000–50,000 units/kg/day IM as a single daily dose or as two divided doses, every 12 hr. *Maximum:* 2 million units/day IM.	Injectables, IM: 300,000, 500,000, 600,000 units/ml; contains povidone.	**Contraindications:** Hypersensitivity to penicillin G procaine, to other penicillins, or to procaine. **ADRs:** See Chapter 5.
Penicillin V Potassium *(Beepen-VK®, Ledercillin VK®, Pen-Vee K®, Phenoxymethylpenicillin Potassium, V-Cillin K®, Veetids®)*	**Bacterial infections** **Note:** Ensure that appropriate culture and sensitivity tests are performed and that the organism is sensitive to penicillin V potassium. **Infection, prophylaxis** (e.g., asplenic patient)/**Rheumatic fever, prophylaxis**	**Children and adolescents:** 25–50 mg/kg/day PO in three or four divided doses, every 6 or 8 hr. *Maximum:* 2 grams/day PO. **Children (<5 years):** 250 mg/day PO in two divided doses, every 12 hr. **Children (≥5 years) and adolescents:** 500 mg/day PO in two divided doses, every 12 hr.	Solutions, oral: 25, 50 mg/ml; may contain aspartame. Suspensions, oral: 25, 35, 50, 60 mg/ml; shake well before use. Tablets, oral: 125, 250, 300, 500 mg **Note:** 250 mg = 400,000 units.	**Contraindications:** Hypersensitivity to penicillin V potassium or to other penicillins. **ADRs:** See "Penicillins" in Chapter 5.
Pentamidine Isethionate *(Pentacarinat®)*	***Pneumocystis carinii* pneumonia, prophylaxis** ***Pneumocystis carinii* pneumonia, treatment**	**Infants and children (<5 years):** 4 mg/kg/dose IV every 2–4 weeks. **Children (≥5 years) and adolescents:** 300 mg/dose by nebulizer once a month. **Infants, children, and adolescents:** 4 mg/kg/day IM or IV as a single daily dose for 14–21 days. **Note:** Reduce dosage for pediatric patients who have renal dysfunction; see Table 14-2.	Injectables, IM, IV: 200, 300 mg/vial Solutions, inhalation (with *Respirgard II®* nebulizer): 60, 300 mg/vial **Note:** The *Respirgard II* nebulizer is for one-time use only and should **not** be reused. Appropriately discard after a single use. **Note:** Each 1.74 mg of pentamidine isethionate is equivalent to 1 mg of pentamidine base. **Note:** Available in Canada as *Pentacarinat* and in the United States as an "orphan drug."	**Contraindications:** Hypersensitivity to pentamidine. **ADRs:** Commonly causes bronchospasm, cough, and nephrotoxicity. Serious ADRs occur in a high percentage of patients. These ADRs, which may be fatal, include cardiac dysrhythmias, hypoglycemia, hypotension (severe), and pancreatitis (acute). **Comments:** Patients should be lying down during IM or IV administration because of the possibility of severe hypotension. Blood pressure should be closely monitored during the administration and until it becomes stable.

Footnotes are on page 558.

TABLE 14-1 continued

DRUG (TRADE AND OTHER NAMES)	INDICATION(S)	USUAL PEDIATRIC DOSAGE AND ADMINISTRATION[a]	DOSAGE FORMS	CONTRAINDICATIONS, ADRs, AND COMMENTS[b]
Pentobarbital (Nembutal®)	**Anxiety or agitation** prior to radiologic examination or surgery **Note:** Has been replaced for the most part with benzodiazepines because of their higher therapeutic index.	**Infants and children (<15 kg):** 2–6 mg/kg IM as a single dose. **Children (≥15 kg):** 2–5 mg/kg IM as a single dose 20–30 min before radiologic examination or surgery; 1/3–1/2 of dose may be repeated 1–2 hr after the initial dose, as needed according to response. *Maximum:* 100 mg total dose IM **or** 2.5 mg/kg (maximum 50 mg) IV over 1 min; wait 1 min, then 1.25 mg/kg (maximum 25 mg) IV over 30 sec; wait 1 min, then 1.25 mg/kg (maximum 25 mg) IV over 30 sec. If required, an additional dose of 1 mg/kg (maximum 20 mg) IV may be given. *Maximum:* 120 mg total dose IV.	Capsules, oral: 50, 100 mg Elixir, oral: 4 mg/ml; contains 18% alcohol. Injectable, IM, IV: 50 mg/ml; contains 10% alcohol and 20% or 40% propylene glycol. Suppositories, rectal: 25, 30, 50, 60, 120, 200 mg **Note:** The 100-mg *Nembutal* capsule contains tartrazine (FD&C yellow No. 5). Tartrazine has been associated with hypersensitivity reactions, including bronchial asthma, among susceptible patients, particularly those who are hypersensitive to aspirin.	**Contraindications:** Acute pulmonary insufficiency and hypersensitivity to pentobarbital or to other barbiturates. **ADRs:** *See* Chapter 5. **Comments:** Generally for infants and children younger than 8 years, administer rectally; for children older than 8 years, administer PO. Do **not** administer pentobarbital IV more rapidly than 30 mg/min. Adjust dosage according to serum concentrations and clinical response.
	Insomnia **Note:** For short-term use (<14 consecutive nights). **Note:** Has been replaced for the most part with benzodiazepines because of their higher therapeutic index.	**Infants (≥2 months):** 30 mg PO as a single bedtime dose. **Children (<5 years):** 30–60 mg PO as a single bedtime dose. **Children (≥5 years):** 60 mg PO as a single bedtime dose. **Adolescents:** 60–200 mg PO as a single bedtime dose.		
	Cerebral edema/Status epilepticus	**Children and adolescents:** Initially, 3–8 mg/kg IV as a single dose. Dose may be repeated if necessary according to response; then 2–5 mg/kg/hr IV by continuous IV infusion or by intermittent IV infusion every 1 hr, as needed according to response. *Maximum:* 500 mg/day IV		
	Agitation/Anxiety **Note:** Has been replaced for the most part with benzodiazepines because of their higher therapeutic index.	**Children and adolescents:** 2–6 mg/kg/day PO or rectal in three divided doses. *Maximum:* 120 mg/day PO or rectal.		
Pericyazine (Neuleptil®, Propericyazine)	**Childhood schizophrenia and other psychotic disorders,** particularly those associated with aggressiveness, hostility, and impulsiveness	**Children (≥5 years):** Initially, 7.5–40 mg/day PO in two divided doses (2.5–10 mg PO in the morning and 5–30 mg PO in the evening). Adjust dosage according to response.	Capsules, oral: 5, 10, 20 mg Drops, oral (with calibrated dropper): 10 mg/ml (peppermint flavored); contains 12% alcohol. **Note:** Not generally available in the United States.	**Contraindications:** Anesthesia (regional or spinal), blood dyscrasias, circulatory collapse, coma (particularly that associated with the use of CNS depressants), hepatic dysfunction, and hypersensitivity to pericyazine or other phenothiazines. **ADRs:** May cause akathisia, constipation, drowsiness, dry mouth, dystonic reactions, extrapyramidal reactions, fecal impaction, hypotension, nasal congestion, paralytic ileus, slowing of reaction time, sweating (excessive), tachycardia, vomiting, voracious appetite, and weight gain.

CHAPTER 14: DRUG DOSING FOR INFANTS, CHILDREN, AND ADOLESCENTS

TABLE 14-1 *continued*

DRUG (*TRADE* AND OTHER NAMES)	INDICATION(S)	USUAL PEDIATRIC DOSAGE AND ADMINISTRATION[a]	DOSAGE FORMS	CONTRAINDICATIONS, ADRs, AND COMMENTS[b]
Pericyazine *continued*				**Note:** Anticholinergic and psychomotor ADRs usually occur initially and remit with continued therapy or with a reduction in dosage. Extrapyramidal reactions usually occur later during pharmacotherapy and with higher dosages.
Permethrin *(Acticin®, Elimite®, Nix Crème Rinse®)*	Head lice *(Pediculosis humanus capitis)* **infestation** and their nits (eggs)	**Infants, children, and adolescents:** After washing the hair and scalp with shampoo and towel drying, apply a sufficient amount of lotion to thoroughly saturate the hair and scalp. Allow to remain in contact with the scalp for 10 min, then rinse thoroughly with water and briskly dry the hair with a clean towel. Repeat in 7 days, if indicated. Dead lice, nits, and nit shells can be removed from the hair with a fine-toothed (nit) comb.	Cream, topical: 5% Lotion, topical *(Nix Crème Rinse)*: 1%; contains 20% isopropyl alcohol and propylene glycol; shake well before use. **Note:** All topical formulations are for external use only. Avoid contact with eyes and mucous membranes (e.g., inside of mouth, nose, or vagina). For eyelash infestation, apply white petrolatum.	**Contraindications:** Hypersensitivity to permethrin. **ADRs:** May cause erythema, pruritus, rash, and stinging. **Comments:** Ensure that all clothes and bedding have been thoroughly washed in hot water or dry cleaned to prevent reinfestation. Assess and treat, as required, **all** household contacts.
	Scabies infestation	**Infants, children, and adolescents:** Apply 15–30 grams of cream to thoroughly cover, in a thin layer, the entire skin surface of the trunk and extremities from the neck to the soles of the feet, including between all digits and skin folds (may also need to apply to the temples and forehead, particularly among infants and young children). Allow to remain in contact with the skin surface for approximately 12 hr, then bathe or shower and thoroughly rinse all areas of application. Repeat once in 7–10 days, if needed. **Note:** Do not bathe or shower before applying the lotion *(Nix Crème Rinse)*.		
Pertussis Vaccine, *see* **Chapter 9**				
Pethidine, *see* **Meperidine**				
Phenazopyridine *(Azo-Gesic®, Azo-Standard®, Pyridium®, Urogesic®)*	Symptomatic relief of burning sensation, irritation, or pain of the lower urinary tract mucosa (caused by catheters, endoscopic procedures, infection, surgery, or trauma) **Note:** Not approved by the HPB for pediatric patients.	**Infants, children, and adolescents:** 12 mg/kg/day PO in three divided doses after meals. *Maximum:* 600 mg/day PO. **Note:** Concomitant phenazopyridine and antibiotic pharmacotherapy for the treatment of a urinary tract infection generally should not exceed 2 days.	Tablets, oral: 95, 100, 200 mg	**Contraindications:** Glomerulonephritis, hepatitis (severe), hypersensitivity to phenazopyridine, renal dysfunction, and uremia. **ADRs:** Generally well tolerated. May cause dizziness, mild GI irritation, headache, pruritus, and rash. **Note:** May cause hemolytic anemia (rare) among patients who have glucose-6-phosphate dehydrogenase deficiency. **Comments:** May discolor tears and urine orange–red and consequently stain contact lenses or undergarments.

Footnotes are on page 558.

TABLE 14-1 continued

DRUG (TRADE AND OTHER NAMES)	INDICATION(S)	USUAL PEDIATRIC DOSAGE AND ADMINISTRATION[a]	DOSAGE FORMS	CONTRAINDICATIONS, ADRs, AND COMMENTS[b]
Phendimetrazine (Adipost®, Bontril®, Prelu-Z®)	Eating disorders, exogenous obesity **Note:** Only indicated for short-term (maximum 12 weeks) therapy.	**Adolescents:** 70–105 mg/day PO in two or three divided doses 1 hr before meals **or** 105 mg/day oral extended-release capsule PO as a single dose 30–60 min before breakfast. *Maximum:* 210 mg/day PO in three divided doses. **Note:** Tolerance to anorexiant action usually develops within a few weeks. When tolerance is noted, discontinue. Do **not** exceed the recommended dosage in an attempt to maintain anorexiant action.	Capsule, oral: 35 mg Capsule, oral extended release: 105 mg Tablet, oral: 35 mg	**Contraindications:** Agitation, arteriosclerosis (advanced), cardiovascular disorders (severe), hypersensitivity to phendimetrazine or sympathomimetic amines (e.g., epinephrine), hypertension (moderate to severe), hyperthyroidism, MAOI therapy (concurrent or within 14 days), and problematic patterns of amphetamine or other abusable psychotropic use (history of). **ADRs:** Long-term regular use may result in addiction and habituation. May exacerbate hypertension among adolescents who have hypertension, even mild hypertension; and alter insulin requirements among adolescents who have insulin-dependent diabetes mellitus. May cause constipation, diarrhea, dizziness, dry mouth, dysphoria, euphoria, GI complaints, headache, hives, hypertension, impotence and changes in sex drive, palpitation, psychotic episodes (rare), restlessness, tachycardia, tremor, and unpleasant taste. **Comments:** Abrupt discontinuation of regular long-term, high-dosage therapy may result in fatigue and mental depression.
Phenobarbital (Phenobarbitone)	Partial and tonic-clonic seizures	**Infants:** 3–6 mg/kg/day PO as a single daily dose in the evening 30 min before bedtime or as two divided doses. **Children:** 1–8 mg/kg/day PO as a single daily dose in the evening 30 min before bedtime or as two divided doses. *Maximum:* 400 mg/day PO.	Capsule, oral: 16 mg Drops, oral: 16, 65 mg/ml Elixirs, oral: 3, 4, 5 mg/ml; contains 10%–13.5% alcohol. Injectables, IM, IV: 30, 60, 65, 120, 130 mg/ml; contains 10% alcohol and ~70% propylene glycol. Suppositories, rectal: 8, 15, 30, 60, 100, 120 mg Tablets, oral: 8.5, 15, 16, 30, 32, 50, 60, 65, 100 mg **Note:** The phenobarbital injectables generally are used for hospitalized patients who require immediate control of seizures. **Note:** The phenobarbital oral drops *(Sedadrops®)* contain tartrazine. Tartrazine may cause hypersensitivity reactions, including bronchial asthma, among susceptible patients, particularly those who have a hypersensitivity to aspirin.	**Contraindications:** Hepatic disease (severe), hypersensitivity to phenobarbital or to other barbiturates, renal disease (severe), porphyria, pregnancy, and respiratory depression (severe). **ADRs:** Caution required for patients who are concurrently receiving oral anticoagulant pharmacotherapy because of associated difficulty stabilizing prothrombin times. May cause mental changes and reduced performance on neuropsychological tests, osteomalacia, respiratory depression, sedation, and skin rash. Also associated with problematic behavior (e.g., disobedience, hyperactivity, irritability, stubbornness) among children. *See* Chapter 5. **Comments:** Long-term therapy may result in addiction and habituation. Sudden discontinuation of long-term therapy may result in the barbiturate-withdrawal syndrome—a medical emergency that can be fatal if not appropriately treated. May increase the hepatic metabolism of other drugs (*see* Chapter 6). **Note:** Therapeutic drug monitoring recommended; *see* Table 14-3.
	Status epilepticus refractory to treatment with other more rapidly acting anticonvulsants	**Infants, children, and adolescents:** 10–20 mg/kg IV. **Note:** Administer IV over at least 15 min. Onset of action generally is <5 min, but peak antiseizure action may not be apparent for ≥15 min. **Note:** Reduce dosage for pediatric patients who have renal dysfunction; *see* Table 14-2.		

TABLE 14-1 *continued*

DRUG (*TRADE* AND OTHER NAMES)	INDICATION(S)	USUAL PEDIATRIC DOSAGE AND ADMINISTRATION[a]	DOSAGE FORMS	CONTRAINDICATIONS, ADRs, AND COMMENTS[b]
Phenobarbitone, *see* **Phenobarbital**				
Phenoxy- benzamine (*Dibenzyline*®)	Pheochromo- cytoma	**Children and adolescents:** Initially, 0.2 mg/kg/day PO as a single daily dose. Increase the dosage gradually as needed to 0.4–1.2 mg/kg/day PO in two or three divided doses. *Maximum:* Initially, 10 mg/day PO; maintenance, 120 mg/day PO.	Capsule, oral: 10 mg **Note:** GI absorption and, therefore, bioavailability generally are limited (20%–30%). **Note:** Not generally available in Canada.	**Contraindications:** Clinical conditions in which a fall in blood pressure is undesirable. **ADRs:** May cause diarrhea, dizziness, headache, lethargy, nasal congestion, postural hypo- tension, syncope, tachycardia, and weakness. **Comments:** Use with caution among pediatric patients with congestive heart failure.
Phenoxymethyl Penicillin Potassium, *see* **Penicillin V Potassium**				
Phentolamine (*Rogitine*®)	Hypertension pre- operatively and dur- ing related surgery among patients with pheochromocytoma	**Children and adolescents:** Initially, 0.05–0.1 mg/kg/dose IV 1–2 hr prior to surgery; repeat as needed according to response. *Maximum:* 5 mg/dose IV. **Note:** Reduce dosage for pediatric patients who have renal dysfunc- tion.	Injectable, IM, IV, SC: 5 mg/vial **Note:** Contains sodium metabisulfite. Sulfites may cause hypersensi- tivity reactions among susceptible patients, particularly those who have a history of asthma. These reactions include life-threatening ana- phylaxis or less severe asthmatic episodes.	**Contraindications:** Angina, coronary artery disease, coronary insufficiency, hypersensitivity to phentolamine, hypotension, and myocardial infarction. **ADRs:** Commonly causes orthostatic hypotension and tachy- cardia. May also cause diarrhea, dizziness, nausea, and vomiting. **Comments:** False-positive test results may occur among hyper- tensive pediatric patients who do not have a pheochromocytoma. The phentolamine test has been largely replaced by urinary and plasma catecholamine tests and the urinary vanillylmandelic acid test.
	Suspected pheo- chromocytoma (diagnostic test) **Note:** Not generally recommended. *See* "Comments."	**Children:** 1 mg IV **or** 3 mg IM once as a single dose. **Adolescents:** 5 mg IM or IV once as a single dose. **Note:** Patient should be kept in a supine position (in a quiet, dark- ened room) and blood pressure monitored throughout the test period.		
	Extravasation associated with vasoactive drug (e.g., norepineph- rine) to prevent tissue necrosis	**Children and adolescents:** 0.1–0.2 mg/kg SC (liberally infiltrate area of extravasation). *Maximum:* 10 mg SC. **Note:** Should be initiated as soon as possible following extravasation of a vasoactive drug. Generally ineffective if administered >12 hr following extravasation.		
Phenylephrine	Hypotension/Shock **Note:** Treatment of hypotension and vas- cular failure in shock **must** be accompa- nied by appropriate blood and other body fluid replacement.	**Children and adolescents:** 0.1 mg/kg/dose IM or SC every 1–2 hr, as needed according to response. **Or** 5–20 μg/kg/dose IV every 10–15 min as needed according to response **or** 0.1–0.5 μg/kg/min by continuous IV infusion. *Maximum:* 5 mg/dose IM or SC; 0.5 mg/dose IV; and 4 μg/min continuous IV infusion.	Injectable, IM, IV, SC: 10 mg/ml **Note:** *Neo-Synephrine* injectable contains sodium metabisulfite. Sulfites may cause hypersensitivity reac- tions among susceptible patients, particularly those who have a his- tory of asthma. These reactions include life-threatening anaphylaxis or less severe asthmatic episodes. **Note:** Not generally available in Canada.	**Contraindications:** Hypersensi- tivity to phenylephrine, hyperten- sion (severe), and ventricular tachycardia. **ADRs:** May cause marked reflex bradycardia (that can be blocked by atropine). **Comments:** Titrate dosage to indi- vidual patient response. Monitor injection sites and avoid extravasation, which has been as- sociated with local tissue necrosis. Treat extravasations immediately with phentolamine.

Footnotes are on page 558.

TABLE 14-1 continued

DRUG (TRADE AND OTHER NAMES)	INDICATION(S)	USUAL PEDIATRIC DOSAGE AND ADMINISTRATION[a]	DOSAGE FORMS	CONTRAINDICATIONS, ADRs, AND COMMENTS[b]
Phenytoin (*Dilantin®*, Diphenylhydantoin) **Note:** *See also* Fosphenytoin.	Partial seizures (psychomotor, temporal lobe) with complex symptomatology/ Tonic-clonic (grand mal) seizures **Note:** Phenytoin is **not** indicated for seizures due to hypoglycemia or other metabolic causes. Tachycardia and dysrhythmias associated with digoxin toxicity **Note:** Not approved by the FDA or HPB for the treatment of cardiac dysrhythmias. Status epilepticus	Infants (≥6 months) and children (≤3 years): 7–9 mg/kg/day PO in two or three divided doses. Children (4–6 years): 6.5 mg/kg/day PO in two or three divided doses. Children (7–9 years): 6 mg/kg/day PO in two or three divided doses. Children (≥10 years) and adolescents: 3–5 mg/kg/day PO in two or three divided doses. *Maximum:* 300 mg/day PO. Children and adolescents: Initially, 15 mg/kg IV over 1 hr **and** 3 mg/kg PO, then 2 mg/kg PO at 6 hr. Initiate maintenance therapy at 12 hr. *Maintenance:* 2–6 mg/kg/day PO as a single daily dose or as four divided doses. *Maximum:* 400 mg/day PO; 1 gram/dose IV. Children and adolescents: 15–20 mg/kg IV at a rate not exceeding 3 mg/kg/min or 50 mg/min, whichever is less. Repeat dose once after 30 min, if required. **Note:** Other appropriate pharmacotherapy (e.g., IV barbiturate or benzodiazepine) may be required for the rapid control of status epilepticus because of the required slow rate of IV phenytoin administration. *Maximum:* 1 gram/dose IV.	Capsules, oral (sodium salt): 30, 100 mg Capsules, oral extended release (sodium salt): 30, 100 mg (*Dilantin Kapseals®*) **Note:** Once the dosage has been stabilized, the oral extended-release capsules can be administered as a single daily dose. Discolored capsules should be safely and appropriately discarded. Injectable (sodium salt): 50 mg/ml; contains 10% alcohol and 40% propylene glycol. Suspensions, oral: 6, 25 mg/ml; contains ≤0.6% alcohol (banana or orange–vanilla flavored); shake well before use. Tablet, oral chewable: 50 mg (*Dilantin Infatabs®*) **Note:** 100 mg of phenytoin sodium = 92 mg of phenytoin.	**Contraindications:** Hypersensitivity to phenytoin or to other hydantoin derivatives. Phenytoin decreases the automaticity of cardiac tissue and, therefore, also is contraindicated for patients who have Adams-Stokes syndrome, AV block (second and third degree), SA block, and sinus bradycardia. **ADRs:** Commonly causes incoordination, mental confusion, and slurred speech. May cause exfoliative dermatitis, gingival hyperplasia, and peripheral neuropathy. *See* Chapter 5. **Comments:** Phenytoin displays nonlinear kinetics. A small change in dosage may result in a large change in phenytoin blood concentrations (*see* Chapter 10). Therapeutic drug monitoring is recommended; *see* Table 14-3. Phenytoin may stimulate (increase) the hepatic metabolism of other drugs (*see* Chapter 6). **Note:** For IV use, *see also* Fosphenytoin. **Note:** Good dental hygiene should be stressed with the patient and parent in order to minimize the development of gingival hyperplasia.
Physostigmine Salicylate (*Antilirium®*, Eserine) **Note:** *See also* Chapter 4.	Anticholinergic drug overdosage	Infants, children, and adolescents: 0.01–0.03 mg/kg IM or IV; may repeat dose after 5–15 min, if needed according to response. *Maximum:* 2 mg/dose IM or IV. *Maximum rate of infusion:* 0.5 mg/min (for children); 1 mg/min (for adolescents).	Injectable, IM, IV: 1 mg/ml; contains benzyl alcohol 2% and sodium bisulfite. **Note:** Sulfites may cause hypersensitivity reactions among susceptible patients, particularly those who have a history of asthma. These reactions include life-threatening anaphylaxis or less severe asthmatic episodes. **Note:** Not generally available in Canada.	**Contraindications:** Asthma, cardiovascular disease, diabetes mellitus, gangrene, mechanical obstruction of the intestinal or urogenital tract, and patients receiving choline esters (e.g., bethanechol, methacholine) or depolarizing neuromuscular blockers (e.g., decamethonium, succinylcholine). **ADRs:** May cause bronchospasm, dyspnea, epigastric distress, lacrimation, miosis, nausea, salivation, vomiting, and weakness. **Comments:** Atropine injectable should be readily available as an antagonist to the muscarinic effects of physostigmine.
Phytonadione (*AquaMEPHYTON®*, *Konakion®*, *Mephyton®*, Vitamin K_1)	Dietary vitamin K_1 deficiency	Infants: 1 mg/dose/month IM or SC. Children: 2.5–25 mg/day PO.	Injectables, IM, IV, SC: 2, 10 mg/ml; contains benzyl alcohol. Tablet, oral: 5 mg **Note:** Oral absorption is variable, depending on presence of bile salts.	**Contraindications:** Hypersensitivity to phytonadione. **ADRs:** Generally well tolerated. *See* Chapter 5. **Comments:** Monitor prothrombin time.

CHAPTER 14: DRUG DOSING FOR INFANTS, CHILDREN, AND ADOLESCENTS

TABLE 14-1 *continued*

DRUG (*TRADE* AND OTHER NAMES)	INDICATION(S)	USUAL PEDIATRIC DOSAGE AND ADMINISTRATION[a]	DOSAGE FORMS	CONTRAINDICATIONS, ADRs, AND COMMENTS[b]
Phytonadione *continued*	**Hypoprothrombinemia** associated with prolonged parenteral nutrition **Oral anticoagulant overdosage**	**Children:** 2–5 mg/week IM. **Adolescents:** 5–10 mg/week IM **or** 1 mg/day IV as a single daily dose. **Infants:** 1–2 mg/dose IM, IV, PO, or SC every 4–8 hr as needed according to response. **Children:** 5–10 mg/dose IM, IV, PO, or SC every 4–8 hr as needed according to response. *Maximum:* 50 mg/dose IM, IV, PO, or SC. **Note:** Inject IV at a rate **not** exceeding 1 mg/min. Rapid IV injection may result in severe hypotension.	**Note:** Benzyl alcohol, which is found in the injectable formulation, is associated with a potentially **fatal** "gasping syndrome" among premature neonates and young infants.	
Pimecrolimus *(Elidel®)*	**Atopic dermatitis** (refractory to conventional therapy), mild to moderate **Note:** May be used for either short-term or intermittent long-term treatment. **Note:** Not indicated for the treatment of clinically infected atopic dermatitis.	**Children (≥2 years) and adolescents:** Apply a thin layer of cream 1% to affected skin site(s) twice daily. Rub cream in gently and completely. Pimecrolimus pharmacotherapy may continue for up to 6 weeks. **Note:** Do **not** use occlusive dressings because they can increase systemic absorption of topical pimecrolimus cream.	Cream, topical: 1% **Note:** For external use only; avoid contact with eyes and mucous membranes. **Note:** Not generally available in Canada.	**Contraindications:** Hypersensitivity to pimecrolimus, Netherton's syndrome (because of risk for increased systemic absorption), and viral skin infections (e.g., chickenpox, herpes). **ADRs:** Generally well tolerated. May cause burning sensation at application site, headache, nasopharyngitis, pyrexia, and viral infection. **Comments:** Patients should be instructed to avoid, or minimize, exposure to both natural and artificial sunlight while receiving treatment with pimecrolimus topical cream. **Note:** Instruct parents to wash their hands with soap and water after applying pimecrolimus topical cream in order to remove any residual cream from their hands.
Pimozide *(Orap®)*	**Tic disorders/ Tourette's disorder** **Note:** Indicated for the suppression of associated motor and phonic tics among patients who have failed to respond to standard drugs (e.g., haloperidol). **Note:** Approved by the FDA but not the HPB for this indication. **Schizophrenia and other psychotic disorders** **Note:** Approved by the FDA but not the HPB for this indication for children.	**Children (≥2 years) and adolescents:** Initially, 0.05 mg/kg/day PO, preferably in a single daily dose at bedtime. Increase the dosage gradually according to response. *Maximum:* 0.2 mg/kg/day PO **or** 10 mg/day PO, whichever is less. **Note:** Do not administer with grapefruit juice; may significantly increase serum concentration of pimozide. **Note:** Because of the availability of several other antipsychotics with a better toxicity profile, we generally do not recommend pimozide for this indication.	Tablets, oral: 2, 4, 10 mg **Note:** Some tablets contain tartrazine (FD&C yellow No. 5). Tartrazine has been associated with hypersensitivity reactions, including bronchial asthma, among susceptible patients, particularly those who are hypersensitive to aspirin. The 2-mg *Orap* tablets do **not** contain tartrazine.	**Contraindications:** Blood dyscrasias, cardiac dysrhythmias, CNS depression (severe), coma, congenital long QT syndrome or concurrent pharmacotherapy with drugs that may prolong the QT interval (pimozide prolongs the QT interval, *see* Chapter 6), depression (moderate to severe), hepatic dysfunction, hypersensitivity to pimozide or related compounds, and renal dysfunction. **ADRs:** Commonly causes extrapyramidal reactions, including akathisia, dystonia (particularly torticollis), and Parkinsonism. Long-term therapy may result in tardive dyskinesia. The neuroleptic malignant syndrome also may occur (*see also* Chapter 5).

Footnotes are on page 558.

TABLE 14-1 continued

DRUG (TRADE AND OTHER NAMES)	INDICATION(S)	USUAL PEDIATRIC DOSAGE AND ADMINISTRATION[a]	DOSAGE FORMS	CONTRAINDICATIONS, ADRs, AND COMMENTS[b]
Piperacillin (*Pipracil®*)	Bacterial infections, severe **Note:** Ensure that appropriate culture and sensitivity tests are performed and that the organism is sensitive to piperacillin. **Note:** Not approved by the FDA or HPB for infants or children.	**Children and adolescents:** 200–300 mg/kg/day IV in four to six divided doses, every 4–6 hr. *Maximum:* 24 grams/day IV. **Note:** Reduce dosage for pediatric patients who have renal dysfunction; see Table 14-2.	Injectables, IM, IV: 2, 3, 4 grams/vial; contains 1.85 mEq of sodium per gram. **Note:** IM therapy is **not** recommended for severe infections.	**Contraindications:** Hypersensitivity to piperacillin or to other penicillins. **ADRs:** *See* Chapter 5.
Piperonyl Butoxide and Pyrethrins (*R&C®, RID®*)	Infestations of head lice (*Pediculus capitis*), Crab/Pubic lice (*Phthirus pubis*), and their nits (eggs)	**Infants, children, and adolescents:** Apply sufficient shampoo to thoroughly soak the hair and skin of the infested area. Allow the shampoo to remain in contact with this area for 10 min. Then add small quantities of water and work the shampoo into a lather. Then rinse the area thoroughly of all shampoo and comb through the hair with a nit (fine toothed) comb to remove the dead lice and their nits before briskly towel drying the area. **Note:** Application of the shampoo may be repeated in 7 days if required. Do not exceed two consecutive applications within 24 hr.	Shampoo, topical: 3% piperonyl butoxide and 0.33% pyrethrins **Note:** For external use only. Avoid contact with eyes and mucous membranes.	**Contraindications:** Hypersensitivity to chrysanthemums, pyrethrins, or synthetic pyrethroids. **ADRs:** Generally well tolerated. Avoid contact with eyes—may cause eye irritation. To prevent re-infestation, wash all bedding and clothing in hot water or have dry cleaned.
Plicamycin (*Mithracin®*, Mithramycin)	Hypercalcemia and hypercalciuria associated with advanced neoplasms (generally reserved for hospitalized patients who are refractory to, or cannot tolerate, conventional pharmacotherapy) **Note:** Not approved by the FDA for children or adolescents.	**Children and adolescents:** 25 μg/kg/day (diluted in 1 liter of 5% dextrose injection or sodium chloride injection) by single daily IV infusion over 4–6 hr for a total of 3 or 4 days. After 1 week off therapy, the 3- or 4-day course may be repeated, as indicated by response. **Note:** Monitor calcium serum and urinary concentrations to guide dosage adjustments.	Injectable, IV: 500 μg/ml (after reconstitution with 4.9 ml sterile water for injection) **Note:** For IV use only. **Note:** Prepare fresh each day. Safely and appropriately discard any unused solution. Because plicamycin is an antineoplastic drug, it should be disposed of in accordance with established guidelines. *See* Chapter 12. **Note:** Not generally available in Canada.	**Contraindications:** Bone marrow suppression, coagulation disorders, hypocalcemia, pregnancy, renal impairment (severe), thrombocytopenia, and thrombocytopathy. **ADRs:** Commonly causes anorexia, diarrhea, nausea, stomatitis, and vomiting. May cause bleeding tendency, thrombocytopenia, and death. **Comments:** Monitor bleeding times, platelet counts, prothrombin time, renal function, calcium serum and urinary concentrations prior to the initiation of, periodically during, and at the conclusion of plicamycin pharmacotherapy. **Note:** Pretreatment with, or concomitant administration of, antiemetics may help to prevent or reduce plicamycin-induced nausea and vomiting.

Pneumococcal Vaccine, *see* **Chapter 9**

Poliomyelitis Vaccines, *see* **Chapter 9**

DRUG (TRADE AND OTHER NAMES)	INDICATION(S)	USUAL PEDIATRIC DOSAGE AND ADMINISTRATION[a]	DOSAGE FORMS	CONTRAINDICATIONS, ADRs, AND COMMENTS[b]
Polyethylene Glycol and Electrolyte Solution (*Co-Lav®, CoLyte®, GoLYTELY®, klean-Prep®, Peglyte®*)	Bowel cleansing prior to GI examination, procedure, or surgery	**Adolescents:** Four liters of polyethylene glycol and electrolyte solution PO according to the following schedule: *After fasting for 3–4 hr:* 240 ml (8 ounces) PO every 10 min until the entire 4 liters are consumed. *After ingesting the 4 liters:* Patient should resume fasting, or only	Solution, oral: polyethylene glycol, 17.6 mmol/liter; bicarbonate, 20 mmol/liter; chloride, 35 mmol/liter; potassium, 10 mmol/liter; sodium, 125 mmol/liter; and sulfate, 40 mmol/liter	**Contraindications:** Gastric retention, GI perforation or obstruction, ileus, megacolon, and toxic colitis. **ADRs:** Commonly causes abdominal bloating and fullness and nausea. **Comments:** Absorption of drugs administered orally within 1 hr of the ingestion of the solution will

TABLE 14-1 continued

DRUG (TRADE AND OTHER NAMES)	INDICATION(S)	USUAL PEDIATRIC DOSAGE AND ADMINISTRATION[a]	DOSAGE FORMS	CONTRAINDICATIONS, ADRs, AND COMMENTS[b]
Polyethylene Glycol and Electrolyte Solution *continued*		ingest clear liquids, until completion of the GI examination, procedure, or surgery.	(after reconstitution with tap water to 4 liters) **Note:** Store the reconstituted solution in the refrigerator and use within 48 hr. Chilling generally improves palatability. Do **not** add any flavoring agents, additional ingredients, or other drugs to the reconstituted solution.	be significantly reduced. Alternate routes of administration should be considered for these drugs.
Polymyxin B Sulfate, systemic	**Infections** caused by susceptible organisms (generally reserved for systemic infections that are resistant to less toxic antibiotics) **Note:** Ensure that appropriate culture and sensitivity tests are performed and that the organism is sensitive to polymyxin B sulfate. *Pseudomonas aeruginosa* meningitis	**Infants:** 15,000–40,000 units/kg/day IV in two divided doses, every 12 hr. **Children and adolescents:** 15,000–25,000 units/kg/day IV in two divided doses, every 12 hr. **Note:** Usually administered as an IV infusion over 60–90 min. **Note:** Pediatric patients with severe renal impairment (creatinine clearance <30 ml/min) will require dosage reduction. **Infants and children (≤2 years):** Initially, 20,000 units/dose intrathecal once daily for 3 or 4 days. Then, 25,000 units/dose intrathecal every other day. **Children (≥2 years) and adolescents:** Initially, 50,000 units/dose intrathecal once daily for 3 or 4 days. Then 50,000 units/dose intrathecal every other day. **Note:** Therapy for meningitis should continue for at least 2 weeks after cerebrospinal fluid cultures are negative for bacteria and cerebrospinal fluid glucose concentration has returned to normal.	Injectable, IM, IV, intrathecal: 500,000 units **Note:** IM administration is associated with severe pain at the injection site and is not recommended. **Note:** *For IV administration*, reconstitute injectable with 300–500 ml of 5% dextrose and water for injection to provide a solution containing 1000–1667 units/ml. **Note:** *For intrathecal administration*, reconstitute injectable with 10 ml of 0.9% sodium chloride for injection to provide a solution containing 50,000 units/ml. **Note:** Not generally available in Canada.	**Contraindications:** Hypersensitivity to polymyxin B sulfate or to other polymyxins. **ADRs:** May cause nephrotoxicity (e.g., albuminuria, azotemia) and neurotoxicity (e.g., apnea, dizziness, drowsiness, irritability, mental confusion, seizures). In addition, may cause meningeal irritation (e.g., fever, headache, stiff neck) following intrathecal administration. **Comments:** Monitor renal function. Use should be restricted to hospitalized patients.
Potassium Chloride	**Potassium deficit** (hypokalemia) **Note:** Ensure adequate urine output **prior** to IV administration.	**Infants, children, and adolescents:** Initial dose is determined by extent of potassium deficit and desired supplementation. Hypokalemia: 1–3 mmol/kg/day IV or PO plus a maintenance requirement of 30–40 mmol/m²/day IV or PO. *Maximum:* 3 mmol/kg/day PO or 200 mmol/day PO, whichever is less. **Note:** Maximum recommended concentration for peripheral IV infusion is 80 mmol/liter. **Note:** Reduce dosage for pediatric patients who have renal dysfunction.	Capsules, oral extended release: 8, 10 mmol Injectables, IV: 1.5, 2, 3 mmol/ml Powders, oral effervescent: 15, 20, 25 mmol/packet Solutions, oral: 1.3, 2, 2.7 mmol/ml Tablet, oral effervescent: 25 mmol Tablets, oral extended release: 6, 7, 8, 10, 12, 20 mmol **Note:** 1 mmol potassium = 1 mEq potassium. **Note:** Oral extended-release capsules and	**Contraindications:** Acute dehydration, Addison's disease (untreated), adynamia episodica hereditaria, extensive tissue breakdown (e.g., severe burns), heat cramps, hyperadrenalism associated with adrenogenital syndrome, hyperkalemia, and renal dysfunction with azotemia or oliguria. **ADRs:** Generally well tolerated. Oral potassium therapy may cause GI irritation. Hyperkalemia is associated with the following signs and symptoms: cardiac dysrhythmias, flaccid paralysis, heart block, hypotension, listlessness, mental confusion, and weakness. *(Continued)*

Footnotes are on page 558.

TABLE 14-1 continued

DRUG (TRADE AND OTHER NAMES)	INDICATION(S)	USUAL PEDIATRIC DOSAGE AND ADMINISTRATION[a]	DOSAGE FORMS	CONTRAINDICATIONS, ADRs, AND COMMENTS[b]
Potassium Chloride *continued*			tablets are **not** generally recommended for use among infants or children.	**Comments:** Monitor potassium serum concentration, ECG, and clinical status during therapy. Continuous ECG monitoring required for any patient receiving >0.5 mmol/kg/hr.
Potassium Iodide (KI, *Pima®, SSKI®, Thyro-Block®*)	Thyrotoxicosis Note: Generally used in combination with other antithyroid pharmacotherapy (e.g., propylthiouracil).	**Infants:** 2–4 mg/kg/day PO in three divided doses. **Children and adolescents:** 4–7 mg/kg/day PO in three divided doses. *Maximum:* 7 mg/kg or 500 mg/dose PO, whichever is less. **Note:** Administer after meals or with food or milk to minimize associated GI irritation.	Solution, oral: 1 gram/ml Syrup, oral: 325 mg/5 ml (black raspberry flavored) Tablet, oral: 130 mg **Note:** Potassium iodide solution contains potassium iodide and free iodine. Potassium iodide is 76.45% iodine by weight. **Note:** Each dose should be diluted in 240 ml (8 ounces) of broth, fruit juice, milk, or water immediately prior to administration to improve palatability.	**Contraindications:** Bronchitis (acute), hypersensitivity to iodides, iodism, and tuberculosis. **ADRs:** Generally well tolerated. May cause acne, arthralgia, and GI irritation. **Comments:** Monitor thyroid function tests.
	Thyroid gland protection from radioactive iodine (prophylaxis for therapeutic exposure to radioactive iodine or treatment for accidental exposure to radioactive iodine associated with a nuclear emergency)	**Infants:** 65 mg/day PO as a single daily dose. **Children and adolescents:** 130 mg/day PO as a single daily dose. Begin therapy prior to, or immediately following, radioactive iodine exposure. **Note:** Duration of therapy depends on type of exposure.		
	Thyroidectomy, adjunctive pharmacotherapy to reduce the vascularity of the thyroid gland prior to its surgical removal	**Children and adolescents:** 2–20 mg/kg/day PO in three divided doses for 10–14 days, immediately prior to surgery. *Maximum:* 750 mg/day PO. **Note:** Administer after meals or with food or milk to minimize associated GI irritation.		
Pralidoxime (*Protopam®*) Note: See also Chapter 4.	Organophosphate poisoning Note: Generally used as adjunctive pharmacotherapy with atropine. See Chapter 4. **Note:** Not approved by the FDA or HPB for infants or children.	**Infants, children, and adolescents:** Initially, 25–50 mg/kg/dose IM, IV, or SC; may repeat dose in 1 hr if necessary; then 25–50 mg IM or IV every 8–12 hr as indicated by response. For severe cases of organophosphate poisoning, 10–25 mg/kg IV as a one-time dose, followed by 10–20 mg/kg/hr by continuous IV infusion for at least 18 hr. *Maximum:* 1 gram/dose IM, IV, or SC. **Note:** Reduce dosage for pediatric patients who have renal dysfunction.	Injectable, IM, IV, SC (1-gram vials for reconstitution): 50 mg/ml (after reconstitution) **Note:** For IV administration, dilute injectable to ≤20 mg/ml and administer over at least 15 min.	**Contraindications:** Hypersensitivity to pralidoxime. **ADRs:** Generally well tolerated. May cause blurred vision, diplopia, dizziness, drowsiness, headache, hypertension, hyperventilation, muscular weakness, pain at the injection site, and tachycardia. **Comments:** Most effective if administered immediately after poisoning.
Praziquantel (*Biltricide®*)	Liver flukes: Clonorchiasis (*Clonorchis sinensis*) and Opisthorchiasis (*Opisthorchis viverrini*)	**Children (≥4 years) and adolescents:** 75 mg/kg/day PO in three divided doses at 4–6-hr intervals. Each dose should be ingested with food or a meal. A single day of praziquantel pharmacotherapy is usually effective for the treatment of clonorchiasis or opisthorchiasis.	Tablet, oral triscored (rectangular tablet): 600 mg **Note:** When broken along score lines, each of the four resulting tablet segments contains 150 mg of praziquantel. **Note:** Tablets are bitter and should be swallowed whole without chewing.	**Contraindications:** Hypersensitivity to praziquantel and ocular cysticercosis. **ADRs:** Generally well tolerated. May cause abdominal discomfort, dizziness, drowsiness, headache, malaise, and nausea.

TABLE 14-1 continued

DRUG (TRADE AND OTHER NAMES)	INDICATION(S)	USUAL PEDIATRIC DOSAGE AND ADMINISTRATION[a]	DOSAGE FORMS	CONTRAINDICATIONS, ADRs, AND COMMENTS[b]
Praziquantel *continued*	**Schistosomiasis** (*Schistosoma haematobium, S. japonicum, S. mansoni,* and *S. mekongi*)	**Children (≥4 years) and adolescents:** 60 mg/kg/day PO in three divided doses at 4–6-hr intervals. Each dose should be ingested with food or a meal. A single day of praziquantel pharmacotherapy is usually effective for the treatment of schistosomiasis. **Note:** Individual doses should be rounded to the nearest 150 mg because praziquantel is only available as 600-mg oral triscored tablets.	Chewing the oral tablets has been associated with gagging and vomiting.	
Prazosin (*Minipress®*)	**Congestive heart failure** **Note:** Generally should be limited to use as short-term therapy for patients who are refractory to traditional pharmacotherapy for the treatment of congestive heart failure (e.g., digoxin).	**Infants, children, and adolescents:** Initially, 5 µg/kg/dose PO in four divided doses, every 6 hr; gradually increase the dosage as needed according to response. *Maximum:* 100 µg/kg/day PO in four divided doses, every 6 hr.	Capsules, oral: 1, 2, 5 mg (USA) Tablets, oral: 1, 2, 5 mg (Canada)	**Contraindications:** Hypersensitivity to prazosin or to other quinazolines (e.g., doxazosin, terazosin). **ADRs:** May cause dizziness, drowsiness, dry mouth, fatigue, headache, malaise, nausea, palpitations, and weakness. Marked hypotension and syncope can occur, particularly in conjunction with the first dose. *See* Chapter 5. **Comments:** May cause excessive postural hypotension and syncope. Long-term therapy is associated with the development of tolerance to therapeutic effects. Therefore, prazosin is indicated for short-term use only.
	Essential hypertension, mild to moderate **Note:** Not approved by the FDA or HPB for infants or children.	**Infants:** Initially, 10 µg/kg/dose PO every 6 hr; increase dosage, according to response, until desired effect is achieved. *Maximum:* Initially, 0.25 mg/dose PO; maintenance, 2.5 mg/day PO. **Children and adolescents:** Initially, 10 µg/kg/dose PO every 6 hr; increase dosage, according to response, until desired effect is achieved. *Maximum:* Initially, 0.5 mg/dose PO; maintenance, 10 mg/day PO.		

Prednisolone, *see also* **Chapter 12**

DRUG (TRADE AND OTHER NAMES)	INDICATION(S)	USUAL PEDIATRIC DOSAGE AND ADMINISTRATION[a]	DOSAGE FORMS	CONTRAINDICATIONS, ADRs, AND COMMENTS[b]
Prednisolone, ophthalmic (*AK-Pred®, Deltahydrocortisone, Econopred®, Inflamase®, Pred Forte®, Pred Mild®*)	**Corneal injury** (associated with chemical, radiation, or thermal burns; or abrasion or penetration with foreign bodies)/ **Steroid-responsive inflammatory conditions** of the exterior eye structures, including the anterior segment of the globe, bulbar conjunctiva, cornea, lid, palpebral conjunctiva, and sclera (specific conditions include acne rosacea, allergic conjunctivitis, anterior	**Children and adolescents:** *Prednisolone Ophthalmic Solution,* instill one or two drops into the conjunctival sac of the affected eye(s) up to every hour while awake and every 2 hr while asleep, depending upon the severity of the inflammatory condition and response. Dosage may be reduced to one drop every 4–6 hr, as indicated by response. *Prednisolone Ophthalmic Suspension,* instill one or two drops into the conjunctival sac of the affected eye(s) two to six times daily depending upon the severity of the inflammatory condition and response. **Note:** Select products with higher concentrations for the treatment	Solutions, ophthalmic: 0.125%, 1% (supplied as prednisolone sodium phosphate in disposable ophthalmic dropper containers) Suspensions, ophthalmic: 0.12%, 0.125%, 1% (supplied as prednisolone acetate in disposable ophthalmic dropper containers); shake well before use. **Note:** Some ophthalmic suspension formulations (e.g., *Pred Mild, Pred Forte*) contain sodium bisulfite. **Note:** In order to minimize cross-infection,	**Contraindications:** After uncomplicated removal of a superficial corneal foreign body, dendritic keratitis, and untreated eye infections. **ADRs:** Generally well tolerated. May cause local adverse reactions, particularly with high dosage and long-term therapy: elevated intraocular pressure (glaucoma), posterior subcapsular cataract formation, and secondary ocular infections. May also mask signs and symptoms of existing eye infections. **Comments:** For patients who require therapy exceeding 9 days, frequently monitor both intraocular pressure and lens condition.

(Continued)

TABLE 14-1 continued

DRUG (TRADE AND OTHER NAMES)	INDICATION(S)	USUAL PEDIATRIC DOSAGE AND ADMINISTRATION[a]	DOSAGE FORMS	CONTRAINDICATIONS, ADRs, AND COMMENTS[b]
Prednisolone, ophthalmic *continued*	uveitis, cyclitis, epinephrine sensitivity, episcleritis, herpes zoster keratitis, iritis, superficial punctate keratitis, and vernal conjunctivitis)	of more severe ophthalmic conditions. **Note:** If therapy has been required for several weeks, discontinue gradually over 3 or 4 days to prevent or minimize risk for relapse, particularly when active chronic lesions are treated.	ensure that separate containers are dispensed for each eye whenever both eyes require prednisolone ophthalmic pharmacotherapy.	**Note:** *See* Chapter 1 for recommended techniques for administering ophthalmic drug formulations to pediatric patients.
Prednisolone, systemic *(Delta-Cortef®, Deltahydrocortisone, Key-Pred®, Pediapred®, Predacort®, Prelone®)*	Corticosteroid-responsive inflammatory conditions (e.g., severe persistent asthma not adequately controlled with conventional pharmacotherapy) **Note:** Prednisolone, because of its minimal mineralocorticoid action, is **not** recommended for the treatment of adrenocortical insufficiency or the adrenogenital syndrome (cortisone, hydrocortisone, or fludrocortisone are generally recommended as the drugs of choice for the pharmacotherapeutic management of these conditions).	**Children:** 0.15–2 mg/kg/day PO in four divided doses. **Adolescents:** 5–60 mg/day PO in two to four divided doses. **Note:** Dosage is dependent upon the severity of the condition being treated and response.	Solution, oral: 5 mg/ml (prednisolone sodium phosphate *[Pediapred]*, raspberry flavored); contains no alcohol. Syrups, oral: 5 mg/ml; 15 mg/ml (cherry flavored); contains up to 5% alcohol and propylene glycol. Tablet, oral: 5 mg **Note:** Prednisolone injectable formulations are available, but other corticosteroid injectables are generally preferred.	**Contraindications:** Hypersensitivity to prednisolone or to other corticosteroids, infections (uncontrolled), and peptic ulcers. **ADRs:** Among children, high dosages have been associated with acute pancreatitis (potentially fatal), pseudotumor cerebri (increased intracranial pressure with resultant headache, papilledema, and visual loss), and steroid psychosis. Pseudotumor cerebri occurs most frequently following dosage reduction. *See* Chapter 5. **Comments:** Periodically monitor blood pressure, height, ocular pressure, and weight of pediatric patients. Avoid long-term therapy because of association with retardation of bone growth. If long-term therapy is necessary, monitor growth velocity. Doubling the therapeutic daily dosage and administering systemic prednisolone only on alternate days (every-other-day therapy) may help to minimize growth suppression.
Prednisone, *see also* **Chapter 12**				
Prednisone *(Deltasone®, Liquid Pred®, Meticorten®, Orasone®, Sterapred®)*	Corticosteroid-responsive inflammatory conditions **Note:** Prednisone, because of its minimal mineralocorticoid action, is **not** recommended for the treatment of adrenocortical insufficiency or the adrenogenital syndrome (cortisone, hydrocortisone, or fludrocortisone are generally recommended as the drugs of choice for the pharmacotherapeutic management of these conditions). **Note:** Prednisone is an inactive prodrug that is metabolized to its active form (prednisolone) in the liver. *See also* Prednisolone.	**Children:** 0.15–2 mg/kg/day PO in four divided doses. **Adolescents:** 5–60 mg/day PO in two to four divided doses. **Note:** Dosage is dependent upon the severity of the condition being treated and response.	Solution, oral: 5 mg/5 ml; contains 5% alcohol and saccharin sodium. Solution, oral concentrate: 5 mg/ml (Prednisone *Intensol®* contains 30% alcohol.) Syrup, oral: 5 mg/ml; contains 5% alcohol. Tablets, oral: 1, 2.5, 5, 10, 20, 50 mg **Note:** Prednisone injectable formulations are available, but other corticosteroid injectables are generally preferred.	**Contraindications:** Hepatic impairment (severe), hypersensitivity to prednisone or to other corticosteroids, infections (uncontrolled), and peptic ulcers. **ADRs:** Among children, high dosages have been associated with acute pancreatitis (potentially fatal), pseudotumor cerebri (increased intracranial pressure with resultant headache, papilledema, and visual loss), and steroid psychosis. Pseudotumor cerebri occurs most frequently following dosage reduction. *See* Chapter 5. **Comments:** Periodically monitor blood pressure, height, ocular pressure, and weight of pediatric patients. Avoid long-term therapy because of association with retardation of bone growth. If long-term therapy is necessary, monitor growth velocity. Doubling the therapeutic daily dosage and administering systemic prednisone only on alternate days (every-other-day therapy) may help to minimize growth suppression.

TABLE 14-1 continued

DRUG (*TRADE* AND OTHER NAMES)	INDICATION(S)	USUAL PEDIATRIC DOSAGE AND ADMINISTRATION[a]	DOSAGE FORMS	CONTRAINDICATIONS, ADRs, AND COMMENTS[b]
Prilocaine and Lidocaine, *see* **Lidocaine and Prilocaine**				
Primaquine	**Malaria, prophylaxis** (optional with chloroquine prophylaxis in the absence of chloroquine-resistant *Plasmodium falciparum*) **Note:** Helps to prevent late-onset malaria due to exoerythrocytic development of *P. vivax* or *P. ovale*.	**Infants, children, and adolescents:** 0.3 mg (primaquine base)/kg/day PO as a single daily dose for 14 days after return from endemic area. *Maximum:* 15 mg (primaquine base)/day PO.	Tablet, oral: 26.3 mg phosphate (equivalent to 15 mg primaquine base)	**Contraindications:** Granulocytopenia, hypersensitivity to primaquine, and concomitant use of quinacrine and other drugs that cause bone marrow suppression. **ADRs:** May cause headache, nausea, pruritus, and vomiting. **Comments:** Use with caution for pediatric patients with favism or glucose-6-phosphate dehydrogenase deficiency. Monitor for possible hemolytic reactions.
	Malaria, treatment (*P. vivax* and *P. ovale*) **Note:** Not effective against asexual erythrocytic forms of plasmodia and, therefore, only should be used in conjunction with a drug that is effective against asexual erythrocytic forms of plasmodia (a blood schizonticidal [e.g., chloroquine]).	**Infants, children, and adolescents:** 0.3 mg (primaquine base)/kg/day PO as a single daily dose for 14 days *after* treatment with chloroquine. **Note:** Administer with food or milk to decrease associated GI irritation. Do not administer on an empty stomach. **Note:** Reduce dosage for pediatric patients who have hepatic dysfunction.		
Primidone (*Mysoline®*)	**Partial seizures with complex symptomatology** (psychomotor seizures)/**Tonic-clonic (grand mal) seizures** **Note:** Abrupt discontinuation may result in status epilepticus; gradually reduce the dosage, unless therapeutically contraindicated, over 2 weeks. Primidone is metabolized to phenobarbital. *See also* Phenobarbital.	**Children (≥8 years) and adolescents:** Initially, 50 mg/day PO at bedtime for days 1–3. Then 100 mg/day PO in two divided doses for days 4–6. Then 200 mg/day PO in two divided doses for days 7–9. Continue with maintenance therapy according to response. *Maintenance:* 375–750 mg/day PO in three divided doses **or** 12–25 mg/kg/day PO in two or three divided doses. *Maximum:* 2 grams/day PO. **Note:** Reduce dosage for pediatric patients who have renal dysfunction; *see* Table 14-2.	Tablets, oral: 50, 250 mg Tablet, oral chewable: 125 mg	**Contraindications:** Hepatic disease (severe), hypersensitivity to primidone or to phenobarbital, and porphyria. **ADRs:** Commonly causes anorexia, ataxia, dizziness, lethargy, nausea, vertigo, and vomiting. *See* Chapter 5. **Note:** Therapeutic drug monitoring is recommended; *see* Table 14-3.
Probenecid (*Benuryl®*)	**Adjunctive therapy with cephalosporin or penicillin therapy for cephalosporin- or penicillin-sensitive infections** **Note:** Probenecid is used with cephalosporins or penicillins to decrease their renal tubular secretion.	**Children (≥2 years):** Initially, 25 mg/kg PO as a single one-time dose, then 40 mg/kg/day PO in four divided doses, every 6 hr. *Maximum:* 1 gram/dose PO and 2 grams/day PO. **Adolescents:** 2 grams/day PO in two divided doses, every 12 hr. **Note:** Reduce dosage for pediatric patients with renal dysfunction; *see* Table 14-2.	Tablet, oral: 500 mg	**Contraindications:** Blood dyscrasias, hypersensitivity to probenecid, and presence of uric acid renal stones. **ADRs:** Generally well tolerated. May cause anorexia, dizziness, flushing, headache, nausea, and vomiting. **Comments:** Salicylates (e.g., aspirin) antagonize the pharmacologic action of probenecid. Concomitant use should generally be avoided.

Footnotes are on page 558.

TABLE 14-1 continued

DRUG (TRADE AND OTHER NAMES)	INDICATION(S)	USUAL PEDIATRIC DOSAGE AND ADMINISTRATION[a]	DOSAGE FORMS	CONTRAINDICATIONS, ADRs, AND COMMENTS[b]
Procainamide (Procan SR®, Procanbid®, Pronestyl®)	**Atrial tachydysrhythmias** (refractory to less toxic antidysrhythmics and other interventions)/ **Supraventricular tachydysrhythmias** (refractory to less toxic antidysrhythmics and other interventions)/ **Ventricular dysrhythmias** (e.g., sustained ventricular tachycardia) **Note:** Generally reserved for the treatment of potentially life-threatening dysrhythmias because of its prodysrhythmic action. **Note:** Not indicated for the treatment of asymptomatic ventricular premature depolarizations. **Note:** Procainamide is generally effective for suppression of dysrhythmias associated with digoxin toxicity/poisoning. However, procainamide pharmacotherapy for this indication may result in ventricular asystole or fibrillation. Therefore, **only** consider use after discontinuation of digoxin pharmacotherapy and demonstrated ineffectiveness of lidocaine, phenytoin, or potassium pharmacotherapy. **Note:** Not approved by the FDA or HPB for infants or children.	**Infants, children, and adolescents:** Loading dose, 3–6 mg/kg by slow IV injection over 5 min; repeat every 5–10 min as needed, according to response, to a maximal total dose of 15 mg/kg **or** 1.2–1.5 mg/kg/hr by continuous IV infusion for up to 75 min. *Maintenance:* 1.2–4.8 mg/kg/hr by continuous IV infusion **or** 15–60 mg/kg/day PO in eight divided doses, every 3 hr. See Note in "Dosage Forms." *Maximum:* Loading dose, 100 mg/dose IV; maintenance, 4 grams/day IM or PO, 2 grams/day IV. **Note:** Reduce dosage for pediatric patients who have renal dysfunction; see Table 14-2. **Note:** May need to decrease dosage for pediatric patients who have severe congestive heart failure (CHF). Monitor ECG. **Note:** Monitor urinary pH. Renal reabsorption of procainamide is increased when urine is alkaline. Closely monitor patient's clinical response and procainamide serum concentrations. Reduce procainamide dosage as needed.	Capsules, oral: 250, 375, 500 mg Injectable, IM, IV: 100 mg/ml Tablets, oral: 250, 375, 500 mg Tablets, oral sustained release: 250, 500, 750, 1000 mg **Note:** Injectable contains sodium bisulfite. Sulfites may cause hypersensitivity reactions, including anaphylactic reactions, among susceptible patients, particularly patients who have asthma. **Note:** Procainamide oral sustained-release tablets are **not** recommended for infants or children. When used for adolescents, the entire daily oral dosage can be administered in either four divided doses, every 6 hr (e.g., *Procan SR®, Pronestyl-SR®*) **or** two divided doses, every 12 hr (e.g., *Procanbid*). **Note:** Injectable solution should be diluted prior to IV administration.	**Contraindications:** Complete heart block, hypersensitivity to procainamide, lupus erythematosus, myasthenia gravis, and torsades de pointes. **ADRs:** Associated with systemic lupus erythematosus, particularly long-term therapy among slow acetylators (*see* Chapter 11). May also cause bradycardia, GI distress, granulocytopenia, hypotension, shock, and ventricular dysrhythmias. *See also* Chapter 5. **Comments:** Metabolized in the liver to produce N-acetylprocainamide (NAPA), an active metabolite. **Note:** Therapeutic drug monitoring is recommended; see Table 14-3. **Note:** Complete blood counts (including white cell, differential, and platelet counts) should be performed at weekly intervals for the first 3 months of procainamide pharmacotherapy and periodically thereafter, because of the potential (~0.5%) risk for **fatal** blood dyscrasias (e.g., agranulocytosis, bone marrow depression, hypoplastic anemia, leukopenia, neutropenia, and thrombocytopenia). Monitor patient for possible signs and symptoms of blood dyscrasias (e.g., bleeding, bruising, chills, fever, sore throat, and stomatitis). **Note:** Continuous ECG monitoring is recommended during IV administration of procainamide. Blood pressure should also be monitored during IV administration (with the patient in a supine position). Temporarily discontinue IV administration if a fall in blood pressure occurs that exceeds 15 mmHg.
Procarbazine, *see* Chapter 12				
Prochlorperazine (Compazine®, Stemetil®)	**Schizophrenia and other psychotic disorders** **Note:** Rarely prescribed for this indication; more commonly prescribed for the treatment of severe nausea and vomiting.	**Children (≥2 years):** Initially, 5–7.5 mg/day PO or rectal in two or three divided doses. Do not administer more than 10 mg during the first day of therapy. Gradually increase the dosage according to response. If IM therapy is required, calculate each dose on the basis of 0.132 mg/kg. Inject each dose deeply into healthy muscle sites. The signs and symptoms of	Capsules, oral: 10, 15, 30, 75 mg Capsules, oral extended release (e.g., *Compazine Spansule*): 10, 15, 30 mg Concentrate, oral: 10 mg/ml Injectable, IM, IV: 5 mg/ml; contains 0.75% alcohol.	**Contraindications:** Blood dyscrasias; cardiovascular dysfunction (severe); CNS depression, including that associated with CNS depressant therapy; circulatory collapse; coma; hepatic dysfunction (severe); hypersensitivity to prochlorperazine or other phenothiazines; and pregnancy. **ADRs:** May cause a higher incidence of extrapyramidal reactions

TABLE 14-1 *continued*

DRUG (*TRADE* AND OTHER NAMES)	INDICATION(S)	USUAL PEDIATRIC DOSAGE AND ADMINISTRATION[a]	DOSAGE FORMS	CONTRAINDICATIONS, ADRs, AND COMMENTS[b]
Prochlor- perazine *continued*		psychosis generally are managed with one dose. Once the signs and symptoms are managed, replace injectable with oral therapy using the same, or higher, dosage according to response. *Maximum:* 20 mg/day PO or rectal for children 2–5 years; 25 mg/day PO or rectal for children 6–12 years.	Injectable, IM (disposable syringe): 5 mg/ml; contains 0.75% alcohol. Suppositories, rectal: 2.5, 5, 10, 25 mg Syrup, oral *(Compazine)*: 1 mg/ml (fruit flavored) Tablets, oral: 5, 10, 25 mg **Note:** Oral and IM administration generally are reserved for the management of psychotic disorders; IV and rectal administration generally are reserved for the medical management of nausea and vomiting. **Note:** *Compazine* injectable contains sodium bisulfite and sodium sulfite. Sulfites may cause hypersensitivity reactions among susceptible patients, particularly those who have a history of asthma. These reactions include life-threatening anaphylaxis or less severe asthmatic episodes. **Note:** Do not administer SC because of possible local irritation. **Note:** 5 mg of prochlorperazine base is approximately equivalent to 7.5 mg of prochlorperazine edisylate or 8 mg of prochlorperazine maleate.	among children and adolescents who are hospitalized for the treatment of psychotic disorders. May cause blood dyscrasias, including agranulocytosis and leukopenia (severe neutropenia may be life threatening); blurred vision; cholestatic jaundice; dizziness; drowsiness; extrapyramidal reactions; hypotension; and skin reactions. *See* "Phenothiazines" in Chapter 5. **Comments:** IV administration may cause hypotension.
	Nausea and vomiting, severe	**Children (9.1–13.2 kg [20–29 lb]):** 2.5 mg/dose PO or rectal **or** 0.132 mg/kg/dose IM. May repeat dose once, if necessary. *Maximum:* 7.5 mg/day PO or rectal. **Children (13.6–17.7 kg [30–39 lb]):** 2.5 mg/dose PO or rectal two or three times daily according to response **or** 0.132 mg/kg/dose IM. May repeat IM dose after 6–12 hr, if necessary. *Maximum:* 10 mg/day PO or rectal. **Children (18.2–38.6 kg [40–85 lb]):** 2.5 mg/dose PO or rectal three times daily **or** 0.132 mg/kg/dose IM. May repeat IM dose after 6–12 hr, if necessary. *Maximum:* 15 mg/day PO or rectal. **Adolescents:** 40 mg/day PO in four divided doses, every 6 hr; **or** 50 mg/day rectal in two divided doses, every 12 hr; **or** 5–10 mg/dose IM. May repeat IM dose after 3–4 hr, if necessary. *Maximum:* 40 mg/day IM.		
Promethazine *(Anergan 50®, Phenergan®, Phenoject-50®)*	Adjunctive pharmacotherapy with other preoperative pharmacotherapy, to provide (or enhance) analgesia, anti-emetic effects, and sedation	**Children (≥2 years) and adolescents:** 0.125–0.25 mg/kg IM or IV as a single dose. **Note:** Generally used in combination with atropine and meperidine. The choice of preoperative pharmacotherapy depends on the clinical condition of the patient, the type of anesthesia to be administered, the type of surgery to be performed, and the duration of the surgery.	Injectables, IM, IV: 25, 50 mg/ml **Note:** For IM or IV use only. Suppositories, rectal: 12.5, 25, 50 mg (in cocoa butter) Syrup, oral: 1.25, 5 mg/ml; contains 1.5%–7% alcohol and saccharin. Tablets, oral: 10, 12.5, 25, 50 mg **Note:** Administer IV at a rate ≤25 mg/min. Caution is required with IV therapy which generally is not recommended because inadvertent intra-arterial injection	**Contraindications:** Acutely ill or dehydrated patients, CNS depression associated with psychotropic pharmacotherapy, coma, and hypersensitivity to promethazine. **ADRs:** Commonly causes confusion and sedation, but may cause CNS excitation in some children. May cause extrapyramidal reactions, particularly among acutely ill children who are dehydrated. *See* Chapter 5. **Comments:** Children should be carefully monitored for adverse effects on cognitive abilities (e.g., school performance) and psychomotor skills (e.g., bike riding, roller blading).
	Motion sickness associated with travel (e.g., automobile, boat, plane), treatment	**Children (≥2 years):** 12.5 mg/dose IM, PO, or rectal every 8–12 hr as needed. *Maximum:* 25 mg/dose IM, PO, or rectal. **Adolescents:** 25 mg/dose IM, PO, or rectal every 8–12 hr as needed. **Note:** Administer first dose 30–60 min prior to travel departure.		

(Continued)

Footnotes are on page 558.

TABLE 14-1 continued

DRUG (TRADE AND OTHER NAMES)	INDICATION(S)	USUAL PEDIATRIC DOSAGE AND ADMINISTRATION[a]	DOSAGE FORMS	CONTRAINDICATIONS, ADRs, AND COMMENTS[b]
Promethazine *continued*	**Nausea and vomiting** (including that associated with anesthesia or surgery), **treatment**	**Children (≥2 years):** 12.5 mg/dose IM, IV, PO, or rectal every 4–6 hr as needed, according to response. **Alternatively,** 0.25 mg/kg/dose IM, IV, PO, or rectal every 4–6 hr as needed, according to response. *Maximum:* 25 mg/dose IM, IV, PO, or rectal; 25 mg/min IV. **Adolescents:** 25 mg/dose IM, IV, PO, or rectal every 4–6 hr as needed, according to response. **Note:** Generally administered IM or IV for postoperative nausea and vomiting.	may result in gangrene of the affected extremity. **Note:** Injectables contain sodium metabisulfite and sodium sulfite. Sulfites may cause hypersensitivity reactions among susceptible patients, particularly patients who have asthma.	
Propafenone *(Rythmol®)*	**Ventricular dysrhythmias** (e.g., sustained ventricular tachycardia), **prevention and suppression** **Note:** Generally reserved for potentially life-threatening dysrhythmias. **Note:** Not approved by the FDA or HPB for infants or children.	**Children and adolescents:** 250–500 mg/m²/day PO in three divided doses, every 8 hr; titrate dosage, according to response, to desired effect and tolerance. **Decrease dosage if widening of the QRS complex or prolongation of the PR interval is noted.** *Maximum:* 900 mg/day PO. **Note:** Reduce dosage for pediatric patients who have hepatic dysfunction.	Tablets, oral: 150, 225, 300 mg **Note:** Administer with food or milk to increase the rate and extent of absorption from the GI tract and to maintain bioavailability as consistent as possible. **Note:** Do not administer oral doses with grapefruit juice. Grapefruit juice may significantly increase the bioavailability of propafenone.	**Contraindications:** AV block, bradycardia, cardiogenic shock, chronic obstructive pulmonary disease, congestive heart failure (uncontrolled), electrolyte imbalance (severe), hypersensitivity to propafenone, hypotension (marked), myasthenia gravis, ritonavir pharmacotherapy (concurrent), and sick sinus syndrome. **ADRs:** May cause congestive heart failure, constipation, dizziness, dysrhythmias, nausea, unusual taste, and vomiting. *See* Chapter 5. **Comments:** Pharmacokinetic differences between fast and slow metabolizers of propafenone contribute to significant variability in plasma concentrations and toxicity. Even low dosages of quinidine, if used concomitantly, completely inhibit the hydroxylation of propafenone (the production of its hydroxy metabolite) and results in the equivalent pharmacokinetic effect as if these patients were slow metabolizers. In addition, propafenone is subject to extensive first-pass hepatic metabolism with a significant degree of interindividual variability. **Note:** Therapeutic drug monitoring is recommended; *see* Table 14-3. **Note:** Decrease digoxin dosage by 50% when initiating propafenone for pediatric patients who are receiving digoxin.
Propantheline *(Propanthel®)*	**Peptic ulcer disease,** adjunctive therapy **Note:** Conclusive evidence supporting the therapeutic efficacy for this indication is lacking.	**Children:** 22.5 mg/day PO in three divided doses, 30 min before meals. If required, an additional 7.5–15 mg may be administered PO at bedtime. **Adolescents:** 45 mg/day PO in three divided doses, 30 min before meals. If required, an additional	Tablets, oral: 7.5, 15 mg	**Contraindications:** GI obstruction, hepatic impairment (severe), hypersensitivity to propantheline or to other anticholinergics, intestinal atony, myasthenia gravis, myocardial ischemia, narrow-angle glaucoma, obstructive neuropathy, paralytic ileus, renal

TABLE 14-1 continued

DRUG (*TRADE* AND OTHER NAMES)	INDICATION(S)	USUAL PEDIATRIC DOSAGE AND ADMINISTRATION[a]	DOSAGE FORMS	CONTRAINDICATIONS, ADRs, AND COMMENTS[b]
Propantheline *continued*	**Note:** Not approved by the FDA or HPB for infants or children.	30 mg may be administered PO at bedtime.		impairment (severe), tachycardia, toxic megacolon, and ulcerative colitis (severe). **ADRs:** May cause a variety of ADRs including blurred vision, bradycardia, constipation, dizziness, drowsiness, dry mouth, fever, headache, insomnia, palpitations, restlessness, and seizures. Children, particularly those who have Down's syndrome or brain damage, appear to be more sensitive to the anticholinergic effects than are adolescents. *See* "Anticholinergics" in Chapter 5.
Proparacaine (*AK-Taine®, Alcaine®, Diocaine®, Ocu-Caine®, Ophthaine®*, Proxymetacaine)	**Ophthalmic anesthesia**, local, for conjunctival scoping for diagnosis, contact lens fitting, gonioscopy, removal of foreign bodies and sutures from the cornea, short surgical procedures involving the conjunctiva and cornea, and tonometry **Note:** Not approved by the FDA or HPB for children.	**Children and adolescents:** *Removal of Foreign Bodies and Sutures from the Cornea*, instill one or two drops 2 or 3 min before beginning the procedure. May repeat initial dose every 5–10 min, as required. *Maximum:* 0.5% ophthalmic solution, 14 drops/day. *Tonometry*, instill one or two drops of 0.5% ophthalmic solution into the affected eye(s) immediately before the procedure.	Solution, ophthalmic: 0.5% **Note:** For ophthalmic use only. **Note:** Store in tightly closed, light-resistant containers at controlled room temperature between 8 and 24°C (46–72°F) until opened. After opening, refrigerate. Safely and appropriately discard any solution that has become discolored.	**Contraindications:** Hypersensitivity to proparacaine. **ADRs:** Generally well tolerated. Some local irritation and stinging may occur several hours after ophthalmic instillation. Prolonged use may result in corneal epithelial erosion and severe keratitis. **Comments:** *See* Chapter 1 for a discussion of recommended techniques for administering ophthalmic drops to pediatric patients. **Note:** To avoid undue injury, instruct patients not to touch the eye(s) until the anesthetic has worn off. In addition, because the blink reflex is temporarily suppressed, an eye patch may be required to protect the eye from inadvertent injury.
Propericyazine, *see* **Pericyazine**				
Propofol (*Diprivan®*)	**Anesthesia, general** (induction and maintenance)	**Children (≥3 years) and adolescents:** *Induction*, 2–2.5 mg/kg IV; titrate dosage to desired effect, according to response. *Maintenance*, initially, 0.1–0.2 mg/kg/min IV (usually combined with 60%–70% nitrous oxide and oxygen). After the first 15–30 min of administration, the maintenance dosage generally can be **reduced** by 30%–50%. *Maximum:* Induction, 3.5 mg/kg IV; maintenance, 0.3 mg/kg/min IV. **Note:** Children of ASA physical status classes III and IV generally require reduced dosage.	Injectable emulsion, IV: 10 mg/ml; shake well before use. **Note:** For IV use only. **Note:** Strict aseptic technique must always be used when handling propofol because it contains no antibacterial preservatives and the vehicle (an emulsion containing egg phosphatide [egg lecithin], glycerol, soybean oil, and water) is capable of supporting rapid growth of microorganisms. Propofol and any syringe containing propofol are for single use only. The propofol vial should be opened just prior to the	**Contraindications:** Hypersensitivity to propofol or to lipid emulsions. **ADRs:** Frequently causes apnea, bradycardia, hypotension, hypertension, movement, rash, and sensation of burning or pain at injection site. **Note:** Apnea may be significantly exacerbated among children with respiratory tract infections. **Comments:** When used with nitrous oxide, propofol therapeutic plasma levels for general anesthesia are approximately 3–7 µg/ml. **Note:** Vital signs should be monitored continuously during the administration of propofol and personnel and equipment capable of providing artificial respiration and circulatory resuscitation must be available.

(Continued)

Footnotes are on page 558.

TABLE 14-1 continued

DRUG (TRADE AND OTHER NAMES)	INDICATION(S)	USUAL PEDIATRIC DOSAGE AND ADMINISTRATION[a]	DOSAGE FORMS	CONTRAINDICATIONS, ADRs, AND COMMENTS[b]
Propofol *continued*			initiation of each individual anesthetic procedure and the contents must be used within 6 hr of opening. Any unused propofol emulsion should be safely and appropriately discarded.	
Propranolol *(Betachron E-R®, Inderal®)*	**Atrial tachydysrhythmias,** which are refractory to standard antidysrhythmic therapy **Note:** Not approved by the FDA or HPB for the treatment of atrial tachydysrhythmias among infants and children.	**Children and adolescents:** Initially, 0.015–0.045 mg/kg IV. Repeat dose, if needed according to response, after 2 min. Additional doses may be administered at 4-hr intervals. Replace IV propranolol pharmacotherapy with oral propranolol pharmacotherapy as soon as feasible. *Maximum:* 3 mg/dose IV. *Maintenance:* 0.45–1.7 mg/kg/day PO in four divided doses, before meals and at bedtime. *Maximum:* 120 mg/day PO. **Note:** Infuse each IV dose over 10 min. *See* Chapter 8.	Capsules, oral sustained release: 60, 80, 120, 160 mg **Note:** Oral sustained-release capsules are not generally used for children. Injectable, IV: 1 mg/ml **Note:** For IV use only. Solutions, oral: 4, 8 mg/ml (strawberry–mint flavored) Solution, oral concentrate: 80 mg/ml Tablets, oral: 10, 20, 40, 60, 80, 90 mg	**Contraindications:** Asthma, bronchospasm, cardiogenic shock, congestive heart failure, heart block, malignant hypertension, myasthenia gravis, Raynaud's syndrome, and sinus bradycardia. **ADRs:** *See* Chapter 5. **Comments:** Considerable variability in oral bioavailability and subject to significant first-pass metabolism. Monitor ECG and blood pressure during IV administration. **Note:** Discontinue slowly over 1–2 weeks, according to response.
	Hypertension **Note:** Often used in combination with other antihypertensives (e.g., peripheral vasodilators, thiazide diuretics). **Note:** Not indicated for the emergency treatment of hypertensive crises.	**Children:** Initially, 1 mg/kg/day PO in two divided doses, every 12 hr. Increase dosage at 3–5-day intervals, as indicated by response, to 4 mg/kg/day PO. *Maximum:* 16 mg/kg/day PO or 320 mg/day PO, whichever is less. **Adolescents:** Initially, 80 mg/day PO as a single dose (if using sustained-release oral capsules) or as two divided doses, every 12 hr. Increase dosage at 3–5-day intervals, as indicated by response. *Maximum:* 640 mg/day PO.		
Propylthiouracil *(Propyl-Thyracil®)*	Hyperthyroidism	**Infants, children, and adolescents:** 5–7 mg/kg/day PO or 150 mg/m²/day PO in three divided doses, every 8 hr; adjust dosage according to thyroid function, usually 1/3 to 1/2 of initial dosage, once patient is euthyroid. *Maximum:* **Children (6–10 years),** initially, 150 mg/day PO; **children (>10 years) and adolescents,** initially, 300 mg/day PO. **Note:** Reduce dosage for pediatric patients who have renal dysfunction; *see* Table 14-2.	Tablets, oral: 50, 100 mg	**Contraindications:** Breast feeding, hypersensitivity to propylthiouracil, and pregnancy. **ADRs:** Generally well tolerated. May cause GI irritation, headache, myalgia, nausea, pruritus, and rash. May rarely cause agranulocytosis, hepatitis, hypothyroidism, jaundice, and thrombocytopenia. **Comments:** Monitor thyroid function. **Note:** Monitor hepatic function periodically. Propylthiouracil pharmacotherapy should be immediately discontinued if signs and symptoms of hepatotoxicity are noted.

Prostaglandin E₁, *see* **Alprostadil**

TABLE 14-1 continued

DRUG (TRADE AND OTHER NAMES)	INDICATION(S)	USUAL PEDIATRIC DOSAGE AND ADMINISTRATION[a]	DOSAGE FORMS	CONTRAINDICATIONS, ADRs, AND COMMENTS[b]
Protamine Sulfate	Heparin overdosage, antidote (reversal of heparinization) **Note:** Not approved by the FDA or HPB for infants or children.	**Infants, children, and adolescents:** 1 mg IV for every 115 units pork intestinal (porcine) heparin or every 90 units beef lung (bovine) heparin administered during previous 3–4 hr. *Maximum:* 50 mg/dose IV. Administer IV at a rate not exceeding 5 mg/min. Rapid IV administration may cause severe hypotension and anaphylacticlike reactions. *See* Chapter 8.	Injectable, IV: 10 mg/ml **Note:** For IV use only. May be administered IV without further dilution.	**Contraindications:** Hypersensitivity to protamine sulfate or to fish (salmon, in particular). **ADRs:** Generally well tolerated. **Comments:** Actual protamine neutralization factor for specific heparin lot is listed on the product label. Protamine sulfate effects persist for ~2 hr. Monitor activated clotting time (ACT), activated partial thromboplastin time (aPPT), or partial thromboplastin time (PTT).
Proxymetacaine, *see* **Proparacaine**				
Pseudoephedrine *(Dimetapp Decongestant Pediatric Drops®, Isoephedrine, PediaCare Infants' Oral Decongestant Drops®, Sudafed®, Triaminic Infant Oral Decongestant Drops®)*	Nasal congestion	**Infants, children, and adolescents:** 4 mg/kg/day PO in four divided doses, every 6 hr (every 12 hr for pseudoephedrine oral sustained-release capsule or tablet). *Maximum:* **Infants and children (<2 years),** 30 mg/day PO; **children (2–5 years),** 60 mg/day PO; **children (≥6 years),** 120 mg/day PO; **adolescents,** 60 mg/dose PO (120 mg/dose for oral sustained-released capsule); 240 mg/day PO. **Note:** Extended- or sustained-release oral formulations are not recommended for infants and children.	Capsule, sustained release: 120 mg Drop, oral: 1 mg/ml Solutions, oral: 15, 30 mg/5 ml Syrup, oral: 30 mg/5 ml Tablets, oral: 30, 60 mg Tablet, oral chewable: 15 mg; contains aspartame. Tablets, oral extended release: 120, 240 mg **Note:** Available in many combination cough and cold products.	**Contraindications:** Coronary artery disease (severe), hypertension (severe), hypersensitivity to pseudoephedrine, and MAOI therapy (concurrent). **ADRs:** Generally well tolerated. May cause mild CNS stimulation (e.g., excitability, insomnia, or nervousness). **Comments:** Use with caution for children with hypertension. Dosage for combination products should be determined by pseudoephedrine content.
Psyllium *(Konsyl®, Metamucil Fiber Laxative®, Serutan®)*	Constipation	**Children (≥6 years):** 5 ml of oral powder (1 teaspoonful), mixed in 240 ml (8 ounces) of water PO. Repeat dose, if required, up to three times per day according to response. **Adolescents:** 15 ml of oral powder (1 tablespoonful), mixed in 240 ml (8 ounces) of water PO. Repeat dose, if required, up to three times per day according to response. **Note:** Administration without adequate liquid may cause the psyllium to expand and block the throat or esophagus upon oral ingestion, resulting in choking.	Powder, oral (for mixing in water or another appropriate beverage **prior** to administration) **Note:** Mix each dose of psyllium powder in 240 ml (8 ounces) of cool water, fruit juice, or milk **prior** to use; ~3.4 grams is the usual dose of psyllium contained in 1 rounded tablespoonful of most manufacturers' products.	**Contraindications:** Fecal impaction, hypersensitivity to psyllium, and intestinal obstruction. **ADRs:** Generally well tolerated. May cause bloating, cramping, and flatulence. **Comments:** Clinical effect may be delayed for 12–72 hr following first dose.
Pteroylglutamic Acid, *see* **Folic Acid**				
Pyrantel Pamoate *(Antiminth®, Combantrin®, Pin-X®, Pin-Rid®, Reese's Pinworm Medicine®)*	Ascariasis (roundworm infestation)	**Infants, children, and adolescents:** 11 mg (pyrantel base)/kg PO as a one-time dose. *Maximum:* 1 gram (pyrantel base)/dose PO.	Capsule, oral soft gel: 62.5 mg (pyrantel base) Solution, oral: 50 mg/ml (pyrantel pamoate) (cherry flavored) Suspension, oral: 250 mg/5 ml (pyrantel base) (caramel–currant flavored); shake well before use. Tablets, oral: 62.5, 125 mg (pyrantel base)	**Contraindications:** Hepatic dysfunction, hypersensitivity to pyrantel pamoate, and pregnancy. **ADRs:** Generally well tolerated. May cause abdominal cramps, anorexia, diarrhea, dizziness, drowsiness, headache, insomnia, nausea, rash, and vomiting. **Comments:** In cases of enterobiasis, it is generally recommended that the entire family be treated with pyrantel pamoate.
	Enterobiasis (pinworm infestation)	**Infants, children, and adolescents:** 11 mg (pyrantel base)/kg PO as a single dose; repeat after 2 weeks. *Maximum:* 1 gram (pyrantel base)/dose PO.		*(Continued)*

Footnotes are on page 558.

TABLE 14-1 continued

DRUG (TRADE AND OTHER NAMES)	INDICATION(S)	USUAL PEDIATRIC DOSAGE AND ADMINISTRATION[a]	DOSAGE FORMS	CONTRAINDICATIONS, ADRs, AND COMMENTS[b]
Pyrantel Pamoate *continued*	Hookworm (*Ancylostoma duodenale* and *Necator americanus*) infestation **Note:** Not approved by the FDA or HPB for infants.	**Infants, children, and adolescents:** 11 mg (pyrantel base)/kg/day PO as a single dose for 3 consecutive days; repeat in 1 month, if necessary. *Maximum:* 1 gram (pyrantel base)/dose PO.	**Note:** 290 mg of pyrantel pamoate is equivalent to ~100 mg of pyrantel base. **Note:** Each dose of suspension may be mixed with milk or fruit juice to facilitate administration.	In addition, thorough cleaning of living quarters (e.g., vacuuming) and washing of all clothes and bed linen in hot water (or dry cleaning) will help to eliminate residual ova and prevent re-infestation.
Pyrazinamide (*Tebrazid®*)	Tuberculosis, adjunctive pharmacotherapy with other effective antitubercular drugs (e.g., isoniazid, rifampin) **Note:** Ensure that appropriate culture and sensitivity tests are performed and that the organism is sensitive to pyrazinamide. **Note:** Not approved by the FDA or HPB for infants or children.	**Children and adolescents:** 15–40 mg/kg/day PO as a single daily dose **or** 40–70 mg/kg PO twice weekly (dosage based on lean body weight). *Maximum:* Daily dosing, 2 grams/dose PO; twice weekly dosing, 4 grams/dose PO. **Note:** Reduce dosage for pediatric patients who have hepatic or renal dysfunction.	Tablet, oral: 500 mg	**Contraindications:** Gout (acute), hepatic dysfunction (severe), and hypersensitivity to pyrazinamide. **ADRs:** May cause anorexia, arthralgia, fever, hepatic dysfunction, hyperuricemia, malaise, nausea, rash, and vomiting. **Comments:** Monitor for hepatotoxicity (e.g., anorexia, darkened urine, fever, jaundice, or malaise), particularly with higher dosages and prolonged usage.
Pyridostigmine Bromide (*Mestinon®, Regonol®*)	Myasthenia gravis **Note:** Not approved by the FDA or HPB for children.	**Children:** Initially, 7 mg/kg/day PO in five or six divided doses. Increase dosage gradually at intervals of 2 days or longer until a further increase in dosage produces no corresponding increase in muscle strength. A reduction to the previous dosage provides the maintenance dosage. *Maximum:* Initial dose, 180 mg/day PO. **Adolescents:** Initially, 180 mg/day PO in three divided doses. Gradually increase the dosage at intervals of 2 days or longer until a further increase in dosage produces no corresponding increase in muscle strength. A reduction to the previous dosage provides the maintenance dosage. *Maximum:* 1500 mg/day PO. **Note:** The timing of divided doses should be individually determined by the needs and clinical condition of the patient. For example, if a patient's muscle fatigue makes eating difficult, then doses should be planned for 30–45 min before meals. **Note:** May need to reduce dosage for pediatric patients who have renal dysfunction.	Injectable, IM, IV: 5 mg/ml (*Regonol* injectable contains benzyl alcohol) Tablet, oral extended release: 180 mg Tablet, oral scored: 60 mg **Note:** Each dose of the extended-release tablet should be swallowed whole and not chewed or crushed. The extended-release tablet is generally recommended only at bedtime and only for those patients who are very weak upon awakening in the morning. **Note:** Pyridostigmine injectable is generally reserved for use during a myasthenic crisis or surgery. One-thirtieth of the oral dose is administered IM or very slowly IV every 2–3 hr as indicated by response. When large injectable doses are required, IV atropine sulfate is indicated to counteract the adverse muscarinic actions associated with pyridostigmine.	**Contraindications:** Hypersensitivity to pyridostigmine, to other anticholinesterases, or to bromides; mechanical intestinal or urinary tract obstruction; and peritonitis. **ADRs:** Generally well tolerated. May cause abdominal cramps, diarrhea, fasciculation, and salivation (increased). **Comments:** Some patients may become refractory after long-term use. Therapeutic response can sometimes be restored by decreasing the dosage or by discontinuing for a few days. Patients must be closely monitored during this period.

TABLE 14-1 continued

DRUG (TRADE AND OTHER NAMES)	INDICATION(S)	USUAL PEDIATRIC DOSAGE AND ADMINISTRATION[a]	DOSAGE FORMS	CONTRAINDICATIONS, ADRs, AND COMMENTS[b]
Pyridoxine (Vitamin B_6) **Note:** See also Chapter 4.	Dietary pyridoxine deficiency Pyridoxine-dependent seizures among patients with an inborn pyridoxine dependency, prophylaxis and treatment **Note:** Maintenance prophylaxis may be life-long.	**Infants, children, and adolescents:** 5–10 mg/day PO. *Maximum:* 20 mg/day PO. **Infants, seizure treatment:** Initially, 10–100 mg/dose IM or IV as a single dose or as several divided doses. **Infants, children, and adolescents, seizure prophylaxis:** 2–5 mg/kg/day PO as a single daily dose. *Maximum:* 100 mg/dose IM or PO.	Capsules, oral extended release: 100, 150 mg Injectable, IM, IV: 100 mg/ml Tablets, oral: 10, 25, 50, 100 mg Tablet, oral extended release: 100 mg	**Contraindications:** Hypersensitivity to pyridoxine. **ADRs:** Generally well tolerated and nontoxic at recommended dosages. **Comments:** Titrate dosage using lowest daily maintenance dose that prevents seizures. Long-term, high-dosage therapy has been associated with ataxia and severe neuropathy.
Pyrimethamine (Daraprim®)	Toxoplasmosis, adjunctive pharmacotherapy generally in combination with a sulfonamide	**Infants, children, and adolescents:** Initially, 2 mg/kg/day PO in two divided doses, every 12 hr, for 3 days. *Maintenance:* 1 mg/kg/day PO as a single daily dose for 4 weeks. *Maximum:* Initially, 100 mg/day PO; maintenance, 25 mg/day PO. **Note:** Administer with food or milk to decrease associated GI irritation. ***Alternatively***, *pyrimethamine pharmacotherapy in combination with sulfadiazine pharmacotherapy:* **Infants (<3 months):** 6.25 mg pyrimethamine PO and 100 mg/kg sulfadiazine (*maximum,* 1000 mg) PO every **other** day in four divided doses. **Infants (3–9 months):** 6.25 mg pyrimethamine and 100 mg/kg sulfadiazine (*maximum,* 1000 mg)/day PO in four divided doses. **Infants (>9 months) and children (<2 years):** 12.5 mg pyrimethamine and 150 mg/kg sulfadiazine (*maximum,* 1500 mg)/day PO in four divided doses. **Children (2–6 years):** Initially, 25 mg pyrimethamine PO, followed by 12.5 mg pyrimethamine and 150 mg/kg sulfadiazine (*maximum,* 2000 mg)/day PO in four divided doses. **Children (>6 years) and adolescents:** Initially, 50 mg pyrimethamine PO, followed by 25 mg pyrimethamine and 150 mg/kg sulfadiazine (*maximum,* 4000 mg)/day PO in four divided doses. **Note:** Duration of pyrimethamine and sulfadiazine combination pharmacotherapy is generally 3–6 weeks. If longer pharmacotherapy is required, a 2-week interval is recommended between treatments.	Tablet, oral: 25 mg	**Contraindications:** Hypersensitivity to pyrimethamine, megaloblastic anemia caused by folate deficiency, and pregnancy (first trimester). **ADRs:** May cause anorexia, diarrhea, and vomiting. **Comments:** May cause folic acid deficiency and associated bone marrow depression. Leucovorin calcium supplementation (2–15 mg/day PO) is recommended every 3 days, or as required, to prevent or reverse blood dyscrasias related to folic acid deficiency. Complete blood cell counts should be performed twice weekly.

Footnotes are on page 558.

TABLE 14-1 continued

DRUG (TRADE AND OTHER NAMES)	INDICATION(S)	USUAL PEDIATRIC DOSAGE AND ADMINISTRATION[a]	DOSAGE FORMS	CONTRAINDICATIONS, ADRs, AND COMMENTS[b]
Pyrithione Zinc (DHS Zinc®, Head & Shoulders®)	Dandruff of the scalp	**Children and adolescents:** Apply a small amount of 1% shampoo to wet hair and massage on scalp into a foamy lather. Rinse thoroughly with water. Repeat application one to three times per week as indicated by response.	Shampoos, topical: 1%, 2% **Note:** For external use only. Avoid contact with eyes.	**Contraindications:** Hypersensitivity to pyrithione or other shampoo formulation ingredients. **ADRs:** Generally well tolerated.
Quinidine (Biquin®, Cardioquin®, Quinidex®)	Atrial tachydysrhythmias/ Supraventricular tachydysrhythmias/ Ventricular dysrhythmias **Note:** Not approved by the FDA or HPB for infants or children.	**Children and adolescents:** 15–30 mg quinidine base/kg/day PO in four to six divided doses every 4–6 hr (every 8 hr for quinidine oral sustained-release tablets), as indicated by response. **Note:** Reduce dosage for pediatric patients who have renal (see Table 14-2) or hepatic dysfunction. **Note:** ECG should be monitored continuously when high dosages are used.	Capsules, oral: 200, 260, 325 mg (as sulfate) Injectables, IV: 80 mg/ml (gluconate); 190, 200 mg/ml (sulfate) Tablets, oral: 100, 200, 260, 300 mg (sulfate); 275 mg (polygalacturonate); 325 mg (gluconate) Tablets, sustained release: 300 mg (sulfate); 324, 330 mg (gluconate); 250 mg (bisulfate) **Note:** Quinidine sulfate is 82.6% quinidine base; quinidine bisulfate is 66% quinidine base; quinidine gluconate is 62.35% quinidine base; quinidine polygalacturonate is 60% quinidine base. **Note:** Injectable formulation is available in Canada through the Special Access Program.	**Contraindications:** AV block, digitalis intoxication, heart failure, hypersensitivity to quinidine or to other cinchona derivatives, heart block, left bundle branch block, long QT syndrome (prolonged QT interval), myasthenia gravis, thrombocytopenia purpura, and torsades de pointes (history of drug induced). **ADRs:** Commonly causes GI distress (anorexia, diarrhea, nausea, and vomiting). See Chapter 5. **Comments:** Therapeutic drug monitoring is recommended; see Table 14-3. Monitor also for signs and symptoms of cinchonism (dizziness, headache, hearing loss, lightheadedness, nausea, tinnitus, vertigo, and visual impairment) that may occur, even after a single dose. Concurrent quinidine and digoxin may significantly increase digoxin to toxic levels (see Chapter 6).
	Plasmodium falciparum malaria, chloroquine resistant **Note:** Generally reserved for potentially life-threatening cases of malaria. Initiate standard oral antimalarial therapy (e.g., quinine sulfate) as soon as clinically feasible. **Note:** Not approved by the FDA or HPB for infants or children.	**Children and adolescents:** 6.2 mg quinidine base/kg IV over 1–2 hr, **then** 12.4 μg quinidine base/kg/min by continuous IV infusion for up to 72 hr. **Note:** For the treatment of malaria, adjust IV infusion so that quinidine blood concentrations remain below 6 μg/ml. Monitor ECG continuously. **Note:** A single 100- or 200-mg oral "test" dose is often recommended to identify quinidine hypersensitivity or idiosyncrasy.		
Quinine Dihydrochloride **Note:** See also Quinine Sulfate.	Chloroquine-resistant *Plasmodium falciparum* malaria (with coma) **Note:** Initiate standard oral antimalarial therapy (e.g., quinine sulfate) as soon as clinically feasible.	**Children and adolescents:** 20 mg/kg IV optional loading dose; then 30 mg/kg/day IV in three divided doses, every 8 hr. **Note:** Infuse each divided dose IV over 4 hr. **Note:** Reduce dosage for pediatric patients who have renal dysfunction; see Table 14-2.	Injectable, IV: Available in Canada only through Health Canada's Special Access Program. **Note:** Not generally available in the United States.	**Contraindications:** Blackwater fever (history of), glucose-6-phosphate dehydrogenase deficiency, hypersensitivity to quinine, optic neuritis, pregnancy, thrombocytopenia purpura (associated with previous quinine use), and tinnitus. **ADRs:** May cause agranulocytosis, confusion, convulsions, fever, GI irritation, hemolysis (acute), rashes, and thrombocytopenia. **Comments:** Monitor for signs and symptoms of cinchonism (dizziness, headache, hearing loss, lightheadedness, nausea, tinnitus, vertigo, and visual impairment) that may occur after a single dose. IV quinine has been generally replaced with IV quinidine therapy.
Quinine Sulfate **Note:** See also Quinine Dihydrochloride.	Chloroquine-resistant *Plasmodium falciparum* malaria	**Children and adolescents:** 30 mg/kg/day PO in three divided doses for 5–7 days. Administer with meals to minimize GI irritation. *Maximum:* 650 mg/day PO; 7 days (total number of days of therapy).	Capsules, oral: 200, 260, 300, 325 mg Tablets, oral: 163, 260, 325 mg	**Contraindications:** Blackwater fever (history of), glucose-6-phosphate dehydrogenase deficiency, hypersensitivity to quinine, optic neuritis, pregnancy, thrombocytopenia purpura (associated with previous quinine use), and tinnitus.

TABLE 14-1 continued

DRUG (TRADE AND OTHER NAMES)	INDICATION(S)	USUAL PEDIATRIC DOSAGE AND ADMINISTRATION[a]	DOSAGE FORMS	CONTRAINDICATIONS, ADRs, AND COMMENTS[b]
Quinine Sulfate *continued*		**Note:** Reduce dosage for pediatric patients who have renal dysfunction; *see* Table 14-2.		**ADRs:** May cause agranulocytosis, confusion, convulsions, fever, GI irritation, rashes, hemolysis (acute), and thrombocytopenia. **Comments:** Monitor for signs and symptoms of cinchonism (dizziness, headache, hearing loss, lightheadedness, nausea, tinnitus, vertigo, and visual impairment) that may occur after a single dose or with prolonged therapy.
Quinupristin and Dalfopristin *(Synercid®)*	Vancomycin-resistant *Enterococcus faecium* (VREF) infection **Note:** Not approved by the FDA or HPB for children or adolescents.	**Children and adolescents:** 22.5 mg/kg/day by IV infusion in three divided doses, every 8 hr. **Note:** Dilute each dose with 250 ml of 5% dextrose in water and infuse IV over 60 min.	Injectable, IV (lyophilized powder for reconstitution): 500 mg (150 mg quinupristin: 350 mg dalfopristin) per 10-ml single-dose vial **Note:** For IV use only. **Note:** Store unopened injectable vials under refrigeration between 2 and 8°C (36–46°F). **Note:** Reconstitute contents of single-dose vial with 5 ml of 5% dextrose in water for injection or sterile water for injection. Gently swirl and invert vial back and forth to ensure dissolution of the powder. Do **not** shake. Let solution stand for a few minutes until all foam has dissipated. Resultant solution should be clear and should contain 100 mg/ml of quinupristin and dalfopristin. The reconstituted solution is stable for 5 hr at room temperature.	**Contraindications:** Hypersensitivity to quinupristin and dalfopristin or to other streptogramins. **ADRs:** May cause arthralgia, diarrhea, myalgia, nausea, and rash. May also cause pain at infusion site, phlebitis, and thrombophlebitis, which account for up to 50% of reasons for the discontinuation of therapy. **Note:** If required, vein may be flushed with 5% dextrose in water solution. Do not flush with heparin or saline solutions because of physical incompatibility with *Synercid*. **Comments:** The combination drug is a potent inhibitor of cytochrome P-450 3A4 and can cause significant drug interactions with a variety of drugs including cyclosporine, midazolam, and nifedipine. (*See* Chapter 6 for further discussion of the drug interactions involving the inhibition of cytochrome P-450 isoenzymes.)

Rabies Immune Globulin, Human, *see* Chapter 9

DRUG	INDICATION(S)	DOSAGE	DOSAGE FORMS	COMMENTS
Ranitidine *(Zantac®)*	Duodenal ulcer/ Peptic ulcer/ Reflux esophagitis **Note:** Not approved by the FDA or HPB for infants or children.	**Children and adolescents:** 2.5–6 mg/kg/day PO in two divided doses, every 12 hr **or** 1–2 mg/kg/dose IM or IV in three or four divided doses, every 6 or 8 hr, according to response. *Maximum:* 50 mg/dose IM or IV; 300 mg/day PO. **Note:** Reduce dosage for pediatric patients who have renal dysfunction; *see* Table 14-2.	Capsules, oral *(Zantac GEL® dose)*: 150, 300 mg Granules, oral effervescent *(Zantac EFFER® dose)*: 150 mg Injectables, IM, IV: 0.5, 25 mg/ml Solution, oral: 15 mg/ml (peppermint flavored); contains 7.5% alcohol and cyclamate sodium.	**Contraindications:** Hypersensitivity to ranitidine. **ADRs:** Generally well tolerated. *See* Chapter 5. **Comments:** Injectable pharmacotherapy is reserved for those patients for whom oral pharmacotherapy is not feasible.
	Excess stomach acid (commonly associated with consumption of food and beverages) and relief of related signs and symptoms (e.g., dyspepsia, hyperacidity,	**Children and adolescents:** 2 mg/kg/dose PO 30–60 min prior to the consumption of food or beverages that are associated with excessive stomach acid and related signs and symptoms. *Maximum:* 75 mg/dose PO; 150 mg/day PO.	Syrup, oral: 15 mg/ml (peppermint flavored); contains 7.5% alcohol and saccharin. Tablets, oral: 75, 150, 300 mg Tablet, oral effervescent *(Zantac EFFER dose)*: 150 mg	

(Continued)

TABLE 14-1 continued

DRUG (TRADE AND OTHER NAMES)	INDICATION(S)	USUAL PEDIATRIC DOSAGE AND ADMINISTRATION[a]	DOSAGE FORMS	CONTRAINDICATIONS, ADRs, AND COMMENTS[b]
Ranitidine *continued*	sour stomach, upset stomach), **prophylaxis**		**Note:** Oral effervescent tablets and granules contain aspartame and phenylalanine.	
	Excess stomach acid, treatment	**Children and adolescents:** 2 mg/kg/dose PO upon the onset of signs and symptoms. May repeat dose once after 1 hr if signs and symptoms persist or return. *Maximum:* 75 mg/dose PO; 150 mg/day PO.		
Remantidin, *see* **Rimantadine**				
Ribavirin (Virazole®)	Respiratory syncytial virus (RSV) infection among high-risk pediatric patients **Note:** Inhalation therapy is usually used as adjunctive therapy with appropriate supportive respiratory therapy and fluid management.	**Infants and children:** 6 grams/day by inhalation diluted in 300 ml sterile water for injection (preservative free) over 12–18 hr/day for 3–7 days. **Note:** Administer by inhalation with a Viratek® small particle aerosol generator (SPAG-2).	Powder, for dilution for aerosol generator inhalation: 6 grams/vial **Note:** Ribavirin aerosol can precipitate in mechanical ventilators and result in ventilator malfunction. The ventilator malfunction has been associated with an increase in pulmonary pressure. Carefully monitor for and minimize accumulation of drug precipitate during inhalation therapy.	**Contraindications:** Hypersensitivity to ribavirin and pregnancy. **ADRs:** Inhalation therapy has been associated with conjunctivitis, rash, and reticulocytosis. In addition, ADRs (including conjunctivitis, headache, lacrimation, and rhinitis) commonly occur among healthcare workers who provide direct care to pediatric patients receiving therapy. *See* Chapter 5. **Comments:** Antagonizes the antiviral activity of zidovudine. Associated with a sudden significant decline in respiratory function. Carefully monitor respiratory function during therapy and discontinue if a sudden significant decline in respiratory function is observed.
Riboflavin (Vitamin B_2)	Dietary riboflavin deficiency	**Children and adolescents:** 2.5–10 mg/day PO as a single daily dose. *Maximum:* 30 mg/day PO.	Tablets, oral: 5, 10, 25, 50, 100, 250 mg	**Contraindications:** None identified. **ADRs:** Generally well tolerated and nontoxic. **Comments:** Large doses may color the urine bright yellow.
Rifampicin, *see* **Rifampin**				
Rifampin (Rifampicin, Rifadin®, Rofact®)	*Haemophilus influenzae* infection, **prophylaxis**	**Infants, children, and adolescents:** 20 mg/kg/day PO as a single daily dose for 4 days. *Maximum:* 600 mg/day PO.	Capsules, oral: 150, 300 mg	**Contraindications:** Hypersensitivity to rifampin and to rifamycins and pregnancy. **ADRs:** Commonly causes GI irritation. *See* Chapter 5. **Comments:** May discolor the urine, sweat, saliva, and tears orange–red. Commonly interacts with other drugs and interactions may be clinically significant (*see* Chapter 6). **Note:** Monitor hepatic function upon initiation of therapy.
	Meningococcal infection (*Neisseria meningitidis*), prophylaxis	**Infants, children, and adolescents:** 20 mg/kg/day PO in two divided doses, every 12 hr, for 2 days. *Maximum:* 600 mg/dose PO; 1200 mg/day PO.		
	Tuberculosis (in combination with at least one other antitubercular drug [e.g., isoniazid])	**Infants, children, and adolescents:** 10–20 mg/kg/day PO as a single daily dose for a minimum of 6 months. *Maximum:* 600 mg/dose PO.		
Rimantadine (Flumadine®, Remantadin)	Respiratory tract infection caused by influenza A virus, prophylaxis and symptomatic treatment	**Children (<10 years), prophylaxis:** 5 mg/kg/day PO as a single daily dose for up to 30 days. **Children (<10 years), treatment:** 5 mg/kg/day PO as a single daily dose for 5 days.	Syrup, oral: 50 mg/5 ml (raspberry flavored) Tablet, oral: 100 mg	**Contraindications:** Hypersensitivity to rimantadine or to amantadine. **ADRs:** Generally well tolerated. May cause dizziness, insomnia, nausea, and nervousness.

CHAPTER 14: DRUG DOSING FOR INFANTS, CHILDREN, AND ADOLESCENTS

TABLE 14-1 continued

DRUG (TRADE AND OTHER NAMES)	INDICATION(S)	USUAL PEDIATRIC DOSAGE AND ADMINISTRATION[a]	DOSAGE FORMS	CONTRAINDICATIONS, ADRs, AND COMMENTS[b]
Rimantadine *continued*	**Note:** Not effective for the treatment of other viral infections (e.g., influenza B).	**Children (≥10 years) and adolescents, prophylaxis.** 200 mg/day PO in two divided doses for up to 30 days. **Children (≥10 years) and adolescents, treatment:** 200 mg/day PO in two divided doses for 5 days. *Maximum:* **Children (<10 years),** 150 mg/day PO; **children (≥10 years) and adolescents,** 200 mg/day PO. **Note:** Reduce dosage for pediatric patients who have hepatic dysfunction.		**Comments:** Therapeutic advantages over the use of amantadine include a significantly lower incidence of ADRs affecting the CNS and not needing to adjust dosage for pediatric patients with renal dysfunction.
Risperidone (Risperdal®)	**Behavioral and conduct disorders,** severe with a significant aggressive component and unresponsive to other conventional treatment interventions/ **Schizophrenia and other psychotic disorders** **Note:** Not approved by the FDA or HPB for children or adolescents.	**Children (≥5 years) and adolescents:** Initially, 0.25 mg/day PO as a single dose at bedtime. Increase dosage by 0.25 mg/day at 7-day intervals as indicated by response. *Maximum:* 5 mg/day PO. **Note:** Reduce dosage for pediatric patients who have renal dysfunction.	Solution, oral: 1 mg/ml Tablets, oral: 0.25, 0.5, 1, 2, 3, 4 mg **Note:** Risperidone oral solution is compatible when mixed with coffee, low-fat milk, orange juice, or water. The oral solution is **not** compatible with cola drinks or tea.	**Contraindications:** Hypersensitivity to risperidone. **ADRs:** May cause agitation, amenorrhea, anxiety, constipation, dizziness, edema, ejaculatory dysfunction, extrapyramidal reactions, headache, hypotension, insomnia, nausea, nervousness, palpitations, psychosis, rash, rhinitis, somnolence, suicide attempt, tachycardia, and weight gain. Rarely causes AV block, cardiac dysrhythmias, neuroleptic malignant syndrome, neutropenia, priapism, QTc interval prolongation, seizures, Stevens-Johnson syndrome, syncope, tardive dyskinesia, and water intoxication.
Ritonavir (Norvir®, Norvir SEC®)	**HIV infection** (usually used in combination with other antiretroviral drugs) **Note:** Patients may continue to develop opportunistic infections and other complications of HIV infection. In addition, ritonavir therapy does not reduce the risk for HIV transmission to others.	**Children:** Initially, 500 mg/m²/day PO in two divided doses. At 2- or 3-day intervals, increase dosage by 100 mg/m²/day, according to response. Usual maintenance dosage is 800 mg/m²/day PO. If this dosage cannot be tolerated, then the highest dosage that can be tolerated should be used as the maintenance dosage. *Maximum:* 1200 mg/day PO. **Note:** Whenever possible, each dose should be administered using a calibrated oral dosing syringe. **Adolescents:** Initially, 600 mg/day PO in two divided doses. Increase dosage by 200 mg/day at 2- or 3-day intervals. Usual maintenance dosage is 1200 mg/day PO. *Maximum:* 1200 mg/day PO. **Note:** Administer each dose with meals (breakfast and dinner). Palatibility of the oral solution may be increased by mixing with chocolate milk or the nutritional supplements Advera® or Ensure® just prior to ingestion.	Capsule, oral soft elastic: 100 mg; contains >10% alcohol. Solution, oral: 80 mg/ml (peppermint–caramel flavored, supplied with oral dosage cup); contains >30% alcohol. **Note:** Oral capsules must be dispensed and stored in their original container; store under refrigeration between 2 and 8°C until dispensed. Once dispensed, refrigeration is still recommended, but not required, provided that the oral capsules are stored at controlled room temperature below 25°C for no longer than 30 days. **Note:** Store oral solution at controlled room temperature between 20 and 25°C. Do not refrigerate,	**Contraindications:** Hypersensitivity to ritonavir and concurrent therapy with the following drugs, which may be negatively affected by drug interactions associated with ritonavir's affinity for several cytochrome P-450 isoenzyme systems, particularly CYP 3A4 (see Chapter 6, Table 6-1): alprazolam, amiodarone, bepridil, bupropion, cisapride, clorazepate, clozapine, diazepam, dihydroergotamine, encainide, ergonovine, ergotamine, estazolam, flecainide, flurazepam, meperidine, methylergonovine, midazolam, pimozide, piroxicam, propafenone, propoxyphene, quinidine, rifabutin, triazolam, and zolpidem. **ADRs:** Commonly causes asthenia, circumoral paresthesia, diarrhea, nausea, peripheral paresthesia, taste distortion, and vomiting. GI irritation and paresthesias generally diminish with continued therapy. May also cause abnormal fat distribution; hepatitis (acute); *(Continued)*

Footnotes are on page 558.

TABLE 14-1 continued

DRUG (*TRADE* AND OTHER NAMES)	INDICATION(S)	USUAL PEDIATRIC DOSAGE AND ADMINISTRATION[a]	DOSAGE FORMS	CONTRAINDICATIONS, ADRs, AND COMMENTS[b]
Ritonavir *continued*			but protect from excessive heat. **Note:** Shake oral solution well before measuring each dose with the oral solution dosage cup that is provided with the product. The cup should be washed immediately after each use with hot sudsy water made with tap water and dish detergent and dried thoroughly. **Note:** Oral solution must be dispensed and stored in its original container.	hyperlipidemia; increased bleeding tendency, particularly among pediatric patients who have hereditary bleeding disorders; and seizures. *See* Chapter 5. **Comments:** Monitor hepatic function and CD4 cell counts upon initiation and periodically during therapy.
Rituximab, *see* Chapter 12				
Rocuronium (*Zemuron®*)	Adjunctive pharmacotherapy with general anesthesia (e.g., halothane) for the facilitation of nonemergency tracheal intubation/**Skeletal muscle relaxation during surgery** **Note:** Provides neuromuscular blockade.	**Infants (≥3 months) and children:** Initial rapid IV injection after patient is unconscious, 0.6 mg/kg IV over 30 sec. *Continuous IV infusion upon spontaneous recovery from the initial rapid IV injection (after ~40 min for infants and ~30 min for children),* 12 μg/kg/min. *Maximum continuous IV infusion rate:* 16 μg/kg/min. **Note:** Do **not** inject initial rapid IV dose until patient is unconscious (*see also* "Comments"). **Adolescents:** *Initial rapid IV injection after patient is unconscious,* 0.6 mg/kg IV over 30 sec. *Continuous IV infusion upon spontaneous recovery from the initial rapid IV injection (after ~22 min),* 12 μg/kg/min. *Maximum continuous IV infusion rate:* 16 μg/kg/min. **Note:** Do **not** inject initial rapid IV dose until patient is unconscious (*see also* "Comments"). **Note:** May need to reduce dosage for pediatric patients who have hepatic dysfunction.	Injectable, IV: 10 mg/ml **Note:** For IV use only.	**Contraindications:** Hypersensitivity to rocuronium, myasthenia gravis, and myasthenic (Eaton-Lambert) syndrome. **ADRs:** Generally well tolerated. ADRs are generally an extension of anticipated pharmacologic actions (e.g., skeletal muscle weakness). **Comments:** Whenever administered, patients should be continuously monitored with a peripheral nerve stimulator to evaluate response, determine the need for additional doses, and measure the adequacy of spontaneous recovery or anticholinesterase (e.g., edrophonium or neostigmine) antagonism (in the event that an antagonist is needed). Additional doses should not be administered before there is a definite response to T1 or to the first twitch. If no response is elicited, the infusion should be discontinued until a response returns.
Rofecoxib (*Vioxx®*)	**Acute pain, mild to moderate,** short-term symptomatic relief **Note:** Evaluated clinically only for pain associated with dental surgery and primary dysmenorrhea.	**Children:** 25 mg/day PO as a single dose. May repeat dose once daily for up to 5 days, according to response. **Adolescents:** 25–50 mg/day PO as a single dose. May repeat dose once daily for up to 5 days, according to response. *Maximum:* 50 mg/day PO.	Suspensions, oral: 12.5, 25 mg/5 ml (strawberry flavored); shake well before use. Tablets, oral: 12.5, 25 mg	**Contraindications:** Hypersensitivity to rofecoxib or to other NSAIDs. **ADRs:** Generally well tolerated. May cause edema of the lower extremities, epigastric irritation, hypertension, and nausea. **Comments:** Published clinical data regarding use for pediatric patients is limited. Until

TABLE 14-1 continued

DRUG (TRADE AND OTHER NAMES)	INDICATION(S)	USUAL PEDIATRIC DOSAGE AND ADMINISTRATION[a]	DOSAGE FORMS	CONTRAINDICATIONS, ADRs, AND COMMENTS[b]
Rofecoxib *continued*	**Note:** Not approved by the FDA or HPB for children.			additional data are available, pediatric therapy requires same cautions afforded other NSAIDs. *See* "Nonsteroidal Anti-inflammatory Drugs" in Chapter 5.
Rosiglitazone *(Avandia®)*	Diabetes, type 2 (used as an adjunct to appropriate diet and exercise for the management of type 2 diabetes) **Note:** Used as either monopharmaco-therapy or adjunctive pharmacotherapy for patients who have inadequate glucose control in response to maximal dosage of metformin. **Note:** Not approved by the FDA or HPB for adolescents.	**Adolescents:** Initially, 4 mg/day PO in two divided doses, morning and evening. If adequate clinical response based on a reduction in fasting blood sugar (FBS) has not been achieved after 12 weeks, then the dosage may be increased to 8 mg/day PO in two divided doses, morning and evening.	Tablets, oral: 2, 4, 8 mg	**Contraindications:** Hepatic impairment (moderate to severe), hypersensitivity to rosiglitazone or to other thiazolidinediones, and New York Heart Association (NYHA) class 3 and 4 cardiac status. **ADRs:** Generally well tolerated. May cause fluid retention (and resultant edema) and hypoglycemia. **Comments:** Monitor hepatic function upon initiation and periodically during therapy.

Rotavirus Vaccine, *see* **Chapter 9**

Rubella Virus Vaccine, *see* **Chapter 9**

Sacrosidase *(Sucraid®)*	Congenital sucrase-isomaltase deficiency (CSID) **Note:** Provides replacement therapy for the sucrase deficiency associated with this syndrome and, thus, allows hydrolysis of the disaccharide, sucrose, into its component monosaccharides. However, dietary starch restriction may still be required.	**Infants (≥5 months) and children (≤15 kg):** 8500 international units (IU)/dose PO with each meal or snack. **Children (>15 kg) and adolescents:** 17,000 IU/dose PO with each meal or snack. **Note:** 8500 IU can be measured by using either the measuring scoop provided with the solution or by counting 22 drops (1 ml) from the container tip.	Solution, oral: 8500 IU/ml (available in a plastic squeeze drop bottle with a measuring scoop) **Note:** Oral solution is fully soluble when mixed in infant formula, milk, and water. However, its enzyme activity is adversely affected when mixed in acidic fruit juices or other acidic beverages, or when heated. **Note:** Store solution under refrigeration between 2 and 8°C (36–46° F). Protect the oral solution from exposure to heat and light. Once the plastic squeeze bottle is opened, the solution should be used within 1 month. After 1 month, any unused oral solution should be safely and appropriately discarded. **Note:** Not generally available in Canada.	**Contraindications:** Hypersensitivity to glycerin (glycerol), sacrosidase, yeast, or yeast products. **ADRs:** Generally well tolerated. May cause nausea or vomiting.

Salicylazosulfapyridine, *see* **Sulfasalazine**

Footnotes are on page 558.

TABLE 14-1 continued

DRUG (TRADE AND OTHER NAMES)	INDICATION(S)	USUAL PEDIATRIC DOSAGE AND ADMINISTRATION[a]	DOSAGE FORMS	CONTRAINDICATIONS, ADRs, AND COMMENTS[b]
Salmeterol Xinafoate (Advair Diskus®, Serevent Diskus®)	Asthma management **Note:** Not indicated for the symptomatic management of acute asthmatic attacks.	Children (≥4 years) and adolescents: 100 µg/day by inhalation in two divided doses, every 12 hr, morning and evening.	Powder, for inhalation (Serevent Diskus): The Serevent Diskus is a specially designed plastic inhalation device that delivers ~50 µg/actuation; contains lactose. Suspension, metered dose inhaler: 25 µg/actuation **Note:** For pulmonary inhalation only.	**Contraindications:** Hypersensitivity to salmeterol xinafoate. **ADRs:** May cause bronchospasms, headache, nausea, sore throat, and tachycardia. **Comments:** When used to prevent exercise-induced bronchospasm, therapeutic effects may last for 9–12 hr.
	Exercise-induced bronchospasm, prophylaxis	Children (≥4 years) and adolescents: One inhalation (50 µg) 30–60 min prior to exercise. **Note:** Patients, who are receiving salmeterol xinafoate for the management of asthma, should **not** receive an additional dose in order to prevent exercise-induced bronchospasm.		
Sargramostim, see Chapter 12				
Scopolamine (Hyoscine, Scopace®, Transderm-Scop®, Transderm-V®)	Inhibition of salivation and excessive respiratory secretions during surgery **Note:** Not approved by the FDA or HPB for children.	Children and adolescents: 6 µg/kg IM, IV, or SC 30–60 min before surgery. *Maximum:* 0.6 mg/dose IM, IV, or SC. **Note:** The choice of preoperative medication depends on the clinical condition of the patient, the type of anesthesia to be administered, the type of surgery to be performed, and the duration of the surgery.	Injectables, IM, IV, SC: 0.3, 0.4, 0.86, 1 mg/ml (hydrobromide) 20 mg/ml (butylbromide) Transdermal drug delivery system (TDDS), topical: 1.5 mg/2.5 cm² (delivers 0.5 mg [Transderm Scop, United States] or 1 mg [Transderm-V, Canada] over 72 hr) **Note:** Wash hands thoroughly after handling the TDDS. Dilation of the pupil and resultant blurred vision may occur if scopolamine comes into contact with the eye(s).	**Contraindications:** Glaucoma and hypersensitivity to scopolamine. **ADRs:** Commonly causes drowsiness and dry mouth. *See* Chapter 5. **Comments:** Infants and children appear to be more susceptible to the adverse anticholinergic effects than are older children and adolescents. Patients exposed to high environmental temperatures may experience hyperthermia and heat prostration.
	Prevention of nausea and vomiting associated with motion sickness **Note:** Not approved by the FDA or HPB for children.	Adolescents: Apply one scopolamine transdermal drug delivery system to a clean, dry, hairless skin site behind the ear approximately 12 hr before the antiemetic effect is required. Replace system, if needed, every 72 hr.		
Secobarbital	Insomnia **Note:** Tolerance to the hypnotic action generally occurs after 2 weeks. Thus, therapy exceeding 2 weeks is not recommended. Re-evaluate patients who appear to require longer therapy. **Note:** Generally replaced with benzodiazepines because of their higher therapeutic index.	Infants (<6 months): 15–30 mg/day rectal at bedtime. Infants (≥6 months) and children (<3 years): 60 mg/day rectal at bedtime. Children (≥3 years): 60–100 mg/day PO at bedtime or 60–100 mg/day rectal at bedtime **or** 3–5 mg/kg/day IM, to a maximum 100 mg, at bedtime. Adolescents: 100 mg/day PO at bedtime.	Capsules, oral: 50, 100 mg Injectable, IM, IV: 50 mg/ml Suppositories, rectal: 30, 60, 100, 120 mg Tablet, oral: 100 mg **Note:** Injectable is highly alkaline; inject IM deeply into healthy muscle sites to minimize possible tissue necrosis. Use extreme care to avoid extravasation during IV injection. IV injection is **not** recommended because of risk for respiratory depression and is generally reserved for hospital settings only.	**Contraindications:** Hepatic dysfunction (severe), hypersensitivity to secobarbital or to other barbiturates, porphyria (severe), renal dysfunction (severe), and respiratory disease (severe) where dyspnea or obstruction is present. **ADRs:** Commonly causes respiratory depression, particularly following IM or IV injection. May also cause bradycardia, GI irritation, headache, hypersensitivity reactions, hypotension, lethargy, skin rash, and suppression of REM sleep. *See* Chapter 5. **Comments:** Some children experience CNS excitation rather than CNS depression. Observed behaviors include aggression, excitability, hyperkinesis, and irritability.

TABLE 14-1 continued

DRUG (TRADE AND OTHER NAMES)	INDICATION(S)	USUAL PEDIATRIC DOSAGE AND ADMINISTRATION[a]	DOSAGE FORMS	CONTRAINDICATIONS, ADRs, AND COMMENTS[b]
Selenium Sulfide (Head & Shoulders Intensive®, Selsun Blue®, Versel®)	**Dandruff of the scalp/Seborrheic dermatitis of the scalp** *Note:* Not approved by the FDA or HPB for children.	**Children and adolescents:** Apply a small amount (5–15 ml) of 1% or 2.5% shampoo to wet hair and massage on scalp into a foamy lather. Allow to remain on scalp for 2–3 min. Then rinse thoroughly with water. Avoid contact with eyes. Repeat application. May use up to two times per week as indicated by response. *Maximum:* 3 grams/application.	Lotion/shampoo, topical: 1%, 2.5% Shampoo, topical: 1% *Note:* For external use only. Avoid contact with eyes and mucous membranes.	**Contraindications:** Hypersensitivity to selenium sulfide or other shampoo formulation ingredients. **ADRs:** Generally well tolerated. May cause local irritation. **Comments:** May cause hair discoloration or skin irritation. May also damage some jewelery—remove before use.
	Tinea versicolor *Note:* Not approved by the FDA or HPB for children.	**Children and adolescents:** Topically apply 2.5% lotion/shampoo with a small amount of water to affected area of the skin to form a lather. Allow to remain on application site for 10 min, then rinse thoroughly. Topically apply once daily for 7 days.		
Senna (Dr. Caldwell Senna Laxative®, Ex-Lax®, Senna X-Prep®, Sennosides, Senokot®)	**Constipation**	**Children and adolescents:** 0.4–1 mg sennosides/kg/day PO as two divided doses or as a single daily dose 30 min before bedtime. *Maximum:* 75 mg/day PO.	Granules, oral: 15 mg/ 3 grams Solution, oral fluid-extract: 3 mg/ml; may contain 4.9% alcohol. Solutions, oral: 6.5%, 7% (with 3%–5% alcohol or alcohol free [*Fletcher's Castoria®*]) Solutions, oral fruit extract: 0.65 mg/ml, 1.8 mg/ml; contains 7% alcohol. Suppository, rectal: 30 mg Syrups, oral: 1.5, 1.7 mg/ml Tablets, oral: 8.6, 10, 15, 17, 20, 25 mg Tablet, oral chewable: 15 mg *Note:* 1 mg sennosides = 21.7 mg standardized senna concentrate. *Note:* All amounts and concentrations are listed in terms of sennosides.	**Contraindications:** Appendicitis, fecal impaction, hypersensitivity to sennosides, intestinal obstruction, and surgical abdomen (acute). **ADRs:** See Chapter 5. **Comments:** Ensure adequate fluid intake. Chronic use of senna may result in laxative dependence (cathartic colon). May discolor acid urine (yellow–brown) and alkaline urine (pink–red).
Sennosides, *see* **Senna**				
Sertraline (Zoloft®)	**Major depressive disorder/Obsessive-compulsive disorder (OCD)** *Note:* Not approved by the FDA or HPB for the treatment of major depressive disorder among children or adolescents.	**Children (≥6 years) and adolescents:** Initially, 25–50 mg/day PO in a single daily dose. Adjust dosage over the next 4 weeks, according to response. *Maximum:* 200 mg/day PO. *Note:* Reduce dosage for pediatric patients who have hepatic dysfunction.	Concentrate, oral: 20 mg/ml (menthol scented, supplied with calibrated dropper); contains 12% alcohol. *Note:* Oral concentrate must be diluted before administration. Immediately before administration, dilute required dose with 120 ml (4 ounces) of either ginger ale, lemon/lime soda, lemonade, orange juice, or water. A slight	**Contraindications:** Hypersensitivity to sertraline and MAOI therapy (concurrent or within 14 days). **ADRs:** May cause agitation, insomnia, nausea, and tremor. See Chapter 5. **Comments:** Clinical improvement may be significantly enhanced by the concurrent use of appropriate depression-specific or OCD-specific cognitive-behavioral therapy.

(Continued)

Footnotes are on page 558.

TABLE 14-1 continued

DRUG (TRADE AND OTHER NAMES)	INDICATION(S)	USUAL PEDIATRIC DOSAGE AND ADMINISTRATION[a]	DOSAGE FORMS	CONTRAINDICATIONS, ADRs, AND COMMENTS[b]
Sertraline *continued*			haze may appear after mixing. Do **not** mix with any other diluents, foods, or products. Tablets, oral: 25, 50, 100 mg	
Sevoflurane *(Sevorane AF®)*	General anesthesia, induction and maintenance	**Children and adolescents:** *Minimal* alveolar concentrations (MAC) are listed, by age, in the following table. **Note:** Sevoflurane has a non-pungent odor and does not cause respiratory irritation; therefore, it can be administered by mask to pediatric patients. **Note:** Sevoflurane can be administered by any type of anesthesia circuit.	Inhalation, solution: 250 ml/bottle (with Quick-Fil® closure) **Note:** Store between 15 and 25°C.	**Contraindications:** Hypersensitivity to sevoflurane or to other halogenated anesthetics, hepatic dysfunction (severe), malignant hyperthermia (known or suspected history), and renal dysfunction (severe, serum creatinine >1.5 mg/100 ml). **ADRs:** Generally well tolerated. May cause agitation, breath holding, cough (increased), hypotension, laryngospasm, nausea, and tachycardia. **Comments:** Fresh gas flow rates in a circle absorber system should be ≥ 2 liters/min.

Minimal Alveolar Concentrations (MACs) by Age

AGE	MAC IN OXYGEN	MAC IN 65% N_2O/35% O_2
Infants		
<6 months	3%	
6–12 months	2.8%	
Children		
<3 years	2.6%	2%
3–12 years	2.5%	
Adolescents		
≥13 years	2.5%	1.4%

DRUG (TRADE AND OTHER NAMES)	INDICATION(S)	USUAL PEDIATRIC DOSAGE AND ADMINISTRATION[a]	DOSAGE FORMS	CONTRAINDICATIONS, ADRs, AND COMMENTS[b]
Simethicone *(Degas®, Flatulex®, Gas-X®, Mylicon®, Phazyme®)*	Infant colic/GI discomfort due to trapped gas (e.g., functional gastric bloating and postoperative gas pain)/**Flatulence** **Note:** Provides symptomatic relief only.	**Infants:** 10–20 mg/dose PO with each meal. Measure each dose with the oral dropper supplied with the product. *Maximum:* 60 mg/day PO. **Children:** 160–320 mg/day PO in four divided doses, after meals and at bedtime. **Adolescents:** 320–640 mg/day PO in four divided doses, after meals and at bedtime.	Capsules, oral soft gel liquid filled: 95, 125, 180 mg Suspension, oral: 40 mg/0.6 ml (peppermint flavored, supplied in plastic dropper bottle); shake well before use. Tablets, oral chewable: 40, 80, 125, 160 mg (cherry or peppermint flavored) Tablets, oral: 62.5, 95 mg	**Contraindications:** None identified. **ADRs:** Generally well tolerated. No specific ADRs have been reported.
Smallpox (Vaccinia) Vaccine *(Dryvax®)* **Note:** *Dryvax®*, although previously marketed as *Dryvax®* by Wyeth-Ayerst, has most recently been under the direct control of the CDC. For additional information or updates regarding smallpox vaccine, contact the CDC at (404) 639-3670.	Prophylactic protection against smallpox infection **Note:** Smallpox vaccine is currently considered to be "investigational" by the FDA and HPB for children and adolescents.	**Children and adolescents:** Using a specially designed presterilized bifurated needle, supplied by the manufacturer, with one drop of vaccine between the prongs, rapidly make 15 punctures with strikes vigorous enough to allow a trace of blood to appear after 15–20 sec. Remove excess vaccine from injection site with a sterile, dry gauze and appropriately dispose in a biohazard container. **Note:** Isopropyl alcohol is **not** generally used to clean the injection site prior to vaccination. If it is used, it must be allowed to dry thoroughly in order to prevent inadvertent inactivation of the vaccine by the alcohol.	Injectable, lyophilized powder with diluent for intradermal use. Also supplied with presterilized, bifurated (pronged) needle. The bifurated needle is inserted vertically into the vaccine vial and removed with a drop of vaccine solution, which will adhere between the prongs (must be visually confirmed). Refrigerate smallpox vaccine between 2 and 8°C (36–46°F). **Note:** Smallpox vaccine contains trace amounts	**Contraindications:** Eczema, HIV infection, hypersensitivity to the vaccine or any of its components, immunodeficiency, and pregnancy. **Note:** Following exposure to smallpox virus (e.g., subsequent to a bioterrorist attack), none of the listed contraindications is considered to be absolute. **ADRs:** Commonly causes fever. May cause malaise and regional lymphadenopathy, particularly with smallpox booster or revaccination. May also cause eczema vaccinatum, generalized vaccinia, postvaccinial encephalitis, and progressive vaccinia. These ADRs occur more frequently

TABLE 14-1 continued

DRUG (TRADE AND OTHER NAMES)	INDICATION(S)	USUAL PEDIATRIC DOSAGE AND ADMINISTRATION[a]	DOSAGE FORMS	CONTRAINDICATIONS, ADRs, AND COMMENTS[b]
Smallpox (Vaccinia) Vaccine *continued*		**Note:** Recommended sites for intradermal smallpox vaccination are healthy skin sites over the deltoid muscle or the posterior aspect of the upper arm over the triceps muscle. **Note:** A dry, sterile porous dressing should be applied to the injection site and should remain in place or be replaced, if needed, until the scab has separated and the underlying tissue has healed. The vaccination site should be kept dry during healing. **Note:** If required, revaccination is generally recommended at 5-year intervals.	of chlortetracycline, neomycin, polymyxin B, and streptomycin.	among infants than among children or adolescents. **Comments:** It should be noted that the expected local response to primary smallpox vaccination is the development of a papule at the vaccination site that will become vesicular, then pustular, and then drying to form a scab that falls off leaving a scar. The entire local response takes approximately 2–3 weeks. **Note:** Vaccinia virus can be cultured from the primary vaccination site from the time that a papule develops to the time that the scab falls off. During this period of time, direct contact may spread the virus to another area of the body or to another person. Ensure that both patient and parent are appropriately cautioned against touching or scratching the vaccination site.

Snake Antivenin, *see* **Antivenin (Crotalidae) Polyvalent**

Sodium Aurothiomalate, *see* **Gold Sodium Thiomalate**

DRUG (TRADE AND OTHER NAMES)	INDICATION(S)	USUAL PEDIATRIC DOSAGE AND ADMINISTRATION[a]	DOSAGE FORMS	CONTRAINDICATIONS, ADRs, AND COMMENTS[b]
Sodium Bicarbonate **Note:** *See also* Chapter 4.	Lactic acidosis/ Adjunctive pharmacotherapy for the treatment of cardiac arrest **Note:** Use for the treatment of cardiac arrest has been recently questioned and it is no longer considered to be standard therapy.	**Children and adolescents:** Initially, 1 mmol/kg IV. *Maintenance* (after blood gases obtained): 1–2 mmol/kg/dose IV every 10–20 min, as needed according to response.	Injectables, IV: 0.5, 0.6, 0.9, 1 mmol/ml (4.2%, 5%, 7.5%, 8.4%) Tablets, oral: 300 mg (3.6 mmol); 600 mg (7.1 mmol) **Note:** 1 mmol bicarbonate = 1 mEq bicarbonate. Each gram of sodium bicarbonate provides 12 mEq each of sodium and bicarbonate ions.	**Contraindications:** Chloride ion loss (excessive from continuous GI suctioning or vomiting), diuretic-induced hypochloremic alkalosis, hypocalcemia, and metabolic or respiratory alkalosis. **ADRs:** May cause edema, hypernatremia, and metabolic alkalosis. *See also* Chapter 5. **Comments:** Adjust dosage according to fluid and electrolyte status (including arterial blood pH and $PaCO_2$ in cases of cardiac arrest). Avoid extravasation during IV administration because of associated tissue necrosis.
	Urinary alkalinization	**Children and adolescents:** 1–2 mmol/kg/day IV by continuous IV infusion or by intermittent IV infusion divided every 6 hr **or** 1–10 mmol/kg/day PO in four divided doses according to response. *Maximum:* 200 mmol/day PO.		

Sodium Chloride, *see* **Chapter 13**

DRUG (TRADE AND OTHER NAMES)	INDICATION(S)	USUAL PEDIATRIC DOSAGE AND ADMINISTRATION[a]	DOSAGE FORMS	CONTRAINDICATIONS, ADRs, AND COMMENTS[b]
Sodium Fluoride (Fluoritab®, Karidium®, Luride®, Pediaflor®)	Dental carie prophylaxis	**Infants and children:** Supplemental fluoride (mg/day) is dosed according to age and fluoride concentration in water supply: (see table below)	Drops, oral: 0.275, 0.55 mg/drop; 1.1 mg/ml (note **difference** in unit of dosage measurement among various products of sodium fluoride oral drops) Solutions, oral: 0.44, 0.5, 2, 2.25, 5.5, 5.9 mg/ml Tablets, chewable: 0.25, 0.55, 1.1, 2.2 mg Tablets, oral: 1, 2.2 mg **Note:** 2.2 mg of sodium fluoride contains 1 mg of fluoride.	**Contraindications:** Fluoride concentration of local water supply exceeds 0.7 ppm, hypersensitivity to fluoride, and low sodium diets. **ADRs:** Generally well tolerated. May cause dermatitis, gastric irritation, headache, and weakness.

AGE	FLUORIDE CONCENTRATION IN LOCAL WATER SUPPLY (PPM)		
	<0.3	0.3–0.7	>0.7
0–2 years	0.25 mg	0	0
2–3 years	0.5 mg	0.25 mg	0
3–12 years	1 mg	0.5 mg	0

Footnotes are on page 558.

TABLE 14-1 continued

DRUG (TRADE AND OTHER NAMES)	INDICATION(S)	USUAL PEDIATRIC DOSAGE AND ADMINISTRATION[a]	DOSAGE FORMS	CONTRAINDICATIONS, ADRs, AND COMMENTS[b]
Sodium Levothyroxine, *see* **Levothyroxine**				
Sodium Nitroprusside (Nitroprusside)	Hypertensive crisis (acute hypertension that is refractory to less potent and less toxic antihypertensive pharmacotherapy)	**Children and adolescents:** Initially, 0.25–0.5 µg/kg/min by continuous IV infusion. Adjust subsequent dosages according to blood pressure and response. *Maximum:* 8 µg/kg/min for a maximum of 10 min. **Note:** May cause profound hypotension; therefore, wait at least 10 min between dosage adjustments.	Injectables, IV: 10, 25 mg/ml **Note:** Not generally available in Canada.	**Contraindications:** Anemia (uncorrected), hepatic or renal disease (severe), hypertension (compensatory), and inadequate cerebral circulation. **ADRs:** *See* Chapter 5. Note that a precipitous drop in blood pressure can result in potentially fatal ischemic conditions (e.g., myocardial infarction and stroke). **Comments:** Continuously monitor blood pressure and heart rate during IV administration. Excessive dosage and/or long-term therapy may result in cyanide toxicity.
Sodium Polystyrene Sulfonate (Kayexalate®, Kionex®)	Hyperkalemia	**Infants, children, and adolescents:** 1 gram/kg/day PO or rectal in four divided doses, every 6 hr as indicated according to response. **Note: Prior** to oral administration, moisten powder for suspension with water, honey, or jam. **Prior** to rectal administration, mix powder for suspension with tap water, dextrose 10% in water, or equal parts tap water and methylcellulose 2%.	Powder (resin) for suspension, oral or rectal: 250 mg/ml after reconstitution **Note:** Each gram of powder (resin) contains 4.1 mmol (100 mg) of sodium. **Note:** Suspension contains 33% sorbitol and 0.3% alcohol. Shake reconstituted powder for suspension well before use.	**Contraindications:** Hypersensitivity to sodium polystyrene sulfonate, obstructive bowel disease, and potassium serum <5 mmol/liter. **ADRs:** May cause hypernatremia, hypocalcemia, hypokalemia, and hypomagnesemia. **Comments:** Sodium polystyrene sulfonate exchanges approximately 1 mmol (1 mEq) potassium/gram of resin. Monitor fluid and electrolyte status.
Sodium Sulfacetamide, *see* **Sulfacetamide Sodium**				
Sodium Thiosulfate, *see* **Chapter 4**				
Sodium Valproate, *see* **Valproic Acid**				
Somatrem (Protropin®, *Somatropin [Human]*) **Note:** *See also* Somatropin and Somatropin, depot.	Growth failure associated with inadequate secretion of normal endogenous growth hormone	**Children:** Initially, 0.54 international units (IU)/kg/week (0.18 mg/kg/week) IM or SC in seven divided daily doses. *Maximum:* 0.9 IU/kg/week (0.3 mg/kg/week) IM or SC.	Injectable, IM, SC (powder for reconstitution): 1 mg/ml (after reconstitution with either 5 or 10 ml of bacteriostatic water for injection) **Note:** To reconstitute powder for injection, slowly add 5–10 ml bacteriostatic water for injection (contains benzyl alcohol). Gently swirl vial and invert back and forth to mix and to ensure dissolution. Do **not** shake vial to mix. Shaking may cause frothing and the protein solution may become cloudy. Only clear solutions should be injected. **Note:** Injectable has a specific activity of 3 IU/mg protein. **Note:** For IM or SC injection only. **Note:** Use **only** one dose per vial and **discard** any unused portion appropriately and safely.	**Contraindications:** Neoplasm (active) and pediatric patients with closed epiphyses. **ADRs:** Generally well tolerated. May cause insulin resistance, pain at the injection site, and peripheral edema. Rarely causes intracranial hypertension. **Comments:** Monitor growth hormone and thyroid hormone serum concentrations. Also monitor patients for insulin resistance.
	Growth failure associated with chronic renal insufficiency (up to the time of renal transplantation) **Note:** Discontinue when desired height is achieved or epiphyseal fusion occurs.	**Children:** Initially, 0.6 IU/kg/week (0.2 mg/kg/week) IM or SC in seven divided daily doses. *Maximum:* 1.05 IU/kg/week (0.35 mg/kg/week) IM or SC.		

TABLE 14-1 continued

DRUG (TRADE AND OTHER NAMES)	INDICATION(S)	USUAL PEDIATRIC DOSAGE AND ADMINISTRATION[a]	DOSAGE FORMS	CONTRAINDICATIONS, ADRs, AND COMMENTS[b]
Somatropin (*Genotropin®*, Human Growth Hormone, *Humatrope®*, *Norditropin®*, *Nutropin®*, *Saizen®*) **Note:** *See also* Somatrem and Somatropin, depot.	**Growth failure associated with inadequate secretion of normal endogenous growth hormone** **Note:** Discontinue when desired height is achieved or epiphyseal fusion occurs.	**Children:** Initially, 0.54 IU/kg/week (0.18 mg/kg/week) IM or SC in seven divided daily doses. Then individualize dosage according to response. *Maximum:* 0.9 IU/kg/week (0.3 mg/kg/week) IM or SC.	Injectable, IM, SC (powder for reconstitution): 1 mg/ml (after reconstitution with 5 ml bacteriostatic water for injection) **Note:** To reconstitute powder, slowly add 5 ml bacteriostatic water for injection (contains benzyl alcohol) and gently swirl and invert vial back and forth to ensure dissolution. Do **not** shake vial to mix. Shaking may cause frothing and the protein solution to become cloudy. Only clear solutions should be injected. **Note:** Diluent provided with some formulations may contain benzyl alcohol. Injectable, IM, SC (solution *[Nutropin AQ®]*): 5 mg/ml (*Nutropin AQ* does **not** require reconstitution or further dilution before injection.) **Note:** *Nutropin AQ* injectable solution does **not** contain benzyl alcohol. **Note:** Injectable formulations have a specific activity of 3 IU/mg protein.	**Contraindications:** Hypersensitivity to m-cresol or glycerin (may be contained in the diluent of some products *[Humatrope]*), neoplasm (active), and pediatric patients with closed epiphyses. **ADRs:** Generally well tolerated. May cause insulin resistance and pain at the injection site. Rarely causes intracranial hypertension. **Comments:** Monitor growth hormone and thyroid hormone serum concentrations. Also monitor for insulin resistance.
	Growth failure associated with chronic renal insufficiency (up to the time of renal transplantation) **Note:** Discontinue when desired height is achieved or epiphyseal fusion occurs.	**Children:** Initially, 0.6 IU/kg/week (0.2 mg/kg/week) IM or SC in seven divided daily doses. Then individualize dosage according to response. *Maximum:* 1.05 IU/kg/week (0.35 mg/kg/week) IM or SC.		
	Turner syndrome	**Children:** 0.54–1.125 IU/kg/week (0.18–0.375 mg/kg/week) SC in three divided doses (on alternate days).		
Somatropin, depot (*Nutropin Depot®*) **Note:** *See also* Somatrem and Somatropin.	**Growth hormone deficiency** (generally used for long-term treatment of growth hormone deficiency) **Note:** Monthly therapy is not approved by the FDA for children.	**Children:** 1.5 mg/kg/dose IM once monthly **or** 0.75 mg/kg/dose IM twice monthly. The injection should be made approximately 15 days apart on the same days each month (e.g., days 1 and 15 of each month). **Note:** Children weighing more than 15 kg require more than one injection per dose. **Note:** Dosage must be determined by response. **Note:** Rotate IM injection sites. When more than one injection per dose is required, make each injection in a different IM injection site. *See* Chapter 1.	Injectables, IM (*Nutropin Depot*): 13.5, 18, 22.5 mg/3-ml single-use vial (supplied with a single-use 1.5-ml vial of diluent, and three sterile 21-gauge, ½-inch needles for reconstitution and IM injection) **Note:** For IM use only. To reconstitute, add 0.8, 1, or 1.2 ml of diluent provided with the product to the respective vial. Swirl the vial vigorously to mix. The resultant suspension should be milky, thick, and uniform in appearance. After reconstitution, use suspension immediately. Do **not** allow suspension to settle prior to withdrawing required dose. Safely and appropriately discard any unused suspension. **Note:** Not generally available in Canada.	*See* Somatropin. **Note:** Ensure that suspension is injected IM. Some children may require injection with a 1-inch, 21-gauge needle, depending on body weight and the amount of subcutaneous tissue over the injection site.

Footnotes are on page 558.

TABLE 14-1 continued

DRUG (TRADE AND OTHER NAMES)	INDICATION(S)	USUAL PEDIATRIC DOSAGE AND ADMINISTRATION[a]	DOSAGE FORMS	CONTRAINDICATIONS, ADRs, AND COMMENTS[b]
Somatropin (Human), *see* **Somatrem**				
Spironolactone (Aldactone®, Novo-Spiroton®)	Ascites/Edema/ Hyperaldosteronism	**Children and adolescents:** Initially, 3 mg/kg/day PO as a single daily dose or as two divided doses. Maintenance, 1–2 mg/kg/day PO as a single daily dose or as two divided doses. *Maximum:* 200 mg/day PO. **Note:** Reduce dosage for pediatric patients who have renal (*see* Table 14-2) and/or hepatic dysfunction.	Tablets, oral: 25, 50, 100 mg	**Contraindications:** Anuria, hyperkalemia, hypersensitivity to spironolactone, and renal dysfunction (severe). **ADRs:** *See* Chapter 5. **Comments:** Metabolized in the liver to produce several metabolites, including canrenone, an active metabolite. Monitor for hyperkalemia, particularly among children who have impaired renal function.
Stavudine (Zerit®)	HIV infection (generally used in combination with other antiretroviral pharmacotherapy) **Note:** Patients may continue to develop opportunistic infections and other complications associated with HIV infection. In addition, stavudine does not reduce the risk for HIV transmission to others. **Note:** Not approved by the FDA for infants or children.	**Infants (≥3 months) and children:** 2 mg/kg/day PO in two divided doses, every 12 hr. *Maximum:* 80 mg/day PO. **Adolescents (<60 kg):** 30 or 60 mg/day PO in two divided doses, every 12 hr. **Adolescents (≥60 kg):** 40 or 80 mg/day PO in two divided doses, every 12 hr. **Note:** Reduce dosage for pediatric patients who have renal dysfunction; *see* Table 14-2.	Capsules, oral: 15, 20, 30, 40 mg	**Contraindications:** Hepatic impairment (severe), hypersensitivity to stavudine, and lactic acidosis. **ADRs:** Commonly causes peripheral neuropathy (may be less common in children). May cause fat redistribution, hepatic impairment, lactic acidosis, and pancreatitis. **Comments:** The use of combination stavudine and didanosine pharmacotherapy for pregnant adolescents may result in **fatal** lactic acidosis.
Streptomycin	Tuberculosis resistant to isoniazid and rifampin **Note:** Ensure that appropriate culture and sensitivity tests are performed and that the organism is sensitive to streptomycin. **Note:** Generally used in combination with another antitubercular drug (e.g., ethambutol).	**Children and adolescents:** 20–40 mg/kg/day IM as a single daily dose or as two divided doses, every 12 hr. *Maximum:* 1 gram/day IM. **Note:** Reduce dosage for pediatric patients who have renal dysfunction; *see* Table 14-2. **Note:** Pharmacotherapy generally continued for a minimum of 1 year.	Injectables, IM: 1, 5 grams/vial **Note:** For IM use only; contains sodium metabisulfite which may cause allergic reactions in susceptible patients. **Note:** Available in Canada through Health Canada Special Access Program.	**Contraindications:** Hypersensitivity to streptomycin or to other aminoglycosides. **ADRs:** *See* Chapter 5. **Comments:** Obtain a baseline audiologic evaluation **prior** to the initiation of therapy in order to monitor for and evaluate any subsequent associated ototoxicity. Therapeutic drug monitoring is recommended; *see* Table 14-3.
Succimer (Chemet®, DMSA) **Note:** *See also* Chapter 4.	Lead poisoning among pediatric patients with lead serum concentration >45 µg/100 ml	**Infants, children, and adolescents:** Initially, 30 mg/kg/day PO in three divided doses, every 8 hr, for 5 days; then 20 mg/kg/day PO in two divided doses, every 12 hr, for 14 additional days.	Capsule, oral: 100 mg	**Contraindications:** Hypersensitivity to succimer. **ADRs:** May cause anorexia, diarrhea, nausea, rash, sulfur odor on the breath, and vomiting. **Comments:** A 2-week interval is recommended between required courses. Monitor lead serum concentration. *See* Chapter 4.
Succinylcholine (Anectine®, Quelicin®, Suxamethonium)	Skeletal muscle **relaxation** to facilitate diagnostic and treatment procedures such as electroconvulsive therapy (ECT), endoscopic examinations, and	**Infants and children (<6 years):** Initially, 2 mg/kg/dose IV or 2.5–4 mg/kg/dose IM. *Maintenance:* 0.03–0.06 mg/kg/min by IV infusion, as needed for longer procedures, according to response. *Maximum:* 150 mg/dose IM.	Injectables, IM, IV: 20, 50, 100 mg/ml	**Contraindications:** Angle-closure (narrow-angle) glaucoma, Duchenne-type muscular dystrophy, homozygosity for the atypical plasma cholinesterase gene, hyperkalemia, hypersensitivity to succinylcholine, low pseudocholinesterase activity or concentration,

TABLE 14-1 continued

DRUG (TRADE AND OTHER NAMES)	INDICATION(S)	USUAL PEDIATRIC DOSAGE AND ADMINISTRATION[a]	DOSAGE FORMS	CONTRAINDICATIONS, ADRs, AND COMMENTS[b]
Succinylcholine *continued*	endotracheal intubation **Note:** Use generally reserved for emergency situations because of potential toxicity.	**Children (≥6 years) and adolescents:** Initially, 1 mg/kg/dose IV or 3–4 mg/kg/dose IM. *Maintenance:* 0.03–0.06 mg/kg/min by IV infusion, as needed for longer procedures, according to response. *Maximum:* 150 mg/dose IM; 10 mg/min IV infusion. **Note:** When possible, succinylcholine is not administered until the patient is unconscious in order to avoid patient distress.		malignant hyperthermia (history of, personal or family), and skeletal muscle myopathies. **ADRs.** May produce apnea (severe), bradycardia, and hyperkalemia, particularly with slow IV injection (IV push) to infants and young children, or rhabdomyolysis (acute). Premedication with atropine may prevent or minimize succinylcholine-induced bradycardia. Be alert to possible development of malignant hyperthermia, particularly with continuous IV infusion, and be prepared to treat appropriately (e.g., with dantrolene). Be alert to possible development of ventricular dysrhythmias or cardiac arrest associated with acute rhabdomyolysis and hyperkalemia and be prepared to immediately treat the hyperkalemia (e.g., with IV calcium, glucose, insulin, and sodium bicarbonate). **Comments:** Adjust dosage according to response.
Sucralfate *(Carafate®, Sulcrate®)*	Duodenal ulcer, active	**Adolescents:** 4 grams/day PO in four divided doses 1 hr before meals and at bedtime. **Note:** Continue for a minimum of 4–8 weeks.	Suspension, oral: 1 gram/5 ml (caramel odor) (Canada); 1 gram/10 ml (United States); shake well before use. Tablet, oral: 1 gram	**Contraindications:** None identified. **ADRs:** Generally well tolerated. May cause constipation.
	Maintenance pharmacotherapy after healing of duodenal ulcer	**Adolescents:** 2 grams/day PO in two divided doses, 1 hr before breakfast and 1 hr before dinner. **Note:** Pharmacotherapy may be continued for up to 1 year. **Note:** Administer on an empty stomach.		

Sulfacetamide, *see* **Sulfacetamide Sodium**

Sulfacetamide Sodium, ophthalmic *(AK-Sulf®, Bleph-10®, Isopto-Cetamide®, Ocusulf-10®, Sodium Sulamyd®)*	Conjunctivitis/Corneal ulcer/Superficial ocular infections caused by susceptible microorganisms **Note:** Ensure that appropriate culture and sensitivity tests are performed and that the organism is sensitive to sulfacetamide sodium, ophthalmic.	**Children and adolescents:** Instill one drop of 30% ophthalmic solution (or one or two drops of 10% ophthalmic solution) into the conjunctival sac of the affected eye(s) every 2–3 hr as indicated by response, usually for 7–10 days. **Alternatively:** Apply a small amount of ophthalmic ointment to the conjunctival sac of the affected eye(s) four times daily and at bedtime. **Note:** The sulfacetamide sodium ophthalmic ointment and ophthalmic solution may be used adjunctively.	Ointment, ophthalmic: 10% (in petrolatum base) Solutions, ophthalmic: 1%, 10%, 15%, 30% **Note:** For ophthalmic use only. In order to avoid cross-infection, a separate container should be dispensed for the treatment of each affected eye. **Note:** Store ophthalmic formulations at 2–30°C; protect from light.	**Contraindications:** Hypersensitivity to sulfacetamide sodium or other sulfonamides. **ADRs:** Generally well tolerated. May cause local eye irritation. **Comments:** Sulfonamides, including sulfacetamide sodium, are inactivated by the para-aminobenzoic acid (PABA) present in purulent exudates. Therefore, eye(s) should be carefully cleansed **prior** to each application.
	Trachoma (as adjunctive pharmacotherapy with systemic sulfonamide pharmacotherapy) **Note:** Not approved by the FDA or HPB for infants or children.	**Children and adolescents:** Instill two drops of 15% or 30% ophthalmic solution into the conjunctival sac of the affected eye(s) every 2 hr.		

Footnotes are on page 558.

TABLE 14-1 continued

DRUG (TRADE AND OTHER NAMES)	INDICATION(S)	USUAL PEDIATRIC DOSAGE AND ADMINISTRATION[a]	DOSAGE FORMS	CONTRAINDICATIONS, ADRs, AND COMMENTS[b]
Sulfacetamide Sodium, topical *(Klaron®, Sebizon®, Sulamyd®)*	Acne vulgaris, topical pharmacotherapy	**Adolescents:** Apply a small amount of 10% topical lotion to affected skin areas twice daily.	Lotion, topical: 10%; contains sodium metabisulfite, which may cause allergic reactions in susceptible patients. **Note:** For external use only. Avoid contact with the eyes.	**Contraindications:** Hypersensitivity to sulfacetamide sodium or to other sulfonamides. **ADRs:** Generally well tolerated. May cause erythema, local edema, and itching at application site.
	Seborrheic dermatitis/Seborrhea sicca (dandruff)	**Adolescents:** Apply a small amount of 10% topical lotion to affected areas of scalp at bedtime and allow to remain overnight. Repeat nightly for 7–14 consecutive nights. Then apply once or twice weekly, as needed. **Note:** Application may be preceded by shampooing and drying the scalp and hair, if necessary (if scalp is excessively oily or has heavy scaling).		
Sulfamethoxazole *(Gantanol®)*	Urinary tract infections **Note:** Ensure that appropriate culture and sensitivity tests are performed and that the organism is sensitive to sulfamethoxazole.	**Children and adolescents:** Initially, 50–60 mg/kg/day PO in two divided doses, every 12 hr. Follow by 25–35 mg/kg/day PO in two divided doses, every 12 hr. *Maximum:* 75 mg/kg/day PO **or** 3 grams/day PO, whichever is less. **Note:** Reduce dosage for pediatric patients who have renal dysfunction; see Table 14-2.	Suspension, oral: 500 mg/5 ml; shake well before use. Tablets, oral: 500 mg, 1 gram **Note:** Not generally available in Canada.	**Contraindications:** Hepatic dysfunction (severe), hypersensitivity to sulfamethoxazole or to other sulfonamides, porphyria, and renal dysfunction (severe). **ADRs:** Associated with Stevens-Johnson syndrome and toxic epidermal necrolysis, particularly among slow acetylators (see Chapter 11). See also Chapter 5. **Comments:** Ensure adequate hydration to prevent associated crystalluria.

Sulfamethoxazole and Trimethoprim, *see* **Trimethoprim and Sulfamethoxazole**

DRUG (TRADE AND OTHER NAMES)	INDICATION(S)	USUAL PEDIATRIC DOSAGE AND ADMINISTRATION[a]	DOSAGE FORMS	CONTRAINDICATIONS, ADRs, AND COMMENTS[b]
Sulfasalazine *(Azulfidine®, Azulfidine EN-tabs®, Salazopyrin®,* Salicylazosulfapyridine, *S.A.S.®)*	Ulcerative colitis, mild to moderate, long-term maintenance **Note:** Long-term maintenance therapy is indicated as an adjunct to standard dietary and supportive therapies. **Note:** Acute attacks of ulcerative colitis are generally more responsive to corticosteroid therapy.	**Children (≥2 years) and adolescents:** Initially, 40–75 mg/kg/day PO in three to six divided doses. Maintenance, 20–40 mg/kg/day PO in four divided doses. *Maximum:* Initially, 4 grams/day PO; maintenance, 2 grams/day PO.	Enema, rectal: 3 grams/100 ml Suspension, oral: 50 mg/ml; shake well before use. Tablet, oral enteric coated delayed release: 500 mg Tablet, oral: 500 mg	**Contraindications:** Blood dyscrasias; hypersensitivity to salicylates, sulfasalazine, or to sulfonamides; hepatic dysfunction (severe); intestinal or urinary obstruction; porphyria; and renal dysfunction (severe). **ADRs:** May discolor skin, tears, and urine orange–yellow. Commonly causes GI irritation including anorexia, diarrhea, nausea, and vomiting. Deaths have been associated with sulfasalazine-induced agranulocytosis, aplastic anemia, fibrosing alveolitis, hepatic and renal damage, hypersensitivity reactions, and irreversible CNS and neuromuscular changes. **Comments:** Monitor for signs and symptoms of blood dyscrasias and hemolysis, which are more likely to occur among slow acetylators (see Chapter 11). **Note:** Complete blood counts, including differential white cell counts, hepatic function tests, renal function tests, and urinalysis should be performed upon initiation of therapy and at regular intervals.
	Juvenile rheumatoid arthritis refractory to conventional pharmacotherapy	**Children (≥6 years) and adolescents:** Initially, 13–20 mg/kg/day PO in two divided doses; increase dosage gradually at 2-day intervals to a maximum of 40–60 mg/kg/day PO. *Maximum:* 2 grams/day PO. **Note:** Administer each oral dose of sulfasalazine with food.		

CHAPTER 14: DRUG DOSING FOR INFANTS, CHILDREN, AND ADOLESCENTS

TABLE 14-1 continued

DRUG (*TRADE* AND OTHER NAMES)	INDICATION(S)	USUAL PEDIATRIC DOSAGE AND ADMINISTRATION[a]	DOSAGE FORMS	CONTRAINDICATIONS, ADRs, AND COMMENTS[b]
Sulfisoxazole	Bacterial infections **Note:** Ensure that appropriate culture and sensitivity tests are performed and that the organism is sensitive to sulfisoxazole.	**Infants (>2 months), children, and adolescents:** 75–150 mg/kg/day PO in four to six divided doses, every 4–6 hr. *Maximum:* 6 grams/day PO. **Note:** Reduce dosage for pediatric patients who have renal dysfunction; *see* Table 14-2.	Suspension, oral: 100 mg/ml; contains 0.3% alcohol; shake well before use. Syrup, oral: 100 mg/ml Tablet, oral: 500 mg **Note:** Not generally available in Canada.	**Contraindications:** Hepatic dysfunction (severe), hypersensitivity to sulfisoxazole or to other sulfonamides, porphyria, and renal dysfunction (severe). **ADRs:** *See* Chapter 5. **Comments:** Ensure adequate hydration.
Suxamethonium, *see* **Succinylcholine**				
Tacrolimus (*Prograf®*)	Prophylaxis of organ rejection among pediatric patients receiving allogeneic liver transplants **Note:** Often used in combination with corticosteroid pharmacotherapy	**Children:** Initially, 0.3 mg/kg/day PO in two divided doses, every 12 hr; should be initiated no sooner than 6 hr post-transplantation. **Alternatively:** Only when the oral route cannot be used, 0.1 mg/kg/day IV by continuous IV infusion. **Adolescents:** Initially, 0.15 mg/kg/day PO in two divided doses, every 12 hr; should be initiated no sooner than 6 hr post-transplantation. **Alternatively:** Only when the oral route cannot be used, 0.05 mg/kg/day IV by continuous IV infusion. **Note:** May need to reduce dosage for pediatric patients who have moderate-to-severe hepatic or renal impairment. **Note:** The total body clearance rate decreases with increasing age during childhood (tacrolimus clearance rates are higher for children younger than 6 years when compared to children older than 6. In turn, clearance rates are higher for children 6 years and older than for adolescents.) Thus, the initial dosages for children are based on a higher milligram-per-kilogram dosage ratio than are dosages for adolescents. Regardless, all pediatric patients require careful monitoring and dosage determinations according to response (*see also* Comments). **Note:** Administer on an empty stomach 1 hr before meals to significantly increase bioavailability.	Capsules, oral: 1, 5 mg Injectable, IV: 5 mg/ml; contains 80% dehydrated alcohol (*see also* Contraindications). **Note:** For IV use only. The injectable must be diluted with 0.9% sodium chloride for injection or 5% dextrose and water for injection to a concentration of between 0.004 and 0.02 mg/ml prior to administration. Do **not** store the diluted infusion solution in IV PVC containers because of decreased stability and potential extraction of phthalates. Diluted solution must be stored in IV glass or polyethylene containers. Safely and appropriately discard any unused diluted solution after 24 hr.	**Contraindications:** Cyclosporine therapy (concurrent or within 24 hr) and hypersensitivity to tacrolimus or to HCO-60 (polyoxyl 60 hydrogenated castor oil used as vehicle for injectable formulation). **ADRs:** Commonly causes headache, hyperkalemia, hypertension, hypomagnesemia, insomnia, nephrotoxicity, pleural effusion, pruritus, rash, and tremor. May also cause diarrhea, hyperglycemia, increased risk of infection, lymphomas, and seizures. **Comments:** Monitor blood pressure, glucose, magnesium, and potassium blood concentrations; hematology (e.g., complete blood counts); hepatic and renal function; and neurological status. **Note:** Therapeutic drug monitoring may be of some assistance in monitoring therapy. *See* Table 14-3.
Tazarotene (*Tazorac®*)	Acne vulgaris	**Adolescents:** Apply a thin layer of cream or gel to the affected area once a day, in the evening. **Note:** Prior to application, gently cleanse skin area with warm soapy water and pat dry with a clean towel.	Cream, topical: 0.1% Gels, topical: 0.05%, 0.1% **Note:** For external use only. Avoid contact with eyes and do not apply to inside mouth, nose, or other mucous membranes. Do not apply to eczematous skin sites.	**Contraindications:** Hypersensitivity to tazarotene or to retinoids, pregnancy, and seborrheic dermatitis. **ADRs:** May cause local skin reactions at site of application including burning or stinging sensation, dry skin, erythema, and pruritus.
	Psoriasis	**Adolescents:** Apply a thin layer of gel to the skin lesion(s) once a day, in the evening. **Note:** Prior to application, bathe or shower and dry the skin gently with a clean towel.		

Footnotes are on page 558.

TABLE 14-1 continued

DRUG (TRADE AND OTHER NAMES)	INDICATION(S)	USUAL PEDIATRIC DOSAGE AND ADMINISTRATION[a]	DOSAGE FORMS	CONTRAINDICATIONS, ADRs, AND COMMENTS[b]
Teniposide, see Chapter 12				
Terbutaline (*Brethaire®, Brethine®, Bricanyl®*)	**Asthma** **Note:** Not approved by the FDA or HPB for infants or children.	**Children (≥6 years) and adolescents:** 0.05–0.15 mg/kg/dose PO three times daily **or** 0.005–0.01 mg/kg/dose SC every 15–20 min for three doses **or** 0.4–0.5 mg/dose by metered-dose inhaler every 4–6 hr as needed. *Maximum:* 0.25 mg/dose SC and 0.5 mg/4-hr period SC; 7.5 mg/day PO; 10 mg/dose by nebulizer; 3 mg/day by metered-dose inhaler.	Injectable, SC: 1 mg/ml **Note:** For SC use only. Solutions, for inhalation by metered-dose inhaler: 0.2, 0.5 mg per actuation Solution, for inhalation by nebulizer: 1 mg/ml Tablets, oral: 2.5, 5 mg	**Contraindications:** Hypersensitivity to terbutaline or to other sympathomimetic amines and tachydysrhythmias. **ADRs:** May cause headache, hyperactivity, hypertension, nausea, nervousness, palpitations, tachycardia, and tremor. *See* Chapter 5. **Comments:** Observe for paradoxical bronchoconstriction, particularly with excessive use of inhaler.
Testosterone Propionate (*Synandrol®*)	**Delayed puberty among boys/ Growth stimulation in Turner syndrome**	**Children (prepubertal boys):** 40–50 mg/m^2/dose IM once every month for 6 months. **Note:** The dorsogluteal site is recommended for deep IM injection. **Note:** Both chronological age and bone (skeletal) age should be considered when determining dosages.	Injectable, IM: 100 mg/ml (in oil); shake well before use. **Note:** For IM use only. **Note:** Not generally available in Canada.	**Contraindications:** Hypersensitivity to testosterone and cardiac, hepatic, or renal impairment (severe). **ADRs:** May cause acne, edema, flushing, gynecomastia, headache, increased sex drive, and nausea.
Tetanus Immune Globulin, Human, see Chapter 9				
Tetanus Toxoid, see Chapter 9				
Tetrabenazine (*Nitoman®*)	**Huntington's chorea/Tardive dyskinesia/ Tic disorders** (e.g., Tourette's disorder) and other hyperkinetic movement disorders	**Children and adolescents:** Initially, 12.5 mg/day PO in two divided doses. Gradually increase the dosage at 3–5-day intervals, if needed, according to response. **Note:** Patients who fail to respond within 7 days are not likely to benefit. *Maximum:* 75 mg/day PO.	Tablet, oral: 25 mg **Note:** Available in Canada by the trade name, *Nitoman*, and in the United States as an "orphan drug."	**Contraindications:** Depression, hypersensitivity to tetrabenazine, and MAOI therapy (concurrent or within 14 days). **ADRs:** Commonly causes depression, drowsiness, fatigue, parkinsonian signs and symptoms, and weakness.
Tetracycline (*Apo-Tetra®, Novo-Tetra®, Nu-Tetra®*)	**Bacterial infections** **Note:** Ensure that appropriate culture and sensitivity tests are performed and that the infecting organism is sensitive to tetracycline. **Inflammatory acne**	**Children (≥8 years) and adolescents:** 25–50 mg/kg/day PO in four divided doses, every 6 hr. *Maximum:* 3 grams/day PO. **Note:** Reduce dosage for pediatric patients who have renal dysfunction; see Table 14-2. (*See also* Comments.) **Adolescents:** Initially, 1 gram/day PO in four divided doses, every 6 hr, for 1 week; then 250–500 mg/day PO as a single daily dose. *Maximum:* 3 grams/day PO.	Capsules, oral: 100, 250, 500 mg Suspension, oral: 25 mg/ml; shake well before use. Syrup, oral: 25 mg/ml Tablets, oral: 250, 500 mg	**Contraindications:** Hypersensitivity to tetracycline or to other tetracyclines, hepatic or renal dysfunction (severe), and pregnancy. **ADRs:** *See* Chapter 5. **Comments:** Avoid use for patients with moderate-to-severe renal dysfunction. Not recommended for children <8 years because of possible growth retardation (generally reversible) and permanent yellow discoloration of teeth. Do not administer oral doses with milk or antacids (*see* Chapter 6).
Tetrahydrocannabinol, see Dronabinol				
Thalidomide (*Thalomid®*)	**Erythema nodosum leprosum** (acute treatment of moderate-to-severe cutaneous lesions) **Note:** Prescription is restricted to prescribers who are registered in the "System for Thalidomide Education and Prescription Safety" (STEPS®) program.	**Adolescents:** 100–300 mg/day PO as a single dose at bedtime (at least 1 hr after the evening meal). **Note:** Pharmacotherapy generally is continued until associated signs and symptoms have subsided (usually ~2 weeks). The dosage is then decreased by decrements of 50 mg every 2–4 weeks until discontinued. Some patients may require long-term maintenance pharmacotherapy in order to prevent recurrence. For these patients, a decrease in	Capsule, oral: 50 mg **Note:** Supplied in prescription packs of 14 or 28 capsules. This drug should **not** be repackaged. **Note:** *Thalomid* is only supplied to pharmacists who are registered with the "System for Thalidomide Education and Prescription Safety" (STEPS®) program. Prior to dispensing, pharmacists must	**Contraindications:** Hypersensitivity to thalidomide and pregnancy. **Note: Thalidomide is a known human teratogen** (*see* Chapter 2). **ADRs:** Commonly causes dizziness, rash, and somnolence. May also cause acne, leukopenia, neutropenia, oral candidiasis, orthostatic hypotension, peripheral neuropathy, and Stevens-Johnson syndrome. **Comments:** A proscribed consent (authorization) form must be

CHAPTER 14: DRUG DOSING FOR INFANTS, CHILDREN, AND ADOLESCENTS

TABLE 14-1 continued

DRUG (TRADE AND OTHER NAMES)	INDICATION(S)	USUAL PEDIATRIC DOSAGE AND ADMINISTRATION[a]	DOSAGE FORMS	CONTRAINDICATIONS, ADRs, AND COMMENTS[b]
Thalidomide *continued*		dosage should be attempted every 3–6 months in decrements of 50 mg every 2–4 weeks.	activate an authorization number on **every** prescription by calling 1-888-4-CELGENE (1-888-423-5436). Careful patient education and counseling with provided data and warnings are required. **Note:** Not generally available in Canada.	signed by the patient and completed by the prescriber before a prescription for thalidomide is issued. In addition, adolescent girls must have a pregnancy test performed within 24 hr prior to the initiation of thalidomide pharmacotherapy. **Note:** Ensure that patients are instructed **not** to donate blood while receiving thalidomide. In addition, adolescent boys should be advised not to donate sperm during thalidomide pharmacotherapy and for 4 additional weeks following its discontinuation.
Theophylline (Theo-24®, T-Phyl®, Uniphyl®)	**Asthma** **Note:** Generally considered to be a secondary choice in the treatment of asthma because of its ADRs, low therapeutic index, and availability of efficacious therapeutic alternatives.	**Note:** Because of higher rates of clearance, older infants (>4 months) and children generally require a higher milligram-per-kilogram dose than adults (see Chapter 11). **Infants, children, and adolescents (not currently receiving aminophylline/ theophylline):** *Loading dose,* 6 mg/kg IV. **Note:** Calculate loading and maintenance dosages according to lean body weight. Slowly inject IV at a rate **not** exceeding 20 mg/min. **Note:** Reduce dosage for pediatric patients who have hepatic dysfunction. Initial IV *maintenance dose* by age: **Infants (2–6 months):** 0.4 mg/kg/hr IV; **Infants (>6 months):** 0.7 mg/kg/hr IV; **children:** 0.8 mg/kg/hr IV; **adolescents (<16 years):** 0.7 mg/kg/hr IV; **adolescents (≥16 years and nonsmoker):** 0.6 mg/kg/hr IV. *Maximum:* 900 mg/day IV (without blood concentration monitoring). **IV maintenance dose for pediatric patients with cardiac decompensation, cor pulmonale, hepatic dysfunction:** Initially, 0.2 mg/kg/hr IV. *Maximum oral maintenance dosage prior to determining theophylline blood concentrations by age:* **Infants (6–52 weeks):** [0.2 × (age in weeks) + 5] mg/kg/day PO in three or four divided doses, every 6 or 8 hr; **children:** 20 mg/kg/day PO in three or four divided doses, every 6 or 8 hr;	Capsules, oral sustained release: 50, 75, 100, 200, 250, 300, 350 mg Elixir, oral: 80 mg/15 ml (may contain up to 20% alcohol) Injectables, IV: 0.8, 4 mg/ml Solution, oral: 5.3 mg/ml Tablets, oral sustained release: 50, 100, 200, 250, 300, 400, 450, 500, 600 mg **Note:** Anhydrous theophylline content in various related drug formulations: anhydrous aminophylline (86%); hydrous aminophylline (80%); oxtriphylline (64%); and theophylline monohydrate (91%). **Note:** Oral sustained-release capsules can be opened and administered as a sprinkle. Oral sustained-release capsules and tablets may be administered once or twice daily according to specific manufacturer's recommendations.	**Contraindications:** Coronary artery disease and hypersensitivity to theophylline or to other xanthines. **ADRs:** See Chapter 5. **Comments:** Therapeutic drug monitoring is recommended; see Table 14-3. For pediatric patients for whom IV therapy is **not** being replaced with oral therapy, begin oral therapy at 50% of recommended dosage and gradually increase dosage according to response. Monitor theophylline blood concentrations during viral infections or when initiating or discontinuing therapy with hepatic microsomal enzyme inducers (e.g., phenobarbital) or inhibitors (e.g., cimetidine) (see Chapter 6).

Footnotes are on page 558.

(Continued)

TABLE 14-1 continued

DRUG (TRADE AND OTHER NAMES)	INDICATION(S)	USUAL PEDIATRIC DOSAGE AND ADMINISTRATION[a]	DOSAGE FORMS	CONTRAINDICATIONS, ADRs, AND COMMENTS[b]
Theophylline *continued*		**adolescents (≤16 years):** 18 mg/kg/day PO in two or three divided doses, every 8 or 12 hr; **adolescents (>16 years):** 13 mg/kg/day PO in two or three divided doses, every 8 or 12 hr. *Maximum:* 900 mg/day/PO.		
Thiabendazole *(Mintezol®)*	**Ascariasis** (large roundworm)/ **Cutaneous larva migrans** (creeping eruption)/**Intestinal roundworms/ Strongyloidiasis** (threadworm)/**Trichostrongyliasis/ Trichinosis/ Trichuriasis** (whipworm)/ **Uncinariasis** (hookworm)/ **Visceral larva migrans** (toxocariasis) **Note:** Not indicated for prophylaxis. In addition, although thiabendazole is effective against enterobiasis (pinworm), it should not be used solely for this indication because of the availability of safer, less toxic drugs (e.g., pyrantel pamoate).	**Children and adolescents:** 50 mg/kg/day PO in two divided doses, every 12 hr after a meal for 2 days (5 days or longer for the treatment of visceral larva migrans or disseminated strongyloidiasis). *Maximum:* 1.5 grams/dose PO; 3 grams/day PO. **Note:** Reduce dosage for pediatric patients who have hepatic dysfunction.	Suspension, oral: 100 mg/ml; shake well before use. Tablet, oral chewable: 500 mg (orange flavored) **Note:** Oral chewable tablets should be thoroughly chewed before swallowing. **Note:** Not generally available in Canada.	**Contraindications:** Hypersensitivity to thiabendazole. **ADRs:** Commonly causes anorexia, dizziness, drowsiness, nausea, and vomiting. Rarely causes life-threatening reactions including hepatic failure and the Stevens-Johnson syndrome. **Comments:** Clinical experience with infants and children (13.6 kg[<30 lb]) is limited.
Thiamazole, *see* **Methimazole**				
Thiamine (Vitamin B₁)	**Beriberi**	**Children and adolescents:** 10–25 mg/day IM or IV, if critically ill **or** 10–50 mg/day PO as a single daily dose for 2 weeks, then 5–10 mg/day PO as a single daily dose for 1 month, for less critical cases. *Maximum:* 50 mg/day IM, IV, or PO.	Injectables, IM, IV: 100, 200 mg/ml Tablets, oral: 5, 10, 25, 50, 100, 250, 500 mg	**Contraindications:** Hypersensitivity to thiamine (vitamin B₁). **ADRs:** May cause feeling of warmth, nausea, pruritus, sweating, urticaria, and weakness. **Comments:** Generally well tolerated. Repeated IV administration occasionally causes angioedema, cardiovascular collapse, and hypersensitivity reactions. Dosages required for the treatment of dietary deficiency can be found on the package labeling for several different multivitamin products.
	Dietary thiamine deficiency **Note:** Whenever possible, adequate dietary intake is preferred over supplementation.	**Infants:** 0.3–0.5 mg/day PO as a single daily dose. **Children:** 0.5–1 mg/day PO as a single daily dose.		
Thioguanine, *see* **Chapter 12**				
Thioproperazine *(Majeptil®)*	**Schizophrenia and other psychotic disorders**	**Children (>10 years) and adolescents:** Initially, 1–3 mg/day PO as a single or divided dose. Increase the daily dosage gradually by the same amount every 2 or 3 days until optimal therapeutic benefit is achieved. *Maximum:* 90 mg/day PO.	Tablet, oral: 10 mg **Note:** Not generally available in the United States.	**Contraindications:** Blood dyscrasias, cardiovascular dysfunction (severe), children <3 years, coma, depression including that associated with CNS depressants, hepatic dysfunction, hypersensitivity to thioproperazine or to other phenothiazines, and Parkinson's disease.

TABLE 14-1 continued

DRUG (TRADE AND OTHER NAMES)	INDICATION(S)	USUAL PEDIATRIC DOSAGE AND ADMINISTRATION[a]	DOSAGE FORMS	CONTRAINDICATIONS, ADRs, AND COMMENTS[b]
Thioproperazine *continued*		**Note:** Children (>10 years) and adolescents who are resistant to antipsychotic therapy may occasionally benefit from discontinuous therapy: 5–10 mg three times/day until the onset of severe extrapyramidal reactions (EPRs); then withhold until there is spontaneous recovery from the EPRs; **then** reinstitute. A total of three consecutive discontinuous treatments is recommended. **Note: Discontinuous pharmacotherapy requires hospitalization and close clinical monitoring.**		**ADRs:** May lower seizure threshold and induce seizures among patients with seizure disorders; may obscure clinical course of patients with suspected or actual brain tumors or GI obstruction due to its antiemetic action. May cause extrapyramidal reactions (EPRs), which are common and dose related. These EPRs usually subside with a decrease in dosage or with the temporary discontinuation of use (*see also* Chapter 5).
Thioridazine (Mellaril®, Novo-Ridazine®)	**Schizophrenia and other psychotic disorders** (generally reserved for patients who are refractory to pharmacotherapy with other antipsychotic drugs)	**Children:** Initially, 75 mg/day PO in three divided doses. Gradually adjust dosage according to response. *Maximum:* 300 mg/day PO. **Note:** Children will generally require hospitalization during initial treatment. **Adolescents:** Initially, 150 mg/day PO in three divided doses. Gradually adjust dosage according to response. *Maximum:* 600 mg/day PO.	Concentrates, oral: 30 mg/ml (cherry odor, contains 3% alcohol); 100 mg/ml (strawberry odor, contains 4.2% alcohol) Solution, oral (with calibrated dropper): 30 mg/ml; contains 2.5% alcohol. Suspensions, oral (*Mellaril-S®*): 2 mg/ml (fruit flavored, contains 0.5% alcohol); 5, 20 mg/ml (buttermint flavored with a peppermint odor) Tablets, oral: 10, 15, 25, 50, 100, 150, 200 mg **Note:** Protect oral formulations from direct exposure to light.	**Contraindications:** Blood dyscrasias; bone marrow depression; cardiovascular dysfunction; coma (severe); CNS depression; concurrent therapy with fluoxetine, fluvoxamine, pindolol, propranolol, and other drugs that either inhibit cytochrome P-450 2D6 or prolong the QTc interval; hepatic dysfunction (severe); hypertension (severe); hypersensitivity to thioridazine or to other phenothiazines. **ADRs:** May cause ADRs affecting virtually every major body system, usually associated with its anticholinergic actions (e.g., confusion, drowsiness, dry mouth, inhibition of ejaculation, tachycardia, urinary retention). Although most ADRs are mild and transient, some may be severe (e.g., prolongation of the QTc interval in a dose-related manner) and permanent (e.g., tardive dyskinesia). (*See* Chapter 5.)
	Severe behavioral problems marked by extreme combativeness and/or explosive behavior. **Note:** Although approved by both the FDA and HPB for the treatment of attention-deficit/hyperactivity disorder (A-D/HD), use for this indication is regarded as inappropriate and is **not** recommended.	**Children (≥2 years):** 0.5–3 mg/kg/day PO in three divided doses. Gradually adjust dosage according to response. **Note:** An initial dose of 30 mg/day PO in three divided doses is generally recommended. *Maximum:* 3 mg/kg/day PO **or** 300 mg/day PO, whichever is less.		

Thiotepa, *see* Chapter 12

Thyroxine, *see* Levothyroxine

DRUG	INDICATION(S)	DOSAGE	DOSAGE FORMS	CONTRAINDICATIONS, ADRs, AND COMMENTS
Tiagabine (Gabitril®)	**Adjunctive pharmacotherapy for the treatment of partial seizures**	**Adolescents:** Initially, 4 mg/day PO in a single dose for the first 2 weeks. Thereafter, increase dosage by 4 mg/day at weekly intervals as indicated by response. Usual maintenance dosage is 32 mg/day PO in four divided doses. *Maximum:* 56 mg/day PO. **Note:** May need to reduce dosage for adolescents who have hepatic dysfunction.	Tablets, oral: 4, 12, 16, 20 mg **Note:** Not generally available in Canada.	**Contraindications:** Hypersensitivity to tiagabine. **ADRs:** Generally well tolerated. May cause asthenia, dizziness, nervousness, and somnolence. **Comments:** May rarely cause episodes of status epilepticus that generally resolve upon reduction of dosage or discontinuation. **Note:** Abrupt discontinuation has been associated with "withdrawal seizures." Discontinue gradually.

Footnotes are on page 558.

TABLE 14-1 continued

DRUG (TRADE AND OTHER NAMES)	INDICATION(S)	USUAL PEDIATRIC DOSAGE AND ADMINISTRATION[a]	DOSAGE FORMS	CONTRAINDICATIONS, ADRs, AND COMMENTS[b]
Ticarcillin and Clavulanate (fixed-ratio combination product) *(Timentin®)*	Bacterial infections **Note:** Ensure that appropriate culture and sensitivity tests are performed and that the organism is sensitive to ticarcillin and clavulanate.	**Infants (≥3 months) and children (<60 kg), for mild-to-moderate infections:** 200 mg/kg/day IV in four divided doses, every 6 hr. **Infants (≥3 months) and children (<60 kg), for severe infections:** 300 mg/kg/day IV in six divided doses, every 4 hr. **Children and adolescents (≥60 kg), for mild-to-moderate infections:** 12 grams/day IV in four divided doses, every 6 hr. **Children and adolescents (>60 kg), for severe infections:** 18 grams/day IV in six divided doses, every 4 hr. **Note:** Reduce dosage for pediatric patients who have renal dysfunction; *see* Table 14-2. **Note:** Administer by intermittent IV infusion over 30 min. Dosage is calculated based on the ticarcillin component.	Injectable, IV: 3.1 grams/vial; contains 3 grams ticarcillin and 0.1 gram clavulanate. **Note:** For IV use only. **Note:** Each gram of ticarcillin contains 4.75 mEq (109 mg) of sodium.	**Contraindications:** Hypersensitivity to clavulanate, to ticarcillin, or to other penicillins or cephalosporins. **ADRs:** *See* Chapter 5.
Tobramycin, inhalation *(TOBI®)* **Note:** *See also* Tobramycin, injectable.	*Pseudomonas aeruginosa* infection among pediatric patients with cystic fibrosis	**Children (≥6 years) and adolescents:** 600 mg/day by inhalation in two divided doses. Continue in cycles of 28 days on followed by 28 days off. **Note:** For pulmonary inhalation only. **Note:** The inhalation solution *(TOBI)* is aerosolized and administered by a special reusable nebulizer (Pari LC Plus®) and compressor (DeVilbiss Pulmo-Aide®). Each treatment requires approximately 10–15 min.	Solution, inhalation: 300 mg/5 ml (in ampule pouches) **Note:** For pulmonary inhalation only. **Note:** Store under refrigeration at 2–8°C (36–46°F). May be safely stored at room temperature up to 25°C (77°F) for up to 28 days. Protect ampule pouches from exposure to intense light.	**Contraindications:** IV aminoglycoside pharmacotherapy (concurrent); hypersensitivity to tobramycin or to other aminoglycosides; and significant hearing, kidney, or neuromuscular dysfunction. **ADRs:** May cause bronchospasm, hoarseness, and tinnitus, which is reportedly self-limiting. *See* Chapter 5.
Tobramycin, injectable *(Nebcin®, Tobrex®)* **Note:** *See also* Tobramycin, inhalation.	Bacterial infections, nonurinary tract Bacterial infections among pediatric patients with cystic fibrosis Urinary tract infections **Note:** Ensure that appropriate culture and sensitivity tests are performed and that the organism is sensitive to tobramycin	**Children and adolescents:** 6–7.5 mg/kg/day IM or IV in three divided doses, every 8 hr, for 7–10 days. *Maximum:* 350 mg/day IM or IV. **Children and adolescents:** 10 mg/kg/day IM or IV in three divided doses, every 8 hr. **Note:** Therapeutic drug monitoring is required. **Children and adolescents:** 3 mg/kg/day IM or IV in two or three divided doses, every 8 or 12 hr. **Note:** Reduce dosage for pediatric patients who have renal dysfunction; *see* Table 14-2.	Injectables, IM, IV: 10 (pediatric), 40 mg/ml **Note:** May contain sodium bisulfite. Sulfites have been associated with hypersensitivity reactions, including anaphylactic reactions, among susceptible patients. Although relatively uncommon, these reactions appear to occur with a higher incidence among patients who have asthma.	**Contraindications:** Hypersensitivity to tobramycin or to other aminoglycosides and significant hearing, kidney, or neuromuscular dysfunction. **ADRs:** *See* Chapter 5. **Comments:** Dosage is determined according to ideal body weight. Some pediatric patients may require higher dosages or more frequent dosing intervals. Therapeutic drug monitoring is recommended; *see* Table 14-3.

Tolmetin, *see* **Tolmetin Sodium**

TABLE 14-1 continued

DRUG (TRADE AND OTHER NAMES)	INDICATION(S)	USUAL PEDIATRIC DOSAGE AND ADMINISTRATION[a]	DOSAGE FORMS	CONTRAINDICATIONS, ADRs, AND COMMENTS[b]
Tolmetin Sodium (*Tolectin®*)	Juvenile rheumatoid arthritis	**Children (≥2 years):** 15–30 mg/kg/day PO in three or four divided doses. *Maximum:* 2 grams/day PO. **Note:** Administer with food or milk to decrease associated GI irritation. **Note:** Reduce dosage for pediatric patients who have hepatic dysfunction.	Capsule, oral: 400 mg Tablets, oral: 200, 600 mg **Note:** Contains 1 mmol (mEq) of sodium per gram of tolmetin sodium.	**Contraindications:** Hypersensitivity to tolmetin or to other NSAIDs and peptic ulcer (history). **ADRs:** *See* Chapter 5.
Tolnaftate (*Aftate®, Genaspor®, NP-27®, Tinactin®, Ting®*)	*Tinea* infections (*T. corporis, T. cruris, T. manuum, T. pedis*)	**Infants, children, and adolescents:** Apply a small amount topically to affected area twice daily, morning and evening. Affected area should be cleansed and dried prior to application. Treatment should generally be continued for 2–4 weeks. May repeat course, if required.	Cream, topical: 1% Gel, topical: 1% Powder, topical: 1% Powder, topical aerosol: 1% Solution, topical aerosol: 1% Solution, topical: 1% **Note:** For external use only. Avoid contact with eyes. **Note:** Topical powder formulations are not recommended for use on the scalp.	**Contraindications:** Hypersensitivity to tolnaftate. **ADRs:** Generally well tolerated. May cause local irritation or sensitization. **Comments:** Ineffective when used alone for the treatment of infections involving hair follicles or nail beds.
Topiramate (*Topamax®*)	Partial onset seizures/Primary generalized tonic-clonic seizures/Seizures associated with Lennox-Gastaut syndrome **Note:** Generally used in combination with other anticonvulsants.	**Children (≥2 years) and adolescents:** Adjust dosage according to response. The following schedule may be used as a guide. | WEEK | AM DOSE | PM DOSE | |---|---|---| | 1 | none | 50 mg | | 2 | 50 mg | 50 mg | | 3 | 50 mg | 100 mg | | 4 | 100 mg | 100 mg | | 5 | 100 mg | 150 mg | | 6 | 150 mg | 150 mg | | 7 | 150 mg | 200 mg | | 8 | 200 mg | 200 mg | **Alternative:** Initially, 1–3 mg/kg/day PO as a single dose 30 min before bedtime. Increase dosage by 1–3 mg/kg/day, at 1- or 2-week intervals according to response, and administer in two divided doses. Usual maintenance dosage is 6 mg/kg/day PO in two divided doses (range: 5–9 mg/kg/day). *Maximum:* 800 mg/day PO. **Note:** Reduce dosage for pediatric patients who have renal dysfunction; *see* Table 14-2.	Capsules, oral: 15, 25 mg Tablets, oral: 25, 100, 200 mg **Note:** The oral capsules may be opened and the contents sprinkled on food for pediatric patients who have difficulty swallowing (*see* Chapter 1).	**Contraindications:** Glaucoma and hypersensitivity to topiramate. **ADRs:** May cause aggressive behavior, anorexia, asthenia, ataxia, cognitive impairment, diplopia, dizziness, drowsiness, fatigue, memory impairment, nausea, nervousness, secondary angle-closure glaucoma, somnolence, tremor, visual impairment, and weight loss.
Topotecan, *see* Chapter 12				
Tranexamic Acid (*Cyklokapron®*)	Prevention and control of bleeding among pediatric patients with hemophilia (primarily in	**Children and adolescents:** 100 mg/kg/day PO in four divided doses beginning 1 day prior to surgery or procedure. Immediately prior to surgery or procedure, administer 10 mg/kg	Injectable, IV: 100 mg/ml Tablet, oral: 500 mg **Note:** Not generally available in the United States.	**Contraindications:** Acquired defective color vision and subarachnoid hemorrhage. **ADRs:** Generally well tolerated. May cause diarrhea, nausea, and vomiting.

(Continued)

Footnotes are on page 558.

TABLE 14-1 continued

DRUG (TRADE AND OTHER NAMES)	INDICATION(S)	USUAL PEDIATRIC DOSAGE AND ADMINISTRATION[a]	DOSAGE FORMS	CONTRAINDICATIONS, ADRs, AND COMMENTS[b]
Tranexamic Acid *continued*	conjunction with tooth extraction) **Note:** For this indication, generally used in conjunction with antihemophilic factors (e.g., factor VIII and factor IX administered prior to dental surgery).	IV; **and** 100 mg/kg/day PO in four divided doses for 6–8 days following surgery or procedure. *Maximum:* 16 grams/day PO. **Note:** Administer IV doses slowly over 5 min. **Note:** Reduce dosage for pediatric patients who have renal dysfunction; *see* Table 14-2		
Trastuzumab, *see* Chapter 12				
Tretinoin, *see* Chapter 12				
Triacetyloleandomycin, *see* **Troleandomycin**				
Triamcinolone, nasal (*Nasacort®, Nasacort AQ®*)	Seasonal and perennial allergic rhinitis signs and symptoms	**Children (6–12 years):** 110 μg/day intranasal (one spray/actuation in each nostril once a day). *Maximum:* 220 μg/day intranasal. **Adolescents:** Initially, 220 μg/day intranasal (two sprays/actuation in each nostril once a day).	Solution, nasal insufflation by metered-dose pump: 55 μg/actuation (does not contain chlorofluorocarbons); shake well before use. Suspension, nasal insufflation by metered-dose inhaler: 55 μg/actuation (contains chlorofluorocarbon propellants) **Note:** For intranasal use only.	**Contraindications:** Hypersensitivity to triamcinolone and local intranasal infections. **ADRs:** In **addition** to those noted for other formulations of triamcinolone, may cause nasal dryness, infection, irritation, pain, stuffiness, and ulceration.
Triamcinolone, oral (*Aristocort®, Kenacort®*)	Adrenal insufficiency **Note:** Usually used in combination with mineralocorticoid therapy.	**Children and adolescents:** 4–12 mg/day PO as a single early morning dose before 9 am.	Syrup, oral: 4 mg/5 ml Tablets, oral: 4, 8 mg	**Contraindications:** Hypersensitivity to triamcinolone. **ADRs:** *See* Chapter 5. **Comments:** In **addition** to those noted for other formulations of triamcinolone, carefully monitor growth and development of children who are receiving long-term therapy because corticosteroid therapy has been associated with the inhibition of skeletal growth.
Triamcinolone, pulmonary (*Azmacort®*)	Prophylactic maintenance pharmacotherapy for chronic asthma **Note:** Not indicated for the treatment of acute asthma attacks (bronchospasms).	**Children (6–12 years):** One or two actuations of metered-dose aerosol (100 or 200 μg) three or four times daily. *Maximum:* 1200 μg/day by inhalation. **Adolescents:** Two actuations of metered-dose aerosol (200 μg) three or four times daily. *Maximum:* 1600 μg/day by inhalation. **Note:** Rinsing the mouth after inhalation is advised to reduce local ADRs (e.g., dry mouth, oral candidiasis) and unnecessary systemic absorption.	Suspension, inhalation by metered-dose inhaler: 200 μg/actuation (however, 100 μg/actuation is delivered from spacer-mouthpiece and stated dosage is based on this amount) **Note:** The inhaler requires priming with two actuations prior to first use and subsequently after each 3-day period of nonuse. **Note:** For pulmonary inhalation only. Take care not to inadvertently spray the aerosol into the eyes. **Note:** Shake the metered-dose inhaler well before use. Do not heat, incinerate, or puncture the canister because the contents are under pressure and it may explode. **Note:** Not generally available in Canada.	**Contraindications:** Hypersensitivity to triamcinolone. **ADRs:** May cause ADRs similar to other corticosteroids (*see* Chapter 5). **Comments:** Pulmonary inhalation may be sufficient to control asthma, but may be insufficient to control the signs and symptoms of adrenal insufficiency due to HPA axis suppression secondary to long-term or high-dosage oral corticosteroid therapy. Patients for whom their oral corticosteroid for asthma has been replaced with inhalation corticosteroid will require monitoring for up to 1 year, particularly during periods of significant mental or physical stress. Resumption of high-dosage oral corticosteroid therapy may be necessary during these periods until recovery of HPA axis function is satisfactory.

TABLE 14-1 continued

DRUG (TRADE AND OTHER NAMES)	INDICATION(S)	USUAL PEDIATRIC DOSAGE AND ADMINISTRATION[a]	DOSAGE FORMS	CONTRAINDICATIONS, ADRs, AND COMMENTS[b]
Triamcinolone, topical *(Aristocort®, Flutex®, Kenalog®, Triaderm®)*	**Dermatologic conditions** responsive to topical corticosteroid pharmacotherapy (e.g., atopic dermatitis, contact dermatitis, seborrheic dermatitis, neurodermatitis)	**Infants, children, and adolescents:** Apply sparingly to affected areas two to four times daily. For relatively chronic or long-term use, **decrease** the frequency of application (e.g., apply sparingly to affected areas twice every other day). **Note:** Occlusive dressings should generally be avoided in order to prevent systemic absorption and associated ADRs (*see* "Comments").	Creams, topical: 0.025%, 0.1%, 0.5% Lotions, topical: 0.025%, 0.1% Ointments, topical: 0.025%, 0.1%, 0.5% **Note:** Topical triamcinolone creams, lotions, and ointments are for external use only. Avoid contact with the eyes.	**Contraindications:** Chickenpox, herpes simplex, fungal dermal lesions, tuberculosis of the skin, vaccinia, and viral dermal lesions. **ADRs:** Generally well tolerated. **Comments:** Infants and young children are relatively more susceptible to HPA axis suppression associated with topical therapy because of their larger skin surface area to body weight ratio.
Triamterene *(Dyrenium®)*	**Edema** **Note:** Not approved by the FDA or HPB for children.	**Children and adolescents:** 1–6 mg/kg/day PO as a single daily dose or as two divided doses. *Maximum:* 300 mg/day PO. **Note:** Administer after meals to decrease associated GI irritation. **Note:** Reduce dosage for pediatric patients who have renal dysfunction; *see* Table 14-2.	Capsules, oral: 50, 100 mg Tablets, oral: 50, 100 mg (contain gluten)	**Contraindications:** Azotemia, hepatic dysfunction (severe), hyperkalemia, and hypersensitivity to triamterene. **ADRs:** *See* Chapter 5. **Comments:** Monitor patient for hyperkalemia or hyponatremia.
Trifluoperazine *(Novo-Flurazine®, Stelazine®, Terfluzine®)*	**Schizophrenia and other psychotic disorders**	**Children (6–12 years):** Initially, 1–2 mg/day PO or IM as a single dose or as two divided doses. Gradually increase the dosage, according to response, until the signs and symptoms of the psychotic disorder are managed. **Note: Not** recommended for children who are 6–12 years or <36.4 kg **unless** they are hospitalized or otherwise closely monitored. *Maximum:* 2 mg/day IM; 15 mg/day PO.	Concentrate, oral: 10 mg/ml (banana–vanilla flavored) Injectable, IM: 2 mg/ml Tablets, oral: 1, 2, 5, 10 mg **Note:** For **IM** injection only. Do **not** inject IV. IM injections generally are well tolerated with little, if any, pain or irritation at the injection site. However, IM route should be used only when necessary for the prompt control of severe signs and symptoms. Replace IM with oral therapy as soon as feasible. Oral therapy is preferred over IM. **Note:** Oral concentrate contains sodium bisulfite. Sulfites have been associated with hypersensitivity reactions, including anaphylactic reactions, among susceptible patients. Although relatively uncommon, these reactions appear to occur with a higher incidence among patients who have asthma. **Note:** Dilute each dose of oral concentrate immediately before ingestion with 60 ml (2 ounces) of a compatible beverage	**Contraindications:** Blood dyscrasias, bone marrow depression, cardiovascular disease (severe), CNS depression (severe, including that associated with the ingestion of alcohol or other CNS depressants [e.g., sedative-hypnotic, opiate analgesic therapy]), coma, hepatic disease (severe), and hypersensitivity to trifluoperazine or to other phenothiazines. **ADRs:** Generally well tolerated. May cause anorexia, blurred vision, dizziness, drowsiness, fatigue, insomnia, overstimulation, and skin rashes. *See* Chapter 5. **Note:** Avoid getting the oral concentrate on the skin or clothing because it is irritating and has been associated with contact dermatitis.

(Continued)

Footnotes are on page 558.

TABLE 14-1 *continued*

DRUG (*TRADE* AND OTHER NAMES)	INDICATION(S)	USUAL PEDIATRIC DOSAGE AND ADMINISTRATION[a]	DOSAGE FORMS	CONTRAINDICATIONS, ADRs, AND COMMENTS[b]
Trifluo-perazine *continued*			(e.g., carbonated soft drink, fruit or tomato juice, milk, water) or gently mix in 60 ml (2 ounces) of soft food (e.g., applesauce, pudding) to increase palatability.	
Trifluridine (*Viroptic®*)	Corneal inflammation (primary keratoconjunctivitis and recurrent epithelial keratitis) caused by herpes simplex virus, types 1 and 2	**Children (≥6 years) and adolescents:** Apply one drop of 1% ophthalmic solution directly to the cornea of the affected eye every 2 hr while awake until the corneal ulcer has completely re-epithelialized (maximum of nine drops per day). Following re-epithelialization, apply one dose of 1% ophthalmic solution to cornea of affected eye every 4 hr while awake (minimum of five drops/day) for 7 days. **Note:** Therapy exceeding 21 days may result in ocular toxicity and is **not** recommended.	Solution, ophthalmic: 1% **Note:** For ophthalmic instillation only. **Note:** In order to minimize cross-infections whenever both eyes require trifluridine ophthalmic pharmacotherapy, ensure that separate containers are dispensed for each eye. **Note:** Not generally available in the United States.	**Contraindications:** Hypersensitivity to trifluridine. **ADRs:** May cause palpebral edema, transient burning or stinging upon instillation, and other eye irritation.
Trimethoprim (*Proloprim®*, *Trimpex®*)	Urinary tract infections **Note:** Ensure that appropriate culture and sensitivity tests are performed and that the organism is sensitive to trimethoprim. **Note:** Not approved by the FDA or HPB for children.	**Children and adolescents:** 4 mg/kg/day PO in two divided doses, every 12 hr. *Maximum:* 200 mg/day PO. **Note:** Reduce dosage for pediatric patients who have renal dysfunction; *see* Table 14-2.	Tablets, oral: 100, 200 mg	**Contraindications:** Hypersensitivity to trimethoprim and megaloblastic anemia due to folate deficiency. **ADRs:** May cause dysgeusia, GI irritation, nausea, pruritus, rash, and vomiting. *See* Chapter 5.
Trimethoprim [T] and Sulfamethoxazole [S] (in a fixed 1:5 ratio) (*Bactrim®*, *Co-Trim®*, *Septra®*, *Sulfatrim®*)	Bacterial infections **Note:** Ensure that appropriate culture and sensitivity tests are performed and that the organism is sensitive to trimethoprim and sulfamethoxazole. *Pneumocystis carinii* **pneumonia, treatment** *Pneumocystis carinii*, **prophylaxis for HIV-infected patients** Gonorrhea, uncomplicated pharyngeal **Note:** Generally reserved for patients who cannot receive cephalosporins or	**Children and adolescents:** 5–10 mg [T] + 25–50 mg [S]/kg/day PO or IV in two divided doses, every 12 hr. **Note:** Reduce dosage for pediatric patients who have renal dysfunction; *see* Table 14-2. **Children and adolescents:** 20 mg [T] + 100 mg [S]/kg/day IV or PO in four divided doses, every 6 hr for 14–21 days. **Children and adolescents:** 150 mg [T] + 750 mg [S]/m²/day PO in two divided doses, every 12 hr, three times weekly. **Children and adolescents:** 640 mg [T] + 3200 mg [S]/1.73 m²/day PO in four divided doses for 2 days.	Injectable: 16 mg [T] + 80 mg [S]/ml; contains 10% alcohol and 40% propylene glycol. Suspensions, oral: 40 mg [T] + 200 mg [S]/5 ml (cherry or grape flavored); shake well before use. Tablets, oral: 20 mg [T] + 100 mg [S], 80 mg [T] + 400 mg [S], 160 mg [T] + 800 mg [S] (double strength) **Note:** Injectable is for IV use only. It contains sodium metabisulfite. Sulfites have been associated with hypersensitivity reactions, including anaphylactic reactions, among susceptible patients. Although relatively uncommon, these reactions appear to occur with a higher incidence	**Contraindications:** Blood dyscrasias, hypersensitivity to sulfonamides or to trimethoprim, and significant hepatic or renal dysfunction. **ADRs:** Commonly causes anorexia, nausea, rash, urticaria, and vomiting. Rarely causes severe potentially fatal reactions including blood dyscrasias and Stevens-Johnson syndrome. *See* Chapter 5. **Comments:** Ensure adequate hydration is maintained. Perform complete blood counts periodically during long-term pharmacotherapy.

CHAPTER 14: DRUG DOSING FOR INFANTS, CHILDREN, AND ADOLESCENTS

TABLE 14-1 continued

DRUG (TRADE AND OTHER NAMES)	INDICATION(S)	USUAL PEDIATRIC DOSAGE AND ADMINISTRATION[a]	DOSAGE FORMS	CONTRAINDICATIONS, ADRs, AND COMMENTS[b]
Trimethoprim [T] and Sulfamethoxazole [S] (in a fixed 1:5 ratio) *continued*	quinolones for gonorrhea. **Note:** Approved by the HPB but not the FDA for this indication.			among patients who have asthma.
	Salmonellosis/ Shigellosis	**Infants (>2 months), children, and adolescents:** 8 mg [T] + 40 mg [S]/kg/day IV or PO in two divided doses, every 12 hr for 5 days.		
	Urinary tract infection, treatment/ Otitis media, acute, treatment **Note:** Ensure that appropriate culture and sensitivity tests are performed and that the organism is sensitive to trimethoprim and sulfamethoxazole.	**Infants (>2 months), children, and adolescents:** 8 mg [T] + 40 mg [S]/kg/day PO in two divided doses, every 12 hr for 10 days. **Note:** Reduce dosage for pediatric patients who have renal dysfunction; see Table 14-2.		
	Urinary tract infection, prophylaxis/ Otitis media, prophylaxis	**Children and adolescents:** 2–5 mg [T] + 10–25 mg [S]/kg/day PO in two divided doses every 12 hr. *Maximum:* 320 mg [T] + 1600 [S]/day PO. **Note:** Reduce dosage for pediatric patients who have renal dysfunction; see Table 14-2. **Note:** Administer IV by infusion over 30–60 min.		
Troleandomycin (*TAO®*, Triacetyloleandomycin)	Infections caused by susceptible organisms **Note:** Ensure that appropriate culture and sensitivity tests are performed and that the organism is sensitive to troleandomycin. **Note:** Rarely used because of the ready availability of equally efficacious but generally less toxic antibiotics including the cephalosporins, erythromycin, and the penicillins.	**Children:** 500–1000 mg/day PO in four divided doses, every 6 hr. **Adolescents:** 1000–2000 mg/day PO in four divided doses, every 6 hr. **Note:** When used for the treatment of *Streptococcus pyogenes* infections of the upper respiratory tract, therapy should generally be continued for 10 days. **Note:** Pediatric patients with moderate-to-severe hepatic or renal dysfunction will require a reduction in dosage.	Capsule, oral: 250 mg **Note:** Not generally available in Canada.	**Contraindications:** Concurrent therapy with ergot alkaloids and hypersensitivity to troleandomycin. **ADRs:** Commonly causes abdominal cramping and discomfort. Cholestatic hepatitis may occur as part of a hypersensitivity reaction. **Comments:** Periodically monitor hepatic function for patients receiving therapy for 2 weeks or longer.
Tubocurarine (d-Tubocurarine)	Muscle relaxation during surgery	**Infants, children, and adolescents:** Initially, 0.2–0.6 mg/kg IV as a single dose. *Maintenance:* 0.04–0.12 mg/kg IV as needed to maintain paralysis during surgery. **Note:** Reduce dosage for pediatric patients who have renal dysfunction; see Table 14-2.	Injectable, IV: 3 mg/ml (contains benzyl alcohol and sodium bisulfite) **Note:** Sulfites have been associated with hypersensitivity reactions, including anaphylactic reactions, among susceptible patients.	**Contraindications:** Hypersensitivity to tubocurarine and patients for whom histamine release is problematic. **ADRs:** May cause bradycardia, cardiac arrest, hypotension, and salivation (excessive). **Comments:** When ether is used as the general anesthetic, only *(Continued)*

Footnotes are on page 558.

TABLE 14-1 continued

DRUG (*TRADE* AND OTHER NAMES)	INDICATION(S)	USUAL PEDIATRIC DOSAGE AND ADMINISTRATION[a]	DOSAGE FORMS	CONTRAINDICATIONS, ADRs, AND COMMENTS[b]
Tubocurarine *continued*		**Note:** *See also* "Comments."	Although relatively uncommon, these reactions appear to occur with a higher incidence among patients who have asthma.	33% of the usual tubocurarine dose is generally required; 66% of the usual dose is required with methoxyflurane; and 80% with cyclopropane or halothane anesthesia.
Undecylenic Acid (*Caldesene®, Cruex®, Desenex®, Pedi-Pro®, Quinsana Plus®*)	*Tinea pedis* infections (athlete's foot) and *T. cruris* infections (jock itch) **Note:** Not indicated for the treatment of fungal infections of the nails or scalp.	**Children and adolescents:** After cleansing and thoroughly drying the affected skin site, apply directly to the affected area according to manufacturer's instructions. Repeat topical application up to four times daily, as indicated by response.	Aerosol spray powder, topical: 25% Creams, topical: 20%, 25% Foam, topical: 10% Ointment, topical: 25% Powders, topical: 10%, 12%, 15%, 19%, 25% **Note:** For external use only. Avoid contact with the eyes and other mucous membranes. Avoid inhalation of the powder.	**Contraindications:** Hypersensitivity to undecylenic acid. **ADRs:** Generally well tolerated. May cause local irritation at application site. **Comments:** For further details and recommended techniques for applying topical pharmacotherapy for pediatric patients, *see* Chapter 1.
Urea Peroxide, *see* **Carbamide Peroxide**				
Valacyclovir (*Valtrex®*)	Genital herpes	**INITIAL EPISODES** **Adolescents:** 2 grams/day PO in two divided doses, every 12 hr, for 10 days. **Note:** Valacyclovir pharmacotherapy should be initiated within 72 hr of the onset of signs and symptoms (efficacy increases significantly if pharmacotherapy is initiated within 48 hr). **RECURRENT EPISODES** **Adolescents:** 1 gram/day PO in two divided doses, every 12 hr, for 3 days. **Note:** Valacyclovir pharmacotherapy should be initiated within 24 hr of the onset of signs and symptoms. **SUPPRESSIVE PHARMACOTHERAPY** **Adolescents:** 1 gram/day PO as a single dose. **Note:** If effective and well tolerated, valacyclovir pharmacotherapy may continue for up to 1 year. For patients who have a history of nine or fewer recurrences of genital herpes annually, a dosage of 0.5 gram/day PO may be of benefit.	Tablet, oral: 500 mg	**Contraindications:** Hypersensitivity to acyclovir or valacyclovir. **ADRs:** May cause abdominal pain, diarrhea, flulike syndrome, infection, nausea, pharyngitis, and rhinitis. **Comments:** Valacyclovir is a prodrug of acyclovir (*see* Acyclovir).
	Herpes zoster	**Adolescents:** 3 grams/day PO in three divided doses for 7 days. **Note:** Valacyclovir pharmacotherapy should be initiated within 72 hr of the onset of signs and symptoms (rash). Efficacy increases significantly if initiated within 48 hr. **Note:** Reduce dosage for pediatric patients who have renal dysfunction; see following table.		

CHAPTER 14: DRUG DOSING FOR INFANTS, CHILDREN, AND ADOLESCENTS

TABLE 14-1 continued

DRUG (TRADE AND OTHER NAMES)	INDICATION(S)	USUAL PEDIATRIC DOSAGE AND ADMINISTRATION[a]	DOSAGE FORMS	CONTRAINDICATIONS, ADRs, AND COMMENTS[b]

Valacyclovir continued

Dosage for Pediatric Patients with Renal Dysfunction

	CREATININE CLEARANCE		
INDICATION	30–49 ml/min	10–29 ml/min	<10 ml/min
Herpes zoster	2000 mg/day PO in two divided doses	1000 mg/day PO in two divided doses	500 mg/day PO as a single dose
Genital herpes, initial episode	2000 mg/day PO in two divided doses	1000 mg/day PO as a single dose	500 mg/day PO as a single dose
Genital herpes, recurrent episode	1000 mg/day PO in two divided doses	500 mg/day PO as a single dose	500 mg/day PO as a single dose
Genital herpes, suppressive therapy	1000 mg/day PO in two divided doses	500 mg/day PO as a single dose	500 mg/day PO as a single dose

Valproate Sodium, *see* **Valproic Acid**

Valproic Acid
(Depacon® [Valproate Sodium], *Depakene®* [Valproic Acid], *Depakote®* [Divalproex Sodium], *Epiject®* [Valproate Sodium], *Epival®* [Divalproex Sodium], Sodium Valproate)

Simple and complex absence seizures, including petit mal seizures

Children (≥2 years) and adolescents: 15 mg/kg/day PO in two or three divided doses. Gradually increase the dosage by 5–10 mg/kg/day every 7 days according to response (until seizures are controlled or ADRs preclude further increase in dosage).
Maximum: 60 mg/kg/day PO.
Note: IV valproic acid pharmacotherapy, on a milligram-per-milligram equivalent basis, may be used to replace oral pharmacotherapy when the latter is temporarily not feasible (e.g., surgery, unconsciousness). Valproic acid IV pharmacotherapy is for short-term use only (usually 48 hr or less) and oral pharmacotherapy should be re-established as soon as feasible.
Note: Administer each IV dose of valproic acid as an intermittent IV infusion over 60 min.
Maximum: 500 mg/dose IV; 2000 mg/day IV; 10 mg/min IV.

Capsules, oral (soft): 250, 500 mg *(Depakene)*
Capsule, oral sprinkle: 125 mg *(Depakote Sprinkle)*
Injectable, IV: 100 mg/ml *(Depacon)*
Solution, oral: 50 mg/ml
Syrup, oral: 250 mg/5 ml *(Depakene)*
Tablets, oral extended release: 125, 250, 500 mg *(Depakene)*
Tablets, oral enteric coated: 125, 250, 500 mg *(Epival)*
Note: Formulations are listed in terms of valproic acid equivalents, even though some (e.g., *Depakote, Epival*) contain the valproic acid producer, divalproex sodium. *Depakote Sprinkle* oral capsules contain coated particles. Capsule contents may be sprinkled on a small amount (5 ml) of cold, soft food (e.g., applesauce, pudding) immediately prior to ingestion. Caution patients against chewing the coated particles. *Depakene* 500-mg oral capsules contain tartrazine (FD&C yellow No. 5). Tartrazine has been associated with hypersensitivity reactions (e.g., bronchial asthma) among susceptible patients, particularly those who have a hypersensitivity to aspirin. Advise patients to ingest valproic acid with food to decrease associated GI irritation. Also advise them, as appropriate, to

Contraindications: Hepatic disease (active), hepatic dysfunction (severe), hypersensitivity to divalproex sodium or valproic acid, and pregnancy.
ADRs: May cause aggression, behavioral deterioration, depression, diplopia, dizziness, edema of the extremities, emotional upset, hyperactivity, incoordination, indigestion, nausea, pancreatitis (potentially fatal), photosensitivity, pruritus, sedation (particularly with concurrent CNS depressant therapy), Stevens-Johnson syndrome, thrombocytopenia (particularly with higher dosages), and vomiting. *See* Chapter 5.
Comments: Adolescents who are or who may become pregnant: FDA Pregnancy Category D. Valproic acid crosses the placenta and achieves higher embryonic, fetal, and neonatal blood concentrations than maternal blood concentrations. Associated teratogenic effects include cardiovascular anomalies, cranial defects, spina bifida, and other defects. *See* Chapter 2. Caution adolescent girls to avoid pregnancy while receiving valproic acid therapy.
Note: Caution is indicated when patients are receiving polydrug pharmacotherapy for the prophylactic and symptomatic management of seizure disorders, have histories of liver dysfunction, or have hepatotoxicity with elevations in liver enzyme tests that may be dose related.
Note: Evaluate hepatic function prior to initiating therapy. Discontinue immediately if hepatic dysfunction is suspected or medically confirmed. Hepatic dysfunction may progress and has been fatal. Therapeutic drug monitoring is recommended; *see* Table 14-3.

(Continued)

Footnotes are on page 558.

TABLE 14-1 *continued*

DRUG (*TRADE* AND OTHER NAMES)	INDICATION(S)	USUAL PEDIATRIC DOSAGE AND ADMINISTRATION[a]	DOSAGE FORMS	CONTRAINDICATIONS, ADRs, AND COMMENTS[b]
Valproic Acid *continued*			swallow each soft oral capsule whole without breaking or chewing to avoid associated local irritation of the mouth and throat.	
Vancomycin (*Vancocin®*)	**Bacterial infections,** severe and not amenable to other antibiotic therapy	**Children and adolescents:** 40 mg/kg/day IV in four divided doses, every 6 hr. *Maximum:* 2 grams/day IV. **Note:** Administer IV over at least 60 min. Intermittent IV infusion is preferred.	Capsules, oral: 125, 250 mg Injectables, IV: 500 mg; 1, 2, 5 grams	**Contraindications:** Hypersensitivity to vancomycin. **ADRs:** *See* Chapter 5. **Comments:** IV administration may cause pain at injection site or thrombophlebitis. Rapid IV administration may result in significant hypotension and the "red man" or "red neck" syndrome (flushing and/or erythematous rash on the face, neck, chest, and upper extremities). Monitor blood pressure during IV administration. Therapeutic drug monitoring is recommended; *see* Table 14-3.
	Pseudomembraneous colitis (antibiotic associated) **Note:** Ensure that appropriate culture and sensitivity tests are performed and that the organism is sensitive to vancomycin.	**Children and adolescents:** 40 mg/kg/day PO in three or four divided doses, every 6 or 8 hr for 7–10 days. *Maximum:* 2 grams/day PO. **Note:** Reduce dosage for pediatric patients who have renal dysfunction; *see* Table 14-2.		

Varicella-Zoster Immune Globulin, Human, *see* **Chapter 9**

Varicella-Zoster Virus Vaccine, *see* **Chapter 9**

DRUG	INDICATION(S)	DOSAGE AND ADMINISTRATION	DOSAGE FORMS	CONTRAINDICATIONS, ADRs, AND COMMENTS
Vasopressin (*Pressyn®*)	**Central diabetes insipidus** (neurogenic diabetes insipidus)	**Children:** 2.5–10 units/dose IM or SC two to four times daily. Adjust dosage until normal urine electrolyte concentrations and osmolality are achieved. **Adolescents:** 5–10 units/dose IM or SC two to four times daily. Adjust dosage until normal urine electrolyte concentrations and osmolality are achieved. **Note:** Administration with one or two glassfuls of water may minimize some ADRs (abdominal cramps, blanching of the skin, and nausea).	Injectable, IM, SC: 20 units/ml; contains 0.5% chlorobutanol.	**Contraindications:** Chronic nephritis accompanied by nitrogen retention and hypersensitivity to vasopressin. **ADRs:** Generally well tolerated. May cause circumoral pallor, cramps, eructation, flatulence, headache, nausea, and vomiting. **Comments:** Adjust dosage according to response; use lowest effective dosage. Monitor fluid intake and output.
Vecuronium (*Norcuron®*)	**Muscle relaxation** during surgery or mechanical ventilation	**Infants, children, and adolescents:** Initially, 0.1 mg/kg IV; maintenance (after 20–40 min), 1 µg/kg/min by continuous IV infusion. Adjust infusion rate according to response. **Note:** A dosage reduction of approximately 15%–30% may be required when used concurrently with general anesthetics (e.g., enflurane, halothane, isoflurane) that potentiate the neuromuscular blocking action. Adjust dosage according to response. Infants may experience more prolonged response to vecuronium and may, thus, require less frequent maintenance dosing. Younger children may require higher dosages initially and during maintenance pharmacotherapy. **Note:** Reduce dosage for pediatric patients with hepatic dysfunction.	Injectables, IV: 10, 20 mg/vial (may contain benzyl alcohol) **Note:** For IV use only. **Note:** Benzyl alcohol, which may be found in the injectable formulation, is associated with a potentially **fatal** "gasping syndrome" among premature neonates and young infants.	**Contraindications:** Hypersensitivity to vecuronium and myasthenia gravis. **ADRs:** Generally well tolerated. Relatively short acting, has minimal cardiovascular effects, and has minimal cumulative effects. May cause respiratory or skeletal muscle weakness and associated pharmacologic effects (e.g., apnea or respiratory insufficiency). **Comments:** IV administration of neostigmine, a cholinesterase inhibitor, antagonizes the neuromuscular blockade produced by vecuronium and should be immediately available to treat overdosage. **Note:** Monitor muscle twitch response to peripheral nerve stimulation during therapy.

TABLE 14-1 continued

DRUG (TRADE AND OTHER NAMES)	INDICATION(S)	USUAL PEDIATRIC DOSAGE AND ADMINISTRATIONa	DOSAGE FORMS	CONTRAINDICATIONS, ADRs, AND COMMENTSb
Venlafaxine (*Effexor®, Effexor XR®*)	**Depression** **Note:** Not approved by the FDA or HPB for adolescents. **Note:** Long-term therapeutic efficacy (beyond 3 months) has not yet been demonstrated in controlled clinical trials.	**Adolescents:** Initially, 37.5 mg/day PO in two divided doses. **Note:** If the venlafaxine extended-release capsules are used, the total daily dosage should be ingested as a single daily dose, either in the morning or evening. **Note:** Each dose should be ingested with food to decrease associated GI distress. **Note:** Reduce initial venlafaxine dosage by 50% for pediatric patients who have hepatic dysfunction. Reduce dosage for pediatric patients who have renal dysfunction; *see* Table 14-2.	Capsules, oral extended release: 37.5, 75, 150 mg Tablets, oral: 37.5, 75 mg	**Contraindications:** Hypersensitivity to venlafaxine and MAOI pharmacotherapy (concurrent or within 2 weeks). **ADRs:** May cause abnormal dreams, abnormal ejaculation, abnormal vision, anorexia, anxiety, asthenia, blurred vision, chills, constipation, depression, dizziness, dry mouth, headache, impotence, insomnia, nausea, nervousness, somnolence, sweating, tremor, vomiting, and yawning. Rarely causes activation of mania, hypertension, hyponatremia, QTc prolongation, and seizures. **Comments:** Assess hepatic function upon initiation of and at regular intervals during therapy. In addition, assess all depressed patients for suicide risk initially and regularly during venlafaxine therapy. All depressed patients who are at risk for suicide need to be dealt with appropriately.
Verapamil (*Calan®, Isoptin®, Verelan®*)	**Cardiac dysrhythmias** (atrial fibrillation and atrial flutter with rapid ventricular response) **Note:** Generally reserved for use when digoxin cannot control the dysrhythmias.	**Infants, children, and adolescents:** Initially, 0.1–0.3 mg/kg/dose IV; may repeat dose once after 15–30 min **or** 4–8 mg/kg/day PO in three or four divided doses (or as a single daily dose or in two divided doses, every 12 hr, using sustained-release formulations). *Maximum:* 5 mg/initial dose IV; 10 mg/repeat dose IV; 480 mg/day PO. **Note:** Administer IV as a slow injection over at least 2 min. **Note:** Reduce dosage for pediatric patients who have hepatic dysfunction.	Capsules, oral sustained release: 120, 240 mg Injectable, IV: 2.5 mg/ml Tablets, oral: 40, 80, 120 mg Tablets, oral sustained release: 180, 240 mg **Note:** Oral sustained-release formulations are **not** approved by the FDA or HPB for infants or children and are not recommended.	**Contraindications:** Acute myocardial infarction, atrial flutter or fibrillation with an accessible bypass tract, AV block (second or third degree), cardiogenic shock, congestive heart failure, hypersensitivity to verapamil, hypotension (marked), left ventricular dysfunction (severe), and sick sinus syndrome. **ADRs:** Generally well tolerated. *See* Chapter 5. **Comments:** Continuously monitor blood pressure and ECG during IV administration. Therapeutic drug monitoring is recommended; *see* Table 14-3. **Note:** Verapamil can increase digoxin serum levels (*see* Chapter 6).
Vigabatrin (*Sabril®*)	**Infantile spasms** (West syndrome), initial monotherapy	**Infants:** 50–100 mg/kg/day PO in two divided doses. Adjust dosage according to response. *Maximum:* 150 mg/kg/day PO. **Note:** For **infants,** dissolve the entire contents (500 mg) of the sachet in 10 ml of fruit juice or water and administer the required dosage using an oral dosing syringe. **Note:** The manufacturer suggests that each oral dose may be administered in milk or the infant's formula; however, this practice is not recommended because of the potential of having infants "go	Powder, oral: 500 mg (in individual sachets for reconstitution) Tablet, oral: 500 mg **Note:** For **children and adolescents,** dissolve the entire contents of the powder sachet(s) in 240 ml (8 ounces) of cold or room temperature juice, milk, or water immediately before ingestion. **Note:** Vigabatrin is available in Canada by the brand or trade name,	**Contraindications:** Breast feeding, hypersensitivity to vigabatrin, and pregnancy. **ADRs:** Generally well tolerated. May cause confusion, depression, dizziness, fatigue, headache, ophthalmological abnormalities, poor concentration, and somnolence. **Comments:** Vigabatrin has been associated with a number of ADRs affecting the ophthalmic system, including permanent visual field defects. Therefore, ophthalmic examinations, including mydriatic peripheral fundus examinations and visual field perimetry (for *(Continued)*

Footnotes are on page 558.

PROBLEMS IN PEDIATRIC DRUG THERAPY

TABLE 14-1 continued

DRUG (TRADE AND OTHER NAMES)	INDICATION(S)	USUAL PEDIATRIC DOSAGE AND ADMINISTRATION[a]	DOSAGE FORMS	CONTRAINDICATIONS, ADRs, AND COMMENTS[b]
Vigabatrin *continued*		"off" (develop an aversion to) their milk or formula (essential source of fluid and nutritional requirements).	*Sabril*, and in the United States as an "orphan drug."	patients ≥9 years of age), are recommended **prior** to the initiation of vigabatrin pharmacotherapy to serve as a baseline and every 3 months during therapy.
	Seizure disorders **Note:** Indicated as adjunctive pharmacotherapy for patients whose seizure disorders have not been satisfactorily controlled by less toxic, conventional anticonvulsant pharmacotherapy alone.	**Children and adolescents:** Initially, 40 mg/kg/day PO as a single dose or as two divided doses. **Alternatively,** may be initiated at a dosage of 500 mg/day PO and increased by 500-mg increments at weekly intervals according to response and body weight:		**Note:** In order to minimize risk of rebound seizures associated with the abrupt discontinuation of vigabatrin pharmacotherapy, gradually reduce the vigabatrin dosage, if possible, by 0.5 gram every 1–2 weeks before completely discontinuing.

BODY WEIGHT	USUAL DAILY DOSAGE
10–15 kg	0.5–1 gram
16–30 kg	1–1.5 grams
31–50 kg	1.5–3 grams
>50 kg	2–3 grams

Maximum: 3 grams/day PO.

Vinblastine, *see* **Chapter 12**

Vincristine, *see* **Chapter 12**

Vitamin B$_1$, *see* **Thiamine**

Vitamin B$_2$, *see* **Riboflavin**

Vitamin B$_6$, *see* **Pyridoxine**

Vitamin B$_{12}$, *see* **Cyanocobalamin**

Vitamin C, *see* **Ascorbic Acid**

Vitamin D, *see* **Calcitriol**

Vitamin D$_2$, *see* **Ergocalciferol**

Vitamin D$_2$ Analog, *see* **Dihydrotachysterol**

Vitamin K$_1$, *see* **Phytonadione**

DRUG (TRADE AND OTHER NAMES)	INDICATION(S)	USUAL PEDIATRIC DOSAGE AND ADMINISTRATION[a]	DOSAGE FORMS	CONTRAINDICATIONS, ADRs, AND COMMENTS[b]
Vitamins, Multiple (*Multi-12*®, USA; *M.V.I.-Pediatric*®, USA; *M.V.I.-12*®, Canada; *M.V.I.-12*®, USA)	Multiple vitamin supplementation for pediatric patients receiving parenteral nutrition (used as a prophylactic maintenance vitamin supplement) **Note:** Although multiple intravenous vitamins products differ among manufacturers (and even the same product between Canada and the United States), the recommended dosage is the same.	**Children (1–10 years):** 10 ml (5 ml of vial #1 and 5 ml of vial #2)/day IV (*M.V.I.-12*®, Canada or *M.V.I.-Pediatric*®, USA). **Children (≥11 years) and adolescents:** 10 ml (5 ml of vial #1 and 5 ml of vial #2)/day IV. (*Multi-12*®, Canada **or** *M.V.I.-12*®, USA). **Note:** Contents of each vial are added directly to 1000 ml of dextrose, saline, or similar intravenous infusion solution.	Injectables, IV: Vitamin components and strengths of multiple vitamin products for IV use differ among various manufacturers; see following table.	

Contents of Multiple Intravenous Vitamins

	MULTI-12® (USA)	M.V.I.-12® (CANADA)	M.V.I.-12® (USA)	M.V.I.-PEDIATRIC® (USA)
Vial #1 (5 ml)				
Ascorbic acid (vitamin C)	100 mg	20 mg	100 mg	80 mg
Dexpanthenol (d-pantothenic acid)	15 mg	3 mg	15 mg	5 mg
Niacinamide	40 mg	8 mg	40 mg	17 mg
Pyridoxine (vitamin B$_6$)	4 mg	0.8 mg	4 mg	1 mg
Riboflavin (vitamin B$_2$)	3.6 mg	0.72 mg	3.6 mg	1.4 mg

TABLE 14-1 continued

DRUG (TRADE AND OTHER NAMES)	INDICATION(S)	USUAL PEDIATRIC DOSAGE AND ADMINISTRATION[a]	DOSAGE FORMS	CONTRAINDICATIONS, ADRs, AND COMMENTS[b]

Contents of Multiple Intravenous Vitamins continued

	MULTI-12® (USA)	M.V.I.-12® (CANADA)	M.V.I.-12® (USA)	M.V.I.-PEDIATRIC® (USA)
Thiamine (vitamin B_1)	3 mg	0.6 mg	3 mg	1.2 mg
Vitamin A	3300 IU	660 IU	3300 IU	2300 IU
Vitamin D	200 IU	40 IU	200 IU	400 IU
Vitamin E	10 IU	2 IU	10 IU	7 IU
Vial #2 (5 ml)*				
Biotin	60 µg	12 µg	60 µg	20 µg
Cyanocobalamin (vitamin B_{12})	5 µg	1 µg	5 µg	1 µg
Folic acid	400 µg	80 µg	400 µg	140 µg

* Contains propylene glycol.

Note: For IV use only. Generally available in sets containing two 5-ml vials that must be diluted in IV solution prior to administration. Do **not** administer multiple intravenous vitamins without prior dilution.

Note: Store unopened vials of multiple intravenous vitamins under refrigeration between 2 and 8°C (36–46°F) until ready for use.

Contraindications: Hypersensitivity to any of the vitamins (e.g., thiamine or vitamin K) and hypervitaminosis.

ADRs: Generally well tolerated. Rarely causes allergic (e.g., erythema, rash, pruritus) and anaphylactic (e.g., angioedema, shortness of breath) reactions.

Comments: Multiple intravenous vitamins generally do not contain vitamin K. Thus, additional vitamin K supplementation may be required.

Note: When long-term multiple intravenous vitamin therapy is required, monitor blood vitamin concentrations and monitor pediatric patients for signs and symptoms of hypovitaminosis and hypervitaminosis.

Warfarin
(Coumadin®, Warfilone®)

Anticoagulation (e.g., prophylaxis and treatment of atrial fibrillation with embolization, heart valve prosthesis, peripheral artery embolism, pulmonary embolism, and venous thrombosis)

Note: Heparin is preferred if rapid anticoagulation is required.

Note: Not approved by the FDA or HPB for pediatric patients.

Infants, children, and adolescents: *Loading dose, day 1:* 0.2 mg/kg PO as a single dose. *Maximum:* Initially, 5 mg/dose. *Loading doses, days 2–7 (based on INR):*

INR	DOSE (PO)
1.1–1.4	0.2 mg/kg
1.5–1.9	0.2 mg/kg
2–3.9	0.1 mg/kg
4–5	0.05 mg/kg
>5	withhold warfarin for one dose, then restart at 0.1 mg/kg

If INR is less than 2 after three doses of 0.2 mg/kg:

DAY	INR	DOSE (PO)
4	<2	0.3 mg/kg
5	<2	0.3 mg/kg
6	<2	0.4 mg/kg
7	<2	0.4 mg/kg

Day 8: Continue to increase warfarin dosage similarly until INR >2. Once the INR >2, decrease loading dose by 50%.

Tablets, oral: 1, 2, 2.5, 3, 4, 5, 6, 7.5, 10 mg

Contraindications: Bacterial endocarditis, blood dyscrasias, hemophilia, hemorrhage, malignant hypertension, pericarditis, pregnancy, spinal puncture, surgery (CNS, eye, traumatic), and thrombocytopenia purpura.

ADRs: May cause bleeding (hemorrhage). *See* Chapter 5.

Comments: Dosage must be individualized. Monitor INR for 5–7 days after any dosage changes. Adjust dosage to maintain an INR between 2 and 3, according to maintenance guidelines. A PT ratio of 1.3–2 is generally equivalent to an INR of 2–4. Observe for signs and symptoms of bleeding (e.g., black tarry stools, easy bruising). Phytonadione is an antidote for warfarin overdosages. Warfarin may interact with other drugs, resulting in significant therapeutic risk for the patient (*see* Chapter 6).

(Continued)

Footnotes are on page 558.

TABLE 14-1 continued

DRUG (TRADE AND OTHER NAMES)	INDICATION(S)	USUAL PEDIATRIC DOSAGE AND ADMINISTRATION[a]	DOSAGE FORMS	CONTRAINDICATIONS, ADRs, AND COMMENTS[b]
Warfarin *continued*		*Maintenance dose:* INR / DOSE 1.1–1.4 / increase (previous dose) by 20% 1.5–1.9 / increase dose by 10% 2–3 / continue current dose 3.1–4 / decrease dose by 10% 4.1–4.5 / decrease dose by 20% >4.5 / withhold one dose, then resume therapy at 20% less than previous dose >5 / withhold dose and monitor INR until <4.5, then resume at 20% less than previous dose **Note:** Reduce dosage for pediatric patients who have hepatic dysfunction.		
Zalcitabine (Dideoxycytidine, Hivid®)	**HIV infection** (as adjunctive therapy with zidovudine) **Note:** Several dosing regimens use a combination of zalcitabine and two other antiretroviral drugs concurrently. **Note:** Patients may continue to develop opportunistic infections and other complications associated with HIV infection. In addition, use does not reduce the risk for HIV transmission to others.	**Adolescents:** 2.25 mg/day PO in three divided doses, every 8 hr. **Note:** May be an adjunct to zidovudine 600 mg/day PO in three divided doses, every 8 hr. **Note:** Reduce dosage for pediatric patients who have renal dysfunction; *see* Table 14-2.	Tablets, oral: 0.375, 0.75 mg	**Contraindications:** Hepatic impairment (severe), hypersensitivity to zalcitabine, pentamidine pharmacotherapy (concurrent), and peripheral neuropathy. **ADRs:** May cause a variety of ADRs, including fatigue, headache, and rash. Major toxicities are peripheral neuropathy and, less commonly, pancreatitis. **Comments:** Monitor patients for signs and symptoms of hepatic impairment, pancreatitis, and peripheral neuropathy. Periodically obtain complete blood counts and monitor blood chemistry.
Zanamivir (Relenza®)	**Influenza A and B virus infection,** treatment of uncomplicated acute illness within 2 days of the initial onset of signs and symptoms **Note:** Not approved by the HPB for children.	**Children (≥7 years) and adolescents:** 20 mg/day by inhalation in two divided doses, every 12 hr, for 5 days. **Note:** On day 1, the two divided doses may be administered between 2 and 12 hr apart.	Inhalation, powder: 5 mg/blister in groups of four on a circular foil disk *(Rotadisks®)*, supplied with a Diskhaler®. **Note:** Contains lactose.	**Contraindications:** Bronchospasm, chronic obstructive pulmonary disease (moderate to severe), and hypersensitivity to zanamivir or to lactose. **ADRs:** Generally well tolerated. May cause transient bronchospasm. **Comments:** For further details and recommended techniques for administering inhalation powder products to pediatric patients, *see* Chapter 1.
Zarfirlukast (Accolate®)	**Asthma,** prophylaxis and long-term chronic management **Note:** Not indicated for the treatment of acute asthma attacks (bronchospasms).	**Children (≥5 years):** 20 mg/day PO in two divided doses on an empty stomach. **Adolescents:** 40 mg/day PO in two divided doses on an empty stomach. **Note:** Food significantly decreases the oral bioavailability.	Tablets, oral: 10, 20 mg	**Contraindications:** Hypersensitivity to zarfirlukast and severe hepatic impairment. **ADRs:** Generally well tolerated. May cause headache. Rarely causes agranulocytosis, bleeding, bruising, edema, and hepatic dysfunction. *See* Chapter 5.

CHAPTER 14: DRUG DOSING FOR INFANTS, CHILDREN, AND ADOLESCENTS

TABLE 14-1 continued

DRUG (TRADE AND OTHER NAMES)	INDICATION(S)	USUAL PEDIATRIC DOSAGE AND ADMINISTRATION[a]	DOSAGE FORMS	CONTRAINDICATIONS, ADRs, AND COMMENTS[b]
Zarfirlukast *continued*		**Note:** Reduce dosage for pediatric patients who have hepatic dysfunction.		**Comments:** Co-administration of warfarin results in a significant increase in prothrombin time. Patients receiving both zarfirlukast and warfarin will require more frequent monitoring of prothrombin times and adjustment of their anticoagulant dosage.
Zidovudine (Azidothymidine, AZT®, Novo-AZT®, Retrovir®)	**HIV infection** **Note:** Although not curative, may delay progression of the disease, reduce the incidence of opportunistic infections, and prolong patient survival time. **Prevention of maternal-to-fetal transmission of HIV**	**Infants:** 480–720 mg/m²/day PO in four divided doses, every 6 hr. **Children:** 400–800 mg/day PO in four divided doses, every 6 hr. *Maximum:* 160 mg/dose IV; 200 mg/dose PO. **Note:** Infuse IV over 1 hr. **Adolescents (pregnant mothers >14 weeks pregnant):** 500 mg/day PO in five divided doses until the start of labor. Then 2 mg/kg IV (over 1 hr), followed by 1 mg/kg/hr IV by continuous infusion until clamping of the umbilical cord. **Neonates and infants (≤6 weeks born to HIV-positive mothers):** 8 mg/kg/day PO in four divided doses, every 6 hr **or** 6 mg/kg/day IV in four divided doses, every 6 hr for 6 weeks.	Capsule, oral: 100 mg Injectable, IV; 10 mg/ml Syrup, oral: 10 mg/ml (strawberry flavored) Tablet, oral: 300 mg	**Contraindications:** Hypersensitivity to zidovudine. **ADRs:** May cause anemia, anorexia, asthenia, constipation, dizziness, dyspepsia, granulocytopenia, headache, malaise, nausea, and vomiting. *See* Chapter 5. **Comments:** Generally used in combination with other antiretroviral drugs. Dosages may vary according to protocol. Monitor blood cell counts and hemoglobin. Not a cure for HIV infection and does not reduce the risk for transmission of HIV to others.
Zileuton (Zyflo®)	**Asthma,** prophylaxis (for long-term, chronic therapy) **Note:** Not indicated for the reversal of bronchospasm (e.g., acute asthmatic attack; status asthmaticus).	**Adolescents:** 2400 mg/day PO in four divided doses, with meals and at bedtime.	Tablet, oral: 600 mg **Note:** Not generally available in Canada.	**Contraindications:** Alcoholism, hepatic disease (active), hepatic impairment (moderate to severe), and hypersensitivity to zileuton. **ADRs:** Generally well tolerated. May cause asthenia, dyspepsia, headache, myalgia, nausea, and rash. May also cause elevated hepatic transaminase serum concentrations. Monitor hepatic function upon initiation of therapy and periodically. **Comments:** Interacts with propranolol, theophylline, and warfarin. These drug interactions appear to be mediated by the cytochrome P-450 isoenzymes CYP1A2, CYP2C9, and CYP3A4, and result in significant increases in the plasma concentrations of these drugs when used concurrently with zileuton. When concurrent use is required, monitor blood concentrations of these drugs and other hepatically metabolized drugs, and reduce their dosage as indicated. *See* Chapter 6.

Footnotes are on page 558.

TABLE 14-1 continued

DRUG (TRADE AND OTHER NAMES)	INDICATION(S)	USUAL PEDIATRIC DOSAGE AND ADMINISTRATION[a]	DOSAGE FORMS	CONTRAINDICATIONS, ADRs, AND COMMENTS[b]
Zinc Oxide (*Borofax SkinProtectant®, Prevex®, Zinaderm®, Zincofax®*)	**Skin irritation and injury,** minor (including abrasions, burns, chafed skin, and diaper rash)	**Infants, children, and adolescents:** After gently cleansing and thoroughly drying affected skin site(s), apply ointment one to four times daily, as indicated by response. For diaper rash, reapply after each diaper change until redness has resolved.	Ointments, topical: 15%, 20%, 68% (ointment base may contain lanolin, mineral oil, and petrolatum) **Note:** For external use only. Avoid contact with the eyes or other mucous membranes.	**Contraindications:** Hypersensitivity to lanolin. **ADRs:** Generally well tolerated. May cause local skin irritation at application site(s).
	Sunburn, prevention **Note:** Zinc oxide topical ointment is cosmetically less preferred when compared to chemical sunscreens because of its white appearance and difficult removal from sensitive skin sites (e.g., face).	**Infants, children, and adolescents:** Uniformly apply generously to exposed skin site(s). **Note:** Use is generally limited to small specific skin sites, such as the ears and nose.		

TABLE 14-2
Modification of Drug Dosage for Infants, Children, and Adolescents with Renal Dysfunction[a]

DRUG	GENERALLY RECOMMENDED ADJUSTMENTS FOR RENAL DYSFUNCTION[b] Creatinine Clearance (ml/min)			SUPPLEMENTAL DOSE REQUIRED AFTER DIALYSIS[c]
	>50	10–50	<10	
Acyclovir	None	For GFR >26–50 ml/min: Increase dosing interval to 12 hr. For GFR 10–25 ml/min: Increase dosing interval to 24 hr.	Increase dosing interval to 24–48 hr.	HD: Yes
Allopurinol	Give 67%–100% of usual daily dosage.	Give 33%–50% of usual daily dosage.	Give 25% of usual daily dosage.	HD: Yes
Amantadine	None	Increase dosing interval to 48–72 hr.	Increase dosing interval to 7 days.	HD: No PD: No
Amikacin	None	Increase dosing interval to 12–18 hr.	Increase dosing interval to 24–48 hr.	HD: Yes PD: Yes
Aminocaproic Acid	Unknown	Unknown	Give 25% of usual daily dosage as single daily dose.	HD: No PD: No
Amoxicillin	None	Increase dosing interval to 8–12 hr.	Increase dosing interval to 12–16 hr.	HD: Yes PD: No
Ampicillin	None	Increase dosing interval to 6–12 hr.	Increase dosing interval to 12–16 hr.	HD: Yes PD: No
Azathioprine	None	Give 75%–100% of usual daily dosage.	Give 50%–75% of usual daily dosage.	HD: Yes
Aztreonam	None	Give 50%–75% of usual daily dosage.	Give 25%–33% of usual daily dosage.	HD: Yes PD: Yes
Captopril	None	Give 75% of usual daily dosage.	Give 50% of usual daily dosage.	HD: Yes
Cefaclor	None	Give 30%–100% of usual daily dosage divided every 8 hr.	Give 20%–50% of usual daily dosage divided every 8 hr.	HD: Yes
Cefadroxil	None	Increase dosing interval to 12–24 hr.	Increase dosing interval to 24–48 hr.	HD: Yes
Cefamandole	None	Increase dosing interval to 6–8 hr.	Increase dosing interval to 8–12 hr.	HD: Yes
Cefazolin	None	Increase dosing interval to 12–36 hr.	Increase dosing interval to 24–72 hr.	HD: Yes PD: No
Cefixime	None	Give 75%–100% of usual daily dosage.	Give 50% of usual daily dosage.	HD: Yes PD: No
Cefotaxime	None	Increase dosing interval to 8–12 hr.	Increase dosing interval to 12–24 hr.	HD: Yes PD: No
Cefoxitin	None	Increase dosing interval to 8–24 hr.	Increase dosing interval to 24–48 hr.	HD: Yes PD: No
Cefprozil	None	Give 50% of usual daily dosage.	Give 25% of usual daily dosage.	HD: Yes
Ceftazidime	None	Increase dosing interval to 12–24 hr.	Increase dosing interval to 24–48 hr.	HD: Yes
Ceftizoxime	Give 50%–100% of usual daily dosage divided every 8 hr or increase dosing interval to 8–12 hr.	Give 15%–50% of usual daily dosage divided every 8 hr.	Give 3%–15% of usual daily dosage divided every 8 hr.	HD: Yes PD: No

[a] Much of the information presented in this table is based on adult data because of a lack of information on dosing in infants, children, and adolescents with renal dysfunction. Dosage reduction in renal dysfunction can be accomplished by decreasing the dose, increasing the dosing interval, or using a combination of these two methods. Individualize dosage, whenever possible, based on serum concentrations (see Table 14-3). Note that omission of a particular drug from this table does not imply that dosage modification is not required in patients with renal dysfunction. The usual dosages and related information listed for each drug have been derived from several sources, including previous editions of Problems in Pediatric Drug Therapy, current product monographs, the references listed at the end of this chapter, and clinical experience. For additional references to original or to earlier citations, please refer to the previous editions of this text.

[b] These adjustments may vary for individual pediatric patients because of possible significant variability in relevant, individual, pharmacotherapeutic factors (e.g., concomitant medical disorders and drug therapy). Thus, therapeutic drug monitoring (see Table 14-3), when possible, and attention to patient response are necessary to help ensure optimal drug therapy.

[c] CrCl = creatinine clearance; GFR = glomerular filtration rate; HD = hemodialysis; PD = peritoneal dialysis.

TABLE 14-2 continued

DRUG	GENERALLY RECOMMENDED ADJUSTMENTS FOR RENAL DYSFUNCTION[b] Creatinine Clearance (ml/min)			SUPPLEMENTAL DOSE REQUIRED AFTER DIALYSIS[c]
	>50	10–50	<10	
Cefuroxime	None	None for >30 ml/min; increase dosing interval to 12–24 hr for 10–30 ml/min.	Increase dosing interval to 24 hr.	HD: Yes
Cephalexin	None	Increase dosing interval to 6–8 hr.	Increase dosing interval to 8–12 hr.	HD: Yes
Cephalothin	None	None	Increase dosing interval to 8–12 hr.	HD: Yes PD: Yes
Cimetidine	None	Give 50% of usual daily dosage.	Give 25% of usual daily dosage.	HD: No PD: No
Clarithromycin	None	None	For GFR <10 ml/min: Increase dosing interval to every 24 hr.	Unknown
Digoxin	Loading and maintenance dosage: None	Loading dose: None Maintenance dose: Give 25%–75% of usual daily dosage.	Loading dose: Give 50% of usual loading dose. Maintenance dose: Give 10%–25% of usual daily dosage.	HD: No PD: No
Disopyramide	None	Increase dosing interval to 8 hr for 30–40 ml/min; increase dosing interval to 12 hr for 15–30 ml/min; increase dosing interval to 24–40 hr for 10–15 ml/min.	Increase dosing interval to 24–40 hr.	HD: No PD: No
Enalapril	None	None for 30–50 ml/min; give 50%–75% of usual daily dosage for 10–30 ml/min.	Give 50% of usual daily dosage.	HD: Yes
Ethambutol	None	Increase dosing interval to 24–36 hr.	Increase dosing interval to 48 hr.	HD: Yes PD: Yes
Famotidine	None	Give 50%–100% of usual daily dosage.	Increase dosing interval to 48 hr.	Unknown
Fluconazole	None	Give 50% of usual daily dosage for CrCl 20–50 ml/min; give 25% of usual daily dosage for CrCl 10–20 ml/min.	Give 25% of usual daily dosage.	HD: Yes
Flucytosine	None	None for CrCl 40–50 ml/min/1.73 m^2; increase dosing interval to 12 hr for CrCl 20–40 ml/min/1.73 m^2; increase dosing interval to 24 hr for CrCl 10–20 ml/min/1.73 m^2.	Increase dosing interval to 24–48 hr.	HD: Yes PD: Yes
Gabapentin	Give 67%–100% of usual daily dosage.	Give 33% of usual daily dosage.	Give 12.5% of usual daily dosage.	HD: Yes
Ganciclovir	50% of usual daily dosage for 50–79 ml/min/1.73 m^2.	Give 50% of usual daily dosage every 24 hr for 25–49 ml/min/1.73 m^2; give 25% of usual daily dosage every 24 hr for 10–25 ml/min/1.73 m^2.	Give 25% of usual daily dosage every 24 hr for <10 ml/min/1.73 m^2.	HD: Yes
Gentamicin	None or increase dosing interval to 12 hr.	Increase dosing interval to 12–24 hr.	Increase dosing interval to 24–48 hr.	HD: Yes PD: Yes
Imipenem + Cilastatin	None	Give 50% of usual daily dosage.	Give 25% of usual daily dosage.	HD: Yes
Lamivudine	None	Give 33% of usual daily dosage.	Give 17% of usual daily dosage.	HD: No
Lepirudin	Give 50%–100% of standard infusion.	Give 15%–30% of standard infusion.	Do not use.	HD: Yes
Lisinopril	None	Give 50% of usual daily dosage.	Give 25% of usual daily dosage.	HD: Yes PD: Yes
Loracarbef	None	Give 50% of usual daily dosage.	Increase dosing interval to every 3–5 days.	HD: Yes
Loratadine	None	Increase dosing interval to 48 hr for CrCl <30 ml/min.	Increase dosing interval to 48 hr.	HD: No
Meperidine	None	Give 75% of usual dosage.	Give 50% of usual dosage.	HD: No

CHAPTER 14: DRUG DOSING FOR INFANTS, CHILDREN, AND ADOLESCENTS

TABLE 14-2 continued

DRUG	GENERALLY RECOMMENDED ADJUSTMENTS FOR RENAL DYSFUNCTION[b] Creatinine Clearance (ml/min)			SUPPLEMENTAL DOSE REQUIRED AFTER DIALYSIS[c]
	>50	10–50	<10	
Methotrexate	None	Give 50%–75% of usual daily dosage.	Give 50% of usual daily dosage or avoid use.	HD: No PD: No
Methyldopa	Use 6–8-hr dosing interval.	Increase dosing interval to 8–18 hr.	Increase dosing interval to 12–24 hr.	HD: Yes PD: No
Metoclopramide	None	Give 75% of usual daily dosage.	Give 50% of usual daily dosage.	HD: No PD: No
Mexiletine	None	None	Give 50%–75% of usual daily dosage.	HD: No PD: No
Mezlocillin	None	Increase dosing interval to 6–8 hr.	Increase dosing interval to 8 hr.	HD: No PD: No
Midazolam	None	None	Give 50% of usual dose.	Unknown
Milrinone	None	Give 50%–75% of usual dose.	Give 40% of usual dose.	Unknown
Morphine	None	Give 40%–75% of usual dose and titrate subsequent dosing to desired effect, avoiding adverse reactions.	Give 50% of usual dose and titrate subsequent dosing to desired effect, avoiding adverse reactions.	HD: No
Nadolol	None	Give 50% of usual daily dosage.	Give 25% of usual daily dosage.	HD: Yes PD: No
Naproxen/Naproxen Sodium	None	None for 20–50 ml/min; do not use for <20 ml/min.	Do not use.	HD: No PD: No
Neostigmine	None	Give 50% of usual daily dosage.	Give 25% of usual daily dosage.	Unknown
Netilmicin	Use 8–12-hr dosing interval.	Increase dosing interval to 12 hr.	Increase dosing interval to 24–48 hr.	HD: Yes PD: Yes
Nitrofurantoin	None	Do not use.	Do not use.	Unknown
Penicillin G	Use 4–8-hr dosing interval.	Increase dosing interval to 8–12 hr.	Increase dosing interval to 12–16 hr.	HD: Yes PD: No
Pentamidine Isethionate	Use 24-hr dosing interval.	Increase dosing interval to 24 hr for CrCl 36–50 ml/min; increase dosing interval to 24–48 hr for CrCl 10–35 ml/min.	Increase dosing interval to 24–48 hr.	HD: No
Phenobarbital	None	None	Increase dosing interval to 12–16 hr.	HD: Yes PD: Yes
Piperacillin	None	Increase dosing interval to 6–8 hr.	Increase dosing interval to 8 hr.	HD: Yes PD: No
Primidone	Use 8-hr dosing interval.	Increase dosing interval to 8–12 hr.	Increase dosing interval to 12–24 hr.	HD: Yes
Probenecid	None	None for GFR ≥30 ml/min; do not use if GFR <30 ml/min.	Do not use.	Unknown
Procainamide	None	Increase dosing interval to 6–12 or individualize dosing based on serum concentrations.	Increase dosing interval to 8–24 hr or individualize dosing based on serum concentrations.	HD: Yes
Propylthiouracil	None	Give 75% of usual daily dosage.	Give 50% of usual daily dosage.	Unknown
Quinidine	None	None	Give 75% of usual daily dosage.	HD: Yes
Quinine	Use 8-hr dosing interval.	Increase dosing interval to 8–12 hr.	Increase dosing interval to 24 hr.	HD: Yes
Ranitidine	None	None for CrCl ≥30 ml/min; give 50% of usual daily dosage for CrCl 10–29 ml/min.	Give 25%–50% of usual daily dosage.	HD: Yes
Spironolactone	None	None	Do not use.	Unknown

Footnotes are on page 757.

TABLE 14-2 continued

DRUG	GENERALLY RECOMMENDED ADJUSTMENTS FOR RENAL DYSFUNCTION[b] Creatinine Clearance (ml/min)			SUPPLEMENTAL DOSE REQUIRED AFTER DIALYSIS[c]
	>50	10–50	<10	
Stavudine	Use low end of dosage range.	Decrease dosage by 50% for CrCl between 26 and 50 ml/min and, in addition, increase dosing interval to 24 hr for CrCl between 10 and 25 ml/min.	Do not use.	Unknown
Streptomycin	Increase dosing interval to 12–24 hr.	Increase dosing interval to 24–72 hr.	Increase dosing interval to 72–96 hr.	HD: Yes
Sulfamethoxazole	Use 12-hr dosing interval.	Increase dosing interval to 12–24 hr.	Increase dosing interval to 24 hr.	HD: Yes
Sulfisoxazole	Use 6-hr dosing interval.	Increase dosing interval to 8–12 hr.	Increase dosing interval to 12–24 hr.	HD: Yes
Tetracycline	Use 8–12-hr dosing interval.	Increase dosing interval to 12–24 hr.	Do not use.	HD: No PD: No
Ticarcillin and Clavulanate	Use 4–6-hr dosing interval for CrCl >60 ml/min; give 66% of usual daily dosage for CrCl 51–60 ml/min.	Give 66% of usual daily dosage for CrCl 30–50 ml/min; give 66% of usual daily dosage and increase dosing interval to 8 hr for CrCl 20–30 ml/min.	Give 66% of usual daily dosage and increase dosing interval to 12 hr.	HD: Yes PD: Yes
Tobramycin	None for CrCl ≥70 ml/min; increase dosing interval to 12 hr for CrCl 51–69 ml/min.	Increase dosing interval to 12 hr for CrCl 40–50 ml/min; increase dosing interval to 18 hr for CrCl 20–39 ml/min; increase dosing interval to 24 hr for CrCl 10–19 ml/min.	Increase dosing interval to 36 hr or longer, use serum concentration as a guide.	HD: Yes PD: Yes
Tranexamic Acid	Give 50% of usual daily dosage.	Give 25% of usual daily dosage.	Give 10% of usual daily dosage.	Unknown
Triamterene	None	None	Do not use.	Unknown
Trimethoprim	Use 12-hr dosing interval.	Use 12-hr dosing interval for CrCl 30–50 ml/min; increase dosing interval to 12–24 hr for CrCl 10–30 ml/min.	Increase dosing interval to 24 hr.	HD: Yes
Trimethoprim + Sulfamethoxazole	None	None for CrCl >30 ml/min; give 50% of usual daily dosage for CrCl 10–≤30.	Increase dosing interval to 24–48 hr.	HD: Yes
Tubocurarine	Give 75% of usual daily dosage.	Give 50% of usual daily dosage.	Do not use.	Unknown
Vancomycin	Increase dosing interval to 24–72 hr or individualize dosing based on serum concentrations.	Individualize dosing based on serum concentrations.	Individualize dosing based on serum concentrations.	HD: No PD: No
Venlafaxine	None	Give 25%–50% of usual daily dosage.	Do not use.	HD: No[d]
Zalcitabine	None	Give 67% of usual daily dosage divided every 12 hr.	Give 33% of usual daily dosage once every 24 hr.	Unknown

[d] Reduce total daily dosage by 50% and administer after completion of dialysis.

TABLE 14-3
Guidelines for Therapeutic Drug Monitoring[a]

DRUG	OPTIMAL SAMPLING TIME[b]	OPTIMAL DRUG SERUM CONCENTRATION RANGE
Amikacin	Peak	20–30 mg/liter (34–51 μmol/liter)
	Trough	<8 mg/liter (<13.7 μmol/liter)
Aminocaproic Acid	Trough	130 mg/liter
Amiodarone	Trough	0.5–2.5 mg/liter (1.5–4 μmol/liter)
Amitriptyline[c]	Trough, 12 hr after last dose	430–900 nmol/liter (110–250 ng/ml) (parent drug + demethylated metabolite [nortriptyline])
Aspirin (Salicylates)	Trough	Juvenile rheumatoid arthritis: 1.2–2.2 mmol/liter (150–300 mg/liter) Kawasaki disease and pericarditis: <2.2 mmol/liter (<300 mg/liter)
Carbamazepine[c]	Trough	17–43 μmol/liter (4–10 μg/ml)
Chloramphenicol	Peak	10–20 mg/liter (31–62 μmol/liter)
	Trough	2–10 mg/liter (6–31 μmol/liter)
Cyclosporine[d]	Trough	Bone marrow transplant: 75–200 μg/liter Heart transplant: 300–400 μg/liter Kidney transplant: 175–200 μg/liter Liver transplant: 100–400 μg/liter
Digoxin	Trough or at least 6 hr after oral dose	1–2.5 nmol/liter (0.8–2.0 ng/ml)
Disopyramide	Trough	6–18 μmol/liter (2–8 mg/liter)
Ethosuximide	Trough	280–710 μmol/liter (40–100 μg/ml)
Flecainide	Trough	0.2–1 mg/liter
Flucytosine	Peak, 2 hr after oral dose or 1 hr after IV dose	50–100 mg/liter
Gentamicin	Peak	6–12 mg/liter (12.5–25 μmol/liter)
	Trough	<2 mg/liter (<4.2 μmol/liter)
Lidocaine	At least 2 hr after loading dose	6–21 μmol/liter (1.5–5 μg/ml)
Lithium	Trough 12 hr after last dose	0.5–1.2 mmol/liter (0.5–1.2 mEq/liter)
Mexiletine	Trough	0.5–2 mg/liter
Muromonab-CD3	Trough	≥800 ng/ml
Netilmicin	Peak	5–12 mg/liter
	Trough	<2 mg/liter
Nortriptyline[c]	Trough, 12 hr after last dose	170–495 nmol/liter (50–150 ng/ml)
Phenobarbital	Trough	43–172 μmol/liter (10–40 μg/ml)
Phenytoin (total)	Trough	40–80 μmol/liter (10–20 μg/ml)

TABLE 14-3 continued

DRUG	OPTIMAL SAMPLING TIME[b]	OPTIMAL DRUG SERUM CONCENTRATION RANGE
Phenytoin (unbound)	Trough	4–8 μmol/liter (1–2 μg/ml)
Primidone	Trough	18–55 μmol/liter (4–12 μg/ml)
Procainamide[e]	Trough or at least 2 hr after start of continuous IV infusion	17–43 μmol/liter (4–10 μg/ml)
Propafenone	Trough	0.5–2 mg/liter
Propranolol	Trough	190–770 nmol/liter (50–200 ng/ml)
Quinidine	Trough	6–15 μmol/liter (2–5 μg/ml)
Streptomycin	Peak	5–20 mg/liter
	Trough	<5 mg/liter
Tacrolimus[f]	Trough, 12 hr after last dose	5–20 μg/liter
Terbutaline[c]	Trough	0.5–4.1 ng/ml
Theophylline	Trough or at anytime during continuous IV infusion	55–110 μmol/liter (10–20 μg/ml)
Tobramycin	Peak	5–12 mg/liter (12.8–21.8 μmol/liter)
	Trough	<2 mg/liter (<4.3 μmol/liter)
Valproic Acid	Trough	280–700 μmol/liter (40–100 μg/ml)
Vancomycin	Peak	20–40 mg/liter
	Trough	5–10 mg/liter
Verapamil	Trough	0.08–0.3 μg/ml

[a] For the purposes of these guidelines, a peak drug serum concentration is defined as a steady-state drug serum concentration measured in a blood sample obtained 30 min after completion of infusion of the IV dose unless otherwise stated. A trough drug serum concentration is defined as a steady-state drug serum concentration measured in a blood sample obtained just prior to the next dose of the drug unless otherwise stated. *See* Chapter 10 for additional related discussion.

[b] Note: For suspected toxicity or overdosage, sample may be obtained at any time.

[c] Therapeutic drug monitoring may be used to assist in the determination of patient compliance and toxicity. However, individual patient response is generally a better guide to dosage modification for this drug.

[d] Optimal drug serum concentration range is dependent upon the clinical status of the patient, type of organ/tissue transplant performed, and time elapsed since the transplantation was performed.

[e] N-Acetylprocainamide (NAPA) concentrations should be measured concurrently. Optimal NAPA serum concentration range = 22–27 μmol/liter.

[f] Standardization of assay methodology for tacrolimus has not yet occurred. Both microparticle enzyme immunoassay (MEIA) and enzyme-linked immunosorbent assay (ELISA) have been used and both utilize the same monoclonal antibody for tacrolimus. Note that results with ELISA during the first week post-transplantation are quite variable and that the levels provided here refer to data obtained from 2 to 52 weeks post-transplantation.

Frequently Used Conversion Formulas

Metric and SI unit conversion formulas:

To determine the conversion factor (CF):

$$CF = \frac{1000}{\text{molecular weight}}$$

To convert from metric to SI units:

$$(\mu g/ml) \times CF = \mu mol/liter$$

To convert from SI units to metric:

$$\frac{(\mu mol/liter)}{CF} = \mu g/ml$$

Milliequivalents (mEq) formula:

$$mEq = \frac{\text{milligrams}}{\text{equivalent weight}}$$

$$\text{Equivalent weight} = \frac{\text{gram molecular weight}}{\text{valence}}$$

Milliequivalents (mEq) per liter formula:

$$\frac{mEq}{liter} = \frac{\text{Weight of salt (grams)} \times \text{valence of ion} \times 1000}{\text{gram molecular weight of salt}}$$

References[9]

Abacavir: New preparation. Risks limit the value. (2000). *Prescrire International, 9*(47), 67–69.

ad-Dab'bagh, Y., Greenfield, B., Milne-Smith, J., et al. (2000). Inpatient treatment of severe disruptive behaviour disorders with risperidone and milieu therapy. *Canadian Journal of Psychiatry, 45*(4), 376–382.

Advisory Committee on Immunization Practices. (2000). Use of anthrax vaccine in the United States. *Morbidity and Mortality Weekly Report, 49*(RR15), 1–20.

Advisory Committee on Immunization Practices. (2001). Vaccinia (smallpox) vaccine recommendations of the Advisory Committee on Immunization practices (ACIP), 2001. *Morbidity and Mortality Weekly Reports, 50*(RR 10), 1–25.

Ahdoot, J., Galindo, A., Alejos, J. C., et al. (2000). Use of OKT3 for acute myocarditis in infants and children. *Journal of Heart and Lung Transplantation, 19*(11), 1118–1121.

Aldaz, A., Ortega, A., Idoate, A., et al. (2000). Effects of hepatic function on vancomycin pharmacokinetics in patients with cancer. *Therapeutic Drug Monitoring, 22*(3), 250–257.

Ambrosini, P. J. (2000). A review of pharmacotherapy of major depression in children and adolescents. *Psychiatric Services, 51*(5), 627–633.

Anderson, J. R., Poklis, A., McQueen, R. C., et al. (1983). Effects of hemodialysis on theophylline kinetics. *Journal of Clinical Pharmacology, 23*, 428–432.

Aoki, F. Y., & Sitar, D. S. (1988). Clinical pharmacokinetics of amantadine hydrochloride. *Clinical Pharmacokinetics, 14*, 35–51.

Appleton, R., Fichtner, K., LaMoreaux, L., et al. (1999). Gabapentin as add-on therapy in children with refractory partial seizures: A 12-week, multicentre, double blind, placebo-controlled study. Gabapentin Paediatric Study Group. *Epilepsia, 40*(8), 1147–1154.

Are rofecoxib and celecoxib safer NSAIDs? (2000). *Drug and Therapeutics Bulletin, 38*(11), 81–86.

Arrieta, A. (1997). Use of meropenem in the treatment of serious infections in children: Review of the current literature. *Clinical Infectious Diseases, 24*(Suppl 2), S207–S212.

Arrowsmith, J., & Campbell, C. (2000). A comparison of local anaesthetics for venepuncture [sic]. *Archives of Disease in Childhood, 82*(4), 309–310.

Asconape, J., Diedrich, A., & DellaBadia, J. (2000). Myoclonus associated with the use of gabapentin. *Epilepsia, 41*(4), 479–481.

Aviner, S., Levy, Y., Yaniv, I., et al. (1999). Anaphylactoid reaction to imiglucerase, but not to alglucerase, in a type I Gaucher patient. *Blood Cells, Molecules, and Diseases, 25*(2), 92–94.

Aweeks, F. T., Gottwald, M. D., Gambertoglio, J. G., et al. (1999). Pharmacokinetics of fosphen-

---

9. The data and suggested guidelines for providing appropriate drug dosages for infants, children, and adolescents contained in this chapter have been derived from several sources. These sources include the three previous editions of *Problems in Pediatric Drug Therapy*, current product monographs (official FDA and HPB drug product labeling), the listed references, other textbooks written by the editors of this reference text, and the authors' clinical experience. Thus, the listed references are meant to provide the reader with some benchmarks only and are not intended to compose an exhaustive reference list. For additional references to original or earlier citations, please refer to the previous editions of this text.

ytoin in patients with hepatic or renal disease. *Epilepsia, 40*(6), 777–782.

Babl, F. E., Cooper, E. R., Damon, B., et al. (2000). HIV postexposure prophylaxis for children and adolescents. *Amercian Journal of Emergency Medicine, 18*(3), 282–287.

Bach, J. F., & Dardenna, M. (1971). The metabolism of azathioprine in renal failure. *Transplantation, 12*, 253–259.

Bailey, J. M., Miller, B. E., Lu, W., et al. (1999). The pharmacokinetics of milrinone in pediatric patients after cardiac surgery. *Anesthesiology, 90*(4), 1012–1018.

Bailey, R. R., Gower, P. E., & Dash, C. H. (1970). The effect of impairment of renal function and hemodialysis on serum and urine levels of cephalexin. *Postgraduate Medical Journal, 46*(Suppl), 60–64.

Bairaktari, E. T., Tzallas, C. S., Tsimihodimos, V. K., et al. (1999). Comparison of the efficacy of atorvastatin and micronized fenofibrate in the treatment of mixed hyperlipidemia. *Journal of Cardiovascular Risk, 6*(2), 113–116.

Baker, K. A., & Ryan, M. E. (1999). RSV infection in infants and young children. What's new in diagnosis, treatment, and prevention? *Postgraduate Medicine, 106*(7), 107–108.

Bakker, A., van Dyck, R., Spinhoven, P., et al. (1999). Paroxetine, clomipramine, and cognitive therapy in the treatment of panic disorder. *Journal of Clinical Psychiatry, 60*(12), 831–838.

Baldree, L. A., & Stapleton, F. B. (1990). Uric acid metabolism in children. *Pediatric Clinics of North America, 37*, 391–418.

Baldwin, D., Bobes, J., Stein, D. J., et al. (1999). Paroxetine in social phobia/social anxiety disorder. Randomised, double-blind, placebo-controlled study. Paroxetine Study Group. *British Journal of Psychiatry, 175*, 120–126.

Balslev, T., Uldall, P., & Buchholt, J. (2000). Provocation of non-convulsive status epilepticus by tiagabine in three adolescent patients. *European Journal of Paediatric Neurology, 4*(4), 169–170.

Banerjee, D., & Stableforth, D. (2000). The treatment of respiratory pseudomonas infection in cystic fibrosis: What drug and which way? *Drugs, 60*(5), 1053–1064.

Barrett, J. F. (2000). SMI's 2nd Annual Superbugs and Superdrugs Conference: Innovations in anti-infectives. *Expert Opinion on Investigational Drugs, 9*(7), 1665–1672.

Bartoloni, A., Strohmeyer, M., Corti, G., et al. (1999). Multicenter randomized trial comparing meropenem (1.5 g daily) and imipenem/cilastatin (2 g daily) in the hospital treatment of community-acquired pneumonia. *Drugs, Experimental and Clinical Research, 25*(6), 243–252.

Batts, D. H. (2000). Linezolid—A new option for treating gram-positive infections. *Oncology, 14*(8, Suppl 6), 23–29.

Beckman, R. A., Siden, R., Yanik, G. A., et al. (2000). Continuous octreotide infusion for the treatment of secretory diarrhea caused by acute intestinal graft-versus-host disease in a child. *Journal of Pediatric Hematology and Oncology, 22*(4), 344–350.

Benedetti, M. S. (2000). Enzyme induction and inhibition by new antiepileptic drugs: A review of human studies. *Fundamental and Clinical Pharmacology, 14*(4), 301–319.

Benson, J. O., McGhee, K., Coplan, P., et al. (2000). Fat redistribution in indinavir-treated patients with HIV infection: A review of postmarketing cases. *Journal of Acquired Immune Deficiency Syndromes, 25*(2), 130–139.

Berard, J. L., Velez, R. L., Freeman, R. B., et al. (1999). A review of interleukin-2 receptor antagonists in solid organ transplantation. *Pharmacotherapy, 19*(10), 1127–1137.

Berardi, R. R., Cornish, L. A., & Hyneck, M. L. (1986). Metoclopramide removal during continuous ambulatory peritoneal dialysis. *Drug Intelligence and Clinical Pharmacy, 20*, 154–155.

Berger, W. E., Fineman, S. M., Lieberman, P., et al. (1999). Double-blind trials of azelastine nasal spray monotherapy versus combination therapy with loratadine tablets and beclomethasone nasal spray in patients with seasonal allergic rhinitis. Rhinitis Study Groups. *Annals of Allergy, Asthma, and Immunology, 82*(6), 535–541.

Berkowitz, R. J., Possidente, C. J., McPherson, B. R., et al. (2000). Anaphylactoid reaction to muromonab-CD3 in a pediatric renal transplant recipient. *Pharmacotherapy, 20*(1), 100–104.

Berry, P. L., & Belsha, C. W. (1990). Hyponatremia. *Pediatric Clinics of North America, 37*, 351–363.

Best Pharmaceuticals for Children Act, House of Representatives, S. 1789, 107th Congress of the United States of America. (2001).

Beydoun, A., Sachdeo, R. C., Rosenfeld, W. E., et al. (2000). *Neurology, 54*(12), 2245–2251.

Bhatt-Mehta, V., & Rosen, D. A. (1991). Management of acute pain in children. *Clinical Pharmacy, 10*, 667–685.

Bialer, M., Johannessen, S. I., Kupferberg, H. J., et al. (2001). Progress report on new antiepileptic drugs: A summary of the Fifth Eilat Conference (EILAT V). *Epilepsy Research, 43*(1), 11–58.

Biban, P., Baraldi, E., Pettenazzo, A., et al. (1993). Adverse effect of chloral hydrate in two young children with obstructive sleep apnea. *Pediatrics, 92*, 461–462.

Bleck, T. P. (1999). Management approaches to prolonged seizures and status epilepticus. *Epilepsia, 40*(Suppl 1), S59–S63; S64–S66.

Bloch, R., Szwed, J. J., Sloan, R. S., et al. (1977). Pharmacokinetics of cefaclor in normal subjects and patients with chronic renal failure. *Antimicrobial Agents and Chemotherapy, 12*, 730–732.

Bloom, B. J. (2000). Development of diabetes mellitus during etanercept therapy in a child with systemic-onset juvenile rheumatoid arthritis. *Arthritis and Rheumatism, 43*(11), 2606–2608.

Blum, M. R., Liao, S. H. T., & DeMiranda, P. (1982). Overview of acyclovir pharmacokinetic disposition in adults and children. *American Journal of Medicine, 73*, 186–196.

Borusiak, P., Korn-Merker, E., Holert, N., et al. (1998). Hyponatremia induced by oxcarbazepine in children. *Epilepsy Research, 30*(3), 241–246.

Bosso, J. A., & Black, P. G. (1991). The use of aztreonam in pediatric patients: A review. *Pharmacotherapy, 11*, 20–25.

Bradley, J. S. (1998). Selecting therapy for serious infections in children: Maximizing safety and efficacy. *Diagnostic Microbiology and Infectious Disease, 31*(2), 405–410.

Breedveld, F. C., & Dayer, J. M. (2000). Leflunomide: Mode of action in the treatment of rheumatoid arthritis. *Annals of the Rheumatic Diseases, 59*(11), 841–849.

Brem, A. S. (1990). Disorders of potassium homeostasis. *Pediatric Clinics of North America, 37*, 419–427.

Brogard, J. M., Pinget, M., Brandt, C., et al. (1977). Pharmacokinetics of cefazolin in patients with renal failure: Special reference to hemodialysis. *Journal of Clinical Pharmacology, 17*, 225.

Brooks, P. M., & Day, R. O. (2000). COX–2 inhibitors. *Medical Journal of Australia, 173*(8), 433–436.

Bryden, K. E., Carrey, N. J., & Kutcher, S. P. (2001). Update and recommendations for the use of antipsychotics in early-onset psychoses. *Journal of Child and Adolescent Psychopharmacology, 11*(2), 113–130.

Bryson, H. M., Palmer, K. J., Langtry, H. D., et al. (1993). Propafenone. A reappraisal of its pharmacology, pharmacokinetics and therapeutic use in cardiac arrhythmias. *Drugs, 45*, 85–130.

Bryson, J. C., Pritchard, J. F., Shurin, S., et al. (1991). Efficacy, pharmacokinetics, and safety of ondansetron in pediatric chemotherapy patients. *Clinical Pharmacology and Therapeutics, 49*, 161.

Buitelaar, J. K. (2000). Open-label treatment with risperidone of 26 psychiatrically-hospitalized children and adolescents with mixed diagnoses and aggressive behavior. *Journal of Child and Adolescent Psychopharmacology, 10*(1), 19–26.

Buitelaar, J. K., van der Gaag, R. J., Cohen-Kettenis, P., et al. (2001). A randomized controlled trial of risperidone in the treatment of aggression in hospitalized adolescents with subaverage cognitive abilities. *Journal of Clinical Psychiatry, 62*(4), 239–248.

Bunchman, T. E., Lynch, R. E., & Wood, E. G. (1992). Intravenously administered labetalol for treatment of hypertension in children. *The Journal of Pediatrics, 120*, 140–144.

Bunke, C. M., Aronoff, G. R., Brier, M. E., et al. (1983). Cefazolin and cephalexin kinetics in continuous ambulatory peritoneal dialysis. *Clinical Pharmacology and Therapeutics, 33*, 66–72.

Burgess, E. D., & Duff, H. J. (1989). Hemodialysis removal of propafenone. *Pharmacotherapy, 9*, 331–333.

Burk, M., & Peters, U. (1983). Disopyramide kinetics in renal impairment. Determinants of interindividual variability. *Clinical Pharmacology and Therapeutics, 34*, 331–334.

Bush, K., & Macielag, M. (2000). New approaches in the treatment of bacterial infections. *Current Opinion in Chemical Biology, 4*(4), 433–439.

Canani, R. B., Spagnuolo, M. I., Cirillo, P., et al. (1999). Ritonavir combination therapy restores intestinal function in children with advanced HIV disease. *Journal of Acquired Immune Deficiency Syndromes, 21*(4), 307–312.

Cannon, C. P. (1999). Low molecular weight heparin in acute coronary syndromes. *Current Cardiology Reports, 1*(3), 206–211.

Cass, L. M., Efthymiopoulos, C., & Bye, A. (1999). Pharmacokinetics of zanamivir after intravenous, oral, inhaled or intranasal administration to healthy volunteers. *Clinical Pharmacokinetics, 36*(Suppl 1), 1–11.

Cassidy, J. T. (1999). Medical management of children with juvenile rheumatoid arthritis. *Drugs, 58*(5), 831–850.

Chakrabarti, P., Wong, H. Y., Scantlebury, V. P., et al. (2000). Outcome after steroid withdrawal in pediatric renal transplant patients receiving tacrolimus-based immunosuppression. *Transplantation, 70*(5), 760–764.

Cheam, E. W., & Chui, P. T. (2000). Randomised double-blind comparison of fentanyl, mivacurium or placebo to facilitate laryngeal mask airway insertion. *Anaesthesia, 55*(4), 323–326.

Chen, H. S., Hwu, C. M., Shih, K. C., et al. (1999). Octreotide effect on hypersecretion of growth hormone in a patient with fibrous dysplasia: A case report. *Chung Hua I Hsueh Tsa Chih (Chinese Medical Journal), 62*(8), 554–559.

Chevalier, P., Rey, J., Pasquier, O., et al. (2000). Pharmacokinetics of quinupristin/dalfopristin in patients with severe chronic renal insufficiency. *Clinical Pharmacokinetics, 39*(1), 77–84.

Chittick, G. E., Gillotin, C., McDowell, J. A., et al. (1999). Abacavir: Absolute bioavailability, bioequivalence of three oral formulations, and effect of food. *Pharmacotherapy, 19*(8), 932–942.

Choy, L., Collier, J., & Watson, A. R. (1999). Comparison of lignocaine–prilocaine cream and amethocaine gel for local analgesia before venepuncture [sic] in children. *Acta Paediatrica, 88*(9), 961–964.

Chu, C. C., Lin, S. M., New, S. H., et al. (2000). Effect of milrinone on postbypass pulmonary hypertension in children after tetralogy of Fallot repair. *Chung Hua I Hsueh Tsa Chih (Chinese Medical Journal), 63*(4), 294–300.

Clay, P. G., Rathbun, R. C., & Slater, L. N. (2000). Management protocol for abacavir-related hypersensitivity reaction. *Annals of Pharmacotherapy, 34*(2), 247–249.

Clemett, D., & Markham, A. (2000). Linezolid. *Drugs, 59*(4), 815–827.

Clotet, B. (1999). Efavirenz: Resistance and cross-resistance. *International Journal of Clinical Practice, 103*(Suppl), 21–25.

Coker, S. B. (1992). Postneonatal vitamin B_6-dependent epilepsy. *Pediatrics, 90,* 221–223.

Compendium of pharmaceuticals and specialties, 35th ed., 2000, L. Welbanks, Ed., Ottawa: Canadian Pharmacists Association.

Comstock, T. J., Sica, D. A., Harford, A., et al. (1989). Ranitidine bioavailability and disposition kinetics in patients undergoing chronic hemodialysis. *Nephron, 52,* 15–19.

Condra, J. H., Petropoulos, C. J., Ziermann, R., et al. (2000). Drug resistance and predicted virologic responses to human immunodeficiency virus type 1 protease inhibitor therapy. *Journal of Infectious Diseases, 182*(3), 758–765.

Conway, B., & Shafran, S. D. (2000). Pharmacology and clinical experience with amprenavir. *Expert Opinion on Investigational Drugs, 9*(2), 371–382.

Couper, R.T. (2000). Methaemoglobinaemia secondary to topical lignocaine/prilocaine in a circumcised neonate. *Journal of Paediatrics and Child Health, 36*(4), 406–407.

Covington, T. R. (1990). Management of head lice infestations. *Drug Newsletter: Facts and Comparisons, 9,* 65–67.

Craig, W. A. (1997). The pharmacology of meropenem, a new carbapenem antibiotic. *Clinical Infectious Diseases, 24*(Suppl 2), S266–S275.

Cutter, R. E., Blair, A. D., & Kelly, M. R. (1978). Flucytosine kinetics in subjects with normal and impaired renal function. *Clinical Pharmacology and Therapeutics, 24,* 333–342.

Dambrin, C., Klupp, J., & Morris, R. E. (2000). Pharmacodynamics of immunosuppressive drugs. *Current Opinion in Immunology, 12*(5), 557–562.

Datta, P. K., & Crawford, P. M. (2000). Refractory epilepsy: Treatment with new antiepileptic drugs. *Seizure, 9*(1), 51–57.

Debruyne, D., & Ryckelynick, J. P. (1988). Pharmacokinetics of zidovudine in a patient on maintenance hemodialysis. *New England Journal of Medicine, 319,* 1606–1607.

Deehan, S., Henderson, D., & Stewart, K. (2000). Intubation conditions and postoperative myalgia in outpatient dental surgery: A comparison of succinylcholine with mivacurium. *Anaesthesia and Intensive Care, 28*(2), 146–150.

de la Serna, G., & Cadarso, C. (1999). Fenofibrate decreased plasma fibrinogen, improves lipid profile, and reduces uricemia. *Clinical Pharmacology and Therapeutics, 66*(2), 166–172.

DeToledo, J. C., & Ramsay, R. E. (2000). Fosphenytoin and phenytoin in patients with status epilepticus: Improved tolerability versus increased costs. *Drug Safety, 22*(6), 459–466.

Diekema, D. I., & Jones, R. N. (2000). Oxazolidinones: A review. *Drugs, 59*(1), 7–16.

Dix, D., Andrew, M., Marzinotto, V., et al. (2000). The use of low molecular weight heparin in pediatric patients: A prospective cohort study. *The Journal of Pediatrics, 136*(4), 439–445.

Doluisio, J. T. (1982). Clinical pharmacokinetics of cefotaxime in patients with normal and reduced renal function. *Review of Infectious Diseases, 4*(Suppl), S333–S345.

Drimmie, F. M., MacLennan, A. C., Nicoll, J. A., et al. (2000). Gigantism due to growth hormone excess in a boy with optic glioma. *Clinical Endocrinology, 53*(4), 535–538.

Dumon, C., Solas, C., Thuret, I., et al. (2000). Relationship between efficacy, tolerance, and plasma drug concentration of ritonavir in children with advanced HIV infection. *Therapeutic Drug Monitoring, 22*(4), 402–408.

Emery, P. (2000). Leflunomide: A new DMARD for rheumatoid arthritis. *Hospital Medicine, 61*(5), 344–347.

Emery, P., Breedveld, F. C., Lemmel, E. M., et al. (2000). A comparison of the efficacy and safety of leflunomide and methotrexate for the treatment of rheumatoid arthritis. *Rheumatology, 39*(6), 655–665.

Eron, J. J., Murphy, R. L., Peterson, D., et al. (2000). A comparison of stavudine, didanosine and indinavir with zidovudine, lamivudine and indinavir for the initial treatment of HIV-1 infected individuals: Selection of thymidine analog regimen therapy (START II). *AIDS, 14*(11), 1601–1610.

Espinos, J. J., Senosiain, R., Aura, M., et al. (1999). Safety and effectiveness of hormonal postcoital contraception: A prospective study. *European Journal of Contraception and Reproductive Health Care, 4*(1), 27–33.

Evans, C. L., Ha, Y., Saisch, S., et al. (1998). *European Journal of Child and Adolescent Psychiatry, 7*(3), 166–167.

Feingold, A. R., Rutstein, R. M., Meislich, D., et al. (2000). Protease inhibitor therapy in HIV-infected children. *AIDS Patient Care and STDs, 14*(11), 589–593.

Feuillan, P. P., Jones, J. V., Barnes, K., et al. (1999). Reproductive axis after discontinuation of gonadotropin-releasing hormone analog treatment of girls with precocious puberty: Long term follow-up comparing girls with hypothalamic hamartoma to those with idiopathic precocious puberty. *Journal of Clinical Endocrinology and Metabolism, 84*(1), 44–49.

Figgitt, D. P., & Plosker, G. L. (2000). Saquinavir

soft-gel capsule: An updated review of its use in the management of HIV infection. *Drugs, 60*(2), 481–516.

Figueroa, Y., Rosenberg, D. R., Birmaher, B., et al. (1998). Combination treatment with clomipramine and selective serotonin reuptake inhibitors for obsessive-compulsive disorder in children and adolescents. *Journal of Child and Adolescent Psychopharmacology, 8*(1), 61–67.

Fillastre, J. P., Leroy, A., Baudoin, C., et al. (1985). Pharmacokinetics of aztreonam in patients with chronic renal failure. *Clinical Pharmacokinetics, 10*, 91–100.

Finch, R. G., Pemberton, K., & Gildon, K. M. (1998). *Journal of Chemotherapy, 10*(1), 35–46.

Findling, R. L., McNamara, N. K., Branicky, L. A., et al. (2000). A double-blind pilot study of risperidone in the treatment of conduct disorder. *Journal of the American Academy of Child and Adolescent Psychiatry, 39*(4), 509–516.

Findling, R. L., Reed, M. D., & Blumer, J. L. (1999). Pharmacological treatment of depression in children and adolescents. *Paediatric Drugs, 1*(3), 161–182.

Findling, R. L., Reed, M. D., Myers, C., et al. (1999). Paroxetine pharmacokinetics in depressed children and adolescents. *Journal of the American Academy of Child and Adolescent Psychiatry, 38*(8), 952–959.

Fiore, P., Donelli, E., Boni, S., et al. (2000). Nutritional status changes in HIV-infected children receiving combined antiretroviral therapy including protease inhibitors. *International Journal of Antimicrobial Agents, 16*(3), 365–369.

Fish, S. S., Pancorbo, S., & Berkseth, R. (1981). Pharmacokinetics of epsilon-aminocaproic acid during peritoneal dialysis. *Journal of Neurosurgery, 54*, 736–739.

Fisher, D. M. (1999). Neuromuscular blocking agents in paediatric anaesthesia. *British Journal of Anaesthesia, 83*(1), 58–64.

Fletcher, C. V., Brundage, R. C., Remmel, R. P., et al. (2000). Pharmacologic characteristics of indinavir, didanosine, and stavudine in human immunodeficiency virus-infected children receiving combination therapy. *Antimicrobial Agents and Chemotherapy, 44*(4), 1029–1034.

Follath, F., Wenk, M., Vozeh, S., et al. (1983). Intravenous cyclosporine kinetics in renal failure. *Clinical Pharmacology and Therapeutics, 34*, 638–643.

Forni, C., Ferrari, S., Loro, L., et al. (2000). Granisetron, tropisetron, and ondansetron in the prevention of acute emesis induced by a combination of cisplatin–Adriamycin and by high-dose ifosfamide delivered in multiple-day continuous infusions. *Supportive Care in Cancer, 8*(2), 131–133.

Fraschini, F., Scaglione, F., Demartini, G. (1993). Clarithromycin clinical pharmacokinetics. *Clinical Pharmacokinetics, 25*, 189–204.

Freed, M. I., Allen, A., Jorkasky, D. K., et al. (1999). Systemic exposure to rosiglitazone is unaltered by food. *European Journal of Clinical Pharmacology, 55*(1), 53–56.

Friedland, I. R., & Lutsar, I. (1998). New antibiotics. *Current Opinion in Pediatrics, 10*(1), 41–45.

Friedman, C. J., Burris, H. A., Yocom, K., et al. (2000). Oral granisetron for the prevention of acute late onset nausea and vomiting in patients treated with moderately emetogenic chemotherapy. *The Oncologist, 5*(2), 136–143.

Fujii, Y., & Tanaka, H. (1999). Granisetron reduces post-operative vomiting in children: A dose-ranging study. *European Journal of Anaesthesiology, 16*(1), 62–65.

Fujii, Y., Saitoh, Y., & Kobayashi, N. (2001). Prevention of vomiting after tonsillectomy in children: Granisetron versus ramosetron. *The Laryngoscope, 111*(2), 255–258.

Fujii, Y., Saitoh, Y., Tanaka, H., et al. (1999). Anti-emetic efficacy of prophylactic granisetron compared with perphenazine for the prevention of post-operative vomiting in children. *European Journal of Anaesthesiology, 16*(5), 304–307.

Fujii, Y., Saitoh, Y., Tanaka, H., et al. (1999). Prevention of postoperative vomiting with granisetron in paediatric patients with and without a history of motion sickness. *Paediatric Anaesthesia, 9*(6), 527–530.

Fung, H. B., Kirschenbaum, H. L., & Hameed, R. (2000). Amprenavir: A new human immunodeficiency virus type 1 protease inhibitor. *Clinical Therapeutics, 22*(5), 549–572.

Furlan, V., Debray, D., Fourre, C., et al. (2000). Conversion from cyclosporin A to tacrolimus in pediatric liver transplantation. *Pediatric Transplants, 4*(3), 207–210.

Gaily, E., Granstrom, M. L., & Liukkonen, E. (1998). Oxcarbazepine in the treatment of epilepsy in children and adolescents with intellectual disability. *Journal of Intellectual Disability Research, 42*(Suppl 1), 41–45.

Gajewski, L. K., Grimone, A. J., Melbourne, K. M., et al. (1999). Characterization of rash with indinavir in a national patient cohort. *Annals of Pharmacotherapy, 33*(1), 17–21.

Gallagher, K. T., & Bernstein, D. (1999). Juvenile rheumatoid arthritis. *Current Opinion in Rheumatology, 11*(5), 372–376.

Gambertoglio, J. G., Azia, N. S., Lin, E. T., et al. (1979). Cefamandole kinetics in uremic patients undergoing hemodialysis. *Clinical Pharmacology and Therapeutics, 26*, 592–599.

Gatell, J. (1999). Coming therapies: Amprenavir. *International Journal of Clinical Practice, 103*(Suppl), 42–44.

Gatti, G., Bonomi, I., Jannuzzi, G., et al. (2000). The new antiepileptic drugs: Pharmacological and clinical aspects. *Current Pharmaceutical Design, 6*(8), 839–860.

Gatti, G., Vigano', A., Sala, N., et al. (2000). Indinavir pharmacokinetics and pharmacodynamics in children with human immunodeficiency virus infection. *Antimicrobial Agents and Chemotherapy, 44*(3), 752–755.

Gerlach, A. T., Pickworth, K. K., Seth, S. K., et al. (2000). Enoxaparin and bleeding complications: A review in patients with and without renal insufficiency. *Pharmacotherapy, 20*(7), 771–775.

Gibson, T. P., Lowenthal, D. T., Nelson, H. A., et al. (1975). Elimination of procainamide in end stage renal failure. *Clinical Pharmacology and Therapeutics, 17,* 321–329.

Gidding, S. S. (1993). The rationale for lowering serum cholesterol levels in American children. *American Journal of Diseases of Children, 147,* 386–392.

Glauser, T. A. (2000). Expanding first-line therapy options for children with partial seizures. *Neurology, 55*(11, Suppl 3), S30–S37.

Glauser, T. A., Nigro, M., Sachdeo, R., et al. (2000). Adjunctive therapy with oxcarbazepine in children with partial seizures. The Oxcarbazepine Pediatric Study Group. *Neurology, 54*(12), 2237–2244.

Gleckman, R., Blagg, N., & Joubert, D. W. (1981). Trimethoprim: Mechanisms of action, antimicrobial activity, bacterial resistance, pharmacokinetics, adverse reactions, and therapeutic indications. *Pharmacotherapy, 1,* 14–20.

Goldstein, J. L. (2000). Significant upper gastrointestinal events associated with conventional NSAID versus celecoxib. *Journal of Rheumatology, 60,* 25–28.

Goldstein, J. L., Silverstein, F. E., Agrawal, N. M., et al. (2000). Reduced risk of upper gastrointestinal ulcer complications with celecoxib, a novel COX-2 inhibitor. *American Journal of Gastroenterology, 95*(7), 1681–1690.

Gooch, W. M., Adelglass, J., Kelsey, D. K., et al. (1999). Loracarbef versus clarithromycin in children with acute otitis media with effusion. *Clinical Therapeutics, 21*(4), 711–722.

Gower, R. E., Kennedy, R. E., & Dash, C. H. (1977). The effect of renal failure and dialysis on the pharmacokinetics of cefuroxime. *Proceedings of the Royal Society of Medicine, 70*(Suppl 9), 151–157.

Grasela, D. M., Stoltz, R. R., Barry, M., et al. (2000). Pharmacokinetics of single-dose oral stavudine in subjects with renal impairment and in subjects requiring hemodialysis. *Antimicrobial Agents and Chemotherapy, 44*(8), 2149–2153.

Gray, J. W., Darbyshire, P. J., Beath, S. V., et al. (2000). Experience with quinupristin/dalfopristin in treating infections with vancomycin-resistant Enterococcus faecium in children. *Pediatric Infectious Disease, 19*(3), 234–238.

Greaves, W. L., Kreeft, J. H., Ogilvie, R. I., et al. (1981). Cefoxitin disposition during peritoneal dialysis. *Antimicrobial Agents and Chemotherapy, 19,* 253–255.

Green, D. W., Fisher, M., & Sockalingham, I. (1998). Mivacurium compared with succinylcholine in children with liver disease. *British Journal of Anaesthesia, 81*(3), 463–465.

Greinacher, A., Volpel, H., Janssens, U., et al. (1999). Recombinant hirudin (lepirudin) provides safe and effective anticoagulation in patients with heparin-induced thrombocytopenia: A prospective study. *Circulation, 99*(1), 73–80.

Gross, M. L., Somani, P., Ribner, B. S., et al. (1983). Ceftizoxime elimination kinetics in continuous ambulatory peritoneal dialysis. *Clinical Pharmacology and Therapeutics, 34,* 673–680.

Guay, D. R. P., Meatherall, R. C., Baxter, H., et al. (1984). Pharmacokinetics of metronidazole in patients undergoing continuous ambulatory peritoneal dialysis. *Antimicrobial Agents and Chemotherapy, 25,* 306–310.

Guay, D. R. P., Meatherall, R. C., Harding, G. K., et al. (1986). Pharmacokinetics of cefixime (CL 284, 635; FK 027) in healthy subjects and patients with renal insufficiency. *Antimicrobial Agents and Chemotherapy, 30,* 485–490.

Gubareva, L. V., Kaiser, L., & Hayden, F. G. (2000). Influenza virus neuraminidase inhibitors. *Lancet, 355*(9206), 827–835.

Halperin, S. A., McGrath, P., Smith, B., et al. (2000). Lidocaine–prilocaine patch decreases the pain associated with the subcutaneous administration of measles–mumps–rubella vaccine but does not adversely affect the antibody response. *The Journal of Pediatrics, 136*(6), 789–794.

Hande, K. R., Noone, R. M., & Stone, W. J. (1984). Severe allopurinol toxicity. Description and guidelines for prevention in patients with renal insufficiency. *American Journal of Medicine, 76,* 47–56.

Hanyok, J. J., Chow, M. S. S., Kluger, J., et al. (1987). Verapamil kinetics and dynamics in chronic hemodialysis patients. *Clinical Pharmacology and Therapeutics, 41,* 224.

Harvey, D. M., & Offord, R. H. (2000). Management of venous and cardiovascular thrombosis: Enoxaparin. *Hospital Medicine, 61*(9), 628–636.

Hayden, F. G., Atmar, R. L., Schilling, M., et al. (1999). Use of the selective oral neuroaminidase inhibitor oseltamivir to prevent influenza. *New England Journal of Medicine, 341*(18), 1336–1343.

Hayden, F. G., Gubareva, L. V., Monto, A. S., et al. (2000). Inhaled zanamivir for the prevention of influenza in families. Zanamivir Family Study Group. *New England Journal of Medicine, 343*(18), 1282–1289.

Hayden, F. G., Treanor, J. J., Fritz, R. S., et al. (1999). Use of the oral neuraminidase inhibitor oseltamivir in experimental human influenza: Randomized controlled trials for prevention and treatment. *Journal of the American Medical Association, 282*(13), 1240–1246.

Hayes, R. P., Grinzaid, K. A., Duffey, E. B., et al. (1998). The impact of Gaucher disease and its treatment on quality of life. *Quality of Life Research, 7*(6), 521–534.

Hays, D. P., Primack, W. A., & Abrams, I. F. (1985). Phenytoin clearance by continuous ambulatory peritoneal dialysis. *Drug Intelligence and Clinical Pharmacy, 19*, 429–431.

Hedrick, J. A., Barzilai, A., Behre, U., et al. (2000). Zanamivir for treatment of symptomatic influenza A and B infection in children five to twelve years of age: A randomized controlled trial. *Pediatric Infectious Disease, 19*(5), 410–417.

Hemmerling, T. M., Schmidt, J., Wolf, T., et al. (2001). Intramuscular versus surface electromyography of the diaphragm for determining neuromuscular blockade. *Anesthesia and Analgesia, 92*(1), 106–111.

Henry, N. K., Hoecker, J. L., & Rhodes, K. H. (2000). Antimicrobial therapy for infants and children: Guidelines for the inpatient and outpatient practice of pediatric infectious diseases. *Mayo Clinic Proceedings, 75*(1), 86–97.

Hervey, P. S., & Perry, C. M. (2000). Abacavir: A review of its clinical potential in patients with HIV infection. *Drugs, 60*(2), 447–479.

Hewitson, P. J., Debroe, S., McBride, A., et al. (2000). Leflunomide and rheumatoid arthritis: A systematic review of effectiveness, safety and cost implications. *Journal of Clinical Pharmacology and Therapeutics, 25*(4), 295–302.

Hiner, L. B., Baluarte, H. J., Polinsky, M. S., et al. (1980). Cefazolin in children with renal insufficiency. *The Journal of Pediatrics, 96*, 335–339.

Hoffmann, F., Notheis, G., Wintergerst, U., et al. (2000). Comparison of ritonavir plus saquinavir- and nelfinavir plus saquinavir-containing regimens as salvage therapy in children with human immunodeficiency type 1 infection. *Pediatric Infectious Disease, 19*(1), 47–51.

Horneff, G., Adams, O., & Wahn, V. (1999). Preliminary experiences with ritonavir in children with advanced HIV infection. *Infection, 27*(2), 103–107.

Hsu, A., Granneman, G. R., Cao, G., et al. (1998). Pharmacokinetic interaction between ritonavir and indinavir in healthy volunteers. *Antimicrobial Agents and Chemotherapy, 42*(11), 2784–2791.

Hugen, P. W., Burger, D. M., Hofstede, H. J., et al. (2000). Dose-finding study of a once-daily indinavir/ritonavir regimen. *Journal of Acquired Immune Deficiency Syndromes, 25*(3), 236–245.

Hughes, W., McDowell, J. A., Shenep, J., et al. (1999). Safety and single-dose pharmacokinetics of abacavir (1592U89) in human immunodeficiency virus type 1-infected children. *Antimicrobial Agents and Chemotherapy, 43*(3), 609–615.

Humbert, G., Eillastre, J. R., Leroy, A., et al. (1979). Pharmacokinetics of cefoxitin in normal subjects and in patients with renal insufficiency. *Reviews of Infectious Diseases, 1*, 118–125.

Hurst, M., & Lamb, H. M. (2000). Meropenem: A review of its use in patients in intensive care. *Drugs, 59*(3), 653–680.

Hurwitz, E. S., Haber, M., Chang, A., et al. (2000). Effectiveness of influenza vaccination of day care children in reducing influenza-related morbidity among household contacts. *Journal of the American Medical Association, 284*(13), 1677–1682.

Hyams, J. S., Markowitz, J., & Wyllie, R. (2000). Use of infliximab in the treatment of Crohn's disease in children and adolescents. *The Journal of Pediatrics, 137*(2), 192–196.

Ida, H., Rennert, O. M., Kobayashi, M., et al. (2001). Effects of enzyme replacement therapy in thirteen Japanese paediatric patients with Gaucher disease. *European Journal of Pediatrics, 160*(1), 21–25.

Infectious Diseases: Tamiflu now comes as a suspension for kids age one and up (document #170105). *Prescriber's Letter, 8*(1), 2.

Ingwersen, S. H., Pedersen, P. C., Groes, L., et al. (2000). Population pharmacokinetics of tiagabine in epileptic patients on monotherapy. *European Journal of Pharmaceutical Sciences, 11*(3), 247–254.

Jacobs, M. R., Bajaksouzian, S., Zilles, A., et al. (1999). Susceptibilities of Streptococcus pneumoniae and Haemophilus influenzae to 10 oral antimicrobial agents based on pharmacodynamic parameters: 1997 U.S. Surveillance study. *Antimicrobial Agents and Chemotherapy, 43*(8), 1901–1908.

Jain, A., Mazariegos, G., Kashyap, R., et al. (2000). Comparative long-term evaluation of tacrolimus and cyclosporine in pediatric liver transplantation. *Transplantation, 70*(4), 617–625.

Jusko, W. J., Ballah, T., Kim, K. H., et al. (1976). Pharmacokinetics of gentamicin during peritoneal dialysis in children. *Kidney International, 9*, 436–438.

Kaiser, L., Henry, D., Flack, N. P., et al. (2000). Short-term treatment with zanamivir to prevent influenza: Results of a placebo controlled study. *Clinical Infectious Disease, 30*(3), 587–589.

Kalviainen, R., Brodie, M. J., Duncan, J., et al. (1998). A double-blind, placebo-controlled trial of tiagabine given three-times daily as add-on therapy for refractory partial seizures. Northern European Tiagabine Study Group. *Epilepsy Research, 30*(1), 31–40.

Kandrotas, R. J., Love, J. M., Gal, P., et al. (1990). The effect of hemodialysis and hemoperfusion on serum valproic acid concentration. *Neurology, 40*, 1456–1458.

Kanra, G., Yalcin, S. S., Ceyhan, M., et al. (2000). Clinical trial to evaluate immunogenicity and safety of inactivated hepatitis A vaccination starting at 2-month-old children. *Turkish Journal of Pediatrics, 42*(2), 105–108.

Kavuru, M. S., Subramony, R., & Vann, A. R. (1998). Antileukotrienes and asthma: Alternative or adjunct to inhaled steroids? *Cleveland Clinical Journal of Medicine, 65*(10), 519–526.

Kearns, G. L., Leeder, J. S., & Wasserman, G. S. (2000). Acetaminophen intoxication during treatment: What you don't know can hurt you. *Clinical Pediatrics, 39*(3), 133–144.

Kilby, J. M., Sfakianos, G., Gizzi, N., et al. (2000). Safety and pharmacokinetics of once-daily regimens of soft-gel capsule saquinavir plus minidose ritonavir in human inmunodeficiency virus-negative adults. *Antimicrobial Agents and Chemotherapy, 44*(10), 2672–2678.

Kleinbloesem, C. H., Van Brummelen, P., Van Harten, J., et al. (1985). Nifedipine: Influence of renal function on pharmacokinetic/hemodynamic relationship. *Clinical Pharmacology and Therapeutics, 37*, 563–574.

Kleinbloesem, C. H., Van Brummelen, P., Woittiez, A. J., et al. (1986). Influence of hemodialysis on the pharmacokinetics of haemodynamic effects of nifedipine during continuous intravenous infusion. *Clinical Pharmacokinetics, 11*, 316–322.

Kline, M. W., Van Dyke, R. B., Lindsey, J. C., et al. (1998). A randomized comparative trial of stavudine (d4T) versus zidovudine (ZDV, AZT) in children with human immunodeficiency virus infection. AIDS Clinical Trials Group 240 Team. *Pediatrics, 101*(2), 214–220.

Kline, M. W., Van Dyke, R. B., Lindsey, J. C., et al. (1999). Combination therapy with stavudine (d4T) plus didanosine (ddI) in children with human immunodeficiency virus infection. The Pediatric AIDS Clinical Trials Group 327 Team. *Pediatrics, 103*(5), E62.

Kneyber, M. C., Moll, H. A., & de Groot, R. (2000). Treatment and prevention of respiratory syncytial virus infection. *European Journal of Pediatrics, 159*(6), 399–411.

Kogan, F. J., Sampliner, R. E., Mayersohn, M., et al. (1983). Cimetidine disposition in patients undergoing continuous ambulatory peritoneal dialysis. *Journal of Clinical Pharmacology, 23*, 252–256.

Komada, Y., Matsuyama, T., Takao, A., et al. (1999). A randomized dose-comparison trial of granisetron in preventing emesis in children with leukaemia receiving emetogenic chemotherapy. *European Journal of Cancer, 35*(7), 1095–1101.

Korn-Merker, E., Borusiak, P., & Boenigk, H. E. (2000). Gabapentin in childhood epilepsy: A prospective evaluation of efficacy and safety. *Epilepsy Research, 38*(1), 27–32.

Korth-Bradley, J. M., Rubin, A. S., Hanna, R. K., et al. (2000). The pharmacokinetics of etanercept in healthy volunteers. *Annals of Pharmacotherapy, 34*(2), 161–164.

Kowalsky, S. F., Echols, R. M., Venezia, A. R., et al. (1983). Pharmacokinetics of ceftizoxime in subjects with various degrees of renal function. *Antimicrobial Agents and Chemotherapy, 24*, 151–155.

Krawiec, M. E., & Wenzel, S. E. (1999). Use of leukotriene antagonists in childhood asthma. *Current Opinion in Pediatrics, 11*(6), 540–547.

Kremer, D., Munar, M. Y., Kohlhepp, S. J., et al. (1992). Zidovudine pharmacokinetics in five HIV seronegative patients undergoing continuous ambulatory peritoneal dialysis. *Pharmacotherapy, 12*, 56–60.

Kugathasan, S., Werlin, S. L., Martinez, A., et al. (2000). Prolonged duration of response to infliximab in early but not late pediatric Crohn's disease. *American Journal of Gastroenterology, 95*(11), 3189–3194.

Lake, K. D., Fletcher, C. V., Love, K. R., et al. (1988). Ganciclovir pharmacokinetics during renal impairment. *Antimicrobial Agents and Chemotherapy, 32*, 1899–1900.

Lamb, H. M., Figgitt, D. P., & Faulds, D. (1999). Quinupristin/dalfopristin: A review of its use in the management of serious gram-positive infections. *Drugs, 58*(6), 1061–1097.

Lanza, F. L., Rack, M. F., Simon, T. J., et al. (1999). Specific inhibition of cyclooxygenase-2 with MK-0966 is associated with less gastroduodenal damage than either aspirin or ibuprofen. *Alimentary Pharmacology and Therapeutics, 13*(6), 761–777.

Larsson, R., Norlander, B., Bodemar, G., et al. (1981). Steady-state kinetics and dosage requirements of cimetidine in renal failure. *Clinical Pharmacokinetics, 6*, 316–325.

Laskin, O. L., Longstreth, J. A., Whelton, A., et al. (1982). Acyclovir kinetics in end-stage renal disease. *Clinical Pharmacology and Therapeutics, 31*, 594–601.

Leese, P. T., Hubbard, R. C., Karim, A., et al. (2000). Effects of celecoxib, a novel cyclooxygenase-2 inhibitor, on platelet function in healthy adults: A randomized, controlled trial. *Journal of Clinical Pharmacology, 40*(2), 124–132.

Lehmann, C. R., Heironimus, J. D., Collins, C. B., et al. (1985). Metoclopramide kinetics in patients with impaired renal function and clearance by hemodialysis. *Clinical Pharmacology and Therapeutics, 37*, 284–289.

Lejus, C., Blanloeil, Y., Le Roux, N., et al. (1998). Prolonged mivacurium neuromuscular block in children. *Paediatric Anaesthesia, 8*(5), 433–435.

Leppik, I. E., Gram, L., Deaton, R., et al. (1999). Safety of tiagabine: Summary of 53 trials. *Epilepsy Research, 33*(2-3), 235–246.

Leroy, A., Humbert, G., Godin, M., et al. (1982). Pharmacokinetics of cefadroxil in patients with impaired renal function. *Journal of Antimicrobial Chemotherapy, 10*(Suppl B), 39–46.

Lindberger, M., Alenius, M., Frisen, L., et al. (2000). Gabapentin versus vigabatrin as first add-on for patients with partial seizures that failed to respond to monotherapy: A randomized, double-blind, dose titration study. GREAT Study Investigators Group. Gabapentin in Refractory Epilepsy Add-on Treatment. *Epilepsia, 41*(10), 1289–1295.

Lindsay, C. A., Barton, P., Lawless, S., et al. (1998). Pharmacokinetics and pharmacodynamics of milrinone lactate in pediatric patients with septic shock. *Journal of Pediatrics, 132*(2), 329–334.

Loiseau, P. (1999). Review of controlled trials of gabitril (tiagabine): A clinician's viewpoint. *Epilepsia, 40*(Suppl 9), S14–S19.

Lorenz, H. M. (2000). Biological agents: A novel approach to the therapy of rheumatoid arthritis. *Expert Opinion on Investigational Drugs, 9*(7), 1479–1490.

Lovell, D. J., Giannini, E. H., Reiff, A., et al. (2000). Etanercept in children with polyarticular juvenile rheumatoid arthritis. Pediatric Rheumatology Collaborative Study Group. *New England Journal of Medicine, 342*(11), 763–769.

Lowe, M. N., & Lamb, H. M. (2000). Meropenem: An updated review of its use in the management of intra-abdominal infections. *Drugs, 60*(3), 619–646.

Luer, M. S., & Rhoney, D. H. (1998). Tiagabine: A novel antiepileptic drug. *Annals of Pharmacotherapy, 32*(11), 1173–1180.

Lundstrom, T. S., & Sobel, J. D. (2000). Antibiotics for gram-positive bacterial infections. Vancomycin, teicoplanin, quinupristin/dalfopristin, and linezolid. *Infectious Disease Clinics of North America, 14*(2), 463–474.

Luong, B. T., Chong, B. S., & Lowder, D. M. (2000). Treatment options for rheumatoid arthritis: Celecoxib, leflunomide, etanercept, and infliximab. *Annals of Pharmacotherapy, 34*(6), 743–760.

Lydiard, R. B., & Bobes, J. (2000). Therapeutic advances: Paroxetine for the treatment of social anxiety disorder. *Depression and Anxiety, 11*(3), 99–104.

Lysakowski, C., Fuchs–Buder, T., & Tassonyi, E. (2000). Mivacurium or vecuronium for paediatric ENT surgery. Clinical experience and cost analysis. *Anaesthesist, 49*(5), 387–391.

MacKenzie, J. J., Amato, D., & Clarke, J. T. (1998). Enzyme replacement therapy for Gaucher's disease: The early Canadian experience. *Canadian Medical Association Journal, 159*(10), 1273–1278.

Maheshwari, H. G., Prezant, T. R., Herman-Bonert, V., et al. (2000). Long-acting peptidomimergic control of gigantism caused by pituitary acidophilic stem cell adenoma. *Journal of Clinical Endocrinology and Metabolism, 85*(9), 3409–3416.

Maini, R. N., & Taylor, P. C. (2000). Anti-cytokine therapy for rheumatoid arthritis. *Annual Review of Medicine, 51*, 207–229.

Makela, M. J., Pauksens, K., Rostila, T., et al. (2000). Clinical efficacy and safety of the orally inhaled neuraminidase inhibitor zanamivir in the treatment of influenza: A randomized, double-blind, placebo-controlled European study. *Journal of Infection, 40*(1), 42–48.

Malay, S., Tizer, K., & Lutwick, L. I. (2000). Current update of pediatric hepatitis vaccine use. *Pediatric Clinics of North America, 47*(2), 395–406.

Mancini, C., Van Ameringen, M., Oakman, J. M., et al. (1999). *Depression and Anxiety, 10*(1), 33–39.

Mann, M., Piazza-Hepp, T., Koller, E., et al. (1999). Unusual distributions of body fat in AIDS patients: A review of adverse events reported to the Food and Drug Administration. *AIDS Patient Care and STDs, 13*(5), 287–295.

Markakis, D. A., Lau, M., Brown, R., et al. (1998). The pharmacokinetics and steady state pharmacodynamics of mivacurium in children. *Anesthesiology, 88*(4), 978–983.

Markham, A., & Lamb, H. M. (2000). Infliximab: A review of its use in the management of rheumatoid arthritis. *Drugs, 59*(6), 1341–1359.

Marquardt, E. D., Ishisaka, D. Y., Batra, K. K., et al. (1992). Removal of ethosuximide and phenobarbital by peritoneal dialysis in a child. *Clinical Pharmacy, 11*, 1030–1031.

Martin, A., Landau, J., Leebens, P., et al. (2000). Risperidone-associated weight gain in children and adolescents: A retrospective chart review. *Journal of Child and Adolescent Psychopharmacology, 10*(4), 259–268.

Martre, H., Sari, R., Jacobs, C., et al. (1985). Haemodialysis does not affect the pharmacokinetics of nifedipine. *British Journal of Clinical Pharmacology, 20*, 155–158.

Martyn, J. A., Goudsouzian, N. G., Chang, Y., et al. (2000). Neuromuscular effects of mivacurium in 2- to 12-yr-old children with burn injury. *Anesthesiology, 92*(1), 31–37.

Masi, G., Cosenza, A., Mucci, M., et al. (2001). Open trial of risperidone in 24 young children with pervasive developmental disorders. *Journal of the American Academy of Child and Adolescent Psychiatry, 40*(10), 1206–1214.

Masi, G., Cosenza, A., Mucci, M., et al. (2001). Risperidone monotherapy in preschool children with pervasive developmental disorders. *Journal of Child Neurology, 16*(6), 395–400.

Mason, E. O., Lamberth, L. B., Kershaw, N. L., et al. (2000). Streptococcus pneumoniae in the USA: In vitro susceptibility and pharmacodynamic analysis. *The Journal of Antimicrobial Chemotherapy, 45*(5), 623–631.

Mayer, P. R., Noonan, H., Gambertoglio, J., et al. (1985). Bioavailability of methylprednisolone in patients with renal insufficiency. *Clinical Pharmacology and Therapeutics, 37*, 184.

Mayer, T., Schutte, W., Wolf, P., et al. (1999).

Gabapentin add-on treatment: How many patients become seizure-free? An open-label multicenter study. *Acta Neurologica Scandinavica, 99*(1), 1–7.

McCune, J. S., Oertel, M. D., Pfeifer, D., et al. (2001). Evaluation of outcomes in converting from intravenous ondansetron to oral granisetron: An observational study. *Annals of Pharmacotherapy, 35*(1), 14–20.

McFadyen, M. L., Folb, P. I., Miller, R., et al. (1983). Pharmacokinetics of ranitidine in patients with chronic renal failure. *European Journal of Clinical Pharmacology, 25,* 347–351.

Meador, K. J., Loring, D. W., Ray, P. G., et al. (1999). Differential cognitive effects of carbamazepine and gabapentin. *Epilepsia, 40*(9), 1279–1285.

Meek, P. D., Davis, S. N., Collins, D. M., et al. (1999). Guidelines for nonemergency use of parenteral phenytoin products: Proceedings of an expert panel consensus process. Panel on Nonemergency Use of Parenteral Phenytoin Products. *Archives of Internal Medicine, 159*(22), 2639–2644.

Mersfelder, T. L. (2001). Phenylpropanolamine and stroke: The study, the FDA ruling, the implications. *Cleveland Clinic Journal of Medicine, 68*(3), 208–209, 213–219, 223.

Michalets, E. L., & Williams, C. R. (2000). Drug interactions with cisapride: Clinical implications. *Clinical Pharmacokinetics, 39*(1), 49–75.

Miller, K. D., Cameron, M., Wood, L. V., et al. (2000). Lactic acidosis and hepatic steatosis associated with use of stavudine: Report of four cases. *Annals of Internal Medicine, 133*(3), 192–196.

Minagawa, M., Yasuda, T., Someya, T., et al. (2000). Effects of octreotide infusion, surgery and estrogen on suppression of height increase and 20K growth hormone ratio in a girl with gigantism due to a growth hormone-secreting macroadenoma. *Hormone Research, 53*(3), 157–160.

Minutello, M., Zotti, C., Orecchia, S., et al. (2000). Dose range evaluation of a new inactivated hepatitis A vaccine administered as a single dose followed by a booster. *Vaccine, 19*(1), 10–15.

Mission, J., Clark, W., & Kendall, M. J. (1999). Therapeutic advances: Leukotriene antagonists for the treatment of asthma. *Journal of Clinical Pharmacy and Therapeutics, 24*(1), 17–22.

Moder, K. G. (2000). New medications for use in patients with rheumatoid arthritis. *Annals of Allergy, Asthma, and Immunology, 84*(3), 280–284.

Moon, Y. S., Chung, K. C., & Gill, M. A. (1997). Pharmacokinetics of meropenem in animals, healthy volunteers, and patients. *Clinical Infectious Disease, 24*(Suppl 2), S249–S255.

Moreland, L. W. (1999). Inhibitors of tumor necrosis factor: New treatment options for rheumatoid arthritis. *Cleveland Clinic Journal of Medicine, 66*(6), 367–374.

Morrison, B. W., Christensen, S., Yuan, W., et al. (1999). Analgesic efficacy of the cyclooxygenase-2-specific inhibitor rofecoxib in post-dental surgery pain: A randomized, controlled trial. *Clinical Therapeutics, 21*(6), 943–953.

Morrison, B. W., Daniels, S. E., Kotey, P., et al. (1999). Rofecoxib, a specific cyclooxygenase-2 inhibitor, in primary dysmenorrhea: A randomized controlled trial. *Obstetrics and Gynecology, 94*(4), 504–508.

Morton, L. D., & Pellock, J. M. (2000). Overview of childhood epilepsy and epileptic syndromes and advances in therapy. *Current Pharmaceutical Design, 6*(8), 879–900.

Mouton, J. W., Touzw, D. J., Horrevorts, A. M., et al. (2000). Comparative pharmacokinetics of the carbapenems: Clinical implications. *Clinical Pharmacokinetics, 39*(3), 185–201.

Moyle, G. (1999). Efavirenz: Practicalities, considerations and new issues. *International Journal of Clinical Practice, 103*(Suppl), 30–34.

Mueller, B. U., Nelson, R. P., Sleasman, J., et al. (1998). A phase I/II study of the protease inhibitor ritonavir in children with human immunodeficiency virus infection. *Pediatrics, 101*(3, Part 1), 335–343.

Myeffin, P. J., Grgurinovich, N., Brooks, P. M., et al. (1983). Ranitidine disposition in patients with renal impairment. *British Journal of Clinical Pharmacology, 16,* 731–734.

Myhre, E., Rugstad, H . E., & Hansen, T. (1982). Clinical pharmacokinetics of methyldopa. *Clinical Pharmacokinetics, 7,* 221–223.

Myre, S. A., Sing, S., Kawamoto, D., et al. (1986). Comment: Metoclopramide kinetics during continuous ambulatory peritoneal dialysis. *Drug Intelligence and Clinical Pharmacy, 20,* 508.

Nachman, S. A., Stanley, K., Yogev, R., et al. (2000). Nucleoside analogs plus ritonavir in stable antiretroviral therapy–experienced HIV-infected children: A randomized controlled trial. Pediatric AIDS Clinical Trials Group 338 Study Team. *Journal of the American Medical Association, 283*(4), 492–498.

Nanto-Salonen, K., Koskinen, P., Sonninen, P., et al. (1999). Suppression of GH secretion in pituitary gigantism by continuous subcutaneous octreotide infusion in a pubertal boy. *Acta Paediatrica, 88*(1), 29–33.

Neuraminidase inhibitors for treatment of influenza A and B infections. (2001). *Morbidity and Mortality Weekly Report, 48*(49), 1–9.

Neuraminidase inhibitors for treatment of influenza A and B infections [Erratum]. (2001). *Morbidity and Mortality Weekly Report, 48*(49), 1139.

Niederau, C., & Haussinger, D. (2000). Gaucher's disease: A review for the internist and hepatologist. *Hepatogastroenterology, 47*(34), 984–997.

Niederau, C., vom Dahl, S., & Haussinger, D. (1998). First long-term results of imiglucerase therapy of type 1 Gaucher disease. *European Journal of Medical Research, 3*(1-2), 25–30.

Nobile, M., Bellotti, B., Marino, C., et al. (2000). An open trial of paroxetine in the treatment of children and adolescents diagnosed with dysthymia. *Journal of Child and Adolescent Psychopharmacology, 10*(2), 103–109.

Norrby, S. R., & Gildon, K. M. (1999). Safety profile of meropenem: A review of nearly 5,000 patients treated with meropenem. *Scandinavian Journal of Infectious Diseases, 31*(1), 3–10.

Odio, C. M., Puig, J. R., Feris, J. M., et al. (1999). Prospective, randomized, investigator-blinded study of the efficacy and safety of meropenem vs. cefotaxime therapy in bacterial meningitis in children. Meropenem Meningitis Study Group. *Pediatric Infectious Disease, 18*(7), 581–590.

Oeullet, D., Hsu, A., Qian, J., et al. (1998). Effect of fluoxetine on pharmacokinetics of ritonavir. *Antimicrobial Agents and Chemotherapy, 42*(12), 107–112.

Orebaugh, S. L. (1999). Succinylcholine: Adverse effects and alternatives in emergency medicine. *American Journal of Emergency Medicine, 17*(7), 715–721.

Osborne, R. J., Jeol, S. P., & Selvin, M. L. (1986). Morphine intoxication in renal failure: The role of morphine-6-glucuronide. *British Medical Journal, 292,* 1548.

Pagliaro, L. A., & Benet, L. A. (1975). Critical compilation of terminal half-lives, percent excreted unchanged, and changes in renal and hepatic dysfunction for studies in humans with references. *Journal of Pharmacokinetics and Biopharmaceutics, 3,* 333–383.

Pagliaro, L. A., & Pagliaro, A. M. (1999). *PNDR: Psychologists' neuropsychotropic drug reference.* Philadelphia, PA: Brunner/Mazel.

Pagliaro, L. A., & Pagliaro, A. M. (1999). *PPDR: Psychologists' psychotropic drug reference.* Philadelphia, PA: Brunner/Mazel.

Pai, V. B., Koranyi, K., Nahata, M. C. (2000). Acute hepatitis and bleeding possibly induced by zidovudine and ritonavir in an infant with HIV infection. *Pharmacotherapy, 20*(9), 1135–1140.

Palmert, M. R., Mansfield, M. J., Crowley, W. F., et al. (1999). Is obesity an outcome of gonadotropin-releasing hormone agonist administration? Analysis of growth and body composition in 110 patients with central precocious puberty. *Journal of Clinical Endocrinology and Metabolism, 84*(12), 4480–4488.

Paradisi, F., Corti, G., & Messeri, D. (2001). Antistaphylococcal (MSSA, MRSA, MSSE, MRSE) antibiotics. *Medical Clinics of North America, 85*(1), 1–17.

Paster, R. Z., McAdoo, M. A., Keyserling, C. H., et al. (2000). A comparison of a five-day regimen of cefdinir with a seven-day regimen of loracarbef for the treatment of acute exacerbations of chronic bronchitis. *International Journal of Clinical Practice, 54*(5), 293–299.

Patel, R. B., & Welling, P. G. (1980). Clinical pharmacokinetics of co-trimoxazole. *Clinical Pharmacokinetics, 5,* 405–423.

Paulson, S. K., Hribar, J. D., Liu, N. W., et al. (2000). Metabolism and excretion of [(14)C] celecoxib in healthy male volunteers. *Drug Metabolism and Disposition, 28*(3), 308–314.

Pellock, J. M. (1999). Managing pediatric epilepsy syndromes with new antiepileptic drugs. *Pediatrics, 104*(5, Part 1), 1106–1116.

Pellock, J. M. & Appleton, R. (1999). Use of new antiepileptic drugs in the treatment of childhood epilepsy. *Epilepsia, 40*(Suppl 6), S29–S38.

Pellock, J. M., & Morton, L. D. (2000). Treatment of epilepsy in the multiply handicapped. *Mental Retardation and Developmental Disability Research Review, 6*(4), 309–323.

Perry, C. M., & Nobel, S. (1999). Didanosine: An updated review of its use in HIV infection. *Drugs, 58*(6), 1099–1135.

Polk, R. E., Crouch, M. A., Israel, D. S., et al. (1999). Pharmacokinetic interaction between ketoconazole and amprenavir after single doses in healthy men. *Pharmacotherapy, 19*(12), 1378–1384.

Posey, D. J., Walsh, K. H., Wilson, G. A., et al. (1999). Risperidone in the treatment of two very young children with autism. *Journal of Child and Adolescent Psychopharmacology, 9*(4), 273–276.

Principi, N., & Marchisio, P. (1998). Meropenem compared with ceftazidime in the empiric treatment of acute severe infections in hospitalized children. Italian Pediatric Meropenem Study Group. *Journal of Chemotherapy, 10*(2), 108–113.

Przepiorka, D., Blamble, D., Hilsenbeck, S., et al. (2000). Tacrolimus clearance is age-dependent within the pediatric population. *Bone Marrow Transplantation, 26*(6), 601–605.

Przepiorka, D., Kernan, N. A., Ippoliti, C., et al. (2000). Daclizumab, a humanized anti-interleukin-2 receptor alpha chain antibody, for treatment of acute graft-versus-host disease. *Blood, 95*(1), 83–89.

Pugh, C. B. (1987). Phenytoin and phenobarbital protein binding alterations in a uremic burn patient. *Drug Intelligence and Clinical Pharmacy, 21,* 264–267.

Punzalan, R. C., Hillery, C. A., Montgomery, R. R., et al. (2000). Low-molecular-weight heparin in thrombotic disease in children and adolescents. *Journal of Pediatric Hematology and Oncology, 22*(2), 137–142.

Racoosin, J. A., & Kessler, C. M. (1999). Bleeding episodes in HIV-positive patients taking HIV protease inhibitors: A case series. *Haemophilia, 5*(4), 266–269.

Raehl, C. L., Moorthy, A. V., Beirne, G. J., et al. (1985). Clearance of procainamide and N-acetylprocainamide in patients undergoing continuous ambulatory peritoneal dialysis. *Clinical Pharmacy, 4*, 669–672.

Rahmah, R., Hayati, A. R., & Kuhnle, U. (1999). Management and short-term outcome of persistent hyperinsulinaemic hypoglycaemia of infancy (nesidioblastosis). *Singapore Medical Journal, 40*(3), 151–156.

Ralph, E. D. (1983). Clinical pharmacokinetics of metronidazole. *Clinical Pharmacokinetics, 8*, 43–62.

Ramamoorthy, C., Anderson, G. D., Williams, G. D., et al. (1998). Pharmacokinetics and side effects of milrinone in infants and children after open heart surgery. *Anesthesia and Analgesia, 86*(2), 283–289.

Ranze, O., Ranze, P., Magnani, H. N., et al. (1999). Heparin-induced thrombocytopenia in paediatric patients—A review of the literature and a new case treated with danaparoid sodium. *European Journal of Pediatrics, 158*(Suppl 3), S130–S133.

Rattya, J., Vainionpaa, L., Knip, M., et al. (1999). The effects of valproate, carbamazepine, and oxcarbazepine on growth and sexual maturation in girls with epilepsy. *Pediatrics, 103*(3), 588–593.

Regeur, L., Colding, H., & Jensen, H. (1977). Pharmacokinetics of amikacin during hemodialysis and peritoneal dialysis. *Antimicrobial Agents and Chemotherapy, 11*, 214–218.

Richter, S. S., Brueggemann, A. B., Huynh, H. K., et al. (1999). A 1997–1998 national surveillance study: Moraxella catarrhalis and Haemophilus influenzae antimicrobial resistance in 34 US institutions. *International Journal of Antimicrobial Agents, 13*(2), 99–107.

Rincon, E., Baker, R. L., Iglesias, A. J., et al. (2000). CNS toxicity after topical application of EMLA cream on a toddler with molluscum contagiosum. *Pediatric Emergency Care, 16*(4), 252–254.

Robb, A. S., Chang, W., Lee, H. K., et al. (2000). Case study. Risperidone-induced neuroleptic malignant syndrome in an adolescent. *Journal of Child and Adolescent Psychopharmacology, 10*(4), 327–330.

Roberts, C. J. C. (1984). Clinical pharmacokinetics of ranitidine. *Clinical Pharmacokinetics, 9*, 211–221.

Rodriguez, W. J. (1999). Management strategies for respiratory syncytial virus infections in infants. *The Journal of Pediatrics, 135*(2, Part 2), 45–50.

Rosenberg, D. R., Stewart, C. M., Fitzgerald, K. D., et al. (1999). Paroxetine open-label treatment of pediatric outpatients with obsessive-compulsive disorder. *Journal of the American Academy of Child and Adolescent Psychiatry, 38*(9), 1180–1185.

Rosenzweig, E. B., Starc, T. J., Chen, J. M., et al. (1999). Intravenous arginine–vasopressin in children with vasodilatory shock after cardiac surgery. *Circulation, 100*(Suppl 19), II182–II186.

Roux, A. F., Moirot, E., Delhotal, B., et al. (1984). Metronidazole kinetics in patients with acute renal failure on dialysis: A cumulative study. *Clinical Pharmacology and Therapeutics, 36*, 363–368.

Rubinstein, E., Prokocimer, P., & Talbot, G. H. (1999). Safety and tolerability of quinupristin/dalfopristin: Administration guidelines. *Journal of Antimicrobial Chemotherapy, 44*(Suppl A), 37–46.

Ruedy, J. (1966). The effects of peritoneal dialysis on the physiological disposition of oxacillin, ampicillin and tetracycline in patients with renal disease. *Canadian Medical Association Journal, 94*, 257.

Ruiz, N. (1999). Clinical history of efavirenz. *International Journal of Clinical Practice, 103*(Suppl), 3–7.

Russell, A. B. (1999). Palivizumab: An overview. *Hospital Medicine, 60*(12), 873–877.

Rutgeerts, P., D'Haens, G., Targan, S., et al. (1999). Efficacy and safety of retreatment with anti-tumor necrosis factor antibody (infliximab) to maintain remission in Crohn's disease. *Gastroenterology, 117*(4), 761–769.

Sabers, A., & Gram, L. (2000). Newer anticonvulsants: Comparative review of drug interactions and adverse effects. *Drugs, 60*(1), 23–33.

Saez-Llorens, X., Nelson, R. P., Emmanuel, P., et al. (2001). A randomized, double-blind study of triple nucleoside therapy of abacavir, lamivudine, and zidovudine versus lamivudine and zidovudine in previously treated human immunodeficiency virus type 1-infected children. The CNAA3006 Study Team. *Pediatrics, 107*(1), E4.

Saltel, E., Angel, J. B., Futter, N. G., et al. (2000). Increased prevalence and analysis of risk factors for indinavir nephrolithiasis. *Journal of Urology, 164*(6), 1895–1897.

Sam, W. J., Aw, M., Quak, S. H., et al. (2000). Population pharmacokinetics of tacrolimus in Asian paediatric liver transplant patients. *British Journal of Clinical Pharmacology, 50*(6), 531–541.

Sandritter, T. (1999). Palivizumab for respiratory syncytial virus prophylaxis. *Journal of Pediatric Health Care, 13*(4), 191–195.

Schachter, S. C., Vazquez, B., Fisher, R. S., et al. (1999). Oxcarbazepine: Double-blind, randomized, placebo-control, monotherapy trial for partial seizures. *Neurology, 52*(4), 732–737.

Schaible, T. F. (2000). Long term safety of infliximab. *Canadian Journal of Gastroenterology, 14*(Suppl C), 29C–32C.

Schiff, M. H., & Whelton, A. (2000). Renal toxicity associated with disease-modifying antirheumatic drugs used for the treatment of rheumatoid arthritis. *Seminars in Arthritis and Rheumatism, 30*(3), 196–208.

Schusziarra, V., Zlekursch, V., Schlamp, R, et al. (1976). Pharmacokinetics of azathioprine under hemodialysis. *International Journal of Clinical Pharmacology and Biopharmaceutics, 14*, 298–302.

Scott, L. J., & Lamb, H. M. (1999). Palivizumab. *Drugs, 58*(2), 305–311.

Shen, D. D., & Azarnoff, D. L. (1978). Clinical pharmacokinetics of methotrexate. *Clinical Pharmacokinetics, 3*, 1–13.

Sherlock, J. E., & Letteri, J. M. (1977). Effect of hemodialysis on methylprednisolone plasma levels. *Nephron, 18*, 208–211.

Shilsby, R. L. (1982). Renal and metabolic toxicities of cancer chemotherapy. *Seminars in Oncology, 9*, 75–83.

Siber, G. R., Gorham, C. C., Ericson, J. F., et al. (1982). Pharmacokinetics of intravenous trimethoprim-sulfamethoxazole in children and adults with normal and impaired renal function. *Reviews of Infectious Diseases, 4*, 566–585.

Simoes, E. A. (1999). Respiratory syncytial virus infection. *Lancet, 354*(9181), 847–852.

Simon, L. S., & Yocum, D. (2000). New and future drug therapies for rheumatoid arthritis. *Rheumatology, 39*(Suppl 1), 36–42.

Sindrup, S. H., & Jensen, T. S. (2000). Pharmacologic treatment of pain in polyneuropathy. *Neurology, 55*(7), 915–920.

Singlas, E., Pioger, J. C., Taburet, A. M., et al. (1989). Zidovudine disposition in patients with severe renal impairment: Influence of hemodialysis. *Clinical Pharmacology and Therapeutics, 46*, 190–197.

Sirinavin, S., McCracken, G. H., & Nelson, J. D. (1980). Determining gentamicin dosage in infants and children with renal failure. *The Journal of Pediatrics, 96*, 331–334.

Skluth, H. A., & Gums, J. G. (1990). Spironolactone: A re-examination. *Drug Intelligence and Clinical Pharmacy, 24*, 52–59.

Skytta, E., Pohjankoski, H., & Savolainen, A. (2000). Etanercept and urticaria in patients with juvenile idiopathic arthritis. *Clinical and Experimental Rheumatology, 18*(4), 533–534.

Slaughter, R. L., Green, L., & Kohli, R. (1982). Hemodialysis clearance of theophylline. *Therapeutic Drug Monitoring, 4*, 191–193.

Smolen, J. S., & Emery, P. (2000). Efficacy and safety of leflunomide in active rheumatoid arthritis. *Rheumatology, 39*(Suppl 1), 48–56.

Spector, S. A., Hsia, K., Yong, F. H., et al. (2000). Patterns of plasma human immunodeficiency virus type 1 RNA response to highly active antiretroviral therapy in infected children. *Journal of Infectious Diseases, 182*(6), 1769–1773.

Spencer-Green, G. (2000). Etanercept (Enbrel): Update on therapeutic use. *Annals of the Rheumatic Diseases, 59*(Suppl 1), i46–i49.

Spyker, D. A., Gober, G. L., Scheld, W. M., et al. (1982). Pharmacokinetics of cefaclor in renal failure: Effects of multiple doses and hemodialysis. *Antimicrobial Agents and Chemotherapy, 21*, 278–281.

St. Peter, W. L., Redic-Kill, K. A., & Halstenson, C. E. (1992). Clinical pharmacokinetics of antibiotics in patients with impaired renal function. *Clinical Pharmacokinetics, 22*, 169–210.

Strong, D. K., Eisenstatki, D. D., Bryson, S. M., et al. (1991). Amantadine neurotoxicity in a pediatric patient with renal insufficiency. *DICP, Annals of Pharmacotherapy, 25*, 1175–1177.

Surveillance for adverse events associated with anthrax vaccination—U. S. Department of Defense, 1998–2000. (2000). *Morbidity and Mortality Weekly Reports, 49*(16), 341–345.

Szigethy, E., Wiznitzer, M., Branicky, L. A., et al. (1999). Risperidone-induced hepatotoxicity in children and adolescents? A chart review study. *Journal of Child and Adolescent Psychopharmacology, 9*(2), 93–98.

Temesgen, Z., & Wright, A. J. (1999). Antiretrovirals. *Mayo Clinic Proceedings, 74*(12), 1284–1301.

Thalhammer, F., Traunmuller, F., El Menyawi, I., et al. (1999). Continuous infusion versus intermittent administration of meropenem in critically ill patients. *Journal of Antimicrobial Chemotherapy, 43*(4), 523–527.

Thomas, M., Bedford-Russell, A., & Sharland, M. (2000). Hospitalisation for RSV infection in ex-preterm infants—Implications for use of RSV immune globulin. *Archives of Disease in Childhood, 83*(2), 122–127.

Thomas, M., Bedford-Russell, A., & Sharland, M. (2000). Prevention of respiratory syncytial virus infection with palivizumab. *Monaldi Archives of Chest Diseases, 55*(4), 333–338.

Thuret, I., Michel, G., Chambost, H., et al. (1999). Combination antiretroviral therapy including ritonavir in children infected with human immunodeficiency. *AIDS, 13*(1), 81–87.

Thyrum, P. T., Yeh, C., Birmingham, B., et al. (1997). Pharmacokinetics of meropenem in patients with liver disease. *Clinical Infectious Diseases, 24*(Suppl 2), S184–S190.

Tomasselli, A. G., & Heinrikson, R. L. (2000). Targeting the HIV–protease in AIDS therapy: A current clinical perspective. *Biochimica et Biophysica Acta, 1477*(1-2), 189–214.

Travel, J. A. (2000). Ongoing trials in HIV protease inhibitors. *Expert Opinion on Investigational Drugs, 9*(4), 917–928.

Treem, W. R., McAdams, L., Stanford, L., et al. (1999). Sacrosidase therapy for congenital sucrase–isomaltase deficiency. *Journal of Pediatric Gastroenterology and Nutrition, 28*(2), 137–142.

Tremblay, C., Merrill, D. P., Chou, T. C., et al. (1999). Interactions among combinations of two and three protease inhibitors against drug-susceptible and drug-resistant HIV-1 isolates. *Journal of Acquired Immune Deficiency Syndromes, 22*(5), 430–436.

Tremont-Lukats, I. W., Megeff, C., & Backonja, M. M. (2000). Anticonvulsants for neuropathic pain syndromes: Mechanisms of action and place in therapy. *Drugs, 60*(5), 1029–1052.

Tsuchida, Y., Hayashi, Y., Asami, K., et al. (1999). Effects of granisetron in children undergoing high-dose chemotherapy: A multi-institutional, cross-over study. *International Journal of Oncology, 14*(4), 673–679.

Uchida, K., Akaza, H., Hattori, K., et al. (1999). Antiemetic efficacy of granisetron: A randomized crossover study in patients receiving cisplatin-containing intraarterial chemotherapy. *Japanese Journal of Clinical Oncology, 29*(2), 87–91.

Uhl, W., Buchler, M. W., Malfertheiner, P., et al. (1999). A randomised, double blind, multicentre trial of octreotide in moderate to severe acute pancreatitis. *Gut, 45*(1), 97–104.

Uldall, P., Bulteau, C., Pedersen, S. A., et al. (2000). Tiagabine adjunctive therapy in children with refractory epilepsy: A single-blind dose escalating study. *Epilepsy Research, 42*(2–3), 159–168.

Update: Interim recommendations for antimicrobial prophylaxis for children and breast-feeding mothers and treatment of children with anthrax, November 2001. (2001). *Morbidity and Mortality Weekly Reports, 50*(45), 1013–1016.

Update: Investigation of bioterrorism-related anthrax and interim guidelines for exposure management and antimicrobial therapy, October 2001. (2001). *Morbidity and Mortality Weekly Reports, 50*(42), 909–919.

Van Bellinghen, M., & De Troch, C. (2001). Risperidone in the treatment of behavioral disturbances in children and adolescents with borderline intellectual functioning: A double-blind, placebo-controlled pilot trial. *Journal of Child and Adolescent Psychopharmacology, 11*(1), 5–13.

Vandercam, B., Gerain, J., Humblet, Y., et al. (2000). Meropenem versus ceftazidime as empirical monotherapy for febrile neutropenic cancer patients. *Annals of Hematology, 79*(3), 152–157.

Venkataramanan, R., Ptachcinski, R. J., Burckart, G. J., et al. (1984). The clearance of cyclosporine by hemodialysis. *Journal of Clinical Pharmacology, 24*, 528–531.

Venuto, R. C., & Plaut, M. (1970). Cephalothin handling in patients undergoing hemodialysis. *Antimicrobial Agents and Chemotherapy, 10*, 50–52.

Vernes, A., Guchelaar, H. J., & Dankert, J. (2000). Flucytosine: A review of its pharmacology, clinical indications, pharmacokinetics, toxicity and drug interactions. *Journal of Antimicrobial Chemotherapy, 46*(2), 171–179.

Villani, P., Regazzi, M. B., Castelli, F., et al. (1999). Pharmacokinetics of efavirenz (EFV) alone and in combination therapy with nelfinavir (NFV) in HIV-1 infected patients. *British Journal of Clinical Pharmacology, 48*(5), 712–715.

Vincent, J., Meredith, P. A., Reid, J. L., et al. (1985). Clinical pharmacokinetics of prazosin. *Clinical Pharmacokinetics, 10*, 144–154.

Vincenti, F., Kirkman, R., Light, S., et al. (1998). Interleukin-2-receptor blockade with daclizumab to prevent acute rejection in renal transplantation. Daclizumab Triple Therapy Study Group. *New England Journal of Medicine, 338*(3), 161–165.

Wain, J. C., Wright, C. D., Ryan, D. P., et al. (1999). Induction immunosuppression for lung transplantation with OKT3. *Annals of Thoracic Surgery, 67*(1), 187–193.

Walters, S. (1999). Paediatric treatment issues. *International Journal of Clinical Practice, 103*(Suppl), 26–29.

Weisberg, S. C. (2000). Pharmacotherapy of asthma in children, with special reference to leukotriene receptor antagonists. *Pediatric Pulmonology, 29*(1), 46–61.

Weller, E. B., Weller, R. A., & Davis, G. P. (2000). Use of venlafaxine in children and adolescents: A review of current literature. *Depression and Anxiety, 12*(Suppl 1), 85–89.

Wermeling, D., Record, K., Bell, R., et al. (1985). Hemodialysis clearance of pentobarbital during continuous infusion. *Therapeutic Drug Monitoring, 7*, 485–487.

Wilde, J. T. (2000). Protease inhibitor therapy and bleeding. *Haemophilia, 6*(5), 487–490.

Wilde, J. T., Lee, C. A., Collins, P., et al. (1999). Increased bleeding associated with protease inhibitor therapy in HIV-positive patients with bleeding disorders. *British Journal of Haematology, 107*(3), 556–559.

Williams, R. (2001). Optimal dosing with risperidone: Updated recommendations. *Journal of Clinical Psychiatry, 62*(4), 282–289.

Winston, D. J., Emmanouilides, C., Kroeber, A., et al. (2000). Quinupristin/dalfopristin therapy for infections due to vancomycin-resistant Enterococcus faecium. *Clinical Infectious Disease, 30*(5), 790–797.

Wiseman, L. R., & Faulds, D. (1999). Daclizumab: A review of its use in the prevention of acute rejection in renal transplant recipients. *Drugs, 58*(6), 1029–1042.

Wiznia, A., Stanley, K., Krogstad, P., et al. (2000). *AIDS Research and Human Retroviruses, 16*(12), 1113–1121.

Woodle, E. S., Millis, J. M., So, S. K., et al. (1998).

Liver transplantation in the first three months of life. *Transplantation, 66*(5), 606–609.

Wu, M. J., Ing, T. S., Soung, L. S., et al. (1982). Amantadine hydrochloride pharmacokinetics in patients with impaired renal function. *Clinical Nephrology, 17*, 19–23.

Yanik, G., Levine, J. E., Ratanatharathorn, V., et al. (2000). Tacrolimus (FK506) and methotrexate as prophylaxis for acute graft-versus-host disease in pediatric allogeneic stem cell transplantation. *Bone Marrow Transplantation, 26*(2), 161–167.

Younes, B. S., McDiarmid, S. V., Martin, M. G., et al. (2000). The effect of immunosuppression on posttransplant lymphoproliferative disease in pediatric liver transplant patients. *Transplantation, 70*(1), 94–99.

Zecca, M., & Locatelli, F. (2000). Management of graft-versus-host disease in paediatric bone marrow transplant recipients. *Paediatric Drugs, 2*(1), 29–55.

Zed, P. J. (2000). Low molecular weight heparins and coronary artery disease. *Current Cardiology Reports, 2*(1) 61–68.

APPENDICES

Appendix A

Abbreviations and Symbols

AAP	American Academy of Pediatrics	C_1	drug plasma concentration at time t_1
AAPCC	American Association of Poison Control Centers	C_2	drug plasma concentration at time t_2
ACE	angiotensin-converting enzyme	CAN	compressed air nebulizer
		CAPD	continuous ambulatory peritoneal dialysis
ACT	activated clotting time		
ACTH	corticotropin (adrenocorticotropic hormone)	C_{ave}	average drug plasma concentration at steady state
ADR	adverse drug reaction	CBC	complete blood count
AGA	appropriate for gestational age	cc	cubic centimeter(s)
AHFS	American Hospital Formulary Service	CDC	Centers for Disease Control and Prevention
AIDS	acquired immune deficiency syndrome	CF	conversion factor; cystic fibrosis
		CHF	congestive heart failure
ALP	alkaline phosphatase	CID	continuous infusion device(s)
ALT	alanine aminotransferase (SGPT)	CK	creatinine kinase
		Cl	clearance
am	morning (ante meridiem)	cm	centimeter(s)
aPTT	activated partial thromboplastin time	C_{max}	maximum drug plasma concentration
AST	aspartate aminotransferase (SGOT)	C_{min}	minimum drug plasma concentration
ATP	adenosine triphosphate	CNS	central nervous system
AUC	area under the curve	CO_2	carbon dioxide
AV	atrioventricular	COPD	chronic obstructive pulmonary disease
AW	atomic weight		
AZT	azidothymidine	CPK	creatinine phosphokinase
		CPS	*Compendium of Pharmaceuticals and Specialties*
BCG	Bacillus Calmette-Guerin (vaccine)		
BSA	body surface area	CrCl	creatinine clearance
BUN	blood urea nitrogen	CR	controlled release/continuous release
C	concentration of drug in plasma	C_{ss}	steady-state drug plasma concentration

D	dose	HBV	hepatitis B virus
$D_{2.5}W$	2.5% dextrose in water	HCl	hydrochloride
D_5W	5% dextrose in water	HCt	hematocrit
$D_{10}W$	10% dextrose in water	HD	hemodialysis
$D_{20}W$	20% dextrose in water	HDCR	human diploid-cell rabies (vaccine)
DA	desmethylamiodarone		
DDAVP	desmopressin acetate	Hib	*Haemophilus influenzae* type b
DDP	n-desmethyldoxepin	HIV	human immunodeficiency virus
DES	diethylstilbestrol	HPA	hypothalamic-pituitary-adrenal
DESAD	diethylstilbestrol adenosis	HPB	Health Protection Branch
dl	deciliter(s) (100 ml) (1×10^{-1} liter)	HRI	human rabies immune globulin
DMSA	succimer (2,3-dimercapto-succinic acid)	^{131}I	iodine-131
		ICU	intensive care unit
DNA	deoxyribonucleic acid	ICW	intracellular water
DTaP	acellular pertussis vaccine combined with diphtheria and tetanus toxoids	IG	immune globulin
		IgA	immunoglobulin A
		IgG	immunoglobulin G
DPT	diphtheria and tetanus toxoids with pertussis (vaccine)	IHL	intermittent heparin lock
		IIC	intermittent infusion control
		INH	isoniazid
e	universal constant (2.718281 . . .)	INR	international normalized ratio
ECG	electrocardiogram	IPPB	intermittent positive pressure breathing
ECRI	Emergency Care Research Institute		
		IPV	inactivated poliomyelitis vaccine
ECT	electroconvulsive therapy		
ECW	extracellular water	IU	international unit(s)
EEG	electroencephalogram	IUGR	intrauterine growth retardation
e.g.	for example		
EICD	electronic infusion-control device	K	first-order elimination rate constant
ESR	erythrocyte sedimentation rate	KCl	potassium chloride
ET	endotracheal	kg	kilogram(s) (1×10^3 grams)
et al.	and others	K_m	plasma concentration at which half of the maximal rate of elimination is reached (Michaelis constant)
ETT	endotracheal tube		
F	bioavailability factor		
FAS	fetal alcohol syndrome	kPa	kilopascal(s)
FDA	Food and Drug Administration		
Fe	iron	LDH	lactate dehydrogenase
fl	femtoliter (1×10^{-15} liter)	LGA	large for gestational age
FSH	follicle-stimulating hormone	LH	luteinizing hormone
		LR	lactated Ringer's solution
GFR	glomerular filtration rate	LSD	lysergic acid diethylamide
G-6-PD	glucose-6-phosphate dehydrogenase		
		m^2	meter(s) squared
		M	molar
HbCV	*Haemophilus influenzae* type b conjugate vaccine	MCH	mean corpuscular hemoglobin
		MCHC	mean corpuscular hemoglobin concentration
HBIG	hepatitis B immune globulin		
HBsAg	hepatitis B surface antigen	mCi	millicurie(s)

MCV	mean corpuscular volume	PGE_2	prostaglandin E_2
MDI	metered dose inhaler	pH	hydrogen ion concentration
MDMA	3,4-methylenedioxymeth-amphetamine	pK_a	degree of ionization
		pm	evening (post meridiem)
mEq	milliequivalent(s)	PPD	purified protein derivative
mg	milligram(s) (1×10^{-3} gram)	ppm	parts per million
MIMAPUAY	Mega Interactive Model of Abusable Psychotropic Use Among Youth	PT	prothrombin time
		PTT	partial thromboplastin time
		PVC	polyvinyl chloride
ml	milliliter(s) (1×10^{-3} liter)		
ML-CVP	multilumen central venous pressure	R	infusion rate: Ringer's solution
mm	millimeter(s)	RBC	red blood cell(s)
mm^3	cubic millimeters	RDS	respiratory distress syndrome
mmol	millimole(s)	RE	retinol equivalent
MMR	measles, mumps, and rubella (vaccine)	RIA	radioimmunoassay
		RIG	rabies immune globulin
mOsm	milliosmole(s)		
MVI	intravenous multiple vitamin	SCr	serum creatinine
MW	molecular weight	SGA	small for gestational age
		SGOT	serum glutamic oxaloacetic transaminase (AST)
NaCl	sodium chloride		
NAPA	N-acetylprocainamide	SGPT	serum glutamic pyruvic transaminase (ALT)
nCi	nanocurie(s)		
ng	nanogram(s) (1×10^{-9} gram)	SI	international system of units (Le Système International)
NG	nasogastric		
nkat	nanokatal	SIDS	sudden infant death syndrome
NLO	nasolacrimal occlusion		
nmol	nanomole(s)	SPAG	small particle aerosol generator
No.	number		
NS	normal saline	SSRI	selective serotonin reuptake inhibitor
NSAIDs	nonsteroidal anti-inflammatory drugs		
		STD	sexually transmitted disease
OPV	oral polio virus (vaccine)		
		t_1	time one
p	probability	t_2	time two
$PaCO_2$	partial pressure (tension) of carbon dioxide, arterial	$T_{½}$	half-life
		T_3	triiodothyronine
PBI	protein-bound iodine	T_4	thyroxine
PCA	patient-controlled analgesia; postconceptional age	TB	tuberculosis
		TBW	total body water
PCP	phencyclidine	Td	combined tetanus and diphtheria toxoids, adult type
PD	peritoneal dialysis		
PDR	*Physicians' Desk Reference*	TGIF	Thank God It's Friday
PEEP	positive end expiratory pressure	THC	tetrahydrocannabinol
		TIBC	total iron-binding capacity
PEFR	peak expiratory flow rate	TIG	tetanus immune globulin
PEL	polyethylene	TPN	total parenteral nutrition
PEMA	phenylethylmalonamide	TSH	thyroid-stimulating hormone
pg	picogram(s) (1×10^{-12} gram)	TT	thrombin time

TTY	teletype for the hearing impaired	WHO	World Health Organization
		×	times (multiplied by)
U.K.	United Kingdom	°C	degrees centigrade
UNICEF	United Nations International Children's Emergency Fund	°F	degrees fahrenheit
		μ	micro (mu)
U.S.	United States	μCi	microcurie(s)
USA	United States of America	μg	microgram(s) (1×10^{-6} gram)
USAN	United States Adopted Names	μmol	micromole(s)
USP	United States Pharmacopeia	>	greater than
UTI	urinary tract infection	≥	greater than or equal to
		<	less than
V	apparent volume of distribution	≤	less than or equal to
VACTREL	vertebra, anus, cardiovascular system, trachea, renal tract, esophagus, and limbs	%	percent
		~	approximately
		−	minus; hyphen, to
VMA	vanillylmandelic acid	±	plus or minus
V_{max}	maximum capacity of enzyme system	+	plus (and)
		=	equal to
V/V	volume-to-volume ratio	#	number
VZIG	varicella zoster immune globulin	/	per
		τ	dosing frequency/interval (tau)
WBC	white blood cell(s)		

Appendix B

Normal Pediatric Laboratory Values [1,2]

COMPOUND[3]	AGE GROUP[4]	METRIC VALUE[5]	SI VALUE[6]	CF[7,8]
Alanine aminotransferase (ALT) (SGPT) (serum)	Neonates & infants	6–60 units/liter	100–1000 nkat/liter	16.67
	Children & adolescents	6–36 units/liter	100–600 nkat/liter	16.67
Albumin (serum)	Neonates	2.9–5.5 grams/dl	29–55 grams/liter	10
	Infants	2.4 grams/dl	24 grams/liter	10
	Children & adolescents	3.3–5.8 grams/dl	33–58 grams/liter	10
Aldolase (plasma or serum)	Neonates	<32 units/liter	<540 nkat/liter	16.9
	Children	<16 units/liter	<270 nkat/liter	16.9
	Adolescents	<8 units/liter	<135 nkat/liter	16.9
Alkaline phosphatase (ALP) (serum)	Neonates	30–275 units/liter	500–4585 nkat/liter	16.67
	Infants & children	40–330 units/liter	666–5500 nkat/liter	16.67
	Adolescents	20–120 units/liter	333–2000 nkat/liter	16.67
Ammonia	Neonates	72–217 µg/dl	40–120 µmol/liter	0.554
	Children	40–120 µg/dl	22–66 µmol/liter	0.554
	Adolescents	18–54 µg/dl	10–30 µmol/liter	0.554
Anion gap (plasma)	Children & adolescents	8–16 mEq/liter	8–16 mmol/liter	1

[1] A compilation of the usual normal ranges of common pediatric laboratory values is presented. However, significant variability is observed as a result of such factors as age, fluid and electrolyte imbalance (e.g., hemoconcentration), and techniques used for obtaining or caring for samples. In addition, variability can also occur among laboratories because of the multiple variations in methods of performing the analyses (e.g., assay methodology, temperature). The values presented, therefore, are meant as only a general guide and the reader should always consult the normal reference ranges provided by the laboratory performing the analysis. In addition, pediatric clinicians are reminded, when interpreting laboratory values, of the numerous factors (e.g., drug interactions, laboratory error, pathophysiology) that can contribute to the occurrence of false positive and false negative laboratory test results.
[2] See Table 14-3 for optimum drug serum concentration ranges.
[3] Measurements are presumed to be taken from venous blood unless otherwise noted.
[4] Neonates (0–30 days of age), infants (1–12 months), children (1–12 years), adolescents (13–19 years).
[5] 1 dl = 100 ml
  1 mg/dl – 1 mg/100 ml = 1 mg %
  1 gram/liter = 100 mg/dl = 1 gram % × 10
  mOsm/liter = [(mg/liter) ÷ MW] × number of dissociation parts
  mEq/liter = [(mg/liter) ÷ AW] × valence
  mmol/liter = (mg/liter) ÷ MW
[6] SI units (Le Système International d'Unites).
[7] Metric and SI unit conversion formulas:
  To determine the conversion factor (CF): CF = 1000/molecular weight
  To convert from metric to SI units: (µg/ml) × CF = (µmol/liter)
  To convert from SI units to metric: (µmol/liter)/CF = µg/ml
[8] Atomic Weights (AW) and Valences of Selected Elements:

ELEMENT	AW	VALENCES(S)	ELEMENT	AW	VALENCES(S)
Calcium	40.08	2	Oxygen	16.00	2
Carbon	12.01	4	Phosphorus	30.97	3, 5
Chloride (Chlorine)	35.45	1	Potassium	39.10	1
Hydrogen	1.00	1	Sodium	22.99	1
Magnesium	24.31	2	Sulfur	32.06	2, 4, 6
Nitrogen	14.01	3, 5			

Normal Pediatric Laboratory Values [1,2] continued

COMPOUND[3]	AGE GROUP[4]	METRIC VALUE[5]	SI VALUE[6]	CF[7,8]
Aspartate aminotransferase (AST) (SGOT) (serum)	Neonates	6–65 units/liter	100–1083 nkat/liter	16.67
	Infants	13–74 units/liter	217–1233 nkat/liter	16.67
	Children	10–50 units/liter	167–833 nkat/liter	16.67
	Adolescents	5–41 units/liter	83–683 nkat/liter	16.67
Billirubin, total (serum)	Neonates	1–12 mg/dl	17–205 µmol/liter	17.1
	Premature: <24 hr	1–6 mg/dl	17–100 µmol/liter	17.1
	1–2 days	6–8 mg/dl	100–140 µmol/liter	17.1
	3–5 days	10–12 mg/dl	170–200 µmol/liter	17.1
	Term: <24 hr	2–6 mg/dl	34–100 µmol/liter	17.1
	1–2 days	6–7 mg/dl	100–120 µmol/liter	17.1
	3–5 days	4–12 mg/dl	70–200 µmol/liter	17.1
	Infants, children, & adolescents	0.1–1.5 mg/dl	1.7–25.7 µmol/liter	17.1
Bilirubin, conjugated (direct) (serum)	Neonates	<1.5 mg/dl	<25.7 µmol/liter	17.1
	Infants, children, & adolescents	<0.5 mg/dl	<8.6 µmol/liter	17.1
Bleeding time (Duke/Ivy/Template methods)	Children & adolescents	1–8 min	60–480 sec	60
Body Water		TBW*	ECW*	ICW*
	Neonates	69–79	34–53	28–40
	Infants & children	52–73	20–30	28–53
	Adolescents	50–64	18–26	40–47
	* expressed as % of body weight			
Calcium, total (serum)	Neonates	7–12 mg/dl	1.75–3 mmol/liter	0.25
	Infants	8.8–11.2 mg/dl	2.2–2.8 mmol/liter	0.25
	Children & adolescents	9–11 mg/dl	2.25–2.75 mmol/liter	0.25
Calcium, ionized		4.4–5.4 mg/dl	1.1–1.4 mmol/liter	0.25
Carbon dioxide content, total (Bicarbonate plus CO_2)	Arterial	19–29 mEq/liter	19–29 mmol/liter	1
	Venous	23–33 mEq/liter	23–33 mmol/liter	1
Chloride	Neonates	93–112 mEq/liter	93–112 mmol/liter	1
	Infants	95–110 mEq/liter	95–110 mmol/liter	1
	Children & adolescents	98–108 mEq/liter	98–108 mmol/liter	1
Cholesterol (plasma)	Neonates	45–170 mg/dl	1.17–4.42 mmol/liter	0.026
	Infants	65–175 mg/dl	1.69–4.55 mmol/liter	0.026
	Children & adolescents	120–200 mg/dl	3.12–5.20 mmol/liter	0.026
Creatine kinase (CK) (creatine phosphokinase [CPK]) (serum)	Neonates	10–450 units/liter	167–7500 nkat/liter	16.7
	Infants	20–200 units/liter	333–3334 nkat/liter	16.7
	Children	10–110 units/liter	167–1833 nkat/liter	16.7
	Adolescents (Male)	<190 units/liter	<3167 nkat/liter	16.7
	(Female)	<170 units/liter	<2834 nkat/liter	16.7
Creatinine (serum)	Neonates	≤ 1.8 mg/dl	≤ 159 µmol/liter	88.4
	Infants	≤ 0.6 mg/dl	≤ 53 µmol/liter	88.4
	Children	≤ 1 mg/dl	≤ 88 µmol/liter	88.4
	Adolescents	≤ 1.2 mg/dl	≤ 106 µmol/liter	88.4
Creatinine clearance (urine)	Children & adolescents	75–125 ml/min	1.28–2.13 ml/sec	0.017
Erythrocyte sedimentation rate (ESR)	Neonates	0–2 mm/hr	0–2 mm/hr	1
	Infants & children	3–13 mm/hr	3–13 mm/hr	1
	Adolescents (Male)	1–10 mm/hr	1–10 mm/hr	1
	(Female)	1–20 mm/hr	1–20 mm/hr	1
Ferritin	Neonates	10–300 ng/ml	10–300 µg/liter	1
	Infants	15–300 ng/ml	15–300 µg/liter	1
	Children	10–140 ng/ml	10–140 µg/liter	1
	Adolescents	15–250 ng/ml	15–250 µg/liter	1
Fibrinogen (plasma)	Neonates	150–300 mg/dl	1.5–3 grams/liter	0.01
	Infants & children	200–400 mg/dl	2–4 grams/liter	0.01
	Adolescents	160–300 mg/dl	1.6–3 grams/liter	0.01
Folate (pteroylglutamic acid) (serum)	Children & adolescents	1.9–14 ng/ml	4.3–23.6 nmol/liter	2.266
Gases (arterial)	pO_2	70–105 mmHg	9.3–13 kPa	0.133
	pCO_2	33–46 mmHg	4.4–6 kPa	0.133

Normal Pediatric Laboratory Values [1,2] continued

COMPOUND[3]	AGE GROUP[4]	METRIC VALUE[5]	SI VALUE[6]	CF[7,8]
Glucose (2-hr postprandial) (blood, plasma, or serum)	Neonates	30–90 mg/dl	1.7–5 mmol/liter	0.056
	Infants, children, & adolescents	60–110 mg/dl	3.4–6.2 mmol/liter	0.056
Glucose (urine)	Infants, children, & adolescents	<150 mg/24 hr		
	Infants, children, & adolescents	<50 mg/liter		
Hematocrit*	Neonates	44%–64%	0.44–0.64	0.01
*expressed as % or fraction of RBCs in whole blood sample	Infants	29%–42%	0.29–0.42	0.01
	Children	31%–43%	0.31–0.43	0.01
	Adolescents	36%–49%	0.36–0.49	0.01
Hemoglobin, total	Neonates	13–22 grams/dl	130–220 grams/liter	10
	Infants	10–17 grams/dl	100–170 grams/liter	10
	Children	11–16 grams/dl	110–160 grams/liter	10
	Adolescents	12–17 grams/dl	120–170 grams/liter	10
Hemoglobin (urine)	Infants, children, & adolescents	0	0	1
Iron (serum)	Neonates	110–270 µg/dl	19.7–48.3 µmol/liter	0.179
	Infants	30–70 µg/dl	5.4–12.5 µmol/liter	0.179
	Children	50–150 µg/dl	9–26.9 µmol/liter	0.179
	Adolescents	60–180 µg/dl	11–32 µmol/liter	0.179
Ketones (urine)	Infants, children, & adolescents	0	0	
Lactate		5–20 mg/dl	0.55–2.2 mmol/liter	0.11
Lactate (lactic) dehydrogenase (LDH) (serum)	Neonates	200–500 units/liter	200–500 units/liter	1
	Infants & children	60–250 units/liter	60–250 units/liter	1
	Adolescents	50–225 units/liter	50–225 units/liter	1
Lipase (serum)	Children	20–140 units/liter	20–140 units/liter	
	Adolescents	<190 units/liter	<190 units/liter	
Magnesium (serum)	Children & adolescents	1.9–2.9 mg/dl	0.8–1.2 mmol/liter	0.411
	Children & adolescents	1.6–2.4 mEq/liter	0.8–1.2 mmol/liter	0.5
Magnesium (urine)	Children & adolescents	<150 mg/24 hr	<6.2 mmol/24 hr	0.0411
Mean Corpuscular Hemoglobin (MCH)	Neonates	31–37 pg	31–37 pg	
	Infants & children	23–33 pg	23–33 pg	
	Adolescents	25–35 pg	25–35 pg	
Mean Corpuscular Hemoglobin Concentration (MCHC)	Neonates	29–37 grams/dl	290–370 grams/liter	10
	Infants & children	23–33 grams/dl	230–330 grams/liter	10
	Adolescents	25–36 grams/dl	250–360 grams/liter	10
Mean Corpuscular Volume (MCV)	Neonates	95–115 µm^3	95–115 femtoliter	1
	Infants & children	74–95 µm^3	74–95 femtoliter	1
	Adolescents	78–96 µm^3	78–96 femtoliter	1
Myoglobin (serum)		0	0	
Osmolality (serum)		275–300 mOsm/kg	275–300 mmol/kg	1
Osmolality (urine)		50–1400 mOsm/kg	50–1400 mmol/kg	1
Oxygen saturation (arterial)		90%–100%	90%–100%	1
pH (arterial)		7.35–7.45	7.35–7.45	1
pH (extracellular fluid)		7.35–7.45	7.35–7.45	1
pH (urine)	Neonates	5–7	5–7	1
	Infants & children	4.5–8	4.5–8	1
	Adolescents	5–7	5–7	1
Phenylpyruvic acid	Neonates (4–14 days of age)	<4 mg/dl	<0.04 gram/liter	0.01
Phosphate (as inorganic phosphorus) (serum)	Neonates	3.5–9 mg/dl	1.13–2.91 mmol/liter	0.323
	Infants	3.8–6.7 mg/dl	1.23–2.16 mmol/liter	0.323
	Children	3.6–5.6 mg/dl	1.19–1.81 mmol/liter	0.323
	Adolescents	2.5–5 mg/dl	0.81–1.62 mmol/liter	0.323
Platelet count (thrombocyte count)	Neonates	$(150–450 \times 10^3)$/mm^3	$(150–450 \times 10^9)$/liter	0.001
	Infants	$(200–600 \times 10^3)$/mm^3	$(200–600 \times 10^9)$/liter	0.001
	Children	$(150–550 \times 10^3)$/mm^3	$(150–550 \times 10^9)$/liter	0.001
	Adolescents	$(150–450 \times 10^3)$/mm^3	$(150–450 \times 10^9)$/liter	0.001

Footnotes are on page 785.

Normal Pediatric Laboratory Values [1,2] *continued*

COMPOUND[3]	AGE GROUP[4]	METRIC VALUE[5]	SI VALUE[6]	CF[7,8]
Potassium (serum)	Neonates	3.5–6 mEq/liter	3.5–6 mmol/liter	1
	Infants	4.1–5.3 mEq/liter	4.1–5.3 mmol/liter	1
	Children	3.5–5 mEq/liter	3.5–5 mmol/liter	1
	Adolescents	3.4–5.6 mEq/liter	3.4–5.6 mmol/liter	1
Protein, total (serum)	Neonates	4.2–7.6 grams/dl	42–76 grams/liter	10
	Infants & children	5.3–8 grams/dl	53–80 grams/liter	10
	Adolescents	6.2–9 grams/dl	62–90 grams/liter	10
Protein (urine)		<5 mg/dl	<0.05 gram/liter	0.01
Protein-bound iodine (PBI)		4–8 µg/dl		
Reticulocyte count (RBC)	Neonates	$(4.1–7.1 \times 10^6)/mm^3$	$(41–71 \times 10^9)/liter$	0.001
	Adolescents	$(4–5.7 \times 10^6)/mm^3$	$(40–57 \times 10^9)/liter$	0.001
Sodium (serum)	Neonates	132–142 mEq/liter	132–142 mmol/liter	1
	Infants	139–146 mEq/liter	139–146 mmol/liter	1
	Children & adolescents	135–145 mEq/liter	135–145 mmol/liter	1
Sodium (sweat)		<55 mEq/liter	<55 mmol/liter	1
Specific gravity (urine)	Neonates	1.001–1.020	1.001–1.020	1
	Infants & children	1.001–1.030	1.001–1.030	1
	Adolescents	1.003–1.030	1.003–1.030	1
Thyroid-stimulating hormone (TSH) (serum)		1–8 µunits/ml	1–8 milliunits/liter	1
Thyroxine (T_4) (radioimmunoassay) (serum)	Neonates	10.1–20.9 µg/dl		12.87
	Infants, children, & adolescents	4.5–12.5 µg/dl		12.87
Transferrin (serum)	Neonates	130–275 mg/dl	1.3–2.75 grams/liter	0.01
	Adolescents	220–400 mg/dl	2.2–4 grams/liter	0.01
Triglycerides (serum)	Neonates	<91 mg/dl	<1 mmol/liter	0.011
	Infants	<171 mg/dl	<1.88 mmol/liter	0.011
	Children	20–130 mg/dl	0.22–1.43 mmol/liter	0.011
	Adolescents	30–200 mg/dl	0.33–2.2 mmol/liter	0.011
Triiodothyronine, total (T_3), by RIA (serum)	Neonates	50–350 ng/dl	0.75–5.25 nmol/liter	0.015
	Infants & children	100–260 ng/dl	1.5–3.9 nmol/liter	0.015
	Adolescents	70–210 ng/dl	1.1–3.15 nmol/liter	0.015
Urea nitrogen (BUN)	Neonates & infants	4–15 mg/dl	1.4–5.4 mmol/liter (urea)	0.357
	Children & adolescents	5–25 mg/dl	1.8–9 mmol/liter (urea)	0.357
Uric acid	Neonates	2–8.3 mg/dl	0.12–0.5 mmol/liter	0.06
	Infants & children (Male)	1.5–7.5 mg/dl	0.09–0.45 mmol/liter	0.06
	(Female)	1.8–7.2 mg/dl	0.11–0.43 mmol/liter	0.06
	Adolescents (Male)	2.9–9 mg/dl	0.17–0.54 mmol/liter	0.06
	(Female)	2.2–7.7 mg/dl	0.13–0.46 mmol/liter	0.06
Vanillylmandelic acid (urine)	Neonates	0–1 mg/24 hr	0–5 µmol/24 hr	5
	Infants	0–2 mg/24 hr	0–10 µmol/24 hr	5
	Children & adolescents	1–5 mg/24 hr	5–25 µmol/24 hr	5
White blood cell count (WBC)	Neonates	$(5–35 \times 10^3)/mm^3$	$(5–35 \times 10^9)/liter$	0.001
	Infants	$(6–18 \times 10^3)/mm^3$	$(6–18 \times 10^9)/liter$	0.001
	Children	$(5–15 \times 10^3)/mm^3$	$(5–15 \times 10^9)/liter$	0.001
	Adolescents	$(4–13 \times 10^3)/mm^3$	$(4–13 \times 10^9)/liter$	0.001
Zinc	Children & adolescents	70–150 µg/dl	10.7–22.9 µmol/liter	0.153

Index

In this index, page numbers in *italics* designate figures; page numbers followed by the letter "t" designate tabular material; page numbers followed by the letter "n" designate material in footnotes; the preposition "in" designates drug dosing; the preposition "with" designates drug interactions. *See also* cross-references designate related topics or the location of detailed subentries.

A

Abacavir, in children and adolescents, 558t
Abbreviations and symbols, 781–784
Abenol®. *See* Acetaminophen
Absence seizures. *See also* Seizures
  acetazolamide in, 558t
  methsuximide in, 676t
  valproic acid in, 749–750t
Absorption, developmental considerations, 495–496
Abusable psychotropic drug use, 347–385
  drug-related variables, 354–370
    CNS depressants, 355–360, 356t, 357t, 358t, 359t
    CNS stimulants, 360–365, 362t, 363t, 365t
    psychedelics, 365–370, 367t, 369t, 370t
  epidemiology, 347–348, 348n, 352
  Mega Interactive Model of, 348–354, *350*
    abusable psychotropic dimension, 354
    background and principles, 348–350
    societal dimension, 353–354
    time dimension, 354
    young person dimension, 351–353
  patterns on use, *371*, 371–373
  polydrug abuse, 370–371
  treatment, 373–375, 375t
Accolate®. *See* Zafirlukast
Accutane®. *See* Isotretinoin
Acebutolol, breast milk excretion, 203t
ACE inhibitors. *See also specific drugs*
  adverse drug reactions, 301t
  with lithium salts, 330
  with potassium-sparing diuretics, 333–334
Acenocoumarol, breast milk excretion, 203t
Acetaminophen
  adverse drug reactions, 292t
  breast milk excretion, 203t
  drug interactions, 319
  hepatotoxicity, 258–260
  in infants, children, and adolescents, 558t
  measurement errors, 10
  in neonates, 532t
  teratogenicity/fetotoxicity, 97–98
  with phenytoin, 331
Acetaminophen poisoning/overdosage, 258–262, *261*
  acetylcysteine in, 254t, 260–262, 559t
  antidotes, 254t
Acetazolamide
  breast milk excretion, 203t
  in children and adolescents, 558
  drug interactions, 319
  intravenous infusion, 390t
  in neonates, 532t
  teratogenicity/fetotoxicity, 98
  with phenytoin, 331
  with primidone, 334
Acetohexamide, teratogenicity/fetotoxicity, 98
Acetylcholine, in children and adolescents, 559t
Acetylcysteine
  in acetaminophen poisoning, 254t, 260–262
  in infants, children, and adolescents, 559t
  intravenous infusion, 390t
Acetylsalicylic acid. *See* Aspirin
N-Acetyltransferases, 481–482, 486. *See also* Pharmacogenetics
Acid(s)
  acetylsalicylic. *See* Aspirin
  aminobenzoic, toxicity, 102
  aminocaproic
    adjustments in renal insufficiency, 757t
    in infants, children, and adolescents, 564t
    intravenous infusion, 391t
    in neonates, 533t
    optimal serum concentrations, 761t
  5-aminosalicylic. *See* Mesalamine
  ascorbic
    adverse drug reactions, 310t
    in infants, children, and adolescents, 572t
  ethacrynic
    adverse drug reactions, 308t
    in children and adolescents, 625t
    in neonates, 540t
  excess stomach, ranitidine in, 723–724t
  folic
    breast milk excretion, 214t
    in children and adolescents, 634t
    deficiency, 541t
    deficiency in pregnancy, 109–110
    drug interactions, 329
    intravenous administration, 407t
    in neonates, 541t
    pyrimethamine-related, 721t
    supplementation in pregnancy, 138
    with phenytoin, 332
  mechanism of poisoning, 266–268
  nalidixic
    adverse drug reactions, 294–295t

Acid(s) *continued*
  breast milk excretion, 220t
  teratogenicity/fetotoxicity, 163
pteroylglutamic. *See* Folic acid
salicylic, aspirin conversion factor, 257t
tranexamic
  adjustments in renal insufficiency, 760t
  in children and adolescents, 743-744t
  intravenous administration, 428t
undecylenic, in children and adolescents, 748t
valproic
  adverse drug reactions, 299t
  breast milk excretion, 228t
  in children and adolescents, 749-750t
  drug interactions, 337
  intravenous administration, 429t
  optimal serum concentrations, 762t
  teratogenicity/fetotoxicity, 196-197
  with phenytoin, 333
  with primidone, 334
Acidification, of urine, 252
Acidosis
  lactic, sodium bicarbonate in, 731t
  metabolic, sodium bicarbonate in, 549t
Acilac®. *See* Lactulose
Acne
  as adverse drug effect, 288t
  inflammatory, tetracycline in, 738t
  isotretinoin in, 655t
  vulgaris
    benzoyl peroxide in, 579t
    chlorhexidine in, 595t
    sulfacetamide sodium topical in, 736t
    tazarotene in, 737t
Acquired immunodeficiency syndrome. *See* AIDS/HIV
Act-D. *See* Dactinomycin
ACTH (corticotropin), teratogenicity/fetotoxicity, 120
Acticin®. *See* Permethrin
Actidose®. *See* Activated charcoal
Actinomycin-D. *See* Dactinomycin
Actiq®. *See* Fentanyl
Activated charcoal
  in children and adolescents, 594t
  in poisoning, 248, 250, 251-252
Acyclovir
  adjustments in renal insufficiency, 757t
  adverse drug reactions, 304t
  in children and adolescents, 559-560t
  intravenous infusion, 390t
  in neonates, 532t
  teratogenicity/fetotoxicity, 98

Adalat®. *See* Nifedipine
Adalat XL®. *See* Nifedipine
Adderall®. *See* Amphetamines: mixed
Addison's disease, fludrocortisone in, 630-631t
Adenocard®. *See* Adenosine
Adenosine
  in children and adolescents, 561
  intravenous infusion, 390t
  in neonates, 532t
Adipost®. *See* Phendimetrazine
Administration, 1-86
  of antineoplastic therapy, 503-505, 504t, 505t
  developmental considerations, 2-6
    adolescents, 5-6t
    infants, 3t
    preschoolers, 4-5t
    school agers, 5t
    toddlers, 3-4t
  inhalation dosage forms, 31-38
    compressed-air and other nebulizers, 31-33
    metered-dose inhalers (MDIs), 33-34
    powder inhalers (insufflators), 35-36
    selection, 36
    spacers and other inhalation devices, 34-35
  injectable dosage forms, 42-83
    developmental considerations, 44-45
    dosage forms and related equipment, 45-48
    general considerations, 42-44
    intramuscular, 53-61, 56, 57, 59, 61
    site preparation, 48-49
    subcutaneous injections, 49-53, 50
  intranasal dosage forms, 28-31
    aerosols, 30-31
    creams and ointments, 29
    drops, 29
  intravenous injections and infusions, 61-83
    activity restriction and, 80-81
    complications, 78-80
    equipment, 62-71, 65
    general considerations, 61-62
    intraosseous, 81-83, 82
    technique, 71-78, 72, 73, 74
  ophthalmic dosage forms, 23-27
    developmental considerations, 25-27
    inserts, 25
    ointments, 25
    solutions and suspensions, 23-25
  oral dosage forms, 7-19
    developmental considerations, 16-19
    liquid, 8-11
    solid, 11-16
  otic dosage forms, 27, *28*

rectal dosage forms, 19-22
  enemas, 22
  gels, 21-22
  suppositories, 20-21
routes of, 2t
special considerations, confused or mentally retarded patients, 6-7
topical dosage forms, 36-42
  buccal, sublingual, and other transmucosal, 38-39
  dermatological for localized effect, 37-38
  transdermal, 39-42
vaginal dosage forms, 22-23
Adolescents
  drug administration in, 5-6t, 17-18
  injections administered to, 45
ADR. *See* Doxorubicin
Adrenalin®. *See* Epinephrine
Adrenaline. *See* Epinephrine
Adrenal insufficiency
  as adverse drug effect, 288t
  hydrocortisone in, 543t
  triamcinolone oral in, 744t
Adrenocortical insufficiency
  betamethasone in, 580t
  cortisone in, 604t
Adrenocorticotropic hormone (ACTH). *See* Corticotropin
Adrucil®. *See* Fluorouracil
Advair Diskus®. *See* Salmeterol xinafoate
Adverse drug reactions (ADRs), 283-313. *See also* Drug interactions; Fetotoxicity; Teratogenesis; and *specific drugs and drug classes*
  classification of, 283-284
  diseases and conditions mimicking, 288-291t
  drugs commonly associated with, 291-311t
  establishing, 285-287
  groups associated with, 284t, 285t, 287t
  ipecac syrup, 249
  nicotine transdermal systems, 41
  predictable, 283-284
    drug interactions, 283-284
    secondary effects, 283
    side effects, 283
    toxicity, 284
  reporting, 287
  risk factors for, 284-285
    abrupt alterations in regimen, 285t
    extremes of age, 283t, 285
    female gender, 285
    hepatic or renal dysfunction, 284
    history of previous ADRs, 284
    polydrug therapy, 284
    special care settings, 285
    special drugs, 285, 285t
    special populations, 285
  scopolamine, 40-41

INDEX

tricyclic antidepressants (TCAs), 300t
unpredictable, 284
  allergic effects, 284
  idiosyncratic effects, 284
  intolerance, 284
  vaccines, 435-437, 437, 439-440, 441, 442, 443-444, 445, 446, 447-448, 449, 450-451, 453, 454, 455-456, 458
Advil®. See Ibuprofen
AeroBid®. See Flunisolide pulmonary
Aerochamber inhalant spacer, 35
Aerosols, intranasal, 30
  nicotine intranasal spray, 30
  rhinyles (rhinals), 30-31
Afrin® products. See Oxymetazoline nasal
Aftate®. See Tolnaftate
Age, as risk factor for ADRs, 284t, 285
Agenerase® oral capsules. See Amprenavir oral capsules
Agenerase® oral solution. See Amprenavir oral solution
Aggressive behavior. See also Behavioral disorders
  as adverse drug effect, 288t
Agitation
  chloral hydrate in, 595t
  chlorpromazine in, 536t
  fentanyl in, 540t
  meperidine in, 670t
  pentobarbital in, 702t
Agoraphobia, paroxetine in, 699t
A-hydroCort®. See Hydrocortisone
AIDS/HIV
  abacavir in, 558t
  atovaquone in, 573t
  cryptococcal meningitis in, fluconazole in, 630t
  efavirenz in, 620t
  immunizations in, 434
  lamivudine in, 657-658t
  Mycobacterium avium complex (MSS) disease in, 599-600t
  nelfinavir in, 687t
  Pneumocystis carinii pneumonia
    atovaquone in, 573t
    pentamidine isethionate in, 701t
    trimethoprim/sulfamethoxazole in, 551t, 746t
  postexposure prophylaxis, 43
  as risk factor for ADRs, 285
  ritonavir in, 725-726t
  stavudine in, 734t
  universal precautions for, 1n
  viral infections in, ganciclovir in, 637t
  zalcitabine in, 754t
  zidovudine in, 755t
    adverse drug reactions, 304t
    teratogenicity/fetotoxicity, 200
Air embolism, as complication of intravenous injections, 78

Ak-Con®. See Naphazoline ophthalmic
AK-Homatropine®. See Homatropine
Akinesia, as adverse drug effect, 288t
AK-Pentolate®. See Cyclopentolate
AK-Pred®. See Prednisolone ophthalmic
AK-Sulf®. See Sulfacetamide sodium ophthalmic
AK-Taine®. See Proparacaine
Alamast®. See Pemirolast
Albumin
  intravenous infusion, 390-391t
  in neonates, 532t
Albuterol
  adverse drug reactions, 305t
  in children and adolescents, 561-562t
  intravenous infusion, 391t
  in neonates, 533t
R-Albuterol. See Levalbuterol
Alcaine®. See Proparacaine
Alcohol (ethanol)
  abuse of, 355-356, 356t, 371
  breast milk excretion, 203t
  drugs used during pregnancy containing, 88
  in ethylene glycol or methanol poisoning, 255t, 274
  teratogenicity/fetotoxicity, 98-101, 99t, 100
Alcohol (toxic), 272-275
  benzyl, 42n
  ethylene glycol, 275-276
  isopropyl alcohol, 273
  methanol, 273-275
Alcohol content, of elixirs, 9
Alcoholism. See also Abusable psychotropic drug use; Alcohol (ethanol) abuse of; Withdrawal
  disulfiram in, 617t
Alcohol poisoning, 255t
Aldactone®. See Spironolactone
Aldomet®. See Methyldopa; Methyldopate
Alesse®. See Ethinyl estradiol and levonorgestrel; Oral contraceptives
Alfentanil, drug interactions, 317t
Alglucerase
  in children and adolescents, 562t
  teratogenicity/fetotoxicity, 101-102
Alkalinization
  in salicylate poisoning, 257-258
  of urine, 252-253
Alkalis. See also Caustic poisoning
  mechanism of poisoning, 266
Alka-Mints®. See Calcium carbonate
Alkeran®. See Melphalan
Allegra®. See Fexofenadine
Allerest® eye drops. See Naphazoline ophthalmic
Allerest 12 Hr Nasal Solution®. See Oxymetazoline nasal

Allergic conjunctivitis. See also Allergy; Conjunctivitis
Allergic effects, 284. See also Anaphylaxis
Allergic rhinitis. See under Rhinitis
Allergy. See also Anaphylaxis; Hypersensitivity
  betamethasone in, 580t
  cetirizine in, 594t
  chlorpheniramine in, 597t
  clemastine in, 600t
  cortisone in, 604t
  cromolyn sodium in, 604t
  cyproheptadine in, 606t
  desloratadine in, 609t
  dimenhydrinate in, 615t
  diphenhydramine systemic in, 616t
  hydroxyzine in, 646t
  to vaccines, 433-434
AllerMax®. See Diphenhydramine
Allograft rejection. See Transplantation
Allopurinol
  adjustments in renal insufficiency, 757t
  breast milk excretion, 203t
  in children and adolescents, 562t
  drug interactions, 319
    with anticoagulants, 320
    with azathioprine, 320
    with mercaptopurine, 320
    with theophylline, 320
All-trans-retinoic acid. See Tretinoin
Alocril®. See Nedocromil ophthalmic
Aloin, breast milk excretion, 203t
Alprazolam
  breast milk excretion, 204t
  drug interactions, 317t
Alprostadil
  intravenous infusion, 391t
  in neonates, 533t
Alteplase
  in children and adolescents, 563t
  intravenous infusion, 391t
Alu-Cap®. See Aluminum hydroxide; Aluminum hydroxide antacids
Aluminum contamination, of total nutritional support formulas, 67n
Aluminum hydroxide, in infants, children, and adolescents, 563t
Aluminum hydroxide antacids, adverse drug reactions, 303t
Alupent®. See Metaproterenol
Alu-Tab®. See Aluminum hydroxide
Amantadine
  adjustments in renal insufficiency, 757t
  adverse drug reactions, 304t
  in children and adolescents, 563-564t
  teratogenicity/fetotoxicity, 102
AmBisone®. See Amphotericin B liposome

Amebiasis. *See also* Parasitic infestations
  iodoquinol in, 651t
  metronidazole in, 678t
  paromomycin in, 698t
Amerge®. See Naratriptan
Americaine®. See Benzocaine
Americaine Anesthetic Lubricant®. See Benzocaine
Americaine Otic®. See Benzocaine
A-methaPred®. See Methylprednisolone sodium succinate
Amethopterin. *See* Methotrexate
Amicar. See Aminocaproic acid
Amifostine,
  dosing, 507t
  intravenous infusion, 391t
Amikacin
  adjustments in renal insufficiency, 757t
  in infants, children, and adolescents, 564t
  in neonates, 533t
  optimal serum concentrations, 761t
Amikacin, adverse drug reactions, 293t
Amikacin sulfate, intravenous infusion, 391t
Amikin®. See Amikacin
Aminobenzoic acid, teratogenicity/fetotoxicity, 102
Aminocaproic acid
  adjustments in renal insufficiency, 757t
  in infants, children, and adolescents, 564t
  intravenous infusion, 391t
  in neonates, 533t
  optimal serum concentrations, 761t
Aminoglutethimide
  drug interactions, 317t
  teratogenicity/fetotoxicity, 102
Aminoglycosides
  adverse drug reactions, 293t
  drug interactions, 319
  with methotrexate, 320
  with neuromuscular blockers, 320
  with penicillins, 320
Aminophylline
  adverse drug reactions, 305t
  intravenous infusion, 391t
  in neonates, 533t
  teratogenicity/fetotoxicity, 102
5-Aminosalicylic acid. *See* Mesalamine
Aminosalicylic acid
  breast milk excretion, 204t
  teratogenicity/fetotoxicity, 102
Amiodarone
  adverse drug reactions, 305t
  breast milk excretion, 204t
  in children and adolescents, 565t
  drug interactions, 317t, 319
  intravenous administration, 392t

  teratogenicity/fetotoxicity, 103
  with anticoagulants, 320
  with digitalis glycosides, 320
Amitriptyline
  in adolescents, 565-566t
  adverse drug reactions, 300t
  breast milk excretion, 204t
  drug interactions, 317t
Amlodipine, drug interactions, 317t
Ammonium chloride
  in children and adolescents, 566t
  intravenous administration, 392t
Amotivational syndrome, marijuana and, 368
Amoxapine, breast milk excretion, 204t
Amoxicillin
  adjustments in renal insufficiency, 757t
  adverse drug reactions, 294t
  breast milk excretion, 204t
  in children and adolescents, 566t
  in neonates, 534t
Amoxicillin and potassium clavulanate, in infants, children, and adolescents, 566-567t
Amoxil®. See Amoxicillin
Amphetamines
  abuse of, 360t, 360-362, 362t
  breast milk excretion, 204t
  mixed
    adverse drug reactions, 307t
    in children and adolescents, 567-568t
Amphojel®. See Aluminum hydroxide
Amphotericin B
  adverse drug reactions, 300t
  in infants, children, and adolescents, 568t
  intravenous administration, 392t
  in neonates, 534t
  teratogenicity/fetotoxicity, 103
Amphotericin B lipid complex, intravenous administration, 392t
Amphotericin B liposome
  in infants, children, and adolescents, 568-569t
  intravenous administration, 392t
Ampicillin
  adjustments in renal insufficiency, 757t
  breast milk excretion, 204-205t
  in children and adolescents, 569t
  intravenous administration, 392-393t
  in neonates, 534t
  teratogenicity/fetotoxicity, 103
Ampicillin/sulbactam, intravenous administration, 393t
Amprenavir
  drug interactions, 317t
  oral capsules, in children and adolescents, 569-570t
  oral solution, in children and adolescents, 570t
Ampules, 46
AMSA®. See Amsacrine

Amsacrine
  dosing, 507t
  intravenous administration, 393t
AMSA P-D®. See Amsacrine
Amyl nitrate inhalant, in cyanide poisoning, 254t
Anabolic steroids
  drug interactions, 319, 320
  with cyclosporine, 327
Analgesics, adverse drug reactions, 292t
Anaphylaxis
  as adverse drug effect, 288t
  diphenhydramine systemic in, 616t
  epinephrine in, 622t
Anaprox®. See Naproxen sodium
Anbesol®. See Benzocaine
Ancef®. See Cefazolin
Ancobon®. See Flucytosine
Ancrod, teratogenicity/fetotoxicity, 103
Anectine®. See Succinylcholine; Succinylcholine chloride
Anemia
  autoimmune hemolytic
    betamethasone in, 580t
    cortisone in, 604t
  drug-related, epoetin alfa in, 623t
  iron-deficiency
    iron dextran injectable in, 653t
    iron oral in, 652t
  iron deficiency, ferrous sulfate in, 541t
  megaloblastic, folic acid in, 541t
Anergan 50®. See Promethazine
Anesthesia
  general
    methohexital in, 675t
    midazolam in premedication, 680t
    propofol in, 717-718t
    rocuronium as adjunct, 726t
    sevoflurane in, 730t
  local
    benzocaine in, 578t
    bupivacaine in, 585t
    ophthalmic, proparacaine in, 717t
    succinylcholine in, 550t
  topical
    for intramuscular injection, 60-61
    lidocaine and prilocaine in, 662t
    for venipuncture, 75-76
Anesthetics, inhalation, teratogenicity, 103-104
Anethole trithione. *See* Anetholtrithion
Anetholtrithion, in adolescents, 570t
Anexate®. See Flumazenil
Angioedema, clemastine in, 600t
Angiotensin-converting enzyme inhibitors. *See* ACE inhibitors; Antihypertensives
Animal data, limitations of extrapolation to humans, 87

INDEX

Anorexia, as adverse drug effect, 288t
Antabuse®. See Disulfiram
Antacids
  adverse drug reactions, 303t
  drug interactions, 319-320
    with phenytoin, 331
    with tetracyclines, 335
Anthrax vaccine, adsorbed, 571t
  in adolescents, 571t
Antiarthritics, adverse drug reactions, 292-293t
Antibiotic-associated diarrhea, 657t
Antibiotic-associated pseudomembranous colitis, vancomycin in, 551t
Antibiotics. *See also specific drugs*
  adverse drug reactions
    aminoglycosides, 293t
    cephalosporins, 293-294t
    fluoroquinolones, 294t
    macrolides, 294t
    miscellaneous, 295-297
    penicillins, 294t
    quinolones, 294-295t
    sulfonamides, 295t
    tetracyclines, 295t
  in caustic poisoning, 269
Anticholinergic drug overdosage, physostigmine salicylate in, 706t
Anticholinergic poisoning, antidotes, 254t
Anticoagulant overdosage, phytonadione in, 707t
Anticoagulants. *See also* Coagulation disorders
  adverse drug reactions, 297-299t
  drug interactions, 320
  in infants, children, and adolescents, 753-754t
  lepirudin, 660t
  with amiodarone, 320
Anticonvulsants
  adverse drug reactions, 298-299t
  drug interactions, 320-321
  measurement of, 11
Antidepressants. *See also specific drugs*
  adverse drug reactions, 299-300t
  selective serotonin reuptake inhibitors (SSRI), 300t
  tricyclic antidepressants (TCAs), 300t
  tricyclic, drug interactions, 322
  tricyclic, with anticonvulsants, 321-322
Antidotes, to common pediatric poisons, 253, 254t-256t
Antidysrhythmics, adverse drug reactions, 305-306t. *See also specific drugs*
Antiemetics, 497-500, 499t
Antifungals. *See also* Antibiotics; Antivirals; *and specific drugs*
  adverse drug reactions, 300-301t
Antihemophilic Factor VIII (Recombinant), in infants, children, and adolescents, 571t

Antihist-1®. See Clemastine
Antihistamine poisoning, 265-266
Antihistamines, adverse drug reactions, 301t
Antihypertensives. *See also* Diuretics
  adverse drug reactions, 301-302t
  ACE inhibitors, 301t
  beta-adrenergic blockers, 301-302t
  miscellaneous, 302t
Antilirium®. See Physostigmine; Physostigmine salicylate
Antimanics, adverse drug reactions, 302-303t
Antiminth®. See Pyrantel pamoate
Antineoplastics
  dolasetron in prevention of vomiting, 618t
  nausea and vomiting, ondansetron in, 693t
Antineoplastic therapy, 493-529
  background and epidemiology, 493-495, 494
  dosing, 507-525t
  guidelines for use, 501-506
    administration, 503-505, 504t, 505t
    post-treatment care, 505-506, 506t
    reconstituting drugs and preparing for transit, 502-503
  pediatric considerations, 495-501
    cardiotoxicity, 497
    disposition in children, 496
    growth and development, 495-496
    intrathecal therapy, 496
    myelotoxicity and infection, 497
    neurotoxicity, 497, 498t
    renal toxicity, 497
    proactive pharmacological intervention, 497-500
    emetogenic potential and antiemetics, 497-500, 498t, 499t
    therapeutic drug monitoring, 500-501, 501t
Antipsychotics. *See also* Psychosis
  adverse drug reactions, 303t
  special formulations, 42n
Antispas®. See Dicyclomine
Anti-Tuss®. See Guaifenesin
Antiulcer drugs, adverse drug reactions, 303-304t
Antivenin (Crotalidae) polyvalent, in children and adolescents, 571-572t
Antivert®. See Meclizine
Antivirals. *See also* Antibiotics; Antifungals
  adverse drug reactions, 304t
Antizol®. See Fomepizole
Anxiety
  diazepam in, 611t

  meperidine in preoperative, 670t
  meprobamate in, 671t
  pentobarbital in, 702t
Anxiety disorders
  chlordiazepoxide in, 595t
  paroxetine in, 699t
Anzemet®. See Dolasetron
Apnea
  aminophylline in, 533t
  caffeine citrate in, 535t
  theophylline in, 550t
Apo-Cloxi®. See Cloxacillin
Apo-Metformin®. See Metformin
Apo-Tetra®. See Tetracyclines
Apresoline®. See Hydralazine
AquaMEPHYTON®. See Phytonadione
Ara-C. See Cytarabine
Aralen®. See Chloroquine
Arava®. See Leflunomide
Aristocort®. See Triamcinolone; Triamcinolone oral; Triamcinolone topical
Arsenic poisoning
  antidotes, 254t
  penicillamine in, 700t
Arsenic trioxide, dosing, 507t
Arthritis
  as adverse drug effect, 288t
  juvenile rheumatoid
    aspirin in, 573t
    betamethasone in, 580t
    celecoxib in, 593t
    cortisone in, 604t
Arthrotec®. See Diclofenac oral
Arylamine *N*-acetyltransferases, 481-482. *See also* Pharmacogenetics
Asacol®. See Mesalamine
Ascariasis. *See also* Parasitic infestations
  mebendazole in, 668t
  pyrantel pamoate in, 719-720t
  thiabendazole in, 740t
Ascites, spironolactone in, 549t, 734t
Ascorbic acid. *See under* Acid(s)
Asparaginase
  dosing, 508t
  intravenous administration, 393t
Aspergillus. See Fungal infections
Aspergum®. See Aspirin
Aspiration, of hydrocarbons, 270-272
Aspirin. *See also* Aspirin poisoning
  adverse drug reactions, 292t
  breast milk excretion, 205t
  in children and adolescents, 572-573t
  conversion factors, 257t
  optimal serum concentrations, 761t
  teratogenicity/fetotoxicity, 104-105
Aspirin poisoning, 253, 256-258, 257t
Assessment, in pediatric poisoning, 247
Astelin®. See Azelastine nasal

Astemizole, 265
  drug interactions, 317t, 319t
Asthma. *See also* Bronchospasm; Inhalation dosage forms; Nebulizers
  as adverse drug effect, 288t
  albuterol in, 561-562t
  beclomethasone in, 577-578t
  budesonide in, 584t
  cromolyn sodium in, 605t
  ephedrine in, 622t
  flunisolide pulmonary in, 632t
  formoterol fumarate in, 635t
  hydrochlorothiazide in, 645t
  ipratropium pulmonary in, 652t
  isoetharine in, 653-654t
  isoproterenol in, 654-655t
  ketotifen in, 657t
  metaproterenol in, 673t
  nedocromil pulmonary in, 687t
  salmeterol xinafoate in, 728t
  terbutaline in, 738t
  theophylline in, 739-740t
  triamcinolone pulmonary in, 744t
  zafirlukast in, 754-755t
  zileuton in, 755t
Atarax®. See Hydroxyzine
Atasol®. See Acetaminophen
Ataxia, as adverse drug effect, 288t
Atenolol
  adverse drug reactions, 301t
  breast milk excretion, 205t
  in children and adolescents, 573t
  teratogenicity/fetotoxicity, 105
Atgam®. See Lymphocyte immune globulin
Ativan®. See Lorazepam
Ativase®. See Alteplase
Atopic dermatitis, pimecrolimus in, 707t
Atorvastatin, drug interactions, 317t
Atovaquone, in adolescents, 573t
ATRA. *See* Tretinoin
Atracurium
  adverse drug reactions, 309t
  in infants, children, and adolescents, 574t
Atracurium besylate, intravenous administration, 393t
Atrial tachydysrhythmias. *See also* Cardiac dysrhythmias
  procainamide in, 714t
  quinidine in, 722t
Atropine. *See also* Atropine poisoning
  adverse drug reactions, 297t
  breast milk excretion, 205t
  in neonates, 534t
  ophthalmic, in children and adolescents, 574t
  systemic, in infants, children, and adolescents, 574t-575t
  teratogenicity/fetotoxicity, 105-106
Atropine-1®. See Atropine: ophthalmic
Atropine-Care®. See Atropine: ophthalmic

Atropine poisoning, antidotes, 254t
Atropine sulfate
  intravenous administration, 393t
  in organophosphate or carbamate poisoning, 256t
Atropisol®. See Atropine ophthalmic
Atrovent®. See Ipratropium bromide
Atrovent Nasal Spray®. See Ipratropium nasal
Attention deficit/hyperactivity disorder (A-D/HD)
  methamphetamine in, 674t
  methylphenidate in, 677t
  mixed amphetamines in, 567t, 610t
  pemoline in, 699-700t
Augmentin®. See Amoxicillin and potassium clavulanate
Auro Ear Drops®. See Carbamide peroxide
Aurolate®. See Gold sodium thiomalate
Autoimmune hemolytic anemia
  betamethasone in, 580t
  cortisone in, 604t
Avapro®. See Irbesartan
AV block, atropine systemic in, 574t
Avelox®. See Moxifloxacin
Aventyl®. See Nortriptyline
Azacitidine, dosing, 508t
Azactam®. See Aztreonam
Azathioprine
  adjustments in renal insufficiency, 757t
  in children and adolescents, 575t
  drug interactions, 322
  intravenous administration, 393-394
  teratogenicity/fetotoxicity, 106
  with allopurinol, 320
Azelastine, nasal, in children and adolescents, 575t
Azidothymidine. *See* Zidovudine
Azithromycin
  adverse drug reactions, 294t
  breast milk excretion, 205t
  in infants, children, and adolescents, 575-576t
  intravenous administration, 394t
Azmacort®. See Triamcinolone pulmonary
Azo-Gesic®. See Phenazopyridine
Azo-Standard®. See Phenazopyridine
AZT. *See* Zidovudine
Aztreonam
  adjustments in renal insufficiency, 757t
  adverse drug reactions, 295t
  breast milk excretion, 205t
  in infants, children, and adolescents, 576t
  intravenous administration, 394t
Azulfidine®. See Sulfasalazine
Azulfidine EN-tabs®. See Sulfasalazine

B

Babee Teething®. See Benzocaine
Bacid®. See Lactobacillus acidophilus
Baciguent®. See Bacitracin
Bacitin®. See Bacitracin
Bacitracin, in children and adolescents, 576t
Baclofen
  breast milk excretion, 205t
  in children and adolescents, 576t
Bacterial endocarditis, ampicillin in, 569t
Bacterial infections
  amikacin in, 564t
  amoxicillin and potassium clavulanate in, 566-567t
  amoxicillin in, 534t, 566t
  ampicillin in, 569t
  aztreonam in, 576t
  carbenicillin indanyl sodium in, 588t
  cefaclor in, 589t
  cefamandole in, 589t
  cefazolin in, 536t, 589t
  cefixime in, 590t
  cefoperazone in, 590t
  cefotaxime in, 590t
  cefoxitin in, 590-591t
  cefprozil in, 592t
  ceftazidime in, 592t
  ceftizoxime in, 592t
  ceftriaxone axetil in, 593t
  ceftriaxone in, 593t
  cephalexin in, 594t
  cephalothin in, 594t
  chloramphenicol in, 536t, 595t
  ciprofloxacin in, 599t
  clindamycin in, 537t, 600t
  cloxacillin in, 537t, 602t
  in cystic fibrosis
    aztreonam in, 576t
    gentamicin in, 637t
    tobramycin inhalation in, 742t
  dicloxacillin in, 612t
  erythromycin in, 624t
  furazolidone in diarrhea, 636t
  gentamicin in, 542t, 637t
  gentian violet in, 638t
  imipenem/cilastatin in, 647t
  immune globulin in, 543t
  linezolid in, 663-664t
  loracarbef in, 665-666t
  meropenem in, 672t
  metronidazole in, 545t, 678-679t
  minocycline in, 681t
  mupirocin nasal in, 683-684t
  nafcillin in, 685t
  neomycin in, 687-688t
  netilmicin in, 688t
  oxacillin in, 695t
  penicillin in, 548t
  penicillin G in, 546t, 547t, 701t
  penicillin G procaine in, 701t
  penicillin V potassium in, 701t
  piperacillin in, 708t
  polymyxin B sulfate systemic in, 709t

quinupristin and dalfopristin in vancomycin-resistant *Enterococcus faecium*, 723t
rifampin in, 724t
sulfacetamide sodium in, 550t
sulfisoxazole in, 737t
tetracycline in, 738t
ticarcillin and clavulanate in, 742t
tobramycin in, 550t
trimethoprim/sulfamethoxazole in, 551t, 746t, 747t
troleandomycin in, 748t
vancomycin in, 551t, 750t
Bacterial meningitis
 ampicillin in, 534t, 569t
 ceftriaxone in, 536t
 chloramphenicol in, 595t
 penicillin G in, 546t
Bacterial vaginosis, metronidazole in, 678t
Bactrim®. See Co-trimoxazole
Bactroban®. See Mupirocin topical
Bactroban Nasal®. See Mupirocin nasal
BAL in Oil®. See Dimercaprol
Balminil®. See Guaifenesin
Barbiturates. See also specific drugs
 adverse drug reactions, 309-310t
 drug interactions, 317t, 322
 with carbamazepine, 323
 with chloramphenicol, 325
 with cyclosporine, 327
 with phenytoin, 331-332
 with primidone, 334
 with theophylline, 335
 with valproic acid, 337
Basiliximab, in children and adolescents, 577t
BCG vaccine
 drug interactions, 322
 teratogenicity/fetotoxicity, 106
Beclomethasone
 adverse drug reactions, 307t
 nasal, in children and adolescents, 577t
 pulmonary, in children and adolescents, 577-578t
 with hydrofluoroalkane propellant, 33n
Bedridden children, drug administration in, 18
Beepen-VK®. See Penicillin V potassium
Behavioral disorders
 as adverse drug effect, 288t
 chlorpromazine in severe, 597t
 risperidone in, 725t
 thioridazine in, 741t
Belladonna, teratogenicity/fetotoxicity, 106-107
Benadryl®. See Diphenhydramine
Bendroflumethiazide
 breast milk excretion, 205t
 teratogenicity/fetotoxicity, 107
BeneFix®. See Factor IX complex
Benemid®. See Probenecid

Benign Rolandic epilepsy, carbamazepine in, 587t
Benoxyl®. See Benzoyl peroxide
Bentyl®. See Dicyclomine
Bentylol®. See Dicyclomine
Benuryl®. See Probenecid
Benylin DM®, See Dextromethorphan
Benzocaine
 anesthetic lubricant, 578t
 otic, 578t
 topical, 578-579t
Benzodiazepine poisoning/overdosage
 antidotes, 254t
 flumazenil in, 541t, 631t
Benzodiazepines. See also specific drugs
 adverse drug reactions, 298t, 310t
 as antiemetics, 499t
 drug interactions, 323
 with valproic acid, 337
Benzoyl peroxide
 in adolescents, 579t
 teratogenicity/fetotoxicity, 107
Benztropine, teratogenicity/fetotoxicity, 107
Benzyl alcohol, 42n
Bepridil, drug interactions, 317t
Beractant, in neonates, 534t
Beriberi, thiamine in, 740t
Beta-adrenergic blockers. See Beta-blockers
Beta-blocker poisoning, antidotes, 254t
Beta-blockers. See also specific drugs
 adverse drug reactions, 301t, 305t
 drug interactions, 323
Betachron E-R®. See Propranolol
Betadine®. See Povidone-iodine
Betaine, in infants, children, and adolescents, 579t
Betaject®. See Betamethasone
Betamethasone
 in children and adolescents, 580t
 injectable, 580t
 oral, 580t
 topical, 580t
Betasept®. See Chlorhexidine
Beta thalassemia, deferoxamine in, 609t
Bethanechol, in children and adolescents, 581t
Biaxin®. See Clarithromycin
Biaxin XL®. See Clarithromycin
Bicillin L-A®. See Penicillin G benzathine
BiCNU®. See Carmustine
Biltricide®. See Praziquantel
Bioallethrin/piperonyl butoxide, in infants, children, and adolescents, 581t
Biotransformation. See Pharmacokinetics
Bipolar disorder. See also Depression
 lithium in, 664-665t

Biquin®. See Quinidine
Bisacodyl
 adverse drug reactions, 309t
 in children and adolescents, 581-582t
Bismuth subsalicylate
 aspirin conversion factor, 257t
 in children and adolescents, 582t
Bleeding/hemorrhage. See also Coagulation disorders *and specific disorders*
 as adverse drug effect, 288t
Blenoxane®. See Bleomycin
Bleomycin
 dosing, 508t
 intravenous administration, 394t
Bleph-10®. See Sulfacetamide sodium ophthalmic
Blepharospasm, botulinum toxin type A in, 582t
Blood dyscrasias. See also Coagulation disorders
 as adverse drug effect, 288t
Blood pressure, restoration and maintenance of, norepinephrine in, 691-692t
Blood replacement therapy, immunizations and, 435
Body surface area (BSA), 495
Bonamine®. See Meclizine
Bone marrow transplant, cyclopentolate in, 605t
Bonine®. See Meclizine
Bontril®. See Phendimetrazine
Borofax Skin Protectant®. See Zinc oxide
Botox®. See Botulinum toxin type A
Bottles, intravenous solution, 63
Botulinum toxin type A, in children and adolescents, 582-583t
Bowel preparation
 bisacodyl in, 581-582t
 magnesium citrate in, 668t
 neomycin in, 688t
 polyethylene glycol and electrolyte solutions in, 708-709t
Bradycardia. See also Cardiac dysrhythmias
 aminophylline in, 533t
 atropine in, 534t
 theophylline in, 550t
Bradycardia and syncope, atropine systemic in, 574t
Breast feeding, immunizations and, 434
Breast milk secretion, 201-243, 227t
 absorption, 202
 drugs excreted, 203-229t. See also specific drugs
 metabolism and excretion, 202
Brethine®. See Terbutaline
Bretylium, breast milk secretion, 205t
Brevibloc®. See Esmolol
Brevicon®. See Ethinyl estradiol/norethindrone; Oral contraceptives

Brevital®. *See* Methohexital
Brevoxyl®. *See* Benzoyl peroxide
Bricanyl. *See* Terbutaline
Bromocriptine
   breast milk excretion, 205t
   drug interactions, 317t
Brompheniramine
   in children and adolescents, 583t
   teratogenicity/fetotoxicity, 107
Bronchitis
   cefpodoxime proxetil in bacterial exacerbation, 591t
   isoetharine in, 653-654t
   loracarbef in, 666t
Bronchodilators, adverse drug reactions, 305t
Bronchopulmonary dysplasia, furosemide in, 541t
Bronchospasm. *See also* Asthma
   as adverse drug effect, 288t
   aminophylline in, 533t
   exercise-induced, salmeterol xinafoate in prophylaxis, 728t
   ipratropium pulmonary in, 652t
   isoetharine in, 653-654t
   levalbuterol in, 660-661t
   theophylline in, 550t
Bronkometer®. *See* Isoetharine
Bronkosol®. *See* Isoetharine
Buccal dosage forms, 38-39
Budesonide
   administration, 31
   nasal, in children and adolescents, 584t
   pulmonary, in infants, children, and adolescents, 584t
Budesonide suspension, contraindications, 31t
Bulimia nervosa, fluoxetine in, 633t
Bumetanide
   in adolescents, 584t
   drug interactions, 323
   intravenous administration, 394t
Bupivacaine
   in children and adolescents, 585t
   teratogenicity/fetotoxicity, 107-108
Bupropion, breast milk excretion, 206t
Burinex®. *See* Bumetanide
Burns
   chlorhexidine in, 596t
   mafenide in, 666-667t
Buspirone, drug interactions, 317t
Busulfan
   dosing, 508t
   teratogenicity/fetotoxicity, 108
Butabarbital, breast milk excretion, 206t
Butenafine, in adolescents, 586t
Butoconazole, in adolescents, 586t
Butorphanol, breast milk excretion, 206t
Butyrophenones, adverse drug reactions, 303t

C

Cafcit®. *See* Caffeine citrate
Caffeine
   breast milk excretion, 206t
   drug interactions, 317t
   teratogenicity/fetotoxicity, 108-109
Caffeine citrate
   intravenous administration, 394t
   in neonates, 535t
Calamine, in temporary itching, 586t
Calan®. *See* Verapamil
Calcijex®. *See* Calcitriol
Calcitriol, in infants, children, and adolescents, 586t
Calcium, in infants, children, and adolescents, 586-587t
Calcium carbonate
   adverse drug reactions, 303t
   in children and adolescents, 587t
Calcium-channel blocker poisoning, antidotes, 254t
Calcium-channel blockers. *See also specific drugs*
   adverse drug reactions, 306-307t
Calcium chloride
   in calcium-channel blocker poisoning, 254t
   intravenous administration, 395t
   in neonates, 535t
Calcium deficiency, prophylaxis in renal disease, 586-587t
Calcium Disodium Versenate®. *See* Edetate calcium disodium (EDTA)
Calcium gluconate
   intravenous administration, 395t
   in neonates, 535t
Calcium salts, teratogenicity/fetotoxicity, 109
Caldesene®. *See* Undecylenic acid
Camptosar®. *See* Irinotecan
Cancer chemotherapy, 493-529. *See also* Antineoplastic therapy
Candida infection. *See* Fungal infections; Vulvovaginal candidiasis
Candistatin®. *See* Nystatin
Canesten®. *See* Clotrimazole
Cannabis. *See* Marijuana
Capoten®. *See* Captopril
Capsules, types of, 14
Captopril
   adjustments in renal insufficiency, 757t
   adverse drug reactions, 301t
   breast milk excretion, 206t
   in infants, children, and adolescents, 587t
   in neonates, 535t
   teratogenicity/fetotoxicity, 109
Carafate®. *See* Sucralfate
Carbamate poisoning, 256t
Carbamazepine
   adverse drug reactions, 298t
   breast milk excretion, 206t
   drug interactions, 317t, 323-324
   in infants, children, and adolescents, 587t
   optimal serum concentrations, 761t
   teratogenicity/fetotoxicity, 109-110
   with theophylline, 335
Carbamide peroxide
   for intra-oral use, in children and adolescents, 588t
   for otic use, in children and adolescents, 588t
Carbenicillin indanyl, adverse drug reactions, 294t
Carbenicillin indanyl sodium, in infants, children, and adolescents, 588t
Carbimazole, breast milk excretion, 206t
Carbolith®. *See* Lithium
Carboplatin
   dosing, 509t
   intravenous administration, 395t
Cardarone®. *See* Amiodarone
Cardene®. *See* Nicardipine
Cardiac arrest
   calcium chloride in, 535t
   epinephrine in, 539t, 622-623t
   sodium bicarbonate in, 731t
Cardiac dysrhythmias. *See also specific dysrhythmias*
   adenosine in, 532t, 561t
   as adverse drug effect, 288t
   aminophylline in, 533t
   amiodarone in, 565t
   atropine in, 534t
   atropine systemic in, 574t
   digoxin in, 538t
   in digoxin toxicity, phenytoin in, 706t
   disopyramide in, 617t
   esmolol in, 625t
   flecainide in, 630t
   lidocaine in, 544t, 662t
   mexiletine in, 679t
   procainamide in, 714t
   propafenone in, 716t
   propranolol in, 548t, 718t
   quinidine in, 722t
   theophylline in, 550t
   verapamil in, 751t
Cardiac failure, as adverse drug effect, 288t
Cardiac insufficiency, sodium nitroprusside in postsurgical, 549t
Cardiogenic shock
   dobutamine in, 617t
   dopamine in, 618t
Cardioquin®. *See* Quinidine
Cardiotoxicity, of antineoplastics, 497, 498t
Cardiovascular collapse, atropine systemic in, 575t
Cardiovascular drugs. *See also specific drugs*
   adverse drug reactions, 305-307t

INDEX

antidysrhythmics, 305-306t
calcium-channel blockers, 306-307t
positive inotropic drugs, 307t
vasodilators, 307t
Carisoprodol
breast milk excretion, 206t
drug interactions, 317t
Carmustine
dosing, 509t
drug interactions, 324
intravenous administration, 395t
with cimetidine, 325
Carvedilol, drug interactions, 317t
Casanthranol, teratogenicity/fetotoxicity, 110
Cascara sagrada
adverse drug reactions, 309t
breast milk excretion, 206t
in infants, children, and adolescents, 588t
teratogenicity/fetotoxicity, 110
Castor oil, in infants, children, and adolescents, 589t
Cataflam®. See Diclofenac oral
Catapres®. See Clonidine
Cataract extraction, complications, diclofenac ophthalmic in, 612t
Cataracts, as adverse drug effect, 289t
Cathartics, in poisoning, 250-251
Catheters. *See also* Extravasation
central venous access, 67-69, 563t
implantable, 69-70
midline, 69
peripherally inserted, 69
for intravenous injections, 69-71. *See also* Venous access devices
irritation from, phenazopyridine in, 703t
Caustic poisoning, 266-270. *See also* Acids; Alkalis; *specific compounds*
antibiotics in, 269
complications of, 269-270
contraindications in, 249-250
corticosteroids in, 268-269
esophageal dilation and surgery in, 269
esophagoscopy in, 268
esophagrams in, 269
immediate treatment, 268
CCNU. *See* Lomustine
Ceclor®. See Cefaclor
CeeNU®. See Lomustine
Cefaclor
adjustments in renal insufficiency, 757t
adverse drug reactions, 293t
in infants, children, and adolescents, 589t
Cefadroxil
adjustments in renal insufficiency, 757t
adverse drug reactions, 293t
breast milk excretion, 206t
in infants, children, and adolescents, 589t
Cefadyl®. See Cephaprin
Cefamandole
adjustments in renal insufficiency, 757t
adverse drug reactions, 293t
in infants, children, and adolescents, 589t
Cefamandole nafate, intravenous administration, 395t
Cefazolin
adjustments in renal insufficiency, 757t
adverse drug reactions, 293t
breast milk excretion, 206t
in infants, children, and adolescents, 589t
Cefepime
in infants, children, and adolescents, 590t
intravenous administration, 396t
Cefixime
adjustments in renal insufficiency, 757t
adverse drug reactions, 293t
in infants, children, and adolescents, 590t
Cefizox®. See Ceftizoxime
Cefobid®. See Cefoperazone
Cefonicid, breast milk excretion, 206t
Cefoperazone
adverse drug reactions, 293t
in infants, children, and adolescents, 590t
intravenous administration, 396t
Cefotaxime
adjustments in renal insufficiency, 757t
adverse drug reactions, 293t
breast milk excretion, 207t
in infants, children, and adolescents, 590t
intravenous administration, 396t
in neonates, 536t
Cefoxitin
adjustments in renal insufficiency, 757t
adverse drug reactions, 293t
in infants, children, and adolescents, 590-591t
intravenous administration, 396t
Cefpodoxime, adverse drug reactions, 293t
Cefpodoxime proxetil, in infants, children, and adolescents, 591t
Cefprozil
adjustments in renal insufficiency, 757t
adverse drug reactions, 293t
breast milk excretion, 207t
in infants, children, and adolescents, 592t
Ceftazidime
adjustments in renal insufficiency, 757t
adverse drug reactions, 293t
breast milk excretion, 207t
in infants, children, and adolescents, 592t
intravenous administration, 396-397t
in neonates, 536t
Ceftin®. See Cefuroxime axetil
Ceftizoxime
adjustments in renal insufficiency, 757t
adverse drug reactions, 293t
in infants, children, and adolescents, 592t
intravenous administration, 397t
Ceftriaxone
adverse drug reactions, 293t
in infants, children, and adolescents, 593t
intravenous administration, 397t
in neonates, 536t
Cefuroxime
adjustments in renal insufficiency, 758t
adverse drug reactions, 293t
intravenous administration, 397t
Cefuroxime axetil
adverse drug reactions, 293t
in infants, children, and adolescents, 593t
Cefzil®. See Cefprozil
Cefzolin
intravenous administration, 396t
in neonates, 536t
Celebrex®. See Celecoxib
Celecoxib
in adolescents, 593t
drug interactions, 317t
Celestoderm®. See Betamethasone topical
Celestoderm-V®. See Betamethasone topical
Celestone®. See Betamethasone oral
Celestone Soluspan®. See Betamethasone injectable
Celontin®. See Methsuximide
Central diabetes insipidus. *See* Diabetes insipidus
Cephalexin
adjustments in renal insufficiency, 758t
adverse drug reactions, 293t
breast milk excretion, 207t
in infants, children, and adolescents, 594t
Cephalosporins. *See also specific drugs*
adverse drug reactions, 293-294t
drug interactions, 325
probenecid as adjunct to, 713t
Cephalothin
adjustments in renal insufficiency, 758t
adverse drug reactions, 293t
breast milk excretion, 207t

Cephalothin *continued*
  in infants, children, and adolescents, 594t
  phlebitis and, 79
  teratogenicity/fetotoxicity, 110-111
Cephapirin, adverse drug reactions, 293t
Cephradine, breast milk excretion, 207t
Ceporacin®. *See* Cephalothin
Ceptaz®. *See* Ceftazidime
Cerebral edema
  mannitol in, 668t
  pentobarbital in, 702t
Cerebyx®. *See* Fosphenytoin
Cerubidine®. *See* Daunorubicin
Cetirizine, 266
  in children and adolescents, 594t
CharcoAid®. *See* Activated charcoal
Charcoal, activated, in poisoning, 248, 250, 251-252
Charcoal-broiled meat, drug interactions, 317t
Charcodote®. *See* Activated charcoal
Chemet®. *See* Succimer
Chewing gums
  medicated, 39
  nicotine, 39
Children's Motrin®. *See* Ibuprofen
Chlamydial infection, erythromycin in, 540t
Chlo-Amine®. *See* Chlorpheniramine
Chloral hydrate
  adverse drug reactions, 310t
  breast milk excretion, 207t
  in infants, children, and adolescents, 594-595t
  in neonates, 536t
  teratogenicity/fetotoxicity, 111
Chlorambucil
  dosing, 509t
  teratogenicity/fetotoxicity, 111
Chloramphenicol
  adverse drug reactions, 295-296t
  breast milk excretion, 207t
  in children and adolescents, 595t
  drug interactions, 325
  intravenous administration, 397t
  in neonates, 536t
  optimal serum concentrations, 761t
  teratogenicity/fetotoxicity, 111
  with phenytoin, 332
Chlordiazepoxide
  adverse drug reactions, 310t
  in children and adolescents, 595t
  teratogenicity/fetotoxicity, 111-112
Chlorhexidine, in children and adolescents, 595-596t, 596t
2-Chlorodeoxyadenosine. *See* Cladribine
Chloroform, teratogenicity/fetotoxicity, 112
Chloroguanide, drug interactions, 317t

Chloromycetin®. *See* Chloramphenicol
Chloroprocaine, teratogenicity/fetotoxicity, 112
Chloroquine
  breast milk excretion, 207t
  in children and adolescents, 596t
  drug interactions, 317t, 325
  teratogenicity/fetotoxicity, 96n, 112-113
Chlorothiazide
  breast milk excretion, 207t
  in infants, children, and adolescents, 596t
  intravenous administration, 397t
  teratogenicity/fetotoxicity, 113
Chlorpheniramine
  adverse drug reactions, 301t
  in children and adolescents, 597t
Chlorpromazine
  adverse drug reactions, 303t
  as antiemetic, 499t
  breast milk excretion, 208t
  in children and adolescents, 597t
  dilution of, 10
  dosage forms, 8
  intravenous administration, 398t
  measurement of, 10-11
  in neonates, 536t
  teratogenicity/fetotoxicity, 113-114
Chlorpropamide, teratogenicity/fetotoxicity, 114
Chlorthalidone, breast milk excretion, 208t
Chlor-Trimeton®. *See* Chlorpheniramine
Chlor-Tripolon®. *See* Chlorpheniramine
Cholecalciferol. *See* Vitamin D
Cholestyramine, in children and adolescents, 598t
Cholestyramine resin
  drug interactions, 325
  with acetaminophen, 319
Choline ester overdosage, atropine systemic in, 575t
Choline salicylate, aspirin conversion factor, 257t
Chorea, Huntington's. *See* Huntington's chorea
Chorionic gonadotropin
  in children, 598t
  teratogenicity/fetotoxicity, 114-115
Choron®. *See* Chorionic gonadotropin
Chronic idiopathic urticaria, loratadine in, 666t
Chronic obstructive pulmonary disease (COPD). *See also* Asthma; Bronchitis; Bronchospasm
  ipratropium pulmonary in, 652t
Chronic renal failure, dihydrotachysterol in, 615t
Ciclopirox, in children and adolescents, 598t

Ciclopirox olamine, in children and adolescents, 598t
Cigarette smoking, epidemiology, 364-365
Cimetidine
  adjustments in renal insufficiency, 758t
  adverse drug reactions, 303-304t
  breast milk excretion, 208t
  in children and adolescents, 598t
  drug interactions, 317t, 325-326
  intravenous administration, 398t
  teratogenicity/fetotoxicity, 115
  with beta-blockers, 323
  with carmustine, 324
  with theophylline, 335-336
  with tricyclic antidepressants, 322
  with warfarin, 284
Cipro®. *See* Ciprofloxacin
Ciprofloxacin
  adverse drug reactions, 294t
  breast milk excretion, 208t
  in children and adolescents, 599t
  drug interactions, 317t, 326
  intravenous administration, 398t
Cisapride
  drug interactions, 319t
  with fluconazole, 284
Cisatracurium
  in children and adolescents, 599t
  intravenous administration, 398t
Cisplatin
  breast milk excretion, 208t
  dosing, 510t
  extravasation care, 506t
  intravenous administration, 398t
13-*Cis*-retinoic acid. *See* Isotretinoin
Citalopram
  breast milk excretion, 208t
  drug interactions, 317t
  teratogenicity/fetotoxicity, 115
Citrate of magnesia. *See* Magnesium citrate
Citro-Mag®. *See* Magnesium citrate
Cladribine
  dosing, 510t
  intravenous administration, 399t
Claforan®. *See* Cefotaxime
Clarinex®. *See* Desloratadine
Clarithromycin
  adjustments in renal insufficiency, 758t
  adverse drug reactions, 294t
  drug interactions, 317t, 326
  in infants, children, and adolescents, 599-600t
  with carbamazepine, 323
  with cyclosporine, 327
Claritin®. *See* Loratadine
Clavulin®. *See* Amoxicillin/potassium clavulanate
Clearasil Maximum Strength®. *See* Benzoyl peroxide
Clear Eyes®. *See* Naphazoline ophthalmic
Clemastine
  breast milk excretion, 208t
  in children and adolescents, 600t

INDEX

in infants, children, and adolescents, 600t
Cleocin®. See Clindamycin
Clindamycin
　adverse drug reactions, 296t
　breast milk excretion, 208t
　in infants, children, and adolescents, 600t
　intravenous administration, 399t
　in neonates, 537t
Clobazam
　adverse drug reactions, 298t
　in infants, children, and adolescents, 600-601t
Clofazimine
　breast milk excretion, 208t
　teratogenicity/fetotoxicity, 115-116
Clomiphene, teratogenicity/fetotoxicity, 116
Clomipramine
　breast milk excretion, 208t
　drug interactions, 317t
　teratogenicity/fetotoxicity, 116
Clonazepam
　adverse drug reactions, 298t
　breast milk excretion, 209t
　in infants, children, and adolescents, 601t
　teratogenicity/fetotoxicity, 116
Clonidine
　adverse drug reactions, 302t
　breast milk excretion, 209t
　drug interactions, 326
　in infants, children, and adolescents, 601t
　teratogenicity/fetotoxicity, 116-117
　with tricyclic antidepressants, 322
Clonorchiasis. See Liver fluke infestation
Clopidogrel, drug interactions, 317t
Clorazepate
　in adolescents, 601-602t
　breast milk excretion, 209t
　teratogenicity/fetotoxicity, 117
Clostridium botulinum, in infant formula, 16
Clostridium difficile enterocolitis, vancomycin in, 551t
Clotrimaderm®. See Clotrimazole
Clotrimazole
　in infants, children, and adolescents, 602t
　teratogenicity/fetotoxicity, 117
Cloxacillin
　adverse drug reactions, 294t
　in children and adolescents, 602t
　in neonates, 537t
Clozapine
　in children, 603t
　drug interactions, 317t
Clozaril®. See Clozapine
CNS depressants, abuse of, 355-360, 356t, 357t, 358t, 359t. See also under Abusable psychotropic drug use

CNS stimulants
　abuse of, 360-365, 362t, 363t, 365t. See also under Abusable psychotropic drug use
　adverse drug reactions, 307t
Coagulation disorders
　aminocaproic acid in, 533t, 564t
　cortisone in, 604t
　Factor IX complex in, 628t
　heparin in, 542t
　lepirudin in, 660t
　phytonadione in, 707t
　tranexamic acid in, 744-745t
Coagulation necrosis, in caustic poisoning, 267
Cocaine
　abuse of, 362-363, 363t
　breast milk excretion, 209t
　in children and adolescents, 586t
　teratogenicity/fetotoxicity, 117-118
Codeine
　breast milk excretion, 209t
　drug interactions, 317t
　in infants, children, and adolescents, 603t
　teratogenicity/fetotoxicity, 118-119
Cognitive dysfunction, as adverse drug effect, 290t
Colace®. See Docusate sodium
Co-Lav®. See Polyethylene glycol and electrolyte solutions
Colchicine
　breast milk excretion, 209t
　teratogenicity/fetotoxicity, 119
Colestipol, drug interactions, 326
Colfosceril palmitate, in neonates, 537t
Colic, simethicone in, 730t
Colitis
　mesalamine in, 672t
　pseudomembranous
　　as adverse drug effect, 290t
　　vancomycin in, 551t, 750t
　ulcerative. See Ulcerative colitis
Colonic evacuation. See also Bowel preparation
　castor oil in, 589t
CoLyte®. See Polyethylene glycol and electrolyte solutions
Coma, hepatic
　neomycin in, 687-688t
　paromomycin in, 698t
Combantrin®. See Pyrantel pamoate
Common cold. See also Rhinitis
　clemastine in sneezing, 600t
　naphazoline nasal in, 686t
Compazine®. See Prochlorperazine
Compendium of Pharmaceuticals and Specialties (CPS), 88
Compressed-air nebulizers (CANs), 13-33
Conception control. See Oral contraceptives and specific drugs
Concerta®. See Methylphenidate

Confused or mentally retarded patients, drug administration in, 6-7
Congenital adrenal hyperplasia, hydrocortisone in, 543t
Congenital cytomegalovirus retinitis, ganciclovir in, 542t
Congenital neutropenia, filgrastim in, 541t
Congenital sucrase-isomaltase deficiency (CSID), sacrosidase in, 727t
Congenital syphilis, penicillin G benzathine in, 547t
Congestive heart failure
　acetazolamide in, 532t
　as adverse drug effect, 288t
　captopril in, 535t, 587t
　digoxin in, 538t, 613-614t
　dobutamine in, 539t
　enalapril in, 621t
　furosemide in, 541t
　hydralazine in, 644-645t
　milrinone in, 681t
　sodium nitroprusside in, 549t
　spironolactone in, 549t
Conjunctivitis
　allergic
　　medrysone in, 669t
　　nedocromil ophthalmic in, 687t
　　pemirolast in, 699t
　fluorometholone in, 633t
　gentamicin ophthalmic in, 637t
　lodoxamide in, 665t
　medrysone in, 669t
　pemirolast in, 699t
　sulfacetamide sodium in, 550t
Constipation
　as adverse drug effect, 289t
　bisacodyl in, 581t
　cascara sagrada in, 588t
　docusate calcium/potassium/sodium in, 618t
　glycerin in, 542t
　glycerin suppositories in, 638t
　lactulose in, 657t
　magnesium hydroxide in, 668t
　mineral oil in, 681t
　psyllium in, 719t
　senna in, 729t
Conversion formulas, 763
Convulsions. See Seizures; Status epilepticus
Copper poisoning, antidotes, 254t
Corgard®. See Nadolol
Corneal inflammation, trifluridine in, 746t
Cort-Dome®. See Hydrocortisone topical
Cortef®. See Hydrocortisone
Corticosteroids. See also specific drugs
　adverse drug reactions, 307-308t
　in caustic poisoning, 268-269
　drug interactions, 326-327
　teratogenicity/fetotoxicity, 119-120
　with barbiturates, 322

Corticosteroids *continued*
  with carbamazepine, 323-324
  with phenytoin, 332
  with rifampin, 334
Corticotropin (ACTH)
  in infants, children, and adolescents, 603-604t
  teratogenicity/fetotoxicity, 120
Cortisol. *See* Hydrocortisone
Cortisone
  in children and adolescents, 604t
  teratogenicity/fetotoxicity, 120
Cortizone®. See Hydrocortisone topical
Cortone®. See Cortisone
Cosmegen®. See Dactinomycin
Cotazym®. See Pancrelipase
Co-trimoxazole
  adverse drug reactions, 296t
  teratogenicity/fetotoxicity, 120
Cough
  as adverse drug effect, 289t
  codeine in, 603t
  dextromethorphan in, 610-611t
Coumadin®. See Warfarin
CPT-11. *See* Irinotecan
13-cRA. *See* Isotretinoin
Crab lice, piperacillin in, 708t
CRF-187. *See* Dexrazoxane
Crixivan®. See Indinavir
Crohn's disease, infliximab in, 648t
Cromolyn sodium
  adverse drug reactions, 305t
  in children and adolescents, 604-605t
  teratogenicity/fetotoxicity, 120
Crotalid serum antivenin, in children and adolescents, 571-572t
Croup, epinephrine in, 623t
Cruex®. See Undecylenic acid
Cryptococcal meningitis, fluconazole in, 630t
Cryptococcus. See Fungal infections
Cryptorchidism, chorionic gonadotropin in prepubertal, 598t
CTX. *See* Cyclophosphamide
Cultural factors, in psychotropic drug abuse, 353-354
Cuprimine®. See Penicillamine
Cushing's syndrome, as adverse drug effect, 289t
Cutaneous infections, bacitracin in, 576t
Cyanide Antidote Kit®, 254t
Cyanide poisoning, antidotes, 254t
Cyanocobalamin
  breast milk excretion, 209t
  in children and adolescents, 605t
Cyclic antidepressant poisoning, antidotes, 254t
Cyclizine, teratogenicity/fetotoxicity, 120-121
Cyclogyl®. See Cyclopentolate
Cyclopedic refraction, atropine ophthalmic in, 574t

Cyclopentolate
  in infants, children, and adolescents, 605t
  in neonates, 537t
Cyclophosphamide
  breast milk excretion, 210t
  dosing, 510t
  intravenous administration, 399t
  teratogenicity/fetotoxicity, 121
Cycloserine, breast milk excretion, 210t
Cyclosporine
  breast milk excretion, 210t
  in children and adolescents, 605-606t
  dosing, 511t
  drug interactions, 317t, 327
  intravenous administration, 399t
  optimal serum concentrations, 761t
  teratogenicity/fetotoxicity, 121
  with carbamazepine, 324
Cyklokapron®. See Tranexamic acid
Cylert®. See Pemoline
Cyproheptadine
  breast milk excretion, 210t
  in children and adolescents, 606t
  teratogenicity/fetotoxicity, 121
Cystadane®. See Betaine
Cystagon®. See Cysteamine
Cysteamine, in children and adolescents, 606-607t
Cystic fibrosis, 17
  bacterial infections
    ceftazidime in, 592t
    tobramycin inhalation in, 742t
    tobramycin injectable in, 742t
  bacterial infections in
    aztreonam in, 576t
    gentamicin in, 637t
  dornase alfa in, 619t
Cystinosis, nephropathic, cysteamine in, 606-607t
Cystinuria, penicillamine in, 700t
Cystitis, loracarbef in, 666t
Cytarabine
  dosing, 511t
  intravenous administration, 399t
  teratogenicity/fetotoxicity, 121-122
Cytochrome P-450 (CYP) enzyme superfamily, 477-481, *478*, 483-486. *See also* Pharmacogenetics
Cytomegalovirus infection. *See also* Viral infections
  ganciclovir in, 637t
Cytomegalovirus retinitis, congenital, ganciclovir in, 542t
Cytosar®. See Cytarabine
Cytosar-U®. See Cytarabine
Cytosine arabinoside. *See* Cytarabine
Cytovene®. See Ganciclovir
Cytoxan®. See Cyclophosphamide

D

Dacarbazine
  dosing, 511t
  intravenous administration, 400t
Dacliximab, in children and adolescents, 607t
Daclizumab. *See* Dacliximab
Dactinomycin
  dosing, 512t
  extravasation care, 506t
  intravenous administration, 400t
  teratogenicity/fetotoxicity, 122
Dalacin C®. See Clindamycin
Danaparoid, in children and adolescents, 607-608t
Danazol
  drug interactions, 317t
  teratogenicity/fetotoxicity, 122
Dandruff
  pyrithione zinc in, 722t
  selenium sulfide in, 729t
  sulfacetamide sodium topical in, 736t
Dantrium®. See Dantrolene
Dantrolene
  in children and adolescents, 608t
  intravenous administration, 400t
Dapsone
  breast milk excretion, 210t
  in children and adolescents, 608t
Daraprim®. See Pyrimethamine
Daunomycin. *See* Daunorubicin
Daunorubicin
  dosing, 512t
  extravasation care, 506t
  intravenous administration, 400t
  teratogenicity/fetotoxicity, 122-123
Dayhist-1®. See Clemastine
DDAVP®. See Desmopressin
Deafness/hearing loss, as adverse drug effect, 289t
Debrox Otic®. See Carbamide peroxide
Decadron®. See Dexamethasone
Declofenac, teratogenicity/fetotoxicity, 126
Deep vein thrombosis. *See* Thrombosis
Deferoxamine
  in children and adolescents, 609t
  teratogenicity/fetotoxicity, 123
Deferoxamine mesylate
  intravenous administration, 400t
  in iron poisoning, 255t, 264-265
Degas®. See Simethicone
Delavirdine, drug interactions, 317t
Delaxin®. See Methocarbamol
Delayed gastric emptying, metoclopramide in, 678t
Delayed puberty
  fluoxymesterone in, 633-634t
  testosterone propionate in, 738t
Delta-Cortef®. See Prednisolone systemic

Deltahydrocortisone. *See*
      Prednisolone ophthalmic;
      Prednisolone systemic
Deltasone®. See Prednisone
Deltoid injection site, 55–56, *56*
Demeclocycline
   breast milk excretion, 210t
   teratogenicity/fetotoxicity, 123
Demerol®. See Meperidine
Dental caries prophylaxis, sodium
      fluoride in, 731t
Depacon®. See Valproic acid
Depakene®. See Valproic acid
Depakote®. See Valproic acid
Depen®. See Penicillamine
Depression
   as adverse drug effect, 289t
   amitriptyline in, 565–566t
   fluoxetine in, 633t
   nortriptyline in, 692t
   paroxetine in, 699t
   sertraline in, 729–730t
   venlafaxine in, 751t
Dermacort®. See Hydrocortisone
      topical
Dermal necrosis. *See* Extravasation
Dermatitis
   as adverse drug effect, 289t
   exfoliative
      betamethasone in, 580t
      cortisone in, 604t
   ketotifen in, 657t
   pimecrolimus in, 707t
   seborrheic, sulfacetamide sodium
      topical in, 736t
   triamcinolone topical in, 745t
   zinc oxide in, 756t
Dermatomycoses. *See also* Fungal
      infections
   miconazole in, 679t
Dermatophytoses
   griseofulvin in, 640t
   miconazole in, 679t
Dermatoses
   betamethasone in, 580t
   hydrocortisone topical in, 645t
Desenex®. See Undecylenic acid
Desenex Prescription Strength®. See
      Miconazole
Desferal®. See Deferoxamine;
      Deferoxamine mesylate
Desferrioxamine. *See* Deferoxamine
Desipramine
   breast milk excretion, 210t
   drug interactions, 317t
   teratogenicity/fetotoxicity, 123
Desloratadine, in adolescents,
      609t
Desmopressin, 30
   breast milk excretion, 210t
   in children and adolescents,
      609t
Desmopressin acetate, intravenous
      administration, 401t
Desoxyephedrine. *See*
      Methamphetamine
Desoxyn®. See Methamphetamine
Desquam-X®. See Benzoyl peroxide

Development
   human gestational, 93–95t
   pharmacokinetics in, 495–496
   teratogenic susceptibility of organ
      systems during, 92
Developmental considerations, in
      drug administration, 2–6, 3–6t
   infants, 3t
Dexamethasone
   adverse drug reactions, 307t
   as antiemetic, 499t
   dosing, 513t
   drug interactions, 317t
   in infants, children, and adolescents, 610t
   in neonates, 537t
   teratogenicity/fetotoxicity, 123–124
Dexamethasone sodium phosphate,
      intravenous administration,
      401t
Dexedrine®. See
      Dextroamphetamine
Dexfenfluramine, drug interactions,
      317t
Dexiron®. See Iron dextran
      injectable
Dexrazoxane
   dosing, 513t
   intravenous administration, 401t
Dextroamphetamine
   abuse of, 361, 362t
   in children and adolescents,
      610t
   teratogenicity/fetotoxicity, 124
Dextromethorphan
   drug interactions, 317t
   in infants, children, and adolescents, 610–611t
   teratogenicity/fetotoxicity, 124
Dextrose
   in infants, children, and adolescents, 611t
   intravenous administration, 401t
   in neonates, 537t, 538t
   teratogenicity/fetotoxicity, 124–125
DHAD. *See* Mitoxantrone
DHAQ. *See* Mitoxantrone
DHT®. See Dihydrotachysterol
Diabetes insipidus
   central, vasopressin in, 750t
   neurohypophyseal, desmopressin
      in, 609t
Diabetes mellitus
   insulin glargine in, 650t
   insulin in, 649–650t
   metformin in, 673t
   roglitazone in, 727t
Diabetic ketoacidosis, insulin in,
      649–650t
Diacetylmorphine (heroin), teratogenicity/fetotoxicity, 141–142
Diaminodiphenyl sulfone. See
      Dapsone
Diamox®. See Acetazolamide
Diaper rash, clotrimazole in, 602t

Diarrhea
   as adverse drug effect, 289t
   antibiotic-associated, 657t
   diphenoxylate and atropine in,
      616–617t
   furazolidone in protozoal or
      bacterial, 636t
   Lactobacillus acidophilus in,
      657t
Diastat®. See Diazepam; Diazepam
      rectal gel
Diazemuls®. See Diazepam
Diazepam. *See also* Benzodiazepines
   adverse drug reactions, 298t,
      310t
   breast milk excretion, 210–211t
   drug interactions, 317t
   in infants, children, and adolescents, 611t
   intravenous administration, 401t
   measurement of, 10–11
   in neonates, 538t
   teratogenicity/fetotoxicity, 125–126
Diazepam rectal gel, 21–22
Diazoxide
   adverse drug reactions, 302t
   injectable, in infants, children,
      and adolescents, 611–612t
   intravenous administration, 401t
   in neonates, 538t
   oral, in infants, children, and
      adolescents, 612t
   teratogenicity/fetotoxicity, 126
DIC. *See* Dacarbazine
Dicarbosil®. See Calcium carbonate
Diclofenac
   drug interactions, 317t
   ophthalmic, in children and
      adolescents, 612t
   oral, in adolescents, 612t
Dicloxacillin
   adverse drug reactions, 294t
   in infants, children, and adolescents, 612t
Dicumarol
   breast milk excretion, 211t
   teratogenicity/fetotoxicity, 126
Dicyclomine
   in infants, children, and adolescents, 613t
   teratogenicity/fetotoxicity, 126–127
Dicycloverine. *See* Dicyclomine
Didanosine
   adverse drug reactions, 304t
   enteric-coated, 14n
Dideoxycytidine. *See* Zalcitabine
Dideoxyinosine. *See* Didanosine
Dienestrol, teratogenicity/
      fetotoxicity, 127
Diethylpropion, teratogenicity/
      fetotoxicity, 127
Diethylstilbestrol (DES), teratogenicity/fetotoxicity, 127–130
Diflucan®. See Fluconazole
Digibind®. See Digoxin immune
      Fab

Digitalis glycosides
  drug interactions, 328
    with amiodarone, 320
    with cholestyramine resin, 325
Digitalis toxicity, lidocaine in, 544t
Digoxin
  adjustments in renal insufficiency, 758t
  adverse drug reactions, 307t
  in infants, children, and adolescents, 613-614t
  intravenous administration, 401t
  in neonates, 538t
  optimal serum concentrations, 761t
  teratogenicity/fetotoxicity, 130
Digoxin immune Fab
  in digoxin poisoning, 255t
  in infants, children, and adolescents, 614t
  intravenous administration, 402t
  in neonates, 538t
Digoxin overdosage/poisoning, 255t
  digoxin immune Fab in, 538t, 614t
  phenytoin in, 706t
Dihydroergotamine, in adolescents, 614t
Dihydrotachysterol, in infants, children, and adolescents, 615t
Dihydroxyanthracenedione. See Mitoxantrone
1α,25-Dihydroxycholecalciferol. See Calcitriol
Diidohydroxyquin. See Iodoquinol
Dilantin®. *See* Phenytoin
Dilaudid®. *See* Hydromorphine
Diltiazem, breast milk excretion, 211t
Dimenhydrinate
  adverse drug reactions, 301t
  in children and adolescents, 615t
  intravenous administration, 402t
  teratogenicity/fetotoxicity, 130
Dimercaprol, 615-616t
  in metal poisoning, 254t
Dimetane®. *See* Brompheniramine
Dimetapp Allergy®. *See* Brompheniramine
Dimetapp Decongestant Pediatric Drops®. *See* Pseudoephedrine
4-Dimethoxy-daunorubicin. See Idarubicin
Diocaine®. *See* Proparacaine
Dioctyl calcium sulfosuccinate. See Docusate calcium
Dioctyl sodium sulfosuccinate. See Docusate sodium
Diodoquin®. *See* Iodoquinol
Diphenhydramine
  adverse drug reactions, 301t
  drug interactions, 317t
  intravenous administration, 402t
  systemic, in infants, children, and adolescents, 616t

  teratogenicity/fetotoxicity, 130
  topical, in children and adolescents, 616t
Diphenhydramine poisoning, 265
Diphenoxylate and atropine, topical, 616t
Diphenylhydantoin. *See* Phenytoin
Diphtheria toxoid vaccine, 437-440
  breast milk excretion, 211t
  teratogenicity/fetotoxicity, 130
Diprivan®. *See* Propofol
Diprolene®. *See* Betamethasone topical
Dipyridamole, teratogenicity/fetotoxicity, 130-131
Disability
  mental. *See* Mental disability; Mental disorders
  physical. *See* Physical disability
Diskhalers, 35
Disopyramide
  adjustments in renal insufficiency, 758t
  adverse drug reactions, 306t
  breast milk excretion, 211t
  in children and adolescents, 617t
  optimal serum concentrations, 761t
  teratogenicity/fetotoxicity, 131
Disposal
  of injection equipment, 48
  of MDI canisters, 34
Disulfiram
  in adolescents, 617t
  drug interactions, 317t, 328
  teratogenicity/fetotoxicity, 131
Ditropan®. *See* Oxybutynin
Diuresis, aminophylline in, 533t
Diuretics. *See also specific drugs*
  adverse drug reactions, 308t
  potassium sparing
    with cyclosporine, 327
    with potassium salts, 333
  thiazide
    drug interactions, 336
    with lithium salts, 330
Diuril®. *See* Chlorothiazide
Divalproex. *See* Valproic acid
Divalproex sodium. *See* Valproic acid
Dixarit®. *See* Clonidine
Dizmiss®. *See* Meclizine
DMSA®. *See* Succimer
DNR. *See* Daunorubicin
Dobutamine
  in infants, children, and adolescents, 617t
  intravenous administration, 402t
  in neonates, 539t
Dobutrex®. *See* Dobutamine
Docetaxel
  dosing, 513t
  intravenous administration, 402t
Docusate, teratogenicity/fetotoxicity, 131
Docusate calcium, adverse drug reactions, 309t

Docusate calcium/potassium/sodium, in children and adolescents, 618t
Docusate sodium, adverse drug reactions, 309t
Dolasetron
  as antiemetic, 499t
  in children and adolescents, 618t
  intravenous administration, 403t
Dome nomogram, 257
Domperidone, in infants, children, and adolescents, 618t
Donnazyme®. *See* Pancreatin
Dopamine
  drug interactions, 328
  in infants, children, and adolescents, 618t
  intravenous administration, 403t
  in neonates, 539t
  with phenytoin, 332
Dopram®. *See* Doxapram
Dornase alfa, in infants, children, and adolescents, 619t
Dorsogluteal injection site, 56-57, 57
Dosage forms. *See also* Administration; Routes of administration; *specific forms*
  inhalation, 31-38
  injectable, 42-83
  intranasal, 28-31
  intravenous injections and infusions, 61-83
  ophthalmic, 23-27
  oral, 7-19
  otic, 27, *28*
  rectal, 19-22
  topical, 36-42
  vaginal, 22-23
Dosing. *See also specific drugs*
  in infants, children, and adolescents, 555-777
    dosage tables, 556-557, 558-756t
    frequently used conversion formulas, 763
    general recommendations in renal dysfunction, 757-760t
    optimal serum concentration ranges, 761-762t
    principles, 555-556
  in neonates, 531, 532-554t
Doxapram, intravenous administration, 403t
Doxepin, breast milk excretion, 211-212t
Doxil®. *See* Doxorubicin liposomal
Doxorubicin
  breast milk excretion, **212t**
  dosing, 514t
  extravasation care, **506t**
  intravenous administration, 403t
  teratogenicity/fetotoxicity, 131-132
Doxorubicin liposomal
  dosing, 514t
  intravenous administration, 403t

Doxychel®. See Doxycycline
Doxycin®. See Doxycycline
Doxycycline
  adverse drug reactions, 295t
  breast milk excretion, 212t
  in children and adolescents, 619t
  with phenytoin, 332
Doxylamine, teratogenicity/
  fetotoxicity, 132-133
Dr. Caldwell Senna Laxative®. See
  Senna
Dramamine®. See Dimenhydrinate
Dramamine II®. See Meclizine
Drink-a-Pill cup, 15n
Drisdol®. See Ergocalciferol
Dristan Long Lasting Nasal Mist/
  Solution®. See Oxymetazoline
  nasal
Dronabinol
  as antiemetic, 499t
  in children and adolescents, 619t
  drug interactions, 317t
Dronulac®. See Lactulose
Droperidol
  as antiemetic, 499t
  in children and adolescents, 619-620t
  intravenous administration, 404t
Drops
  intranasal, 29
  ophthalmic, 23-25, 26
Drug factors, in teratogenesis, 91
Drug interactions, 283-284, 315-345. *See also* Adverse drug
  reactions (ADRs)
  pharmacokinetic vs.
    pharmacodynamic, 316
  QT prolongation and, 316-318, 319t
  sites of, 315-316, *316*
  of specific drugs, 319-337
Drug intolerance, 284
Drug storage, 8
Drug toxicity. *See* Toxicity
Dryvax®. See Smallpox vaccine
DTIC. *See* Dacarbazine
DTIC-Dome®. See Dacarbazine
d-Tubocurarine. *See* Tubocurarine
Dulcolax®. See Bisacodyl
Duodenal ulcer. *See also* Peptic ulcer
  ranitidine in, 723-724t
Duphalac®. See Lactulose
Duramorph®. See Morphine
Duricef®. See Cefadroxil
Dyna-hex Skin Cleanser®. See
  Chlorhexidine
Dynamic equinus foot deformity,
  botulinum toxin type A in,
  582-583t
Dyrenium®. See Triamterene
Dysmenorrhea, naproxen sodium in, 687t
Dyspepsia, calcium carbonate in, 587t
Dysplasia, bronchopulmonary,
  furosemide in, 541t
Dysrhythmias. *See* Cardiac
  dysrhythmias

E
Ear wax removal, carbamide
  peroxide in, 588t
Easprin®. See Aspirin
Eating disorders, phendimetrazine
  in, 704t
Eclampsia, magnesium sulfate in, 668t
Econazole, in children and adolescents, 620t
Econopred®. See Prednisolone
  ophthalmic
Ecostatin®. See Econazole
Ecotrin®. See Aspirin
Ecstasy. *See* Methylenedioxy
  methamphetamine
Edecrin®. See Ethacrynic acid
Edema
  acetazolamide in, 532t, 559t
  bumetanide in, 584t
  captopril in, 535t
  cerebral
    mannitol in, 668t
    pentobarbital in, 702t
  chlorothiazide in, 596t
  ethacrynic acid in, 625t
  furosemide in, 636t
  hydrochlorothiazide in, 543t, 645t
  spironolactone in, 549t, 734t
  triamterene in, 745t
Edetate calcium disodium (EDTA),
  in lead poisoning, 255t
Edrophonium chloride, intravenous
  administration, 404t
Edrophonium, in infants, children,
  and adolescents, 620t
E.E.S.®. See Erythromycin
Efavirenz
  in children and adolescents, 620t
  drug interactions, 317t
Effexor®. See Venlafaxine
Effexor XR®. See Venlafaxine
Elavil®. See Amitriptyline
Elimite®. See Permethrin
Elixirs, alcohol content of, 9
Elspar®. See Asparaginase
Eltroxin®. See Levothyroxine
Embryo/fetal factors affecting
  teratogenesis, 90
EMLA®. See Lidocaine/prilocaine
EMLA Patch®, 61
Emollient laxatives, adverse drug
  reactions, 309t
Emotional distress, in dermatologic
  disorders, 37
Enalapril
  adjustments in renal insufficiency, 758t
  adverse drug reactions, 301t
  breast milk excretion, 212t
  in infants, children, and adolescents, 621t
  teratogenicity/fetotoxicity, 133
Enalaprilat, intravenous administration, 404t
Enbrel®. See Etanercept
Encainide, drug interactions, 317t

Encephalitis, herpes simplex,
  acyclovir in, 559t
Encephalopathy, as adverse drug
  effect, 289t
Endocarditis, bacterial, ampicillin in, 569t
Endoscopy, midazolam in
  premedication, 680t
Endotracheal intubation. *See*
  Intubation
Enemas, administration, 22
Ener-B®. See Cyanocobalamin
Enlon®. See Edrophonium;
  Edrophonium chloride
Enoxaparin, in children and adolescents, 621-622t
Enteric-coated tablets, 13
Enterobiasis. *See also* Parasitic
  infestations
  mebendazole in, 668t
  pyrantel pamoate in, 719-720t
Enterocolitis
  necrotizing, vancomycin in, 551t
  staphylococcal, vancomycin in, 551t
  streptococcal, as adverse drug
    effect, 290t
Entozyme®. See Pancreatin
Enuresis, desmopressin in, 609t
Environmental factors, in
  teratogenesis, 90-91
Enzyme inducers. *See also*
  Anticoagulants
  drug interactions, 321, 328
Enzyme inhibitors. *See also*
  Anticoagulants
  drug interactions, 328
  with anticoagulants, 321
Epaxal Berna®. See Hepatitis A
  vaccine, inactivated, virosome
  formulated
Ephedrine
  in children and adolescents, 622t
  teratogenicity/fetotoxicity, 133
Epidemiology, of pediatric
  poisoning, 245-247, 246t
Epigastric distress, as adverse drug
  effect, 289t
Epiject®. See Valproic acid
Epiject IV®. See Valproate sodium
Epilepsy. *See also* Seizures
  benign Rolandic, carbamazepine
  in, 587t
Epinephrine
  adverse drug reactions, 305t
  breast milk excretion, 212t
  in infants, children, and adolescents, 622-623t
  intravenous administration, 404t
  in neonates, 539t
  teratogenicity/fetotoxicity, 133-134
Episcleritis, medrysone in, 669t
Epival®. See Valproic acid
Epivir®. See Lamivudine
Epivir-HBV®. See Lamivudine

INDEX

Epoetin alfa
  in infants, children, and adolescents, 623t
  intravenous administration, 404t
Epogen®. See Epoetin alfa
Epsom salt. *See* Magnesium sulfate
Equanil®. See Meprobamate
Equipment disposal. *See* Disposal
Ergocalciferol, in neonates, 540t
Ergot alkaloids, breast milk excretion, 212t
Ergotamine, teratogenicity/fetotoxicity, 134
E.R.O. Ear®. See Carbamide peroxide
EryPed®. See Erythromycin
Ery-Tab®. See Erythromycin
Erythema nodosum leprosum, thalidomide in, 738-739t
Erythrocin®. See Erythromycin
Erythromycin
  adverse drug reactions, 294t
  breast milk excretion, 212t
  drug interactions, 328
  in infants, children, and adolescents, 624t
  in neonates, 540t
  teratogenicity/fetotoxicity, 134
  with carbamazepine, 324
  with cyclosporine, 327
  with theophylline, 336
Erythromycin ethylsuccinate, in infants, children, and adolescents, 624t
Erythromycin lactobionate, intravenous administration, 404t
Eryzole®. See Erythromycin ethylsuccinate
Eserine. *See* Physostigmine salicylate
Esidrix®. See Hydrochlorothiazide
Eskalith CR®. See Lithium
Esmolol
  in children and adolescents, 625t
  intravenous administration, 404t
Esophageal dilation, in caustic poisoning, 269
Esophagitis. *See also* Gastroesophageal reflux disease (GERD)
  omeprazole in refractory, 693t
  related to tablet sticking, 14n
Esophagoscopy, in caustic poisoning, 268
Estradiol, teratogenicity/fetotoxicity, 134-135
Estrogens, teratogenicity/fetotoxicity, 135
Etanercept, in children and adolescents, 625t
Ethacrynate sodium. *See* Ethacrynic acid
Ethacrynic acid
  adverse drug reactions, 308t
  intravenous administration, 404t
  in neonates, 540t
Ethambutol
  adjustments in renal insufficiency, 758t

breast milk excretion, 212t
  in children and adolescents, 625t
  teratogenicity/fetotoxicity, 135
Ether, breast milk excretion, 213t
Ethinyl estradiol
  drug interactions, 317t
  teratogenicity/fetotoxicity, 135
Ethinyl estradiol/levonorgestrel. *See also* Oral contraceptives
  in adolescents, 626t
Ethinyl estradiol/norethindrone. *See also* Oral contraceptives
  in adolescents, 626t
Ethionamide
  in children and adolescents, 627t
  teratogenicity/fetotoxicity, 135-136
Ethisterone, teratogenicity/fetotoxicity, 136
Ethosuximide
  adverse drug reactions, 298t
  breast milk excretion, 213t
  in infants, children, and adolescents, 627t
  optimal serum concentrations, 761t
  teratogenicity/fetotoxicity, 136
Ethotoin, teratogenicity/fetotoxicity, 136
Ethyl aminobenzoate. *See* Benzocaine
Ethylenediamine, teratogenicity/fetotoxicity, 102
Ethylene glycol poisoning, 255t, 275-276
Ethyol®. See Amifostine
Etibi®. See Ethambutol
Etopophos®. See Etoposide
Etoposide
  breast milk excretion, 213t
  dosing, 515t
  extravasation care, 506t
  intravenous administration, 405t
Etretinate, teratogenicity/fetotoxicity, 136-137
Evac-Q-Mag®. See Magnesium citrate
Exercise-induced bronchospasm. *See under* Bronchospasm
Exfoliative dermatitis
  betamethasone in, 580t
  cortisone in, 604t
Exidine Skin Cleanser®. See Chlorhexidine
Ex-Lax®. See Senna
Expectoration, guaifenesin in facilitation of, 640t
Extracorporeal membrane oxygenation (ECMO), in hydrocarbon poisoning, 271
Extrapyramidal reactions, as adverse drug effect, 289t
Extravasation
  hyaluronidase in, 542t
  of intravenous drugs, 78
  phentolamine in, 547t, 705t
Extubation preparation, aminophylline in, 533t
Eye conditions. *See* Ocular *entries*

F

Factor IX (human)
  in infants, children, and adolescents, 627t-628t
  intravenous administration, 405t
Factor IX complex
  in infants, children, and adolescents, 628t
  intravenous administration, 405t
Factrel®. See Gonadorelin
Famotidine
  adjustments in renal insufficiency, 758t
  adverse drug reactions, 304t
  breast milk excretion, 213t
  in children and adolescents, 628t
  intravenous administration, 405t
FAMP. *See* Fludarabine
Fat emulsions
  intravenous administration, 406t
  in neonates, 540t
Fat intake, inadequate, medium chain triglyceride oil in neonates, 544t
FDA teratogenesis codes, 97
Febrile neutropenia, cefepime in, 590t
Felbamate, drug interactions, 317t
Female gender, as risk factor for ADRs, 285
Femstat®. See Butoconazole
Fenofibrate, in children and adolescents
  microcoated, 628-629t
  micronized, 629t
Fentanyl
  breast milk excretion, 213t
  in children and adolescents, 629t
  in neonates, 540t
  teratogenicity/fetotoxicity, 137
Fentanyl citrate, intravenous administration, 406t
Fermalac®. See Lactobacillus acidophilus
Ferrous sulfate, in neonates, 541t
Fetal alcohol syndrome (FAS), 98-101, 99t, *100*
Fetotoxicity. *See also specific drugs and drug classes*
  factors affecting teratogenesis, 89-96, *90*, 92-95t
  drug factors, 91
  embryo/fetal factors, 90
  environmental factors, 90-91
  maternal factors, 89-90
  placental factors, 90
  maternal pharmacotherapy and drug use during pregnancy, 88-89, *89*
Fever
  acetaminophen in, 532t, 558t
  as adverse drug effect, 289t
  aspirin in, 572-573t
  ibuprofen in, 646t
Fexofenadine, in children and adolescents, 629t
Fexofenadine poisoning, 266

Filgrastim
  dosing, 515t
  intravenous administration, 406t
  in neonates, 541t
Flagyl®. See Metronidazole
Flarex®. See Fluorometholone
Flatulence, simethicone in, 730t
Flatulex®. See Simethicone
Flecainide
  adverse drug reactions, 306t
  breast milk excretion, 213t
  in children and adolescents, 630t
  drug interactions, 317t
  optimal serum concentrations, 761t
  teratogenicity/fetotoxicity, 137
Fleet Babylax®. See Glycerin
Flonase®. See Fluticasone nasal
Florinef®. See Fludrocortisone
Flovent®. See Fluticasone pulmonary
Flovent Rotadisk®. See Fluticasone pulmonary
Fluconazole
  adjustments in renal insufficiency, 758t
  adverse drug reactions, 300t
  drug interactions, 317t, 328
  in infants, children, and adolescents, 630t
  intravenous administration, 406t
  with cisapride, 284
Flucytosine
  adjustments in renal insufficiency, 758t
  adverse drug reactions, 300t
  in children and adolescents, 630t
  in neonates, 541t
  optimal serum concentrations, 761t
Fludara®. See Fludarabine
Fludarabine
  dosing, 515t
  intravenous administration, 406t
Fludrocortisone, in infants, children, and adolescents, 630t-631t
Fluid overload, 78
  ethacrynic acid in, 540t
Fluid retention. *See* Edema
Flumazenil
  in benzodiazepine poisoning, 254t
  in children and adolescents, 631t
  intravenous administration, 407t
  in neonates, 541t
Flunarizine, in adolescents, 631t
Flunisolide, in children and adolescents
  nasal, 631t
  pulmonary, 632t
Fluocinolone, in infants, children, and adolescents, 632t
Fluocinonide, in infants, children, and adolescents, 632t
Fluoderm®. See Fluocinolone
Fluonex®. See Fluocinonide
Fluonid®. See Fluocinolone
Fluoride. *See* Sodium fluoride

Fluoritab®. See Sodium fluoride
Fluorocytosine. *See* Flucytosine
5-Fluorocytosine. *See* Flucytosine
Fluorometholone, in children and adolescents, 633t
Fluor-Op®. See Fluorometholone
Fluoroquinolone, adverse drug reactions, 294t
Fluoroquinolones
  drug interactions, 328
  with antacids, 320-321
  with theophylline, 336
Fluorouracil
  dosing, 515t
  intravenous administration, 407t
  teratogenicity/fetotoxicity, 137-138
Fluoxetine
  adverse drug reactions, 300t
  breast milk excretion, 213t
  in children and adolescents, 633t
  drug interactions, 317t, 328-329
  teratogenicity/fetotoxicity, 138
  with carbamazepine, 324
Fluoxymesterone, in adolescents, 633-634t
Fluphenazine
  food interactions, 10
  teratogenicity/fetotoxicity, 138
Flurbiprofen
  breast milk excretion, 214t
  drug interactions, 317t
Flurosyn®. See Fluocinolone
Flutamide, drug interactions, 317t
Flutex®. See Triamcinolone topical
Fluticasone, in children and adolescents
  nasal, 634t
  pulmonary, 634t
Fluvastatin, drug interactions, 317t
Fluvoxamine
  breast milk excretion, 214t
  drug interactions, 317t
FML®. See Fluorometholone
Folic acid
  breast milk excretion, 214t
  in children and adolescents, 634t
  deficiency in pregnancy, 109-110
  drug interactions, 329
  intravenous administration, 407t
  in neonates, 541t
  supplementation in pregnancy, 138
  with phenytoin, 332
Folic acid deficiency
  folic acid supplementation in, 541t
  pyrimethamine-related, 721t
Fomepizole
  in children and adolescents, 634t
  in ethylene glycol or methanol poisoning, 255t
  in methanol poisoning, 274
Foradil®. See Formoterol fumarate
Formoterol fumarate, in children and adolescents, 635t
Fortaz®. See Ceftazidime

Fosphenytoin. *See also* Phenytoin
  in children and adolescents, 635t
  intravenous administration, 407t
Fostex®. See Benzoyl peroxide
Frisium®. See Clobazam
Frusemide. *See* Furosemide
Fulvicin®. See Griseofulvin
Fungal infections
  as adverse drug effect, 288t
  amphotericin B in, 534t, 568t
  butenafine in, 586t
  butoconazole in, 586t
  ciclopirox in, 598t
  ciclopirox olamine in, 598t
  clotrimazole in, 602t
  econazole in, 620t
  fluconazole in, 630t
  flucytosine in, 541t, 630t
  gentian violet in, 638t
  miconazole in, 679t
  nystatin in, 546t, 692t
Fungizone®. See Amphotericin B
Furazolidone
  in infants, children, and adolescents, 636t
  teratogenicity/fetotoxicity, 138
Furosemide. *See also* Diuretics
  adverse drug reactions, 308t
  breast milk excretion, 214t
  drug interactions, 329
  in infants, children, and adolescents, 636t
  intravenous administration, 407t
  in neonates, 541t
  teratogenicity/fetotoxicity, 138-139
  with cholestyramine resin, 325
  with phenytoin, 332
Furoxone®. See Furazolidone

G

Gabapentin
  adjustments in renal insufficiency, 758t
  in children and adolescents, 636t
Gabitril®. See Tiagabine
Gallium citrate, breast milk excretion, 214t
Gamimune N®. See Immune globulin
Gamma benzene hydrochloride. *See* Lindane
Gamma-gard®. See Immune globulin
Gammar-P®. See Immune globulin
Ganciclovir
  adjustments in renal insufficiency, 758t
  adverse drug reactions, 304t
  in children and adolescents, 637t
  drug interactions, 329
  intravenous administration, 407t
  in neonates, 542t
Gantanol®. See Sulfamethoxazole
Gantrisin®. See Sulfamethoxazole
Garamycin®. See Gentamicin
Gasoline ingestion, 270-272
Gasping syndrome, 42n

Gastric emptying, delayed, metoclopramide in, 678t
Gastric hyperacidity, aluminum hydroxide in, 563t
Gastric lavage, 249–250
Gastrocrom®. See Cromolyn sodium
Gastroesophageal reflux disease (GERD)
　bethanechol in, 581t
　calcium carbonate in, 587t
　domperidone in, 618t
　famotidine in, 628t
　omeprazole in, 693t
　ranitidine in, 548t, 723–724t
Gastrostomy tubes, drug administration and, 18–19
Gas-X®. See Simethicone
Gaucher's disease
　alglucerase in, 562t
　imiglucerase in type 1, 647t
G-CSF. *See* Filgrastim
Gee Gee®. See Guaifenesin
Gels, rectal, administration, 21–22
Genaspor®. See Tolnaftate
Gen-Fenofibrate Micro®. See Fenofibrate micronized
Genital herpes simplex
　acyclovir in, 559t
　valacyclovir in, 748–749t
Genoptic®. See Gentamicin ophthalmic
Genotropin®. See Somatropin
Gentacidin®. See Gentamicin ophthalmic
Gentamicin
　adjustments in renal insufficiency, 758t
　adverse drug reactions, 293t
　breast milk excretion, 214t
　intravenous administration, 408t
　in neonates, 542t
　ophthalmic, in infants, children, and adolescents, 637t
　optimal serum concentrations, 761t
　systemic, in infants, children, and adolescents, 637t
　teratogenicity/fetotoxicity, 139
　topical, in infants, children, and adolescents, 637t
Gentian violet, in children and adolescents, 638t
GenXene®. See Clorazepate
Geocillin®. See Carbenicillin indanyl
Geodon®. See Ziprasidone
Giardiasis. *See also* Parasitic infestations
　metronidazole in, 678t
GI decontamination, in poisoning, 248–251
Gigantism, octreotide in, 693t
Gingival hyperplasia, as adverse drug effect, 289t
Gingivitis, as adverse drug effect, 289t
GI tract smooth muscle spasms, dicyclomine in, 613t

Glaucoma
　acetazolamide in, 559t
　as adverse drug effect, 289t
Gliadel Wafer®. See Carmustine
Glimepiride, drug interactions, 317t
Glucagon
　in beta-blocker poisoning, 254t
　in children and adolescents, 638t
　intravenous administration, 408t
　in neonates, 542t
Glucophage®. See Metformin
Glucose intolerance. *See also* Diabetes mellitus
　insulin in, 544t
Glucuronosyl transferases, 481, 486. *See also* Pharmacogenetics
Glue, inhalant drug abuse, 358t, 360
Glukor®. See Chorionic gonadotropin
Glutethimide, teratogenicity/fetotoxicity, 139
Glyburide, teratogenicity/fetotoxicity, 139
Glycerin
　in infants, children, and adolescents, 638t
　in neonates, 542t
Glycerin rectal suppositories, adverse drug reactions, 309t
Glycerol guaiacolate. *See* Guaifenesin
Glyceryl guaiacolate carbamate. *See* Methocarbamol
Glyceryl trinitrate. *See* Nitroglycerin
Glycon®. See Metformin
Glycopyrrolate
　adverse drug reactions, 297t
　in children and adolescents, 639t
　intravenous administration, 408t
Gly-Oxide®. See Carbamide peroxide
GM-CSF. *See* Sargramostim
G-myticin®. See Gentamicin topical
Goiter/hypothyroidism, as adverse drug effect, 289t
Gold, breast milk excretion, 214t
Gold poisoning
　antidotes, 254t
　dimercaprol in, 615–616t
Gold salts, teratogenicity/fetotoxicity, 139–140
Gold sodium thiomalate
　adverse drug reactions, 293t
　in children and adolescents, 639t
GoLYTELY®. See Polyethylene glycol and electrolyte solutions
Gonadorelin, intravenous administration, 408t
Gonorrhea
　amoxicillin in, 566t
　cefpodoxime proxetil in, 591t
　ceftriaxone axetil in, 593t
　ceftriaxone in, 593t
　doxycycline in, 619t
　probenecid in, 566t
　trimethoprim/sulfamethoxazole in, 746–747t
Grand mal. *See* Convulsions

Granisetron
　as antiemetic, 499t
　in children and adolescents, 639–640t
　intravenous administration, 408t
Granules, administration, 14
Gravol®. See Dimenhydrinate
Gray baby syndrome, as adverse drug effect, 289t
Grifulvin V®. See Griseofulvin
Grisactin®. See Griseofulvin
Griseofulvin
　adverse drug reactions, 300t
　in children and adolescents, 640t
　drug interactions, 317t
　teratogenicity/fetotoxicity, 140
Gris-PEG®. See Griseofulvin
Growth failure
　somatrem in, 732t
　somatropin depot in, 733t
　somatropin in, 733t
Growth hormone
　breast milk excretion, 214t
　human. *See* Somatropin
Growth hormone deficiency, 732t, 733t. *See also* Growth failure
Growth suppression, as adverse drug effect, 289t
Guaiacolate. *See* Guaifenesin
Guaifenesin
　in children and adolescents, 640t
　teratogenicity/fetotoxicity, 140
Gynazole-1®. See Butaconazole

H

Haemophilus influenzae infection, rifampin in prophylaxis, 724t
Haldol®. See Haloperidol
Hallucinations, as adverse drug effect, 289t
Haloperidol
　adverse drug reactions, 303t
　breast milk excretion, 214t
　in children and adolescents, 640–641t
　dilution of, 10
　drug interactions, 317t
　teratogenicity/fetotoxicity, 140
Halotestin®. See Fluoxymesterone
Halothane, teratogenicity/fetotoxicity, 140
Halprogin, in children and adolescents, 641t
Headache, as adverse drug effect, 289t
Head lice
　bioallethrin and piperonyl butoxide in, 581t
　lindane in, 663t
　permethrin in, 703t
　piperacillin in, 708t
Head & Shoulders Intensive®. See Selenium sulfide
Heart transplant, cyclopentolate in, 606t
Helminthic infestations. *See* Parasitic infestations *and specific organisms*

Hemochromatosis, as adverse drug effect, 289t
Hemodialysis
  in methanol poisoning, 275
  in poisoning, 253
Hemolytic anemia, autoimmune, betamethasone in, 580t
Hemolytic jaundice, immune globulin in, 543t
Hemonyne®. See Factor IX complex
Hemoperfusion, in poisoning, 252-253
Hemophilia
  Factor IX complex in, 628t
  immunizations and, 435
  tranexamic acid in, 744-745t
Hemophilia A, antihemophilic Factor VIII in, 571t
Hemophilus influenzae type B vaccine, 440-441, 441t
Hemorrhage. See also Bleeding
  aminocaproic acid in, 533t
  aminocaproic acid in life-threatening, 564t
  subarachnoid, aminocaproic acid in, 564t
Heparin
  adverse drug reactions, 297t
  breast milk excretion, 214t
  in infants, children, and adolescents, 641t
  intravenous administration, 409t
  in neonates, 542t
  teratogenicity/fetotoxicity, 140-141
Heparin-induced coagulation disorders, lepirudin in, 660t
Heparin-induced thrombocytopenia, 51n
  danaparoid in, 607-608t
Heparin locks, 66
Heparin overdosage, protamine sulfate in, 548t, 719t
Hepatic coma
  neomycin in, 687-688t
  paromomycin in, 698t
Hepatic dysfunction, as adverse drug effect, 289t
Hepatitis, as adverse drug effect, 289t
Hepatitis A and B vaccine, in infants, children, and adolescents, 642t
Hepatitis A vaccine, 441-442
  in children and adolescents
    inactivated, 641-642t
    inactivated purified, 642t
    inactivated virosome formulated, 642t
Hepatitis B
  interferon alfa-2b in, 650-651t
  lamivudine in, 658t
Hepatitis B vaccine, 442-444
  teratogenicity/fetotoxicity, 141
Hepatolenticular degeneration (Wilson's disease), penicillamine in, 700t
Hepatotoxicity, of acetaminophen, 258-260

Heptovir®. See Lamivudine
Herceptin®. See Trastuzumab
Heroin, 356-357, 357t
  breast milk excretion, 215t
  teratogenicity/fetotoxicity, 141-142
Herpes simplex encephalitis, acyclovir in, 559t
Herpesvirus infections
  acyclovir in, 532t, 559t
  valacyclovir in, 748-749t
Hexachlorophane. See Hexachlorophene
Hexachlorophene
  in infants, children, and adolescents, 643t
  teratogenicity/fetotoxicity, 142
Hibiclens®. See Chlorhexidine
Hibitane®. See Chlorhexidine
Hiccups, related to tablet sticking, 14n
Hiprex®. See Methenamine; Methenamine hippurate
Hirsutism, as adverse drug effect, 289t
Hismanal®. See Astemizole
Histrelin, in children and adolescents, 643-644t
HIV/AIDS
  amprenavir in, 569-570t
  bacterial infections in, immune globulin in prevention, 648t
  didanosine in, 613t
  indinavir in, 648t
  zidovudine in, 551t
Hi-Vegi-Lip®. See Pancreatin
HMS®. See Medrysone
Hodgkin's lymphoma, antineoplastic drug regimens, 506t
Homatropine, in children and adolescents, 644t
Homocystinuria, betaine in, 579t
Hookworm. See also Parasitic infestations
  mebendazole in, 668t
  pyrantel pamoate in, 720t
Hormones. See specific hormones
H.P. Acthar®. See Corticotropin
H_2 receptor antagonists. See also specific drugs
  adverse drug reactions, 303-304t
Human chorionic gonadotropin (hCG), teratogenicity/fetotoxicity, 114-115
Human diploid-cell rabies (HDCR) vaccine, with chloramphenicol, 325
Human growth hormone. See Somatropin
Human immunodeficiency virus. See AIDS/HIV
Humatin®. See Paromomycin
Humatrope®. See Somatropin
Humulin®. See Insulin
Huntington's chorea, tetrabenazine in, 738t

Hyaluronidase
  in infants, children, and adolescents, 644t
  in neonates, 542t
Hycamtin®. See Topotecan
Hydralazine
  adverse drug reactions, 302t
  breast milk excretion, 215t
  in children and adolescents, 644-645t
  intravenous administration, 409t
  in neonates, 543t
  teratogenicity/fetotoxicity, 142-143
Hydrea®. See Hydroxyurea
Hydrocarbons, 270-272
  aspiration, 270-271
  aspiration pneumonia, 271-272
  ingestion, 270
  skin exposure, 272
Hydrochlorothiazide
  adverse drug reactions, 308t
  breast milk excretion, 215t
  in infants, children, and adolescents, 645t
  in neonates, 543t
  teratogenicity/fetotoxicity, 143
Hydrocodone, drug interactions, 317t
Hydrocort®. See Hydrocortisone topical
Hydrocortisone
  adverse drug reactions, 307t
  in children and adolescents, systemic, 645t
  in infants, children, and adolescents, topical, 645t
  in neonates, 543t
Hydrocortisone sodium phosphate, intravenous administration, 409t
Hydrocortisone sodium succinate, intravenous administration, 409t
Hydrocortone®. See Hydrocortisone sodium phosphate
HydroDIURIL®. See Hydrochlorothiazide
Hydroflumethiazide, teratogenicity/fetotoxicity, 143
Hydrogen peroxide, in children and adolescents, 646t
Hydromorphone
  in adolescents, 646t
  intravenous administration, 409t
Hydroxychloroquine
  breast milk excretion, 215t
  in children and adolescents, 646t
Hydroxydaunorubicin. See Doxorubicin
Hydroxyprogesterone, teratogenicity/fetotoxicity, 143
Hydroxyurea
  breast milk excretion, 215t
  dosing, 516t
Hydroxyzine
  adverse drug reactions, 301t
  in children and adolescents, 646t
  teratogenicity/fetotoxicity, 143

INDEX

dl-Hyocyamine. *See* Atropine systemic
Hyoscine. *See* Scopolamine
Hyperaldosteronism, spironolactone in, 549t, 734t
Hypercalcemia
 as adverse drug effect, 289t
 plicamycin in, 708t
Hypercalciuria, plicamycin in, 708t
Hypercholesterolemia
 cholestyramine in, 598t
 fenofibrate in
  microcoated, 628t
  micronized, 629t
Hypercoagulability. *See also* Coagulation disorders
Hyperemia
 naphazoline ophthalmic in, 686t
 oxymetazoline ophthalmic in, 696t
Hyperglycemia. *See also* Diabetes mellitus
 as adverse drug effect, 289t
Hyperkalemia
 calcium chloride in, 535t
 calcium gluconate in, 535t
 insulin in, 544t
 sodium polystyrene sulfonate in, 549t
Hyperphosphatemia, aluminum hydroxide in, 563t, 732t
Hypersensitivity. *See also* Allergy; Anaphylaxis
 as adverse drug effect, 289t
 to intravenous drugs, 79
 to iodine, 48-50
 to oil formulations, 42, 42n
 to sulfites, 8n
Hyperstat®. *See* Diazoxide; Diazoxide injectable
Hypertension
 as adverse drug effect, 289t
 atenolol in, 573t
 bumetanide in, 584t
 captopril in, 535t, 587t
 chlorothiazide in, 596t
 clonidine in, 601t
 diazoxide in, 611-612t
 enalapril in, 621t
 hydralazine in, 543t, 644-645t
 irbesartan in, 652t
 labetalol in, 657t
 lisinopril in, 664t
 methyldopa in, 676t
 minoxidil in, 681-682t
 nadolol in, 685t
 nifedipine in, 690t
 nitroglycerin in, 691t
 phentolamine in, 705t
 propranolol in, 548t, 718t
 pulmonary. *See* Pulmonary hypertension
Hypertensive crisis, sodium nitroprusside in, 732t
Hyperthermia, malignant. *See* Malignant hyperthermia
Hyperthyroidism
 methimazole in, 674t
 propylthiouracil in, 718t

Hyperuricemia, allopurinol in, 562t
Hypervitaminosis A, 198-199
Hypoadrenalism, hydrocortisone in, 645t
Hypocalcemia
 calcium chloride in, 535t
 calcium gluconate in, 535t
 calcium in, 586t
Hypodermoclysis, hyaluronidase in, 644t
Hypogammaglobinemia, immune globulin in, 648t
Hypoglycemia, 300t
 as adverse drug effect, 290t
 dextrose in, 538t
 diazoxide in, 538t
 diazoxide oral in, 612t
 epinephrine in, 539t
 glucagon in, 542t, 638t
Hypoglycemia prophylaxis, dextrose in, 537t
Hypoglycemic coma, dextrose in, 611t
Hypokalemia
 as adverse drug effect, 290t
 potassium chloride in, 548t, 709-710t
Hypomagnesemia
 magnesium sulfate in, 544t, 668t
Hyponatremia, sodium chloride in, 549t
Hypoparathyroidism, dihydrotachysterol in, 615t
Hypoproteinemia, albumin in, 532t
Hypoprothrombinemia, phytonadione in, 707t
Hypotension
 epinephrine in, 539t
 phenylephrine in, 705t
Hypothermia, as adverse drug effect, 290t
Hypothyroidism
 as adverse drug effect, 289t, 290t
 levothyroxine in, 661-662t
Hytakerol®. *See* Dihydrotachysterol
Hytone®. *See* Hydrocortisone topical

I

Ibuprofen
 breast milk excretion, 215t
 drug interactions, 317t
 in infants, children, and adolescents, 646-647t
 teratogenicity/fetotoxicity, 143-144
Ibuprofen poisoning, 262-263
IDA. *See* Idarubicin
Idamycin®. *See* Idarubicin
Idarubicin
 dosing, 516t
 extravasation care, 506t
 intravenous administration, 410t
Idiopathic thrombocytopenic purpura, 648t
Idiosyncratic drug effects, 284
Ifex®. *See* Ifosfamide
IFOS. *See* Ifosfamide

Ifosfamide
 dosing, 516t
 intravenous administration, 410t
Iletin®. *See* Insulin
Imidazole carboxamide. *See* Dacarbazine
Imiglucerase, in children and adolescents, 647t
Imipenem/cilastatin
 adjustments in renal insufficiency, 758t
 adverse drug reactions, 296t
 in infants, children, and adolescents, 647t
 intravenous administration, 410t
Imipramine
 breast milk excretion, 215t
 drug interactions, 317t
 teratogenicity/fetotoxicity, 144
Immune globulin
 in children and adolescents, 648t
 intravenous administration, 410t
 in neonates, 543t
Immunin VH®. *See* Factor IX complex (human)
Immunizations, 433-458. *See also* Vaccines
 general cautions, 433-437
  adverse drug reactions (ADRs), 435-437, 437
  AIDS/HIV, 434
  allergy, 433-434
  blood replacement therapy, 435
  breast feeding, 434
  contraindications, 433
  hemophilia, 435
  immunosuppressive therapy, 434
  live viral vaccines, 434
  neurologic disorders, 434
  pregnancy, 434
  record-keeping, 435
  storage and handling, 435
  timing, 435
  vaccine combinations, 435
 schedules and monographs, 437-458, 438t, 439t
  diphtheria toxoid, 437-440
  Hemophilus influenzae type B, 440-441, 441t
  hepatitis A, 441-442
  hepatitis B, 442-444
  influenza virus, 444-445
  measles virus, 445-447
  meningococcus, 447-448
  mumps virus, 448-449
  passive immunization, 449-450
  pertussis, 450-452, 452t
  pneumococcus, 452-453
  poliomyelitis, 453-455
  rotavirus, 455
  rubella virus, 455-456
  tetanus toxoid, 456-457
  varicella zoster, 457-458
Immunocompromise, acyclovir in, 559-560t
Immunosuppressive therapy, immunizations and, 434

INDEX

Imodium®. *See* Loperamide
Impetigo, mupirocin topical in, 684t
Inapsine®. *See* Droperidol
Increased intracranial pressure, as adverse drug effect, 290t
Inderal®. *See* Propranolol
Indinavir
   adverse drug reactions, 304t
   in children and adolescents, 648t
Indocid®. *See* Indomethacin
Indocin®. *See* Indomethacin
Indomethacin
   in adolescents, 648t
   breast milk excretion, 215t
   drug interactions, 317t
   intravenous administration, 411t
   in neonates, 543t
   teratogenicity/fetotoxicity, 144-145
Infantile spasms (West syndrome)
   corticotropin in, 603-604t
   vigabatrin in, 751t
Infants
   drug administration in, 3t, 16
   injections administered in, 44
Infections. *See also* Antibiotics; Bacterial infections; Fungal infections
   ampicillin in, 534t
   cefazolin in prophylaxis, 536t
   in antineoplastic therapy, 497
   intravenous-administration/ related, 79
   parasitic. *See* Parasitic infestations; Protozoal infestations; *specific diseases*
   skin, cefpodoxime proxetil in, 591t
INFeD®. *See* Iron dextran
Inflamase®. *See* Prednisolone ophthalmic
Inflammatory acne, tetracycline in, 738t
Inflammatory bowel disease (IBD). *See* Crohn's disease; Ulcerative colitis
Inflammatory bowel syndrome, cromolyn sodium in, 604-605t
Infliximab, in children and adolescents, 648-649t
Influenza
   oseltamivir in, 694-695t
   rimantadine in, 724-725t
   zanamivir in, 754t
Influenza virus vaccine, 444-445
   teratogenicity/fetotoxicity, 144-145
Infusion. *See also* Intravenous administration
   continuous, 77
   intermittent, 76-77
   opiate analgesic, 52-53
   subcutaneous opiate, 52-53
   types of intravenous, 388
Infusion pumps, 70-71
Infusion rate, calculation of, 64n
INH®. *See* Isoniazid

Inhalant drug abuse, 357-360, 358t, 359t
Inhalation dosage forms, 31-38
   compressed-air and other nebulizers, 31-33
   metered-dose inhalers (MDIs), 33-34
   powder inhalers (insufflators), 35-36
   selection, 36
   spacers and other inhalation devices, 34-35
Injectable dosage forms, 42-83
   developmental considerations, 44-45
   dosage forms and related equipment, 45-48
      ampules, 46
      disposal of eqipment, 48
      needles, 47-48
      syringes, 48
      vials, 46-47
   general considerations, 42-44
   intramuscular, 53-61, *56, 57, 59, 61*
      equipment selection, 54-55
      sites, 55-60, *56, 57, 59*. *See also* Injection sites
      technique, 60-61
   site preparation, 48-49
   subcutaneous, 49-53, *50*
      equipment selection, 49
      sites, 49-50, *50*
      technique, 50-53
Injection sites, 55-60
   deltoid, 55-56, *56*
   dorsogluteal, 56-57, *57*
   quadriceps contracture, 59-60
   vastus lateralis, 58, *59*
   ventrogluteal, *57*, 57-58
Inotropic drugs, adverse drug reactions, 307t
Inserts, ophthalmic, 25
Insomnia
   as adverse drug effect, 290t
   chloral hydrate in, 595t
   diphenhydramine systemic in, 616t
   pentobarbital in, 702t
   secobarbital in, 728t
Insufflators (powder inhalers), 35-36
Insulin
   absorption rates, 51n
   adverse drug reactions, 300t
   breast milk excretion, 215t
   in children and adolescents, 649-650t
   drug interactions, 329
   intravenous administration, 411t
   in neonates, 544t
   teratogenicity/fetotoxicity, 145-146
   with anabolic steroids, 320
   with beta-blockers, 323
Insulin syringes, 49
Intal®. *See* Cromolyn sodium
Intensol® concentrated mixtures, 10, 11

Interferon alfa-2b, in children and adolescents, 650-651t
Intestinal moniliasis, nystatin in, 692t
Intralipid®. *See* Fat emulsions
Intramuscular injections
   equipment selection, 54-55
   sites, 55-60, *56, 57, 59*. *See also* Injection sites
   technique, 60-61
      topical anesthesia, 60-61
      Z-track, 61, *61*
Intranasal dosage forms, 28-31
   aerosols, 30-31
   creams and ointments, 29
   drops, 29
Intraosseous injections and infusions, 81-83, *82*
   complications, 82-83
   technique, 81-82, *82*
Intrathecal antineoplastic therapy, 496
Intravenous drugs, 387-431
   administration guidelines, 390-431t
   general considerations, 387-389
      clinician skills and training, 388-389
      dilution and fluid restriction, 388
      equipment and cost, 387-388
      physicochemical properties, 388
      rate and method of delivery, 388
Intravenous injections and infusions, 61-83
   activity restriction and, 80-81
   complications, 78-80
      air embolism and thrombus, 78
      extravasation, 78. *See also* Extravasation
      fluid overload and drug toxicity, 78-79
      hypersensitivity, 79
      infection, 79
      phlebitis, 79-80
   equipment, 62-71, *65*
      needleless and other alternative systems, 64-65
      solutions and containers, 63
      tubing and drip chambers, 64
      venous access devices, *65*, 65-71. *See also* Venous access devices
   general considerations, 61-62
   intraosseous, 81-83, *82*
   special precautions, 78n
   technique, 71-78, *72, 73, 74*
      continuous infusion, 78
      intermittent infusion, 76-77
      scalp vein technique, *73*, 73-74
      sites for children and adolescents, 74
      slow and rapid injection (IV push), 76
      topical anesthesia, 75-76
      venipuncture, *72*, 72-73

Intron® A. See Interferon alfa-2b
Intropin®. See Dopamine
Intubation
  cisatracurium in, 599t
  mivacurium in, 682t
  pancuronium in, 546t
  small bowel, metoclopramide in, 678t
  in status epilepticus, pancuronium bromide in, 698t
  succinylcholine in, 550t
  theophylline in 550t
Iodide, teratogenicity/fetotoxicity, 146
Iodine, breast milk excretion, 215t
Iodoquinol in children and adolescents, 651t
  teratogenicity/fetotoxicity, 146
I-PAM. *See* Melphalan
Ipecac syrup
  contraindications, 249, 274, 276
  in infants, children, and adolescents, 651t
  in poisoning, 248-249
Ipratropium, in children and adolescents
  nasal, 651t, 652t
  pulmonary, 652t
Ipratropium bromide, adverse drug reactions, 297t
Irbesartan, in children and adolescents, 652t
Irinotecan
  dosing, 516t
  intravenous administration, 411t
Iron
  breast milk excretion, 216t
  drug interactions, 329
  oral
    adverse drug reactions, 310-311t
    in children and adolescents, 652-653t
    with antacids, 321
    with tetracyclines, 335
Iron-deficiency anemia
  iron dextran injectable in, 653t
  iron oral in, 652t
Iron dextran
  injectable
    adverse drug reactions, 310t
    in infants, children, and adolescents, 653t
    intravenous administration, 411t
Iron poisoning, 263-265. *See also* Metal poisoning
  deferoxamine in, 609t
Iron salts, teratogenicity/fetotoxicity, 146-147
Irrigation, whole bowel, in poisoning, 251
Isoephedrine. *See* Pseudoephedrine
Isoetharine, in children and adolescents, 653-654t
Isoniazid
  adverse drug reactions, 296t
  breast milk excretion, 216t
  in children and adolescents, 654t

drug interactions, 317t, 329
teratogenicity/fetotoxicity, 147
with BCG vaccine, 322
with carbamazepine, 324
with phenytoin, 332
with primidone, 334
Isoniazid poisoning, 255t
Isoniazid-resistant tuberculosis, streptomycin in, 734t
Isonicotinic acid hydrazide. *See* Isoniazid
Isophedrine. *See* Pseudoephedrine
Isoprel®. See Isoproterenol
Isoprenaline. *See* Isoproterenol
Isopropyl alcohol, 273
Isoproterenol
  adverse drug reactions, 305t
  in children and adolescents, 654-655t
  intravenous administration, 411t
  in neonates, 544t
Isoptin®. See Verapamil
Isopto-Atropine®. See Atropine ophthalmic
Isopto-Cetamide®. See Sulfacetamide sodium ophthalmic
Isopto Homatropine®. See Homatropine
Isotretinoin
  in adolescents, 655t
  in cancer, 517t
  teratogenicity/fetotoxicity, 147-148
Itching. *See also* Allergy; Dermatitis
  calamine in, 586t
  cetirizine in, 594t
  clemastine in, 600t
  diphenhydramine topical in, 616t
  hydroxyzine in, 646t
  ocular, naphazoline ophthalmic in, 686t
Itraconazole
  drug interactions, 317t, 329
  with antacids, 321
  with cimetidine, 325
Iveegam®. See Immune globulin
Ivermectin, breast milk excretion, 216t
IV push, 76

J

Jaundice
  as adverse drug effect, 290t
  immune globulin in, 543t
Juvenile rheumatoid arthritis
  aspirin in, 573t
  betamethasone in, 580t
  celecoxib in, 593t
  cortisone in, 604t
  diclofenac oral in, 612t
  etanercept in, 625t
  gold sodium thiomalate in, 639t
  hydroxychloroquine in, 646t
  ibuprofen in, 646t
  indomethacin in, 648-649t
  leflunomide in, 659t

methotrexate in, 675-676t
nabumetone in, 685t
naproxen sodium in, 686t
penicillamine in, 700t
sulfasalazine in, 736t
tolmetin sodium in, 743t

K

Kanamycin
  breast milk excretion, 216t
  intravenous administration, 412t
  teratogenicity/fetotoxicity, 148
Kantrex®. See Kanamycin
Kaolin, teratogenicity/fetotoxicity, 148
Kaolin-pectin, with digitalis glycosides, 328
Karidium®. See Sodium fluoride
Kawasaki disease (mucocutaneous lymph node syndrome)
  aspirin in, 573t
  immune globulin in, 648t
Kayexalate®. See Sodium polystyrene sulfonate
Keflex®. See Cephalexin
Keflin®. See Cephalothin
Kefzol®. See Cefazolin
Kenacort®. See Triamcinolone oral
Kenalog®. See Triamcinolone topical
Keratitis, vernal, lodoxamide in, 665t
Kerosene ingestion, 270-272
Ketalar®. See Ketamine
Ketamine
  in children and adolescents, 656t
  teratogenicity/fetotoxicity, 148
Ketoacidosis, diabetic, insulin in, 649-650t
Ketoconazole
  adverse drug reactions, 301t
  breast milk excretion, 216t
  in children and adolescents
    oral systemic, 656t
    topical cream, 656t
    topical shampoo, 656-657t
  drug interactions, 317t, 329
  with antacids, 321
  with cimetidine, 325-326
  with cyclosporine, 327
Ketorolac tromethamine, breast milk excretion, 216t
Ketotifen, in infants and children, 657t
Key-Pred®. See Prednisolone systemic
Kidrolase®. See Asparaginase
Kionex®. See Sodium polystyrene sulfonate
Klaron®. See Sulfacetamide sodium topical
Klean-Prep®. See Polyethylene glycol and electrolyte solutions
Klonopin®. See Clonazepam
Kogenate®. See Antihemophilic Factor VIII (Recombinant)
Konakion®. See Phytonadione
Kondremul®. See Mineral oil

INDEX

Konsyl®. See Psyllium
Konyne®. See Factor IX complex
Kreteks (cigarettes with spices), 364n
Kyo-Dophilus®. See Lactobacillus acidophilus
Kytril®. See Granisetron

L

Labetalol
　adverse drug reactions, 301t
　breast milk excretion, 216t
　in children and adolescents, 657t
　intravenous administration, 412t
　teratogenicity/fetotoxicity, 149
Laboratory values, pediatric, 785-788t
Labyrinthitis, meclizine in, 669t
Lactic acidosis, sodium bicarbonate in, 731t
Lactinex®. See Lactobacillus acidophilus
Lactobacillus acidophilus, 657t
Lactulose, in children and adolescents, 657
Lamictal®. See Lamotrigine
Lamivudine
　adjustments in renal insufficiency, 758t
　breast milk excretion, 216t
　in infants, children, and adolescents, 657-658t
Lamotrigine, in children and adolescents, 658-659t
Lanoxin®. See Digoxin
Lansoprazole, drug interactions, 317t
Largactil®. See Chlorpromazine
Lariam®. See Mefloquine
Lasix®. See Furosemide
Lavage, gastric, 249-250
Laxatives. *See also specific products*
　adverse drug reactions, 309t
Laxilose®. See Lactulose
Lead, breast milk excretion, 216t
Lead poisoning, 255t
　antidotes, 254t
　dimercaprol in, 616t
　penicillamine in, 700t
　succimer in, 734t
Learning impairment
　as adverse drug effect, 290t
　marijuana and, 368
Ledercillin VK®. See Penicillin G potassium
Leflunomide, in adolescents, 659t
Leishmaniasis, visceral, amphotericin B liposome in, 568-569t
Lennox-Gastaut syndrome
　clonazepam in, 601t
　lamotrigine in
　topiramate in, 743t
Lepirudin
　adjustments in renal insufficiency, 758t
　in children and adolescents, 660t
Leprosy, dapsone in, 608t

Leucovorin calcium
　dosing, 517t
　intravenous administration, 412t
Leukemias, antineoplastic drug regimens, 506t
Leukeran®. See Chlorambucil
Leukine®. See Sargramostim
Leukotriene antagonists, adverse drug reactions, 305t
Leuprolide, in children, 660t
Leustatin®. See Cladribine
Levalbuterol, in children and adolescents, 660-661t
Levarterenol. *See* Epinephrine; Norepinephrine
Levodopa/carbidopa, breast milk excretion, 216t
Levomepromazine. *See* Methotrimeprazine
Levonorgestrel
　in adolescents, 661t
　breast milk excretion, 216-217t
Levonorgestrel/ethinyl estradiol emergency contraceptive combination, in adolescents, 661t
Levophed®. See Norepinephrine; Norepinephrine bitartrate
Levoprome®. See Methotrimeprazine
Levotec®. See Levothyroxine
Levothyroxine
　adverse drug reactions, 309t
　in infants, children, and adolescents, 661-662t
　intravenous administration, 412t
　teratogenicity/fetotoxicity, 149
Lidemol®. See Fluocinolone
Lidex®. See Fluocinonide
Lidocaine
　adverse drug reactions, 306t
　breast milk excretion, 217t
　in children and adolescents, 662t
　intravenous administration, 413t
　in neonates, 544t
　optimal serum concentrations, 761t
　teratogenicity/fetotoxicity, 149
Lidocaine/prilocaine, topical, in infants, children, and adolescents, 662t
Life-threatening conditions, methylprednisolone sodium succinate in, 677t
Lignocaine. *See* Lidocaine
Lincocin®. See Lincomycin
Lincomycin
　breast milk excretion, 217t
　intravenous administration, 413t
　teratogenicity/fetotoxicity, 149
Lindane
　breast milk excretion, 217t
　in infants, children, and adolescents, 663t
Linezolid, in children and adolescents, 663-664t
Lioresal®. See Baclofen
Lipidil Micro®. See Fenofibrate micronized

Lipidil Supra®. See Fenofibrate microcoated
Liposome formulations, 43
Liquid oral dosage forms, 8-11. *See also under* Oral dosage forms
Liquid Pred®. See Prednisone
Lisinopril
　adjustments in renal insufficiency, 758t
　in adolescents, 664t
Lithane®. See Lithium
Lithium
　in adolescents, 664-665t
　adverse drug reactions, 302-303t
　breast milk excretion, 217t
　drug interactions, 329
　optimal serum concentrations, 761t
　teratogenicity/fetotoxicity, 149-151
　with carbamazepine, 324
　with phenytoin, 332
Lithobid®. See Lithium
Liver fluke infestation. *See also* Parasitic infestations; Protozoal infestations
　praziquantel in, 710t
Liver transplantation. *See also* Transplantation
　muromonab-CD3 in, 684t
　tacrolimus in, 737t
Lodoxamide, in children, 665t
Lomine®. See Dicyclomine
Lomotil®. See Diphenoxylate and atropine
Lomustine, dosing, 518t
Loniten®. See Minoxidil
Lonox®. See Diphenoxylate and atropine
Loop diuretics. *See also specific drugs*
　adverse drug reactions, 308t
Loperacap®. See Loperamide
Loperamide
　breast milk excretion, 217t
　in infants, children, and adolescents, 665t
　teratogenicity/fetotoxicity, 151
Lorabid®. See Loracarbef
Loracarbef
　adjustments in renal insufficiency, 758t
　in infants, children, and adolescents, 665-666t
Loratadine, 266
　adjustments in renal insufficiency, 758t
　breast milk excretion, 217t
　in children and adolescents, 666t
Lorazepam
　adverse drug reactions, 298t, 310t
　as antiemetic, 499t
　breast milk excretion, 217t
　in children and adolescents, 666t
　in neonates, 544t
　sublingual, 39
　teratogenicity/fetotoxicity, 151
Losartan, drug interactions, 317t

Losec®. See Omeprazole
Lotions, 37-38
Lotrimin®. See Clotrimazole; Miconazole
Lovenox®. See Enoxaparin
Lubricant laxatives. *See also* Oils
  adverse drug reactions, 309t
Lupron®. See Leuprolide
Lupron Depot®. See Leuprolide
Lupron Depot-PED®. See Leuprolide
Luride®. See Sodium fluoride
Luxiq®. See Betamethasone topical
Lyderm®. See Fluocinonide
Lyme disease, doxycycline in, 619t
Lymphadenopathy, as adverse drug effect, 290t
Lymphocyte immune globulin, intravenous administration, 413t
Lymphoma, antineoplastic drug regimens, 506t
Lysergic acid diethylamide (LSD), 368, 371
  teratogenicity/fetotoxicity, 151-152

M

Maalox®. See Aluminum hydroxide antacids
Maalox Antacid Caplets®. See Calcium carbonate
MacroBID®. See Nitrofurantoin
Macrodantin®. See Nitrofurantoin
Macrolides. *See also specific drugs*
  adverse drug reactions, 294t
Mafenide, in infants, children, and adolescents, 666-667t
Magnesium citrate
  adverse drug reactions, 309t
  in children and adolescents, 668t
Magnesium hydroxide
  adverse drug reactions, 303t, 309t
  breast milk excretion, 219t
  in children and adolescents, 668t
Magnesium salicylate, aspirin conversion factor, 257t
Magnesium sulfate
  breast milk excretion, 218t
  in children and adolescents, 668t
  intravenous administration, 413t
  in neonates, 544t
  teratogenicity/fetotoxicity, 152
Majeptil®. See Thioproperazine
Major depressive disorder. *See* Depression
Malaria
  chloroquine in, 596t
  doxycycline in prophylaxis, 619t
  mefloquine in, 669-670t
  Plasmodium falciparum
    chloroquine resistant
    quinidine in, 722t
    quinine dihydrochloride in, 722t
    quinine sulfate in, 722-723
  primaquine in, 713t
Malignant hyperthermia, dantrolene in prophylaxis, 608t

Mandelamine®. See Methenamine; Methenamine mandelate
Mandol®. See Cefamandole; Cefamandole nafate
Mania, lithium in, 664t
Mannitol
  in children and adolescents, 668t
  intravenous administration, 413t
Marbaxin®. See Methocarbamol
Marcaine®. See Bupivacaine
Marijuana, 366-368
  amotivational syndrome and, 368
  breast milk excretion, 227t
  driving impairment and, 367-368
  learning impairment and, 368
  respiratory disease and, 367
  teratogenicity/fetotoxicity, 152-153
Marinol®. See Dronabinol
Maternal factors affecting teratogenesis, 89-90
Matulane®. See Procarbazine
Maxipime®. See Cefepime
M.C.T. Oil®. See Medium chain triglyceride oil
MDMA, 369n, 369-370, 370t
Measles virus vaccine, 445-447
Measurement devices, for oral drugs, 10-11
Mebendazole
  in children and adolescents, 668t
  teratogenicity/fetotoxicity, 153
Mechanical ventilation. *See also* Intubation
  pancuronium bromide in, 698t
Mechlorethamine
  dosing, 518t
  extravasation care, 506t
  intravenous administration, 414t
  teratogenicity/fetotoxicity, 153
Meclizine
  in children and adolescents, 668-669t
  teratogenicity/fetotoxicity, 153
Medihaler-Iso®. See Isoproterenol
Medicorten®. See Prednisone
Medium chain triglyceride oil, in neonates, 544t
Medroxyprogesterone
  breast milk excretion, 218t
  teratogenicity/fetotoxicity, 153-154
Medrysone, in children and adolescents, 669t
Mefloquine
  breast milk excretion, 218t
  in infants, children, and adolescents, 669-670t
Mefoxin®. See Cefoxitin
Mega Interactive Model of abusable psychotropic drug use, 348-354, 350. *See also under* Abusable psychotropic drug use
Megaloblastic anemia, folic acid in, 541t
Mellaril®. See Thioridazine

Melphalan
  dosing, 518t
  intravenous administration, 414t
Meniere's syndrome, meclizine in, 669t
Meningitis
  bacterial
    ampicillin in, 534t, 569t
    ceftriaxone in, 536t
    chloramphenicol in, 595t
    dexamethasone in, 610t
    penicillin G in, 546t
  cryptococcal, fluconazole in, 630t
  fungal, amphotericin B in, 534t
  neonatal, cefotaxime in, 536t
  Pseudomonas aeruginosa, polymyxin B sulfate systemic in, 709t
Meningococcus vaccine, 447-448
Mental disability, drug administration and, 6-7, 18
Mentax®. See Butenafine
Meperidine, 9
  adjustments in renal insufficiency, 758t
  breast milk excretion, 218t
  in children and adolescents, 670t
  intravenous administration, 414t
  in neonates, 544t
  teratogenicity/fetotoxicity, 154
Mephenytoin
  in children and adolescents, 671t
  drug interactions, 317t
  teratogenicity/fetotoxicity, 154-155
Mephobarbital
  in children and adolescents, 671t
  teratogenicity/fetotoxicity, 155
Mephyton®. See Phytonadione
Mepivacaine, teratogenicity/fetotoxicity, 155
Meprobamate
  in anxiety disorders, 671t
  teratogenicity/fetotoxicity, 155-156
Mepron®. See Atovaquone
Meprospan®. See Meprobamate
Mercaptopurine
  dosing, 518t
  drug interactions, 330
  teratogenicity/fetotoxicity, 156
  with allopurinol, 320
Mercury poisoning
  antidotes, 254t
  dimercaprol in, 615-616t
Meropenem
  in infants, children, and adolescents, 672t
  intravenous administration, 414t
Merrem®. See Meropenem
Mesalamine
  breast milk excretion, 218t
  in children and adolescents, 672t
  toxicity, 102
Mesasal®. See Mesalamine
Mesna
  dosing, 519t
  intravenous administration, 415t

Mesnex®. See Mesna
Mesoridazine, in children and adolescents, 672-673t
Mestinon®. See Pyridostigmine bromide
Mestranol, breast milk excretion, 218t
Mesuximide. *See* Methsuximide
Metabolic acidosis, sodium bicarbonate in, 549t
Metadate®. See Methylphenidate
Metal poisoning, 254t, 255t. *See also specific metals*
  dimercaprol in, 615-616t
  penicillamine in, 700t
  succimer in, 734t
Metamucil®. See Psyllium
Metamucil Fiber Laxative®. See Psyllium
Metaproterenol
  adverse drug reactions, 305t
  in children and adolescents, 673t
Metered-dose inhalers (MDIs), 33-34
  open-mouth vs. closed-mouth technique, 33n
  spacers, 34-35, 36
Metformin, in children and adolescents, 673t
Methadone
  breast milk excretion, 218t
  teratogenicity/fetotoxicity, 156-157
Methamphetamine
  abuse of, 361-362, 362t
  in children and adolescents, 674t
  drug interactions, 317t
  teratogenicity/fetotoxicity, 157
Methanol poisoning, 255t, 273-275
Methemoglobinemia, 255t
  prilocaine-induced, 76n
Methenamine
  adverse drug reactions, 296t
  teratogenicity/fetotoxicity, 157-158
Methenamine hippurate, in children and adolescents, 674t
Methenamine mandelate, in children and adolescents, 674t
Methicillin-resistant *Staphylococcus aureus,* mupirocin nasal in, 683-684t
Methimazole
  breast milk excretion, 218t
  in children and adolescents, 674t
  teratogenicity/fetotoxicity, 158
Methocarbamol, in children and adolescents, 675t
Methohexital
  in children and adolescents, 675t
  intravenous administration, 415t
Methohexitone. *See* Methohexital
Methotrexate
  adjustments in renal insufficiency, 759t
  adverse drug reactions, 293t
  breast milk excretion, 219t

in children and adolescents, 675-676t
  dosing, 519t
  drug interactions, 330
  intravenous administration, 415t
  teratogenicity/fetotoxicity, 158
  with aminoglycosides, 320
  with penicillins, 331
  with sulfonamides, 335
Methotrimeprazine
  in children and adolescents, 676t
  teratogenicity/fetotoxicity, 158
Methsuximide
  in children and adolescents, 676t
  teratogenicity/fetotoxicity, 159
Methyldopa
  adjustments in renal insufficiency, 759t
  adverse drug reactions, 302t
  breast milk excretion, 219t
  in children and adolescents, 676t
  teratogenicity/fetotoxicity, 159
Methyldopate, intravenous administration, 415t
Methylene blue
  in children and adolescents, 677t
  intravenous administration, 415t
  in methemoglobinemia, 255t
  teratogenicity/fetotoxicity, 159-160
Methylenedioxy methamphetamine (Ecstasy, MDMA), teratogenicity/fetotoxicity, 160
Methylergonovine, breast milk excretion, 219t
Methylmorphine. *See* Codeine
Methylprenisolone sodium succinate
Methylphenidate
  adverse drug reactions, 307t
  in children and adolescents, 677t
  controlled-release tablets, 12-13
  teratogenicity/fetotoxicity, 160
Methylphenobarbital. *See* Mephobarbital
Methylprednisolone, in cancer, 519t
Methylprednisolone sodium succinate
  in children and adolescents, 677-678t
  intravenous administration, 416t
Methyl salicylate, aspirin conversion factor, 257t
Methyltestosterone, teratogenicity/fetotoxicity, 160-161
S-Methyltransferase. *See* Pharmacogenetics
S-Methyltransferase gene, antineoplastics and, 496
Metoclopramide
  adjustments in renal insufficiency, 759t
  as antiemetic, 499t
  breast milk excretion, 219t
  in infants, children, and adolescents, 678t
  intravenous administration, 416t
  teratogenicity/fetotoxicity, 161

Metoprolol
  breast milk excretion, 219t
  drug interactions, 317t
  intravenous administration, 416t
  teratogenicity/fetotoxicity, 161
Metric and SI conversion formulas, 763
Metronidazole
  adverse drug reactions, 296t
  breast milk excretion, 219t
  in children and adolescents, 678-679t
  drug interactions, 330
  intravenous administration, 416t
  in neonates, 545t
  teratogenicity/fetotoxicity, 161
Mexate®. See Methotrexate
Mexiletine
  adjustments in renal insufficiency, 759t
  adverse drug reactions, 306t
  breast milk excretion, 219t
  in children and adolescents, 679t
  drug interactions, 317t
  optimal serum concentrations, 761t
Mexitil®. See Mexiletine
Mezlin®. See Mezlocillin
Mezlocillin
  adjustments in renal insufficiency, 759t
  adverse drug reactions, 294t
Mibefradil, drug interactions, 317t
Micatin®. See Miconazole
Miconazole
  in children and adolescents, 679t
  teratogenicity/fetotoxicity, 161-162
Midazolam
  adjustments in renal insufficiency, 759t
  adverse drug reactions, 310t
  breast milk excretion, 219t
  in infants, children, and adolescents, 680-681t
  intravenous administration, 416t
  in neonates, 545t
Migraine headache
  dihydroergotamine in, 614t
  flunarizine in prophylaxis, 632t
  ibuprofen in, 647t
  naratriptan contraindicated in adolescents, 687t
Milliequivalents (mEq) conversion formula, 763
Milliequivalents per liter (mEq/l) conversion formula, 763
Milrinone
  adjustments in renal insufficiency, 759t
  in children and adolescents, 681t
  intravenous administration, 417t
Miltown®. See Meprobamate
MIMAPUY. *See* Mega Interactive Model of abusable psychotropic drug use

Mineral oil
  adverse drug reactions, 309t
  breast milk excretion, 220t
  in children and adolescents, 681t
Minipress®. See Prazosin
Minocin®. See Minocycline
Minocycline
  adverse drug reactions, 295t
  breast milk excretion, 220t
  in children and adolescents, 681t
  intravenous administration, 417t
Min-Ovral®. See Ethinyl estradiol/
    levonorgestrel; Oral
    contraceptives
Minox®. See Minoxidil
Minoxidil
  adverse drug reactions, 302t
  breast milk excretion, 220t
  in children and adolescents, 681–682t
  teratogenicity/fetotoxicity, 162
Mintezol®. See Thiabendazole
Miosis of iris, acetylcholine in, 559t
Misoprostol, teratogenicity/
    fetotoxicity, 162
Mithracin®. See Plicamycin
Mithramycin. See Plicamycin
Mitomycin, intravenous administration, 417t
Mitoxantrone
  breast milk excretion, 220t
  dosing, 520t
  intravenous administration, 417t
Mivacurium, in children and adolescents, 682t
MMDA. See Methylenedioxy methamphetamine (Ecstasy, MDMA)
Modadon®. See Nitrazepam
Molifen Ear Wax Removing Formula®. See Carbamide peroxide
Mometasone furoate monohydrate, in children and adolescents, 682t
Monazole®. See Miconazole
Moniliasis. See also Fungal infections
  intestinal, nystatin in, 692t
Monistat®. See Miconazole
Mononine®. See Factor IX (human); Factor IX complex (human)
Montelukast
  adverse drug reactions, 305t
  in children and adolescents, 683t
  drug interactions, 317t
Morbitec®. See Morphine
Morphine
  abuse of, 356–357, 357t
  adjustments in renal insufficiency, 759t
  breast milk excretion, 220t
  in children and adolescents, 683t
  concentrated solutions, 43
  drug interactions, 317t
  intravenous administration, 417t
  measurement of, 10–11
  in neonates, 545t
  teratogenicity/fetotoxicity, 162

Mortality, in pediatric poisoning, 246t
M.O.S.®. See Morphine
Motilium®. See Domperidone
Motion sickness
  dimenhydrinate in, 615t
  meclizine in, 669t
  promethazine in, 715t
  scopolamine in, 728t
Motrin®. See Ibuprofen
Mouth irritation, benzocaine in, 578–579t
Movement disorders, tetrabenazine in, 738t
Moxalactam, breast milk excretion, 220t
Moxifloxacin, drug interactions, 319t, 330
6-MP. See Mercaptopurine
MS Contin®. See Morphine
MTX. See Methotrexate
Mucocutaneous lymph node syndrome (Kawasaki disease)
  aspirin in, 573t
  immune globulin in, 648t
Mucomyst®. See Acetylcysteine
Multi-12®. See Vitamins, multiple
Mumps virus vaccine, 448–449
  teratogenicity/fetotoxicity, 162–163
Mupirocin
  nasal, in adolescents, 683–684t
  topical, in infants, children, and adolescents, 684t
Murine Ear Drops®. See Carbamide peroxide
Muromonab-CD3
  in infants, children, and adolescents, 684t
  intravenous administration, 418t
  optimal serum concentrations, 761t
Muscle relaxation. See also Neuromuscular blockade
  succinylcholine in, 550t
Muscles, sensory properties, 55n
Mustargen®. See Mechlorethamine
Mutamycin. See Mitomycin
M.V.I. 12®. See Vitamins, multiple
M.V.I. Pediatric®. See Vitamins, multiple
Myambutol®. See Ethambutol
Myasthenia gravis
  edrophonium in diagnosis, 620t
  neostigmine in diagnosis of, 688t
  pyridostigmine bromide in, 720t
Mycifradin®. See Neomycin
Mycobacterium avium complex (MAC) disease, clarithromycin in, 599–600t
Mycobutin®. See Rifabutin
Mycostatin®. See Nystatin
Mycotic infections. See Fungal infections
Mydriasis, cyclopentolate in, 537t, 605t
Mylanta®. See Aluminum hydroxide antacids

Mylanta Lozenges®. See Calcium carbonate
Myleran®. See Busulfan
Mylicon®. See Simethicone
Mylocel®. See Hydroxyurea
Myocardial failure. See also Cardiac arrest; Congestive failure
  dopamine in, 539t
Myochol-E®. See Acetylcysteine
Myochrysine®. See Gold sodium thiomalate
Myoglobinuria, 252
Mysoline®. See Primidone

N

Nabumetone, in children and adolescents, 685t
N-Acetylcysteine. See Acetylcysteine
N-Acetyltransferases, 481–482, 486. See also Pharmacogenetics
  in infants, children, and adolescents, 685t
Nadolol
  adjustments in renal insufficiency, 759t
  adverse drug reactions, 301t
  breast milk excretion, 220t
  in children and adolescents, 685t
Nafcil®. See Nafcillin
Nafcillin
  adverse drug reactions, 294t
  drug interactions, 317t
  intravenous administration, 418t
  in infants, children, and adolescents, 685t
Nalbuphine
  in children and adolescents, 685t
  teratogenicity/fetotoxicity, 163
Nalcrom®. See Cromolyn sodium
Nalidixic acid
  breast milk excretion, 220t
  teratogenicity/fetotoxicity, 163
Naloxone
  in infants, children, and adolescents, 685–686t
  intravenous administration, 418t
  in neonates, 545t
  in opiate poisoning, 256t
Nalpen®. See Nafcillin
Naphazoline
  nasal, in infants, children, and adolescents, 686t
  ophthalmic, in infants, children, and adolescents, 686t
Naprosyn®. See Naproxen sodium
Naproxen sodium
  adjustments in renal insufficiency, 759t
  breast milk excretion, 220t
  in children and adolescents, 686–687t
  drug interactions, 317t
  teratogenicity/fetotoxicity, 163
Naratriptan, contraindicated in adolescents, 687t
Narcan®. See Naloxone
Narcolepsy, mixed amphetamines in, 567t, 610t

Nasacort®. See Triamcinolone nasal
Nasacort AQ®. See Triamcinolone nasal
Nasal congestion. *See also* Rhinitis
   naphazoline nasal in, 686t
   oxymetazoline nasal in, 696t
   pseudoephedrine in, 719t
Nasalide®. See Flunisolide nasal
Nasal polyps, budesonide in, 584t
Nasarel®. See Flunisolide nasal
Nascobal®. See Cyanocobalamin
Nasogastric tubes, drug administration and, 18-19
Nasolacrimal occlusion, 24-25
Nausea. *See also* Vomiting
   as adverse drug effect, 290t
   in antineoplastic therapy, 497-500, 498t, 499t
   chlorpromazine in, 597t
   meclizine in, 668-669t
   ondansetron in, 693t
   prochlorperazine in severe, 715t
   promethazine in, 715-716t
   prophylaxis
      dronabinol in, 619t
      droperidol in, 619-620t
      granisetron in, 639-640t
      scopolamine in motion sickness, 728t
Naxen®. See Naproxen sodium
Nebcin®. See Tobramycin; Tobramycin injectable
Nebulizers, compressed-air and other, 31-33, 36
Necrolysis, toxic epidermal, as adverse drug effect, 291t
Necrotizing enterocolitis, vancomycin in, 551t
Nedocromil
   ophthalmic, in children, 687t
   pulmonary, in children and adolescents, 687t
Nedromycin. See Netilmicin
Needleless intravenous delivery systems, 64-65, 67
Needles, 47-48
   gauge of, 48n
   length and therapeutic efficacy, 54n
Needle-stick injuries, 48
Nefazodone
   drug interactions, 330
   with cyclosporine, 327
Negran®. See Nalidixic acid
Neisseria meningitidis, rifampin in prophylaxis, 724t
Nelfinavir
   adverse drug reactions, 304t
   in children and adolescents, 687t
Nembutal®. See Pentobarbital
Neo-Fradin®. See Neomycin
Neomycin
   adverse drug reactions, 293t
   in children and adolescents, 687-688t
Neonatal meningitis, cefotaxime in, 536t

Neonatal opiate analgesic withdrawal syndrome, 87
Neonatal respiratory distress syndrome, beractant in, 534t
Neonatal thyrotoxicosis, propranolol in, 548t
Neonates, dosing in, 531, 532-554t.
   See also specific drugs
Neoral®. See Cyclosporine
Neosar®. See Cyclophosphamide
Neostigmine
   adjustments in renal insufficiency, 759t
   in infants, children, and adolescents, 688t
   in neonates, 545t
Neostigmine methylsulfate, intravenous administration, 418t
Nephropathic cystinosis, cysteamine in, 606-607t
Netilmicin
   adjustments in renal insufficiency, 759t
   adverse drug reactions, 293t
   in infants, children, and adolescents, 688t
   optimal serum concentrations, 761t
Netilmicin sulfate, intravenous administration, 418t
Netromycin®. See Netilmicin; Netilmicin sulfate
Neuleptil®. See Pericyazine
Neupogen®. See Filgrastim
Neuroblastoma, antineoplastic drug regimens, 506t
Neurogenic bladder, oxybutynin in, 696t
Neurohypophyseal diabetes insipidus, desmopressin in, 609t
Neuroleptic malignant syndrome, as adverse drug effect, 290t
Neuromuscular blockade
   mivacurium in, 682t
   neostigmine in reversal, 545t, 688t
   rocuronium in, 726t
   succinylcholine in, 734-735t
   tubocurarine in, 748-749t
   vecuronium in, 750t
Neuromuscular blockers
   adverse drug reactions, 309t
   drug interactions, 331
   with aminoglycosides, 320
Neurontin®. See Gabapentin
Neutrogena Acne Mask®. See Benzoyl peroxide
Neutropenia
   febrile, cefepime in, 590t
   of immaturity, filgrastim in, 541t
   immune globulin in, 543t
Nevirapine, in infants, children, and adolescents, 689t
Nicardipine, intravenous administration, 418t
Niclosamide, teratogenicity/fetotoxicity, 163

Nicorette®. See Nicotine chewing gums
Nicotine. *See also* Tobacco smoking
   in adolescents, 689-690t
   breast milk excretion, 220t
Nicotine chewing gums, 39
Nicotine intranasal spray, 30
Nicotine transdermal systems, 41-42, 363n, 689-690t
Nicotrol NS®. See Nicotine nasal spray
Nifedipine
   adverse drug reactions, 306t
   breast milk excretion, 221t
   in children and adolescents, 690t
   controlled-release, 12
   teratogenicity/fetotoxicity, 163-164
Nightmares/night terrors, as adverse drug effect, 290t
Nilstat®. See Nystatin
Nimbex®. See Cisatracurium
Nimodipine, breast milk excretion, 221t
Nitoman®. See Tetrabenazine
Nitrate/nitrite poisoning, 255t
Nitrazepam
   adverse drug reactions, 298t
   in children, 691t
   teratogenicity/fetotoxicity, 164
Nitrofurantoin
   adverse drug reactions, 296t
   breast milk excretion, 221t
   in infants, children, and adolescents, 691t
   teratogenicity/fetotoxicity, 164
Nitrogen mustard. *See* Mechlorethamine
Nitroglycerin
   adverse drug reactions, 307t
   in children and adolescents, 691t
   intravenous administration, 419t
   in neonates, 546t
   toxicities, IV tubing and, 64
Nitropress®. See Sodium nitroprusside
Nitroprusside. *See* Sodium nitroprusside
Nitrous oxide, teratogenicity/fetotoxicity, 164
Nix Creme Rinse®. See Permethrin
Nizatidine, breast milk excretion, 221t
Nizoral®. See Ketoconazole
Nocturnal enuresis, oxybutynin in, 696t
Non-Hodgkin's lymphoma, antineoplastic drug regimens, 506t
Nonoxynol 9, teratogenicity/fetotoxicity, 165
Nonsteroidal anti-inflammatory drugs. *See* NSAIDs *and specific drugs*
Noradrenaline. *See* Norepinephrine
Norcuron®. See Vecuronium
Norditropin®. See Somatropin

Norepinephrine
  in children and adolescents, 691-692t
  in neonates, 546t
Norepinephrine bitartrate, intravenous administration, 419t
Norethindrone
  drug interactions, 317t
  teratogenicity/fetotoxicity, 165-166
Norethindrone/ethinyl estradiol. *See* Ethinyl estradiol/norethindrone
Norethynodrel, breast milk excretion, 221t
Normodyne®. *See* Labetalol
Norpace®. *See* Disopyramide
Nortriptyline
  in adolescents, 692t
  breast milk excretion, 221t
  drug interactions, 317t
  optimal serum concentrations, 761t
  teratogenicity/fetotoxicity, 166
Norvir®. *See* Ritonavir
Novahistex DM®. *See* Dextromethorphan
Novantrone®. *See* Mitoxantrone
Novarel®. *See* Chorionic gonadotropin
Novo-AZT®. *See* Zidovudine
Novo-Clopate®. *See* Clorazepate
Novo-Cloxin®. *See* Cloxacillin
Novo-Difenac-K®. *See* Diclofenac oral
Novo-Flurazine®. *See* Trifluoperazine
Novolin®. *See* Insulin
Novo-Lorazem®. *See* Lorazepam
Novo-Meprazine®. *See* Methotrimeprazine
Novo-Mepro®. *See* Meprobamate
Novo-Metformin®. *See* Metformin
Novo-Pen® insulin devices, 51-52
Novo-Ridazine®. *See* Thioridazine
Novo-Spiroton®. *See* Spironolactone
Novo-Tetra®. *See* Tetracycline
Nozinan®. *See* Methotrimeprazine
NP-27®. *See* Tolnaftate
NSAID poisoning, 262-263
NSAIDs
  drug interactions, 331
  fetal toxicities, 87
  with beta-blockers, 323
  with cyclosporine, 327
  with folic acid, 329
  with lithium salts, 330
  with methotrexate, 330
Nubain®. *See* Nalbuphine
Nu-Cloxi®. *See* Cloxacillin
Nu-Loraz®. *See* Lorazepam
Nu-Medrol®. *See* Methylprednisolone sodium succinate
Nu-Metformin®. *See* Metformin
Nuprin®. *See* Ibuprofen
Nu-Tetra®. *See* Tetracycline
Nutropin®. *See* Somatropin
Nutropin Depot®. *See* Somatropin depot

Nydrazid®. *See* Isoniazid
Nystagmus, as adverse drug reaction, 290t
Nystatin
  adverse drug reactions, 301t
  in infants, children, and adolescents, 692-693t
  in neonates, 546t
  teratogenicity/fetotoxicity, 166

O

Obesity
  orlistat in, 694t
  phendimetrazine in, 704t
Obsessive-compulsive disorder
  fluoxetine in, 633t
  paroxetine in, 699t
  sertraline in, 729-730t
Obstructive hypertrophic subaortic stenosis, propranolol in, 548t
Occlusion
  of central venous catheters, 68, 563t
  heparin in prophylaxis, 542t
  nasolacrimal, 24-25
Octostim®. *See* Desmopressin
Octreotide, in children and adolescents, 693t
Ocu-Caine®. *See* Proparacaine
OcuClear® eyedrops. *See* Oxymetazoline ophthalmic
Ocular congestion, naphazoline ophthalmic in, 686t
Ocular infections
  gentamicin ophthalmic in, 637t
  lodoxamide in, 665t
  sulfacetamide sodium in, 550t
Ocular inflammation
  diclofenac ophthalmic in, 612t
  fluorometholone in, 633t
  prednisolone ophthalmic in, 711t
  trifluridine in, 746t
Ocular irritation
  naphazoline ophthalmic in, 686t
  oxymetazoline ophthalmic in, 696t
Ocular refraction, homatropine in, 644t
Ocusulf-10®. *See* Sulfacetamide sodium ophthalmic
Ofloxacin
  breast milk excretion, 221t
  teratogenicity/fetotoxicity, 166
Oil(s)
  castor, in infants, children, and adolescents, 589t
  medium chain triglyceride, in neonates, 544t
  mineral
    adverse drug reactions, 309t
    breast milk excretion, 220t
    in children and adolescents, 681t
    petroleum (hydrocarbon) ingestion, 270-272
Oil formulations
  hypersensitivity to, 42, 42n
  of oral drugs, 9

Ointments
  intranasal, 29
  ophthalmic, 25, 27
Omeprazole
  in children and adolescents, 693t
  drug interactions, 317t
  teratogenicity/fetotoxicity, 166
Omnipen®. *See* Ampicillin
Oncaspar®. *See* Pegaspargase
Oncovin®. *See* Vincristine
Ondansetron
  as antiemetic, 499t
  in children and adolescents, 693t
  drug interactions, 317t
  intravenous administration, 419t
Ophthaine®. *See* Proparacaine
Ophthalmia neonatorum prophylaxis, erythromycin in, 540t
Ophthalmic dosage forms, 23-27
  developmental considerations, 25-27
  inserts, 25
  ointments, 25
  solutions and suspensions, 23-25
Opiate analgesic withdrawal syndrome, neonatal, 87
Opiate overdosage/poisoning, 256t
  naloxone in, 545t, 685-686t
Opiates
  abuse of, 356-357, 357t
  adverse drug reactions, 292t
  phenobarbital in withdrawal from, 547t
  subcutaneous analgesic infusion, 52-53
Opisthorchiasis. *See* Liver fluke infestation
Optimal serum concentrations, 761-762t
Orabase Gel®. *See* Benzocaine
Orajel Mouth-Aid®. *See* Benzocaine
Orajel Perioseptic®. *See* Carbamide peroxide
Oral candidiasis (thrush). *See also* Fungal infections
  nystatin in, 692t
Oral contraceptives. *See also specific drugs*
  breast milk excretion, 221t
  dosing, 626t
  drug interactions, 326
  emergency postintercourse
    levonorgestrel/ethinyl estradiol, 661t
    levonorgestrel, 661t
  teratogenicity/fetotoxicity, 166-168
  with anticonvulsants, 322
Oral dosage forms, 7-19
  developmental considerations, 16-19
  liquid, 8-11
    concentrated, 11
    measuring devices, 10-11
    palatability, 9-10
    types, 8-9

powders and granules, 14
solid, 11-16
  administering, 14-16
  capsules, 14
  developmental considerations and, 16-19
  powders and granules, 14
  tablets, 11-13
Oral inflammation, carbamide peroxide in, 588t
Oral suspensions, 9
Oramorph SR®. See Morphine
Orap®. See Pimozide
Orasone®. See Prednisone
Orciprenaline. *See* Metaproterenol
Organophosphate poisoning, 256t
  pralidoxime in, 710t
Oristat, in adolescents, 694t
Orniprenaline. *See* Metaproterenol
Oropharyngeal candidiasis. *See also* Fungal infections
  fluconazole in, 630t
Ortho®. See Ethinyl estradiol/norethindrone; Oral contraceptives
Orthoclone OKT3®. See Muromonab-CD3
Oseltamivir, in children and adolescents, 694-695t
Osmitrol®. See Mannitol
Otic dosage forms, 27, 28
Otitis externa, benzocaine in, 578t
Otitis media
  amoxicillin and potassium clavulanate in, 566-567t
  azithromycin in, 575t
  benzocaine in, 578t
  cefpodoxime proxetil in, 591t
  clarithromycin in, 599t
  erythromycin ethylsuccinate in, 624t
Oxacillin
  adverse drug reactions, 294t
  in infants, children, and adolescents, 695t
  intravenous administration, 419t
Oxazepam
  breast milk excretion, 222t
  teratogenicity/fetotoxicity, 168
Oxcarbazepine, in children and adolescents, 695-696t
Oxeze®. See Formoterol fumarate
Oxprenolol, teratogenicity/fetotoxicity, 168
Oxybutynin, in children, 696t
Oxycodone
  breast milk excretion, 222t
  drug interactions, 317t
Oxygen weaning, dexamethasone in, 537t
Oxymetazoline
  in children and adolescents
    nasal, 696t
    ophthalmic, 696t
  teratogenicity/fetotoxicity, 168
Oxytetracycline, teratogenicity/fetotoxicity, 168

Oxytocin
  breast milk excretion, 222t
  teratogenicity/fetotoxicity, 168-169

P

Pacerone®. See Amiodarone
Paclitaxel
  dosing, 520t
  extravasation care, 506t
  intravenous administration, 419t
Pain. *See also* Headache; Spasm
  acetaminophen in, 532t, 558t
  aspirin in, 572-573t
  codeine in, 603t
  fentanyl in, 540t, 629t
  hydromorphone in, 646t
  ibuprofen in, 647t
  meperidine in, 544t, 670t
  methocarbamol in muscle spasm, 675t
  morphine in, 545t, 683t
  nalbuphine in, 685t
  naproxen sodium in, 687t
  promethazine as adjunct in, 715t
  rofecoxib in, 726-727t
Palatability, of oral drugs, 9-11
Palivizumab, in infants and children, 697t
Pamelor®. See Nortriptyline
Pancrease®. See Pancrelipase
Pancreatin, in children and adolescents, 697t
Pancreatitis, as adverse drug effect, 290t
Pancrelipase
  in infants, children, and adolescents, 697t
  powder formulation, 14
Pancrezyme®. See Pancreatin
Pancuronium bromide
  in infants, children, and adolescents, 698t
  intravenous administration, 420t
Panic disorder, paroxetine in, 699t
PanOxyl®. See Benzoyl peroxide
Pantoprazole, drug interactions, 317t
PARA®. See Bioallethrin and piperonyl butoxide
Para-aminosalicylic acid (PABA). *See* Aminosalicylic acid
Parabromdylamine. *See* Brompheniramine
Paracetaldehyde. *See* Paraldehyde
Paracetamol. *See* Acetaminophen
Paraldehyde
  adverse drug reactions, 298-299t
  in children, 698t
  intravenous administration, 420t
  in neonates, 546t
Paralysis, as adverse drug effect, 290t
Paramethadione, teratogenicity/fetotoxicity, 169
Paranoia, as adverse drug effect, 290t
Paraplatin®. See Carboplatin

Paraplatin-AQ®. See Carboplatin
Parasitic infestations
  iodoquinol in, 651t
  lindane in, 663t
  Lyme disease, doxycycline in, 619t
  mebendazole in, 668t
  metronidazole in, 678t
  paromomycin in, 698t
  permethrin in, 703t
  piperacillin in, 708t
  praziquantel in, 710-711t
  pyrantel pamoate in, 719-720t
  thiabendazole in, 740t
Paromomycin
  in children and adolescents, 698t
  teratogenicity/fetotoxicity, 169
Paroxetine
  in adolescents, 699t
  adverse drug reactions, 300t
  breast milk excretion, 222t
  drug interactions, 317t
Parvolex®. See Acetylcysteine
Passive immunization, 449-450
Patent ductus arteriosus, indomethacin in, 543t
Paxil®. See Paroxetine
PCZ. *See* Procarbazine
Peak expiratory flow rate (PEFR), 32-33
Pedapred®. See Prednisolone systemic
Pediacare Infants' Oral Decongestant Drops®. See Pseudoephedrine
Pediaflor®. See Sodium fluoride
Pediatric laboratory values, 785-788t
Pediatrix®. See Acetaminophen
Pediazole®. See Erythromycin ethylsuccinate
Pediculus capitis. See Head lice
Pediculus pubis. See Crab lice
Pedi-Pro®. See Undecylenic acid
Pefloxacin, breast milk excretion, 222t
Pegaspargase, dosing, 520t
Peglyte®. See Polyethylene glycol and electrolyte solutions
Pemirolast, in children and adolescents, 699t
Pemoline
  adverse drug reactions, 307t
  in children and adolescents, 699-700t
Penerject-50®. See Promethazine
Penicillamine
  adverse drug reactions, 293t
  in infants, children, and adolescents, 700t
  in metal poisoning, 254t
  teratogenicity/fetotoxicity, 169-170
Penicillin
  adverse drug reactions, 294t
  drug interactions, 331
  probenecid as adjunct to, 713t
  with aminoglycosides, 320

Penicillin G
　adjustments in renal insufficiency, 759t
　adverse drug reactions, 294t
　breast milk excretion, 222t
　in children and adolescents, 701t
　in neonates, 546t
　teratogenicity/fetotoxicity, 170
Penicillin G benzathine, in neonates, 547t
Penicillin G potassium, intravenous administration, 420t
Penicillin G procaine, in infants, children, and adolescents, 701t
Penicillin V
　adverse drug reactions, 294t
　breast milk excretion, 222t
　drug interactions, 331
　with aminoglycosides, 320
Penicillin V potassium, in children and adolescents, 701t
Pentacarinat®. *See* Pentamidine isethionate
Pentamidine, drug interactions, 317t
Pentamidine isethionate
　adjustments in renal insufficiency, 759t
　in infants, children, and adolescents, 701t
　intravenous administration, 420t
Pentamycetin®. *See* Chloramphenicol
Pentasa®. *See* Mesalamine
Pentazocine, teratogenicity/fetotoxicity, 170
Pentobarbital
　adverse drug reactions, 309t
　breast milk excretion, 222t
　in infants, children, and adolescents, 702t
　intravenous administration, 420t
　teratogenicity/fetotoxicity, 170-171
Pentolair®. *See* Cyclopentolate
Pentoxyfylline, breast milk excretion, 222t
Pen-Vee K®. *See* Penicillin G potassium
Pepcid®. *See* Famotidine
Peptic ulcer
　as adverse drug effect, 290t
　calcium carbonate in, 587t
　cimetidine in, 598t
　famotidine in, 628t
　propantheline in, 716-717t
　ranitidine in, 548t, 723-724t
Pepto-Bismol®. *See* Bismuth subsalicylate
Periactin®. *See* Cyproheptadine
Pericyazine, in children and adolescents, 702-703t
Peripheral neuropathy, as adverse drug effect, 290t
Peripheral venous access devices, 65-67. *See also under* Venous access devices
Permethrin, in infants, children, and adolescents, 703t

Permitil®. *See* Fluphenazine
Perphenazine
　drug interactions, 317t
　teratogenicity/fetotoxicity, 171
Persa-Gel®. *See* Benzoyl peroxide
Pertussis vaccine, 450-452, 452t
Pethidine. *See* Meperidine
Petit mal. *See* Absence seizures
pH, alteration of urine, in poisoning, 252-253
Pharmacogenetics, 475-491
　pediatric considerations, 483-487
　　cytochrome P-450 enzymes, 483-486
　　glucuronyl transferases, 486
　　N-acetyltransferase-2, 486
　　thiopurine *S*-methyltransferase, 486-487
　principles, 475-477
　of specific drug-metabolizing enzymes, 477-483, 483t
　　arylamine *N*-acetyltransferases, 481-482
　　cytochrome P-450 (CYP) superfamily, 477-481, 478
　　glucuronosyl transferases, 481
　　thiopurine *S*-methyltransferase, 482
Pharmacokinetics, 459-473
　alterations in, 468-470
　　in cystic fibrosis, 469
　　in liver disease/dysfunction, 469
　　in renal disease/dysfunction, 468-469
　　with concurrent drug therapy, 469-470
　developmental considerations, 495-496
　drug effect and, 459-463
　　absorption, 460-461
　　distribution, 461, 461-463
　　excretion, 464
　　metabolism, 463-464
　principles, 464-468
　　disposition parameters, 464-466, 465, 466
　　dosing, 466-468, 467
Pharmacokinetic vs. pharmacodynamic drug interactions, 316
Pharyngitis. *See also* Tonsillitis
　azithromycin in, 576t
　cefprozil in, 592t
　clarithromycin in, 599t
　loracarbef in, 666t
Phazyme®. *See* Simethicone
Phenacemide, teratogenicity/fetotoxicity, 171
Phenazopyridine
　in infants, children, and adolescents, 703t
　teratogenicity/fetotoxicity, 171
Phencyclidine
　breast milk excretion, 222t
　teratogenicity/fetotoxicity, 171-172
Phendimetrazine, in adolescents, 704t

Phenergan®. *See* Promethazine
Pheniramine, teratogenicity/fetotoxicity, 172
Phenmetrazine, teratogenicity/fetotoxicity, 172
Phenobarbital. *See also* Anticonvulsants
　adjustments in renal insufficiency, 759t
　adverse drug reactions, 299t, 309-310t
　breast milk excretion, 222t
　in infants, children, and adolescents, 704t
　intravenous administration, 420t
　in neonates, 547t
　optimal serum concentrations, 761t
　teratogenicity/fetotoxicity, 172-173
Phenobarbitone. *See* Phenobarbital
Phenolphthalein, breast milk excretion, 222t
Phenothiazines. *See also specific formulations*
　adverse drug reactions, 303t
　teratogenicity/fetotoxicity, 173
Phenoxybenzamine, in children and adolescents, 705t
Phenoxymethylpenicillin potassium. *See* Penicillin G potassium; Penicillin V potassium
Phentolamine
　in children and adolescents, 705t
　extravasation care, 547t
　in neonates, 547t
Phenylephedrine, intravenous administration, 421t
Phenylephrine
　in children and adolescents, 705t
　teratogenicity/fetotoxicity, 173-174
Phenylpropanolamine, teratogenicity/fetotoxicity, 174
Phenyl salicylate, aspirin conversion factor, 257t
Phenytoin. *See also* Fosphenytoin
　adverse drug reactions, 299t, 306t
　breast milk excretion, 223t
　drug interactions, 317t, 331-333
　in infants, children, and adolescents, 706t
　intravenous administration, 421t
　in neonates, 547t
　optimal serum concentrations, 761-762t
　teratogenicity/fetotoxicity, 174-176
　with cimetidine, 326
　with cyclosporine, 327
　with fluconazole, 328
Pheochromocytoma, phentolamine in suspected, 705t
pHisoHex®. *See* Hexachlorophene
Phlebitis. *See also* Extravasation
　intravenous-administration/related, 79-80

INDEX

Photosensitivity, as adverse drug effect, 290t
Phyllocontin®. See Aminophylline
Physical disability, drug administration and, 18
Physicians' Desk Reference (PDR), 88
Physostigmine
  in antihhistamine poisoning, 265
  intravenous administration, 421t
Physostigmine salicylate
  in anticholinergic poisoning, 254t
  in infants, children, and adolescents, 706t
Phytonadione
  adverse drug reactions, 311t
  breast milk excretion, 223t
  in infants, children, and adolescents, 706-707t
  intravenous administration, 421t
Pimecrolimus, in children and adolescents, 707t
Pimozide
  in children and adolescents, 707t
  drug interactions, 319t, 333
Pin-X®. See Pyrantel pamoate
Pindolol, teratogenicity/fetotoxicity, 176
Pink Bismuth®. See Bismuth subsalicylate
Pin-Rid®. See Pyrantel pamoate
Piperacillin
  adjustments in renal insufficiency, 759t
  adverse drug reactions, 294t
  in children and adolescents, 708t
  intravenous administration, 421t
  in neonates, 548t
Piperacillin/tazobactam, intravenous administration, 421t
Piperazine, teratogenicity/fetotoxicity, 176
Piperonyl butoxide/pyrethrins, in infants, children, and adolescents, 708t
Pipracil®. See Piperacillin
Piroxicam
  breast milk excretion, 223t
  drug interactions, 317t
Pivampicillin, teratogenicity/fetotoxicity, 176
Placental drug transfer, 89, 91n
Placental factors affecting teratogenesis, 90
Plague vaccine, teratogenicity/fetotoxicity, 176
Plan B®. See Levonorgestrel
Plasmodium falciparum
  chloroquine resistant malaria
    quinidine in, 722t
    quinine dihydrochloride in, 722t
    quinine sulfate in, 722-723t
Platinol-AQ®. See Cisplatin
Plicamycin
  in children and adolescents, 708t
  intravenous administration, 421t

PMS-Fenofibrate Micro®. See Fenofibrate micronized
Pneumococcus vaccine, 452-453
Pneumocystis carinii pneumonia
  atovaquone in, 573t
  pentamidine isethionate in, 701t
  trimethoprim/sulfamethoxazole in, 551t, 746t
Pneumonia
  azithromycin in, 576t
  cefpodoxime proxetil in, 591t
  hydrocarbon, 271-272
  linezolid in, 663-664t
  loracarbef in, 666t
  Pneumocystis carinii. See Pneumocystis carinii pneumonia
Pneumonitis, as adverse drug effect, 290t
Poison control centers, 246-247
Poisoning, 245-281
  activated charcoal in, 594t
  antidotes, 253, 254-256t
  arsenic, penicillamine in, 700t
  epidemiology, 245-247
  general considerations, 247-253
    assessment, 247
    management, 247
    supportive medical care, 247-248
  ipecac syrup in, 651t
  lead
    penicillamine in, 700t
    succimer in, 734t
  organophosphate, pralidoxime in, 710t
  prevention of GI absorption, 248-251
  promotion of elimination, 251-253
  treatment, 253-276
    acetaminophen, 258-262, 261
    antihistamines, 265-266
    aspirin and other salicylates, 253, 256-258, 257t
    caustics, 249-250, 266-270
    hydrocarbons, 270-272
    iron, 263-265
    NSAIDs other than aspirin, 262-263
    toxic alcohols and glycols, 272-275, 276t
Poliovirus vaccine, 453-455
  inactivated (Salk), teratogenicity/fetotoxicity, 176-177
  live oral (Sabin)
    breast milk excretion, 223t
    teratogenicity/fetotoxicity, 177
Polycillin®. See Ampicillin
Polyethylene glycol and electrolyte solutions, in adolescents, 708-709t
Polygam S/D®. See Immune globulin
Polymorphisms, antineoplastics and, 496

Polymyxin B sulfate, systemic, in infants, children, and adolescents, 709t
Polyps, nasal, budesonide in, 584t
Porphyria, as adverse drug effect, 290t
Positive inotropic drugs, adverse drug reactions, 307t
Postexposure prophylaxis, 43
Post-traumatic stress disorder, paroxetine in, 699t
Potassium chloride
  in infants, children, and adolescents, 709-710t
  intravenous administration, 422t
  in neonates, 548t
  toxicities, phlebitis, 79
Potassium deficit. *See* Hypokalemia
Potassium iodide, in infants, children, and adolescents, 710t
Potassium phosphate, intravenous administration, 422t
Potassium salicylate, aspirin conversion factor, 257t
Potassium sparing diuretics
  adverse drug reactions, 308t
  drug interactions, 333-334
  with cyclosporine, 327
  with potassium salts, 333
Powder inhalers (insufflators), 35-36
  Diskhaler, 35
  Rotahaler, 35
  Spinhaler, 36
Powders, topical, 37-38
Powders and granules, administration, 14
Pralidoxime
  in infants, children, and adolescents, 710t
  intravenous administration, 422t
Pralidoxime chloride, in organophosphate poisoning, 256t
Praziquantel, in children and adolescents, 710-711t
Prazosin
  adverse drug reactions, 302t
  drug interactions, 334
  in infants, children, and adolescents, 711t
  with beta-blockers, 323
Precocious puberty
  histrelin in, 643-644t
  leuprolide in, 660t
Predacort®. See Prednisolone systemic
Pred Forte®. See Prednisolone ophthalmic
Pred Mild®. See Prednisolone ophthalmic
Prednisolone
  adverse drug reactions, 308t
  breast milk excretion, 223t
  in cancer, 520t
  in children and adolescents
    ophthalmic, 711-712t
    systemic, 712t

Prednisone
  adverse drug reactions, 308t
  breast milk excretion, 223t
  in cancer, 521t
  in children and adolescents, 712t
  teratogenicity/fetotoxicity, 177
Pre-eclampsia, magnesium sulfate in, 668t
Pregmyl®. See Chorionic gonadotropin
Pregnancy
  classification of drugs for use in, 88-89
  drug use during, 88-89. *See also* Fetotoxicity; Teratogens
  immunizations and, 434
Prelone®. See Prednisolone systemic
Prelu-2®. See Phendimetrazine
Pre-operative bowel preparation. *See* Bowel preparation
Prepulsid®. See Cisapride
Preschoolers
  drug administration in, 4-5t, 17
  injections administered in, 44
Pressyn®. See Vasopressin
Prevalite®. See Cholestyramine
Preven®. See Levonorgestrel/ethinyl estradiol
Prevex®. See Zinc oxide
Prilocaine, methemoglobinemia caused by, 76n
Prilocaine/lidocaine. *See* Lidocaine/prilocaine
Prilosec®. See Omeprazole
Primacor®. See Milrinone
Primaquine, in infants, children, and adolescents, 713t
Primaxin®. See Imipenem/cilastatin
Primidone
  adjustments in renal insufficiency, 759t
  adverse drug reactions, 299t
  breast milk excretion, 223-224t
  in children and adolescents, 713t
  drug interactions, 317t, 334
  optimal serum concentrations, 762t
  teratogenicity/fetotoxicity, 177-178
  with phenytoin, 332
Principen®. See Ampicillin
Prinivil®. See Lisinopril
Privine®. See Naphazoline nasal
Probenecid
  adjustments in renal insufficiency, 759t
  in children and adolescents, 713t
  drug interactions, 334
  with cephalosporins, 325
  with methotrexate, 330
Procainamide
  adjustments in renal insufficiency, 759t
  adverse drug reactions, 306t
  breast milk excretion, 224t
  drug interactions, 334
  in infants, children, and adolescents, 714t
  optimal serum concentrations, 762t
  teratogenicity/fetotoxicity, 178
  with cimetidine, 326
Procaine, teratogenicity/fetotoxicity, 178-179
Procanbid®. See Procainamide
Procan SR®. See Procainamide
Procarbazine
  dosing, 521t
  teratogenicity/fetotoxicity, 179
Procardia®. See Nifedipine
Procardia XL®. See Nifedipine
Prochlorperazine
  as antiemetic, 499t
  in children and adolescents, 714-715t
  teratogenicity/fetotoxicity, 179
Procytox®. See Cyclophosphamide
Profasi®. See Chorionic gonadotropin
Profilnine®. See Factor IX complex
Progestogen/estrogen oral contraceptives, teratogenicity/fetotoxicity, 166-168
Progestogens, teratogenicity/fetotoxicity, 179-180
Proglycem®. See Diazoxide
Prograf®. See Tacrolimus
Proloprim®. See Trimethoprim
Promazine, teratogenicity/fetotoxicity, 180
Promethazine
  adverse drug reactions, 301t
  as antiemetic, 499t
  in children and adolescents, 715-716t
  intravenous administration, 422t
  teratogenicity/fetotoxicity, 180
Pronestyl®. See Procainamide
Propafenone
  adverse drug reactions, 306t
  breast milk excretion, 224t
  in children and adolescents, 716t
  drug interactions, 317t, 334
  optimal serum concentrations, 762t
Propanthel®. See Propantheline
Propantheline, 716-717t
Proparacaine, in children and adolescents, 717t
Propericyazine. *See* Pericyazine
Proplex®. See Factor IX complex
Propofol
  in children and adolescents, 717-718t
  intravenous administration, 422t
Propoxyphene
  breast milk excretion, 224t
  drug interactions, 317t
  teratogenicity/fetotoxicity, 180-181
  with carbamazepine, 324
Propranolol
  adverse drug reactions, 301t
  breast milk excretion, 224t
  in children and adolescents, 718t
  drug interactions, 317t
  intravenous administration, 423t
  in neonates, 548t
  optimal serum concentrations, 762t
  teratogenicity/fetotoxicity, 181
Propulsid®. See Cisapride
Propyl-Thyracil®. See Propylthiouracil
Propylthiouracil
  adjustments in renal insufficiency, 759t
  breast milk excretion, 224t
  in infants, children, and adolescents, 718t
  teratogenicity/fetotoxicity, 181-182
Prostaglandin E_2. *See* Alprostadil
Prostaphlin®. See Oxacillin
Prostep®. See Nicotine
Prostigmin®. See Neostigmine; Neostigmine methylsulfate
Prostin VR®. See Alprostadil
Protamine sulfate
  in infants, children, and adolescents, 719t
  intravenous administration, 423t
  in neonates, 548t
Protease inhibitors, adverse drug reactions, 304t
Protoprim®. See Trimethoprim
Protozoal infestations
  furazolidone in diarrhea, 636t
  praziquantel in, 710-711t
Protropin®. See Somatrem
Proxymetacaine. *See* Proparacaine
Prozac®. See Fluoxetine
Pruritus. *See* Itching
Pseudoephedrine
  breast milk excretion, 224t
  in infants, children, and adolescents, 719t
  teratogenicity/fetotoxicity, 182
Pseudomembranous colitis
  as adverse drug effect, 290t
  vancomycin in, 750t
Pseudomonas aeruginosa infection. *See also* Bacterial infections
  in cystic fibrosis, tobramycin in, 742t
Pseudomonas aeruginosa meningitis, polymyxin B sulfate systemic in, 709t
Pseudotumor cerebri, as adverse drug effect, 290t
Psoriasis
  betamethasone in, 580t
  tazarotene in, 737t
Psychedelics, abuse of, 365-370, 367t, 369t, 370t. *See also under* Abusable psychotropic drug use
Psychological variables, in psychotropic drug abuse, 352-353

Psychosis. *See also* Schizophrenia
  as adverse drug effect, 290t
  clozapine in, 603t
  haloperidol in, 640
  mesoridazine in, 672-673t
  methotrimeprazine in, 676t
  pericyazine in, 702-703t
  pimozide in, 707t
  prochlorperazine in, 714-715t
  risperidone in, 725t
  thioproperazine in, 740-741t
  thioridazine in, 741t
Psychotic patients. *See* Mental disorders
Psychotropic drugs, abuse of, 347-385. *See also* Abusable psychotropic drug use *and specific drugs*
Psychotropics
  abusable vs. nonabusable, 348
  major abusable, 348t
Psyllium, in children and adolescents, 719t
Psyllium powder, formulations of, 15
Pteroylglutamic acid. *See* Folic acid
Puberty
  delayed, testosterone propionate in, 738t
  precocious
    histrelin in, 643-644t
    leuprolide in, 660t
Pulmicort®. *See* Budesonide
Pulmicort Nebuamp®. *See* Budesonide pulmonary
Pulmicort Turbuhaler®. *See* Budesonide pulmonary
Pulmonary hypertension, nitroglycerin in, 546t
Pumps, infusion, 70-71
Purinethol®. *See* Mercaptopurine
Purpura, idiopathic thrombocytopenic, 648t
Pyelonephritis, loracarbef in, 666t
Pyrantel pamoate
  in infants, children, and adolescents, 719-720t
  teratogenicity/fetotoxicity, 182
Pyrazinamide
  breast milk excretion, 224t
  in children and adolescents, 720t
Pyridium®. *See* Phenazopyridine
Pyridostigmine, breast milk excretion, 224t
Pyridostigmine bromide, in children and adolescents, 720t
Pyridoxine
  breast milk excretion, 224t
  drug interactions, 334
  in infants, children, and adolescents, 721t
  intravenous administration, 423t
  in isoniazid poisoning, 255t
  in neonates, 548t
  with phenytoin, 332-333
Pyridoxine-dependent seizures, 721t
Pyrimethamine
  breast milk excretion, 225t
  in infants, children, and adolescents, 721t
  teratogenicity/fetotoxicity, 182-183
Pyrithione zinc, in children and adolescents, 722t

Q

QT prolongation, drug interactions and, 316-318, 319t
Quadriceps contracture injection site, 59-60
Quelicin®. *See* Succinylcholine
Questran®. *See* Cholestyramine
Quinacrine, drug interactions, 317t
Quinidex®. *See* Quinidine
Quinidine
  adjustments in renal insufficiency, 759t
  adverse drug reactions, 306t
  breast milk excretion, 225t
  in children and adolescents, 722t
  drug interactions, 317t, 334
  optimal serum concentrations, 762t
  teratogenicity/fetotoxicity, 183
  with cimetidine, 326
  with digitalis glycosides, 328
Quinidine gluconate, intravenous administration, 423t
Quinine
  adjustments in renal insufficiency, 759t
  breast milk excretion, 225t
  teratogenicity/fetotoxicity, 183-184
Quinine dihydrochloride, in children and adolescents, 722t
Quinine sulfate, in children and adolescents, 722-723t
Quinolones, adverse drug reactions, 294-295t
Quinsana Plus®. *See* Undecylenic acid
Quinupristin/dalfopristin, in children and adolescents, 723t

R

Rabeprazole, drug interactions, 317t
Radiation sickness, meclizine in, 669t
Radioactive iodine, thyroid gland protection from, potassium iodide in, 710t
R-Albuterol. *See* Levalbuterol
Ranitidine
  adverse drug reactions, 304t
  breast milk excretion, 225t
  in children and adolescents, 723-724t
  intravenous administration, 423t
  in neonates, 548t
  teratogenicity/fetotoxicity, 184
Raves (drug parties), 369n
R&C®. *See* Piperonyl butoxide and pyrethrins

Recombinate®. *See* Antihemophilic Factor VIII (Recombinant)
Record-keeping, for immunizations, 435
Rectal dosage forms, 19-22
  enemas, 22
  gels, 21-22
  suppositories, 20-21
Red man syndrome, as adverse drug effect, 290t
Reese's Pinworm Medicine®. *See* Pyrantel pamoate
Refludan®. *See* Lepirudin
Reflux esophagitis. *See also* Gastroesophageal reflux disease (GERD)
  ranitidine in, 548t
Regional enteritis. *See* Crohn's disease
Regitine®. *See* Phentolamine
Reglan®. *See* Metoclopramide
Regonol®. *See* Pyridostigmine bromide
Relafen®. *See* Nabumetone
Relenza®. *See* Zanamivir
Remantidin. *See* Rimantidine
Remicade®. *See* Infliximab
Renal failure, chronic
  dihydrotachysterol in, 615t
  epoetin alfa in anemia, 623t
Renal insufficiency
  as adverse drug effect, 290t
  calcium deficiency prophylaxis in, 586t
  dopamine in, 618t
  dosage adjustments for, 757-760t
  general dosage recommendations, 757-560t
  growth failure in
    somatrem in, 732t
    somatropin depot in, 733t
    somatropin in, 733t
Renal toxicity, of antineoplastics, 497
Renal transplantation. *See also* Transplantation
  azathioprine in, 575t
  basiliximab in, 577t
  cyclopentolate in, 606t
  dacliximab in, 607t
  muromonab-CD3 in allograft rejection, 684t
Reporting, of ADRs, 287
Reserpine, teratogenicity/fetotoxicity, 184
Respimat® inhaler, 33n
Respiratory depression, naloxone in, 545t
Respiratory disease, marijuana and, 367
Respiratory dysfunction, as adverse drug effect, 290t
Respiratory syncytial virus, palivizumab in prophylaxis, 697t
Respiratory tract infection. *See also* Common cold; Influenza
  rimantadine in, 724-725

Retinitis, congenital
cytomegalovirus, ganciclovir in, 542t
13-*Cis*-Retinoic acid. *See* Isotretinoin
all-*trans*-Retinoic acid. *See* Tretinoin
Reversol®. See Edrophonium chloride
Reyes' syndrome, as adverse drug effect, 290t
Rezulin®. See Troglitazone
Rhabdomyolysis, 252
Rheumatic fever, aspirin in, 573t
Rheumatic fever prophylaxis, penicillin V potassium in, 701t
Rheumatoid arthritis, juvenile. *See* Juvenile rheumatoid arthritis
Rheumatrex®. See Methotrexate
Rhinalar®. See Flunisolide nasal
Rhinitis
 allergic
  azelastine nasal in, 575t
  brompheniramine in, 583t
  clemastine in, 600t
  cromolyn sodium in, 604t
  fexofenadine in, 629t
  flunisolide nasal in, 632t
  ipratropium nasal in, 651t
  loratadine in, 666t
  mometasone furoate monohydrate in, 682t
  naphazoline nasal in, 686t
  triamcinolone nasal in, 744t
 beclomethasone nasal in seasonal, 577t
 budesonide in, 584t
 desloratadine in, 609t
 ipratropium nasal in, 651t
 loratadine in, 666t
 mometasone furoate monohydrate in, 682t
 naphazoline nasal in, 686t
 oxymetazoline nasal in, 696t
 pseudoephedrine in, 719t
Rhinocort Aqua®. See Budesonide nasal
Rhinocort Turbohaler®. See Budesonide nasal
Ribavirin
 adverse drug reactions, 304t
 in infants and children, 724t
Riboflavin, in children and adolescents, 724t
Rickets
 as adverse drug effect, 290t
 vitamin D-resistant, dihydrotachysterol in, 615t
RID®. See Piperonyl butoxide/pyrethrins
Rifabutin, drug interactions, 334
Rifadin®. See Rifampin
Rifampicin. *See* Rifampin
Rifampin
 adverse drug reactions, 297t
 breast milk excretion, 225t
 drug interactions, 317t, 334-335
 in infants, children, and adolescents, 724t

 intravenous administration, 424t
 teratogenicity/fetotoxicity, 184
 with cyclosporine, 327
 with isoniazid, 329
 with oral contraceptives, 326
 with theophylline, 336
Rifampin-resistant tuberculosis, streptomycin in, 734t
Rimantadine, in children and adolescents, 724-725t
Riphenidate®. See Methylphenidate
Risk factors, for ADRs, 284t, 284-285, 285t
Risperidone
 in children and adolescents, 725t
 drug interactions, 317t
Ritalin®. See Methylphenidate
Ritalin-SR®. See Methylphenidate
Ritonavir
 adverse drug reactions, 304t
 in children and adolescents, 725-726t
 drug interactions, 317t
Rituxan®. See Rituximab
Rituximab
 dosing, 521t
 intravenous administration, 424t
Rivotril®. See Clonazepam
Robaxin®. See Methocarbamol
Robinul®. See Glycopyrrolate
Robitussin®. See Guaifenesin
Robomol®. See Methocarbamol
Rocaltrol®. See Calcitriol
Rocephin®. See Ceftriaxone
Rocuronium
 in infants, children, and adolescents, 726t
 intravenous administration, 424t
Rofact®. See Rifampin
Rofecoxib, in children and adolescents, 726-727t
Rogitine®. See Phentolamine
Roglitazone
 in adolescents, 727t
 drug interactions, 317t
Romazicon®. See Flumazenil
Ropinitide, drug interactions, 317t
Rotahaler, 35
Rotavirus vaccine, 455
Roundworms. *See also* Parasitic infestations
 thiabendazole in, 740t
Rowasa®. See Mesalamine
Rubella virus vaccine, 455-456
 breast milk excretion, 225t
 teratogenicity/fetotoxicity, 184-185
Rubex®. See Doxorubicin
Rubidomycin. *See* Daunorubicin
Rumack/Matthew nomogram, for acetaminophen poisoning, 261
Rythmodan®. See Disopyramide
Rythmol®. See Propafenone

S

Sabril®. See Vigabatrin
Sacrosidase, in infants, children, and adolescents, 727t

Saizen®. See Somatropin
Salazopyrin®. See Sulfasalazine
Salbutamol. *See* Albuterol
Salicylate poisoning, 253, 256-258, 257t
Salicylates. *See also* Aspirin
 drug interactions, 335
 with anticoagulants, 321
 with corticosteroids, 326-327
 with methotrexate, 330
 with phenytoin, 333
Salicylazosulfapyridine. *See* Sulfasalazine
Salicylic acid, aspirin conversion factor, 257t
Saline laxatives, adverse drug reactions, 309t
Salivation, perisurgical inhibition of, atropine systemic in, 574t
Salmeterol xinafoate, in children and adolescents, 728t
Salmonellosis. *See also* Bacterial infections
 trimethoprim/sulfamethoxazole in, 747t
Salt-losing adrenogenital syndrome, fludrocortisone in, 632t
Salts
 calcium, teratogenicity, 109
 epsom. *See* Magnesium sulfate
 gold
  breast milk excretion, 214t
  teratogenicity/fetotoxicity, 139-140
 iron, teratogenicity/fetotoxicity, 146-147
 lithium. *See* Lithium
Sandimmune®. See Cyclosporine
Sandoglobulin. See Immune globulin
Sandostatin®. See Octreotide
Santmyer swallow reflex, 16
Sarcoma, antineoplastic drug regimens, 506t
Sargramostim
 dosing, 522t
 intravenous administration, 424t
S.A.S.®. See Sulfasalazine
Scabies infestation. *See also* Parasitic infestation
 permethrin in, 703t
Schistosomiasis. *See also* Parasitic infestation
 praziquantel in, 711t
Schizophrenia. *See also* Psychosis
 clozapine in, 603t
 haloperidol in, 640
 mesoridazine in, 672-673t
 methotrimeprazine in, 676t
 pericyazine in, 702-703t
 pimozide in, 707t
 prochlorperazine in, 714-715t
 risperidone in, 725t
 thioproperazine in, 741t
 thioridazine in, 741t
 trifluoperazine in, 745-746t
School-agers
 drug administration in, 5t, 17-18
 injections administered in, 44-45

Scopace®. See Scopolamine
Scopolamine
  adverse drug reactions, 297t
  as antiemetic, 499t
  in children and adolescents, 728t
  intravenous administration, 425t
  teratogenicity/fetotoxicity, 185
  toxicities, 40n
Scopolamine transdermal system, 40–41
Scurvy
  prophylaxis, ascorbic acid in, 572t
  treatment, ascorbic acid in, 572t
Sebizon®. See Sulfacetamide sodium topical
Seborrhea sicca. *See* Dandruff
Seborrheic dermatitis, sulfacetamide sodium topical in, 736t
Secobarbital
  in infants, children, and adolescents, 728t
  intravenous administration, 425t
  teratogenicity/fetotoxicity, 185
Secondary effects, of drug therapy, 283
Secretions
  guaifenesin in facilitation of expectoration, 640t
  reduction of glycopyrrolate in, 639t
  scopolamine in inhibition, 728t
Sedation. *See also* Anesthesia; *specific drugs*
  chloral hydrate in, 594t
  mephobarbital in, 671t
  midazolam in, 545t, 680–681t
  promethazine as adjunct in preoperative, 715t
Sedative-hypnotics, adverse drug reactions, 309–310t
  barbiturates, 309–310t
  benzodiazepines, 310t
  miscellaneous, 310t
Seizures
  absence. *See* Absence seizures
  as adverse drug effect, 289t
  carbamazepine in, 587t
  clobazam in, 600t
  clonazepam in, 601t
  clorazepate in, 602t
  diazepam in, 538t, 611t
  ethosuximide in, 627t
  fosphenytoin in, 635t
  gabapentin in, 636t
  lorazepam in, 544t, 666t
  magnesium sulfate in, 668t
  mephenytoin in, 671t
  oxcarbazepine in, 695–696t
  pancuronium bromide in intubation during, 698t
  paraldehyde in, 546t, 698t
  phenobarbital in, 547t, 704t
  phenytoin in, 547t, 706t
  primidone in, 713t
  pyridoxine-dependent, 721t
  pyridoxine in, 548t
  tiagabine in, 741t
  topiramate in, 743t

Seldane®. See Terfenadine
Select®. See Ethinyl estradiol/norethindrone; Oral contraceptives
Selective serotonin reuptake inhibitors (SSRIs). *See also* Antidepressants *and specific drugs*
  adverse drug reactions, 300t
  as antiemetics, 499t
  with tricyclic antidepressants, 322
Selenium sulfide, in children and adolescents, 729t
Selsun Blue®. See Selenium sulfide
Senna
  adverse drug reactions, 309t
  breast milk excretion, 225t
  in children and adolescents, 729t
Senna X-Prep®. See Senna
Sennosides. *See* Senna
Senokot®. See Senna
Sensorcaine®. See Bupivacaine
Sepsis, immune globulin in, 543t
Septra®. See Co-trimoxazole
Serentil®. See Mesoridazine
Serevent Diskus®. See Salmeterol xinafoate
Sertraline
  adverse drug reactions, 300t
  breast milk excretion, 225t
  in children and adolescents, 729–730t
Serum concentration ranges, 761–762t
Serutan®. See Psyllium
Serzone®. See Nefazodone
Sevoflurane, in children and adolescents, 730t
Sevorane AF®. See Sevoflurane
Sexually transmitted diseases
  AIDS/HIV. *See* AIDS/HIV
  chlamydial infection, erythromycin in, 540t
  congenital syphilis, penicillin G benzathine in, 547t
  genital herpes simplex
    acyclovir in, 559t
    valacyclovir in, 748–749t
  gonorrhea
    amoxicillin in, 566t
    cefpodoxime proxetil in, 591t
    ceftriaxone axetil in, 593t
    ceftriaxone in, 593t
    doxycycline in, 619t
    probenecid in, 566t
    trimethoprim/sulfamethoxazole in, 746–747t
Shigellosis. *See also* Bacterial infections
  trimethoprim/sulfamethoxazole in, 747t
Shock
  dobutamine in, 539t
  methylprednisolone sodium succinate in, 677t
  norepinephrine in, 546t
  phenylephrine in, 705t

Short bowel syndrome, ranitidine in, 548t
Sibelium®. See Flunarizine
Sickle cell disease, morphine in vaso-occlusive crisis, 683t
SI conversion formulas, 763
Simethicone, in infants, children, and adolescents, 730t
Simply Sleep®. See Diphenhydramine
Sinarest 12 Hr Nasal Solution®. See Oxymetazoline nasal
Singulair®. See Montelukast
Sinusitis
  cefpodoxime proxetil in, 591t
  cefprozil in, 592t
  loracarbef in, 666t
  naphazoline nasal in, 686t
Skeletal muscle relaxation. *See* Neuromuscular blockade
Skin cleansing
  hexachlorophene in, 643t
  hydrogen peroxide in, 646t
Skin disorders. *See also* Dermatitis; Dermatoses; Itching; *specific conditions*
  fluocinolone in, 632t
Skin infections
  cefpodoxime proxetil in, 591t
  gentamicin topical in, 637t
Skin preparation, chlorhexidine in, 596t
Skin rash, as adverse drug effect, 290t
Small bowel intubation, metoclopramide in, 678t
Smallpox vaccine
  in children and adolescents, 730–731t
  teratogenicity/fetotoxicity, 186
S-Methyltransferase, 482, 486–487. *See also* Pharmacogenetics
S-Methyltransferase gene, antineoplastic therapy and, 496
Smoking. *See* Tobacco smoking
Snake bite, antivenin (Crotalidae) polyvalent in, 571–572t
Social anxiety disorder, paroxetine in, 699t
Social variables, in psychotropic drug abuse, 353
Societal dimensions, of psychotropic drug abuse, 353–354
Sodium aurothiomalate. *See* Gold sodium thiomalate
Sodium bicarbonate
  in children and adolescents, 731t
  in cyclic antidepressant poisoning, 254t
  intravenous administration, 425t
  in neonates, 549t
  in poisoning, 252
  in salicylate poisoning, 257–258
  in urine alkalinization, 252
Sodium chloride
  intravenous administration, 425t
  in neonates, 549t

Sodium cromoglycate. *See* Cromolyn sodium
Sodium fluoride
  breast milk excretion, 213t
  in infants and children, 731t
Sodium iodide
  breast milk excretion
    I 125, 225t
    I 131, 226t
  teratogenicity/fetotoxicity, 186
Sodium levothyroxine. *See* Levothyroxine
Sodium 2-mercaptoethanesulfonate. *See* Mesna
Sodium nitrite IV, in cyanide poisoning, 254t
Sodium nitroprusside
  adverse drug reactions, 302t
  in children and adolescents, 732t
  intravenous administration, 425t
  in neonates, 549t
Sodium polystyrene sulfonate
  in infants, children, and adolescents, 732t
  in neonates, 549t
Sodium salicylate
  aspirin conversion factor, 257t
  teratogenicity/fetotoxicity, 186
Sodium Sulamyd®. See Sulfacetamide sodium ophthalmic
Sodium sulfacetamide. *See* Sulfacetamide sodium
Sodium thiosulfate IV, in cyanide poisoning, 254t
Sodium valproate. *See* Valproic acid
Solu-Cortef®. *See* Hydrocortisone
Solu-Cortef®. *See* Hydrocortisone sodium succinate
Solu-Medrol®. *See* Methylprenisolone sodium succinate
Solutions
  intravenous, 63
  ophthalmic, 23-25, 26
Solvent or inhalant drug abuse, 357-360, 358t, 359t
Somatrem, in children, 732t
Somatropin
  in children, 733t
  human. *See* Somatrem
Somatropin depot, in children, 733t
Sotalol, breast milk excretion, 226t
Sparfloxacin, drug interactions, 335
Spasms
  GI tract smooth muscle, dicyclomine in, 613t
  infantile (West syndrome)
    corticotropin in, 603-604t
    vigabatrin in, 751t
  methocarbamol in, 675t
Spasticity, baclofen in, 576t
Spectazole®. See Econazole
Spinal cord injury, methylprednisolone sodium succinate in, 678t
Spinhaler, 36

Spironolactone
  adjustments in renal insufficiency, 759t
  adverse drug reactions, 308t
  breast milk excretion, 226t
  in children and adolescents, 734t
  in neonates, 549t
Sporanox®. See Itraconazole
Sprays. *See* Aerosols
SSKI®. See Potassium chloride
Stalor®. See Anetholtrithion
Staphylococcus aureus. See also Bacterial infections
  methicillin-resistant, mupirocin nasal in, 683-684t
Status asthmaticus, methylprednisolone sodium succinate in, 678t
Status epilepticus. *See also* Seizures
  diazepam in, 538t, 611t
  fosphenytoin in, 635t
  lorazepam in, 666t
  paraldehyde in, 698t
  pentobarbital in, 702t
  phenobarbital in, 704t
  phenytoin in dysrhythmias related to, 706t
Stavudine
  adjustments in renal insufficiency, 760t
  in infants, children, and adolescents, 734t
Steatorrhea
  pancreatin in, 697t
  pancrelipase in, 697-698t
Stelazine®. See Trifluoperazine
Stemetil®. See Prochlorperazine
Sterapred®. See Prednisone
Steroids. *See* Anabolic steroids; Corticosteroids
Stevens-Johnson syndrome, as adverse drug effect, 291t
Stimate®. See Desmopressin
Stimulant laxatives, adverse drug reactions, 309t
Stomach acid, excess. *See also* Gastroesophageal reflux disease (GERD)
  ranitidine in, 723-724t
Stomatitis, ulcerative, as adverse drug effect, 291t
Storage of drugs, 8
Strabismus, botulinum toxin type A in, 583t
Streptase®. See Streptokinase
Streptococcal enterocolitis, as adverse drug effect, 290t
Streptococcus pyogenes, mupirocin topical in impetigo caused by, 684t
Streptokinase
  intravenous administration, 426t
  teratogenicity/fetotoxicity, 186
Streptomycin
  adjustments in renal insufficiency, 760t
  adverse drug reactions, 293t
  breast milk excretion, 226t

  in children and adolescents, 734t
  optimal serum concentrations, 762t
  teratogenicity/fetotoxicity, 186-187
Strongyloidiasis. *See also* Parasitic infestations
  thiabendazole in, 740t
Subaortic stenosis, obstructive hypertrophic, propranolol in, 548t
Subarachnoid hemorrhage, aminocaproic acid in, 564t
Subcutaneous injections
  equipment selection, 49
  sites, 49-50, 50
  technique, 50-53
    heparin injections, 51
    insulin delivery devices, 51-52
    opiate analgesic infusion, 52-53
    subcutaneous intermittent drug administration, 52
Subglottic stenosis, dexamethasone in, 537t
Sublingual dosage forms, 38-39
Succimer (DMSA)
  in infants, children, and adolescents, 734t
  in lead poisoning, 255t
Succinylcholine
  in infants, children, and adolescents, 734-735t
  in neonates, 550t
Succinylcholine chloride, intravenous administration, 426t
Sucralfate, in adolescents, 735t
Sucrase-isomaltase deficiency, congenital (CSID), sacrosidase in, 727t
Sulamyd®. See Sulfacetamide sodium; Sulfacetamide sodium topical
Sulcrate®. See Sucralfate
Sulfacetamide. *See* Sulfacetamide sodium
  in neonates, 550t
  ophthalmic, in children and adolescents, 735t
  teratogenicity/fetotoxicity, 187
  topical, in adolescents, 736t
Sulfamethoxazole
  adjustments in renal insufficiency, 760t
  adverse drug reactions, 295t
  in children and adolescents, 736t
  in infants, children, and adolescents, 737t
  teratogenicity/fetotoxicity, 187-188
Sulfamethoxazole/trimethoprim. *See* Trimethoprim/sulfamethoxazole
Sulfamylon®. See Mafenide
Sulfasalazine
  breast milk excretion, 226t
  in children and adolescents, 736t
  teratogenicity/fetotoxicity, 187

Sulfinpyrazone, drug interactions, 317t
Sulfisoxazole
  adverse drug reactions, 295t
  contraindicated in neonates, 550t
Sulfonamides. *See also specific drugs*
  adverse drug reactions, 295t
  drug interactions, 335
  teratogenicity/fetotoxicity, 188
  with phenytoin, 333
Sumatriptan, breast milk excretion, 226t
Sunburn prevention, zinc oxide in, 756t
Superdophilus. See Lactobacillus acidophilus
Supportive care, in pediatric poisoning, 247-248
Suppositories
  rectal, administration, 20-21
  vaginal, 22-23
Supprelin®. See Histrelin
Supraventricular tachycardia. *See also* Cardiac dysrhythmias
  adenosine in, 532t, 561t
  esmolol in, 625t
Suprax®. See Cefixime
Surfak®. See Docusate calcium
Survanta®. See Beractant
Suspensions, oral, 9
Sustiva®. See Efavirenz
Suxamethonium. *See* Succinylcholine
Symbols and abbreviations, 781-784
Symmetrel®. See Amantadine
Sympathomimetics. *See also* Antidepressants: tricyclic; Beta-blockers
  drug interactions, 335
  with beta-blockers, 323
  with tricyclic antidepressants, 322
Synagis®. See Palivizumab
Synalar®. See Fluocinolone
Synandrol®. See Testosterone propionate
Synercid®. See Quinupristin and dalfopristin
Synflex®. See Naproxen sodium
Synphasic®. See Ethinyl estradiol/norethindrone; Oral contraceptives
Synthroid®. See Levothyroxine
Syphilis
  congenital, penicillin G benzathine in, 547t
  doxycycline in, 619t
Syringes, 48
  insulin, 49, 49n
  oral drug, 10
Systemic lupus erythematosus, as adverse drug effect, 291t

T

Tablet crushers, 15
Tablets
  buccal and sublingual, 13
  chewable, 12
  controlled-release, 12-13
  effervescent, 13
  enteric-coated, 13
  "quick-dissolve," 13
  sublingual, 39
Tabloid®. See Thioguanine
Tacrine, drug interactions, 317t
Tacrolimus
  in children and adolescents, 737t
  optimal serum concentrations, 762t
  teratogenicity/fetotoxicity, 188
Tagamet®. See Cimetidine
Tambocor®. See Flecainide
Tamiflu®. See Oseltamivir
TAO®. See Troleandomycin
Tapazole®. See Methimazole
Tardive dyskinesia
  as adverse drug effect, 291t
  tetrabenazine in, 738t
Tavist®. See Clemastine
Taxicef®. See Ceftazidime
Taxol®. See Paclitaxel
Taxotere®. See Docetaxel
Tazarotene, in adolescents, 737t
Tazidime®. See Ceftazidime
Tazorac®. See Tazarotene
Tebrazid®. See Pyrazinamide
Technetium Tc 99m, breast milk excretion, 226t
Technetium Tc 99m albumin, aggregated, breast milk excretion, 226t
Tegopen®. See Cloxacillin
Tegretol®. See Carbamazepine
Telterodine, drug interactions, 317t
Temazepam, breast milk excretion, 227t
Temporal arteries, penetration of in venipuncture, 75n
Tempra®. See Acetaminophen
Teniposide
  dosing, 522t
  extravasation care, 506t
  intravenous administration, 426t
Tenormin®. See Atenolol
Tensilon®. See Edrophonium; Edrophonium chloride
Teratogenesis
  drug monograph codes, 97
  drug monographs, 96-200. *See also specific drugs and drug classes*
  factors affecting, 89-96, *90*, *92-95t*
    embryo/fetal, 90
    environmental, 90-91
    maternal, 89-90
    placental, 90
  maternal pharmacotherapy and drug use during pregnancy, 88-89, *89*
Teratogenicity, 87-200. *See also* Fetotoxicity *and related entries*
  defined, 87
Teratogenic susceptibility of developing organ systems, *92*
Terbinafine, drug interactions, 317t
Terbutaline
  adverse drug reactions, 305t
  breast milk excretion, 227t
  in children and adolescents, 738t
  optimal serum concentrations, 762t
Terfenadine, drug interactions, 319t, 335
Terfenadine poisoning, 266
Terfluzine®. See Trifluoperazine
Terpin hydrate, teratogenicity/fetotoxicity, 188-189
Testosterone, teratogenicity/fetotoxicity, 189
Testosterone propionate, in children, 738t
Tests, pediatric laboratory values, 785-788t
Tetanus
  chlorpromazine in, 597t
  methocarbamol in, 675t
Tetanus toxoid vaccine, 456-457
  teratogenicity/fetotoxicity, 189
Tetrabenzamine, in children and adolescents, 738t
Tetracyclines. *See also specific drugs*
  adjustments in renal insufficiency, 760t
  adverse drug reactions, 295t
  breast milk excretion, 227t
  in children and adolescents, 738t
  drug interactions, 335
  teratogenicity/fetotoxicity, 189-190
Tetraethylperazine, teratogenicity/fetotoxicity, 191
Tetrahydrocannabinol. *See* Marijuana
Tetralogy of Fallot, propranolol in, 548t
6-TG. *See* Thioguanine
Thalidomide
  in adolescents, 738-749t
  teratogenicity/fetotoxicity, 87, 190-191
Thalomid®. See Thalidomide
Theo-24®. See Theophylline
Theobromine, breast milk excretion, 227t
Theolair®. See Theophylline
Theophylline
  adverse drug reactions, 305t
  breast milk excretion, 227t
  drug interactions, 317t, 335-336
  in infants, children, and adolescents, 739-740t
  in neonates, 550t
  optimal serum concentrations, 762t
  teratogenicity/fetotoxicity, 102, 191
  with allopurinol, 320
  with phenytoin, 333
Theophylline ethylene diamine. *See* Aminophylline

Thiabendazole, in children and adolescents, 740t
Thiamazole. *See* Methimazole
Thiamine
 breast milk excretion, 227t
 in infants, children, and adolescents, 740t
 intravenous administration, 426t
Thiamine deficiency, supplementation in, 740t
Thiazide diuretics. *See also specific drugs*
 adverse drug reactions, 308t
 drug interactions, 336
 with lithium salts, 330
Thioguanine, dosing, 522t
Thiopental
 breast milk excretion, 227t
 intravenous administration, 427t
 teratogenicity/fetotoxicity, 191-192
Thioperazine, in children and adolescents, 740-741t
Thioplex®. See Thiotepa
Thioproperazine, in children and adolescents, 740-741t
Thiopurine *S*-methyltransferase, 482, 486-487. *See also* Pharmacogenetics
Thioridazine
 in children and adolescents, 741t
 drug interactions, 317t, 319t, 336
 measurement of, 10
Thiotepa
 dosing, 522t
 intravenous administration, 427t
Thiouracil, breast milk excretion, 227t
Thorazine®. See Chlorpromazine
3-*TC®. See* Lamivudine
Thrombocytopenia
 heparin-induced, 51n
  danaparoid in, 607-608t
 hydrocortisone in, 543t
Thrombocytopenic purpura, idiopathic, 648t
Thrombophlebitis, as adverse drug effect, 291t
Thrombosis
 as complication of intravenous injections, 78
 danaparoid in, 607t
 enoxaparin in, 621-622t
Thyro-Block®. See Potassium iodide
Thyroidectomy, potassium iodide in, 710t
Thyroid hormones
 adverse drug reactions, 309t
 drug interactions, 336
 with anticoagulants, 321
 with cholestyramine resin, 325
Thyrotoxicosis
 neonatal, propranolol in, 548t
 potassium iodide in, 710t
Thyroxine. *See* Levothyroxine
Tiagabine, in adolescents, 741t

Ticar®. See Ticarcillin
Ticarcillin, adverse drug reactions, 294t
Ticarcillin/clavulanate
 adjustments in renal insufficiency, 760t
 in infants, children, and adolescents, 742t
Ticarcillin disodium/clavulanate potassium, intravenous administration, 427t
Tic disorders
 pimozide in, 707t
 tetrabenazine in, 738t
Ticlopidine, drug interactions, 317t
Tilade®. See Nedocromil pulmonary
Time dimension, in psychotropic drug abuse, 353-354
Timentin®. See Ticarcillin disodium/clavulanate potassium
Timolol
 breast milk excretion, 228t
 drug interactions, 317t
Tinactin®. See Tolnaftate
Tinea infections. *See also* Fungal infections
 butenafine in, 586t
 clotrimazole in, 602t
 griseofulvin in, 640t
 selenium sulfide in, 729t
 tolnaftate in, 743t
 undecylenic acid in, 748t
Ting®. See Tolnaftate
Tinnitus, as adverse drug effect, 291t
TOBI®. See Tobramycin inhalation
Tobacco smoking, 363-365, 365t
 drug interactions, 317t
 teratogenicity/fetotoxicity, 192-193
 variations of cigarettes, 364n
Tobramycin
 adjustments in renal insufficiency, 760t
 adverse drug reactions, 293t
 breast milk excretion, 228t
 in children and adolescents
  inhalation, 742t
  injectable, 742t
 intravenous administration, 427t
 in neonates, 550t
 optimal serum concentrations, 762t
Tobrex®. See Tobramycin; Tobramycin injectable
Tocainide, breast milk excretion, 228t
Toddlers
 drug administration in, 3-4t, 16-17
 injections administered in, 44
Tolbutamide
 breast milk excretion, 228t
 drug interactions, 317t
 teratogenicity/fetotoxicity, 193-194
Tolectin®. See Tolmetin sodium

Tolmectin. *See* Tolmetin sodium
Tolmetin sodium
 breast milk excretion, 228t
 in children, 743t
Tolnaftate, in infants, children, and adolescents, 743t
Toluene, teratogenicity/fetotoxicity, 194
Tonsillitis. *See also* Pharyngitis
 cefprozil in, 592t
 loracarbef in, 666t
Tooth discoloration, as adverse drug effect, 291t
Topactin®. See Fluocinonide
Topical dosage forms, 36-42
 buccal, sublingual, and other transmucosal, 38-39
 dermatological for localized effect, 37-38
 transdermal, 39-42
Topiramate, in children, 743t
Topamax®. See Topiramate
Topotecan, intravenous administration, 428t
Topsyn®. See Fluocinonide
Torsenide, drug interactions, 317t
Totacillin®. See Ampicillin
Total body water (TBW), 495
Total nutritional support, aluminum contamination in, 67n
Tourette's syndrome
 as adverse drug effect, 291t
 pimozide in, 707t
Toxic epidermal necrolysis, as adverse drug effect, 291t
Toxicities. *See also* Fetotoxicity; Poisoning; Teratogenicity
 of antineoplastics, 497, 498t
 of intravenous drugs, 78-79
Toxoplasmosis, pyrimethamine in, 721t
T-Phyl®. See Theophylline
Tracheal intubation. *See* Intubation
Traconazole, with antacids, 321
Tramadol, drug interactions, 317t
Trandate®. See Labetalol
Tranexamic acid
 adjustments in renal insufficiency, 760t
 in children and adolescents, 743-744t
 intravenous administration, 428t
Transderm®. See Scopolamine
Transdermal drug delivery systems (TDDSs), 39-42, *40*
 nicotine transdermal system, 41-42
 scopolamine transdermal system, 40-41
Transderm Scop®. See Scopolamine
Transderm-V®. See Scopolamine
Transmucosal dosage forms, 38-39
Transplantation. *See also specific type*
 cyclopentolate in, 605-606t
 muromonab-CD3 in, 684t
 tacrolimus in, 737t

Tranxene®. See Clorazepate
Trastuzamab
   dosing, 523t
   intravenous administration, 428t
Trauma, naproxen sodium in skeletal, 687t
Trazodone
   breast milk excretion, 228t
   drug interactions, 317t
Tretinoin. *See also* Isotretinoin
   dosing, 523t
Triacetyloleandomycin. *See* Troleandomycin
Triaderm®. See Triamcinolone topical
Triamcinolone
   adverse drug reactions, 308t
   in children and adolescents
      nasal, 744t
      oral, 744t
      pulmonary, 744t
   teratogenicity/fetotoxicity, 194
   topical, in infants, children, and adolescents, 745t
Triaminic Infant Oral Decongestant Drops®. See Pseudoephedrine
Triaminic Softchews Cough®. See Dextromethorphan
Triamterene
   adjustments in renal insufficiency, 760t
   adverse drug reactions, 308t
   in children and adolescents, 745t
   teratogenicity/fetotoxicity, 194
Trichinosis. *See also* Parasitic infestations
   thiabendazole in, 740t
Trichomonas vaginalis, metronidazole in, 679t
Tricor®. See Fenofibrate micronized
Tricyclic antidepressants. *See also* Depression *and specific drugs*
   adverse drug reactions, 300t
   with anticonvulsants, 321-322
Triethanolamine salicylate, aspirin conversion factor, 257t
Triethylenethiophosphamide. *See* Thiotepa
Trifluoperazine
   in children, 745-746t
   teratogenicity/fetotoxicity, 194-195
Trifluridine, in children and adolescents, 746t
Trileptal®. See Oxcarbazepine
Trimeprazine, teratogenicity/fetotoxicity, 195
Trimethadione, teratogenicity/fetotoxicity, 195
Trimethobenzamide, teratogenicity/fetotoxicity, 195-196
Trimethoprim
   adjustments in renal insufficiency, 760t
   adverse drug reactions, 297t
   in children and adolescents, 746t
   drug interactions, 337

teratogenicity/fetotoxicity, 196
   with phenytoin, 333
Trimethoprim/sulfamethoxazole
   adjustments in renal insufficiency, 760t
   in children and adolescents, 746-747t
   drug interactions, 317t, 337
   intravenous administration, 428t
   in neonates, 551t
   with cyclosporine, 327
Trimox®. See Amoxicillin
Tripelennamine, teratogenicity/fetotoxicity, 196
Triphasil®. See Ethinyl estradiol/levonorgestrel; Oral contraceptives
Triprolidine, teratogenicity/fetotoxicity, 196
Triquilar®. See Ethinyl estradiol/levonorgestrel; Oral contraceptives
t-RNA. *See* Tretinoin
Troglitazone, drug interactions, 336
Troleandomycin
   in children and adolescents, 747t
   drug interactions, 337
   with carbamazepine, 324
   with theophylline, 336
Tuberculin test (TB test), breast milk excretion, 228t
Tuberculosis
   ethambutol in pulmonary, 625t
   ethionamide in, 627t
   isoniazid in, 654t
   pyrazinamide in, 720t
   rifampin in, 724t
   streptomycin in, 734t
Tubes
   nasogastric and feeding, 18-19
   selection of feeding, 19
Tubing, for intravenous administration, 64
Tubocurarine
   adjustments in renal insufficiency, 760t
   in infants, children, and adolescents, 747-748t
   intravenous administration, 428t
Tumors, antineoplastic drug regimens, 506t
Tums®. See Calcium carbonate
Turbuhaler, 36
Turner syndrome, testosterone propionate in growth delay, 738t
Twinrix®. See Hepatitis A and B vaccine
Typhoid vaccine, teratogenicity/fetotoxicity, 196
Typhus vaccine, teratogenicity/fetotoxicity, 196

U

Ulcerative colitis
   mesalamine in, 672t
   sulfasalazine in, 736t

Ulcerative stomatitis, as adverse drug effect, 291t
Ulcers. *See* Duodenal ulcer; Peptic ulcer
Ultrase®. See Pancrelipase
Unasyn®. See Ampicillin/sulbactam
Uncinariasis. *See also* Parasitic infestations
   thiabendazole in, 740t
Undecylenic acid, in children and adolescents, 748t
Unipen®. See Nafcillin
Uniphyl®. See Theophylline
Uni-Tussin®. See Guaifenesin
Urea peroxide. *See* Carbamide peroxide
Urex®. See Methenamine hippurate
Urinary acidification
   ammonium chloride in, 566t
   ascorbic acid in, 572t
Urinary retention, bethanecol in, 581t
Urinary tract infections
   cefpodoxime proxetil in, 592t
   methenamine hippurate in, 674t
   methenamine mandelate in, 674t
   sulfamethoxazole in, 736t
   tobramycin in, 742t
   trimethoprim in, 746t
   trimethoprim/sulfamethoxazole in, 747t
Urinary tract mucosal irritation, phenazopyridine in, 703t
Urine pH, alteration in poisoning, 252
Urogesic®. See Phenazopyridine
Urokinase
   injection precautions, 68n
   teratogenicity/fetotoxicity, 196
Uromitexan®. See Mesna
Urticaria. *See also* Allergy; Itching
   cetirizine in, 594t
   chronic idiopathic, loratadine in, 666t
   clemastine in, 600t
   desloratadine in, 609t
U.S. Food and Drug Administration. *See* FDA *entries*
Uveitis
   atropine ophthalmic in, 574t
   homatropine in, 644t

V

Vaccines
   anthrax, adsorbed, 571t
   BCG, drug interactions, 322
   diphtheria, 437-440
      breast milk excretion, 211t
   Hemophilus influenzae type B, 440-441, 441t
   hepatitis A, 441-442
      inactivated, 641-642t
      inactivated purified, 642t
      inactivated virosome formulated, 642t
   hepatitis A and B, 642t
   hepatitis B, 442-444

Vaccines *continued*
  human diploid-cell rabies (HDCR), with chloramphenicol, 325
  influenza virus, 444-445
  measles virus, 445-447
  meningococcus, 447-448
  mumps virus, 448-449
  passive immunization, 449-450
  pertussis, 450-452, 452t
  pneumococcus, 452-453
  poliovirus, 453-455
    breast milk excretion, 223t
  rotavirus, 455
  rubella virus, 455-456
    breast milk excretion, 225t
  smallpox, 730-731t
  teratogenicity/fetotoxicity
    BCG, 106
    diphtheria vaccine, 130
    hepatitis B vaccine, 141
    influenza virus vaccine, 144-145
    mumps virus vaccine, 162-163
    plague vaccine, 176
    poliovirus
      inactivated (Salk), 176-177
      live oral (Sabin), 177
    rubella virus vaccine, 184-185
    smallpox vaccine, 186
    tetanus vaccine, 189
    typhoid vaccine, 196
    typhus vaccine, 196
    yellow fever, 200
  tetanus, 456-457
Vaginal dosage forms, 22-23
Vaginosis. *See also* Vulvovaginosis
  bacterial, metronidazole in, 678t
Valacyclovir, in adolescents, 748-749t
Valium®. *See* Diazepam
Valproate sodium. *See* Valproic acid
Valproic acid
  adverse drug reactions, 299t
  breast milk excretion, 228t
  in children and adolescents, 749-750t
  drug interactions, 337
  intravenous administration, 429t
  optimal serum concentrations, 762t
  teratogenicity/fetotoxicity, 196-197
  with phenytoin, 333
  with primidone, 334
Valtrex®. *See* Valacyclovir
Vancenase®. *See* Beclomethasone
Vanceril®. *See* Beclomethasone
Vancomycin
  adjustments in renal insufficiency, 760t
  adverse drug reactions, 297t
  breast milk excretion, 228t
  in children and adolescents, 750t
  intravenous administration, 429t
  in neonates, 551t

optimal serum concentrations, 762t
Vancomycin-resistant infections
  linezolid in, 663-664t
  quinupristin and dalfopristin in, 723t
Vantin®. *See* Cefpodoxime; Cefpodoxime proxetil
Vaqta®. *See* Hepatitis A vaccine
Varicella zoster (chickenpox), acyclovir in, 559t
Varicella zoster vaccine, 457-458
Vasoclear®. *See* Naphazoline ophthalmic
Vasocon®. *See* Naphazoline ophthalmic
Vasodilators, adverse drug reactions, 307t
Vasopressin, in children and adolescents, 750t
Vasotec®. *See* Enalapril
Vastus lateralis injection site, 58, 59
V-Cillin K®. *See* Penicillin G potassium
VCR. *See* Vincristine
Vecuronium bromide, intravenous administration, 429t
Veetids®. *See* Penicillin G potassium
Velban®. *See* Vinblastine
Venipuncture, 71-76
  scalp vein, 72, 72
  sites for children and adolescents, 74
Venlafaxine
  adjustments in renal insufficiency, 760t
  in adolescents, 751t
  breast milk excretion, 229t
  drug interactions, 317t
Venoglobulin-S®. *See* Immune globulin
Venous access devices, 65-71
  central, 67-71, 563t
    complications of, 71
    electronic infusion control devices, 70
    gravity controllers, 70
    implantable, 69-70
    infusion pumps, 70-71
    midline catheters, 69
    peripherally inserted venous catheters, 69
  peripheral, 65, 65-67
Ventilator weaning, dexamethasone in, 537t
Ventolin®. *See* Albuterol
Ventricular dysrhythmias. *See also* Cardiac dysrhythmias
  amiodarone in, 565t
  disopyramide in, 617t
  flecainide in, 630t
  lidocaine in, 544t
  mexiletine in, 679t
  procainamide in, 714t
  propafenone in, 716t
  quinidine in, 722t

Ventricular fibrillation, lidocaine in, 662t
Ventricular tachycardia. *See also* Cardiac dysrhythmias
  lidocaine in, 662t
Ventrogluteal injection site, 57, 57-58
VePesid®. *See* Etoposide
Verapamil
  adverse drug reactions, 306t
  breast milk excretion, 229t
  drug interactions, 337
  in infants, children, and adolescents, 751t
  intravenous administration, 429t
  optimal serum concentrations, 762t
  teratogenicity/fetotoxicity, 197-198
  with carbamazepine, 324
  with digitalis glycosides, 328
  with theophylline, 336
Vercuronium, in infants, children, and adolescents, 750t
Verelan®. *See* Verapamil
Vermox®. *See* Mebendazole
Vernal conjunctivitis, medrysone in, 669t
Vernal keratitis, lodoxamide in, 665t
Versed®. *See* Midazolam
Versel®. *See* Selenium sulfide
Vertigo, meclizine in, 668-669t
Vertigo/vestibular dysfunction, as adverse drug effect, 291t
Vesanoid®. *See* Tretinoin
Vials, 46-47
Vibramycin®. *See* Doxycycline
Vibra-Tabs®. *See* Doxycycline
Videx®. *See* Didanosine
Videx EC®. *See* Didanosine
Vigabatrin
  breast milk excretion, 229t
  in infants, 751-752t
Vinblastine
  dosing, 524t
  extravasation care, 506t
  intravenous administration, 429t
  teratogenicity/fetotoxicity, 198
Vincaleukoblastine sulfate. *See* Vinblastine
Vincristine
  dosing, 524t
  extravasation care, 506t
  intravenous administration, 430t
  teratogenicity/fetotoxicity, 198
Viokase®. *See* Pancrelipase
Vioxx®. *See* Rofecoxib
Viracept®. *See* Nelfinavir
Viral infections. *See also* AIDS/HIV; Hepatitis; Influenza
  amantadine in, 563-564t
  ganciclovir in, 637t
  palivizumab in prophylaxis, 697t

ribavirin in respiratory syncytial virus, 724t
zanamivir in, 754t
Virazole®. See Ribavirin
Visceral leishmaniasis, amphotericin B liposome in, 568-569t
Visine L.R.® eyedrops. *See* Oxymetazoline ophthalmic
Visual dysfunction, as adverse drug effect, 291t
Vitamin A. *See also* Retinoic acid; Tretinoin
  adverse drug reactions, 311t
  teratogenicity/fetotoxicity, 198-199
Vitamin B_1. *See* Thiamine
Vitamin B_2. *See* Riboflavin
Vitamin B_6. *See* Pyridoxine
Vitamin B_{12}. *See* Cyanocobalamin
Vitamin C. *See* Ascorbic acid
Vitamin D
  adverse drug reactions, 311t
  breast milk excretion, 229t
  teratogenicity/fetotoxicity, 199
Vitamin D_2. *See* Ergocalciferol
Vitamin D_2 analog. *See* Dihydrotachysterol
Vitamin D deficiency, calcitriol in, 586t
Vitamin D-resistant rickets, dihydrotachysterol in, 615t
Vitamin E, with iron, 329
Vitamin K_1. *See* Phytonadione
Vitamin K_1 deficiency, phytonadione in, 706t
Vitamins, multiple
  in children and adolescents, 752-753t
  intravenous administration, 430t
Vitamins and minerals, adverse drug reactions, 310-311t
VLB. *See* Vinblastine
VM-26. *See* Teniposide
Volatile solvent or inhalant drug abuse, 357-360, 358t, 359t
Voltaren®. See Diclofenac
Vomiting. *See also* Nausea
  as adverse drug effect, 291t
  chlorpromazine in, 597t
  dolasetron in prevention, 618t
  granisetron in prevention, 639-640t
  meclizine in, 668-669t
  ondansetron in, 693t
  prochlorperazine in severe, 715t
  prophylaxis
    dronabinol in, 619t
    droperidol in, 619-620t
VP-16. *See* Etoposide

Vulvovaginal candidiasis. *See also* Fungal infections
  butoconazole in, 586t
  clotrimazole in, 602t
  miconazole in, 679t
  nystatin in, 692t
Vumon®. See Teniposide

W

Warfarin
  adverse drug reactions, 297-298t
  breast milk excretion, 229t
  drug interactions, 317t
  in infants, children, and adolescents, 753-754t
  teratogenicity/fetotoxicity, 199-200
  with cimetidine, 284
Warfilone®. See Warfarin
Weight gain, cyproheptadine in promotion of, 606t
Wellcovorin®. See Leucovorin calcium
West syndrome (infantile spasms)
  corticotropin in, 603-604t
  vigabatrin in, 751t
Whole bowel irrigation, in poisoning, 251
Wilson's disease (hepatolenticular degeneration), penicillamine in, 700t
WinRho SDF. See Immune globulin
Withdrawal
  alcohol, clorazepate in, 601-602t
  neonatal opiate analgesic syndrome, 87
  nicotine, 689-690t. *See also* Nicotine; Nicotine transdermal systems
Withdrawal seizures, phenobarbital in, 547t
Wycillin®. See Penicillin G procaine
Wydase®. See Hyaluronidase
Wymox®. See Amoxicillin

X

Xenical®. See Orlistat
Xerostomia, as adverse drug effect, 291t
Xopenex®. See Levalbuterol
Xylocaine®. See Lidocaine
Xylocard®. See Lidocaine

Y

Yellow fever vaccine, teratogenicity/fetotoxicity, 200
Yodoxin®. See Iodoquinol
Y-site injection port, 76

Z

Zaditen®. See Ketotifen
Zafirlukast
  adverse drug reactions, 305t
  in children and adolescents, 754-755t
  drug interactions, 317t
Zagam®. See Sparfloxacin
Zalcitabine
  adjustments in renal insufficiency, 760t
  in adolescents, 754t
Zanamivir, in children and adolescents, 754t
Zantac®. See Ranitidine
Zarontin®. See Ethosuximide
Zemuron®. See Rocuronium
Zerit®. See Stavudine
Zestril®. See Lisinopril
Ziagen®. See Abacavir
Zidovudine
  in adolescents, neonates, and infants, 755t
  adverse drug reactions, 304t
  drug interactions, 337
  intravenous administration, 430t
  in neonates, 551t
  teratogenicity/fetotoxicity, 200
  with ganciclovir, 329
Zileuton
  in adolescents, 755t
  drug interactions, 317t
Zinacef®. See Cefuroxime
Zinaderm®. See Zinc oxide
Zincofax®. See Zinc oxide
Zinc oxide, in infants, children, and adolescents, 756t
Zinecard®. See Dextrazoxane
Ziprasidone, drug interactions, 319t, 337
Zithromax®. See Azithromycin
Zofran®. See Ondansetron
Zoloft®. See Sertraline
Zolpidem, breast milk excretion, 229t
Zopiclone, teratogenicity/fetotoxicity, 200
ZORprin®. See Aspirin
Zosyn®. See Piperacillin/tazobactam
Zovirax®. See Acyclovir
Z-track injection technique, 61, *61*
Zyflo®. See Zileuton
Zyloprim®. See Allopurinol
Zymase®. See Pancrelipase
Zyrtec®. See Cetirizine
Zyvox®. See Linezolid
Zyvoxam®. See Linezolid